Volume One / Book 1

Radiology of the skull and brain

THE SKULL

Volume One / Book 1

Radiology of the skull and brain

THE SKULL

EDITED BY

Thomas H. Newton, M.D.

Professor of Radiology, Neurology and Neurosurgery; Chief, Section of Neuroradiology, University of California School of Medicine, San Francisco Medical Center, San Francisco, California

D. Gordon Potts, M.D.

Professor of Radiology, Cornell Medical College; Attending Radiologist, The New York Hospital, New York, New York

With 2,314 illustrations

The C. V. Mosby Company

Saint Louis 1971

Printed in the United States of America

International Standard Book Number 0-8016-3646-9

Library of Congress Catalog Card Number 78-173600

Distributed in Great Britain by Henry Kimpton, London

Contributors

R. THOMAS BERGERON, M.D.

Associate Professor of Radiology and Neuroradiology, Los Angeles County–University of Southern California Medical Center, Los Angeles, California

E. H. BURROWS, M. Rad., D.M.R.D.

Consultant Neuroradiologist, Wessex Neurological Centre; Senior Lecturer in Neuroradiology, University of Southampton, Southampton, England

JOHN A. CAMPBELL, M.D.

Professor and Chairman, Department of Radiology, Indiana University Medical Center, Indianapolis, Indiana

C. G. COIN, M.D.

Chairman, Department of Radiology, Lovelace-Bataan Medical Center, Albuquerque, New Mexico; formerly Assistant Professor of Radiology, University of California Center for the Health Sciences, Los Angeles, California

DAVID O. DAVIS, M.D.

Professor of Radiology, University of Utah College of Medicine, Salt Lake City, Utah

JOHN P. DORST, M.D.

Professor of Radiology and Associate Professor of Pediatrics, The Johns Hopkins Medical Institutions, Baltimore, Maryland

GEORGE H. du BOULAY, M.B., B.S., M.R.C.P., D.M.R.D., F.F.R.

Radiologist, The National Hospital for Nervous Diseases, Queen Square, and Nuffield Institute of Comparative Medicine, The Zoological Society of London, London, England

ROMEO ETHIER, M.D.

Associate Professor of Radiology, Neurosurgery and Neurology, McGill University; Director, Department of Radiology, Neurological Institute, Montreal, Quebec, Canada

CHARLES A. GOODING, M.D.

Assistant Professor of Radiology and Pediatrics; Chief, Pediatric Radiology, University of California School of Medicine, San Francisco Medical Center, San Francisco, California

HERMAN GROSSMAN, M.D.

Associate Professor of Radiology and Pediatrics, Cornell University Medical College; Associate Attending Radiologist Pediatrician, The New York Hospital–Cornell Medical Center; Pediatric Radiologist, Memorial Hospital for Cancer and Allied Diseases, New York, New York; presently Professor of Radiology and Pediatrics, Duke University School of Medicine, Durham, North Carolina

JOHN HALE, Ph.D.

Professor of Radiological Physics, Hospital of the University of Pennsylvania, Philadelphia, Pennsylvania

FRED J. HODGES, III, M.D.

Associate Professor of Radiology (Neuroradiology), The Johns Hopkins Hospital, Baltimore, Maryland

PETER E. KANE, M.D.

Associate Radiologist, Children's Hospital Medical Center, Oakland, California; Assistant Clinical Professor of Radiology, University of California School of Medicine, San Francisco, California

STEPHEN A. KIEFFER, M.D.

Associate Professor of Radiology, University of Minnesota Health Sciences Center; Chief, Radiology Service, Minneapolis Veterans Administration Hospital, Minneapolis, Minnesota

E. LEON KIER, M.D.

Associate Professor of Radiology; Chief, Section of Neuroradiology, Yale University School of Medicine, New Haven, Connecticut

ERIK LINDGREN

Professor of Radiology and Neuroradiology, Karolinska Institutet, Stockholm, Sweden

J. T. LITTLETON, M.D., F.A.C.R.

Co-Chairman, Department of Radiology, The Guthrie Clinic and Robert Packer Hospital, Guthrie Square, Sayre, Pennsylvania

GUIDO LOMBARDI, M.D.

Chief Radiologist, Istituto Neurologico di Milano; Consultant Radiologist, Istituto Oftalmico di Milano, Milan, Italy

DENNIS R. MALKASIAN, Ph.D.

Acting Instructor in Anatomy, University of California Center for the Health Sciences, Los Angeles, California

DONALD L. McRAE, M.D.

Professor of Radiology, University of Toronto; Radiologist in Chief, Sunnybrook Hospital, Toronto, Ontario, Canada

HIDEYO MINAGI, M.D.

Assistant Professor of Radiology, University of California School of Medicine, San Francisco Medical Center, San Francisco, California

JOHN E. MOSELEY, M.D.

Associate Clinical Professor of Radiology, Mount Sinai School of Medicine of the City University of New York; Associate Attending Radiologist, The Mount Sinai Hospital; Director, Department of Radiology, Sydenham Hospital, New York, New York

ARNOLD M. NOYEK, M.D., F.R.C.S.(C), F.A.C.S.

Assistant Professor of Otolaryngology, University of Toronto; Attending Otolaryngologist, New Mount Sinai Hospital and Sunnybrook Hospital; Consultant Otolaryngologist, Baycrest Hospital and Jewish Home for the Aged, Toronto, Ontario, Canada

M. B. OZONOFF, M.D.

Director of Radiology, Newington Children's Hospital, Newington, Connecticut; formerly Assistant Chief of Radiology, San Francisco General Hospital, and Assistant Professor of Radiology, University of California School of Medicine, San Francisco, California

JAMES A. POLLOCK, M.D.

Neuroradiologist, Sutter Community Hospitals, Sacramento, California; Assistant Clinical Professor of Radiology, University of California School of Medicine, San Francisco, California

GUY D. POTTER, M.D.

Associate Professor of Radiology, Columbia University College of Physicians and Surgeons, and Columbia-Presbyterian Medical Center, New York, New York

HENRY W. PRIBRAM, M.D.

Chief, Radiology Service, Veterans Administration Hospital, Long Beach, California; Clinical Professor of Radiology, University of California, Irvine, California

RICHARD H. RASKIND, M.D.

Clinical Assistant Professor, Cornell University Medical College; Associate Attending Ophthalmologist, The New York Hospital; Associate Attending Surgeon, Manhattan Eye, Ear and Throat Hospital, New York, New York

RICHARD J. RIZZUTI, M.D.

Fellow in Radiology, Cornell University Medical College, New York, New York

CALVIN L. RUMBAUGH, M.D.

Associate Professor of Radiology and Neuroradiology, Los Angeles County–University of Southern California Medical Center, Los Angeles, California

FRED K. SONDHEIMER, M.D.

Neuroradiologist and Assistant Chief of Radiology, Mount Zion Hospital and Medical Center; Assistant Clinical Professor of Radiology, University of California School of Medicine, San Francisco; Consultant in Neuroradiology, St. Mary's Hospital and Kaiser Foundation Hospitals, San Francisco, California

HOWARD L. STEINBACH, M.D.

Chief, Department of Radiology, French Hospital; Clinical Professor of Radiology, University of California School of Medicine, San Francisco, California, and Stanford University School of Medicine, Palo Alto, California

HOOSHANG TAYBI, M.D., M.Sc.

Chief, Department of Radiology, Children's Hospital Medical Center, Oakland, California; Clinical Professor of Radiology, University of California School of Medicine, San Francisco, California

STEPHEN L. TROKEL, M.D.

Instructor in Ophthalmology, Columbia University College of Physicians and Surgeons; Assistant Ophthalmologist, The Presbyterian Hospital, New York, New York

JOSEPH P. WHALEN, M.D.

Professor of Radiology, Cornell University Medical College; Attending Radiologist, The New York Hospital, New York, New York

PATRICIA H. WINCHESTER, M.D.

Assistant Professor of Radiology and Pediatrics, Cornell University Medical College; Assistant Attending Radiologist and Pediatrician, The New York Hospital–Cornell Medical Center; Pediatric Radiologist, Memorial Hospital for Cancer and Allied Diseases, New York, New York

JUDAH ZIZMOR, M.D.

Director of Radiology, Manhattan Eye, Ear and Throat Hospital; Attending Radiologist, The New York Hospital–Cornell University Medical Center, New York, New York

Preface

This volume is the first of a three-volume set intended primarily for physicians interested in the roentgenologic diagnosis of neurologic problems. The set is intended to be a reference source for those training in the fields of neuroradiology, neurology, and neurosurgery, as well as for the experienced radiologist and clinician.

Neuroradiology has made impressive progress in recent years. The use of smaller focal spots, subtraction techniques, more sophisticated tomography, and selective methods of angiography has improved the display of anatomic details. Roentgenographic techniques have been more widely applied during the postmortem examination, often after the opacification of the vessels, ventricles, and cisterns. For the first time we have accurate descriptions of almost every anatomic structure that can be demonstrated by the finest techniques available. Neuroradiologists have also obtained physiologic information from their studies. The dynamics of the cerebral circulation have been studied by angiography, and cerebrospinal fluid physiology has been analyzed by pneumography. New methods of investigation have been devised—the application of radioactive isotopes, echoencephalography, and thermography.

This volume and those to follow bring together a large amount of new information. Many authors who have contributed to the expanding knowledge in the field of neuroradiology have been invited to share in the writing of the three volumes: volume 1 on the skull, volume 2 on angiography, and volume 3 on pneumography, neuropathology, and isotopic and other diagnostic techniques. Each volume contains a section devoted to a discussion of the technical problems relating to a particular examination as well as the gross and radiologic anatomy; and, when indicated, separate chapters are devoted to a detailed analysis of the roentgen features of specific pathologic entities.

Whenever possible, we have tried to analyze each anatomic structure exhaustively, based on a review of the gross and radiologic normal anatomy, the variants of normal, and the effects of pathologic change on the anatomic structure under discussion. This sequence parallels the process of analysis of clinical neuroradiologic problems. Each chapter is provided with an extensive list of references for the reader who wishes to explore the subject further. Since radiology is based on an analysis of visual evidence, liberal use of illustrations has been made.

Neuroradiologic procedures are no longer performed in a standardized and stereotyped manner. Modification of the study based on clinical findings, as well as on roentgenographic information obtained during the study, has increased the diagnostic value of these examinations. This is an important change in the philosophy of neuroradiology, which is difficult to convey in this work.

A discussion of the spine and spinal cord has not been included, not because these topics are considered to be of less importance but because they are well covered in available textbooks. Perhaps the greatest recent advance in this area has been the angiographic examination of the spinal cord, extensively described by Djindjian, Doppman, Di Chiro, and their co-workers.

The editors wish to express their sincere thanks to the authors who contributed so generously to this work. We also wish to thank our editorial assistant, Miss Hildegarde Braun, and our secretaries, Mrs. Geri Murphy, Mrs. Pauline Pitman, Miss Sally Woodring, and Miss Piroska Szabo, who helped us extensively in the preparation of the manuscript.

Thomas H. Newton
D. Gordon Potts

Contents

Book 1

Book 2

CHAPTER 1

A history of neuroradiology

Erik Lindgren

The term neuroradiology, properly, should apply to both diagnosis and therapy of diseases of the nervous system, but it is often used as if it referred only to diagnosis. This interpretation can be readily understood, since diagnosis must be considered the more important of the two fields. The present chapter deals only with the diagnostic aspects, and aims to give a general picture of the development of neuroradiology. Details regarding individual contributions will not be discussed beyond those necessary to illustrate ideas and trains of thought. Particular emphasis will be placed on the examination procedures and less attention given to the results achieved. During the past few years echoencephalographic and thermographic examinations have also been carried out to a certain extent at departments of neuroradiology. These procedures will not be treated here, however, since as yet their significance can hardly be estimated. In any case it is too early to discuss their historical aspects.

Few discoveries can have attracted as much attention as the discovery of roentgen rays, and few can have been so rapidly utilized in so many fields. As early as the end of the nineteenth century, roentgenograms of the skull had been obtained in several different countries, and attempts to demonstrate or localize brain tumors had been made.

Church (1899), for instance, described a case in which views taken at the Fuchs X-Ray Laboratory showed what appeared to be a nodular tumor. At necropsy a tumor of the same appearance was found. In November of that year, Oppenheim (1899), in Berlin, reported a case of pituitary tumor that had been roentgenographically demonstrated. Already, in 1896, Arthur Schuster, a physicist, had at the request of a Dr. Little, in a small town in northwest England, demonstrated four bullets in the head of a patient with a gunshot wound, at an examination in the patient's home (Schuster, 1962). On September 10, 1896, the Swedish physician Stenbeck (1900) obtained a lateral view of the skull of a patient suffering from headaches after an earlier gunshot wound. A bullet was shown in the occipital region. Later he also succeeded in obtaining a frontal view and was thus able to localize the bullet exactly. An operation on this patient performed by Lennander on February 2, 1897, revealed that the bullet was in the position suggested in the occipital region. It was situated at a depth of 1 cm and 4.5 cm to the right of the median line, close to the calcarine fissure. This case was reported by Henschen (1897) at a congress in Moscow. It was probably the first case in which an intracranial lesion was localized exactly with roentgen rays and treated successfully by surgery.

The central nervous system forms the subject for neuroradiologic study, since no method is available for the investigation of the peripheral nerves. The brain and spinal cord lie for the most part enclosed in a shell formed by the skeleton. Expanding processes within this shell may affect its appearance. On the other hand, diseases originating in the bones of the skull or vertebral column may give rise to signs or symptoms of brain or spinal cord involvement. As important as investigations of the skull and vertebral column may be, however, they can seldom provide more than indirect signs of disease in the central nervous system.

Investigation of the skull and vertebral column forms part of the general practice of roentgen diagnostics. The technique must be mastered by all radiologists, even though these examinations are also included in a neuroradiologic analysis of symptoms or signs from the brain or spinal cord. Only after the introduction of contrast media, which permit a more direct demonstration of the pathologic condition, can it be said that neuroradiology was born. Thus neuroradiology came into existence, according to this view, with the introduction of pneumography. The next important date in the development of neuroradiology was 1927, when a method for examination of the blood vessels was added to the other possibilities. The last period of development began in 1947, when radioactive isotopes were first applied as a supplement to the earlier diagnostic methods.

EARLY PERIOD

Before neuroradiology proper was developed, there was a long period in which the skeleton in normal and various pathologic states was studied intensively. During that period special attention was directed to the complex anatomy of the skull, with respect both to the general roentgenographic appearances and to the most suitable projections for best defining details. Several important discoveries about the appearance of the bones in different diseases were also made during this period. In the view of some radiologists (Bull and Fischgold, 1967), this era of development belongs to neuroradiology; but in my opinion the period belongs to the general development of the entire field of diagnostic radiology.

As already mentioned, roentgenograms of the skull were obtained at an early stage, despite the long exposures that were necessary. At first these exposure times were as long as 30 minutes with intervals of 1 minute of direct exposure alternating with 1 minute's cooling of the tube. In 1902, however, Pfahler, using an exposure time of 4 minutes and a tube distance of 18 inches, obtained a view that "showed good detail of all structures, namely the scalp, the outer table of the skull, the diploe and the inner table, the frontal sinuses, the ethmoidal, sphenoidal and mastoid cells, the coronal suture, the groove of the posterior meningeal artery, the outline of the base of the skull and the depressions of the frontal convolutions." In a patient with symptoms and signs suggestive of brain tumor, Pfahler also found what appeared to be a dumbbell-shaped tumor. At operation a tumor was located in the place suggested. He also conducted experiments on cadavers. A part of the brain was removed and replaced with embalmed tumor, simulating as nearly as possible the conditions in the living subject. In his experiments on some live subjects, he was able to demonstrate transparent areas "which corresponded with the areas of degeneration subsequently found at autopsy." The cautious optimism aroused by these experiments soon proved to be premature, however, for most of the intracranial pathologic processes could not be directly demonstrated.

The investigator mainly responsible for elucidating the roentgenographic anatomy of the skull and the best projections to show its various structures was Schüller. Several reports had already been published in this field at the end of the nineteenth and the beginning of the twentieth century. The two works by Schüller, "Die Schädelbasis im Röntgen-Bilde," in 1905, and *Röntgen-Diagnostik der Erkrankungen des Kopfes,* in 1912, must be accorded fundamental significance, however. In regard to projections, Schüller mentioned twelve suitable directions for the rays even in the first of these two publications. In the preface to his "Apparatus and Technique for Roentgen Examination of the Skull," Lysholm (1931) stated: "It is surprising to note how little new in the way of different ways of projections has been published. It is true that the literature on skull roentgenology has been simply flooded by a vast number of different projections and variations of projections mostly named after those who have suggested them. A great number of them can be traced back to Schüller and many are probably only used in the institutions where they originated. This idea of naming the projections after their authors has as a result that the name will come to vary according to the language in which the publication has been issued. This naturally results in great confusion."* Although in general these statements may be correct, many of the more recently introduced modifications nevertheless have provided increased possibilities for detailed diagnosis. This statement applies also to the wholly new projections, especially those for the petrous bone and the nasal sinuses.

Schüller, who was the first to demonstrate calcifications in the pineal body, in 1906, stated in his work from 1912: "Auch kann man beispielsweise bei Verlagerung des Schattens der Zirbeldrüse, nach rechts oder links von der Medianebene bei symmetrisch geformten Schädeln, auf eine Verschiebung durch Druck von Seite eines Tumors oder Zug von Seite einer Hirnnarbe schliessen."† Thus, even in this early report, Schüller pointed out the significance of the position of the pineal body. The bone diseases that are usually known under his name—Schüller-Christian disease, osteoporosis circumscripta cranii and cephalhematoma deformans—are, however, of less interest from the aspect of neuroradiology. Because of his work on the skull early in this century, Schüller is considered by some authors, e.g., Bull and Fischgold (1967), as the father of neuroradiology. In my opinion he ought rather to be described as one

---

*From Lysholm, E.: Apparatus and technique for roentgen examination of the skull, Acta Radiol., supp. 12, pp. 1-120, 1931.

†"One may, for instance, conclude that displacement of the pineal shadow to the right or left of midline in symmetric skulls is due to pressure by a tumor or to traction from cerebral scarring." From Schüller, A.: Röntgen-Diagnostik der Erkrankungen des Kopfes, Vienna, 1912, A. Hölder.

of its forerunners. At no time did he express interest in the contrast medium studies that are a characteristic of true neuroradiology. The view advanced by Bingel, in 1921, namely, that before that time one could speak of roentgenology of the skull but not of the brain—"wohl von einer Röntgenologie des Schädels nicht aber von einer des Gehirns sprechen (kann)," seems to me more in accord with the real situation.

In 1902, Béclère, in Paris, showed roentgenograms of the skull of a young healthy woman and roentgenograms of a 24-year-old patient with acromegaly. By comparing the two, he demonstrated three characteristic roentgenographic changes in acromegaly: "(1) un épaississement irrégulier des parois crâniennes, (2) un développement extraordinairement exagéré en hauteur et en profondeur des sinus frontaux auxquels se joint d'ailleurs un développement analogue des sinus maxillaires, (3) une augmentation très notable, dans le sens vertical et surtout dans le sens antéropostérieur, des dimensions de la fosse pituitaire."*

Thus in the first decade of the twentieth century, knowledge had been acquired regarding the most important projections for different anatomic structures in the skull. By that time the normal appearance of these structures had been established. It was also known that intracranial tumors were demonstrable if they distorted the sella turcica (pituitary tumors), contained calcifications, encroached on the sinuses, or destroyed any part of the skull. At the beginning of the next decade, the importance of the position of the pineal body began to be realized. Demonstration of tumors of the acoustic nerve also became possible at this time. Henschen (1912) had observed at autopsies that these tumors nearly always widened the internal auditory meatus. He therefore referred a patient with a possible acoustic tumor to the radiologist Forssell. An oblique lateral view was obtained, with the ray directed slightly from the vault so that the internal meatus was superimposed over the external meatus. A dilatation on the affected side was visible when compared with the appearance on the opposite side. Why a more suitable projection was not used is strange, in view of the knowledge then available about the anatomy of the skull and the direction of the rays for demonstrating different structures.

By the middle of the second decade, the roentgenographic appearance of the skull as well as some of the changes produced by intracranial tumors were known in several countries. A review by Heuer and Dandy in 1916, however, revealed that of 100 consecutive brain tumors proved at operation the tumor was distinguishable in only six cases. An additional nine had been detected because of bone destruction.

Air in the ventricular system was demonstrated for the first time in 1912. A 47-year-old man was admitted with a head injury to a hospital in New York. He was under the care of W. Luckett, who submitted him to radiography, which was performed by W. H. Stewart. Skull fractures involving the posterior wall of the frontal sinuses were detected. Three weeks later the patient was again examined because of deterioration. Immediately before the examination he had had an attack of sneezing followed by a terrific pain in the head. At the second examination Stewart found what appeared to be air or gas in dilated ventricles. The patient was operated on by Luckett, and since the fluid in the ventricle proved to be sterile, air and not gas was assumed to be present (Luckett, 1913). This case thus was the first of what later was called traumatic pneumatocele. During the next few years similar cases were observed and described.

PNEUMOGRAPHY

Despite the fact that air had been observed in the cranium following fractures and Williams as early as 1901 had described various radiologic procedures based on injection of air, the use of air as a contrast medium for examination of the intracranial spaces was not suggested until 1918.

The limited possibilities for detection of intracranial tumors at roentgenography of the skull led to further experiments by Dandy (1918). By injecting "the various solutions and suspensions used in pyelography" into the ventricles of dogs, he tried to depict the ventricular system. He stated that these were "always with fatal results, owing to the injurious effects on the brain." A contrast medium, Dandy (1919a) wrote, "must satisfy two very rigid exactions, (1) it must be absolutely non-irritating and non-toxic; and (2) it must be readily absorbed and excreted." Dandy worked at the Johns Hopkins Hospital, in the Department of Surgery with W. S. Halsted. Dandy's report, "Ventriculography Following the Injection of Air into the Cerebral Ventricles," may be said to have signified the birth of neuroradiology (Fig. 1-1). In it he stated:

> It is largely due to the frequent comment by Doctor Halsted on the remarkable power of intestinal gas to "perforate bone" that my attention was drawn to its practical possibilities in the brain. . . . The stomach and intestines are often outlined by the contained air, even more sharply than when filled with bismuth. . . . The paranasal sinuses and mastoid cells show up

*"(1)an irregular thickening of the cranial vault; (2) an extraordinary and exaggerated development in height and depth of both the frontal and the maxillary sinuses; (3) a distinct increase in size vertically, and particularly in the anteroposterior dimensions, of the pituitary fossa." From Béclère, A.: L'exposé des travaux scientifiques du docteur Antoine Béclère, médecin de l'Hôpital Saint-Antoine, Paris, 1907, Masson & Cie.

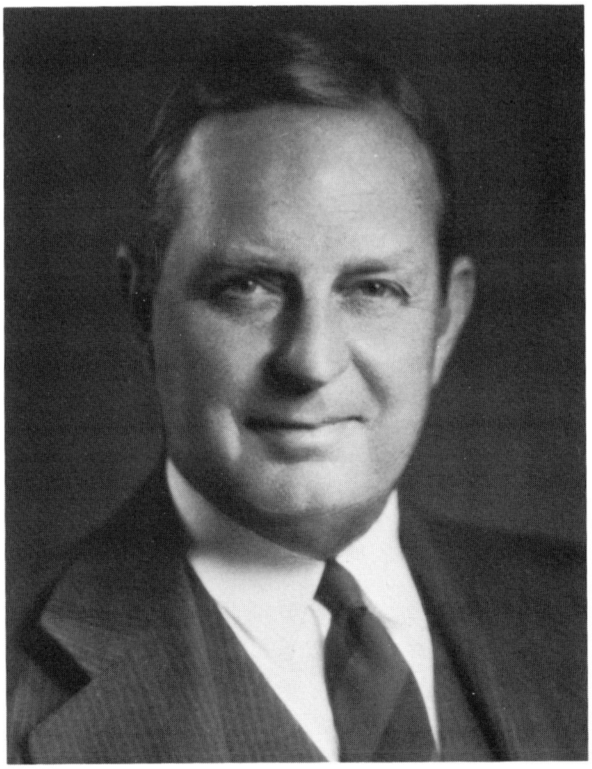

Fig. 1-1. Walter Dandy (1886-1946).

in a thick skull by virtue of the air, and pathological conditions of the sinuses are evident because inflammatory or tumor tissue replaces the air. From these and many other normal and pathological clinical demonstrations of the radiographic properties of air, it is but a step to the injection of gas into the cerebral ventricles—pneumoventriculography.*

In this first description of ventriculography, Dandy reported his experiences from "at least twenty" injections. In some instances the injections had been repeated. All of the injections had been made in children of from 6 months to 12 years of age. The amount of air injected had varied from 40 to 300 ml. In only one child was any reaction observed. The lateral ventricles were sharply outlined in all the patients, and in two the third ventricle was visible as well. The aqueduct of Sylvius and the fourth ventricle were never observed. A diagram illustrated that more fluid could be removed when a single ventricular puncture was made anteriorly and the forehead was depended. Dandy summarized his observations as follows: "Even in the few cases here reported, ventriculography has proved of great practical value." The value was expected to lie mainly in the assessment of the lateral ventricles, since demonstration of the third and fourth ventricles with any regularity seemed unlikely.

*From Dandy, W. E.: Ventriculography following the injection of air into the cerebral ventricles, Amer. J. Roentgen. **6**:26-36, 1919.

Dandy had noticed that air injected into the ventricular system sometimes passed out into the subarachnoid space over the cerebral convexity. In another report (1919b) he wrote:

> These observations at once gave promise of new possibilities in intracranial diagnostic studies. After the injection of air into a cerebral ventricle, a certain amount will soon appear on the external surface of the brain, if the head is carefully manipulated so that the air is guided to the small aqueduct of Sylvius and the fourth ventricle. . . . The problem therefore before us was: How can we in every case be sure of obtaining a complete injection of the subarachnoid space? The solution lies in the direct injection of air into the spinal canal. A small quantity of spinal fluid is withdrawn and an equal amount of air injected into the spinal canal. This process of substitution is repeated until the fluid ceases to appear on aspiration.*

Dandy's original technique consisted of placing the patient recumbent with the head elevated at least 20° above the lumbar region. To avoid excessive pressure intracranially, the needle was left open for 2 or 3 minutes after the last injection of air. In his first publication (1918) he reported on eight cases without any bad effect. He also drew the conclusion that "from the data obtainable from the combination of intraventricular and intraspinous injections, it is difficult to see how intracranial tumors can escape localization." This comment reveals the great significance Dandy himself placed on these two methods of examination. Many decades were required, however, for improvement and elaboration of the technique and for development of a systematization of the results before ventriculography and encephalography became tolerably safe. We also know today that, despite the highly developed technique, brain tumors cannot always be demonstrated or correctly localized by pneumography.

Time was ripe, so to speak, for the injection of air into the ventricular system or the subarachnoid space. Observations and speculations similar to those advanced by Dandy had been reported by other investigators without previous knowledge of Dandy's work. Bingel (Fig. 1-2), for instance, wrote in 1921: "Nachdem wir wissen, dass luftgefüllte Gebilde, Trachea, Lunge, Pneumothorax, aufgeblähter Magen und Darm sich gut differenzieren und nachdem wir gelernt haben, dass Lufteinblasungen in die Gelenke oder in die Bauchhöhle den Kontrastreichtum der Röntgenbilder ganz bedeutend heben und ausserdem gut vertragen werden, lag es nahe zu versuchen, ob Ähnliches nicht auch beim Gehirn

*From Dandy, W. E.: Roentgenography of the brain after the injection of air into the spinal canal, Ann. Surg. **70**:397-403, 1919.

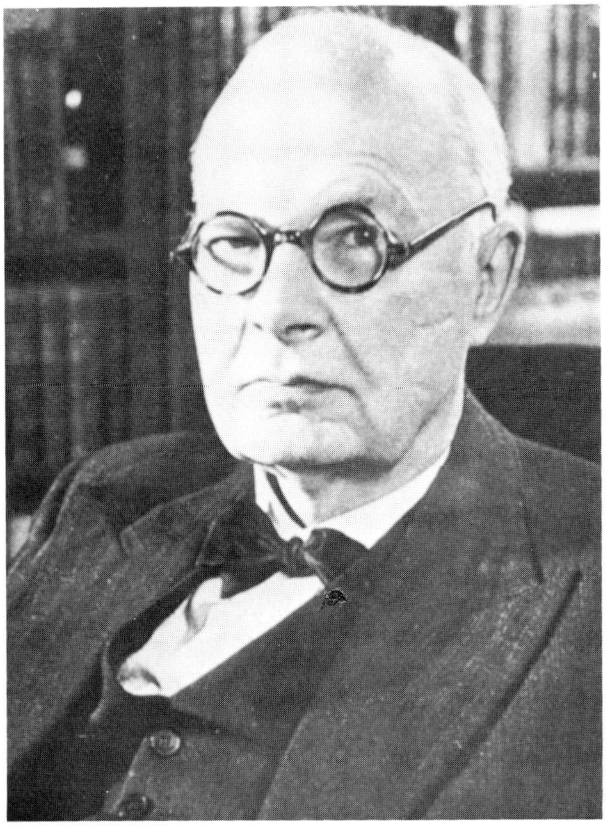

Fig. 1-2. Adolf Bingel (1879-1963).

möglich ist. Die Röntgenbilder der intrakraniellen Pneumatocele geben einen Hinweis." In that article Bingel stated that Dandy, on the basis of similar reasoning, had suggested a procedure, which he had named ventriculography, and continued: "Ich bin ohne Kenntnis der amerikanischen Arbeit anders vorgegangen."* Bingel first injected air after lumbar puncture and withdrew a few milliliters of spinal fluid. In his attempt to demonstrate spinal expanding processes by this method, he was successful in two cases. Shortly afterwards he drew attention to a report by Wideröe (1921), who also had tried to localize spinal tumors after the injection of air into the lumbar region. In these studies Wideröe observed that the intracranial subarachnoid space, but not the ventricular system, was filled with air. Bingel had begun with trials in human cadavers. He had observed that the air, after lumbar puncture, was distributed both through the ventricular system and in the sulci on the convexity. Later he demonstrated this same distribution to be achieved in the living. "Es ist klar, dass eine Lumbalpunktion einen wesentlichen geringeren Eingriff bedeutet, als eine Hirnpunktion und ausserdem bringt die intralumbale Lufteinblasung erheblich mehr zur Darstellung, nämlich ausser den Ventrikel die grosse Längshirnspalte und die Oberfläche des Gehirns."* Bingel suggested that ventriculography and encephalography might be combined when a pathologic process prevented the air from passing into the ventricular system. He injected 40 to 60 ml of air into the sitting patient by fractionated exchange in amounts of 5 to 10 ml after the withdrawal of corresponding amounts of cerebrospinal fluid. Maintenance of pressure was considered of great importance, and a simple device was therefore used to record continuous pressure. He asserted that the dangers of the method associated with increases in intracranial pressure could in this way be reduced ("dass man. . . . die Gefahren erheblich verringern kann"). The films were exposed after the patient had been placed in the recumbent position. Fluoroscopy was also used to obtain a general view of how the air was distributed. Bingel further demonstrated that the air could be made to flow between the lateral ventricles if the position of the patient's head was altered. Side effects of headache and vomiting were noted, and measures for reducing these were suggested. One of the first forty patients reported had diabetes and clinical signs of a cerebellar tumor. No air passed into the ventricular system at encephalography. From the appearance of the air on the convexity, Bingel concluded that an expanding process was present in the left cerebellar hemisphere. Ventriculography was also performed a few weeks later in this patient. An amount of 120 ml of air was injected into the ventricular system, and considerable dilatation of the lateral ventricles was revealed. Bingel commented on his results: "Die amerikanische Methode der direkten Lufteinblasung in die Ventrikel hatte also den Hydrocephalus internus elegant ad oculos demonstriert.

*"Since we know that air-filled structures, trachea, lungs, pneumothorax, inflated stomach and intestine are well demonstrated and since we have learned that air insufflations into joints or abdominal cavity not only markedly enhance the roentgenographic contrast but are also well tolerated, it seemed reasonable to attempt to determine whether a similar process was not also possible in the brain. The roentgenograms of an intracranial pneumatocele gave a suggestion."

"I proceeded, using a different technique, without prior knowledge of the American work."

From Bingel, A.: Zur Technik der intralumbalen Lufteinblasung insbesondere zum Zwecke der "Encephalographie," Deutsch. Med. Wschr. **47**:1492-1493, 1921.

*"It is clear that lumbar puncture represents a much less serious intervention than cerebral puncture, and besides that, the lumbar injection of air gives much better demonstration not only of the ventricles but also of the interhemispheric fissure and the surface of the brain." From Bingel, A.: Intralumbale Lufteinblasung zur Höhendiagnose intraduraler extramedullärer Prozesse und zur Differentialdiagnose gegenüber intramedullären Prozessen, Deutsch. Z. Nervenheilk. **72**:359-370, 1921.

Durch meine Methode war ebenfalls die Behinderung des Liquorabflusses dargetan, die Beachtung der Medulla-Kleinhirnbucht gab aber ausserdem noch einen wichtigen Hinweis auf den Sitz der Erkrankung im linken Kleinhirn."* The term encephalography, which he applied to his examination method, has been generally accepted since then. In my opinion his procedure was more logical than Dandy's. It was also more suitable from the technical point of view since the intracranial distribution of the air was more symmetric. Subsequently, in fact, the encephalographic method has been developed along the lines suggested by Bingel's technique.

Whereas American and British investigators seem to have been fairly restrictive in their use of encephalography, several reports of the procedure appeared in the German literature (Weigeldt, 1922, 1923; Wartenberg, 1924-1925; Fischer, 1926-1927, 1927-1928; Heidrich, 1927, 1928; Flügel, 1930). In addition to air in the lumbar region, these workers injected air after cisternal puncture. They noted that the ventricular system was often more completely filled after cisternal puncture than after lumbar puncture. After lumbar puncture the sulci and cisterns, instead, were better filled. In Europe also a definite tendency toward the use of smaller amounts of air than in America was especially noticeable with cisternal puncture. Schaeffer (1929) stated that besides less air being needed with cisternal punctures, the patient's reaction was less severe than with a lumbar injection. Schaltenbrand (1932, 1933) held that 30 to 40 ml were sufficient for a cisternal puncture as compared with approximately 100 ml by the lumbar route. Denk (1923) stressed the danger of encephalography when brain tumor was suggested and maintained that ventriculography should be employed in these cases. Bingel endorsed this view in 1928, after several deaths had followed the injection of gas in the lumbar region in patients with brain tumor. The Americans Martin and Uhler (1922), however, considered that only tumors of the posterior fossa constituted contraindications to encephalography. Heidrich (1928) used this method to demonstrate the presence of suprasellar extension of pituitary tumors. Flügel (1930) expressed the belief that a possible brain tumor should not preclude encephalography; but he injected only 20 ml of air by cisternal puncture. Gardner and Nichols (1933) described encephalography with large amounts of air in thirty-three patients with increased intracranial pressure. Complications arose in only one, but the respiratory disturbances disappeared after a ventricular puncture. These authors, however, stressed that encephalography should be used only if preparations for immediate craniotomy had been made in advance.

This period in the history of encephalography was characterized mainly by various suggestions concerning the technical aspects of air injection. As Davidoff and Dyke (1946) have pointed out, two groups whose techniques differed were distinguishable. The first group injected air with a syringe through the inserted needle via a single lumbar puncture. The second group used a more complicated method, which also included measurement of the pressure. This group used one lumbar needle (Bingel's original method, 1921; Schinz, 1922; Wartenberg, 1924-1925) or two lumbar needles (Bingel's modified method, 1928; von Storch, 1936). With the latter technique, air was injected through the upper needle and the cerebrospinal fluid flowed out through the lower one. The purely roentgenologic technique, in contrast, did not receive the same attention, either in ventriculography or in encephalography. The reason for this difference in emphasis may have been that most of those engaged in such investigations were clinicians, usually neurologists or neurosurgeons. Radiologists were not particularly interested in the problem. The exposure of the films after the air injection was not done in accordance with clear-cut principles. Some investigators obtained anteroposterior, posteroanterior, and lateral views with vertically directed rays and the patient always recumbent; other investigators took views with the patient always in the sitting position; still others obtained views with the patient in both the recumbent and the sitting positions. For the most part, views were obtained immediately after the termination of the air injection; but a few investigators (Friedman et al., 1928) took them on the following day. Pancoast and Fay (1929), however, attempted a standardization of the roentgenologic technique.

Encephalography is often an unpleasant experience for the patient. Headache, nausea, vomiting, pallor, perspiration, a fall in blood pressure, and faintness may occur both during and after the examination. Even in the early days, Bingel (1922) noted that with certain conditions such reactions were much milder and in some instances even absent. This was especially true in patients with generalized cerebral disease. The postencephalographic reactions usually persisted for up to 3 days, but in some cases they lasted as long as a week. Many theories were advanced to account for this phenomenon. Gradually the view became accepted that the severity and duration of the reactions depended mainly on the amount of air injected. If the amount of air was small

*"The American method of direct injection of air into the ventricle had also elegantly demonstrated internal hydrocephalus. With my method likewise, a hindrance to the cerebrospinal fluid outflow was shown, but, in addition, an evaluation of the posterior fossa cisterns indicated the presence of an abnormality of the left cerebellar hemisphere." From Bingel, A.: Encephalographie, eine Methode zur röntgenographischen Darstellung des Gehirns, Fortschr. Roentgenstr. **28**:205-217, 1921.

and was injected by cisternal puncture, reactions often failed to appear at all when only the ventricular system was filled. Consequently, Laruelle (1933) at an early stage devised the most drastic changes. He injected the air with the patient sitting, because air rises through the cerebrospinal fluid as high as it can reach. The head was slightly flexed so that air would pass into the ventricular system. Too much flexion or too upright a position of the head usually caused the air to flow out into the subarachnoid space; or, in the upright position, the air could become concentrated below the tentorium cerebelli. The first film was exposed immediately after the injection had been completed, so that the third ventricle could be studied. Laruelle (1933) stated that an anteroposterior view obtained after injection of 2 to 5 ml of air would show whether the ventricular system was normal. If this view suggested the possibility of pathologic conditions, more air was injected. An amount of 10 ml was considered sufficient to permit assessment of the size of the lateral ventricles even when hydrocephalus was present. By changing the position of the head, the air could be distributed within the ventricular system so that different parts were outlined in turn. Six different positions of the head were used for this purpose. Thus Laruelle was the first to draw attention to the simple fact that gas rises upward in a liquid. He also showed that the distribution of air within the cranium depends on the position of the head during the injection. Furthermore he demonstrated that a large amount of air was not needed. A small amount of air, maneuvered about in the ventricular system by repositioning of the patient's head, offered just as much information as a large amount. Many years were to pass, however, before the significance of these two essential principles was fully recognized. In the beginning the small amount of air was the main subject of discussion. The risks involved in the examination as well as the discomfort to the patient could undoubtedly be reduced by keeping the amount of air low. Conversely, the general consensus seemed to be that the diagnostic effectiveness of the method was decreased.

In general the pneumographic diagnosis was based on the interpretation of roentgenograms obtained in certain standard projections. These projections differed in different clinics, and the result naturally depended on the suitability in the individual case and on the experience of the interpreter. Consequently the results from the different clinics were hardly comparable. Opinions regarding the value of the pneumographic method would thus still have differed, even if the primary material had been published in detail. As with the examination of the skull bones, the precision of the positioning left much to be desired. An apparatus was needed that could be of assistance in obtaining exactly

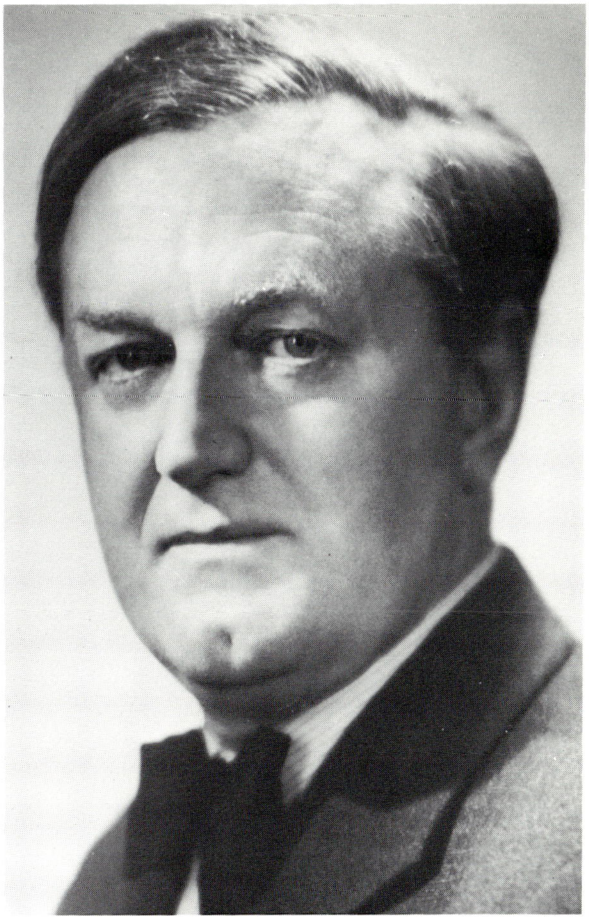

Fig. 1-3. Erik Lysholm (1891-1947).

projected films and could ensure their exact reproduction. After a few preliminary experiments Lysholm (Fig. 1-3) presented the first skull table in 1931, which represented the first precision apparatus for roentgenography (Fig. 1-4). The requirements of the pneumographic examinations soon necessitated alterations in the design of the table, however. The new apparatus, which is known today as Lysholm's skull table and whose underlying principle has been copied in many countries, was presented in 1935 (Fig. 1-5). The basic idea of the design was that the roentgen tube could be moved along the surface of a sphere. Its central ray was always directed toward the center of the sphere. The position of the tube could be determined by reading off different angles, and the focus film distance was constant. When the direction of the roentgen ray was changed, the result of the altered direction could be calculated. With the aid of this apparatus, a large number of pneumographic examinations (ventriculography, encephalography) were performed in the early 1930's by the "Stockholm school," at that time led by Lysholm. The principle of the technique was to localize the collections of air and determine their shape by roentgenograms in at least two projections obtained at right angles to each other without change of position of the head. This technique meant, among other things, that to a large extent the rays were horizontally directed even in the recumbent patient. The air in turn was moved to different parts of the ventricular system by alteration of the positions of the head. The amount of air and the observations during examination as well as the clinical problem determined the projections used and the order of their application. It may be said that the guiding principle was to "place the air against the tumor area." Accordingly, despite the fact that certain standard projections were used, each case constituted a special problem that required variation and individualization of the positioning and exposure techniques. Since the focus film distance was always constant, the different sectional views could be joined to make a composite drawing of the appearance of the whole ventricular system. This three-dimensional sketch facilitated analysis of the material at a later stage.

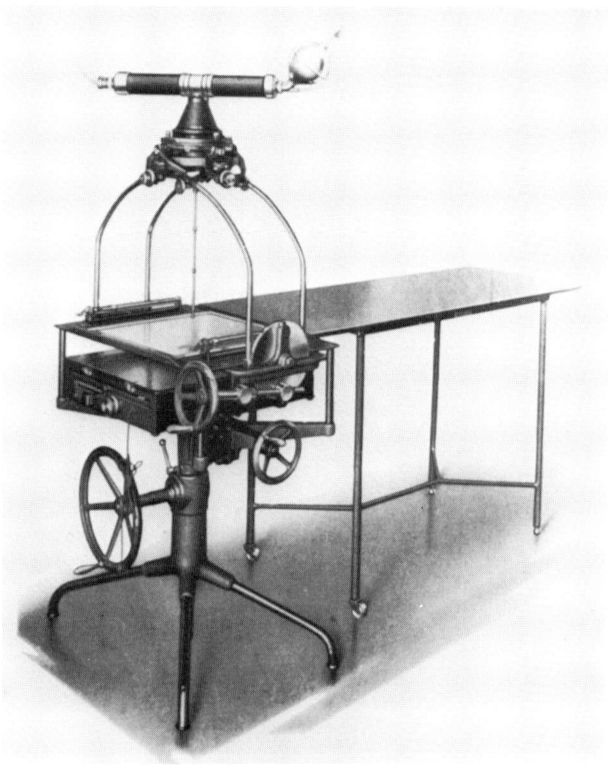

Fig. 1-4. Lysholm's original apparatus for roentgen examination of the skull (1931). It was developed from his earlier apparatus and was designed for examination of nasal sinuses and the ear (1925). It was found unsuitable for examination of other parts of skull. Water cooled the roentgen tube. Note the simple table for the patient.

Lysholm and co-workers presented results of their investigations on this subject in "Das Ventrikulogramm," from 1935 to 1937. The first part dealt with the apparatus, the examination technique, and the normal roentgenologic appearances of the ventricular system; the second part considered tumors in the third and fourth ventricles and the aqueduct; and the third part dealt with supratentorial tumors. Their work, now a classic, formed the foundation for all subsequent pneumographic diagnosis of tumors. Only a few details have required readjustment and expansion since that time. All the essential changes in the ventricular system, related to tumors in different sites, are to be found in these volumes. The book was written in German, and unfortunately its existence became known only slowly in English-speaking countries. It was not mentioned in the bibliography of Davidoff and Dyke's second edition of *The Normal Encephalogram* (1946). Had the fundamental knowledge in Lsyholm's book been known and applied in wider circles, the literature from the following 20 years would have been different. My statement (in 1948) would then not have been justified: "A certain amount of knowledge may be taken over from literature studies, but in the field of neuroradiology there is less to be gained than one would a priori expect."

One detail, but an essential one, that was not described adequately in Lysholm's book, however, was the temporal horn. Torkildsen said in 1933: "Some parts of the ventricles are difficult to fill well, and one should not attach, consequently, too much importance to the findings concerning such positions. This is especially true of the inferior horns." Even in 1937, Childe and Penfield remarked: "In published pneumographic studies the temporal or inferior horn of the lateral cerebral ventricle has received scant attention, and there is a persisting misconception of its shape to be found in textbooks of anatomy." Their investigation was the first attempt at a thorough study of this part

Fig. 1-5. Lysholm skull table. **A,** In 1935, apparatus appears same with only small changes of details. It is this design that usually is called Lysholm's skull table. Primary diaphragms are seen on the stand. **B,** Use of shock-proof and ray-proof tube housings made heavier counterweight necessary and U-shaped foot stand instead of earlier T-shaped one. **C,** Last development: tilting device for tube and floor-wall–mounted apparatus (1950). Note the more convenient patient table. Types of Lysholm skull table represent general development of apparatuses for roentgen examination of skull until 1960.

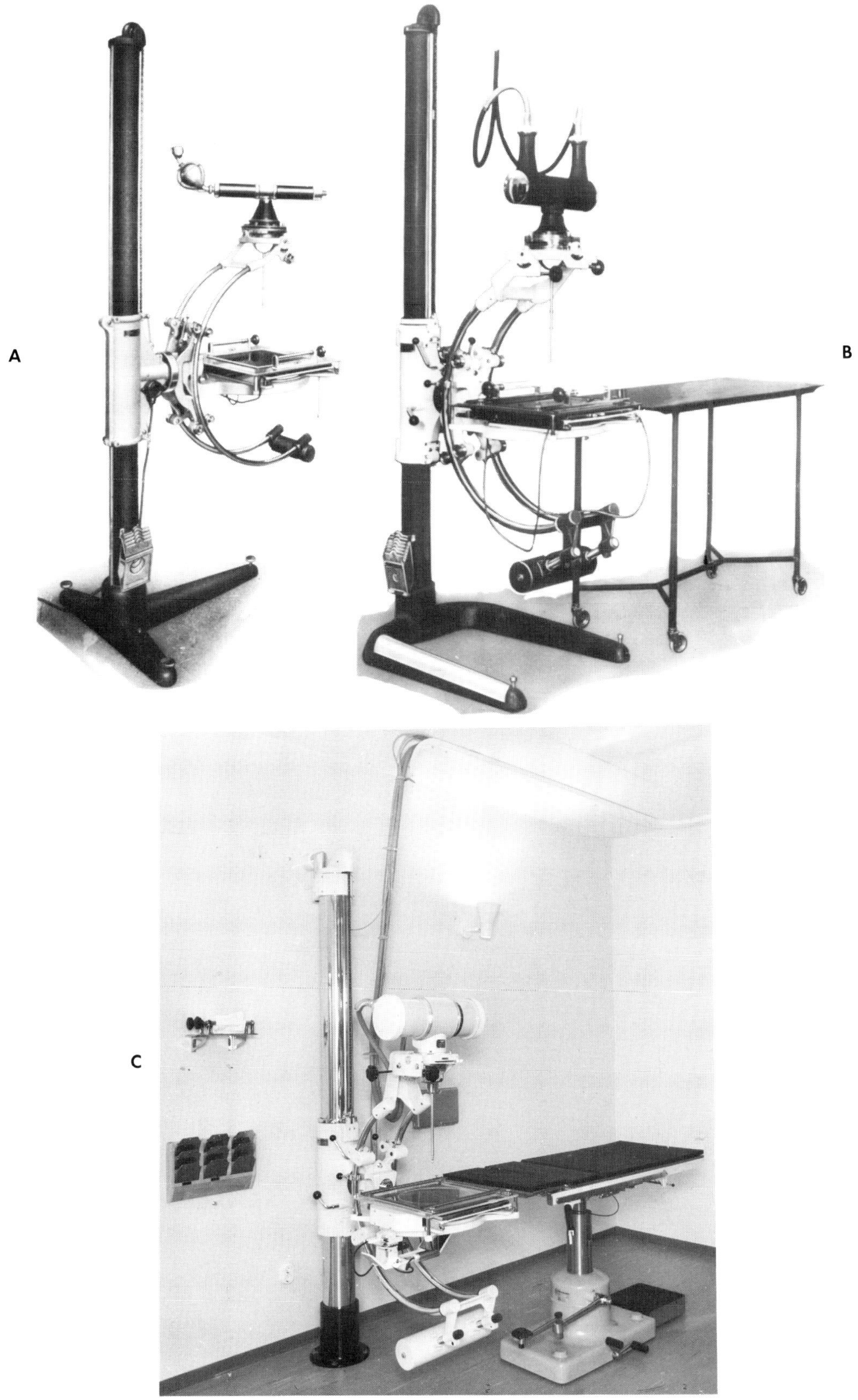

Fig. 1-5. For legend see opposite page.

of the lateral ventricle. Their description, however, seems to have been partly misunderstood even by Davidoff and Dyke (in 1946). The deficiency that had existed until then was rectified in some measure by Childe and Penfield (1937); but the definitive report was first presented by the Stockholm school (Lindgren, 1948). It included descriptions of the anatomic and roentgenographic appearances of the temporal horn and the technique for its roentgenographic demonstration. The appearance of the temporal horn in various types of tumor was described. The significance of its position not only for the localization of temporally situated tumors was discussed. That report stated among other things that some tumors in the middle cranial fossa do not cause general displacement or distortion of the ventricular system. Such tumors therefore cannot be demonstrated unless the temporal horn is investigated adequately. This finding could explain to some extent the statements in the literature that cerebral tumors may be present even when the ventricular system is judged to be normal. In many cases, however, the ventricles had not been examined with an adequate roentgenologic technique. The statements were based only on anteroposterior or posteroanterior views possibly supplemented with lateral views obtained with a vertically directed ray (Pennybacker and Meadows, 1938). By and large, the role of radiologists in pneumographic examinations both earlier and at that time was, with few exceptions, minor. This lack of involvement by radiologists may explain why the roentgenographic technique often left much to be desired. Although conditions have gradually changed in this respect, they still remain as before in many quarters.

Robertson (1941) studied the intracranial movements of the air at encephalography in some detail. He confirmed Laruelle's statement (1931, 1933) in regard to the significance of the position of the head during the injection of air. He also pointed out that the fourth ventricle and aqueduct were more easily studied while the air passed into the ventricular system than when it flowed out. Injection of the air before the withdrawal of cerebrospinal fluid was advised. Robertson stated that 20 ml were sufficient for an examination of the ventricular system. For the cisterns and the subarachnoid space on the convexity, he used up to 100 ml. His first monograph on encephalography was published in 1941, but knowledge of his views seems to have been delayed. Probably the conditions that prevailed immediately after World War II accounted for this delay.

Flügel had already pointed out, in 1930, that cisternal puncture with the patient seated and the head in forward flexion was the best method to accomplish filling of the ventricular system: "Wir haben den Eindruck, dass bei dieser Position die Luft besonders leicht in das Ventrikelsystem gelangt."* He also obtained a lateral view of the posterior cranial fossa after the injection of 5 to 6 ml of air. The fourth ventricle and the aqueduct could then be observed. The forward flexion of the head needed for cisternal puncture automatically created a position that would facilitate the passage of air into the fourth ventricle. Probably in many instances, when air was injected by the lumbar route, less attention was paid to the position of the head. Often the head may have been more or less erect. This disregard of head position may explain why investigators of that time considered lumbar puncture the method of choice for examination of the convexity. On the basis of these observations and those of Laruelle, the Stockholm school developed a technique for directing the air to different parts of the intracranial space. It consisted of alteration of the position of the head during, as well as after, the injection of air into the lumbar region (Lindgren, 1949). This technique does not differ in essentials from that of Robertson (1941). Both are based on the fact that gas rises in liquid. To ensure distention by fluid of the different parts of the subarachnoid space, the air should be injected before withdrawal of cerebrospinal fluid. The Stockholm school used about 15 ml in an undilated ventricular system and about the same amount for the convexity in a normal case. They considered that amounts exceeding 50 ml were seldom necessary, even when considerable dilatation of the cerebrospinal fluid spaces was present. Robertson (1941) also used encephalography if tumor was suspected and signs of increased pressure were absent. Observations made at autopsy after ventriculographies disclosed that the puncture needle had caused hemorrhage of various sizes in the brain substance of some patients. Roentgen examinations of patients who had previously undergone ventriculography showed that calcifications had formed in the needle track (Falk, 1951). For this reason encephalography was tried by the Stockholm school in an increasing number of patients even when intracranial pressure was increased. At first (1948, 1949) cisternal puncture was always performed in these patients. Information was then obtainable immediately regarding any obliteration of the cisterna magna resulting from herniation. If cerebrospinal fluid was obtained, 5 to 10 ml of air were injected slowly. The situation that was revealed in the immediately exposed roentgenograms governed the decision as to continuation or termination of the examination. Later, however, lumbar

---

*"We have the impression that in this position the air enters the ventricular system with particular ease." From Flügel, F. E.: Zur Methodik und Verwertbarkeit der Encephalographie in der Tumordiagnostik, Deutsch. Z. Nervenheilk. **112**:251-265, 1930.

A B C

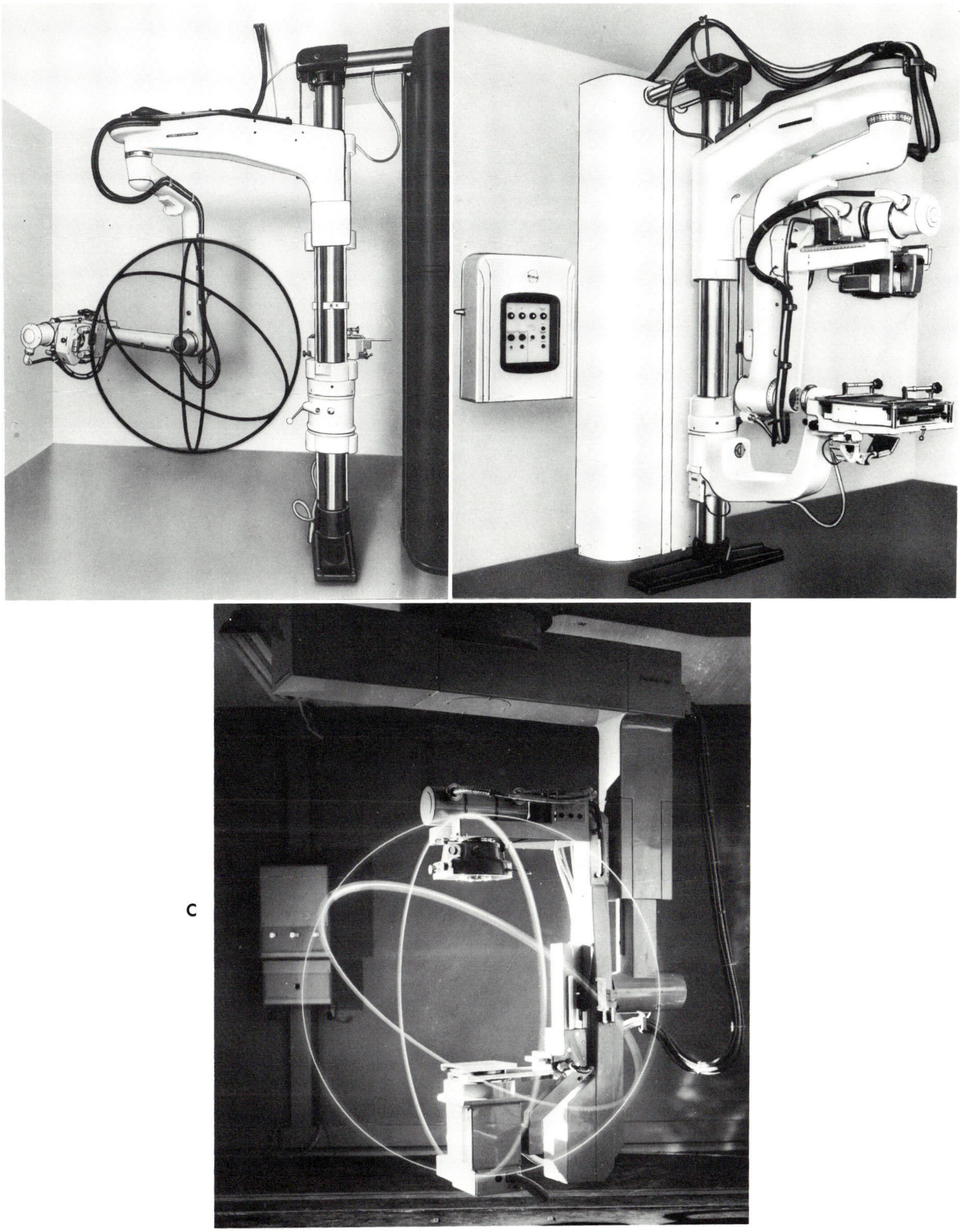

Fig. 1-6. A, First Mimer (1960). Ranges of rotation of roentgen tube are indicated by three circles. **B,** Mimer II adopted for use of Lysholm technique. **C,** Latest type (Mimer III, 1967) with image intensifier.

injection was also used in patients with increased intracranial pressure. Either no cerebrospinal fluid was removed in these patients or, after the completed injection of air, a smaller amount of fluid was removed than the amount of air injected. Encephalography is sometimes superior to ventriculography, especially when extracerebral expanding processes in the posterior cranial fossa and suprasellar region are to be evaluated (Lindgren, 1950b). Some of these tumors cannot be demonstrated or exactly localized, nor can their extent be determined, without the aid of encephalography. The reason that encephalography may be superior is that sometimes the subarachnoid space is changed earlier than the ventricular system. Tumors in the cerebellopontine angle, for instance, may have this effect (Liliequist, 1959a). A combination of ventriculography and encephalography may be of value in a few instances as pointed out by Bingel (1928) and later by Hyndman (1938). Although the appearance of the cisterns had been described earlier, a complete description was first published in 1959 (Liliequist, 1959b). As a result of this increased knowledge about the cisterns, the presence of an expanding intracranial lesion could be ascertained even when air did not pass into the ventricular system at encephalography.

An expanding intracranial process affects the appearance of the ventricular system and subarachnoid space not only through its own expanding growth; it also affects the appearance of these components by displacement of adjacent brain tissue with herniation of cerebral tissue into the foramen magnum, through the tentorium cerebelli, or over the sphenoid ridge. The changes thus produced by the tentorial herniation were described systematically for the first time by the Stockholm school at the Fourth Symposium Neuroradiologicum in London, in 1955 (Lindgren et al., 1956).

Many investigators have preferred ventriculography with positive contrast media when tumors lie in the posterior cranial fossa or posterior part of the third ventricle. Probably the reason for this preference is that in many cases the examination with air places great demands on the efficiency of the technique. Also this type of examination usually requires a relatively large amount of air, which in turn may cause deleterious effects; but Azambuja and his co-workers (1956) directly injected a small amount of air through a catheter inserted in the third ventricle. Azambuja later described his 6 years' experience with this technique at the Symposium Neuroradiologicum in Rome, in 1961. Unfortunately, however, the report was not included among the Symposium papers published subsequently, and the method is described only in the South American literature. This omission probably accounts for the unfamiliarity with the direct injection method.

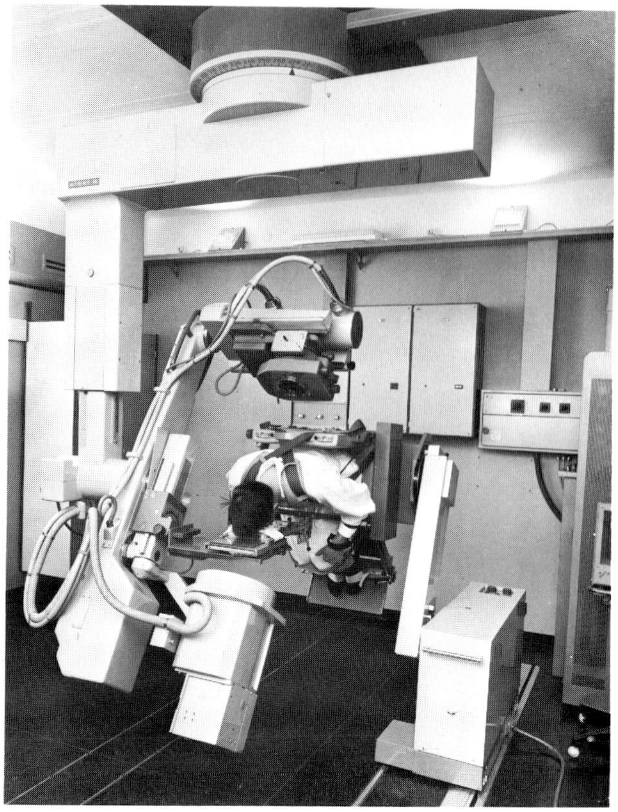

Fig. 1-7. Mimer III in use together with a rotating chair-couch for patient. Similar units were also constructed later in other countries.

The underlying principle of the Lysholm skull table is that every oblique projection causes a distortion that becomes greater with increasing obliquity in the direction of the rays. Dulac (1953, 1956) presented another principle. The tube and film plane were firmly fixed to an arm that was rotatable around a center. This center could be localized to a selected point in the head, which was entirely separate from the tube-film apparatus.

The original skull table was excellent for skull investigations and ventriculography. It proved to be less suitable, however, for angiography and encephalography as practiced by the Stockholm school. This deficiency led to the creation of another apparatus, the Mimer I (1959) (Fig. 1-6, *A*). Later the Mimer III (Fig. 1-6, *C*) was introduced in conjunction with the development of television screening. This apparatus allowed the examiner a free choice between the Lysholm principle and the Dulac principle. Similar types of apparatus were designed subsequently in other countries. During the past decade, a rotating chair has been used in several countries as an aid at encephalographic examinations. With this device the examiner may direct the air by bringing the patient into any desired position. Even somersaulting can be achieved (Fig. 1-7).

POSITIVE CONTRAST VENTRICULOGRAPHY

The first positive contrast medium employed in neuroradiology was an iodized oil (Lipiodol), introduced by Sicard and Forestier (1922) for myelography. Balado (1928) seems to have been the first to use it for investigation of the ventricular system. The Stockholm school also used Lipiodol in the middle 1930's but discontinued it after a few years. It was discarded partly because it was not resorbable and in some cases caused arachnoiditis. Also, with increasing experience, the pneumographic technique, if applied correctly, proved capable of giving equally good results. In the early 1940's a contrast medium was introduced that was a mixture of ethyl esters of isomeric iodophenyl undecylenic acid and was marketed as Pantopaque. It was much less viscous than Lipiodol at body temperature and also tended less to droplet formation. At the end of the examination, the positive contrast medium has to be maneuvered out of the ventricular system into the lumbosacral sac. Pantopaque or similar contrast media have since then been used in various clinics. They have served for investigation of the ventricular system, especially of the third and fourth ventricles. During recent years they have been used in examination of the cisterns in the posterior cranial fossa, particularly when acoustic neurinoma is suspected. I am in agreement, however, with a statement made by Bull at the Symposium Neuroradiologicum in Rotterdam, in 1949: "There is no doubt that air or oxygen is the contrast material of choice. The degree of success one obtains with air is an index of one's ability as a neuroradiologist. In my view the more often one falls back on positive contrast material, the less capable one proves oneself as a neuroradiologist."*

Even at present the iodized oils, particularly Pantopaque, are still widely used, especially in America. Their continued use is surprising since this form of contrast medium undoubtedly gives rise to arachnoiditis. The significance of arachnoiditis is admittedly open to discussion; but even if the inflammation should prove to be inconsiderable, the fact remains that because of the physical properties of these contrast media, the iodized oils cannot depict the anatomic relations with exactitude. For this reason alone they are unsuitable.

Bleasel, in 1961, used emulsified Pantopaque for lumbar myelography. His results stimulated Portera (1966) to use this myelographic method and also to employ the same emulsion for ventriculography. In his view the advantages were the elimination of special equipment and the shorter time needed for the examination than with air or Pantopaque techniques. The method has not been generally accepted, however.

*From Bull, J., and Fischgold, H.: A short history of neuroradiology, VIIIth Symposium Neuroradiologicum, Paris, 1967.

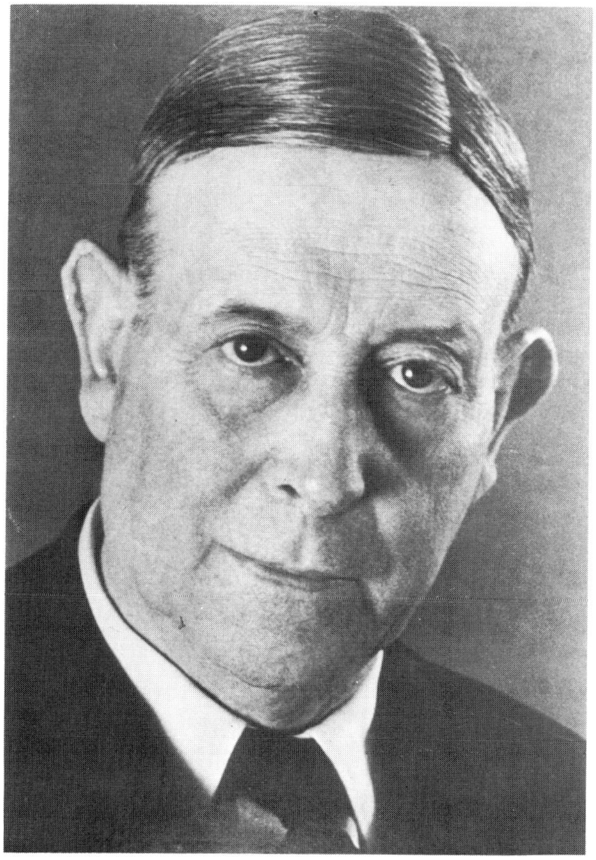

Fig. 1-8. Egas Moniz (1874-1955).

ANGIOGRAPHY

Although Dandy (1918) had introduced pneumography, the technique was far from faultless and for a long time the results were unsatisfactory. A survey of the literature by the American neurosurgeon Grant (1925) revealed that among 392 patients examined by ventriculography a correct diagnosis was obtained in only 124. In 1927 Olivecrona wrote in his monograph, *Die chirurgische Behandlung der Gehirntumoren:* "Für eine kritische Bewertung der Ventrikulographie bzw. Encephalographie als diagnostische Hilfsmittel bei Tumor cerebri und damit verwandten Symptomenkomplexen ist es aber noch zu früh."* Encephalography was considered by most workers to be contraindicated with increased intracranial pressure or when an intracranial

*"It is, however, too early for a critical evaluation of ventriculography and encephalography as aids in diagnosis of cerebral tumors and related symptom complexes." From Olivecrona, H.: Die chirurgische Behandlung der Gehirntumoren. Eine kleíne Studie, Berlin, 1927, Julius Springer, p. 243.

expanding process was suggested clinically. The Portuguese neurologist Moniz (1927) proposed that instead of attempts at improving the diagnostic possibilities of pneumography, a different method of examination be devised (Fig. 1-8). He suggested the introduction of a substance in large doses, either intravenously or by mouth, by which the brain would become directly visible in the roentgenogram. After trying lithium bromide and strontium bromide without success, he attempted the demonstration of blood vessels of the brain instead.

The outlining of blood vessels had been desired for almost as long a time as roentgen rays had been used in medicine, but all the radiopaque substances tried proved either to give unsatisfactory contrast in the roentgenograms or to be too toxic in man. The Argentinian radiologist Heuser (1919) was probably the first to fill blood vessels in human beings with a contrast medium. In a report in 1919, he stated that he had injected potassium iodide into a vein in a dog. He could "observe great opacity in all the veins of the limb." At that time syphilis was treated with potassium iodide or sodium iodide, and he obtained roentgenograms of the veins of the arm when these substances were injected intravenously. In addition, he observed the iodide in a roentgenogram of the heart of a child with congenital syphilis. Heuser concluded his paper with a recommendation "to those who have hospital services, for here is a new method for examining the pulmonary artery and vein." A few years later Osborne discovered that injected sodium iodide was rapidly excreted through the kidneys. This observation gave Rowntree the idea for the examination known today as urography. Osborne and his coworkers had described the method in 1923. They had also examined a patient's arm fluoroscopically and had observed that the vein into which the iodide was injected had "the appearance of steel wire" during the injection. Wide use of the method for the roentgenographic demonstration of blood vessels was predicted. Apparently without any knowledge of this paper, Dünner and Calm (1923) reported that when water-soluble iodide compounds were injected the arteries and veins became visible. None of these investigators aimed at the demonstration of the cerebral vessels. Sicard and Forestier (1922), on the other hand, had tried Lipiodol to demonstrate cerebral arteries of animals, but all the animals had died. Moniz investigated the toxicity of various substances (bromide and iodide of lithium, sodium, potassium, ammonium, strontium, and rubidium) in animal experiments. He also injected human cadavers to study the vascular anatomy. In experiments on dogs, he succeeded in outlining the cerebral vessels on roentgenograms with the aid of strontium bromide and lithium bromide. He then began trials in man with strontium bromide; his subjects were insane patients or others with grave neurologic disturbances. Percutaneous injection was used at first, but a severe reaction and fever developed in the fourth patient. Moniz attributed this reaction to paravasal injection and altered the technique to exposure of the artery instead. The sixth patient died 8 hours after the injection. Thereupon the substance was changed to sodium iodide 25%. Not until the ninth case did he succeed in obtaining a satisfactory view of the brain vessels. He presented a paper under the title "L'encéphalographie artérielle: son importance dans la localization des tumeurs cérébrales" at a meeting in Paris in 1927. His book *Diagnostic des tumeurs cérébrales et épreuve de l'encéphalographie artérielle,* in 1931, described his experiences with ninety patients, of whom two died.

The first attempts at cerebral angiography are an example of a stubborn adherence to an idea and the endeavor toward its realization. At that time the ethical demands prevalent in most countries today, concerning experiments on human beings, were disregarded entirely. Doubts as to the advisability of angiography increased in several quarters as reports of serious complications began to be published. Those regarding cerebral angiography reported epileptic attacks, transitory and permanent hemiplegia, and even death (after two injections of 5 ml of sodium iodide). Moniz, in 1931, changed to Thorotrast (colloidal thorium dioxide), which in his view could be used without risk (1932). This preparation had been introduced in Germany in 1928-1929, for hepatolienography. In Europe angiography was performed with Thorotrast, mainly in Germany. Among others, Löhr and Jacobi also applied the method in the investigation of head injuries to demonstrate possible intracranial complications. These investigators published monographs in the early 1930's on a combination of encephalography and angiography (Löhr and Jacobi, 1932, 1933). The titles were misleading, however, since the authors themselves reported abandonment of the method because it was troublesome and had not improved the diagnostic possibilities.

Strong doubts were also expressed, especially in America, regarding the harmlessness of Thorotrast. All investigators agreed that little risk of complications existed during the actual examination procedure. Filling of the blood vessels by the contrast medium also was satisfactory; but opinions differed widely regarding the possibility of late damage. As early as 1932, the Council of Pharmacy and Chemistry in the United States issued a warning against the use of Thorotrast. Some workers (Jessen and de Fine Licht, 1934) discarded cerebral angiography after epileptic attacks followed angiographic examinations with sodium iodide. Despite theoretical calculations of the radiation doses from thorium dioxide deposited in the reticuloendothelium, and the warning against its use, Thorotrast continued to be used in many clinics. Arguments were presented that late damage was improbable, at least with the small amounts used for cerebral angiography. In general, until the middle of the 1930's, cerebral angiography was employed relatively seldom except in certain clinics. Probably it was not used more often because of lack of a suitable contrast medium and the necessity of surgical exposure of the carotid artery. A report, in 1936, by Loman and Myerson represented a big step forward. They had performed direct puncture of the carotid artery for therapeutic purposes, and it occurred to them to adopt this method also for injection of Thorotrast. In their procedure the patient was placed in supine position with the head flexed backward to facilitate the puncture. This position seems to have been maintained during the exposure of the films, which consequently must have been accomplished with a horizontal projection. Exact lateral views were thus obtained. Previously the roentgenograms had been obtained with the patient in the supine position but with the head turned to the side. Exact lateral views were then often difficult or impossible to obtain. Assessment of the exact position of the blood vessels therefore was also most difficult. Anteroposterior views were seldom obtained at that time, since many investigators expressed the belief that these views did not impart much information of importance. Without knowledge of Loman and Myerson's work, Shimidzu published a paper in the following year (1937) in which he proposed a percutaneous approach. Since Loman and Myerson's article appeared in the English literature and that of Shimidzu in the German, each author is regarded as the initiator of the percutaneous method.

The one factor that initially hindered wider acceptance of cerebral angiography, and especially the percutaneous method, was the lack of a suitable contrast medium. The hesitation about using Thorotrast became increasingly widespread. That local tissue was damaged ("thorotrastoma") by the paravasal injection of the medium had been proved beyond doubt. Uncertainty existed whether late damage would arise because of the radioactivity of Thorotrast despite the fact that experiments in animals pointed clearly to this possibility. As late as 1950, Kuntzmann and his co-workers maintained that not even a theoretical risk of late damage could be expected after cerebral angiography. An excellent review of the distribution, retention, and late effects of thorium dioxide, which demonstrated clearly that this contrast medium should not be used, appeared in the Annals of the New York Academy of Sciences in 1967. Because of the possible damage to local tissue, the Stockholm school also tended to withhold the percutaneous method. Cerebral angiography therefore was used only in those patients in whom vascular changes (aneurysm, arteriovenous malformation, thrombosis) were suggested clinically or when pneumography did not give definite information regarding the presence of an expanding process. In the early 1940's we also obtained necropsy proof that Thorotrast could cause cirrhosis of the liver. In view of this finding, we restricted our use of the method even more, except in patients too old for late effects to develop.

The risks from the use of Thorotrast served as an incentive to produce other contrast media. In Germany a colloidal ethyl triiodostearate, introduced under the name of Vasoselectan, was used to some extent during the early 1940's. Because of difficulties in its preparation, it was soon abandoned and never attained wide use. In 1939 Gross had published an article on Diodrast as a contrast medium for cerebral angiography. It was soon followed by trials with similar preparations of the diiodized diethanol amine salt type (Perabrodil, Umbradil, Joduron). These agents also proved to be somewhat toxic. They gave rise in some patients to epileptic attacks, confusional states, paresis, and aphasia. Usually the symptoms subsided after a few minutes, hours, or days, but unfortunately in a few instances they became permanent. Broman and Olsson (1948, 1950) demonstrated in animal experiments that these media were capable of producing damage to the blood-brain barrier. They stated that the toxicity depended on the concentration of the contrast medium and the time during which it acted on the vessel wall. Their conclusions were that high concentrations and repetition of injections at close intervals should be avoided and that the amount of contrast medium be kept as low as possible. Not until the introduction of the water-soluble iodinated contrast media did the percutaneous puncture technique come into more general use. These two factors (the puncture method and improvement of the contrast medium) were the basic requirements for a general application of carotid angiography. Serious complications related to the examination could still arise, but they were relatively rare and late effects were precluded. Therefore, in view of the diagnostic advantages offered by the method as experience in its use increased, the risks were considered justified. Research on contrast media continues and has resulted in the production of agents that cause fewer and fewer side effects. At present the triiodized contrast media produced by the pharmaceutical industry for use in cerebral angiography may be said to cause virtually no side effects.

Although depiction of both arterial and venous phases at angiography were attempted at a relatively early date, in practice the examination long remained an arteriography. With the angiographic method, localization of an expanding process, because of its displacement of vascular branches, became possible. An idea of the nature of the process also was gained because the vascular structure of tumors often differs from the normal vascularity of the brain. In some cases these divergences proved to be visible only for very short periods. This observation, as well as the desirability to observe the circulation in patients with vascular malformations and thrombosis, emphasized the need for serial views.

Serial views of the different phases of angiography were attempted also in the early stages (Caldas, 1934). The number of views, however, were usually limited to three or four because of the lack of suitable film and cassette changers. The Stockholm school had designed a manual cassette changer for three views. Two injections were made and the two series of films were shifted with regard to time. Thus six views were obtained that showed the passage of the contrast medium through the cerebral vessels. The result was serial angiography. Rapid serial angiography came into use in the late 1940's. In general the development of cerebral angiography has been more closely connected with techical developments. These pertained to roentgen tubes with smaller focal areas and an increased capacity, cassette or film changers, secondary diaphragms, contrast media, and the subtraction technique introduced by Ziedses des Plantes (1961). These technical improvements made possible the study of smaller and smaller blood vessels. In the beginning it was the Stockholm school in particular whose evaluation of their anatomic and angiographic studies increased our knowledge of the field. This development, which has continued up to the present day, has subsequently been augmented by other investigators.

As early as 1937, Moniz commented on the uniform appearance of the central veins and the deep dural sinuses of the brain. In many cases, he stated, this appearance could provide valuable information and serve as a basis for diagnosis. Other authors, however (Riechert, 1939; Engeset, 1944; List and Hodges, 1946), expressed the view that these veins varied so much that determination of displacement was difficult. Lima (1950) expressed the opinion that they "may sometimes be useful for confirming arteriograms but have no special value by themselves." Lorenz (1951), on the other hand, reasoned that the condition of the veins had seldom been studied not so much because their importance had been underestimated as because technical difficulties prevented their satisfactory demonstration. The first fundamental study regarding the normal position and appearance of these veins was presented by Johanson in 1952 at the Symposium Neuroradiologicum. Their relation in the presence of different expanding or atrophying processes was described at this symposium and in a monograph in 1954. Their importance as aids to diagnosis was clearly demonstrated in these papers.

Rapid serial angiography is a necessity for exact demonstration of the circulatory conditions. The term rapid serial angiography was adopted by the Stockholm school. It referred to a film frequency of not less than one exposure per second for 20 seconds. As a rule two to three views per second were obtained during the arterial phase. A longer interval was allowed between the views in the venous phase. Reports that stated that these requirements had been met were published around 1950 (Curtis, 1949; Lewin, 1950; Schurr and Wickbom, 1952). Statements regarding the speed of the normal cerebral circulation varied, however. The reason for this variation is obvious. The determinations were too strongly influenced by the amount of contrast medium used and the length of the injection time. Many investigators, furthermore, held that angiography was not a suitable examination method for circulatory studies. Greitz (1956) cleared up the sources of error related to the method, however. He suggested more clearly defined points for determination of the circulation time, which would permit exact assessment and comparison in different subjects. By comparisons with an isotope method of his own, Greitz showed that by angiography the circulation time could be determined if certain definite criteria were set. Even with the contrast media then available, which in some cases affected the general circulation, pulse rate, and blood pressure, these angiographic determinations were possible. The method also yielded information not obtainable in other ways. Neuroradiologists in general now recognize the necessity for rapid serial angiography whenever an intracranial expanding process or a cerebrovascular lesion is suspected. As technical improvements continue to appear, cinematography is being tried by an increasing number of workers. Although this method has its advocates, most authors have stated that it does not give sufficiently detailed information.

At autopsies of subjects who had had clinical signs of a cerebrovascular lesion, often no changes could be detected in the intracranial vessels. Changes were seen in the major vessels of the neck, however. This observation led to the idea of angiographic examination of these vessels both during life and postmortem. Interest in this procedure increased, especially after operative removal of stenosing processes in the cervical vessels had become possible. Because atherosclerotic changes are often situated at the site where the neck vessels leave the aorta, these angiographic examinations should be in the form of an aortocervical angiography. Injection into the brachial artery or retrograde injection into the common carotid artery, however, has also been used. The brachial artery may be punctured just above the antecubital fossa, or the needle may be inserted anywhere up to the axilla. The injection may be performed either with or without insertion of a catheter. The method was first described by Gould and co-workers (1955). Pygott and Hutton used percutaneous puncture (1959). The method has been applied for examination of the neck vessels and the intracranial vessels. The Stockholm school, in contrast, favored aortocervical angiography, which permits simultaneous demonstration of all four major arteries in the neck. It also gives a certain amount of information about the intracranial vessels. As a rule, however, a sufficiently detailed view of the intracranial vessels cannot be obtained, and the examination must be combined with a selective study of these vessels. The impression gained from the extensive literature in recent years is that of an overemphasis on the changes in the extracranial vessels. The American literature, particularly, has given the impression that sufficiently exhaustive studies of the intracranial vessels have not been undertaken. When changes are present in the neck vessels, intracranial changes are also present in about 75% of the patients. Without changes in the neck vessels, intracranial changes are noted in about 40%.

Venous angiography has been used to some extent in these patients. Because they are often in the older age groups, they are frequently poor risks and catheterization is impossible. Methods for venous angiography have been devised by, among others, Viallet and his co-workers (1956), Schramel and co-workers (1961), and Scatliff and Greenspan (1963). The Stockholm school at present employs a modified technique described by Ahlberg and his co-workers (1968).

Intracerebral functional disturbances may be present even if morphologic angiographic changes are absent. Such disturbances are easily overlooked at angiography, particularly if the examination has not been performed in accordance with the rules for rapid serial angiography. We have Cronqvist (1968) and Cronqvist and Greitz (1969), in particular, to thank for having drawn attention to this situation. They did so through their comparative studies between angiography and flow rate determinations by the isotope clearance method.

The preceding discussion has dealt mainly with carotid angiography; but the examination of vessels in the posterior cranial fossa presented greater difficulty for a long time. Among others, Sjöqvist (1938), with varying success, exposed the vertebral artery proximal to its entry into the canal formed by the transverse foramina. Berczeller and Kugler (1937) suggested exposure of the artery at the sulcus atlantis. The best results seem to have been obtained after operative exposure of the subclavian artery and retrograde injection of the contrast medium (Moniz et al., 1933; List, 1946). Shimidzu punctured the subclavian artery percutaneously instead (1937). Takahashi, in 1940, described a method for direct percutaneous puncture of the vertebral artery proximal to its entry into the bone canal. This method does not seem to have been used much. In a contribution to the discussion on List's presentation of cerebral angiography, Freeman (1946) implied that he had succeeded in puncturing the vertebral artery percutaneously. With reference to percutaneous carotid angiography, he stated: "Sometimes a picture of the posterior fossa can be obtained by injecting the vertebral artery through the same type of puncture in the neck. It is a little deeper, a little closer to the bone." Apparently he did not develop the method further, nor did he use it to any great extent. Successive trials with the earlier methods all produced unsatisfactory results. These failures led the Stockholm school to devise a method for direct percutaneous puncture of the vertebral artery in the bony canal, which was presented at the Symposium Neuroradiologicum in Rotterdam, in 1949 (Lindgren, 1950a). This method proved usable in about two thirds of the cases. With further experience and an improved technique (Sjögren, 1953a), success with the examination was achieved without difficulty in 70%. In a further 15% it could be performed with difficulty. Quite independently of these trials, Sugar and co-workers also developed a similar procedure (1949).

Radner (1951) noticed that a catheter inserted via the radial artery for thoracic aortography often slid into the vertebral artery or some other branch of the subclavian artery. This observation led him to develop a catheterization method for vertebral angiography, which was finally perfected in 1951. The technique involved operative exposure and ligation of the radial artery. Despite the fact that the percutaneous method could be carried out with approximately the same rate of success as this catheter method, it placed great demands on the examiner's skill and experience. Also arteriovenous fistulae sometimes arose, especially after repeated attempts at puncture, because of the venous plexus lying around the vertebral artery. Conversely, with Radner's method, spastic vascular contractions often occurred around the catheter and caused difficulties during the examination. These contractions probably explain the fairly numerous complications that could arise (Hauge, 1954). The fact that the radial artery had to be ligated was another reason that many workers considered this method not wholly suitable. These factors led the Stockholm school to present another catheterization method (Lindgren, 1956). The catheter was introduced percutaneously into the femoral artery and was then passed up to the subclavian artery, where the contrast medium was injected. At a later date it was also passed up into the vertebral artery. Gould and co-workers exposed the brachial artery instead and injected the contrast medium in a retrograde direction (1955). They considered the method especially suitable for children. Later the artery was punctured percutaneously and the contrast medium was injected with a pressure syringe. Many authors have reported excellent results with this method. Kuhn (1960) recommended injection into the right brachial artery as a substitute for percutaneous puncture of the carotid and vertebral arteries on that side. The method for intravenous angiography presented by Viallet and his co-workers (1956) does not seem to have been used by other authors for investigation of the intracranial vessels. With recent developments in the technique for catheterization of blood vessels, the different vessel areas may be catheterized in turn on one side and on both sides during the same examination. The technique is aided by suitably shaped catheters placed in position via the femoral artery. Selective examination of the external carotid artery has been greatly facilitated through the use of a catheter inserted preferably via the common carotid artery.

Our knowledge about the arteries of the posterior cranial fossa and the most important pathologic changes related to expanding lesions has been gained mainly through the work of the Stockholm school and from Radner's investigations. Recent studies by Huang and Wolf (1965, 1967, 1969) have established the relation of the posterior fossa veins in normal and pathologic states.

THE SPINE

Investigation of the bones is a relatively important measure in the examination of a patient with symptoms and signs suggestive of an intracerebral lesion. Such an investigation is of less significance when the possibility of a spinal tumor exists. In the former case examination of the skull bones often reveals whether an intracranial expanding process is present. In other cases it also supplies information on the site of the lesion, and in still others on the nature of the lesion. An investigation of the spine gives information mainly as to whether a malignant process with skeletal destruction is present. In 1933 Camp and his co-workers drew attention to the fact that extramedullary benign processes often caused pressure changes at the pedicles whereas changes in the vertebral bodies arose late. The following year Elsberg and Dyke (1934) showed that the interpedicular space was a usable measure of the diameter of the vertebral canal. Furthermore they showed that spinal tumors caused widening of the canal in many cases. The significance of these changes must now be considered slight, for the diagnosis ought to be established before these changes develop if good results by operation are to be achieved.

Jacobaeus wrote in 1921:

> As early as 1909 or 1910 . . . I attempted influencing the process of the disease [tuberculous meningitis] through replacing, to as large an extent as possible, the pathologically changed cerebrospinal fluid with air. It was not unusual that nearly 100 ml of cerebrospinal fluid were removed which were then replaced with a corresponding quantity of air. As no therapeutic effect, apart from a quite whimsical improvement during the first 24 to 48 hours, could be proved, these experiments of mine have not been published, nor have they been continued.*

Had Jacobaeus allowed his patients to be examined roentgenographically, both air myelography and intracranial pneumography would probably have come to light much sooner.

Several authors (e.g., Jacobaeus, 1921; Wideröe, 1921; Josefson, 1922) reported on patients with spinal tumor localized by small amounts of air in whom the tumor caused absolute blocks.

After Dandy had injected air into the lumbar region for investigation of the intracranial subarachnoid space, he began to use air for examination of the spinal subarachnoid space. In 1925 he described thirty-six cases of spinal cord tumor localized with air, of which all except two were subsequently verified at operation. In the same article he mentioned that he had changed to Lipiodol, and he reported on ten cases examined with that medium. Despite the objections raised against Lipiodol by several American investigators, Dandy recommended its use instead of air, for he had noticed no adverse results. He pointed out, however, that the oil remained as a foreign body that might cause trouble later, if not initially. Moreover, he added that "the value of Lipiodol in cases where it is indicated overwhelms these objections which then become of minor concern. . . . Its employment makes the diagnosis and localization almost foolproof. And doubtless one can exclude spinal cord tumors with equal certainty."

Lipiodol had been used since 1901 in the treatment of different infections. When injected subcutaneously or intravascularly, it was observed to remain in the tissues for a long time. Several reports during the first two decades discussed the possibility of misinterpretation of residual Lipiodol deposits at roentgen examinations and how they could be differentiated from pathologic processes. As early as 1909, Sicard suggested that the opacity of Lipiodol could be used in the radiologic field. Not until Forestier became associated with Sicard was this suggestion more closely investigated (Sicard and Forestier, 1922). Forestier began a series of experiments on animals, and since Sicard was interested in neurologic problems, especially diseases of the spinal cord, these two workers directed their attention to the diagnosis of spinal tumors. Lipiodol was an iodized oil and thus did

*From Jacobaeus, H. C.: On insufflation of air into the spinal canal for diagnostic purposes in cases of tumors in the spinal canal, Acta Med. Scand. 55:555-564, 1921.

not mix with the cerebrospinal fluid. Following the animal experiments, trials were carried out with Lipiodol in patients. By alteration of the patient's position, the Lipiodol could be moved into the subarachnoid space, and any obstruction to its passage could be readily observed. This observation was possible, even with the roentgen equipment then in use, because of the high capacity of the Lipiodol to absorb the rays.

Lipiodol could be observed more easily than air, and its use soon became widespread. In Germany, in 1926, air as a contrast medium for myelography was considered to be forever discarded "endgültig verlassen." Since Lipiodol, however, was retained in the subarachnoid space, the question arose whether it might not give rise to arachnoiditis. The production of other iodized oils that would be resorbed more easily was attempted in several countries, but with little success; nor were attempts to withdraw the oil by puncture after the examination particularly effective. Thorotrast was also tried in the early 1930's (Radovici and Meller, 1932; Lucherini, 1934). In the United States, Nosik (1938) and Nosik and Mortenson (1938) tried forced spinal drainage techniques after the examination. They succeeded in flushing out 70% to 90% of the injected amount of Thorotrast, but this method did not prove suitable either.

In 1934 van Wagenen described three patients in whom the site of the lesion had been demonstrated with small quantities of air. The same year, however, Coggeshall and von Storch presented a greatly improved technique. They filled the sac with air by lumbar puncture while the patient was in the Trendelenburg position. They thereby introduced the principle that has been a decisive factor in the development of myelography with negative contrast medium. The next significant step was taken by Young and Scott (1938). If an absolute obstruction was present, they proceeded in accordance with the earlier method; in other words, they used a few milliliters of air to localize the block. When the block was only partial, they employed cisternal puncture. The patient was placed in the Trendelenburg position and 65 to 85 ml of air were introduced to fill the spinal subarachnoid space.

Observation had proved that iodized oil could produce arachnoiditis, which in a few cases had caused difficulty in removal of a tumor (Olivecrona, 1936), when for some reason the operation could not be undertaken directly after the examination. For this reason the Stockholm school tried gas myelography during the same period. Their results with the first fourteen spinal tumors, thirteen of which were localized exactly, were described by Lindgren in 1939. The one exception was a tumor at the level of the first and second cervical vertebrae. Earlier authors had drawn off cerebrospinal fluid, which they replaced with the same amount of air. The Stockholm school, instead, injected gas to produce an excess pressure of 300 to 500 mm of water. The subarachnoid space then became completely filled with gas. The increased pressure did not remain permanent but leveled rapidly. The air was exchanged for oxygen that had been warmed to body temperature to reduce the discomfort of the patient. The method reached its final form with the introduction of tomography. Gas myelography requires a more highly perfected roentgenographic technique than does myelography with a positive contrast medium. It supplies information that cannot be obtained with the latter method, and it eliminates the sources of error related to the use of iodized oil. Gas myelography is used exclusively in Sweden today for examination in cases of possible spinal tumors. It has also been employed widely in Europe, but, strangely, it has not gained ground in English-speaking countries. The improvement of the technique introduced by Westberg (1966) has made possible the differentiation of cystic processes from solid tumors.

Water-soluble iodinated contrast media were also tried for ventriculography and myelography, but they proved highly irritative. Arnell had been experimenting with such contrast media ever since 1931 and finally reached the conclusion that Abrodil could be used in the lumbar region after lumbar anesthesia. This method was improved in the early 1940's by Lindblom. As a rule the root sleeves and nerves cannot be demonstrated distinctly with gas. Consequently myelography with water-soluble contrast media has been used mainly when a rupture of a disk in the lumbar spine is suggested. Complications have been described by some authors, especially when the method first came into use. Undoubtedly these complications are avoidable with the correct technique. During the last few years another positive contrast medium, three-iodinated meglumine iothalamate (Conray), has been tried in several quarters. The results indicate that this contrast material can be used in the lumbar region without a lumbar anesthetic.

Coloring agents had been injected into the nucleus pulposus in anatomic studies of the intervertebral disks. Therefore the introduction of a water-soluble contrast medium into disks followed by roentgenograms seemed logical. Such roentgenograms would demonstrate ruptures and prolapsed disks directly. This method, diskography, was especially advocated by Lindblom (1948), who first used a transdural puncture method; Erlacher (1951), who called the method nucleography, described an extradural technique. Lindblom (1950) and others later also presented an extradural method. Several enthusiastic reports on diskography appeared in the late 1940's and early 1950's, but warnings were also voiced. de Sèze and Levernieux (1951, 1952) examined fifty-nine patients 1 year after diskography. They found a lesion, which they described as "discites nécrosants," or greatly reduced height of the intervertebral disk, in thirteen. As judged by the literature, diskography lost considerable ground during the 1960's.

Although angiography is important in the study of intracranial processes, it is not as valuable in the study of spinal tumors. Spinal angiography, technically speaking, is much more difficult to perform. The spinal cord, furthermore, is more sensitive than the brain to the toxic side effects of contrast media. Arteriovenous malformations develop in this area too, however. Real progress in spinal angiography began only during the 1960's, with the development of selective catheterization of the fine blood vessels and the use of subtraction. Pioneer work in this field has been carried out by Di Chiro (Di Chiro and Fischer, 1964; Doppman and Di Chiro, 1965) and particularly by Djindjian and his co-workers (Djindjian, 1962; Djindjian et al., 1970).

RADIOACTIVE ISOTOPES

Moore and his co-workers (1948, 1950) theorized that negatively charged dyes, in contrast to those positively charged, generally do not possess the power to pass the blood-brain barrier under normal conditions. If this barrier is penetrated locally (through the presence of a tumor, for instance), the dyes can pass into the lesion. Moore's group applied this theory during operation to localize and determine the extent of the lesion. They used fluorescein, since even at low concentrations it was detectable because of the fluorescent properties of the dye under ultraviolet light (1948). Later they used sodium diiodofluorescein tagged with ^{131}I for preoperative localization of brain tumors (1950). Approximately 30 minutes after the intravenous injection, symmetric regions of the head were investigated with a shielded Geiger-Müller counter. If the uptake in the lesion was at least 10% higher than in the surrounding areas, it could be detected. The isotope technique was considered, especially in the United States, to offer wide possibilities, and many reports on the good results were published. Brownell and Sweet (1956) devised a new method based on the use of positron emitters, such as ^{52}Mn, ^{64}Cu, ^{74}As, and coincidence-counting techniques with collimated detectors. Kramer and co-workers (1956) considered that: "the results obtained . . . are likely to influence the final diagnosis for only a limited number of patients. . . . Yet from the positive results we have obtained we may reasonably conclude that with some technical improvement radioactive localization will be added to the diagnostic methods finally available." Automatic scanning was introduced later.

In the late 1950's and the early 1960's the most commonly used substances were gamma-emitting RISA (^{131}I-tagged human serum albumin) and ^{203}Hg neohydrin. Sjögren (1953b) suggested a scheme for the measuring points. Later Planiol (1959) worked out a similar but more detailed scheme that was used fairly widely, at least in Europe. Around this time, however, investigators were beginning to use scintillography to an increasing extent. With the latest technical improvement, the gamma camera, the length of examination has been shortened considerably, allowing conditions of blood flow to be recorded as well. The radiation doses to patients have been reduced with the more short-lived isotopes ^{99m}Tc and ^{113m}In. However, recording of rapid regional flow, by means of ^{133}Xe or ^{85}Kr, gives the most exact result at present.

Extracranial evaluation of brain lesions has developed into a valuable neuroradiologic method. Its advantages do not lie solely in the fact that it constitutes a suitable screening procedure that causes no discomfort to the patient. In some cases it also results in demonstration of lesions that have escaped detection by other radiologic methods, or it corroborates uncertain findings. In addition, the extent of a lesion detected in another way can be determined more exactly in some instances. Information is obtainable as to whether multiple processes are present. In some cases also, preoperative assessment of the nature of the process is facilitated. Conversely, exact information about the relation of a lesion to the ventricular system and blood vessels is never obtainable. According to most surgeons such relation should be known before surgical intervention is undertaken.

The RISA-cisternography procedure introduced by Di Chiro (1964, 1966) has increased our knowledge of the circulation of cerebrospinal fluid. The consequences of incisural block and convexity block are becoming more evident. Comparison of the results of isotope examinations with those of encephalography means that distinction between low-pressure hydrocephalus and cerebral atrophy is now becoming possible, with all the therapeutic consequences this implies.

FUTURE IN THE LIGHT OF HISTORY

Neuroradiology, as the preceding pages have demonstrated, is based on ideas contributed from many different quarters, in the beginning mainly from clinicians (neurologists, neurosurgeons, internists). To a large extent, examinations were also performed by clinicians, a situation still prevalent in many clinics. Radiologists, in contrast, showed little interest in this field. The long neglect of the purely radiodiagnostic aspects of the technique is clear evidence of this disinterest. The investigator mainly responsible for changing this state of affairs was Lysholm, the radiologist. He worked at the hospital in Stockholm where Antoni, the neurologist, and

Olivecrona, the neurosurgeon, were also engaged. In other countries the radiologic work was previously conducted, and still is to some extent, by clinicians in other specialities. In Sweden this has never been the case. The founder of Swedish radiology, Gösta Forssell, realized that for the clinical specialities to derive full benefit from radiology, physicians who devoted themselves exclusively to this new field were needed. All radiologic activities were then concentrated in central radiologic departments under the leadership of qualified radiologists. When the neurologic and neurosurgical clinics were established at Serafimerlasarettet, their radiologic investigations were assigned to the central department of radiology. The director of this department at that time was Forssell, but Lysholm was in charge of the neuroradiologic section. Later Lysholm was appointed director of the entire department. Thus what has been called the Stockholm school in the preceding sections consists of the radiologists trained at the radiology department of this hospital. From 1947 to 1964, this department was under my leadership, and after 1964 it was under the leadership of Torgny Greitz. This system, of separating clinical and radiologic activities, has given excellent results. That such a system has not been more generally accepted is strange. As early as 1908 at a meeting of the American Roentgen Ray Society, a prominent New York surgeon, Reginald H. Sayre, declared: "I was one of those who early tried the Roentgen rays, but I found that if I was to do as good x-ray work as was being done by others I could not practice surgery. . . . I concluded that I would let somebody who had become more competent than I carry on the work and that I would seek his advice." And he continued: ". . . call in the assistance of a competent radiologist. We must work hand in hand if we expect to get good results and accurate results. This is the day for specialism." With these words, Sayre gave expression to the same line of thought.*

Some clinicians are engaged in radiologic work for a few years and then return to clinical work. A lack of continuity will then result in the work at the radiologic unit. The technical ability among the staff may be inadequate. If radiologic and clinical activities are conducted by one and the same physician, a failure of objectivity may result. This last point was expressed by Charles D. Enfield (1932) in the following way: "The amateur roentgenologist tends to make his x-ray interpretations conform to his clinical impressions. He inclines to interpret what he sees in the light of physical findings, history and laboratory reports. Only the most strikingly contradictory appearances on the films or screen can lead him away from his already made tentative diagnosis."* Without doubt the best result is obtained if both clinician and radiologist, each working independently of the other, carries his own investigations as far as possible. A combination and comparison of both sets of observations will then result in a final opinion of the condition. In this way the clinician and the radiologist also may check each other. Advancement in one field also brings improvements in the other, and progress is thus promoted.

Diagnostic radiology has developed rapidly, particularly during recent years, and one radiologist cannot master the whole field. The need for specialization within this field is becoming increasingly evident. If diagnostic radiology is to be able to satisfy the demands of the different relatively new clinical specialities, such as thoracic surgery or neurosurgery, it must be divided into subsections. One of these must be neuroradiology.

The first period in the history of neuroradiology was concerned with investigations of the skull and with pneumography. The latter method differs from other procedures of diagnostic radiology in that the problems are mainly mechanical. The skull is a hard shell, and within it, in the space divided into compartments by the falx and tentorium, lies the brain. In the living human being the brain is a mass more or less semifluid. In the center is the fluid-filled and air-filled ventricular system. The distortion and displacement produced in this system by expanding or atrophic lesions allow conclusions about the site and size of the lesions. Then angiography came into use. At first the observations were interpreted in the same way. Vascular displacements were recorded, and the site of the lesion was assessed from these. Soon, however, the different processes were seen to differ in degree of vascularization and vascular structures. With this observation a biologic factor entered the interpretation. In recent years a physiologic factor has been introduced as the significance of the circulation rate, both general and local, has become increasingly recognized. Radioactive isotopes are now being used as well, and with this form of diagnostic interpretation all three aspects are involved, anatomic, biologic, and physiologic.

The neuroradiologist must possess an excellent foundation in general radiology, including a satisfactory knowledge of radiophysics, radiobiology, and nuclear medicine. He must also know the anatomy and the pathologic processes of the central nervous system and must master the special examination procedures. The procedures include cisternal and lumbar punctures, vascular punctures and catheterizations, myelographic

*From Brecher, R., and Brecher, E.: The rays, Baltimore, 1969, The Williams & Wilkins Co.

*From Enfield, C. D.: Is roentgenology, as a specialty, destined to survive? Radiology **18**:1039-1043, 1932.

methods, and isotope diagnosis of cerebral and spinal processes.

The standard of neuroradiology differs considerably in different countries. One reason for this difference is that neuroradiology has in many quarters not yet achieved the standing of a separate speciality, not even the standing of a radiologic subsection. In consequence, training has not received sufficient attention. In the second edition (1951) of *A Textbook of X-ray Diagnosis by British Authors,* Cairns and Jupe remarked: "The perfection of technique and increasing popularity of radiological examination are revealing more and more novel appearances on and inside the skull. There is a strong temptation to regard appearances that are novel as abnormal, and thus as the cause of the patient's symptoms. . . . We have stressed this point because in recent years there have been more negative operative explorations for intracranial tumor resulting from faulty radiological diagnosis than from any other cause."* It is to be hoped that in the near future the importance of neuroradiology as an independent medicoradiologic specialty will be recognized everywhere. Its own special training requirements must be available for those who wish to make use of it. Such recognition and training would create better conditions for research and promote progress in the science of neuroradiology as a service to patients in need of medical assistance.

---

*From Cairns, H., and Jupe, M. H.: In Shanks, S. C., and Kerley, P., editors: A textbook of x-ray diagnosis by British authors, ed. 2, London, 1951, H. K. Lewis & Co., vol. 1, p. 6.

REFERENCES

Ahlberg, N. E., Bartley, O., and Chidekel, N.: Venous arteriography. A modified technique and indications for its use, Acta Radiol. [Diagn.] **7**:321-330, 1968.

Arnell, S.: Weitere Erfahrungen über Myelographie mit Abrodil, Acta Radiol. **25**:408-413, 1944.

Azambuja, N., Arana Iniguez, R., Sande, M. T., and Garcia Guelfi, A.: Central ventriculography, Acta Neurol. Latinoamer. **2**:58-64, 1956.

Balado, M.: Radiografia del tercer ventriculo mediante la inyeccion intraventricular de Lipiodol, Arch. Argent. Neurol. **2**: 69-77, 1928.

Béclère, A.: La radiographie du crâne et le diagnostic de l'acromégalia, Bull. Mem. Soc. Med. Hop. Paris, Dec. 5, 1902.

Béclère, A.: L'exposé des travaux scientifiques du docteur Antoine Béclère, médecin de l'Hôpital Saint-Antoine, Paris, 1907, Masson & Cie.

Berczeller, A., and Kugler, H.: Freilegung der Arteria vertebralis am Sulcus atlantis, Arch. Klin. Chir. **190**:810-815, 1937.

Bingel, A.: Zur Technik der intralumbalen Lufteinblasung insbesondere zum Zwecke der "Encephalographie," Deutsch. Med. Wschr. **47**:1492-1493, 1921a.

Bingel, A.: Intralumbale Lufteinblasung zur Höhendiagnose intraduraler extramedullärer Prozesse und zur Differentialdiagnose gegenüber intramedullären Prozessen, Deutsch. Z. Nervenheilk. **72**:359-370, 1921b.

Bingel, A.: Encephalographie, eine Methode zur röntgenographischen Darstellung des Gehirns, Fortschr. Roentgenstr. **28**:205-217, 1921c.

Bingel, A.: Neben- und Nachwirkungen bei Gaseinblasungen in den Lumbalkanal, Deutsch. Z. Nervenheilk. **75**:230-249, 1922.

Bingel, A.: Todesfälle nach Gaseinblasungen in den Lumbalkanal, bezw. in die Gehirnventrikel, Med. Klin. **19**:637-640, 1923.

Bingel, A.: Encephalographische Erfahrungen, Z. Ges. Neurol. Psychiat. **114**:323-475, 1928.

Bleasel, K.: Nerve root radiography, Brit. J. Radiol. **34**:596-601, 1961.

Brecher, R., and Brecher, E.: The rays, Baltimore, 1969, The Williams & Wilkins Co.

Broman, T., Forssman, B., and Olsson, O.: Further experimental investigations of injuries from contrast media in cerebral angiography, Acta Radiol. **34**:135-143, 1950.

Broman, T., and Olsson, O.: The tolerance of cerebral bloodvessels to a contrast medium of the Diodrast group, Acta Radiol. **30**:326-342, 1948.

Brownell, G. L., and Sweet, W. H.: Scanning of positron-emitting isotopes in diagnosis of intracranial and other lesions, Acta Radiol. **46**:425-434, 1956.

Bull, J.: Positive contrast ventriculography, Acta Radiol. **34**: 253-268, 1950.

Bull, J., and Fischgold, H.: A short history of neuroradiology, VIIIth Symposium Neuroradiologicum, Paris, 1967.

Cairns, H., and Jupe, M. H.: In Shanks, S. C., and Kerley, P., editors: A textbook of x-ray diagnosis by British authors, ed. 2, London, 1951, H. K. Lewis & Co., vol. 1.

Caldas, J. P.: Artériographie en série avec l'appareil radiocarrousel, J. Radiol. Electr. **18**:34-39, 1934.

Camp, J. D.: Contrast myelography, past and present. Carman lecture, Radiology **54**:477-506, 1950.

Camp, J. D., Adson, W. W., and Shugrue, J. J.: Roentgenographic findings associated with tumors of the spinal column, spinal cord and associated tissues, Amer. J. Cancer **17**:348-372, 1933.

Childe, A. E., and Penfield, W.: Anatomic and pneumographic studies of the temporal horn, Arch. Neurol. Psychiat. **37**: 1021-1034, 1937.

Church, A.: Cerebellar tumor; recognized clinically, demonstrated by the x-ray, and proved by autopsy, Amer. J. Med. Sci. **117**:126-130, 1899.

Coggeshall, H. C., and von Storch, T. J. C.: Diagnostic value of myelographic studies of caudal dural sac, Arch. Neurol. Psychiat. **31**:611-613, 1934.

Cronqvist, S.: Transitory hyperemia in focal cerebral ischemic lesion. In Proceedings of the research group on cerebral circulation, Salzburg, 1966, Springfield, Ill., 1968, Charles C Thomas, Publisher.

Cronqvist, S., and Greitz, T.: Cerebral circulation time and cerebral blood flow. Comparison of angiography and the ^{133}Xe technique, Acta Radiol. [Diagn.] **8**:296-304, 1969.

Curtis, J. B.: Rapid serial angiography. Preliminary report, J. Neurol. Neurosurg. Psychiat. **12**:167-181, 1949.

Dandy, W. E.: Ventriculography following the injection of air into the cerebral ventricles, Ann. Surg. **68**:4-11, 1918.

Dandy, W. E.: Ventriculography following the injection of air into the cerebral ventricles, Amer. J. Roentgen. **6**:26-36, 1919a.

Dandy, W. E.: Roentgenography of the brain after the injection of air into the spinal canal, Ann. Surg. **70**:397-403, 1919b.

Dandy, W. E.: The diagnosis and localization of spinal cord tumors, Ann. Surg. **81**:223-254, 1925.

Davidoff, L. M., and Dyke, C. G.: The normal encephalogram, ed. 2, Philadelphia, 1946, Lea & Febiger.

Denk, W.: Ueber die Gefahr der lumbalen Encephalographie bei Hirntumoren, Zbl. Chir. **50**:471-472, 1923.

Di Chiro, G.: Movement of the cerebrospinal fluid in human beings, Nature **204**:290-291, 1964.

Di Chiro, G.: Observations on the circulation of the cerebrospinal fluid, Acta Radiol. [Diagn.] **5**:988-1002, 1966.

Di Chiro, G., and Fischer, R. L.: Contrast radiography of the spinal cord, Arch. Neurol. **11**:125-143, 1964.

Djindjian, R.: Discussion to Thurel, R.: Hématome intramédullaire, Rev. Neurol. **106**:704-707, 1962.

Djindjian, R., Hurth, M., and Houdart, R.: L'angiographie de la moelle épinière, Paris, 1970, Masson & Cie.

Doppman, J., and Di Chiro, G.: Subtraction-angiography of spinal cord vascular malformations, J. Neurosurg. **23**:440-443, 1965.

Dulac, J.: Appareil pour l'exploration radiographique du crâne et de la face, Ann. Otolaryng. **70**:770-774, 1953.

Dulac, J.: Applications du craniographe C.G.R., J. Radiol. Electr. **37**:852-855, 1956.

Dünner, L., and Calm, A.: Die Röntgenologie der Gefässe, insbesondere Lungengefässe am lebenden Menschen, Fortschr. Roentgenstr. **3**:635, 1923.

Elsberg, C. A., and Dyke, C. G.: Diagnosis and localization of tumors of spinal cord by means of measurements made on x-ray films of vertebrae and correlation of clinical and x-ray findings, Bull. Neurol. Inst. N. Y. **3**:359-394, 1934.

Enfield, C. D.: Is roentgenology, as a speciality, destined to survive? Radiology **18**:1039-1043, 1932.

Engeset, A.: Cerebral angiography with perabrodil (carotid angiography), Acta Radiol., supp. 56, pp. 1-207, 1944.

Erlacher, P.: Direkte Kontrastdarstellung des Nucleus pulposus, zugleich ein Beitrag zur Pathologie der Bandscheibe, Z. Orthop. **80**:40-57, 1951.

Falk, B.: Calcification in the track of the needle following ventricular puncture, Acta Radiol. **35**:304-308, 1951.

Fischer, M.: Grenzen und Möglichkeiten der Encephalographie, Arch. Psychiat. **79**:96-130, 1926-1927.

Fischer, M.: Encephalographische Befunde bei Schädelverletzungen, Arch. Psychiat. **82**:403-421, 1927-1928.

Flügel, F. E.: Zur Methodik und Verwertbarkeit der Encephalographie in der Tumordiagnostik, Deutsch. Z. Nervenheilk. **112**:251-265, 1930.

Freeman, W.: Discussion to List, C. F.: Trans. Amer. Neurol. Ass. **71**:63-67, 1946.

Friedman, E. D., Snow, W., and Kasanin, J.: Experiences with encephalography via the lumbar route, Arch. Neurol. Psychiat. **19**:762-791, 1928.

Fürnrohr, W.: Die Röntgenstrahlen im Dienste der Neurologie, Berlin, 1906, S. Karger, AG.

Gardner, W. J., and Nichols, B. H.: Encephalography in surgical lesions of the brain: report of fifty consecutive cases, Amer. J. Cancer **17**:342-347, 1933.

Gould, P. L., Peyton, W. T., and French, L. A.: Vertebral angiography by retrograde injection of the brachial artery, J. Neurosurg. **12**:369-374, 1955.

Grant, F. C.: Ventriculography: review based on an analysis of 392 cases, Arch. Neurol. Psychiat. **14**:513-522, 1925.

Greitz, T.: A radiologic study of the brain circulation by rapid serial angiography of the carotid artery, Acta Radiol., supp. 140, pp. 1-123, 1956.

Gross, S. W.: Cerebral arteriography in the dog and in man with a rapidly excreted organic iodine, Proc. Soc. Exp. Biol. **42**:258-259, 1939.

Hauge, T.: Catheter vertebral angiography, Acta Radiol., supp. 109, pp. 1-129, 1954.

Heidrich, L.: Die Encephalographie und Ventrikulographie, Ergebn. Chir. Orthop. **20**:156-265, 1927.

Heidrich, L.: Zur Chirurgie der Hypophyse, insbesondere die Darstellung von Hypophysentumoren im Encephalogramm, Bruns Beitr. Klin. Chir. **142**:837-841, 1928.

Henschen, F.: Die Akustikustumoren, eine neue Gruppe radiographisch darstellbarer Hirntumoren, Fortschr. Roentgenstr. **18**:207-216, 1912.

Henschen, S. E.: Die Röntgen-Strahlen im Dienste der Hirnchirurgie, Comptes rendus du XII Congrès International de Médecine, Moscow, 1897.

Heuer, G., and Dandy, W. E.: Roentgenography in the localization of brain tumor, based upon a series of one hundred consecutive cases, Bull. Johns Hopkins Hosp. **27**:311-322, 1916.

Heuser, C.: Pieloradiografiá con ioduro potásico y las inyecciones intravenosas de ioduro potásico en radiografía, Sem. Med. **26**:424, 1919.

Huang, Y. P., and Wolf, B. S.: The veins of the posterior fossa-superior or Galenic draining group, Amer. J. Roentgen. **95**:808-821, 1965.

Huang, Y. P., and Wolf, B. S.: The veins of the lateral recess of the fourth ventricle and its tributaries. Roentgen appearance and anatomical relationships, Amer. J. Roentgen. **101**:1-21, 1967.

Huang, Y. P., Wolf, B. S., and Okudera, T.: Angiographic anatomy of the inferior vermian vein of the cerebellum, Acta Radiol. [Diagn.] **9**:327-344, 1969.

Hyndman, O. R.: Cerebral pneumography, Arch. Surg. **36**: 245-291, 1938.

Jacobaeus, H. C.: On insufflation of air into the spinal canal for diagnostic purposes in cases of tumors in the spinal canal, Acta Med. Scand. **55**:555-564, 1921.

Jessen, H., and de Fine Licht, E.: Arteriel encephalografí, Nord. Med. T. **7**:7-16, 1934.

Johanson, C.: The central veins and deep dural sinuses of the brain, Acta Radiol., supp. 107, pp. 1-184, 1954.

Josefson, A.: Ueber Verschluss des Rückenmarkkanales, durch Lufteinblasungen in den Spinalkanal festgestellt, und über ein neues Absperrungssymptom, Munchen Med. Wschr. **68**: 555, 1922.

Kolle, K.: Die Geschichte der Neuroradiologie, Fortschr. Neurol. **33**:145-157, 1965.

Kramer, S., Burton, L. K., and Trott, N. G.: Radioactive isotopes in the localisation of brain tumours, Acta Radiol. **46**: 415-424, 1956.

Kuhn, R. A.: The normal brachial cerebral angiogram, Amer. J. Roentgen. **84**:78-87, 1960.

Kuntzmann, J., Gross, C. M., and Meyer, J.: A propos de deux cas de thorotrastome à manifestation clinique tardive, J. Chir. **66**:201-212, 1950.

Laruelle, L.: Le repérage des ventricules cérébraux par un procédé de routine, Presse Med. **39**:1888-1891, 1931.

Laruelle, L.: Le repérage ventriculaire, Rev. Neurol. **40**:129-149, 1933.

Lewin, W.: Rapid serial angiography, Acta Radiol. **34**:319-320, 1950.

Liliequist, B.: Pontine angle tumour. Encephalographic appearances, Acta Radiol., supp. 186, pp. 1-96, 1959a.

Liliequist, B.: The subarachnoid cisterns, Acta Radiol. supp. 185, pp. 1-108, 1959b.

Lima, P. A.: Cerebral angiography, London, 1950, Oxford University Press.

Lindblom, K.: Diagnostic puncture of intervertebral disks in sciatica, Acta Orthop. Scand. **17**:231-239, 1948.

Lindblom, K.: Technique and results in myelography and disc puncture, Acta Radiol. **34**:321-330, 1950.

Lindgren, E.: On the diagnosis of tumours of the spinal cord by the aid of gas myelography, Acta Chir. Scand. **82**:303-318, 1939.

Lindgren, E.: A pneumographic study of the temporal horn with special reference to tumours in the temporal region, Acta Radiol., supp. 69, pp. 1-151, 1948.

Lindgren, E.: Some aspects on the technique of encephalography, Acta Radiol. **31**:161-177, 1949.

Lindgren, E.: Percutaneous angiography of the vertebral artery, Acta Radiol. **33**:389-404, 1950a.

Lindgren, E.: Encephalographic examination of tumours in the posterior fossa, Acta Radiol. **34**:331-338, 1950b.

Lindgren, E.: Another method of vertebral angiography, Acta Radiol. **46**:257-261, 1956.

Lindgren, E., Azambuja, N., and Sjögren, S. E.: Tentorial herniations, Acta Radiol. **46**:215-223, 224-231, 232-241, 1956.

List, C. F.: The differential diagnosis of expanding intracranial lesions by cerebral angiography, Trans. Amer. Neurol. Ass. **71**:63-67, 1946.

List, C. F., and Hodges, F. J.: Angiographic diagnosis of expanding intracranial lesions by vascular displacement, Radiology **47**:319-333, 1946.

Löhr, W., and Jacobi, W.: Die kombinierte Encephalo-Arteriographie, Arch. Klin. Chir. **173**:399-420, 1932.

Löhr, W., and Jacobi, W.: Gefässkrankheiten des Gehirns in arteriographischer Darstellung, Arch. Klin. Chir. **177**:510-527, 1933a.

Löhr, W., and Jacobi, W.: Die kombinierte Encephalo-Arteriographie; ihre Technik und ihre Gefahren, Chirurg **5**:81-90, 1933b.

Löhr, W., and Jacobi, W.: Die kombinierte Encephalo-Arteriographie, Leipzig, 1933c, Georg Thieme.

Loman, J., and Myerson, A.: Visualization of cerebral vessels by direct intra-carotid injection of thorium dioxide, Amer. J. Roentgen. **35**:188-193, 1936.

Lorenz, R.: Die Bedeutung der Phlebographie für die Tumordiagnostik des Gehirns, Acta Neurochir. **1**:392-433, 1951.

Lucherini, T.: La radicolo-mielografia col thorotrast, Riv. Osp. **24**:475-484, 1934.

Luckett, W. H.: Air in the ventricles of the brain, following a fracture of the skull, Surg. Gynec. Obstet. **17**:237-240, 1913.

Lysholm, E.: Apparatus and technique for roentgen examination of the skull, Acta Radiol, supp. 12, pp. 1-120, 1931.

Lysholm, E., Ebenius, B., and Sahlstedt, H.: Das Ventrikulogramm, part 1, Acta Radiol., supp. 24, pp. 1-75, 1935.

Lysholm, E., Ebenius, B., Lindblom, K., and Sahlstedt, H.: Das Ventrikulogramm, part 3, Acta Radiol, supp. 25, pp. 1-124, 1935.

Lysholm, E.: Ebenius, B., and Sahlstedt, H.: Das Ventrikulogramm, part 2, Acta Radiol., supp. 26, pp. 1-199, 1937.

Martin, C. L., and Uhler, C. V.: Roentgenography of intracranial passages following spinal air injections, Amer. J. Roentgen. **9**:543-549, 1922.

Moniz, E.: L'encéphalographie artérielle, son importance dans la localisation des tumeurs cérébrales, Rev. Neurol. **2**:72-89, 1927.

Moniz, E.: Diagnostic des tumeurs cérébrales et épreuve de l'encéphalographic artérielle, Paris, 1931, Masson & Cie.

Moniz, E.: Sur la vitesse du sang dans l'organisme. Détermination de la vitesse de la circulation dans le cerveau, les méninges et les parties molles de la boîte crânienne par l'artériographie, Ann. Med. **32**:193-220, 1932.

Moniz, E., Pinto, A., and Alves, A.: Artériographie du cervelet et des autres organes de la fosse postérieure, Bull. Acad. Med. **109**:758-760, 1933.

Moore, G. E.: The use of radioactive diiodofluorescein in the diagnosis and localization of brain tumors, Science **107**:569-571, 1948.

Moore, G. E., Kohl, D. A., Marvin, J. F., Wang, J. C., and Caudric, C. M.: Biophysical studies of methods utilizing fluorescein and its derivatives to diagnose brain tumors, Radiology **55**:344-362, 1950.

Nosik, W. A.: Clinical application of thorotrast myelography and subsequent forced drainage, Cleveland Clin. Quart. **5**:262-266, 1938.

Nosik, W. A., and Mortenson, O. A.: Myelography with thorotrast and subsequent removal by forced drainage, an experimental study. Preliminary report, Amer. J. Roentgen. **39**:727-730, 1938.

Olivecrona, H.: Die chirurgische Behandlung der Gehirntumoren. Eine kleine Studie, Berlin, 1927, Julius Springer.

Olivecrona, H.: Personal communication, 1936.

Oppenheim, H.: Cited by Bull, J., and Fischgold, H.: VIIIth Symposium Neuroradiologicum, Paris, 1967.

Osborne, E. D., Sutherland, C. G., Scholl, A. J., Jr., and Rowntree, L. G.: Roentgenography of urinary tract during excretion of sodium iodide, J.A.M.A. **80**:368-373, 1923.

Pancoast, H. K., and Fay, T.: Encephalography: roentgenological and clinical considerations for its use, Amer. J. Roentgen. **21**:421-447, 1929.

Pennybacker, J., and Meadows, S. P.: Normal ventriculograms in tumours of the cerebral hemispheres, Lancet **1**:186-190, 1938.

Pfahler, G. E.: Cerebral skiagraphy, Trans. Amer. Roentgen Ray Soc., pp. 175-181, 1905.

Planiol, T.: Diagnostic des lesions intracrâniennes par les radioisotopes, Paris, 1959, Masson & Cie.

Planiol, T.: Radioisotopes et affections du système nerveux central, Paris, 1965, Masson & Cie.

Portera, A.: Pan-ventriculography, Acta Radiol. [Diagn.] **5**:693-704, 1966.

Pygott, F., and Hutton, C. F.: Vertebral angiography by percutaneous brachial artery catheterization, Brit. J. Radiol. **32**:114-119, 1959.

Radner, S.: Vertebral angiography by catheterization: new methods employed in 222 cases, Acta Radiol., supp. 87, pp. 1-134, 1951.

Radovici, A., and Meller, O.: Essai de liquidographie céphalorachidienne. Encéphalo-myélographie par le thorotrast sousarachnoidien, Bull. Acad. Med. **107**:314-320, 1932.

Riechert, T.: Zur Phlebographie der Hirngefässe, Zbl. Chir. **66**:662-674, 1939.

Robertson, E. G.: Encephalography, Melbourne, 1941, Macmillan & Co.

Scatliff, J. H., and Greenspan, R. H.: Radiographic evaluation of major arteries of the neck by intravenous aortography, Acta Radiol. [Diagn.] **1**:404-416, 1963.

Schaeffer, R.: Ueber die diagnostische und therapeutische Verwendbarkeit der Encephalographie durch Subokzipitalpunktion, Deutsch. Arch. Klin. Med. **165**:23-40, 1929.

Schaltenbrand, G.: Die Abhängigkeit des Encephalogramms vom äusseren Atmosphärendruck, Deutsch. Z. Nervenheilk. **124**:158-164, 1932a.

Schaltenbrand, G.: Spontane Luftfüllung der Ventrikel bei Zysternenpunktion im Sitzen, Med. Klin. **28**:609-611, 1932b.

Schaltenbrand, G.: Richtlinien für die Luftfüllung der Liquorräume zum Zwecke ihrer röntgenographischen Darstellung, Deutsch. Med. Wschr. **59**:1039-1040, 1933.

Schinz, H. R.: Ein kleiner Apparat zur Ventrikulographie und Encephalographie, Zbl. Chir. **49**:1367-1368, 1922.

Schramel, R., Creech, O., Llewellyn, R., and Corales, R.: Visualization of the extracranial cerebral circulation by cardioangiography, J.A.M.A. **175**:804-805, 1961.

Schüller, A.: Die Schädelbasis im Röntgen-Bilde, Fortschr. Roentgenstr., supp. vol. 11, 1905.

Schüller, A.: Röntgen-Diagnostik der Erkrankungen des Kopfes, Vienna, 1912, A. Hölder.

Schurr, P. H., and Wickbom, I.: Rapid serial angiography. Further experience, J. Neurol. Neurosurg. Psychiat. **15**:110-118, 1952.

Schuster, N. H.: Early days of roentgen photography in Britain, Brit. Med. J. **2**:1164-1166, 1962.

de Sèze, S., and Levernieux, J.: L'injection directe du nucleus pulposus par voie paravertébrale, Sem. Hop. Paris **27**:1230-1231, 1951.

de Sèze, S., and Levernieux, J.: Les accidents de la discographie, Rev. Rhum. **19**:1027-1033, 1952.

Shimidzu, K.: Beiträge zur Arteriographie des Gehirns. Einfache percutane Methode, Arch. Klin. Chir. **188**:295-316, 1937.

Sicard, J. A., and Forestier, J. E.: Méthode générale d'exploration radiologique par l'huile iodée (Lipiodol), Bull. Soc. Med. Hop. Paris **46**:463-'69, 1922.

Sicard, J. A., and Forestier, J. E.: L'huile iodée en clinique; applications therapeutiques et diagnostiques, Bull. Soc. Med. Hop. Paris **47**:309-314, 1923.

Sjögren, S. E.: Percutaneous vertebral angiography, Acta Radiol. **40**:113-127, 1953a.

Sjögren, S. E.: Experiences in localisation of brain tumours by means of diiodo 131 fluorescein, Acta Radiol. **40**:356-360, 1953b.

Sjöqvist, O.: Arteriographische Darstellung der Gefässe der hinteren Schädelgrube, Chirurg **10**:377-380, 1938.

Stenbeck, T.: Röntgenstrålarna i medicinens tjänst, Stockholm, 1900, Wahlström & Widstrand.

von Storch, T. J. C.: On the technique of encephalography: with special reference to the use of apparatus, Amer. J. Roentgen. **35**:78-92, 1936.

Sugar, O., Holden, L. B., and Powell, C. B.: Vertebral angiography, Amer. J. Roentgen. **61**:166-182, 1949.

Takahashi, K.: Die percutane Arteriographie der Arteria vertebralis und ihrer Versorgungsgebiete, Arch. Psychiat. **3**: 373-379, 1940.

Torkildsen, A.: The gross anatomy of the lateral ventricles, J. Anat. **68**:480-491, 1933-1934.

Torkildsen, A.: An analysis of shadows seen in pneumograms of cerebral ventricles, Acta Psychiat. **9**:465-488, 1934.

Viallet, P., Sendra, L., Chevrot, L., Combe, P., Descuns, P., and Aubry, P.: Nouvelle méthode d'angiographie cérébrale simultanée totale par injection intraveineuse rapide, Acta Radiol. **46**:273-278, 1956.

van Wagenen, W. P.: The roentgenological localization of spinal subarachnoid block by use of air in the subarachnoid space, Ann. Surg. **99**:939-943, 1934.

Wartenberg, R.: Encephalographische Erfahrungen, Z. Neurol. Psychiat. **94**:585-628, 1924-1925.

Weigeldt, W.: Die röntgenographische Darstellung des Gehirns durch Luftfüllung der liquorführenden Räume, Munchen. Med. Wschr. **69**:1764-1767, 1922.

Weigeldt, W.: Die Bedeutung der Lufteinblasung für Hirn- und Rückenmarkdiagnostik, Deutsch. Z. Nervenheilk. **77**: 165-173, 1923.

Westberg, G.: Gas myelography and percutaneous puncture in the diagnosis of spinal cord cysts, Acta Radiol., supp. 252, pp. 1-67, 1966.

Wideröe, S.: Ueber die diagnostische Bedeutung der intraspinalen Luftinjektionen bei Rückenmarksleiden besonders bei Geschwülsten, Zbl. Chir. **48**:394-397, 1921.

Williams, F. H.: The roentgen rays in medicine and surgery, New York, 1901, The Macmillan Co.

Young, B., and Scott, M.: Air myelography. The substitution of air for lipiodol in roentgen visualization of tumours and other structures in the spinal canal, Amer. J. Roentgen. **39**:187-192, 1938.

Ziedses des Plantes, B. G.: Subtraktion, Stuttgart, 1961, Georg Thieme Verlag.

PART I

Technical aspects of skull roentgenography

LEON M. NEAL, M.D.

CHAPTER 2

Radiographic techniques and projections

D. Gordon Potts

The first roentgenographic examination of a patient with possible disease of the skull or of its contents normally consists of a series of roentgenograms of the entire skull. These roentgenograms may be supplemented with further views of a particular region when the clinical examination or the initial skull roentgenograms indicate that additional views are needed. For example, if the clinical evidence suggests an optic glioma, views of the optic canals are obtained; or if the routine roentgenograms of the skull suggest that the internal auditory canal is eroded, further views are obtained to define this structure more clearly.

SKULL PROJECTIONS, GENERAL CONSIDERATIONS

Many skull projections have been described in the years since the first roentgenographic examination of the skull. Sometimes the same view has been described and named independently in different countries at about the same time. Eponyms are common, and views with trivial differences have been given different names. At least two roentgenographic base lines are in common use, and no completely satisfactory system for conversion from one base line to another has been widely applied.

In addition to the standard views that have been defined, a new projection is sometimes necessary to produce the ideal roentgenogram of a structure. For example, the best view of an aneurysm may project the aneurysm through the center of the orbit; or a precise tangential view of a lesion of the cranial vault may require an unusual projection.

Base lines and planes

Increasing concern over the lack of uniformity of skull projections led to a conference of the World Federation of Neurology, Problem Commission of Neuroradiology, in 1961. The Commission sought to achieve:

1. Precise projections for skull radiology
2. A clarification of similarities or differences in techniques that are not significantly important
3. A divorce of numerous eponyms (proper names) belonging to an era when unknowingly, due to lack of contact between countries, similar discoveries were made simultaneously

The following base lines and planes were chosen by the Commission:

1. The anthropologic base line: this joins the infraorbital point to the superior border of the external auditory meatus; the anthropologic plane contains both anthropologic base lines
2. The orbitomeatal base line: this joins the outer canthus of the eye to the central point of the external auditory meatus; the orbitomeatal plane contains both orbitomeatal base lines

Although the work of this commission eliminated many inconsistencies and increased the clarity of definitions related to skull radiology, some problems still remained. For example, the *anteroposterior half-axial view* is defined as follows:

> The head rests on the occiput. The median-sagittal plane is perpendicular to the film. If the orbito-meatal plane is perpendicular to the film, the central ray makes an angle of 25 to 30 degrees craniocaudally to the plane. If the anthropological plane is perpendicular to the film, the central ray makes an angle of 35 to 45 degrees craniocaudally. The true half-axial projection will by definition be obtained by using an angle of 45 degrees. The central ray, which coincides with the median-sagittal plane, passes through the midpoint of a line which joins the two external auditory meatuses.*

This definition does not establish a single projection but rather a range of possible angulations between the central ray and the orbitomeatal or anthropologic plane. The range of angulations is 5° when the orbitomeatal plane is used, whereas the acceptable range is 10° when the anthropologic plane is used. The definition includes a statement that the true half-axial projection requires a 45° angle; but the base line to be used is not indicated. A fairly wide range of projections therefore would appear to meet the Commission's definition of the "anteroposterior, half-axial projection." Similar problems arise with some of the other definitions suggested by the Commission.

Even with the constructive suggestions of the Commission, any projection of the skull, standard or nonstandard, remains difficult to define with brevity and precision.

Most radiologists include the following considerations in their definitions of skull projections.

Position of central ray in relation to roentgenographic base plane and median-sagittal plane

The part of the definition dealing with position of the ray is most important because it determines almost exclusively the direction from which the various skull structures are viewed and their relation to one another.

The view obtained will be modified slightly by two other factors.

Anode-skull distance. Alterations in the distance between the anode and the skull will alter the relation between structures close to the film and structures more distant from the film (Fig. 2-1). This change is more marked for structures farther away from the central ray.

Centering point. See the ensuing discussion.

Position of head in relation to film

The forehead and nose touch the film—as in the Commission's definition of the posteroanterior projection (inclined).

*From World Federation of Neurology, Problem Commission of Neuroradiology: Study meeting on projections and nomenclature, Milan, 1961, Brit. J. Radiol. 35:501-503, 1962.

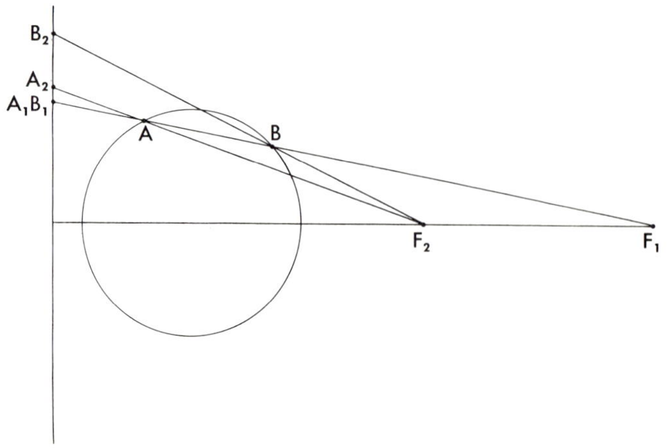

Fig. 2-1. Effect of alteration of anode-film distance on structures at varying distances from film. When tube is at F_1, structures A and B are projected to same point (A_1B_1) on film. When tube is at F_2 (closer to skull and film), A is projected to A_2 and B to B_2 on film.

A more accurate definition of the position of the head in relation to the film is possible. The roentgenographic base plane and the median-sagittal plane, rather than the forehead and nose, are related to the film. In fact, if the position of the head in relation to the tube and central ray is defined, an altered position of the film in relation to the head or the central ray merely alters the degree of magnification or distortion. The silhouette obtained will otherwise be the same.

Area to be included in film

Normally the area included in the projection is the area of interest. Coning or collimation includes that area and no more.

Centering point

In general the centering point will be at the center of the area of interest. One possible exception is the lateral view of the skull. In this case it is desirable to center over the sella turcica, which lies below the center of the intracranial cavity and the surrounding vault and base. Some radiologists center on the sella turcica but increase the size of the collimator or cone to include the whole vault and base. They therefore also include the facial bones, mandible, and upper neck, which may be of no great interest. If a long anode-patient distance is used, the rays diverge relatively little; and even when the central ray passes through the center of the cranial vault and base (above the sella), the obliquity of the rays passing through the sella is minor. A still more satisfactory system is one in which the central ray passes through the sella turcica and the coning or collimation is eccentrically placed around the central ray to include the vault and base. Such collimators are now available.

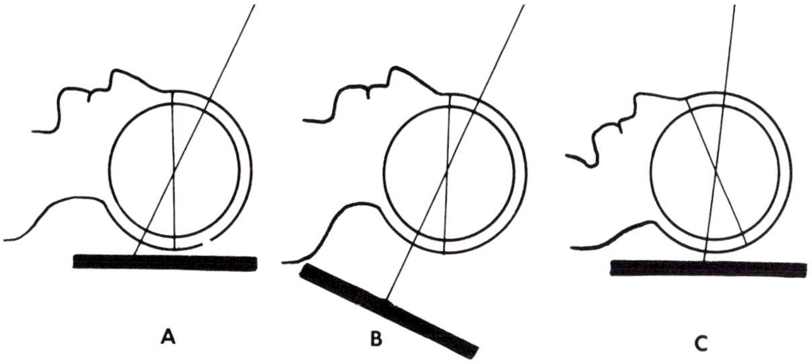

Fig. 2-2. Anteroposterior projection with caudal angulation of central ray. **A,** Radiographic base plane is perpendicular to film. **B,** Central ray is perpendicular to film. **C,** Head is flexed maximally and central ray is angled appropriately in relation to roentgenographic base plane.

In many commonly used projections the definition of centering point is rather empirical. For example in the Kemp Harper view of the jugular foramina (Kemp Harper, 1957; Merrill, 1967), the central ray is directed "to a point about 1 inch distal to the mandibular symphysis."

Because the commonly used system presents so many problems, even with improvements suggested by the Commission, a new system (Potts, 1970) is described here. The suggested system permits conversion from a view defined in relation to the anthropologic base plane to one that is defined with relation to the orbitomeatal base plane, or vice versa. The definitions will be supplemented with diagrams and eponyms when these are helpful. The relation of the film to the head or the central ray will not be included in the definition. It is excluded not because it is unimportant but because it may be varied according to circumstances, even for the same projection. For example, the elimination of rectilinear distortion may be important, in which case the film will be perpendicular to the central ray; or the film may need to be as close as possible to the area of interest, in which case the rectilinear distortion may be considerable (Fig. 2-2).

The centering point will not be included in the definition. The technician can learn the surface projections of structures such as the sella turcica, internal auditory canal, and jugular fossa, or he can derive them from the initial whole skull series. The latter method is simpler than to learn a large number of empirical surface landmarks for the various projections.

The size of the collimator or cone also will not be included in the definition. Presumably the technician will include the area of interest and no more.

The position of any point in space may be defined by spherical polar coordinates. In this system the direction of any radius of the sphere may be defined by two angles (Fig. 2-3). These angles are (1) the longitude

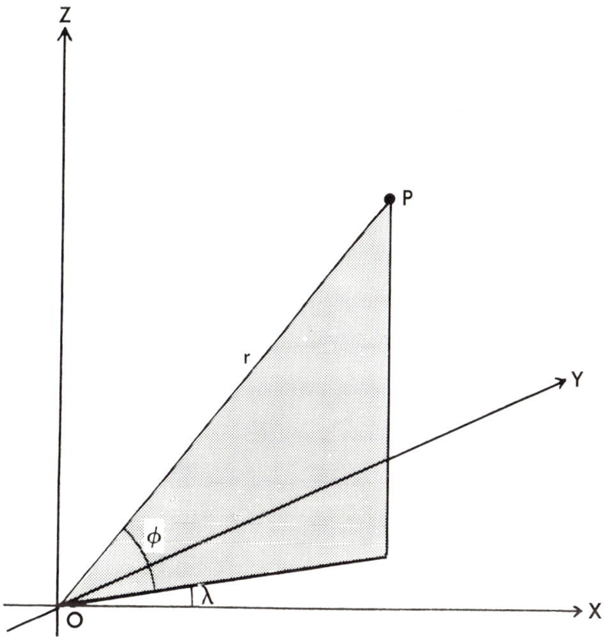

Fig. 2-3. Method of definition of a point *(P)* in space with spherical polar coordinates. (See text.)

(λ), the angle formed by the radius (projected on the XY plane) and the X axis, and (2) the latitude (ϕ), the angle formed by the radius vector and the XY plane. If we wish to define the position of a point, P, in space, we must also know the length, r, of the radius measured from the origin.

USE OF SPHERICAL POLAR COORDINATES TO DEFINE DIRECTION OF CENTRAL RAY FOR SKULL RADIOGRAPHY

Spherical polar coordinates can be applied to skull projections in both nonrotated (anteroposterior and posteroanterior) and rotated views.

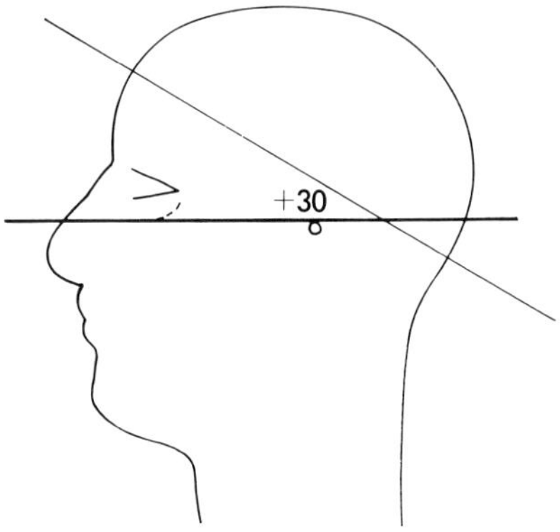

Fig. 2-4. Positive angulation (+30°). Central ray is angled 30° to anthropologic base plane and passes through center of area of interest.

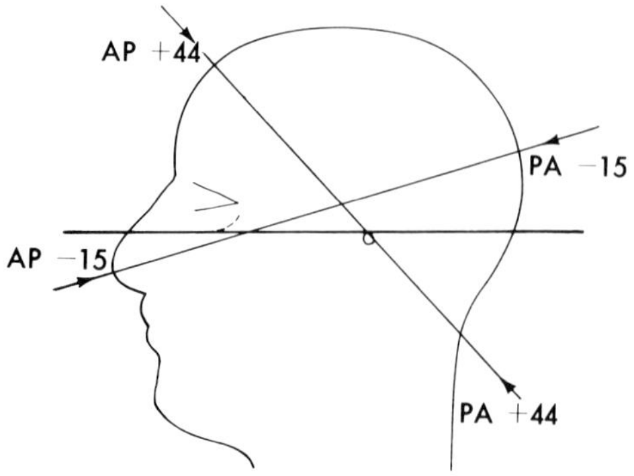

Fig. 2-6. Diagram shows examples of anteroposterior and posteroanterior frontal projections of skull.

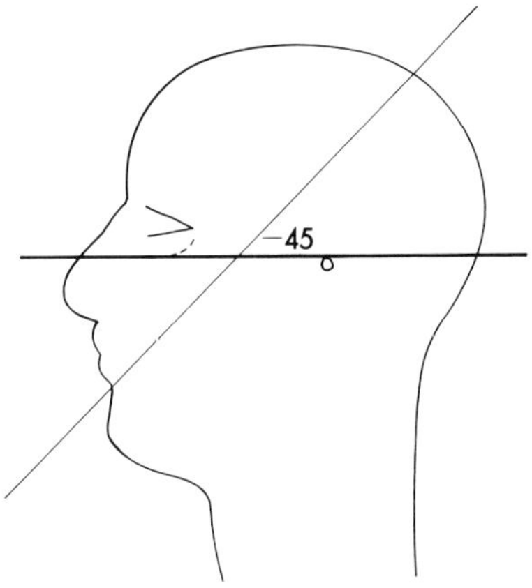

Fig. 2-5. Negative angulation (−45°). Central ray is angled 45° to anthropologic base plane and passes through center of area of interest.

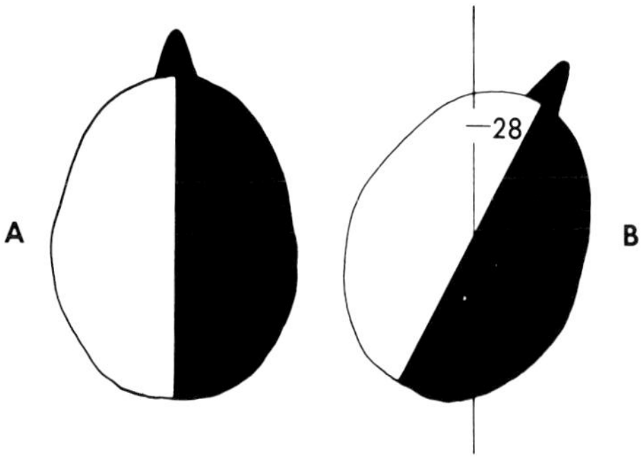

Fig. 2-7. Skull viewed from above. **A,** Not rotated. **B,** Nose turned 28° toward side of interest (−28°). Side of interest is shaded.

Nonrotated views

Positive (+) angulation. If we view the skull from the side (Fig. 2-4) and the central ray is angled so that its anterior part is superior to the base line and its posterior part is inferior to the base line, the angulation will be regarded as positive (+). Thus positive angulation is in the direction of the Towne or half-axial projection. The angle is given in degrees.

Negative (−) angulation. If we view the skull from the side (Fig. 2-5) and the central ray is angled so that its anterior part is inferior to the base line and its posterior part is superior to the base line, the angulation will be regarded as negative (−). Thus negative angulation is in the direction of the Waters projection. The angle is given in degrees.

The direction of the central ray may be posteroanterior or anteroposterior, indicated by the prefix PA or AP respectively (Fig. 2-6).

Rotated views. A second angle must be defined in rotated views. If we view the skull from above (Fig. 2-7) with the nose rotated away from the side of interest, the rotation is regarded as positive (+). When the nose is rotated toward the side of interest, the rotation is regarded as negative (−).

If, for example, during a right carotid angiogram a projection is obtained with the tube in front of the patient, the film behind (anteroposterior), the central ray angled 25° caudally, and the nose rotated 35° to the left (i.e., away from the side of interest), then the view is defined as AP +25, +35.

CONVERSION FROM ONE BASE PLANE TO ANOTHER

Nonrotated views. The World Federation of Neurology, Problem Commission of Neuroradiology (1962), indicated that the anthropologic and orbitomeatal base planes meet at about 10°. Therefore if conversion is desired from one base plane to the other, the correction factor is 10°. As an example, a projection is given in relation to the anthropologic base plane. To obtain the projection in relation to the orbitomeatal base plane, the 10° correction factor must be subtracted (Fig. 2-8).

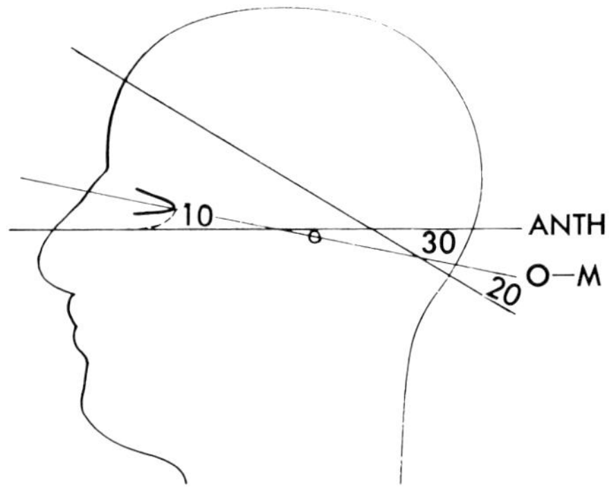

Fig. 2-8. This projection in relation to anthropologic base plane is +30°; central ray is at 20° to orbitomeatal base plane (i.e., *O-M* = *ANTH* –10, where *O-M* is angle in relation to orbitomeatal base plane and *ANTH* is angle in relation to anthropologic base plane).

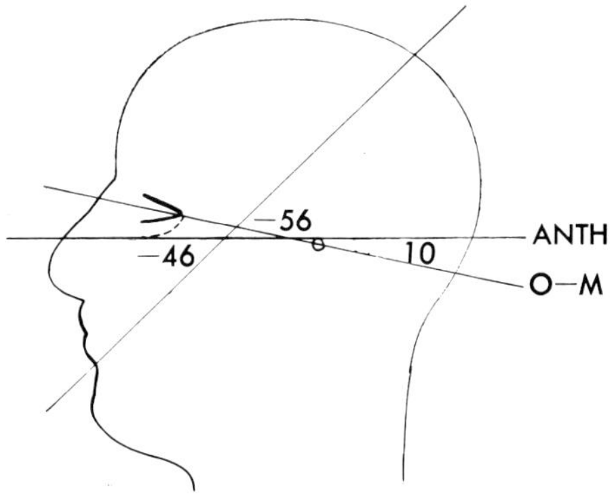

Fig. 2-9. When projection is defined in relation to orbitomeatal base plane, projection may be calculated in relation to anthropologic base plane: *ANTH* = *O-M* +10°. (In this case –56° +10° = –46°.)

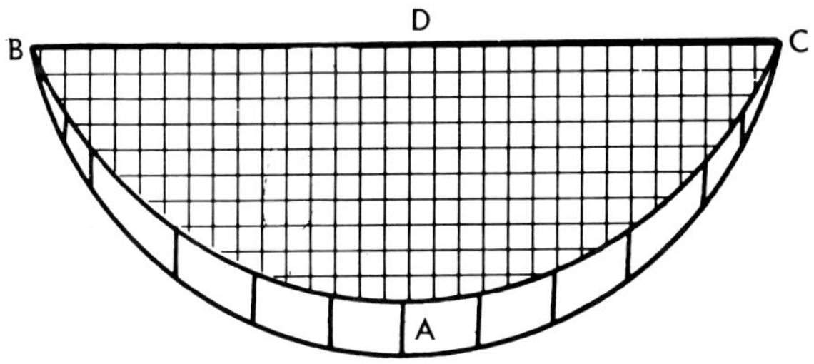

Fig. 2-10. Two semicircular disks separated by angle of 10°. Lines that join corresponding points on circumferences become shorter toward common diameter of two disks.

If the projection is related to the orbitomeatal base plane, the 10° correction factor must be added to obtain the projection in relation to the anthropologic base plane (Fig. 2-9).

Rotated views. To convert the definitions of rotated views from one base plane to the other, the correction factor is less than 10°. If the head is rotated 90°, a lateral view is obtained and the view is PA 0, +90, the same when either base plane is used. In other words, the correction factor for tube angulation is 0°. For other degrees of rotation between 0° and 90°, the correction factor is 10° (cos β), where β is the angle of rotation of the head in degrees (Potts, 1970). The approximate correction factors for various degrees of head rotation are given in Table 2-1. When the head is rotated, it must be turned on an axis perpendicular to the base plane.

Table 2-1. Rotation correction factors

Angle of rotation of head (degrees)	*Correction factor (degrees)*
0	10
10	10
20	9
30	9
40	8
50	6
60	5
70	3
80	2
90	0

The reason for this correction factor is perhaps best explained by Fig. 2-10, which shows two semicircular disks separated by an angle of 10°. Imagine that each disk corresponds with one of the roentgenographic base planes. The x-ray tube travels around the lower semicircle when one base line is used and around the upper semicircle when the other base line is used. Vertical lines that join the two semicircles at different points become shorter as the tube moves out from point *A* to points *B* and *C*, where the two semicircles intersect. Therefore the angles subtended by these lines at the center, *D*, of the semicircles become smaller as the tube passes from *A* toward *C* or *D*. These angles represent the correction factor at any point (Table 2-1).

PRACTICAL APPLICATION OF SYSTEM

In general, skull roentgenographic units may be divided into two types: (1) those in which the tube has a circular movement and the patient is rotated to obtain rotated views and (2) those in which the tube can move anywhere on the surface of a sphere.

In the first type of unit, rotated views may be obtained by either of two methods: (1) the head and neck of the patient are turned while he sits in a standard chair; (2) the patient sits in a rotating chair and the head is immobilized in a head support attached to the chair so that the entire patient is turned. The degree of chair rotation may be indicated on a protractor incorporated in the chair.

In the type of unit with a spherical tube movement, the rotated views are obtained by the tube movement

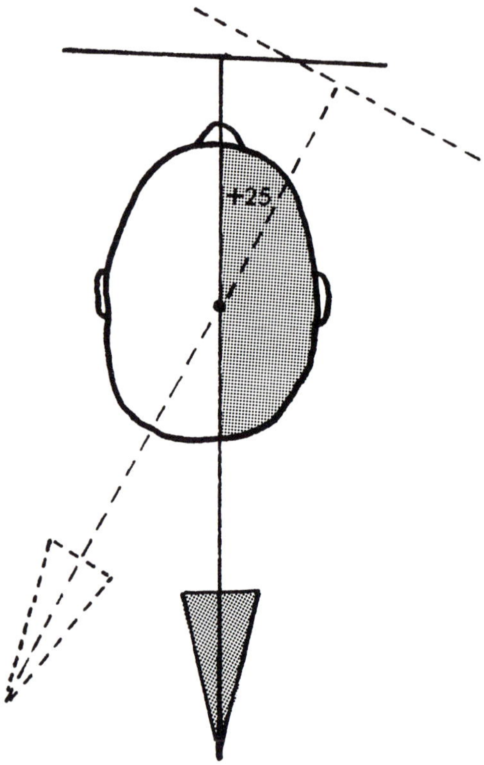

Fig. 2-11. Positive rotated view. Film is in front of patient and is rotated toward side of interest (shaded).

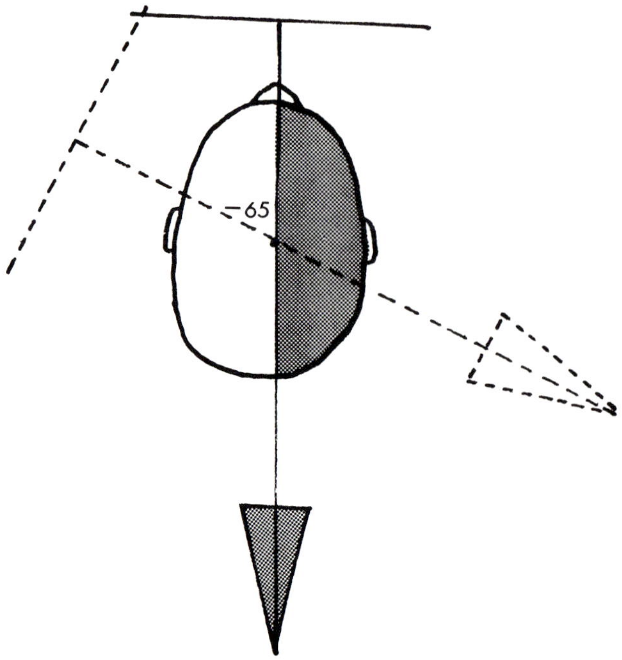

Fig. 2-12. Negative rotated view. Film is in front of patient and is rotated away from side of interest (shaded).

(Fig. 2-11). The movement is equivalent to the head rotation indicated in the definition of the projection. For a positive rotation the tube or film, whichever is anterior, is rotated toward the side of interest. For a negative rotation the tube or film, whichever is anterior, is rotated away from the side of interest (Fig. 2-12).

The system does not parallel exactly the mathematical system of polar coordinates because to do so would require a head rotation or tube rotation of almost 360° for some views.

The definition of any nonrotated view consists of two parts, a prefix (AP or PA) and one angle (the tube angulation). The rotated view consists of the prefix AP or PA and two angles; the first angle indicates the tube angulation, and the second the patient rotation (or equivalent tube movement if a spherical tube movement is employed).

The definition may be regarded as a series of instructions for producing the view. For example, if the view is defined as PA −25, +90 (Fig. 2-13), the tube and film will first be positioned with the tube behind, and the film in front of, the patient. The central ray passes through the sagittal plane and parallel to the roentgenographic base plane (i.e., positioned for a straight posteroanterior view). The tube and film will then be

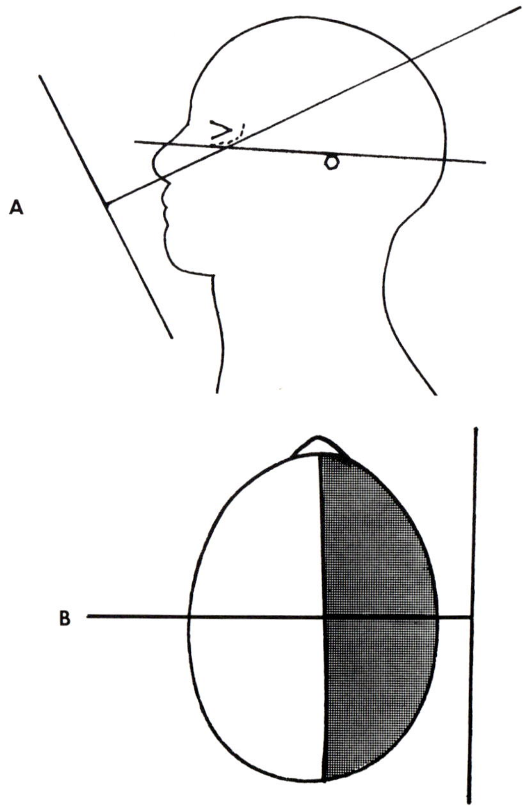

Fig. 2-13. PA −25°, +90° view. **A,** Film is in front of patient and central ray is angled 25° caudally (i.e., *PA* −25). **B,** Nose is then turned 90° away from side of interest (shaded). Skull is viewed from above.

angled so that the central ray passes 25° caudally, and the patient will be rotated 90° away from the side of interest. Adjustment of the position of the patient may then be necessary to permit perfect centering over the area of interest. The adjustment may be a change in the right-left, anteroposterior, or superoinferior directions in relation to the roentgenographic unit. The adjustment must be made without rotation of the head or alteration of the position of the base plane in relation to the roentgenographic unit.

Other instructions may be added to the definition, and in general these should be given in the order in which they will be acted upon by the technician.

Position of patient. The position of the patient is particularly important in air studies. For example, a brow down series could be defined as prone PA +15, prone PA +30, and prone lateral (or prone PA 0, +90).

Centering instructions. For example, AP +15, +35, center on mastoid process away from the film.

To show fluid levels, the instructions must include horizontal ray.

Miscellaneous instructions. For example, film at 90° to central ray, or an air gap of 18 inches.

SKULL PROJECTIONS USED FREQUENTLY

Frequently used skull projections, referred to the orbitomeatal and anthropologic base planes, are summarized in Table 2-2. In most radiology departments all projections are referred to one of these base planes and therefore the base plane need not be stated for every projection. *Unless otherwise stated in this book, views will be defined in relation to the anthropologic base plane.*

Routine skull projections

No set of projections of the skull for intracranial disease has been universally accepted, but the following represents a typical skull series (Fig. 2-14): lateral (or

Table 2-2. Frequently used skull projections (referred to orbitomeatal and anthropologic base lines)

Structure	Name of projection	*Suggested name*		Comments
		O-M base line*	*Anth* base line*	
Skull	Lateral	Lateral (or PA 0, +90)	Lateral or PA 0, +90	See text
Skull	Anteroposterior half-axial	AP +25	AP +35	
Skull	Straight anteroposterior	AP 0	AP +10	
Skull	Inclined anteroposterior	AP −15	AP −5	
Skull	Subaxial	AP −90	AP −80	
Skull	Axial	AP −100	AP −90	
Skull	Posteroanterior half-axial	PA +25	PA +35	Identical to Haas view of sella
Skull	Straight posteroanterior	PA 0	PA +10	
Skull	Inclined posteroanterior	PA −15	PA −5	Identical to modified Caldwell of facial bones and sinuses
Petrous temporal bone	Stenvers	PA +5, +45	PA +12, +45	
Petrous temporal bone	Valdini	PA +30	PA +40	
Petrous temporal bone	Mayer	AP +38, −45	AP +45, −45	
Petrous temporal bone	Arcelin	AP +3, +45	AP +10, +45	
Petrous temporal bone	Chaussé III	AP +20, +15	AP +30, +15	
Optic foramen	Pfeiffer	PA −30, +37	PA −22, +37	
Facial bones, sinuses	Waters	PA −53	PA −43	
Facial bones, sinuses	Exaggerated Waters	PA −45	PA −35	
Sphenoid sinus	Posteroanterior	PA +10	PA +20	Identical to view of inferior orbital fissure
Jugular foramina	Anteroposterior	AP +50	AP +60	
Jugular foramina	Eraso	AP −65	AP −55	
Jugular foramina	Kemp Harper	AP −70	AP −60	
Jugular foramina	Porcher	AP −35, +15	AP −25, +15	
Sphenoid strut	Hough	PA −16, +20	PA −7, +20	
Superior orbital fissure	Posteroanterior	PA −20	PA −10	
Mastoid	Law	PA −18, +75	PA −15, +75	
Mastoid	Hickey	AP +7, +35	AP +15, +35	
Mastoid	Henschen	PA −15, +90	PA −15, +90	
Mastoid	Schüller	PA −25, +90	PA −25, +90	
Mastoid	Lysholm	PA −35, +90	PA −35, +90	
Hypoglossal canal	Miller	AP +5, +45	AP +12, +45	Mouth open

**O-M*, Orbitomeatal; *Anth*, anthropologic.

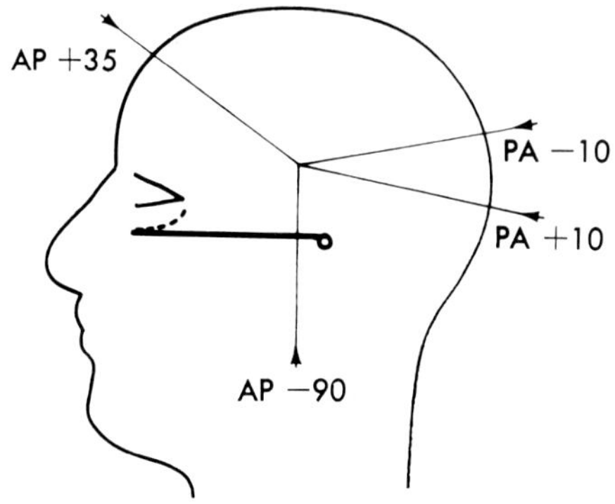

Fig. 2-14. Routine projections of skull.

PA 0, +90); AP +35 (AP half-axial); PA +10; PA −10; AP −90 (axial).

Lateral. The lateral view should be obtained with a horizontal central ray. The patient may be either erect or supine. The head and neck should not be rotated in relation to the body, for important changes in the upper cervical region may be obscured. The central ray should be perpendicular to the median-sagittal plane, and the film placed on the side of the suspected lesion. The lateral view may be defined as PA 0, +90. For this view the film is placed in front of the skull and the central ray is positioned parallel to the base line. The nose is rotated 90° away from the side of interest. The term lateral, however, is so simple and so specific that nothing is gained by substituting the suggested system for this view.

AP +35 (AP half-axial). The head and neck are flexed as much as possible, with the median-sagittal plane perpendicular to the film. The central ray is angled 35° caudally in relation to the anthropologic base plane. Some definitions of this view have stipulated that the roentgenographic base plane should be perpendicular to the film. The system of flexing the head as much as possible, as suggested here, has a dual advantage: it allows for the patient who cannot flex the head and neck sufficiently to bring the base plane perpendicular to the film; it provides reduced rectilinear distortion (and possibly finer detail) in the patient who can flex the head and neck more than usual (Fig. 2-2).

PA +10. The film is placed in front of the patient, and the central ray is angled 10° rostrally in relation to the anthropologic base plane. The view should project the internal auditory canal through the lower half of the orbit. (Note: some radiologists prefer the AP +10 view instead of the PA +10 because, with the film behind the patient, the orbit is more highly magnified; projection of the petrous temporal bone through the orbit is therefore a little easier.)

PA −10. The film is placed in front of the patient and the central ray is angled 10° caudally in relation to the anthropologic base plane. This view should project the entire petrous temporal bone below the orbit.

AP −90 (axial). Starting from the AP 0 position, the head is fully extended and the central ray is angled at 90° in relation to the anthropologic base plane.

After head trauma both right and left lateral projections should be obtained. If a pituitary lesion or a brain tumor or increased intracranial pressure is suspected, a coned lateral view of the sella turcica should be obtained.

Centering point

When the lesions of the brain or the cranial vault are suspected, the area of interest in routine skull roentgenograms is roughly spherical. The top half of the sphere is formed by the upper vault (Fig. 2-15). The central ray should be directed toward the center of this area of interest.

Other commonly used skull projections

Entire skull. The nonrotated views of the entire skull shown in Table 2-2 are summarized in Fig. 2-16.

Petrous temporal bone

PA +12, +45 (Stenvers, 1917). Starting from the straight PA position, the central ray is angled 12° rostrally and the head is rotated 45° away from the side of interest (Fig. 2-17, *A*). Taveras and Wood (1964) used the orbitomeatal base plane, but Merrill (1967) used the anthropologic base plane for the projection defined by these angles. Since the anthropologic base plane results in a more satisfactory projection with +12° tube angulation, it is suggested here.

The central ray passes through the petrous temporal bone.

PA +40 (Valdini, 1928) (Fig. 2-17, *B*). Merrill (1967) suggested this projection for the demonstration of the labyrinths and internal auditory canals. PA +50 is suggested for the demonstration of the external auditory canals, the tympanic cavities, and the bony parts of the eustachian tubes (Merrill, 1967). PA +40 may include both temporal bones, or each temporal bone may be examined separately.

AP +45, −45 (Mayer, 1926) (Fig. 2-17, *C*) (Merrill, 1967).

AP +10, +45 (Arcelin, 1923) (Fig. 2-17, *D*) (Merrill, 1967). This view is similar to the Stenvers view except that the central ray passes in the opposite direction. It displays the temporal bone away from the film.

AP +30, +15 (Chaussé III, 1950) (Fig. 2-17, *E*). Center on the mastoid as shown in the diagram. This view demonstrates the mastoid process and lateral part of the petrous temporal bone.

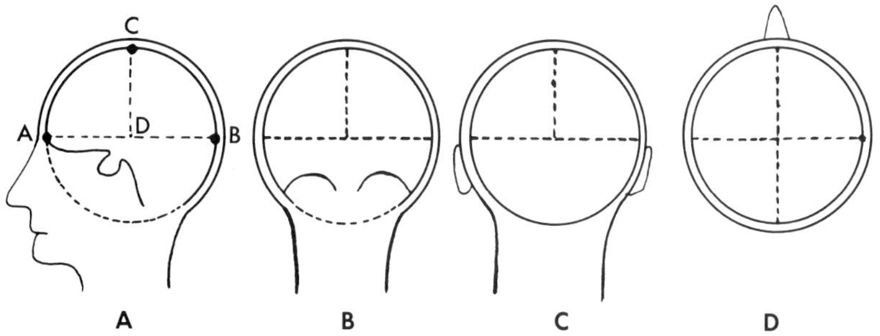

Fig. 2-15. Views of skull. **A,** Lateral. Diameter *AB* of sphere is bisected at *D* by radius *CD*. In practice, centering point *D* is half the anteroposterior diameter of skull—below top of head and halfway between front and back of skull. **B,** Anterior. **C,** Posterior. **D,** Superior. Area of interest is roughly spherical.

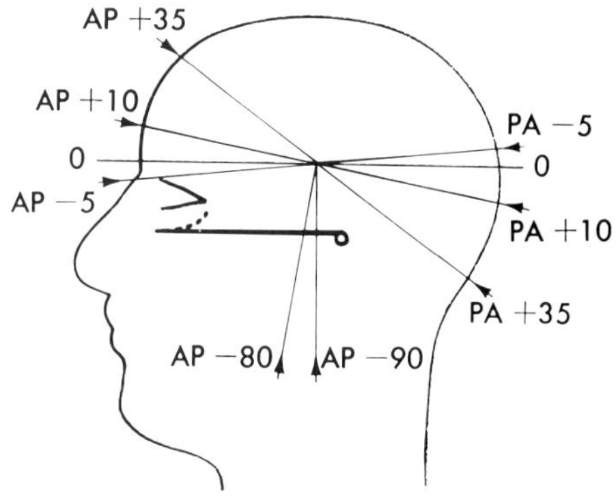

Fig. 2-16. Other commonly employed projections of nonrotated skull.

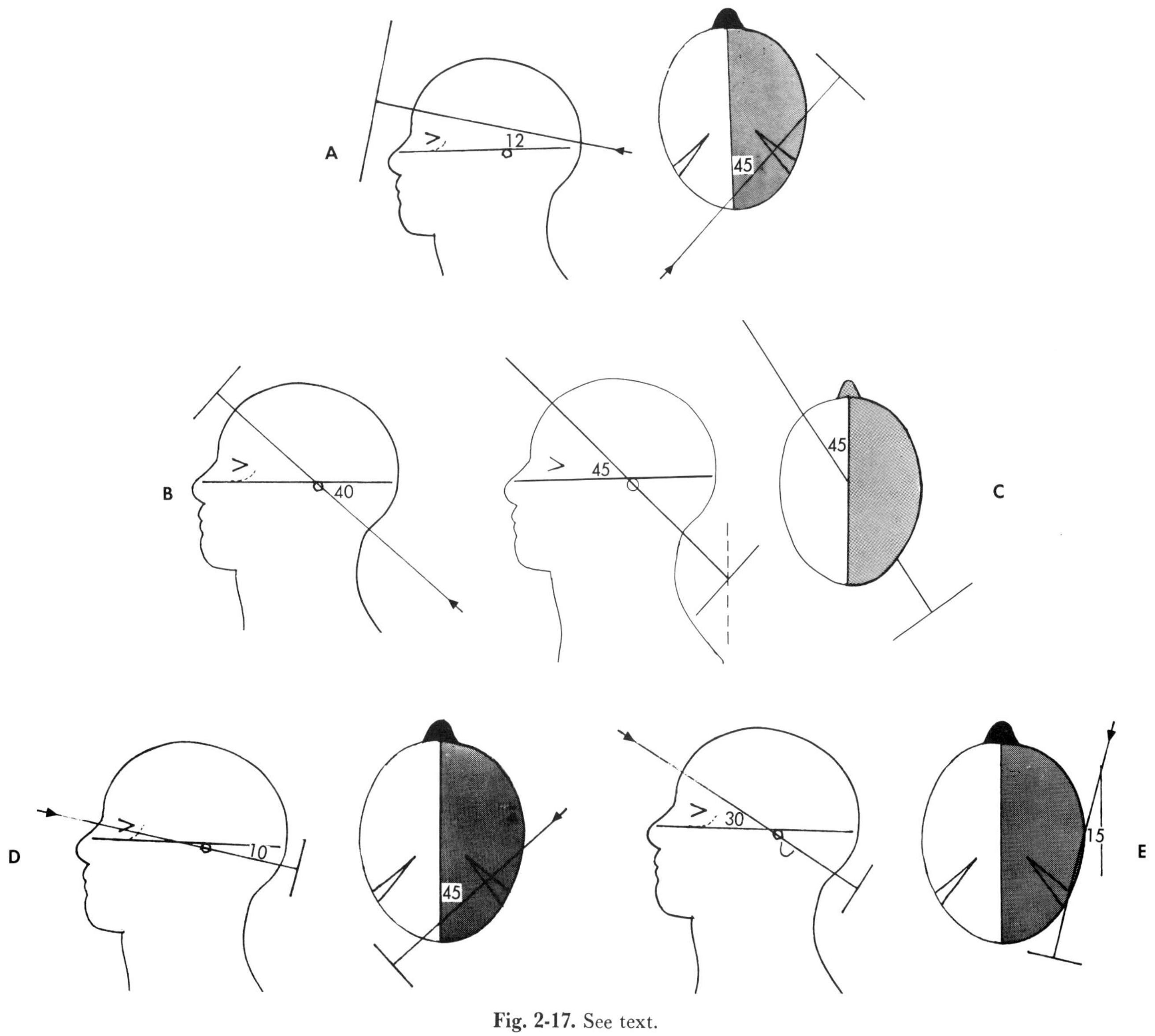

Fig. 2-17. See text.

Optic canal

PA −22, +37 (Pfeiffer, 1933) (Fig. 2-18). The optic foramen should be projected into the lower and lateral quadrant of the orbit.

Facial bones and sinuses

PA −43 (Waters, 1915) (Fig. 2-19, *A*) (Merrill, 1967). This view projects the petrous temporal bones below the maxillary antra and demonstrates the antra together with the frontal and ethmoid sinuses. (Note: this view was defined by Potts [1970] as PA −37; when referred to the orbitomeatal plane, it should be defined as PA −53; and when referred to the anthropologic plane, it is PA −43.)

PA −35 (exaggerated Waters) (Fig. 2-19, *B*).

PA +20 (Fig. 2-19, *C*). This projection is used to demonstrate the sphenoid sinus.

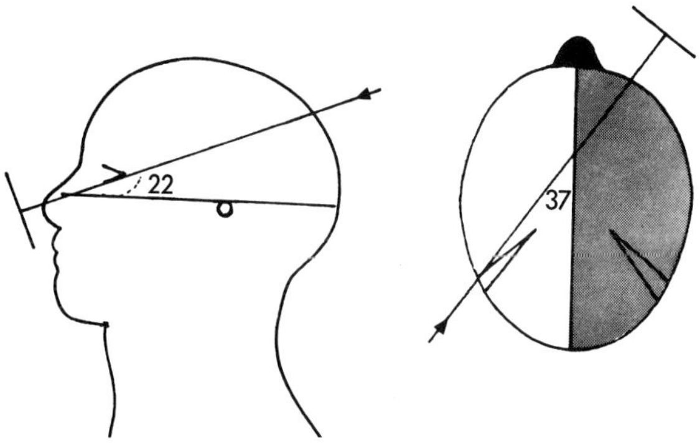

Fig. 2-18. See text.

Jugular foramina

AP +60 (Fig. 2-20, *A*).

AP −55 (Eraso, 1961) (Fig. 2-20, *B*).

AP −60 (Kemp Harper, 1957) (Fig. 2-20, *C*).

AP −25, +15 (Porcher et al., 1952) (Fig. 2-20, *D*).

Sphenoid strut

PA −7, +20 (Hough) (Fig. 2-21) (Merrill, 1967).

Superior orbital fissure

PA −10 (Fig. 2-22).

Mastoid

PA −15, +75 (Law, 1913) (Fig. 2-23, *A*).

AP +15, +35 (Hickey, 1914) (Fig. 2-23, *B*).

PA −15, +90 (Henschen, 1912) (Fig. 2-23, *C*).

PA −25, +90 (Schüller) (Fig. 2-23, *D*) (Merrill,, 1967).

PA −35, +90 (Lysholm, 1931) (Fig. 2-23, *E*).

Hypoglossal canal

AP +12, +45 (Miller) (Fig. 2-24) (Merrill, 1967). The central ray passes through the open mouth.

OTHER ASPECTS OF SPHERICAL POLAR COORDINATE SYSTEM USED FOR SKULL ROENTGENOGRAPHY

A matter important to note is that head units with a spherical tube movement may have one of two different types of movement (Fig. 2-25). Units with the motion shown in Fig. 2-25, *A* (e.g., the Mimer III), are more satisfactory for the suggested system than those with the tube motion shown in Fig. 2-25, *B* (e.g., the

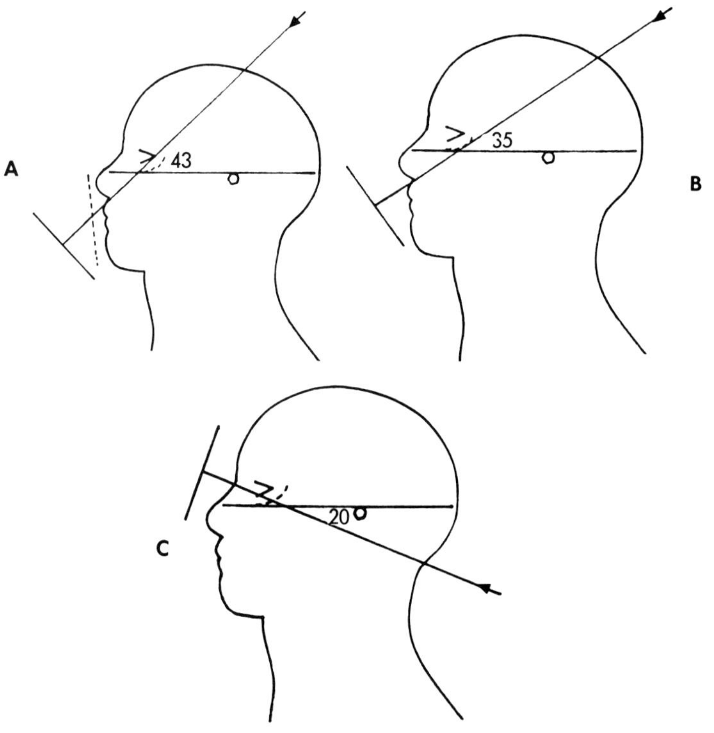

Fig. 2-19. See text.

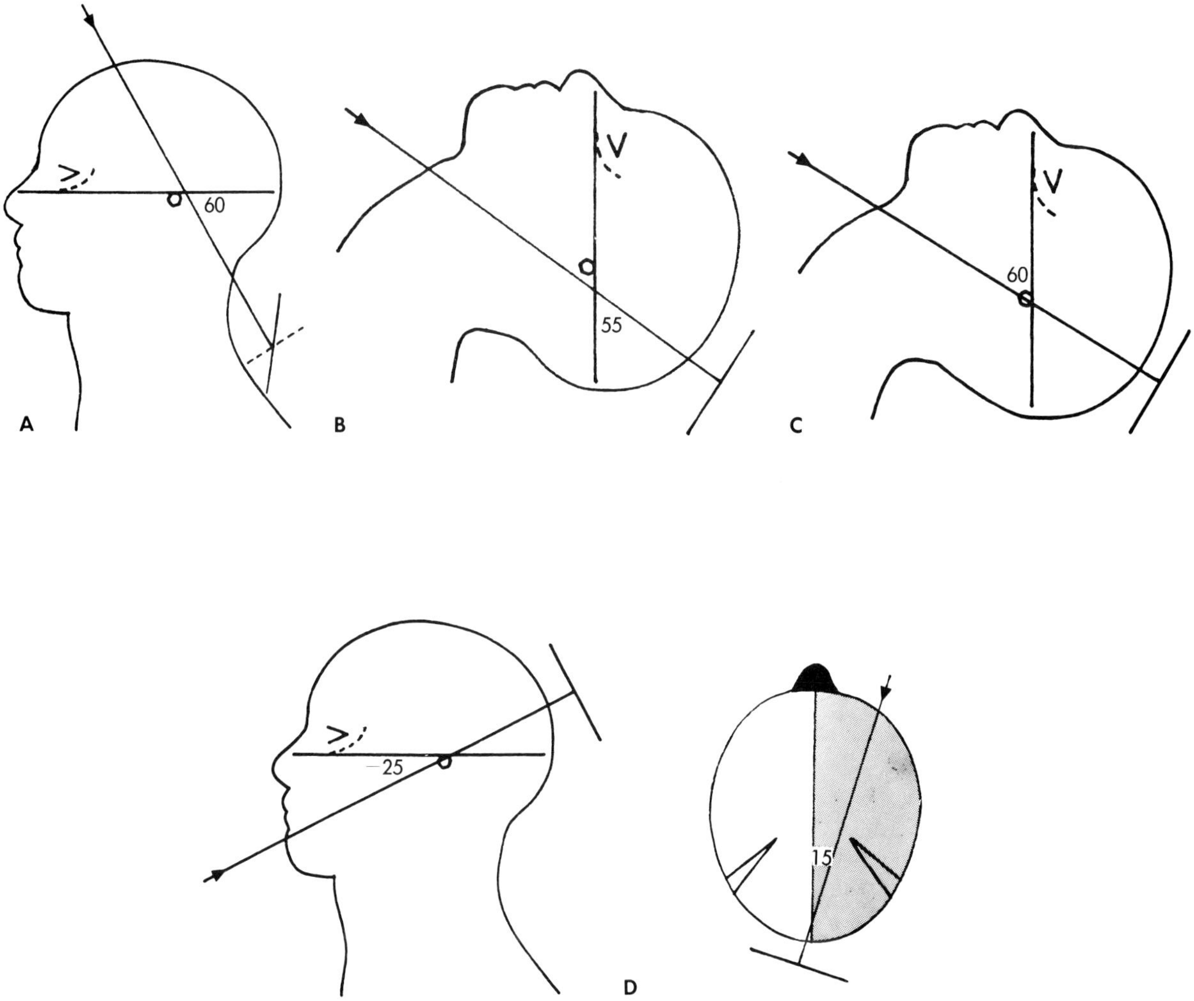

Fig. 2-20. See text.

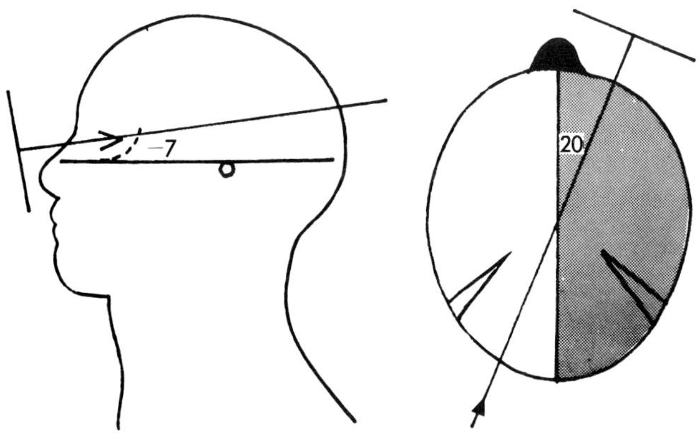

Fig. 2-21. See text.

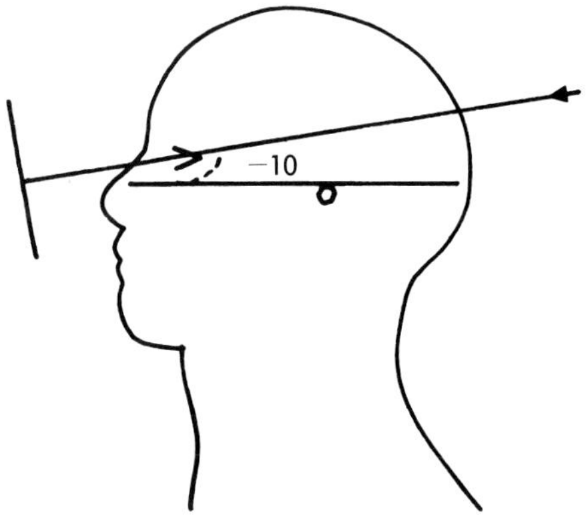

Fig. 2-22. See text.

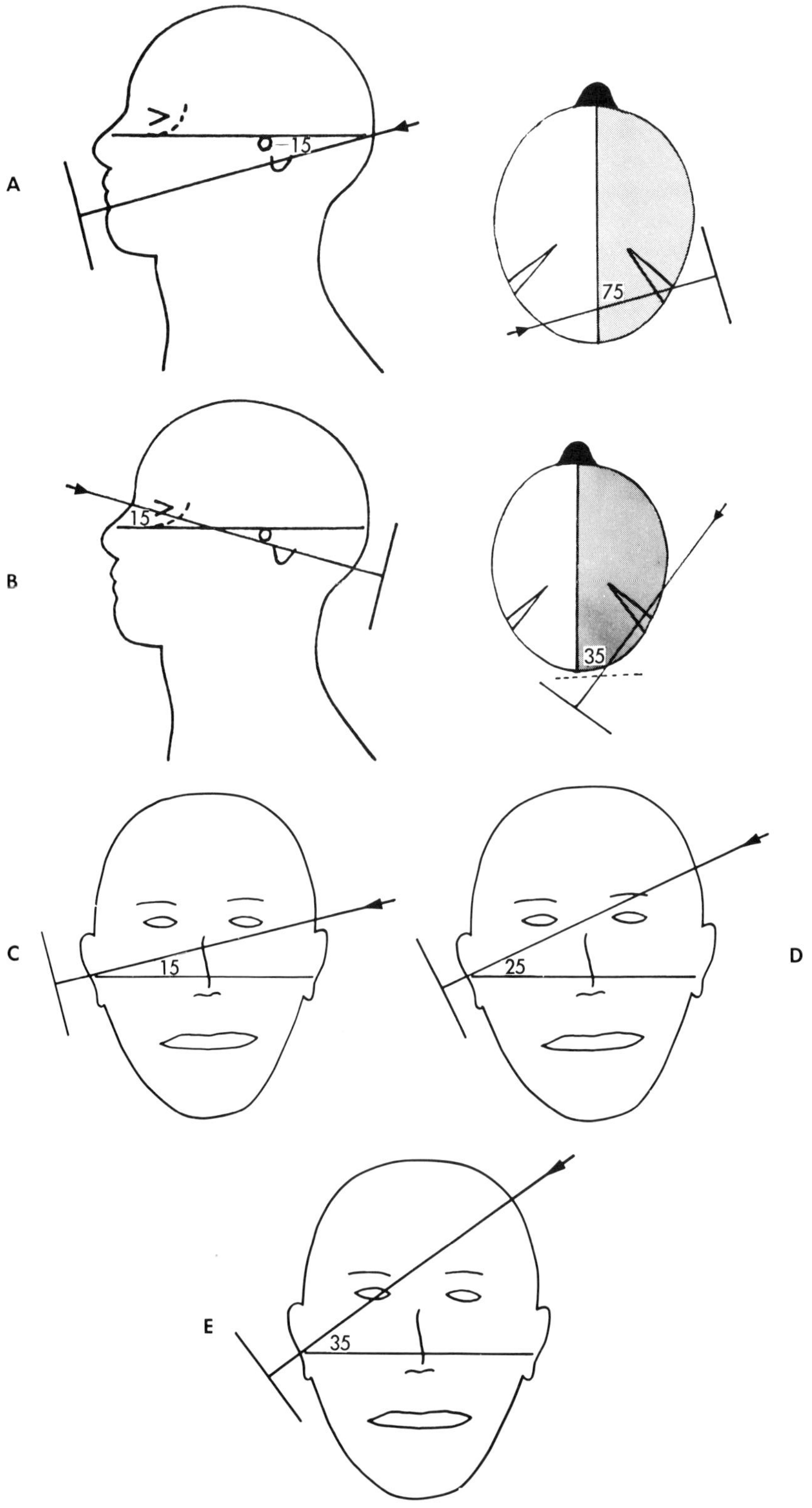

Fig. 2-23. See text.

Schonander and Princeps head units). The latter units, when used for angled and rotated views (e.g., PA +45, +45), reduce the first angle when the tube is moved around the head to simulate head rotation.

Either type of unit may be used for the system by rotating the patient when necessary for rotated views.

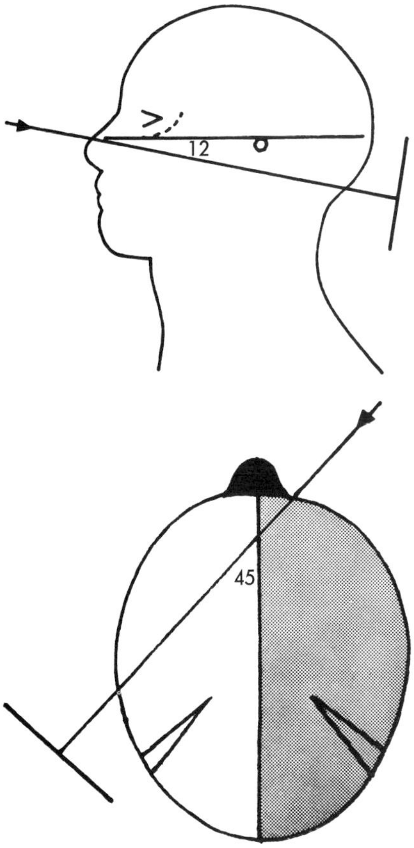

Fig. 2-24. See text.

DIRECTION OF CENTRAL RAY

Many of the nonrotated skull views may be obtained by anteroposterior or posteroanterior projections. Generally, in the past, placement of the film as close as possible to the area of interest was suggested. Thus if the orbit was the main area of interest, the view was obtained as a posteroanterior projection; and if the occipital bone was to be demonstrated, the view was obtained as an anteroposterior projection. Experience both with smaller focal spots that are now available and with magnification techniques suggests that the demonstrated details may actually be increased by separating the structure of interest a moderate distance from the film. Thus many projections are possible either anteroposteriorly or posteroanteriorly without loss of detail on the parts of the skull away from the film.

When the film is placed behind the patient (i.e., anteroposteriorly) and angulation is positive, it is usually not possible to have the film perpendicular to the central ray unless the film is separated considerably from the skull (Fig. 2-26, *A*). If the film is placed close to the

Text continued on p. 51.

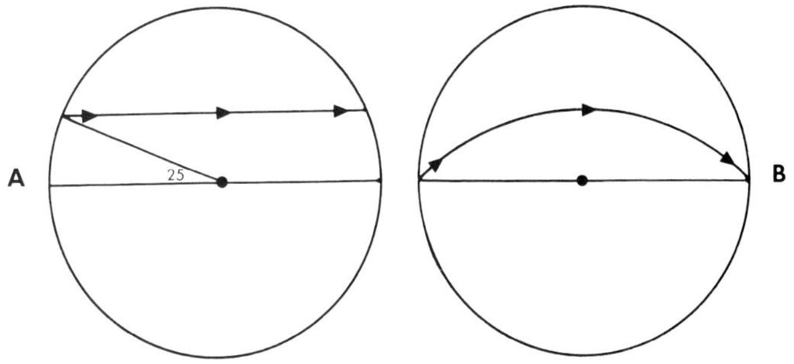

Fig. 2-25. Diagram illustrating the two types of tube movement commonly employed in roentgenographic units for skull.

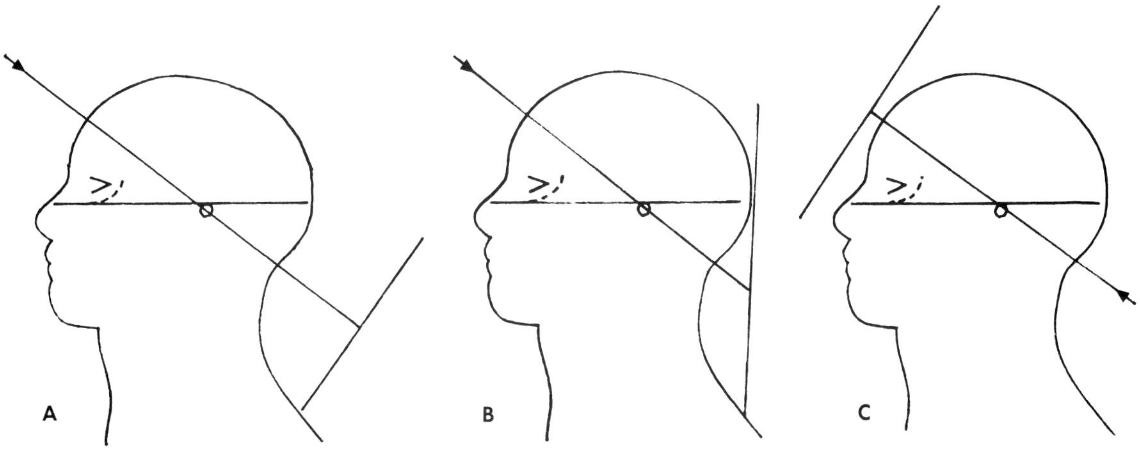

Fig. 2-26. A, Anteroposterior view with positive tube angulation and film perpendicular to central ray. Film is separated from head. **B,** Same projection as in **A** but with film close to head. Considerable rectilinear distortion results. **C,** Same view as in **A** and **B** but posteroanterior. Film is perpendicular to central ray and close to skull.

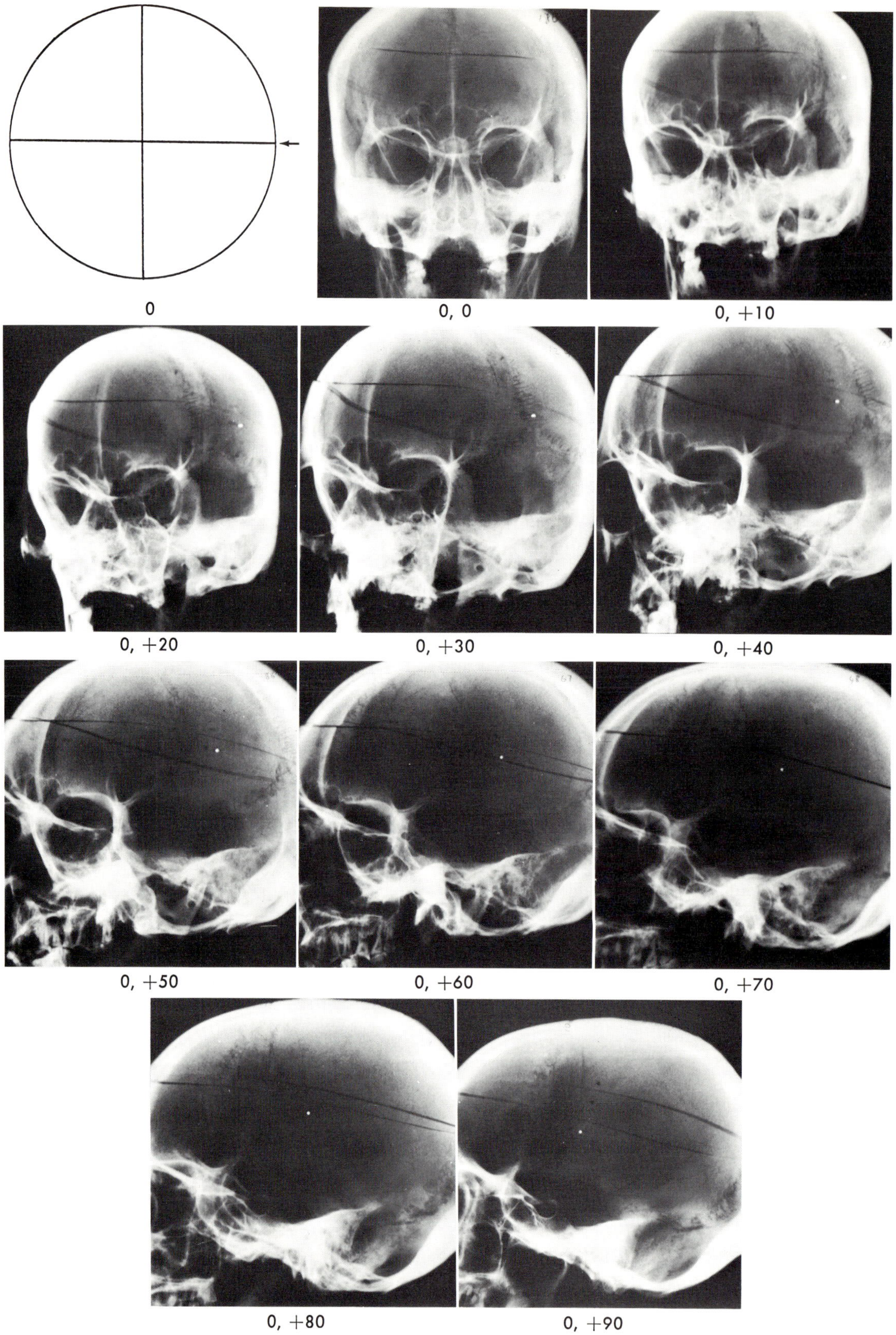

Fig. 2-27. Series of posteroanterior skull projections at 10° intervals for which spherical polar coordinate system was employed. Arrow in each diagram indicates latitude of sphere around which tube moves. Skull is at center of sphere. Rotated views (with positive head rotation) are of left side of skull. If right side of skull had been side of interest, these angles would be same except that second angle in all rotated views (angle of head rotation) would be negative. Small metallic density is visible in left side of cranial vault.

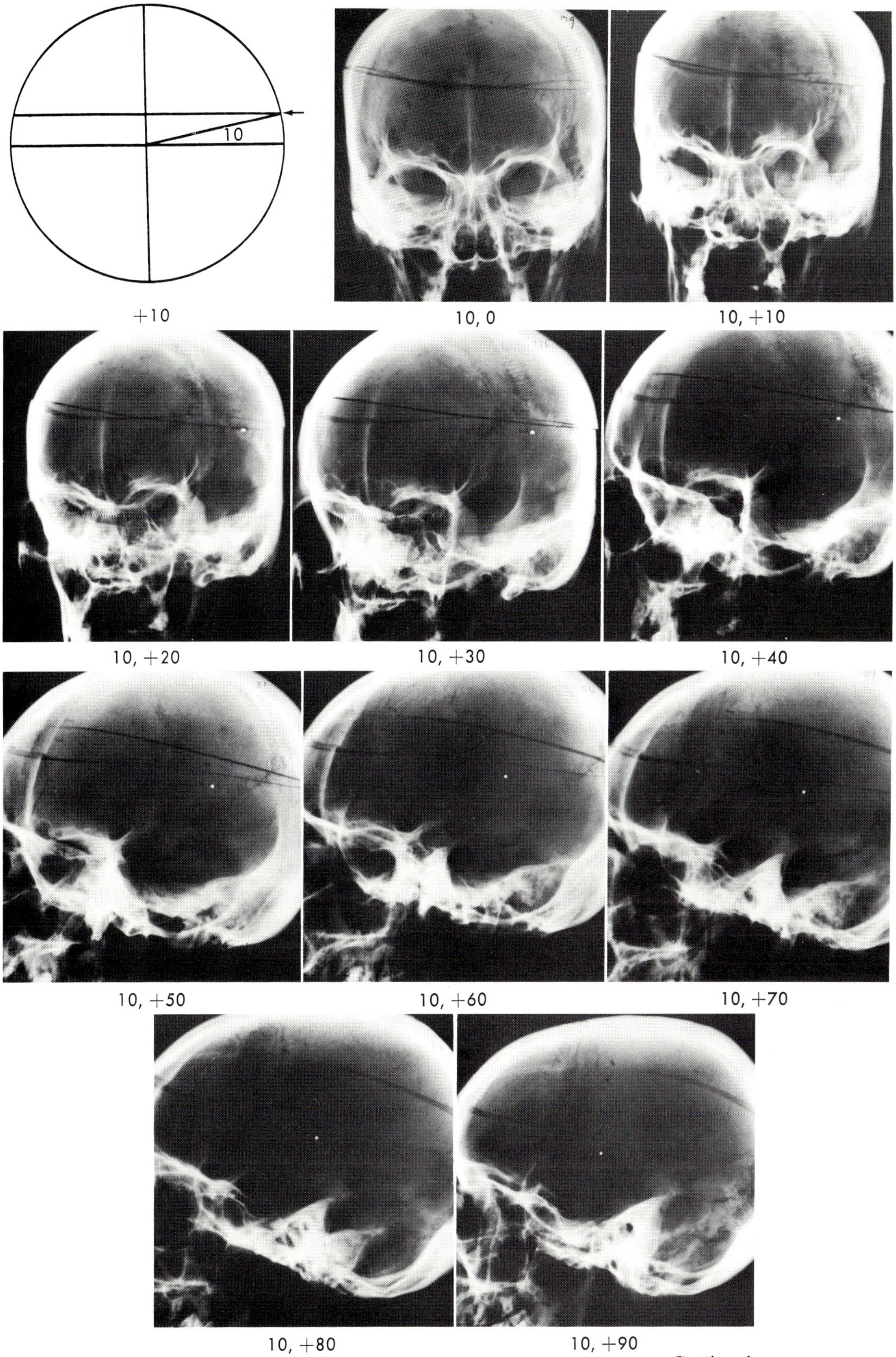

Continued.

Fig. 2-27, cont'd. For legend see opposite page.

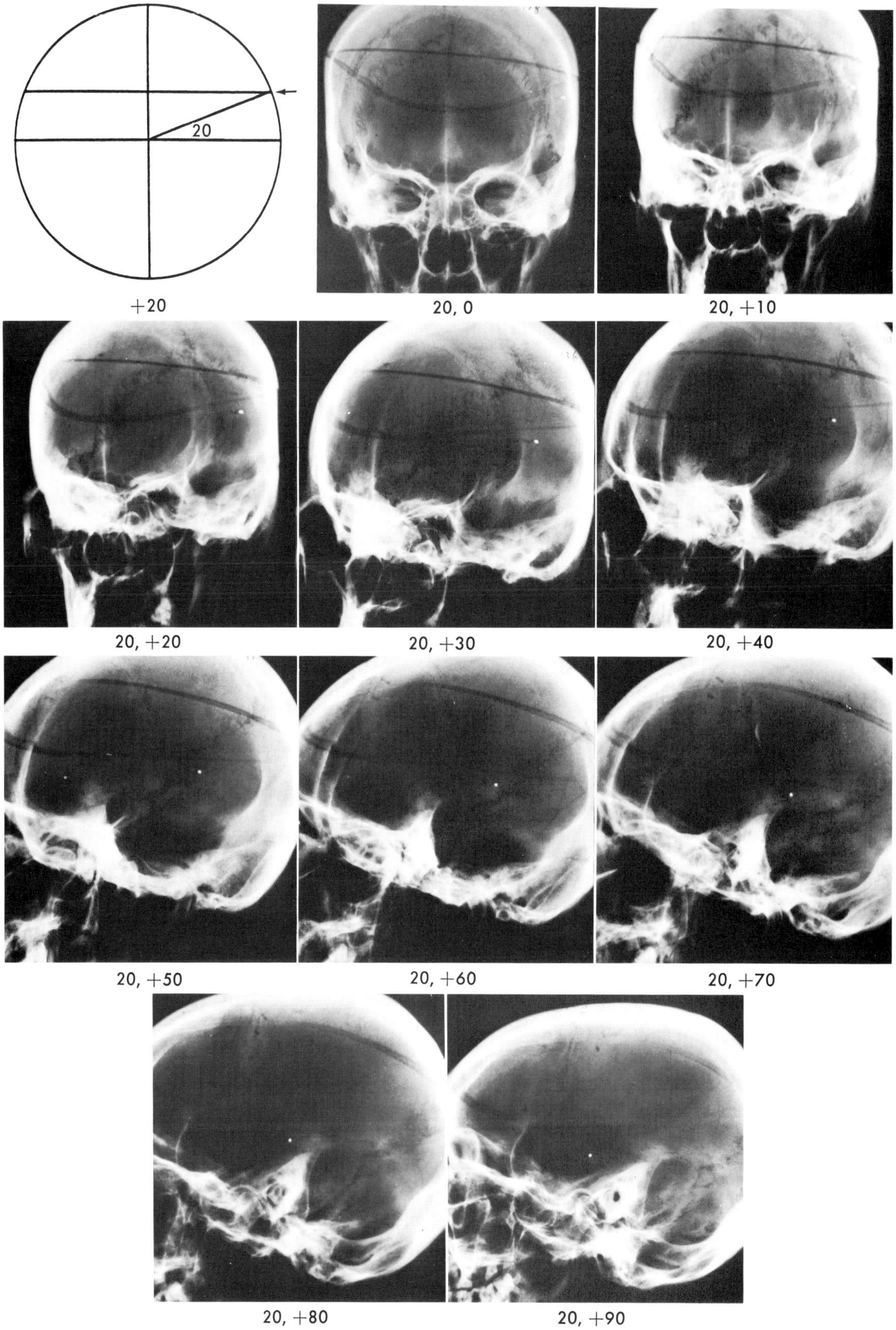

Fig. 2-27, cont'd. For legend see p. 42.

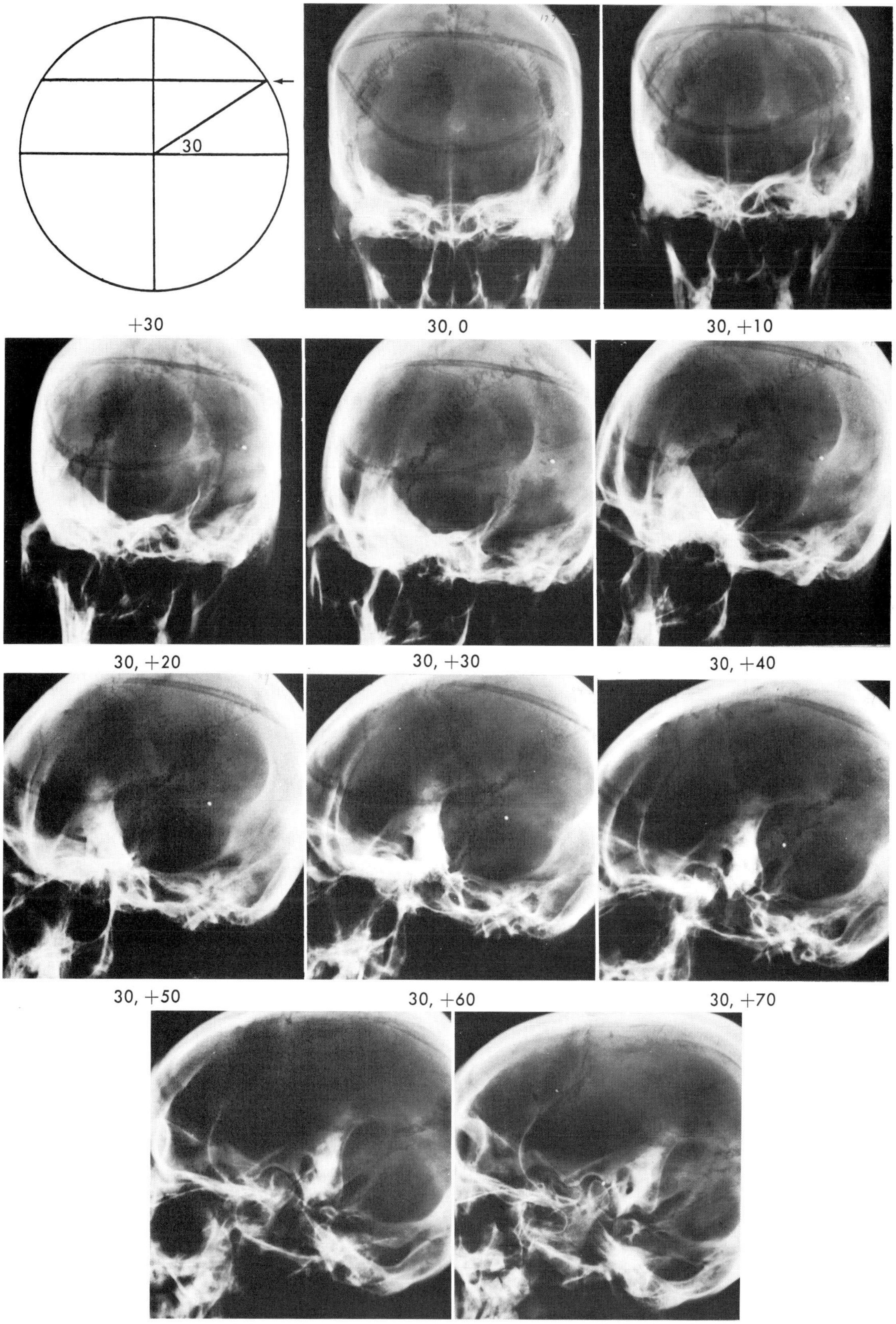

Continued.

Fig. 2-27, cont'd. For legend see p. 42.

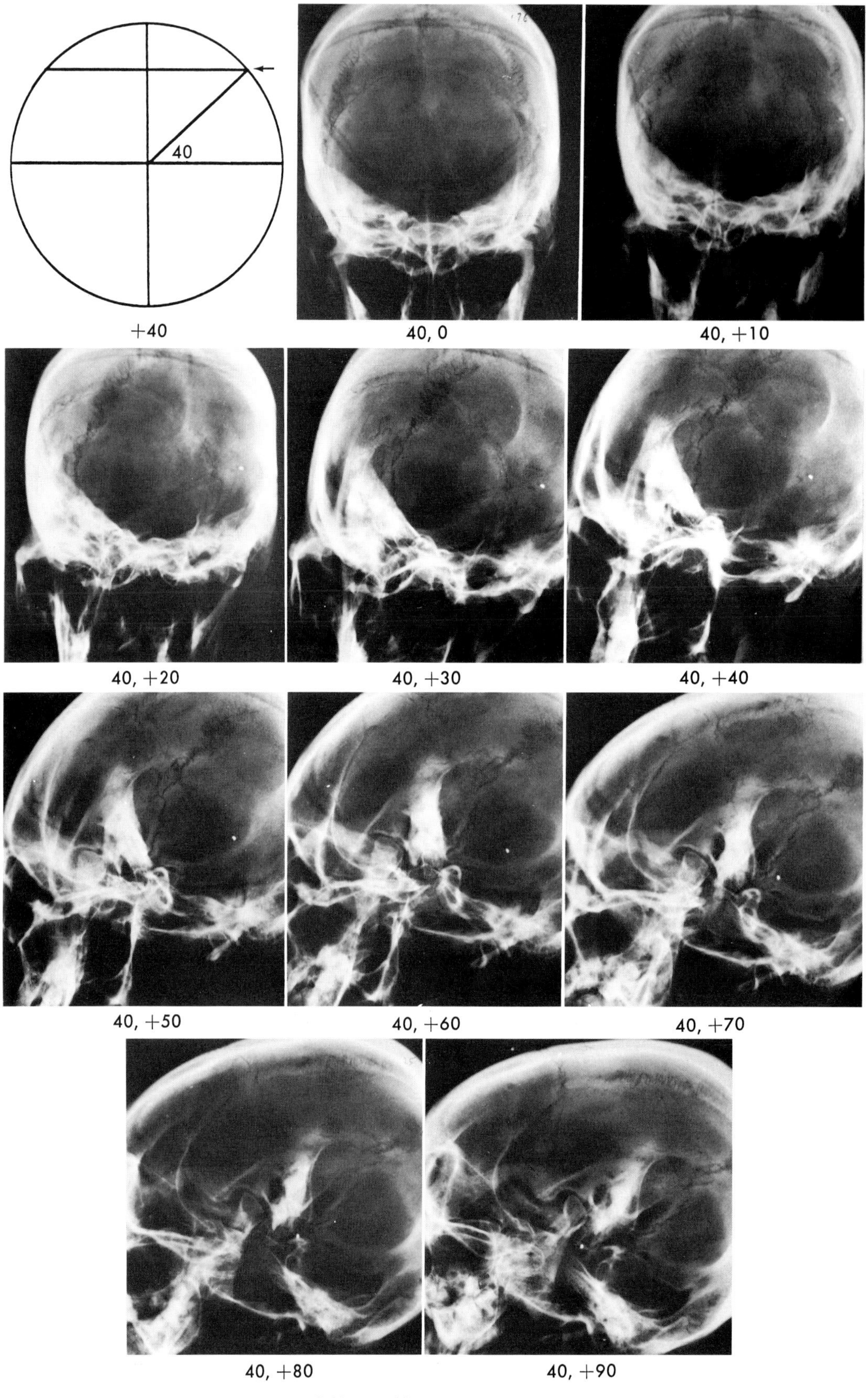

Fig. 2-27, cont'd. For legend see p. 42.

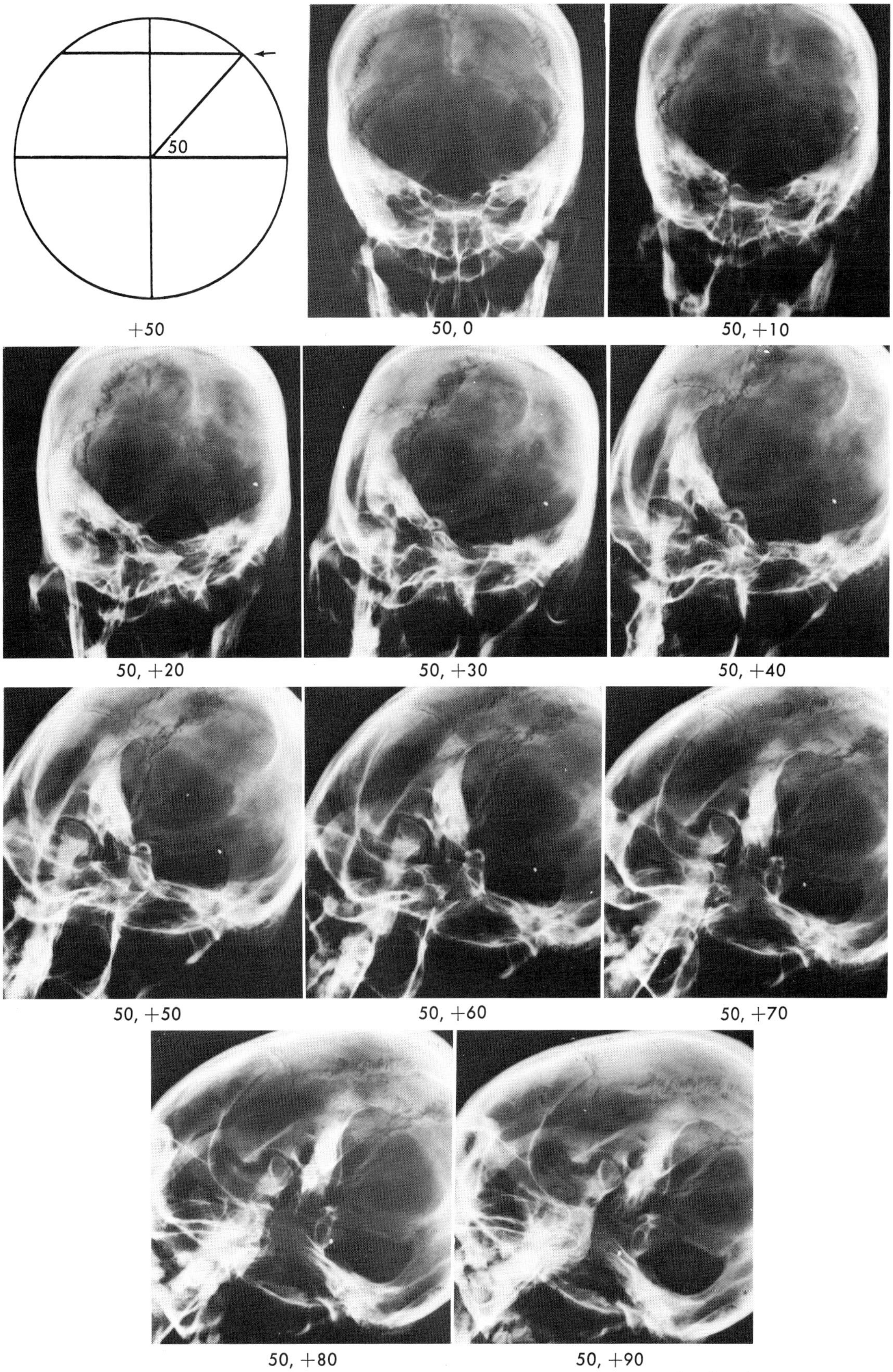

Continued.

Fig. 2-27, cont'd. For legend see p. 42.

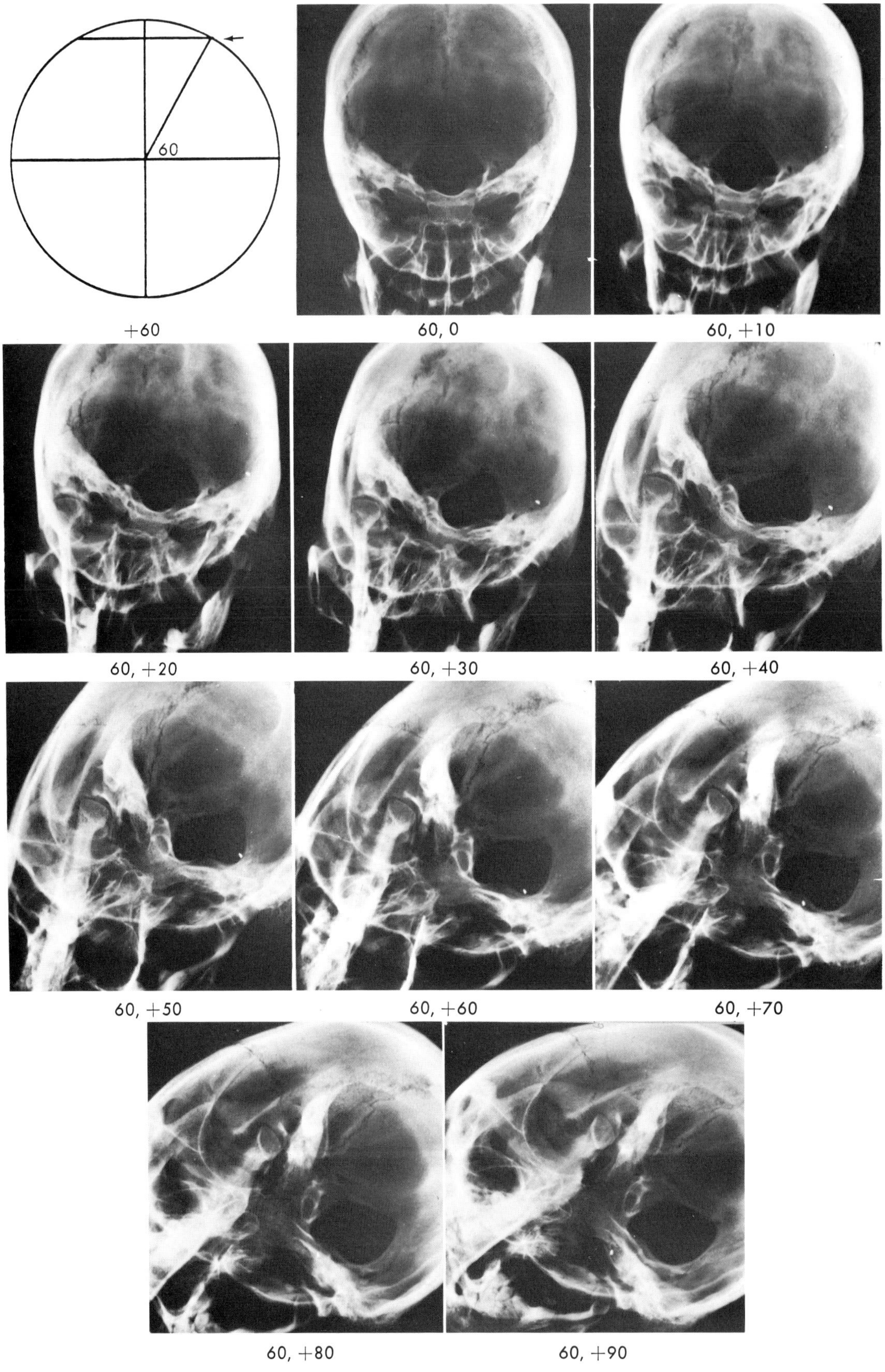

Fig. 2-27, cont'd. For legend see p. 42.

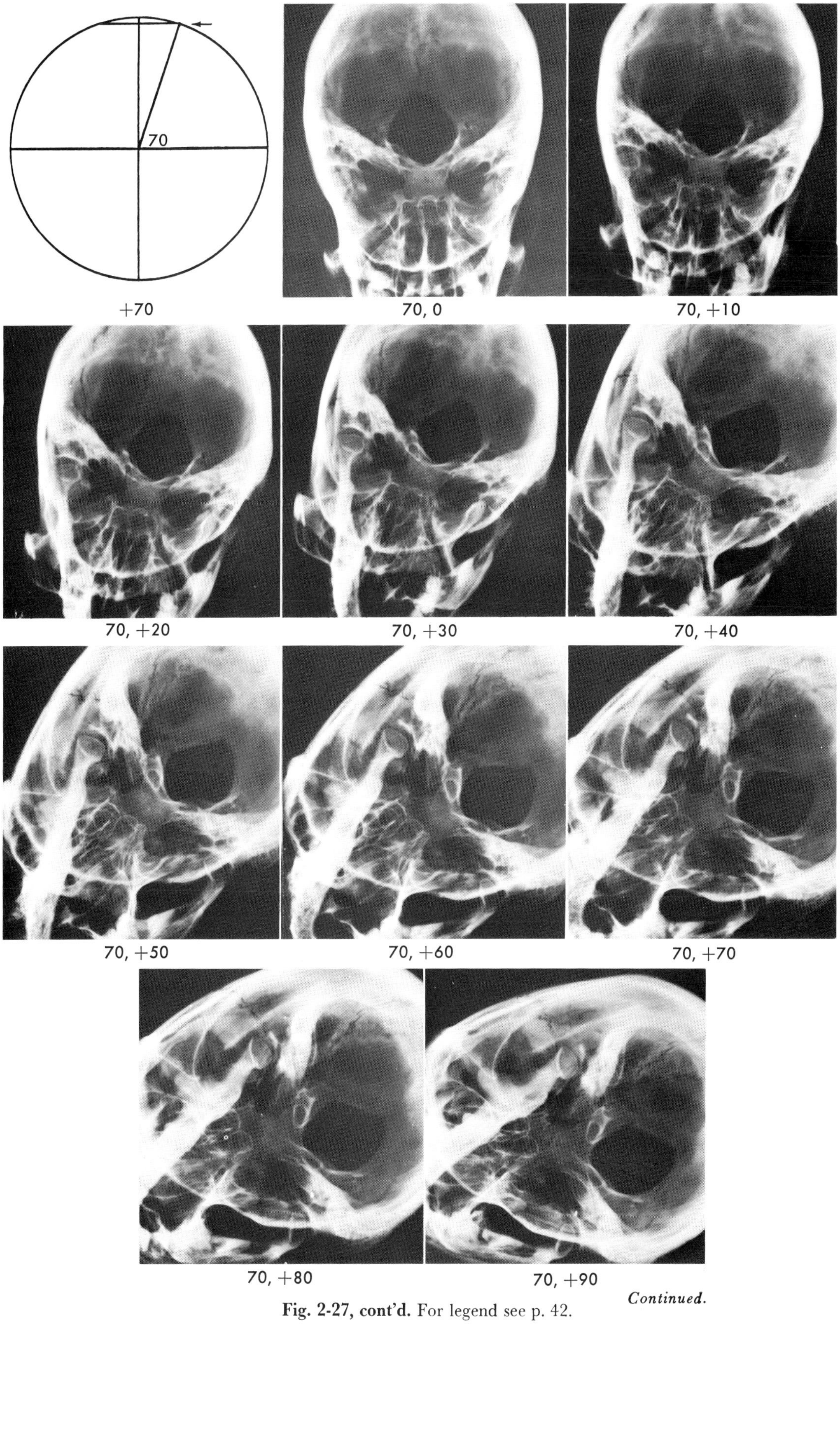

Fig. 2-27, cont'd. For legend see p. 42.

Continued.

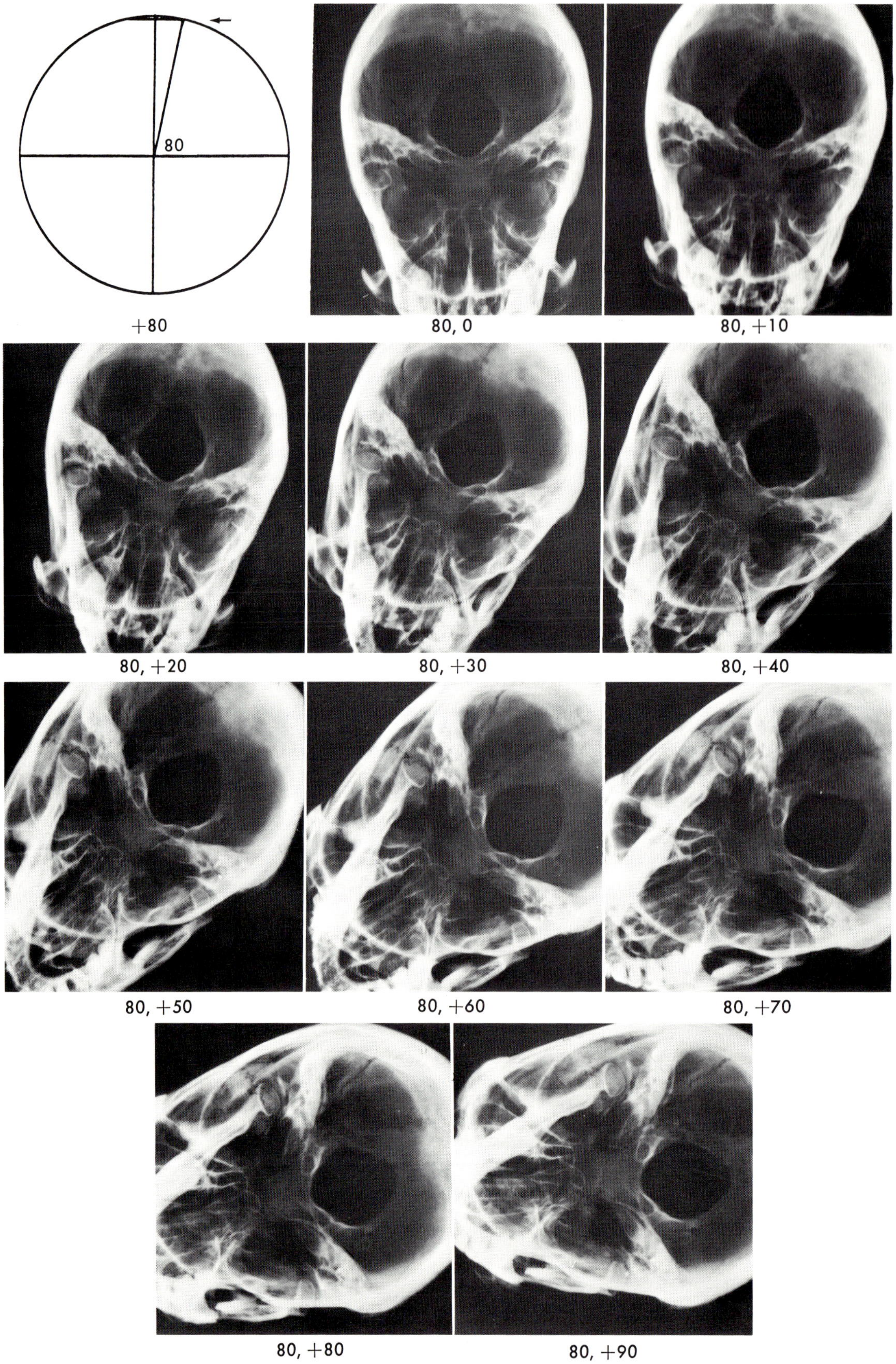

Fig. 2-27, cont'd. For legend see p. 42.

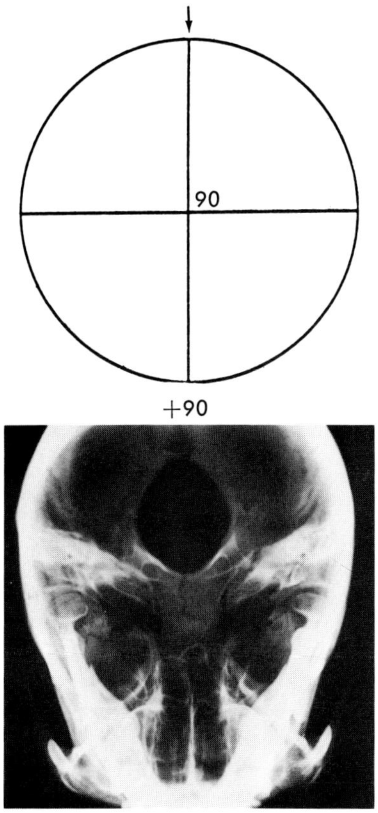

90, 0 *Continued.*

Fig. 2-27, cont'd. For legend see p. 42.

skull in this situation, a considerable degree of rectilinear distortion must be accepted, with magnification of the superior-inferior dimensions of the skull (Fig. 2-26, *B*). Alternatively this view may be taken posteroanteriorly; and placement of the film perpendicular to the central ray, without undue separation of the film from the skull, is then possible (Fig. 2-26, *C*).

FACTORS THAT MAY CONTRIBUTE TO QUALITY OF ROENTGENOGRAM OF SKULL

Tube focal spot

A small focal spot is desirable for skull roentgenography, and a satisfactory combination of sizes is 0.3 mm and 1 or 1.2 mm. The various factors that determine detail in the roentgenogram are discussed in detail in Chapter 4.

Anode-film distance

In the past a short anode-film distance (of about 24 to 28 inches) was considered an advantage. The structures on the side of the skull close to the film were said to be shown with a high degree of detail and structures away from the film would be blurred. Such a short distance may be of value to show the side of a fissure fracture of the cranial vault. In general, however, this technique has the serious disadvantage that structures near the center of the skull are also blurred to some degree.

A long anode-film distance requires that the exposure time be increased to obtain an adequate exposure. This increase in exposure, in turn, increases the possibility of blurring because of movement of the patient. When the anode-film distance is long, the skull unit must be large and massive, particularly if a spherical tube movement is employed.

In actual practice most modern units use an anode-film distance of 32 to 46 inches.

Intensifying screens

In general, screens of relatively high definition should be used for plain views of the skull. For specific views screens of the highest definition (low-speed) may be necessary.

Patient immobilization

Blurring results if the patient moves in relation to the film and tube during exposure. Movement is often the most important reason that detail is lost in roentgenograms of the skull. The skull should therefore be adequately immobilized with head clamps, headbands, or some other means during the examination.

Grid

du Boulay (1965) recommended a grid ratio of up to 8:1 or 10:1. He expressed the belief that a grid with sixty or more lines per inch interferes little with bone detail. A stationary grid may give better detail than a moving grid because of vibrations associated with the latter system. He therefore recommended a well-coned view with a stationary grid to give the finest detail in the bony cortex of the sella turcica.

STEREOSCOPIC VIEWS

Undoubtedly stereoscopic roentgenograms offer a great deal of information about the spatial relation of different structures within the skull. Different workers vary in their enthusiasm for these stereoscopic views, however. Most roentgenologists prefer to see a structure in two views with the central rays at right angles. If a structure is seen with certainty only in one view, then stereoscopy may be of considerable value. With stereoscopy faint intracranial calcification may become more readily visible. Stereoscopy is also particularly valuable for analysis of the complex structures that are seen in the base view. The relation between shift of the tube, the interpupillary distance, the focus-film distance, and the viewing distance is given by the following equation (du Boulay, 1965):

$$\frac{\text{Tube shift}}{\text{Interpupillary distance}} = \frac{\text{Focus-film distance}}{\text{Viewing distance}}$$

Text continued on p. 60.

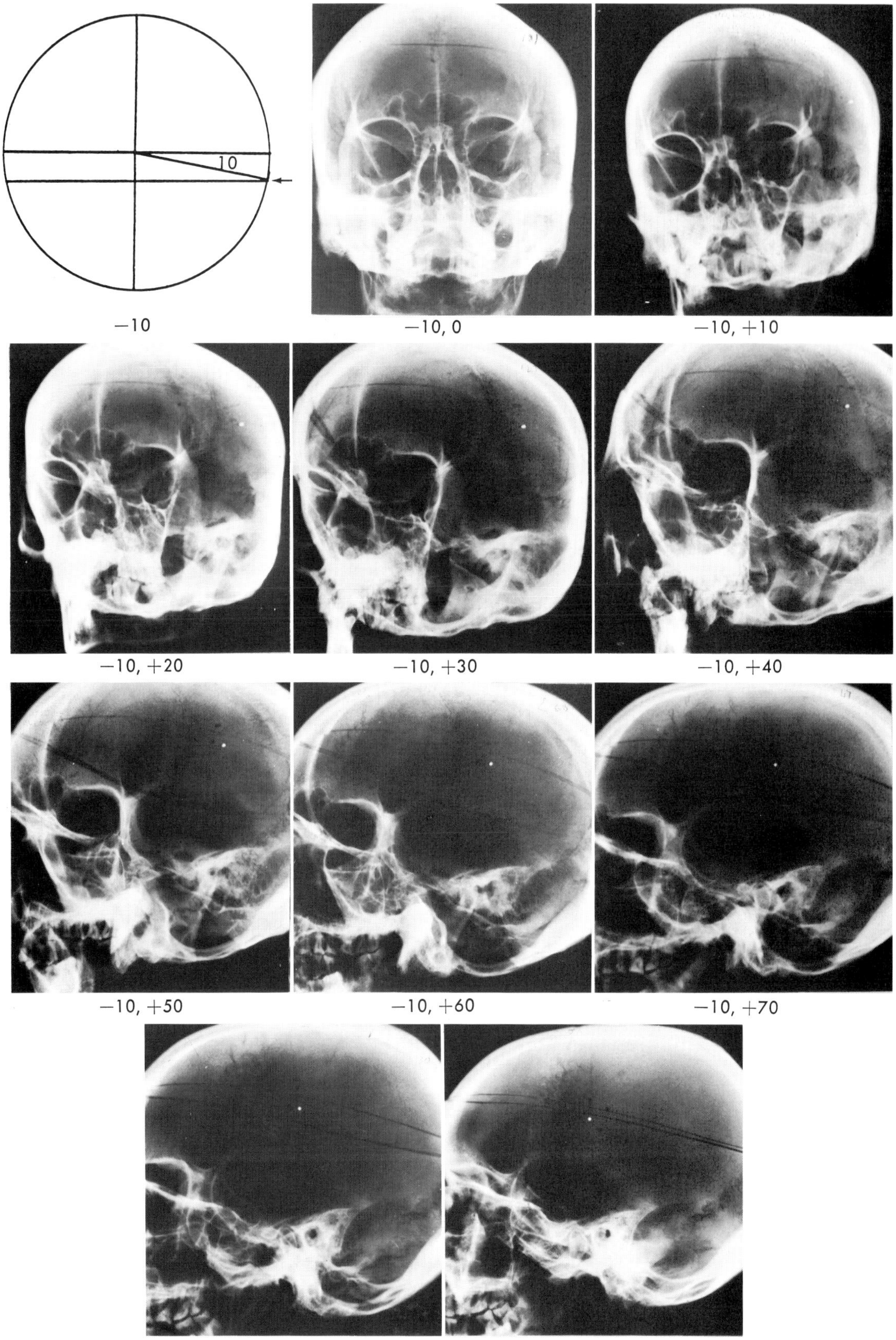

Fig. 2-27, cont'd. For legend see p. 42.

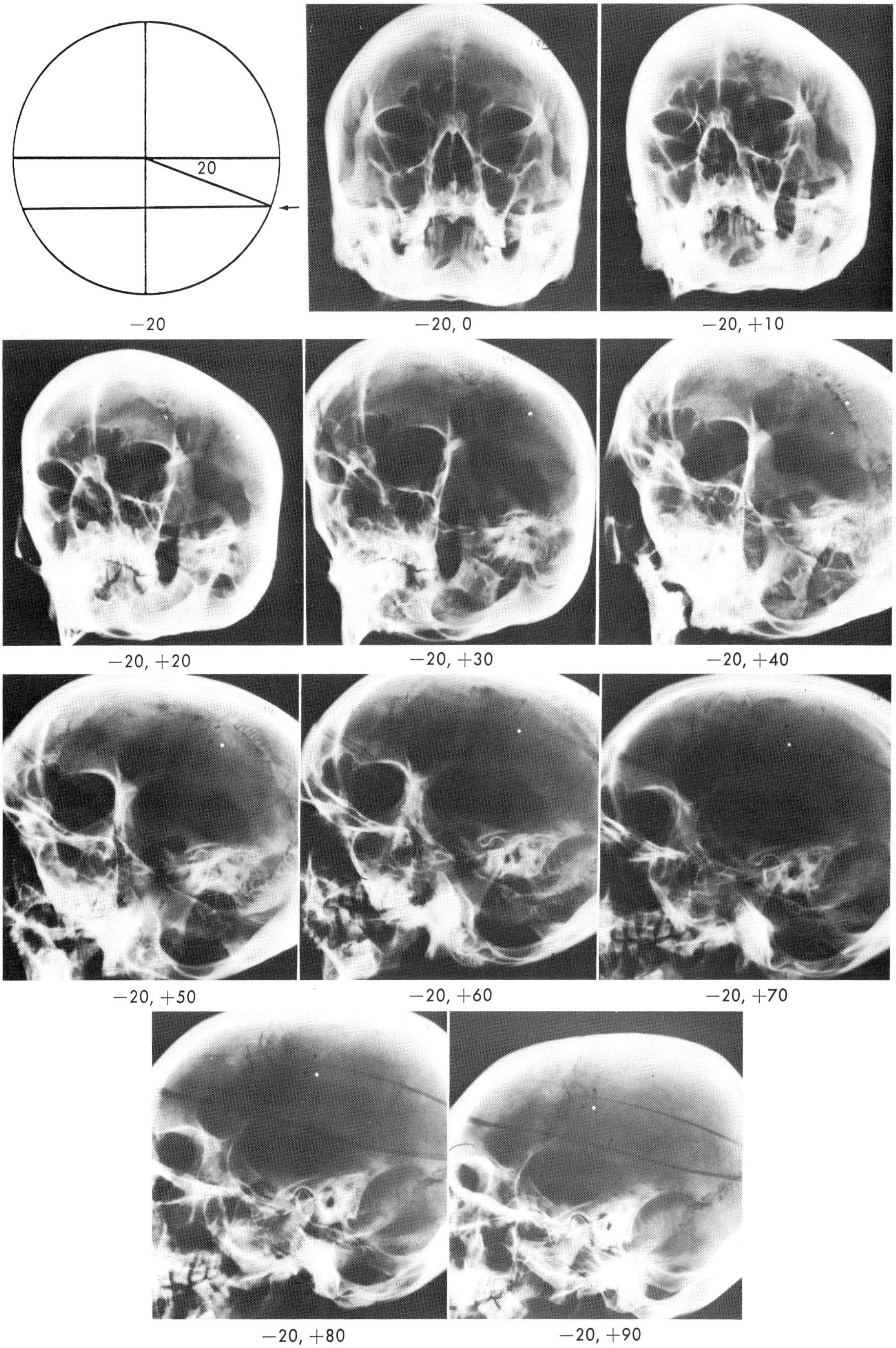

Continued.

Fig. 2-27, cont'd. For legend see p. 42.

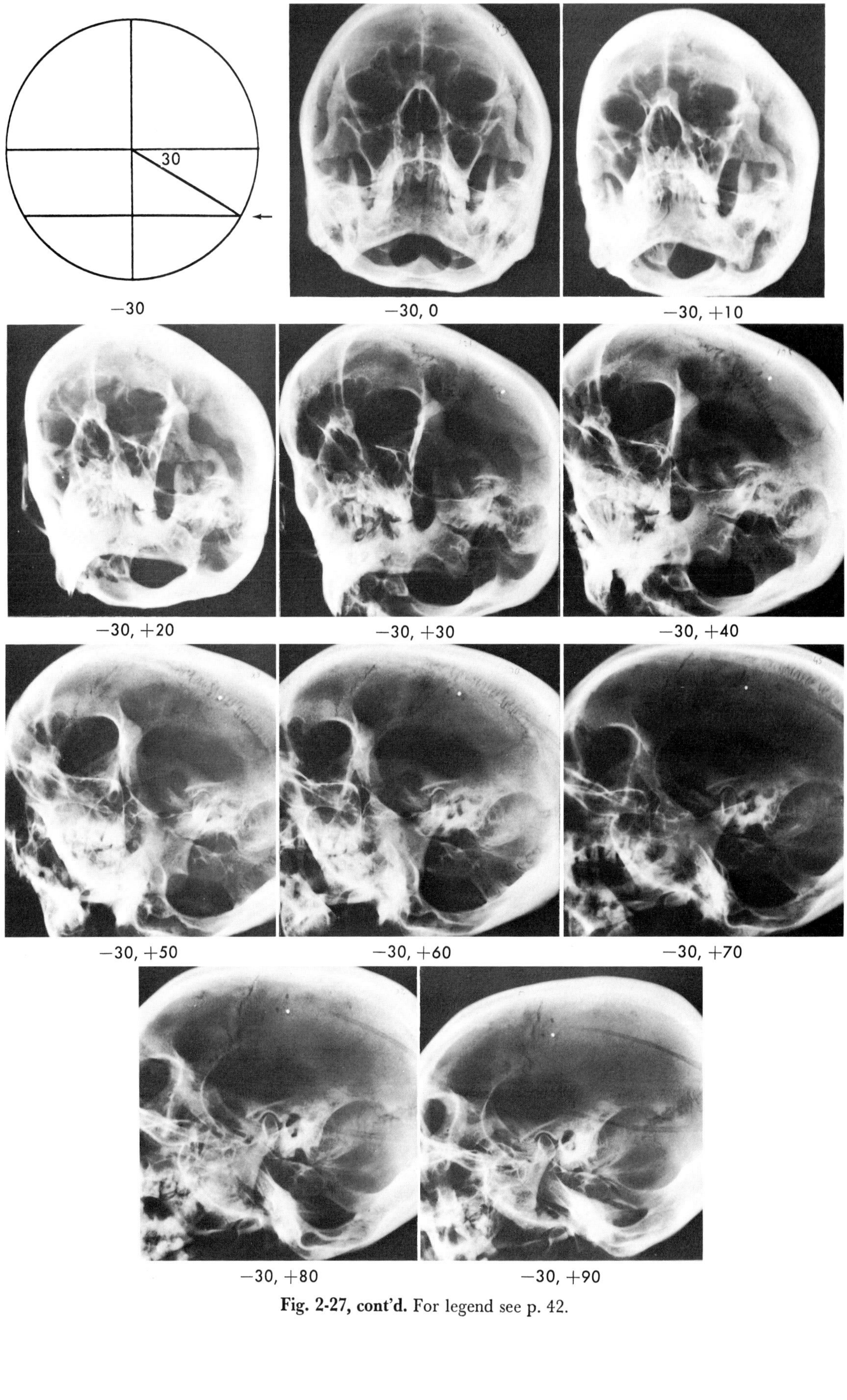

Fig. 2-27, cont'd. For legend see p. 42.

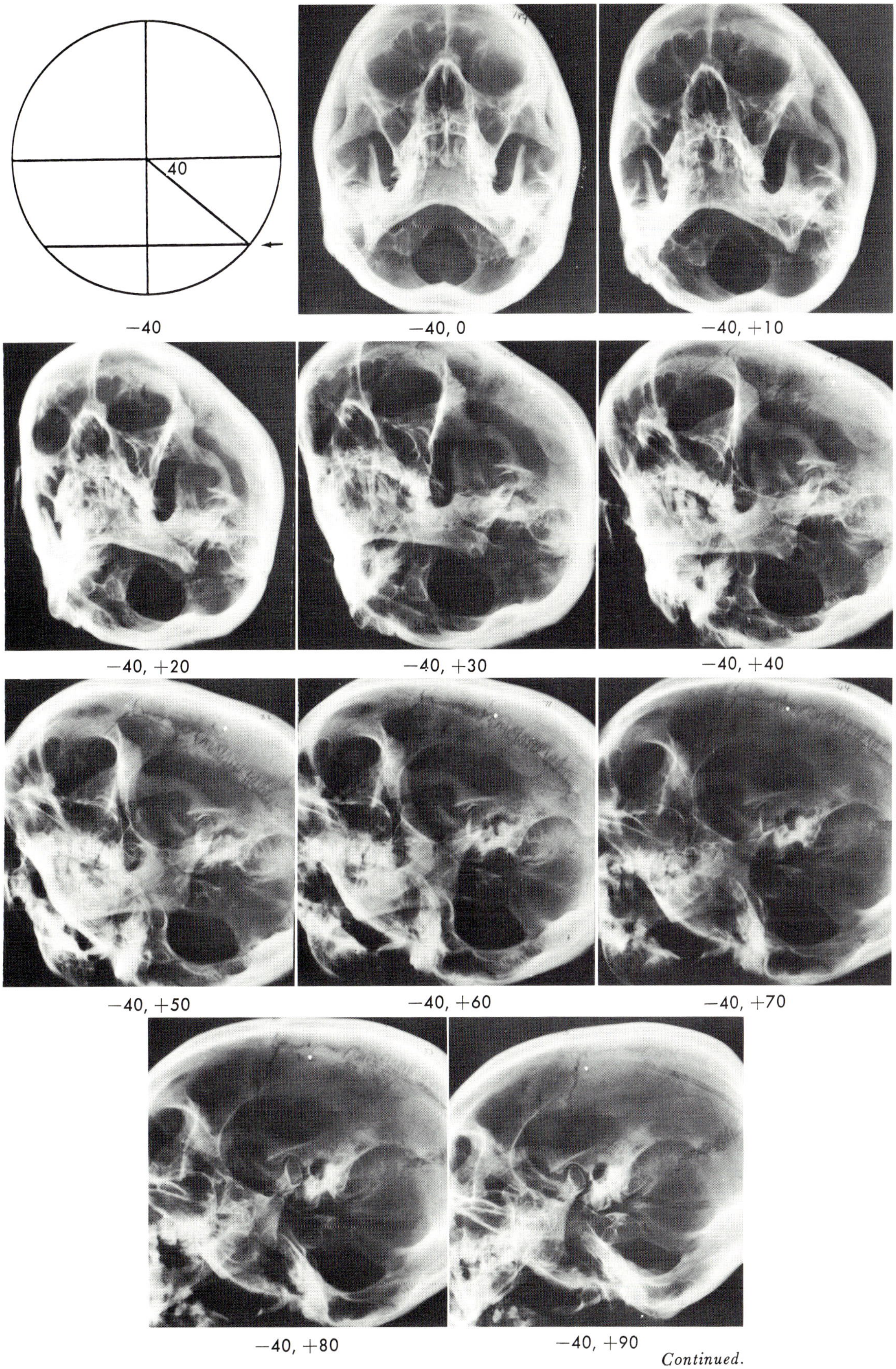

Continued.

Fig. 2-27, cont'd. For legend see p. 42.

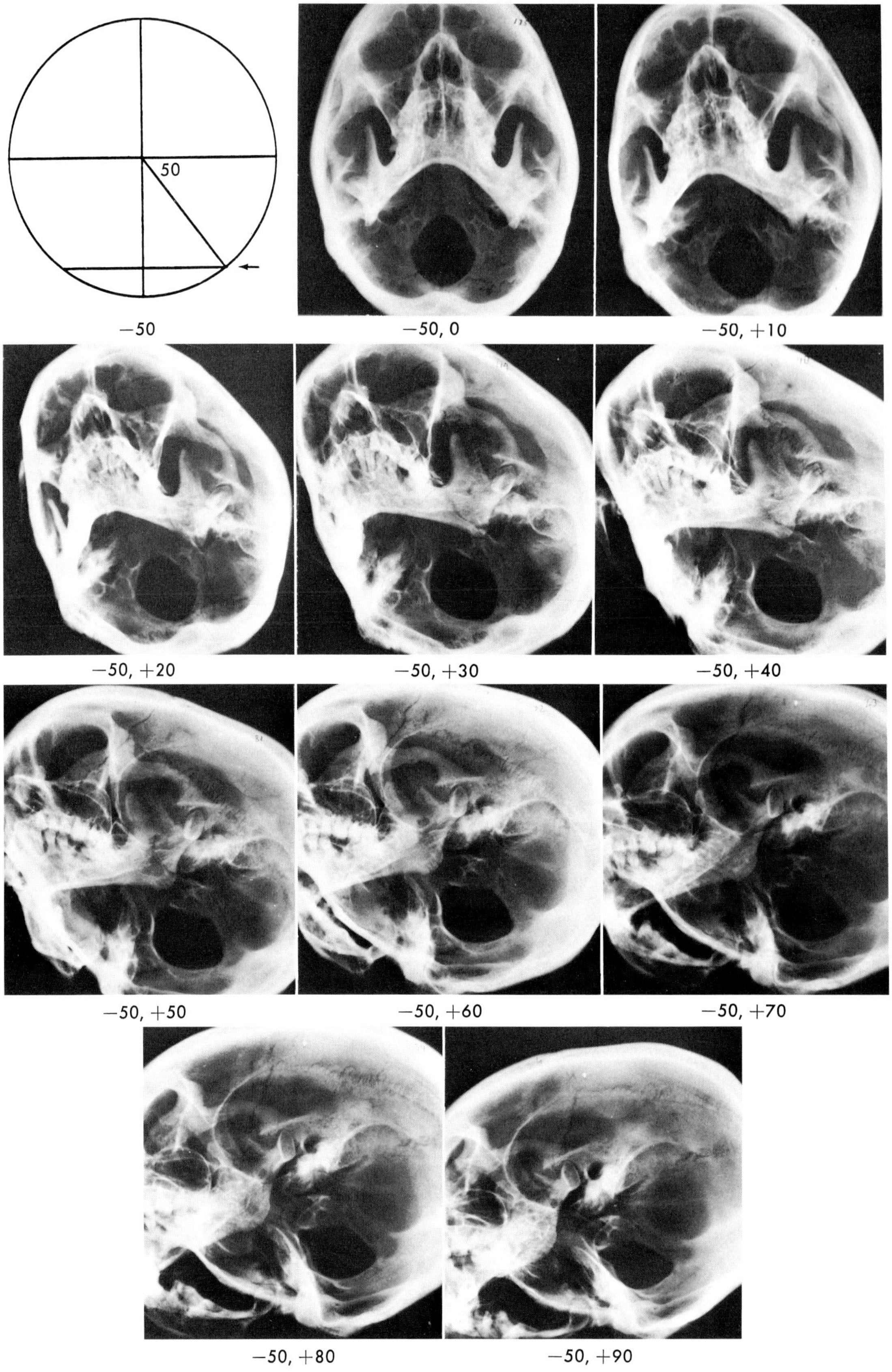

Fig. 2-27, cont'd. For legend see p. 42.

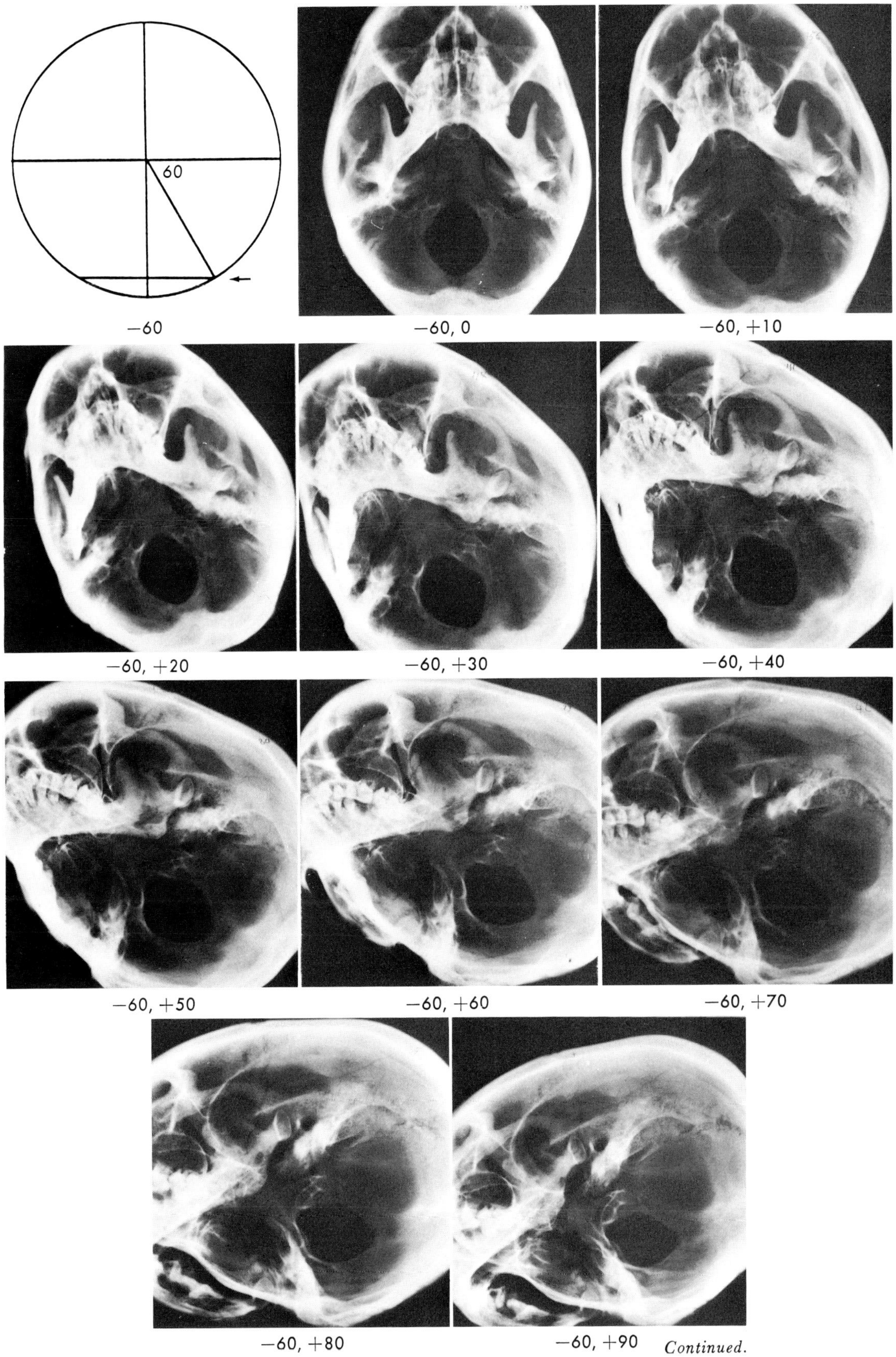

Continued.

Fig. 2-27, cont'd. For legend see p. 42.

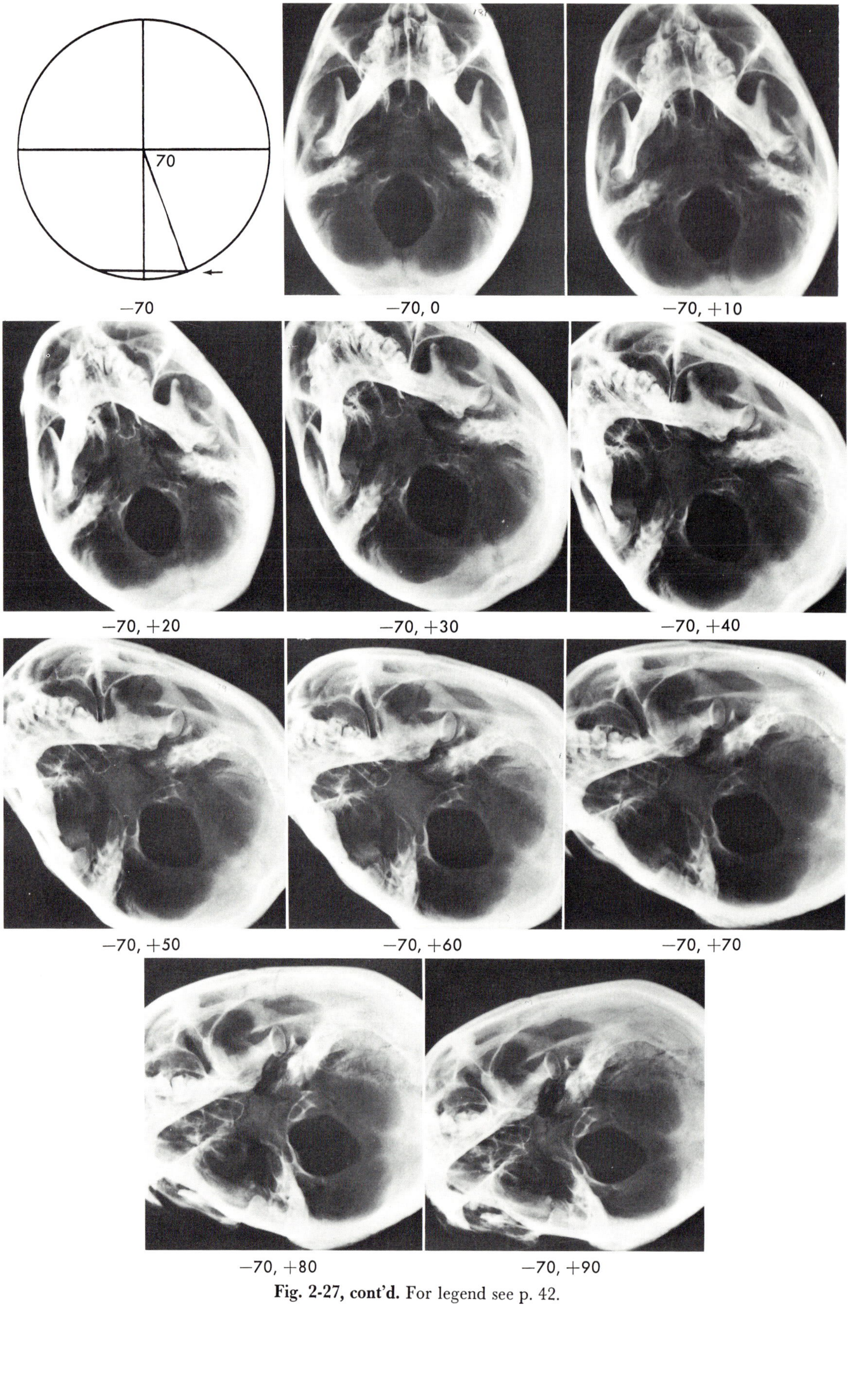

Fig. 2-27, cont'd. For legend see p. 42.

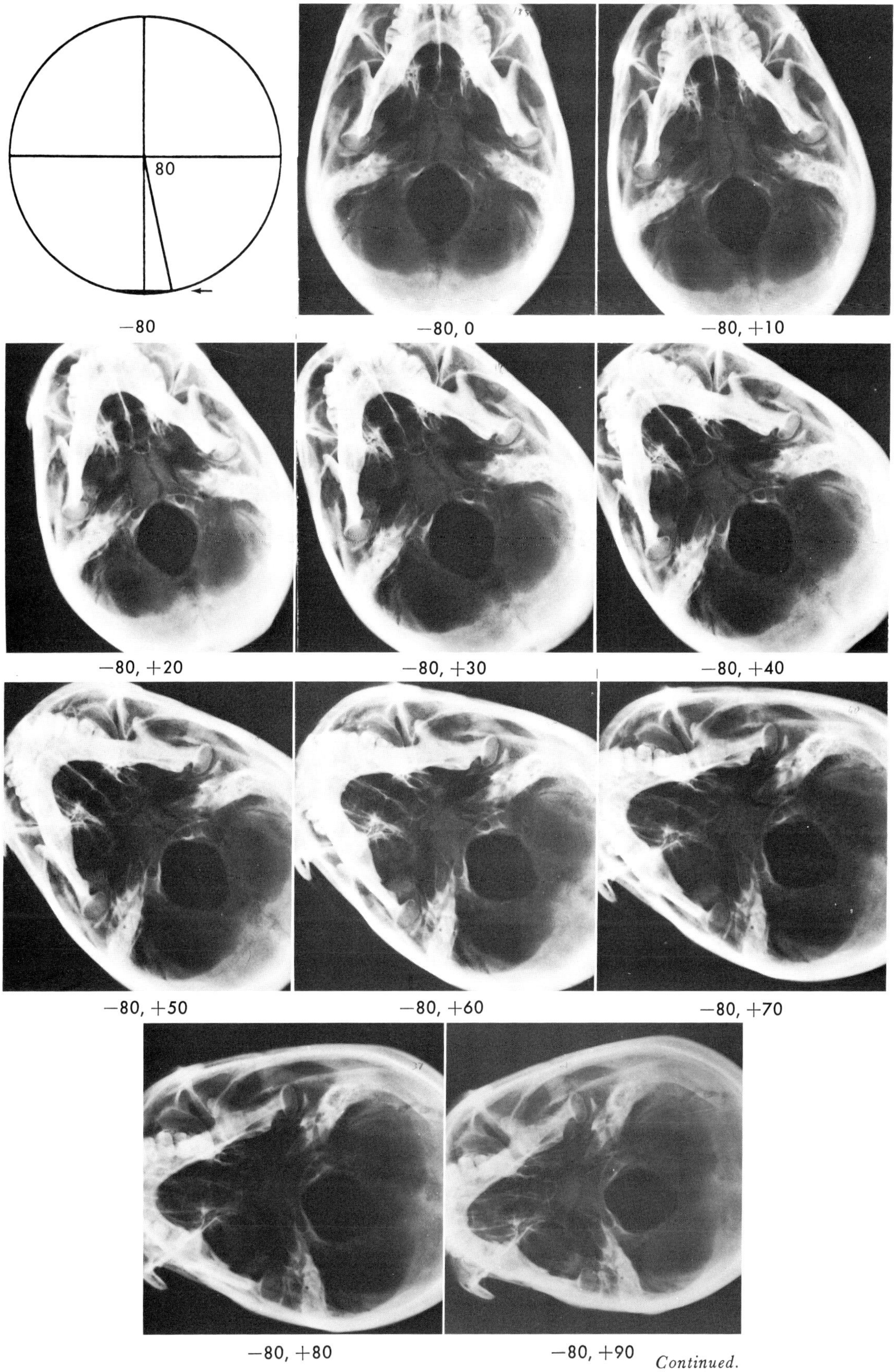

Continued.

Fig. 2-27, cont'd. For legend see p. 42.

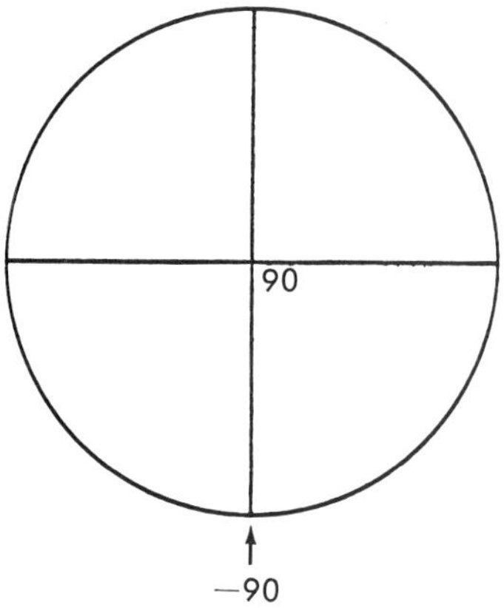

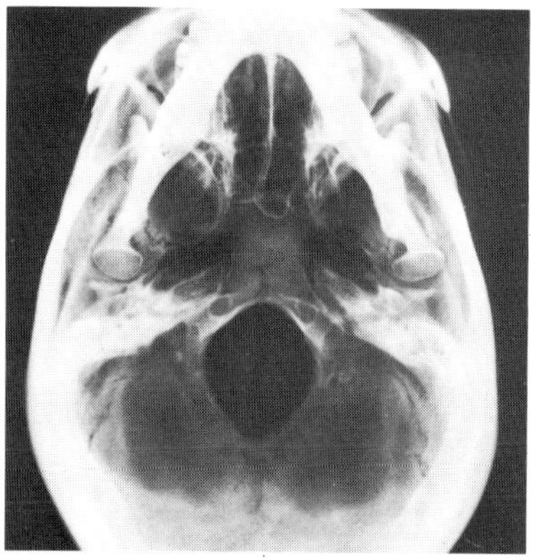

−90, 0

Fig. 2-27, cont'd. For legend see p. 42.

COMPLETE SERIES OF ROENTGENOGRAMS OF SKULL AT 10° INTERVALS

To demonstrate the application of the spherical polar coordinate system and to provide a fairly complete series of roentgenograms for reference purposes, the left side of the skull is examined with rotation of the head at 10° intervals from 0° to +90° (Fig. 2-27). If in these roentgenograms we consider that the right side of the head is the side of interest, then the angle of head rotation would be the same but in a negative direction.

REFERENCES

Arcelin, F.: L'exploration radiologique du rocher, J. Radiol. Electr. **7**:507, 1923.

Chaussé, C.: Trois incidences pour l'examen du rocher, Acta Radiol. **34**:274-287, 1950.

du Boulay, G. H.: Principles of x-ray diagnosis of the skull, London, 1965, Butterworth & Co., Ltd.

Eraso, S. T.: Roentgen and clinical diagnosis of glomus jugulare tumors, Radiology **77**:252-256, 1961.

Henschen, F.: Die Akusticus Tumoren, eine neue Gruppe radiographisch darstellbarer Hirntumoren, Fortschr. Roentgenstr. **18**:207-216, 1912.

Hickey, P. M.: The anteroposterior position for the mastoid, Amer. J. Roentgen. **1**:321, 1914.

Kemp Harper, R. A.: Glomus jugulare tumors of the temporal bone, J. Fac. Radiologists **8**:325-334, 1957.

Law, F. M.: Radiography as an aid in the diagnosis of mastoid disease, Ann. Otol. Rhinol. Laryng. **22**:635-637, 1913.

Lysholm, E.: Apparatus and technique for roentgen examination of the skull, Acta Radiol., supp. 12, pp. 67-93, 1931.

Mayer, E. G.: The technic of the roentgenologic examination of the temporal bone, Radiology **7**:306-317, 1926.

Merrill, V.: Atlas of roentgenographic positions, ed. 3, St. Louis, 1967, The C. V. Mosby Co., vol. 2.

Pfeiffer, R. L.: A new technique for roentgenography of the optic canals, Amer. J. Roentgen. **29**:410-415, 1933.

Porcher, P., Porot, J., and Rossand, L.: L'incidence transmaxillaire (incidence facile et sûre pour la mise en evidence de la pyramide pétreuse et du trou déchiré postérieur), J. Radiol. Electr. **33**:379-382, 1952.

Potts, D. G.: A system of skull radiography, Radiology **94**:25-33, 1970.

Stenvers, H. W.: Roentgenology of the os petrosum, Arch. Radiol. Electr. **22**:97-112, 1917.

Taveras, J. M., and Wood, E. H.: Diagnostic neuroradiology, Baltimore, 1964, The Williams & Wilkins Co.

Valdini, L.: La sella turcica in proiezione occipito-frontale, Radiol. Med. **15**:881-886, 1928.

Waters, C. A.: A modification of the occipitofrontal position in the roentgen examination of the accessory nasal sinuses, Arch. Radiol. Radiother. **20**:15-17, 1915.

World Federation of Neurology, Problem Commission of Neuroradiology: Study meeting on projections and nomenclature, Milan, 1961, Brit. J. Radiol. **35**:501-503, 1962.

CHAPTER 3

Equipment for skull radiography

D. Gordon Potts

SKULL RADIOGRAPHIC DEVICES

Several devices have been specifically designed for skull roentgenography. In general they may be divided into two groups: those with a circular tube movement and those in which the tube may be moved on the surface of a sphere. Some of the devices in common use will be described.

Circular tube movement

*Franklin head unit**

The Franklin head unit (Fig. 3-1) is typical of those in which the tube moves around a circle. The film holder Bucky tray is at the center of the circle around which the tube rotates.

This unit may be modified to perform linear tomography. When it is used for pneumoencephalography, a second tube is normally required for lateral projections.

Concentric†

In the Concentric unit (Fig. 3-2) the tube for frontal views moves around a circle with the cassette holder and image amplifier on the same arm so that they also move around a circle with the same fulcrum. The patient is mounted on a somersaulting chair, and the center of his head is at the center of rotation of the frontal tube. The lateral tube is fixed in position so that it is always centered on the head (Potts, 1965).

The patient may be inverted through a complete somersault with the center of the head at a fixed point in space; or he may be rotated around his long axis without loss of centering. Linear tomography may be performed with the frontal tube, and the chair may be rotated for autotomography.

*Liebel-Flarsheim, Cincinnati, Ohio.

†Picker Medical Products Division, Cleveland, Ohio.

Spherical tube movement

*Diagnost N**

The Diagnost N unit (Fig. 3-3) consists of a massive vertical support on which a second massive arm moves up and down. This arm has tracks on its lower aspect and on the side away from the vertical support. The tracks allow the pivot that carries the tube arm to move around part of a circle (about 120°) centered on the skull. The tube arm also carries a cassette holder and an image amplifier; these are centered on the skull when the tube arm rotates.

The unit may be used with a somersaulting chair or a standard convertible chair-table, and it will perform linear tomography.

*Schonander CRT-4**

The Schonander CRT-4 unit (Figs. 1-5, *C*, and 3-4) has a tube that is supported on two parallel semicircular arches. These arches permit the tube to move around part of the surface of a sphere. The film is at the center of the sphere, and the anode-film distance is usually about 72 cm. The tube and film may be angled together or independently. This unit will not perform tomography. It has been used widely for skull roentgenography, pneumoencephalography, and angiography. During angiography it is used with a manual film changer.

*N. V. Philips, Eindhoven, Netherlands.

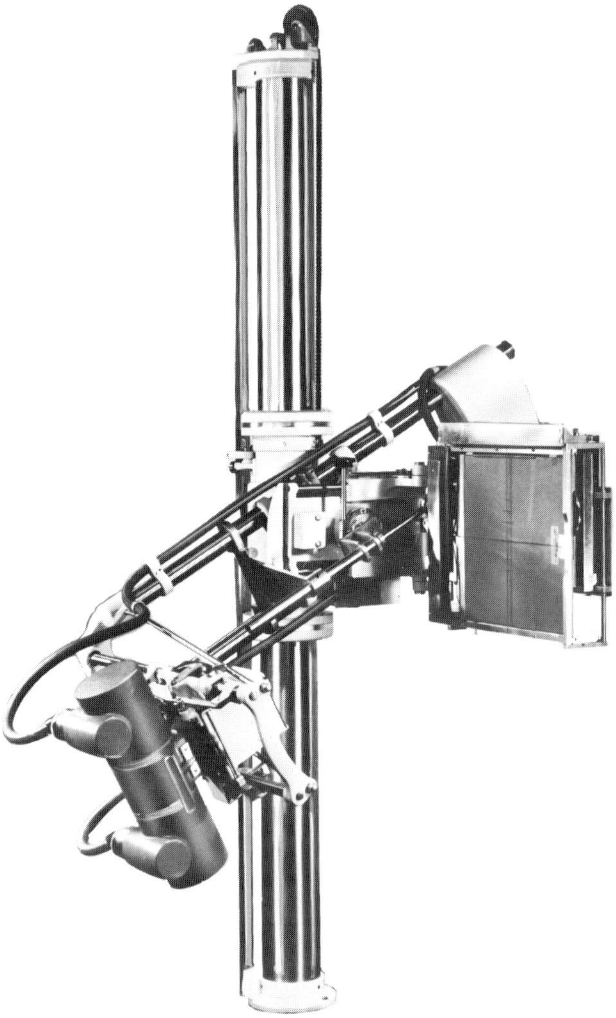

Fig. 3-1. Franklin head unit.

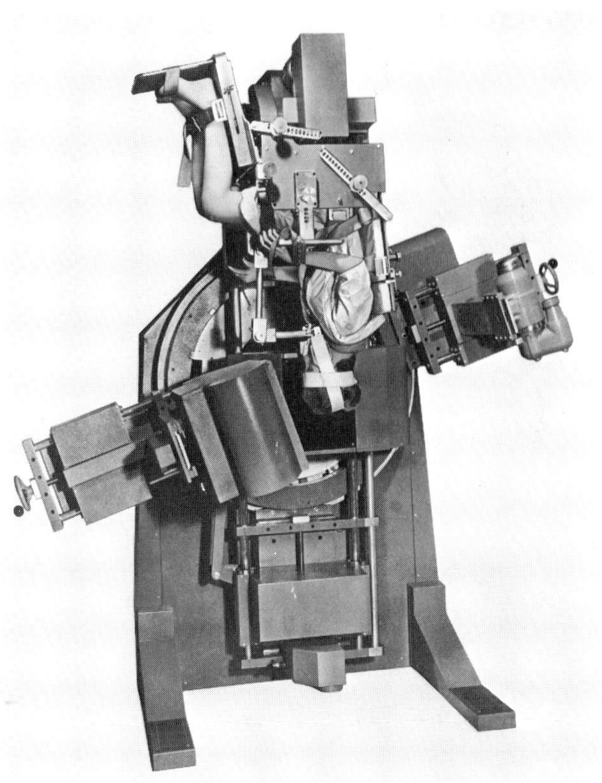

Fig. 3-2. Concentric unit shown with biplane film changers.

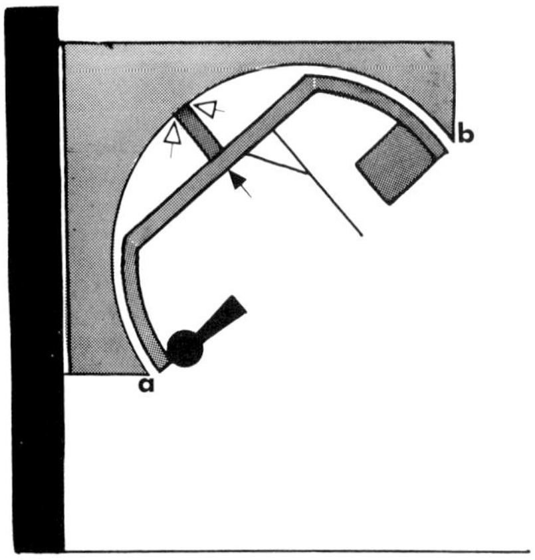

Fig. 3-3. Diagnost N diagram. Solid arrow indicates axis of rotation. Assembly (open arrows) carrying tube, film tray, and image amplifier moves around curved track from *a* to *b*.

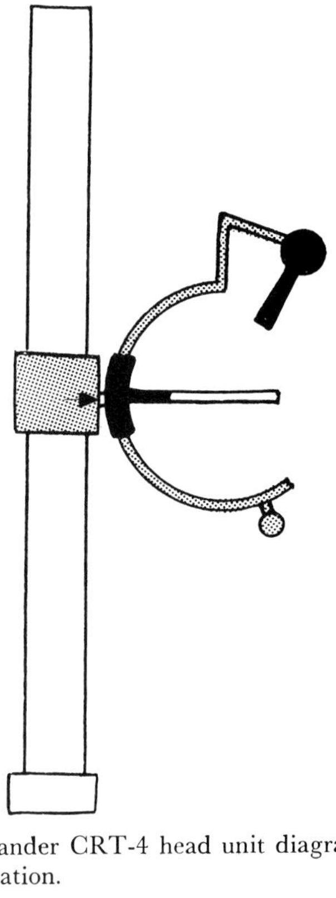

Fig. 3-4. Schonander CRT-4 head unit diagram. Arrow indicates axis of rotation.

Fig. 3-5. Princeps head unit. **A**, Diagram of basic movements. Arrows indicate axes of rotation. **B**, Unit with somersaulting chair. **C**, Unit used for axial projection.

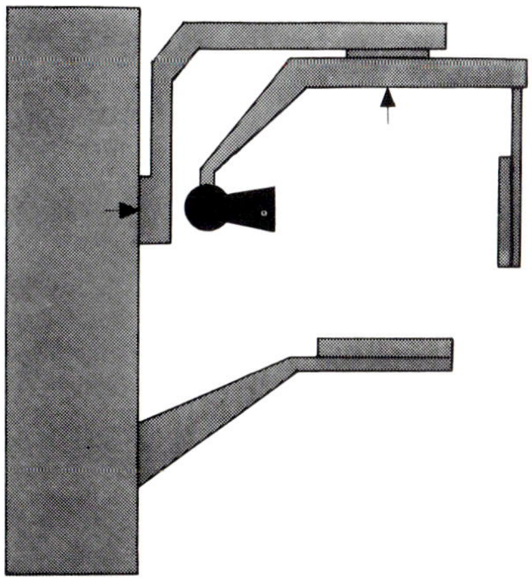

A

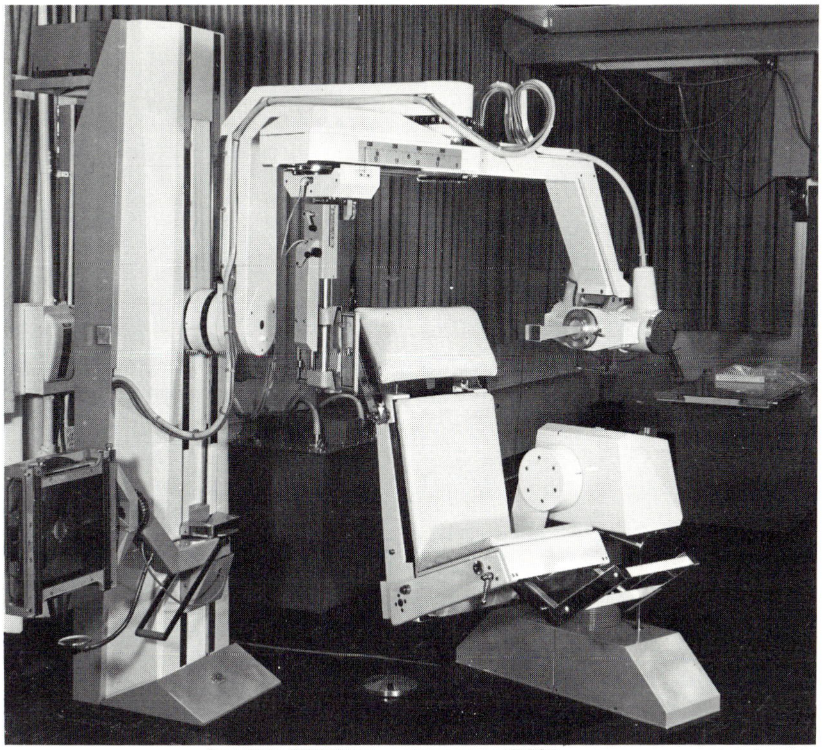

B

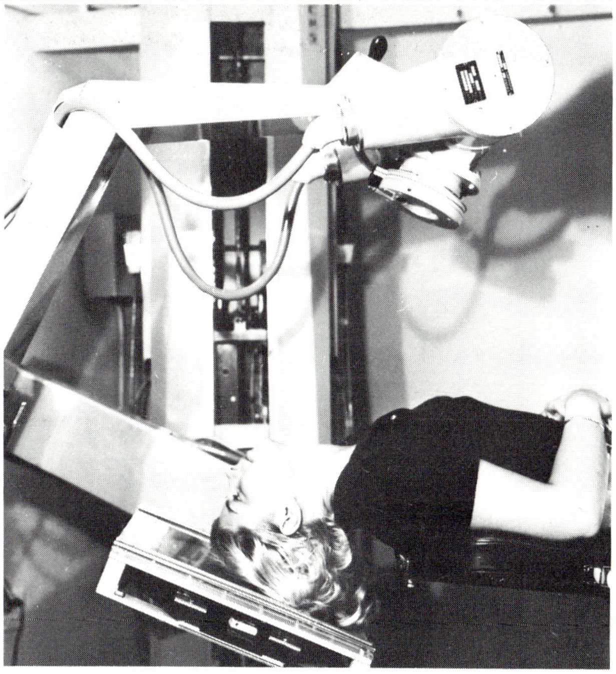

C

*Schonander CRT-7**

The Schonander CRT-7 unit is similar in construction to the Schonander CRT-4 except that its floor column is much more massive. The semicircular arches that support the tube are also heavier and stronger. It will perform linear longitudinal tomography, by tilting the arches, or linear transverse tomography, by sliding the arches through their support. The angle of each of these motions is ±7.5° and that of exposure ±7.0°. By combining these two motions, circular tomography is possible. When used with the standard Bucky tray, the anode-film distance is 31½ inches. This tray is retracted during tomography. The unit has been suggested for all skull examinations, including pneumoencephalography and angiography (with a manual film changer).

Princeps†

In the Princeps unit (Fig. 3-5) the tube also carries a simple cassette holder. The holder may be used at the axis of rotation or beyond this axis (i.e., farther from the tube). The tube arm is supported by a pivot attached to a second arm that moves up or down a support column or pivots around a horizontal axis. By means of the motion of the two arms and pivots, the tube may be moved around the surface of a sphere. The unit may be used in conjunction with a somersaulting chair, and it will perform linear tomography. A Bucky tray is also provided with this unit and may be swung into position on a horizontal arm that extends from the support column.

*Elema-Schonander, Solna 1, Sweden.

†Compagnie Générale de Radiologie, Paris, France.

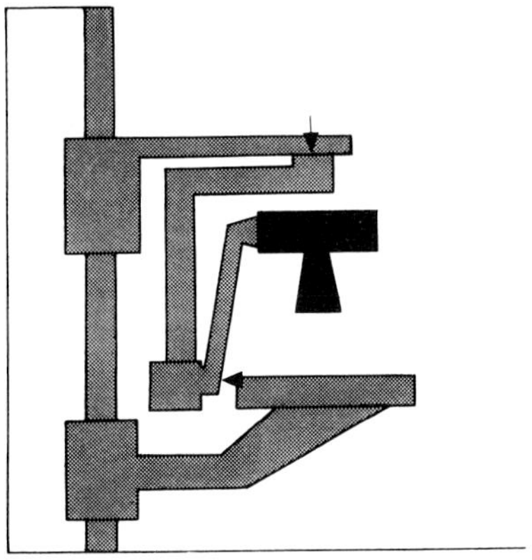

Fig. 3-6. Mimer I diagram. Arrows indicate axes of rotation.

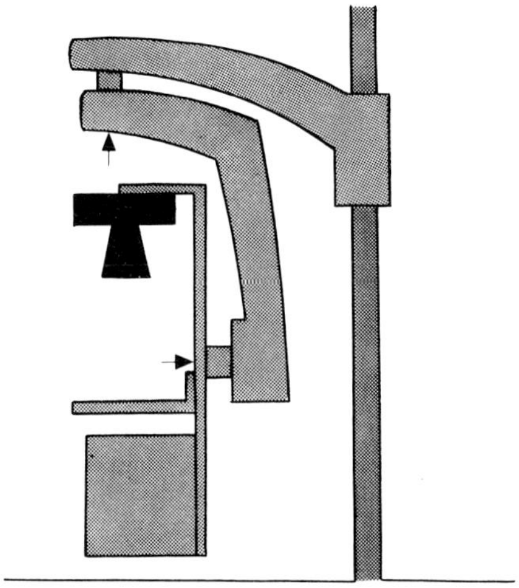

Fig. 3-7. Mimer II diagram. Arrows indicate axes of rotation.

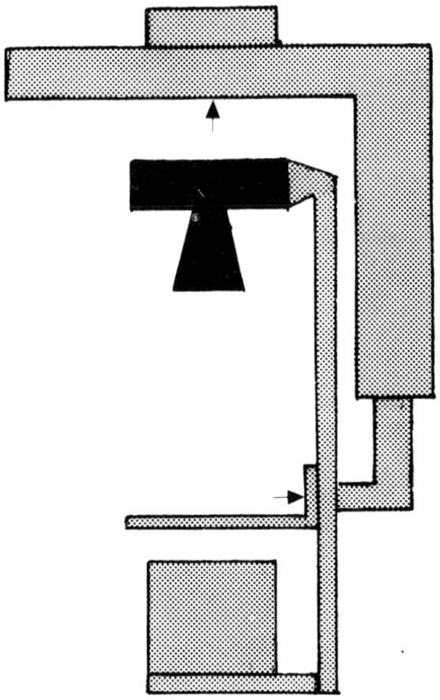

Fig. 3-8. Mimer III diagram. Arrows indicate axes of rotation.

*Mimer I**

The Mimer I unit (Fredzell and Lindgren, 1960) (Figs. 1-6, *A,* and 3-6) consists of a tube arm that carries the roentgen tube and pivots around a horizontal axis. The tube arm, in turn, is supported by a vertical arm that pivots around a vertical axis. This vertical arm is supported at the free end of a cantilever that travels up and down a vertical column mounted on the floor. The upper end of the column is attached to the wall. Another arm mounted on the lower part of the vertical column supports the object table. This arm may be swung away to obtain free floor space beneath the roentgen tube. Here a film changer, stretcher, or mobile examination couch may be placed if necessary.

The radius of the sphere around which the tube moves is 80 to 90 cm. A fluoroscopic screen with cassette holder can be attached to the tube arm. The whole tube-screen assembly may be turned around the patient so that fluoroscopy and roentgenography can be performed from any desired direction. The center of the sphere is normally at the same level as the center of the object table. Tomography may be performed by substitution of tomographic equipment for the object table.

*Mimer II**

The Mimer II unit (Figs. 1-6, *B,* and 3-7) consists of a U arm (the tube arm) that carries the roentgen tube at one end and the cassette holder at the other. The arm rotates about a horizontal axis and is supported by a vertical arm that rotates about a vertical axis. The central ray can therefore be directed from any point on the surface of a sphere to the center of the sphere. The center corresponds with the intersection of the two axes. The radius of the sphere is 80 cm. The focus-film distance can be varied from 80 to 110 cm, according to the position of the cassette holder along the tube arm. An image intensifier may be attached to the tube arm. The unit performs linear tomography with magnification of 40%.

A somersaulting chair (RCT-2) may be used with this unit and may be converted into a flat tabletop. During a somersault the center of the patient's head does not remain at a fixed point in space.

The entire unit is suspended in a heavy cantilever, which travels up and down a vertical column attached to the floor and wall.

*Mimer III**

The Mimer III unit (Fredzell et al., 1968) (Figs. 1-6, *C,* and 3-8) is similar to the Mimer II except that it is supported from the ceiling.

---

*Elema-Schonander, Solna 1, Sweden.

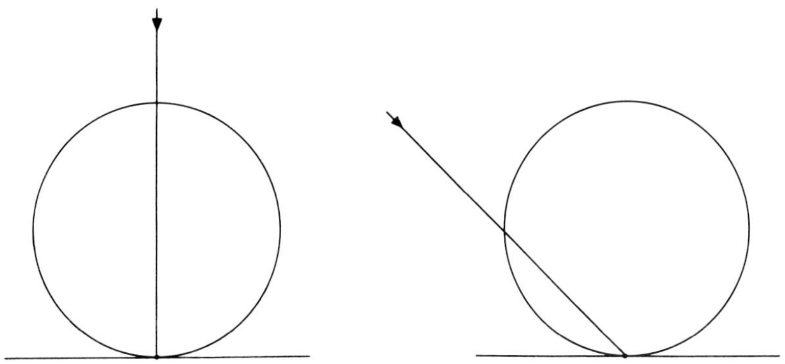

Fig. 3-9. Diagram to show effect of changes of tube angulation when fulcrum of tube rotation passes through center of film. In diagram on left, central ray is perpendicular to film and passes through center of skull. In diagram on right, central ray no longer passes through center of skull.

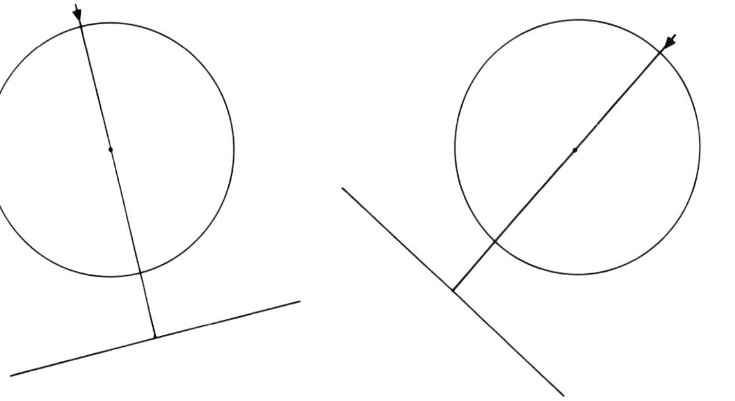

Fig. 3-10. Diagram to show fulcrum of rotation of tube and film passing through center of skull. Correct centering is achieved even when tube angulation is altered.

COMPARISON OF SKULL RADIOGRAPHIC DEVICES

In most of the earlier devices the tube rotated around a point close to the center of the film. This type of rotation was employed in the Schonander CRT-4 and CRT-7, Franklin, and Mimer I units when they were operated in the usual manner. Because the fulcrum of tube rotation did not pass through the center of the patient's head, the patient had to be recentered when the tube angulation was altered (Fig. 3-9). Many of the newer devices, such as the Mimer II and III, Princeps, Diagnost N, and Concentric units, permit rotation of the tube and film around an axis near the center of the patient's head. In these units correct centering is maintained even when the tube angulation is varied (Fig. 3-10).

Those units with a linear tomographic movement may be divided into two groups. The first group includes the Mimer I, II, and III units and the Concentric, in which the tomographic motion is around a horizontal axis. The second group includes the Princeps and Diagnost N, in which the axis of the tomographic motion may be at any angle from horizontal to vertical. The variability of the tomographic axis seen in the second group permits a greater choice of direction of tube motion for tomographic sections. For example, when the patient is erect, tomography can be performed with a horizontal motion of the tube and film by the units of the second group but not by the units of the first group. This consideration may be important during pneumoencephalography, when the position of the air is determined by the position of the patient.

REFERENCES

Fredzell, G., Greitz, T., Grepe, A., and Holmström, L.: Mimer III and rotating chair, Acta Radiol. **7:**543-552, 1968.

Fredzell, G., and Lindgren, E.: Mimer, Acta Radiol. **53:**209-214, 1960.

Potts, D. G.: A new universal head unit, Amer. J. Roentgen. **95:**957-961, 1965.

CHAPTER 4

Physical factors affecting radiographic images

John Hale

The concept of quality in radiology is in an unsatisfactory state. Science progresses in an orderly fashion only if (1) the phenomena observed in the universe are organized into well-defined concepts and (2) units are devised that measure these phenomena accurately. As an example, the concept of length, the extent in space between two points, is well understood and its unit of measurement, the meter, is a means of accurate measurement; or, as another example, in radiology, the concept of electrical potential is accompanied by its unit of measurement, the volt. At present, image quality is not satisfactorily defined. We know that it is important, however, and we can judge whether a radiographic image is of poor quality, perhaps because of underexposure or improper development. The converse problem, of specifying the excellence of an image, is more difficult.

Quantitative measurement of some visual phenomena has been attempted. An example is the measurement of the periphery of specific anatomic regions of a beauty queen. These numbers would be interesting but would not tell the whole story. The situation in radiology is somewhat similar. We can measure some factors that degrade image quality, but undoubtedly much is unknown.

What, then, can we measure? First, we can measure density. When an x-ray film is developed, a pattern of silver is deposited that corresponds with the pattern of light from the intensifying screens. When the roentgenogram is placed on a view box, the pattern of silver interferes with the transmission of the visible light from the fluorescent tube to the eyes of the viewer. Density is a measure of the amount of incident light transmitted through the metallic silver on the roentgenogram. A uniformly exposed roentgenogram would not be useful. The patterns of interest are formed because of the differential attenuation of the light by various parts of the roentgenogram. We speak, then, of the density of one area compared with the density of some other area. This difference in density is the concept of contrast.

The second aspect of a roentgenogram that we can measure is the resolving power, a measure of the size of the smallest object that is perceptible. This concept is usually called detail.

CONTRAST AND DETAIL

The first application of these ideas in radiology to problems of image quality was reported by Chamberlain (1942) in his Carman lecture. He was concerned with the reason for the poorer image quality in fluoroscopy than in radiography. He argued that the difference could be explained by data on the physiology of the retina. Fig. 4-1, taken from his lecture, shows the minimum perceptible change in light intensity as a function of the luminance. The $\Delta I/I$ is essentially minimum detectable contrast. The *X*'s on the curve are data that Dr. George Henny obtained to show the light levels under various conditions of fluoroscopy. The ability of the eye to perceive contrast is poor at low light levels. In Fig. 4-2, which is also from Chamberlain's lecture, visual acuity is shown as a function of luminance. Visual acuity is defined in the optical sense as the smallest of a set of pairs of decreasingly smaller dots that are recognizable as discrete. This idea is closely related to what we would now call detail size. These data show that the visual acuity of the eye is much poorer at the low light levels of conventional fluoroscopy than at the high levels produced by an illuminator used for viewing a roentgenogram.

The experimental determination of visual acuity is

Supported in part by United States Public Health Service Dosimetry Grant Number RC-00099-17.

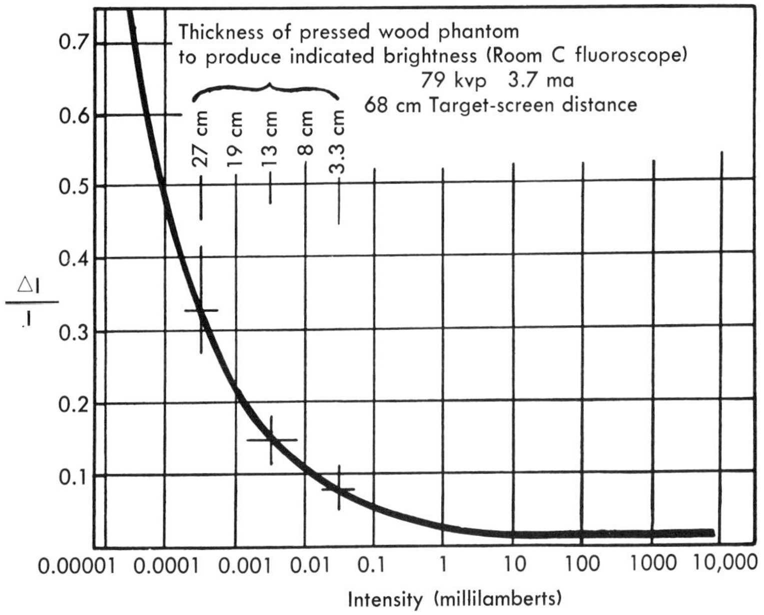

Fig. 4-1. Intensity discrimination $(\Delta I/I)$ expressed as fraction by which given light intensity must be added to for difference to be visible at that particular light level. (From Chamberlain, W.: Radiology **38**:383-425, 1942.)

simpler in light optics than in radiology. For visible light a test object of 100% contrast and sharp edges is easily made. However, in radiology the contrast in the region of interest is much less than 100%; and, in addition, roentgen rays always produce images with unsharp edges. Furthermore, the size of the smallest perceptible detail is related to its contrast. This idea was first demonstrated by Burger (1950) with a special test object. A roentgenogram of a test object of this type, now called a Burger phantom, is shown in Fig. 4-3. The phantom is essentially an aluminum step wedge except that a series of holes of decreasing diameter have been drilled through each step. Thus, as the phantom thickness increases, the contrast between the test object and the background increases. At any phantom thickness level the detail size changes at a fixed contrast. At an intermediate contrast level there is some detail size that is just perceptible; and as contrast decreases, the smallest perceptible detail size increases.

Measurements made with this technique are useful. As an example, Fig. 4-4 shows some experimental data obtained by Webster and Wipselder (1964) plotted to form a contrast-detail diagram. In their experiment a series of observers were presented a set of Burger-type test objects of varying contrast and detail. The observers were graded according to their ability to perceive the images of the holes under conditions simulating fluoroscopy. From these data a line was constructed to represent the minimum detail diameter that the observers could perceive as a function of image contrast. Details

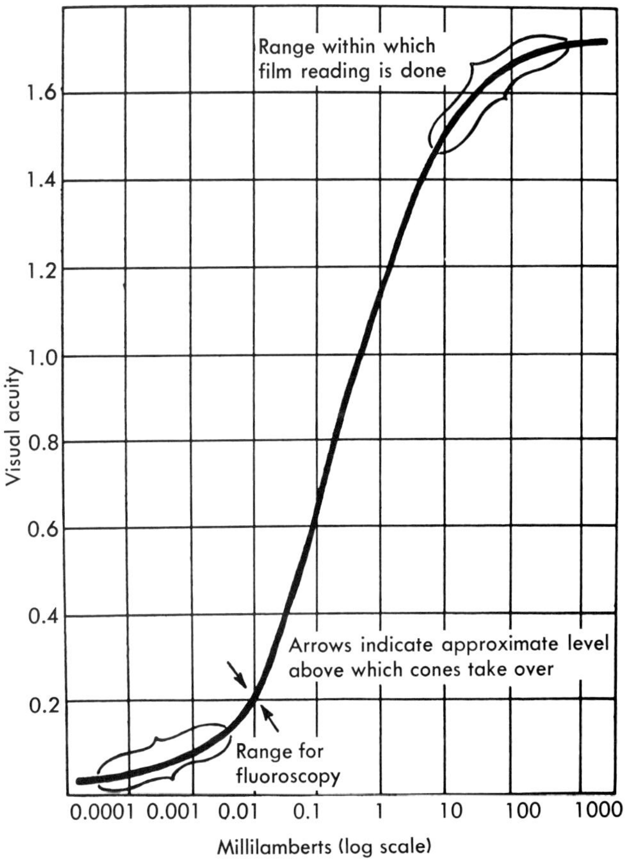

Fig. 4-2. Visual acuity as function of brightness. Visual acuity is reciprocal of angular separation that must separate two contours so that they may be recognized as discrete, the unit of separation being 1 minute of arc. (From Chamberlain, W.: Radiology **38**:383-425, 1942.)

Fig. 4-3. Roentgenogram of a Burger phantom. (See text for discussion of construction.)

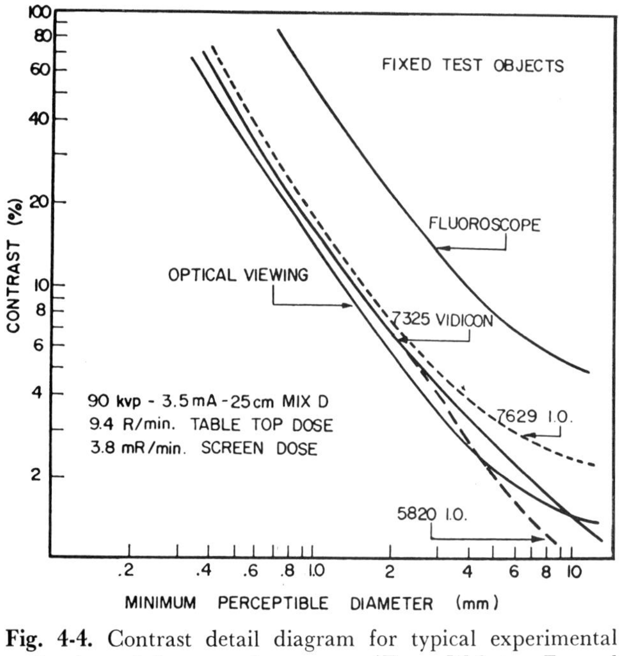

Fig. 4-4. Contrast detail diagram for typical experimental evaluation of fluoroscopic systems. (From Webster, E., and Wipselder, R.: J.S.M.P.T.E. **73:**617-621, 1964.)

of smaller size are seen to require higher contrast for perception. In this particular example the direct viewing of the output phosphor of an image intensifier tube is compared with the viewing of a vidicon or image orthicon (IO) television chain. The data show that any of the intensified systems is better than conventional fluoroscopy but that the three methods of viewing the image intensifier are not significantly different.

FACTORS AFFECTING CONTRAST

Fig. 4-5 represents the principal physical factors that reduce contrast in a roentgenogram. The uniform flux of roentgen rays generated at an infinitely small focal spot passes through a wave-shaped test object with a subject contrast of 25%. All sources of unsharpness in the roentgenographic system, however, combine to produce on the film an image with degraded contrast. This contrast governs the photon flux that illuminates the retina of the observer. Listed in the box representing the radiographic system are the four classic factors of unsharpness: focal spot size, magnification resulting from object-film distance, the finite size of the grains in film and intensifying screens, and motion.

Unsharpness that results from focal spot size can be illustrated geometrically. Fig. 4-6 demonstrates unsharpness caused by focal spot size and magnification. The test object is a simple line created by two edges of gold foil separated by a narrow gap. The drawing is exaggerated for clarity, but the relative sizes and distances are correct. In this example a 1 mm focal spot is assumed to be used with a conventional magnification factor of 1.1. In the upper left corner is a roentgenogram of the test object, and below it is a microdensitometer tracing of the roentgenogram. An ideal radiographic system would produce a perfectly sharp image of the line. The effect of the finite size of the focal spot is seen to round the edges of the object. The microdensitometer trace pattern, which measures how much the line has been spread by the system unsharpness, is called the line spread-function. On the right side of the figure, the situation with a 0.3 mm focal spot is illustrated. Little difference is seen in the line spread-functions of the two focal spots with this magnification factor.

The situation is different when a magnification technique is used. The right side of Fig. 4-7 shows a 0.3 mm focal spot used with a magnification factor of 1.6. Because the focal spot is so small, the penumbra is small, even with this large magnification factor. Thus the line spread-function has not changed much, compared with that produced by conventional magnification. The left side of the figure shows what may be expected if a 1 mm focal spot is used with a large magnification factor. The penumbra enlarges, almost covering the whole image. The microdensitometer tracing of the roentgenogram shows that the line has been spread significantly and that, in addition, the contrast of the image has decreased dramatically. Furthermore, comparison of the right side of Figs. 4-6 and 4-7 shows no significant

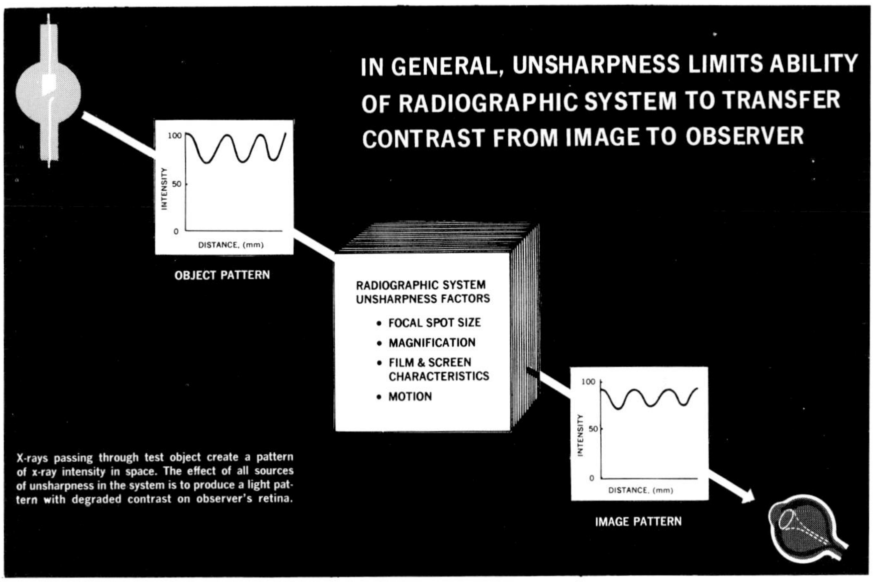

Fig. 4-5. Schematic illustration of factors in radiographic unsharpness.

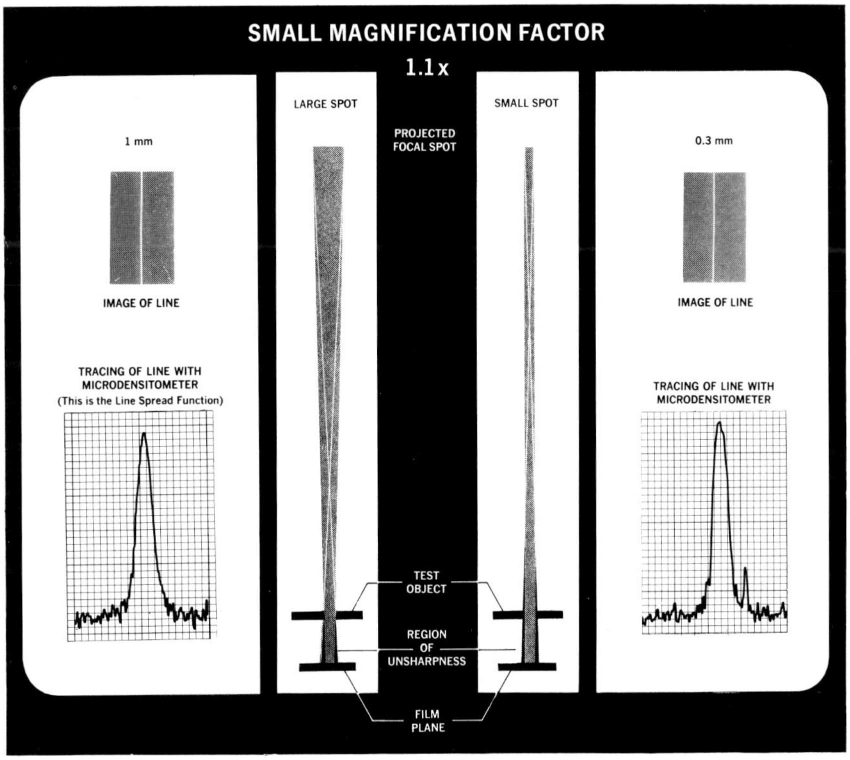

Fig. 4-6. Illustration of geometric unsharpness, the result of focal spot size for small magnification factor. For conventional object-film distance, focal spot unsharpness is not major factor in total image unsharpness.

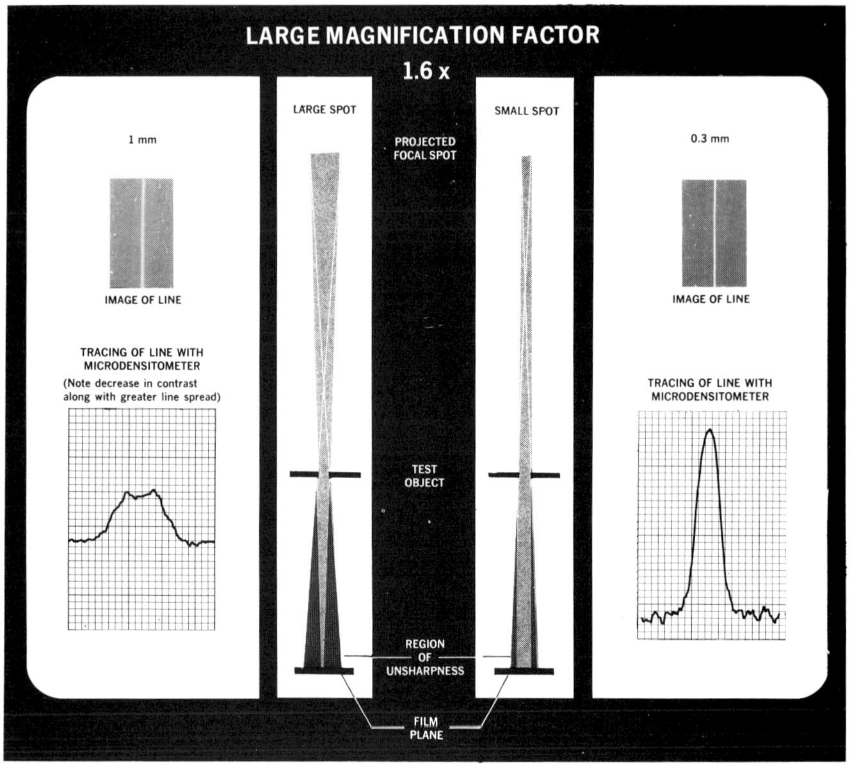

Fig. 4-7. Illustration of geometric unsharpness, the result of focal spot size for large magnification factors. For magnification techniques, focal spot unsharpness may be prominent contributor to total unsharpness and thus limit ability of system to record small detail.

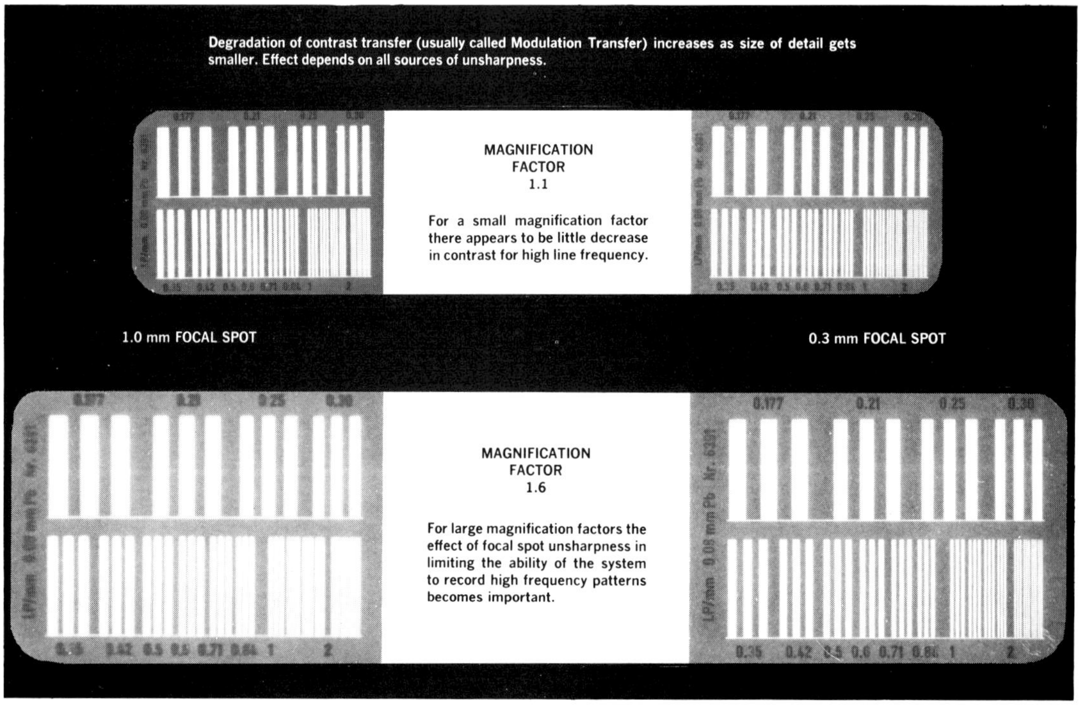

Fig. 4-8. Roentgenogram of lead line test object under various conditions to illustrate effect of focal spot unsharpness in decreasing contrast of closely spaced lines.

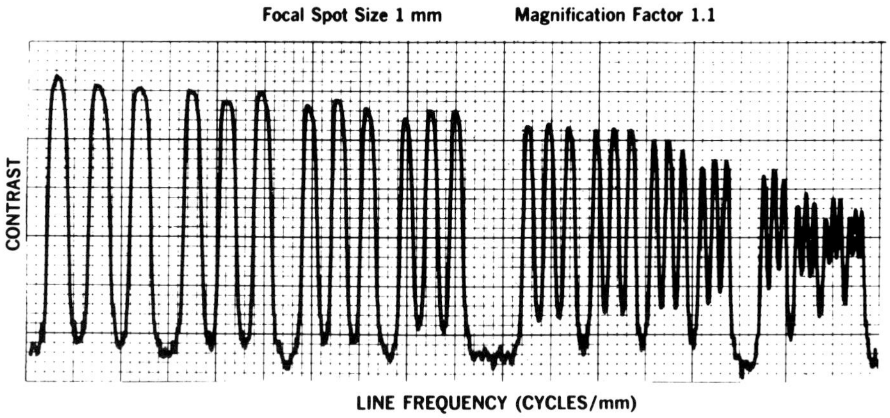

Fig. 4-9. Microdensitometer tracing of part of one roentgenogram shown in Fig. 4-8. Contrast is seen to decrease markedly as line frequency increases.

change in contrast in the image of the line with the small focal spot when magnification is changed from 1.1 to 1.6.

The decrease in image contrast caused by unsharpness and quantified by the line spread-function depends on the size of the object. Fig. 4-8 is a roentgenogram of a test object obtained under the exposure conditions of Figs. 4-6 and 4-7. The test object is constructed by carefully cutting lines in a piece of lead foil. The numbers on the top of the pattern indicate the number of line pairs per millimeter. The frequency of line pairs in this test object varies from 0.177 line pairs per millimeter, at the upper left, to 5 line pairs per millimeter, at the lower right. Changing the frequency of the line pairs corresponds to changing detail size: high-frequency line pairs correspond to small detail. With a magnification factor of 1.1, both focal spots are seen to image the test pattern accurately. The contrast between the density underneath the space in the test pattern and the density underneath the lead in the test pattern does not seem to change much until the frequency exceeds about 0.5 line pairs per millimeter. Above this frequency the contrast falls, but either system resolves the highest-frequency line pairs. The situation is different for the 1.0 mm focal spot with a magnification factor of 1.6. Now the poor line spread-function seen in Fig. 4-7 blurs the image so that line pairs above about 1.5 per millimeter cannot be resolved.* Even with the high magnification factor, however, the highest-frequency lines are resolved by the system with the smaller focal spot. Note that this experiment confirms the conclusions reached from the measurements of the line spread-function in Figs. 4-6 and 4-7.

*The apparent reappearance of lines above the frequency of 2 lines per millimeter is an example of "spurious" resolution. This artifact is the result of overlap of penumbra caused by the periodic pattern of the test object.

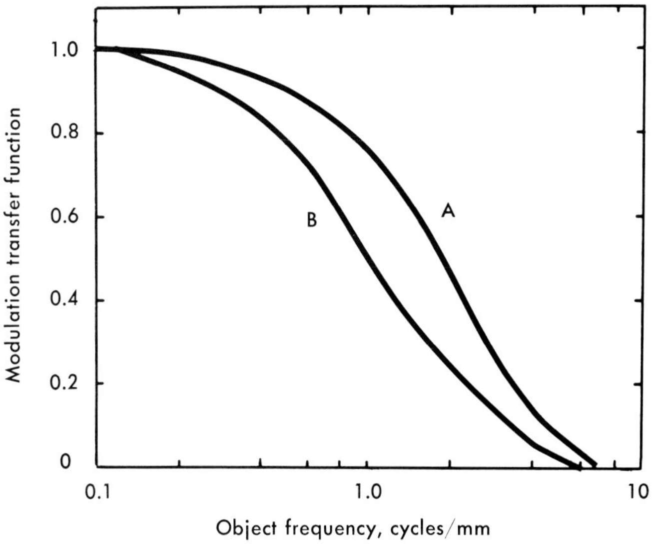

Fig. 4-10. Typical modulation transfer function of two roentgenographic systems. (See text.)

MODULATION TRANSFER FUNCTION

The relationship between line contrast and frequency can be quantified by scanning the roentgenogram of the test pattern with a microdensitometer. Fig. 4-9 is a typical tracing of the right side of the bottom row of the upper left image in Fig. 4-8. The ordinate of this graph is density, so the difference between the density level at the top and the density level at the bottom of the wave is a measure of image contrast. The scale along the bottom is frequency in line pairs (or cycles) per millimeter. The pronounced decrease in the ability of the roentgenographic system to transfer contrast from object to image as the frequency of the object increases is evident.

A graphic representation of these data is called the modulation transfer function (MTF). Fig. 4-10 is a typical graph with contrast of the images produced by the two roentgenographic systems plotted on the y-axis as a function of object frequency on the x-axis. From the standpoint of the MTF theory, system *A* would be considered the better system because it would image any object with higher contrast than would system *B*. This concept is called the modulation transfer function since the method was originally developed in electrical engineering, where the word modulation means alteration of the amplitude of an electric signal. This approach to specifying imaging properties in radiology was first proposed by Coltman (1957). The terminology seems appropriate. For example, if a uniform photon flux enters the anterior aspect of a patient's thorax, the difference between the attenuation coefficients of soft tissue and of bone in the chest of the patient modulates the amplitude of the photon flux as the beam emerges from the patient. The ability of the roentgenographic system to reproduce this pattern of amplitude modulation in the photon flux and record it can be quantified by the modulation transfer function.

UNSHARPNESS RESULTING FROM INTENSIFYING SCREENS

Intensifying screens also have a significant effect in spreading the image of a line. The bottom half of Fig. 4-11 shows a roentgenogram obtained by placing the line test object directly on a cardboard cassette. The microdensitometer tracing and a 21× enlargement of the roentgenogram show accurate imaging of the sharp edges of the test object. The upper half of Fig. 4-11 is a roentgenogram of the test object placed directly on an intensifying screen cassette. The tracing shows the effect of the size of the grains in the intensifying screen in rounding edges of the image of the test object. In the enlargement of the roentgenogram, the blurring of the edges of the object is obvious.

APPLICATION OF MODULATION TRANSFER FUNCTION THEORY

From the foregoing discussion it appears that the concepts of line spread-function and modulation transfer function (MTF) appear closely related. Actually they are related in the mathematical sense: the MTF is the Fourier transform of the line spread-function. This relationship is useful. The MTF is most easily obtained experimentally by measuring the line spread-function with a microdensitometer and then calculating the MTF from these data.

The primary reason the MTF is a powerful method of analysis of roentgenographic systems is that the effect of each component of the system can be examined individually. As an example, the top curve in Fig. 4-12 is the MTF of high-speed film alone (Rossmann and Lubberts, 1966); the second curve is the MTF due to motion alone. In this example motion of 1 mm/sec with a magnification factor of 1.6 and exposure time of 1/20 second was assumed. These conditions should be conservative for techniques in cerebral angiography.* The third curve is the MTF of a pair of high-speed intensifying screens alone (Rossmann and Lubberts, 1966). Note, for example, that at a frequency of 1 cycle/

*This curve was calculated from a formula derived by Morgan (1962).

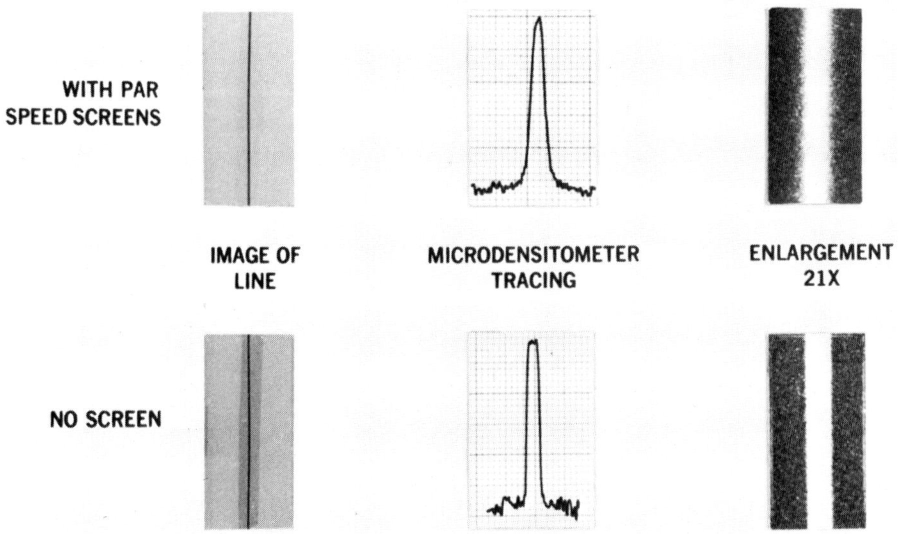

Fig. 4-11. Illustration of effect of intensifying screens in blurring image of a line.

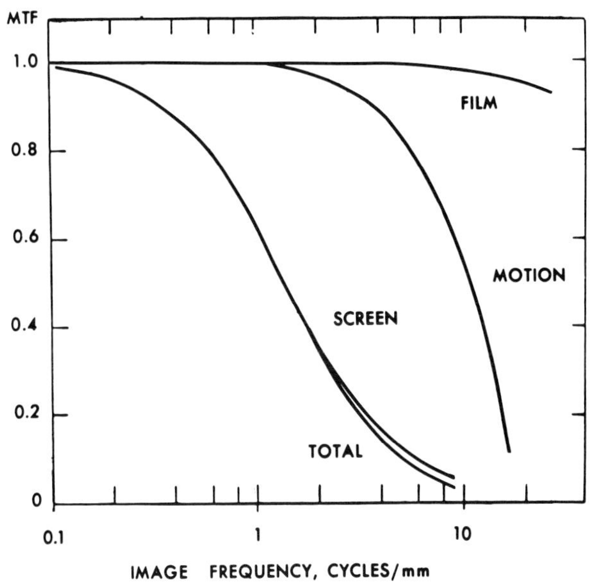

Fig. 4-12. Modulation transfer functions for high-speed film alone, motion alone (1 mm/sec) with magnification factor of 1.6 and exposure time of 1/20 sec, and high-speed screen alone.

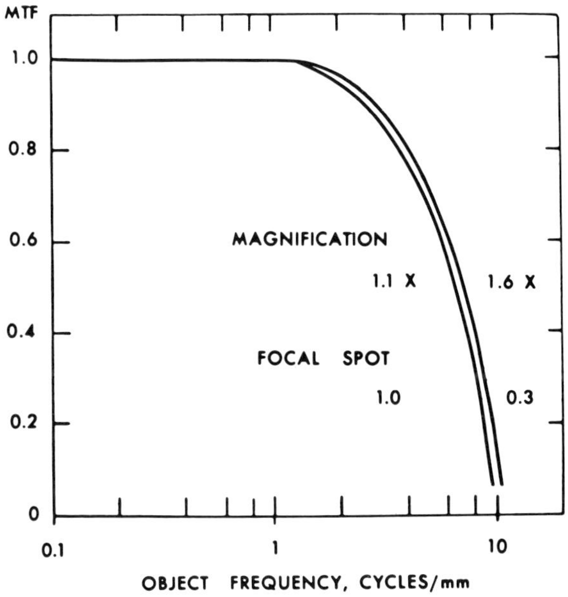

Fig. 4-13. Modulation transfer function resulting from focal spot size alone. MTF of 1 mm focal spot with magnification factor of 1.1 is compared with that of 0.3 mm focal spot with magnification factor 1.6.

mm, the contrast of the image would be reduced to 0.64 of the contrast of the object because intensifying screens were used. Neither the film MTF nor the motion MTF has any effect on image contrast at this frequency.

The power of the MTF system analysis lies in the fact that the MTF of the total system is obtained simply by point multiplication of the individual MTF's. The

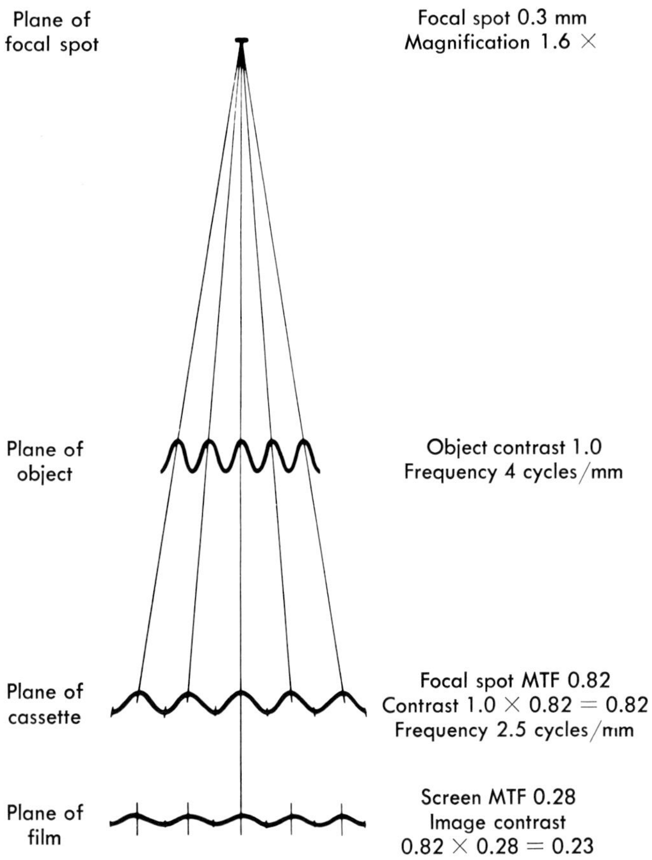

Fig. 4-14. Diagram to illustrate steps in calculation of total system modulation transfer function.

bottom curve in Fig. 4-12, labeled *Total,* was obtained by this method. It is essentially the same as the MTF curve for the high-speed intensifying screens.

The MTF approach can also be applied to the study of the effect of focal spot size. Fig. 4-13 shows the MTF of a 1 mm focal spot used with a conventional magnification factor of 1.1 compared to the MTF of a 0.3 mm focal spot with a magnification factor of 1.6* The MTF's of these two focal spots under these conditions are similar and would be expected to produce similar images. This observation agrees with the results illustrated in Fig. 4-8 and the comparison of line spread-functions in Figs. 4-6 and 4-7.

Fig. 4-14 represents an example of how the MTF for a complete roentgenographic system can be calculated. A test object is assumed to have a contrast of 1.0 and a frequency of 4 cycles/mm. It is placed between the plane of a 0.3 mm focal spot and the plane of the film so that the magnification factor is 1.6. From Fig. 4-13 the MTF of the 0.3 mm focal spot under these condi-

*These curves were calculated from a formula derived by Morgan (1962).

Table 4-1. Calculation of MTF for an object with a frequency of 4 cycles/mm (1.1× magnification with 1.0 mm focal spot and 1.6× magnification with 0.3 mm focal spot)

	Focal spot	
	0.3 mm	*1.0 mm*
Assumed contrast at object plane	1.0	1.0
Frequency at object plane, cycles/mm	4	4
Focal spot MTF	0.82	0.78
Contrast at cassette plane	0.82	0.78
Frequency at cassette plane, cycles/mm	2.5	3.6
Screen MTF	0.28	0.18
Contrast at image plane	0.23	0.14

tions is found to be 0.82. The contrast of the object when projected on the film plane, therefore, has been decreased from 1.0 to 0.82 because of focal spot unsharpness. The frequency of the image is smaller because of the magnification. The magnification factor is 1.6, so the frequency of the photon pattern just before the photons strike the intensifying screen is 4/1.6 = 2.5 cycles/mm. Next the MTF curve for intensifying screens from Fig. 4-12 is entered at the appropriate frequency, 2.5 cycles/mm. The MTF of the screens, film, and motion* is then found to be 0.28. The total system MTF for an object of 4 cycles/mm and a magnification factor of 1.6, then, is the product of these various factors. In this example the contrast of the image will be 1 × 0.82 × 0.28 = 0.23. This is the complete system MTF at an object frequency of 4 cycles/mm. In Table 4-1 is shown the same calculation for a larger focal spot with conventional magnification. The numbers in the second column (0.3 mm) are those just discussed. The numbers in the third column (1.0 mm) are pertinent to a 1 mm focal spot used with a conventional magnification factor of 1.1. As noted before, the MTF of these two roentgenographic systems is about the same as far as focal spot unsharpness is concerned. The difference between them is that the frequency of the image of the test object is significantly greater with conventional magnification. Thus the MTF curve for the intensifying screens must be entered at the higher frequency of 4/1.1 = 3.6 cycles/mm.† The screen MTF for the conventional magnification factor is significantly lower, 0.18, compared with that for the magnification technique. This difference is reflected in the overall system MTF, 0.14, compared with the MTF calculated for the magnification technique.

A full MTF curve is determined by repeating this calculation for a number of different test frequencies. The results of a calculation of this kind are shown on Fig. 4-15. The MTF of the roentgenographic system with a 1 mm focal spot and a conventional magnification factor of 1.1 is compared with that of a 0.3 mm focal spot used with a magnification factor of 1.6. The magnification technique provides a greater contrast at all frequencies. Of particular importance in cerebral angiography is the greater contrast transfer of the small focal spot–magnification technique at the high frequencies, which corresponds to small blood vessels.

The MTF of a 0.3 mm focal spot used with high-speed screens does not depend very much on the magnification factor. Two phenomena occur at the same time, but their effects are opposite. (1) As the magnification factor increases, the MTF resulting from the finite size of the focal spot becomes poorer. At the same time, however, (2) the frequency of the image decreases so that the image contrast caused by the MTF of the intensifying screens improves with greater magnification. This effect is demonstrated in Table 4-2, which shows that the MTF for a 0.3 mm focal spot does not change significantly as the magnification factor increases from 1.1 to 1.6. Above a magnification factor of about 1.6, however, the degradation of the image quality resulting from focal spot unsharpness becomes apparent for high frequencies. The contrast transfer for lower frequencies continues to improve gradually. These calculations indicate, then, that the optimum magnification factor for this focal spot size is probably somewhere between 1.6 and 2.

EFFECT OF SCATTERED RADIATION

On comparison of enlargement techniques with conventional techniques, one further factor should be considered. Scattered radiation certainly affects image contrast, and the ratio of secondary exposure to primary exposure at the film may be different for the air gap used in enlargement techniques compared with the grid used in conventional techniques. Fig. 4-16 shows the results of a study of this effect made with a 15 cm diameter cylindric water phantom to simulate the scattering from the patient's head. Exposures were made at 105 kvp. The distance from focal spot to film was 40 inches. Primary exposure was determined, using the characteristic curve of the film, by measuring the density produced by a series of exposures; a very small field was used with the water phantom as far as possible from

*Magnification has been taken into account in the calculation of the motion MTF.

†The motion MTF for the smaller magnification will be even better than that shown in Fig. 4-12 since motion unsharpness is inversely proportional to object-film distance. In this example, therefore, it will have no significant effect on image quality; the film motion MTF is as high as 0.90 at 6 cycles/mm.

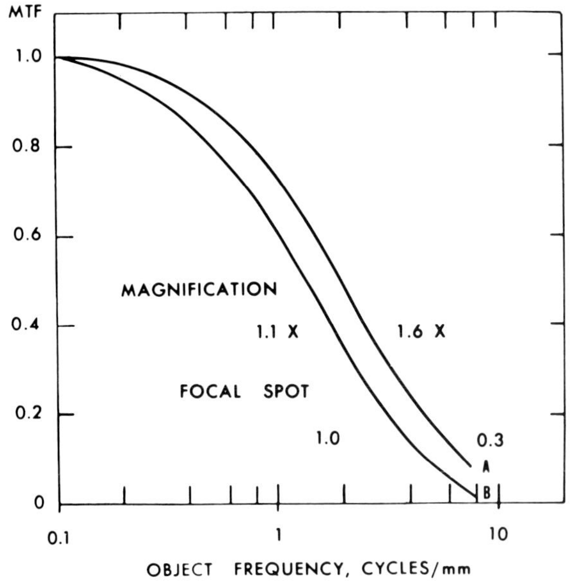

Fig. 4-15. Modulation transfer function of roentgenographic system with focal spot of 1 mm and magnification factor of 1.1 compared with that of system using 0.3 mm focal spot with magnification factor of 1.6. Other physical factors are as shown in Fig. 4-12. MTF of smaller focal spot with magnification technique is better at all frequencies.

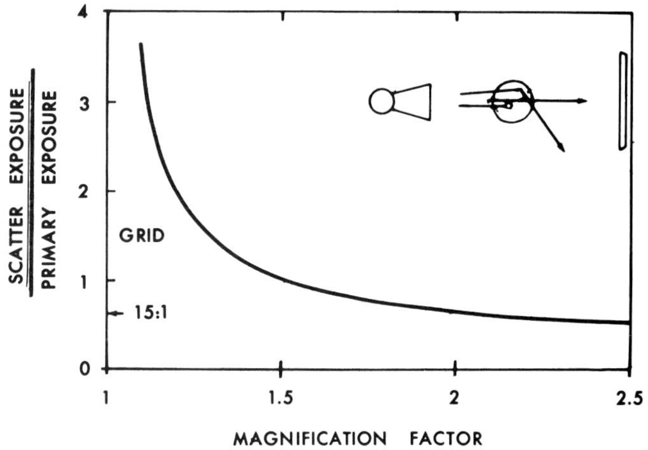

Fig. 4-16. Experimental data on ratio of scatter exposure to primary exposure of roentgen film as function of magnification factor. Reduction of scatter exposure, consequent to introduction of air gap with technique using magnification factor of 2, is about equivalent to reduction of scatter caused by a 15:1 grid.

Table 4-2. Modulation transfer function for 0.3 mm focal spot used with high-speed screens

Object frequency (cycles/mm)	*Magnification factor* 1.1			1.4			1.6			1.8			2.0		
	Modulation transfer function														
	S	*F*	*T**	*S*	*F*	*T*	*S*	*F*	*T*	*S*	*F*	*T*	*S*	*F*	*T*
0.5	0.77	1.0	0.77	0.83	1.0	0.83	0.86	1.0	0.86	0.89	1.0	0.89	0.90	1.0	0.90
1.0	0.54	1.0	0.54	0.63	1.0	0.63	0.68	0.99	0.67	0.71	0.99	0.70	0.75	0.98	0.74
2.0	0.27	1.0	0.27	0.36	0.99	0.36	0.41	0.92	0.38	0.46	0.87	0.40	0.50	0.85	0.43
3.0	0.15	1.0	0.15	0.20	0.98	0.20	0.25	0.82	0.20	0.30	0.75	0.23	0.36	0.69	0.25
4.0	0.09	1.0	0.09	0.14	0.92	0.13	0.17	0.69	0.12	0.20	0.58	0.11	0.24	0.51	0.12
5.0	0.05	0.99	0.05	0.09	0.88	0.08	0.12	0.55	0.07	0.15	0.41	0.06	0.17	0.28	0.05
6.0	0.04	0.98	0.04	0.06	0.82	0.05	0.08	0.38	0.03	0.10	0.23	0.02	0.13	0.09	0.01

**S*, High-speed screen MTF; *F*, focal spot MTF; *T*, system total MTF, $S \times F$.

the cassette. To determine primary plus secondary exposure, a series of exposures were made with the distance from absorber to cassette being varied but with a fixed 9-inch-square field at the cassette. The decrease in photon energy of the scattered radiation was neglected because an average photon, in this technique, has an energy of about 30 kev and the energy shift for a 30° scatter angle will be less than 1%. In addition, the intensification factor of screens is not sensitive to variations of photon energy (Johns, 1961). The ratio of the scatter exposure to the primary exposure for a 15:1 grid at 100 kvp was calculated from data derived by Boldingh (1961) and from data in Fig. 4-16. The reduction in scattered radiation with a magnification factor of 2.0 is about the same as that from a 15:1 (900 mg/cm^2) grid.

CONCLUSIONS AND SUMMARY

The methods proposed to study the effect of changes in roentgenographic variables on image quality have been reviewed. As an example, the theory of modulation transfer function has been applied to the problem of optimum magnification for cerebral angiography with a small focal spot. The theory predicts that the optimum magnification factor is between 1.6 and 2.0 when an x-ray tube with a 0.3 mm focal spot is used together with high-speed film and intensifying screens. The MTF of such a system is compared with that of an x-ray tube whose focal spot is 1.0 mm with a conventional magnification factor of 1.1. Calculations predict that better contrast may be expected with the smaller focal spot and greater magnification at all object frequencies.

The technique of greater magnification has an additional advantage. It increases the contrast, by reducing the ratio of film exposure caused by scattered and primary radiation. Data show that in magnification studies of the skull, the air gap with a magnification factor of 2.0 is about as effective as with a 15:1 grid.

Much is still to be learned about the specification of image quality. Present techniques, for example, do not directly include the statistics of quantum mottle (Rossmann, 1963). Nevertheless, the MTF theory is useful for analysis of the effect on image quality of changing system variables.

REFERENCES

Boldingh, W. H.: Quality and choice of Potter Bucky grids, Acta Radiol. **55:**225-235, 1961.

Burger, G. C. E.: Phantom tests with x-rays, Philips Tech. Rev. **11:**291-298, 1950.

Chamberlain, W. E.: Fluoroscopes and fluoroscopy, Radiology **38:**383-413, 1942.

Coltman, J. W.: The specification of imaging properties by response to a sine wave input, J. Opt. Soc. Amer. **44:**468-471, 1954.

Johns, H. E.: The physics of radiology, Springfield, Ill., 1961, Charles C Thomas, Publisher.

Morgan, R. H.: The frequency response function, Amer. J. Roentgen. **88:**175-186, 1962.

Rossman, K.: Spatial fluctuations of x-ray quanta and the recording of radiographic mottle, Amer. J. Roentgen. **90:** 863-869, 1963.

Rossman, K., and Lubberts, G.: Some characteristics of the line spread-function and modulation transfer function of medical radiographic films and screen film systems, Radiology **86:**235-241, 1966.

Webster, E. W., and Wipselder, R.: Contrast and detail perception in television and cine systems for medical fluoroscopy, J.S.M.P.T.E. **73:**617-621, 1964.

CHAPTER 5

Film analysis

D. Gordon Potts

To build a complete three-dimensional picture of the structures shown in a radiograph, the radiologist should be able to recognize a structure in more than one projection. He may also be required to estimate the magnification or degree of rectilinear distortion and relate structures demonstrated radiographically to external landmarks. An architect's plans of a building usually include three views of known scale mutually at right angles without rectilinear distortion. This system cannot always be applied to the skull. Often there is rectilinear distortion; the magnification may not be known accurately; and at times it is impossible to obtain three views mutually at right angles. For these reasons the transposition of information from one radiograph to another may be relatively complex.

CALCULATION OF ANGULATION OF A FRONTAL PROJECTION

If frontal and lateral views are available, the tube angulation required to produce the frontal view may usually be calculated with fair accuracy. To do this, it is necessary to identify two structures in different planes that are superimposed or at approximately the same height in the frontal view (Fig. 5-1). Ideally one of these structures should be located posteriorly in the skull and the other should be anterior, but a less marked separation of the structures used is still acceptable. If the two structures are at the same height or superimposed in the frontal view, they are joined in the lateral view to give the direction of the central ray required to produce the frontal view. If they are at different heights in the frontal view, they are transposed to the lateral view as in Fig. 5-2. The positions of the inferior orbital margins and the superior aspects of the external auditory meatuses usually can be determined with fair accuracy on the lateral view. Therefore it is possible to indicate the anthropologic base plane in this view. The angle between this plane and the direction of the central ray can then be determined.

PROJECTION OBTAINED FROM EXTERNAL LANDMARKS

An example of the use of external landmarks is the projection of the internal auditory canals through the orbits. The internal auditory canals lie almost directly medial to the external auditory canals. If a line is drawn from the center of the external auditory canal to the center of the orbit, it will correspond with the direction of the central ray required to project the internal canals close to the centers of the orbits.

SPECIFIC FRONTAL PROJECTION OBTAINED FROM LATERAL PROJECTION

If, for example, it is desired to project a calcified pineal between the posterior margin of the foramen magnum and the posterior arch of the first cervical vertebra, a lateral film is obtained. A line is drawn on this film joining the pineal to the point through which it is to be projected. This line will correspond with the direction of the central ray for the desired projection (Fig. 5-3).

EXTERNAL PROJECTION OF STRUCTURE DEMONSTRATED RADIOLOGICALLY

The structure must be related to landmarks that can be identified both radiologically and by external examination of the head. This manipulation is needed when tightly coned views are required, when the plane of a structure for tomographic cuts must be determined, or

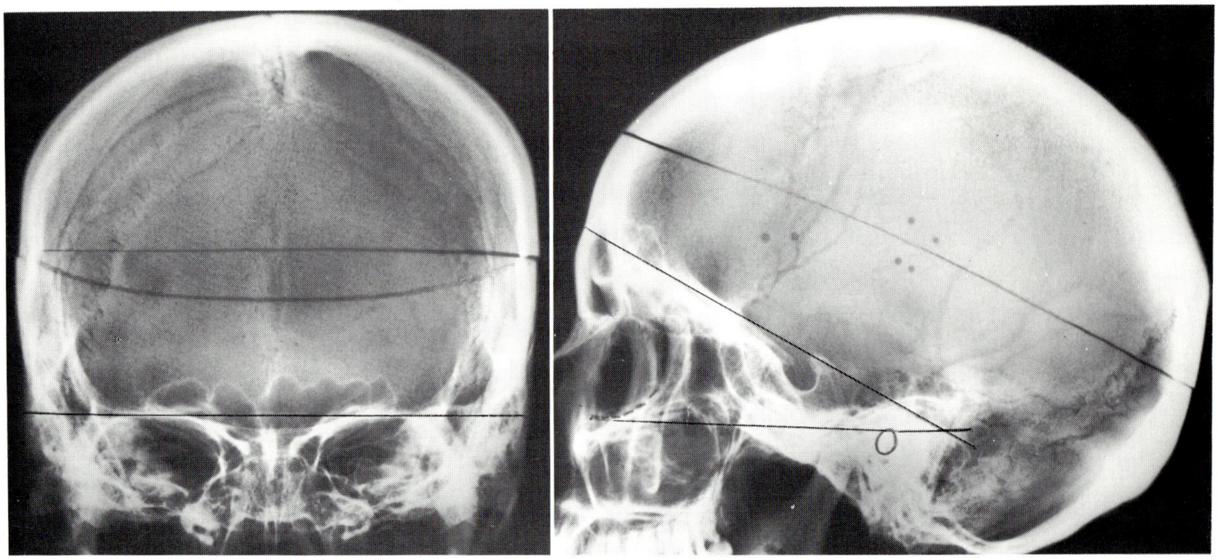

Fig. 5-1. In the frontal view, roofs of the orbits are projected close to superior aspects of petrous temporal bones. Line joining roofs of orbits and superior aspects of petrous temporal bones in lateral projection indicates direction of central ray required for this frontal projection. Anthropologic base line may be drawn on lateral projection by joining inferior orbital margin to superior aspect of petrous temporal bone. Angulation of central ray in relation to base line may then be measured.

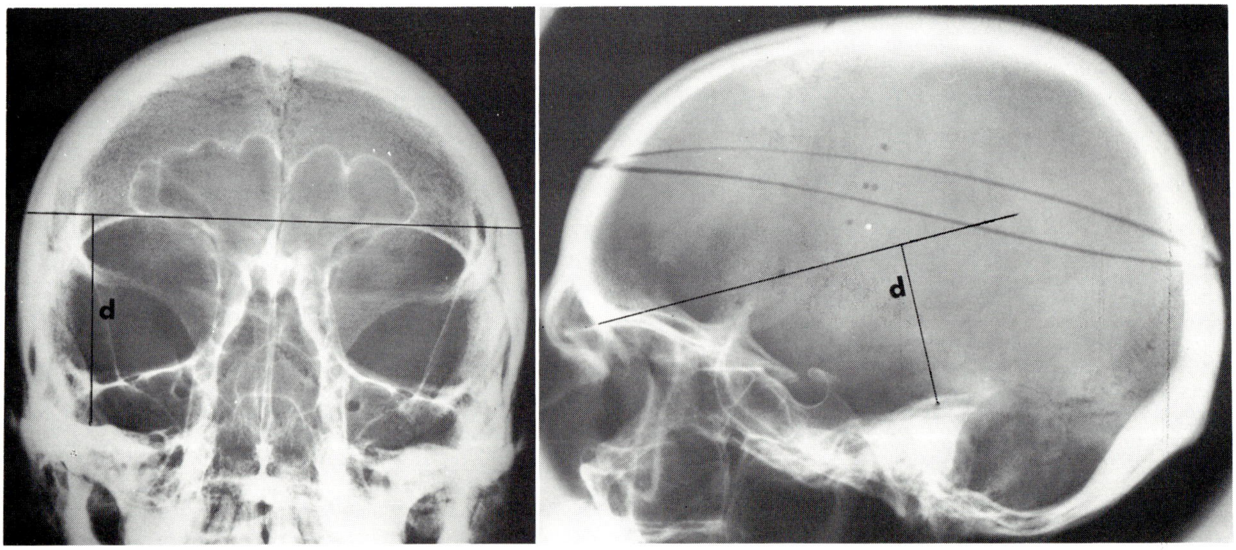

Fig. 5-2. In frontal view, distance *d* of orbital roofs above ridges of petrous temporal bones is measured. Direction of central ray required to produce this frontal projection passes through orbital roof and also passes distance *d* above petrous temporal bones. If there is rectilinear distortion in frontal view, allowance must be made for distortion, or method is inaccurate.

when radiotherapy is to be directed to a circumscribed lesion demonstrated radiologically. The structure shown on a lateral radiograph is commonly related to the anthropologic base line on one side (Fig. 5-4). If there is a significant magnification, the degree of magnification of structures near the sagittal plane is determined by making the same measurements on both radiograph and patient (for example, the maximum anteroposterior measurement including the soft tissues). The true measurement on the patient divided by the radiographic measurement gives the correction factor. All radiographic measurements must be multiplied by this correction

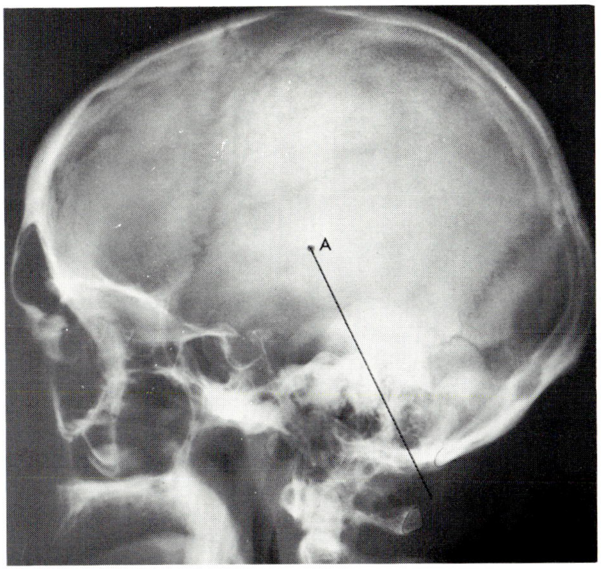

Fig. 5-3. There is faint pineal calcification at *A*. If this is to be projected between posterior margin of foramen magnum and posterior arch of first cervical vertebra on frontal view, direction of central ray is indicated by line shown. Provided position of patient remains unchanged and one edge of this lateral film is parallel to floor, tube may be angled correctly for this projection without reference to roentgenographic base plane. View would be very difficult to obtain with patient in this position because of extreme tube angulation, which would project area of interest close to back of cervical and upper dorsal spine.

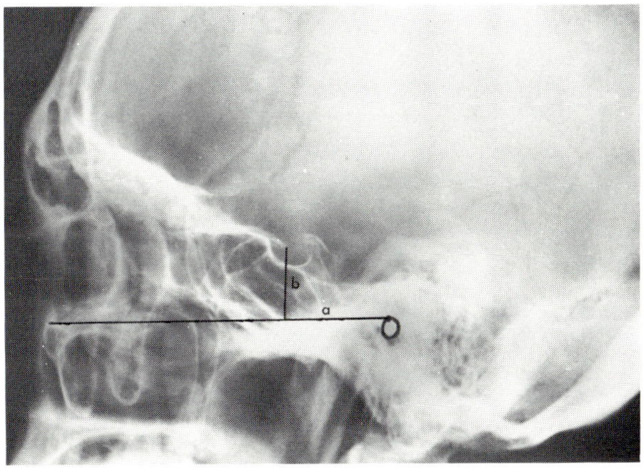

Fig. 5-4. External projection of tip of anterior clinoid process is determined by relation of tip to anthropologic base line on side of interest. Anterior clinoid is distance *a* in front of external auditory meatus and distance *b* above anthropologic base line. These measurements may be made on patient in same manner. If there is significant magnification in roentgenogram, reduction of measurements may be necessary.

factor to obtain the true measurement. The distance of the structure from the midline may be measured on a frontal radiograph in the same way. For accurate measurements of this kind, the frontal projection should have no rectilinear distortion.

COMPARISON OF MAGNIFICATION OF DIMENSION SHOWN IN DIFFERENT PROJECTIONS

The maximum width of the skull may be measured in any nonrotated view (including the AP –90 or submentovertical view). A correction factor derived from these measurements may be needed when *side-to-side* measurements are transposed from one film to another and when films differ in the degree of magnification. In frontal films, when the film is not perpendicular to the central ray, there is rectilinear distortion and the degree of magnification of superoinferior dimensions may vary widely.

CALCULATION OF ACTUAL SIZE OF STRUCTURE

The method for correcting measurements made on a radiograph for magnification (mentioned in regard to external projection of a structure demonstrated radiologically) presumes that all structures in the skull are magnified equally. In fact, structures in the skull closer to the film are magnified less than structures further from the film. The true measurement of a structure can be calculated if the anode-film distance and the distance of the structure from the film are known.

CORRELATION OF LANDMARK IN LATERAL AND FRONTAL PROJECTIONS

It is not unusual for the pineal to be easily recognizable in a lateral projection. However, the gland may be difficult to detect in a frontal projection. The height of the pineal in the frontal projection may be calculated as in Fig. 5-5.

ANALYSIS OF STEREOSCOPIC FILMS

Apparently stereoscopy was used first in 1898 (Davidson, 1916). In addition to the information that may be gained by viewing radiographs stereoscopically, the positions of objects shown on a stereoscopic pair of films may be assessed objectively (Daves and Dalrymple, 1962).

If a pair of stereoscopic films are superimposed so that the two images of an object are aligned, the images of all objects in a plane parallel to the plane of the film and including the initial object will also be in alignment. Daves and Dalrymple reported that the images of the object used for the initial alignment must have at least two points of alignment so that the films are not rotated on each other. For example, if a stereoscopic pair of lateral skull radiographs are superimposed, the sella turcica may be used for the initial alignment. Any calcification near the sagittal plane will also be superimposed.

The degree of shift of two stereoscopic images of an object with respect to the films is directly proportionate

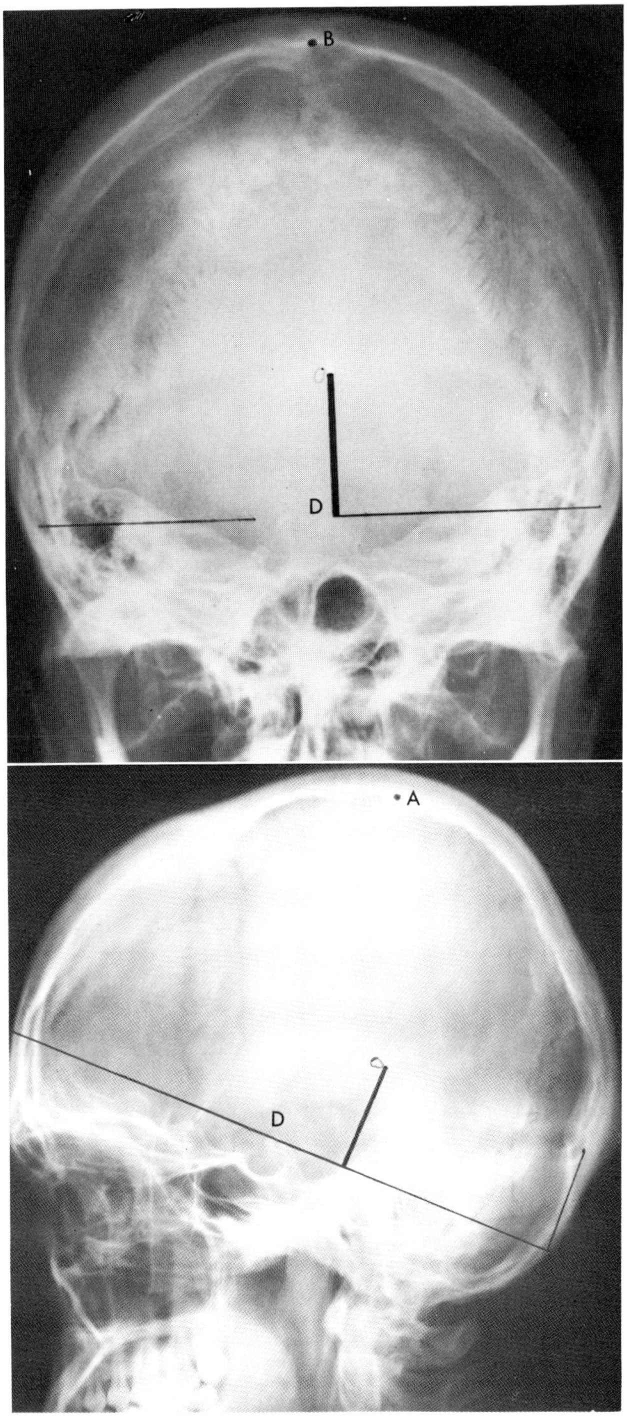

Fig. 5-5. Faintly calcified pineal is shown in lateral projection but is difficult to identify in frontal projection. In the frontal projection, top of dorsum sellae is 3.6 cm below center of venous groove at torcular. There is some rectilinear distortion, and this dimension is magnified. The magnification here as compared with magnification in lateral projection can be determined approximately by measuring distance of top of dorsum *(D)* to most distant part of inner aspect of skull (to point *A* in lateral and point *B* in frontal). *DA* divided by *DB* is correction factor required to transpose superoinferior measurements from frontal to lateral projection. In this case *DA* is 11 cm, *DB* is 12 cm, and correction factor is 0.92. Thus direction of central ray on lateral projection required to give this frontal projection is indicated by a line through top of dorsum and a point 3.6 cm × 0.92 or 3.3 cm below torcular. Pineal is 3.3 cm above this line in lateral view. When measurement is transposed back to frontal projection, it is 3.3 cm divided by 0.92 (or 3.6 cm); i.e., pineal must be on line 3.6 cm above dorsum, or projected over venous groove at torcular. Pineal is outlined in both projections.

to the distance of the object from the film. For this reason a side marker is usually placed on the radiographic table close to the head and the images of this marker are used for the initial alignment. If the film is close to the side of the head when the stereoscopic lateral skull films are obtained, if the distance of the sella turcica from the film is known (measured on a frontal projection), and if the shift of the structure is less than that of the sella turcica, then the structure must be closer to the film than the sella turcica. If the shift of the structure is greater than the shift of the sella turcica, then the structure must be further from the film than the sella turcica.

Daves and Dalrymple also stated that if a pair of stereoscopic films are superimposed so that the images in the midline of the subject are aligned, and then they are moved over each other until images from an object beneath the subject are aligned, during this process: (1) images of structures above the midline of the subject will diverge and (2) images of structures below the midline of the subject will converge and cross. The value of this principle may be illustrated when a skull fracture is seen in a lateral radiograph in the parietal region but the side of the fracture is uncertain. Stereoscopic lateral films are first superimposed so that the images of the sella turcica are aligned. The films are then moved over one another until the images of the side markers are aligned. If during this process the images of the fracture diverge, the fracture is on the side of the skull away from the film. If the images of the fracture converge and cross, then the fracture is on the side of the skull near the film.

REFERENCES

Daves, M. L., and Dalrymple, G. V.: Objective stereoscopy, Radiology **78**:802-805, 1962.

Davidson, J. M.: Localization by x-rays and stereoscopy, New York, 1916, Paul B. Hoeber, Inc.

CHAPTER 6

Tomography of the skull

J. T. Littleton

Roentgenography of the skull presents many technical problems, of which the primary one is the wealth of superimposition of disturbing shadows on the area of interest. As examples, sinus shadows obscure middle fossa structures in anteroposterior views, and the petrous pyramids obscure temporomandibular joints in lateral views. Precise positioning, special head units, attention to film quality, stereoscopy, and other techniques have been employed to improve detail; but none is as effective as tomography in separation of disturbing shadows. Properly employed pluridirectional body-section radiography can significantly increase the retrievable information from roentgen studies of the skull by selectively isolating specific areas of interest. This modality actually represents a new dimension in diagnostic radiology and elevates tomography from an ancillary method to a primary roentgen approach.

I wish to express my appreciation to Mrs. Mary Lou Durizch, R.T. She contributed immeasurably to the scientific and technical aspects of this material, prepared the illustrations, and reviewed the manuscript. At her own insistence, she is not listed as a coauthor.

The intelligent use of this modality requires a basic understanding of the physical principles that influence the development of a tomographic image. In simplest form a tomogram is a roentgen image of a predetermined plane of tissue. The image is recorded by having the tube and film in motion in opposite directions at the time of filming. Only those structures in the plane of focus will be sharply recorded while elements outside the focal plane will be displaced on the film and hence blurred out. The optimal tomogram presents the clearest picture of the focal plane with the least interference from superimposed blur. The direction of the tube-film motion during the tomographic movement has a greater influence on the resulting tomograms than does any other single element of the tomographic system. In general, two basic types of blurring movement are recognized: linear movement and nonlinear or pluridirectional movement.

Recent studies (Littleton, 1964; Stieve, 1964; Littleton and Winter, 1965) would suggest that a linear obscuring movement does not actually develop a tomographic image. Therefore, tomography of the skull should be performed only with a device that provides a satisfactory pluridirectional movement.

BASIC BLURRING PATTERNS

As previously indicated, a tomogram is composed of the *image of the focal plane* plus *blur*. The blur represents any component that contributes to the unsharpness of the resultant picture or in any way distorts the image of the plane of focus. The optimal effect from the blur, therefore, is to accomplish maximum effacement of disturbing shadows outside the focal plane with a minimal disturbance of the focal plane image. A number of blurring movements are available in present tomographic devices. These are linear (in any direction), elliptic, circular (with small and large angles), hypocycloidal (or variations thereof), various spirals, and pseudosinusoidals. In previous communications Littleton (1964) and Littleton and Winter (1965) described a simple phantom on which the effectiveness of the different types of obscuring movements can be determined. By separating the blur from the image of the focal plane, separate examination of the picture of the focal plane and of the quality of the blur is possible. The phantom consists of two identical simple geometric patterns made of 0.010-inch copper wire. One pattern is located in the plane of focus (Fig. 6-1, *A*), and the other (Fig. 6-1, *B*) is positioned outside the focal level. In a tomogram of the test object, the first pattern is located in the focal plane and represents an image of this plane. The second pattern is effaced and represents the blur pattern of any element layer outside the focal plane.

The most basic axiom of tomography implies that *objects perpendicular to the plane of section are maximally blurred whereas those portions of the object parallel to the plane of section are not blurred but are merely elongated.* When a linear obscuring movement is employed (Fig. 6-2, *B*), these basic axioms may be appreciated visually. The wires that are perpendicular to the obscuring ray are blurred maximally. The parallel wires are not blurred but are merely elongated, with progressive blurring of the arcs. Further, the blur pattern

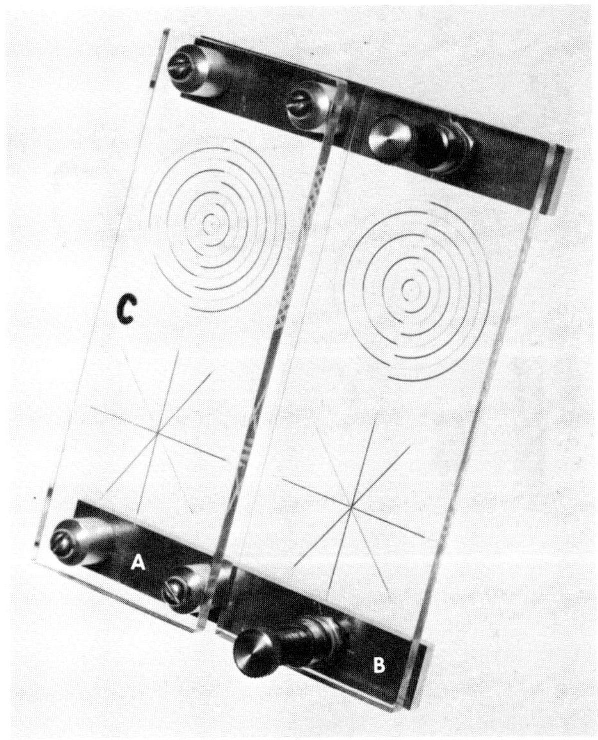

Fig. 6-1. Linear phantom consisting of two identical patterns, one of which, **A,** is permanently located in plane of focus and marked *C*. The other, **B,** can be moved on micrometer scale for a distance of 1.0 cm on either side of plane of focus.

of the arcs of different radii differs. If we change the relation of the phantom to the long axis of the obscuring movement, a different blurring pattern results. This pattern is again related to the obliquity of the object to the obscuring ray. The blurring pattern created by a linear tube-film movement depends therefore on the orientation of the object in the linear blurring system. The blur pattern will always reflect the predominant direction of the obscuring movement.

An elliptic movement (Fig. 6-2, *C*) retains the linear element in its blurring pattern. Increased blur results from the additional change of direction of the tube-film blurring system, but the basic linear elements still prevail.

A circular movement provides a uniform blur (Fig. 6-2, *D*). A sharp cutoff line develops, however, at the margin of the blur, consistent with the constant radius of the circle. If the radius of the object to be blurred happens to coincide with the radius of the obscuring movement, a false shadow may be created by virtue of the incomplete blur. Also, as the separation increases, the blur pattern from the circular movement widens until the sharp cutoff margins fuse. A picture is thereby created that is the mirror image of the object being blurred (Fig. 6-3). This phenomenon explains the occurrence of false shadows in circular blurring systems, particularly with respect to regularly recurring objects to be blurred, such as the teeth.

A uniform blur with significant marginal dissociation of the blur is seen with a hypocycloidal movement (Fig. 6-2, *E*). A similar type of marginal blur is seen with spiral movements of more than one and one half spirals. With a pseudosinusoidal movement a somewhat similar pattern is also seen.

FOCAL PLANE IMAGE

The second factor to consider in the development of the tomogram is the quality of the focal plane image. The roentgen image of the focal plane is governed by the same principles that affect formation of an x-ray image in any system. One aspect of image formation, however, is not well appreciated; yet it does influence the appearance of the tomographic image in the focal plane significantly. This aspect concerns the *law of tangents* as described by Ziedses des Plantes (1932). For example, in any x-ray system the image is formed by the differential absorption of roentgen rays as they pass through tissues of variable density. Although this absorption creates a difference in grayness on the film, it does not actually produce a picture. Those elements of the objects that are tangential to the roentgen ray (such as rays *A, B, C,* and *D* in Fig. 6-4) record marginal shadows that actually represent the image-forming elements of the roentgenogram. In effect, the steepest contrast gradi-

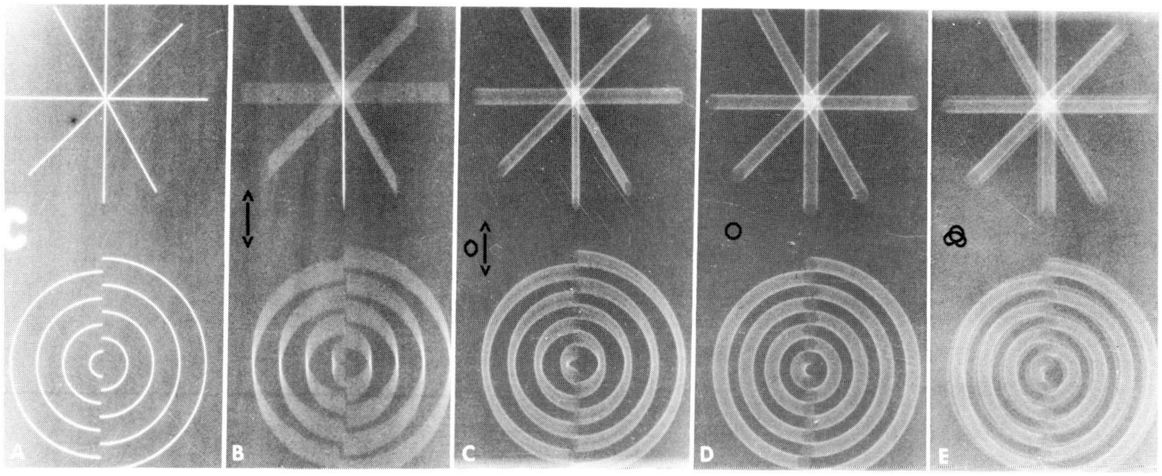

Fig. 6-2. Basic blur pattern of four obscuring movements are as follows: **A,** Focal plane image. **B,** Linear blur pattern. **C,** Elliptic. **D,** Circular. **E,** Hypocycloidal. Note the sharp cutoff margin of the circular movement and the excellent marginal dissociation of blur pattern of the hypocycloidal movement.

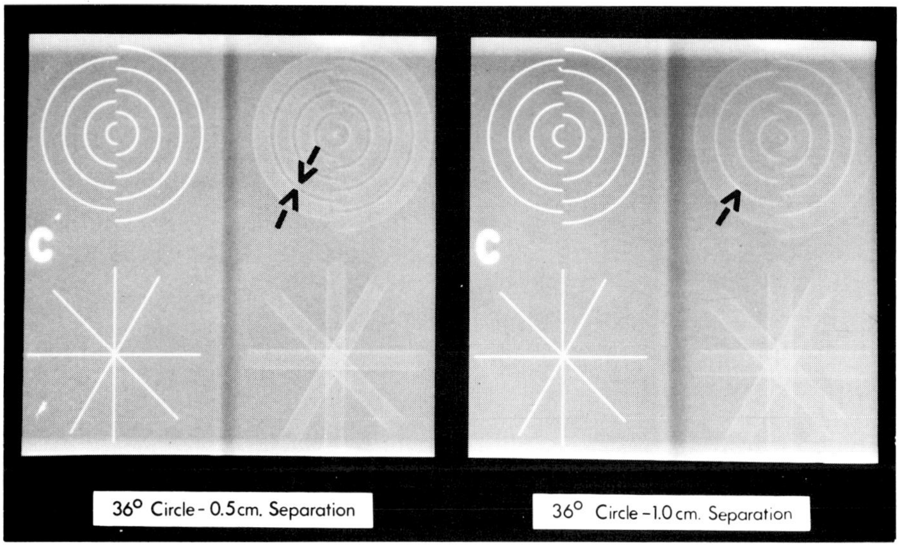

Fig. 6-3. When test pattern *B* (Fig. 6-1) is separated 0.5 to 1.5 cm from focal plane, circular blur pattern widens to cause fusion of sharp cutoff margins to develop false shadows, which in this instance are mirror image of original pattern *C*. These are factitious shadows created by circular blurring movements.

ents at the tangential margins of the object are recorded. A plastic cone (Fig. 6-5) may serve as a simple example. When filmed from above, the shape of the object or whether the cone is inverted or everted cannot be determined. The resultant roentgenograms (Fig. 6-6, *A* and *B*) are identical because the tangential margins are the same and the amount of absorbing material is identical. The differences in grayness are the same between the two films. The true geometry of the cone is not visualized until the object is placed in the full lateral position (Fig. 6-6, *C*), when the geometric shape is recorded as tangential shadows. Therefore the movement with an obscuring ray that undergoes the greatest change in direction will experience the greatest number of tangential occurrences. Hence this movement provides the most complete image of the elements of the focal plane. In 1964 Stieve illustrated this point with a small plastic phantom. Holes were drilled radially in this phantom at 5° increments to a maximum inclination of 20°. A tomogram through the midplane of this phantom gave a

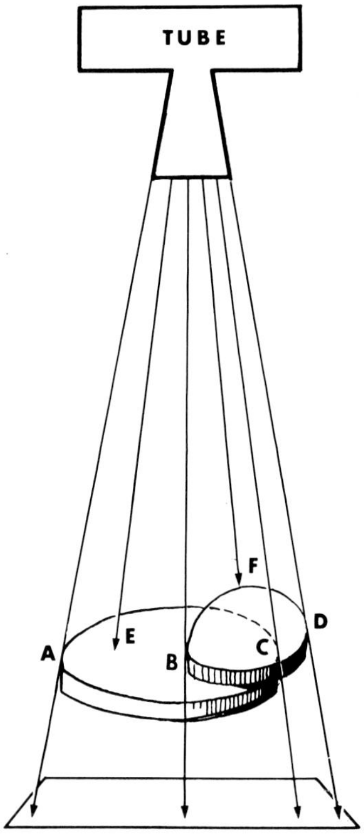

Fig. 6-4. Simple diagrammatic representation of law of tangents. Rays *E* and *F* are absorbed in mass of object and contribute only to variations in grayness. Picture-forming elements are tangents *A, B, C,* and *D.*

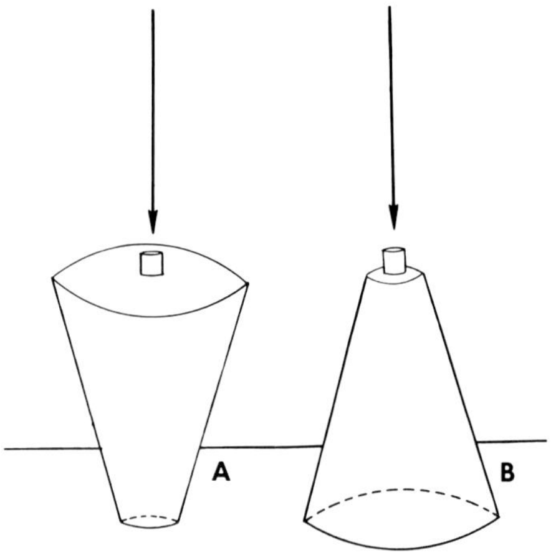

Fig. 6-5. Line drawing of plastic cone in everted position, **A,** and inverted position, **B.**

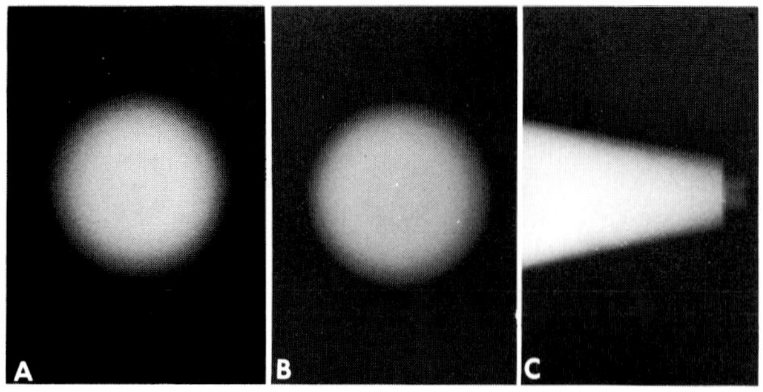

Fig. 6-6. Roentgenograms of plastic cone in everted position, **A,** and inverted position, **B.** Shape or position of object cannot be determined from resultant roentgenograms. Only in lateral position, **C,** is correct geometry of cone recorded in roentgen image.

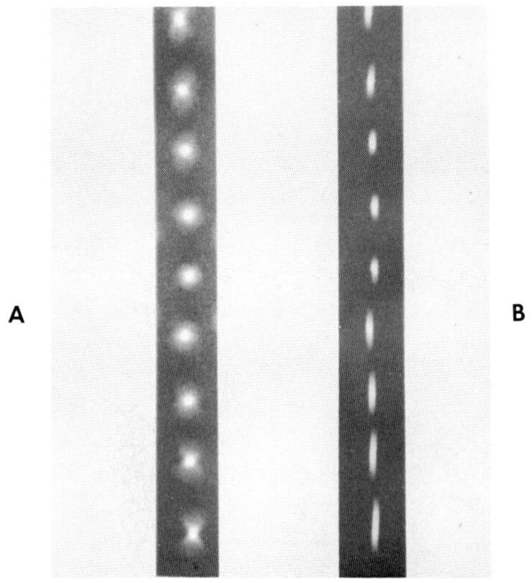

Fig. 6-7. Two segments from Stieve phantom to illustrate fundamental limitations of image formation. With hypocycloidal movement, **A,** increased tangential occurrences of x-ray beam during this compound movement result in an accurate record of cut surface of drill holes at all angles. **B,** Linear obscuring movements incompletely record tangential image of object in focal plane. In no position is complete marginal image of drill holes recorded.

circular image for perpendicular holes and an ellipse for the inclined holes at the periphery. A linear tomogram through the central plane of the test object showed incomplete blurring and elongation of the roentgen images of the drilled holes (Fig. 6-7, *B*). A hypocycloidal movement (Fig. 6-7, *A*) produced an accurate image that consisted of simple cross sections of the hole with a circular image in the central portion and an oval appearance of the inclined holes at the periphery. Of all the available blurring systems, the linear movement provides the least number of marginal occurrences and, consequently, provides the poorest record of the image of the focal plane.

The application of these principles to tomography of the skull is striking. A human skull (Fig. 6-8, *A*) was embedded in plastic and sectioned into multiple coronal sections each 2 mm thick (Fig. 6-8, *B*). A plain plastic phantom was constructed of opal plastic dummies of each layer (Fig. 6-8, *C*). By substituting the dummy plastic layers for anatomic layers, the influence of the

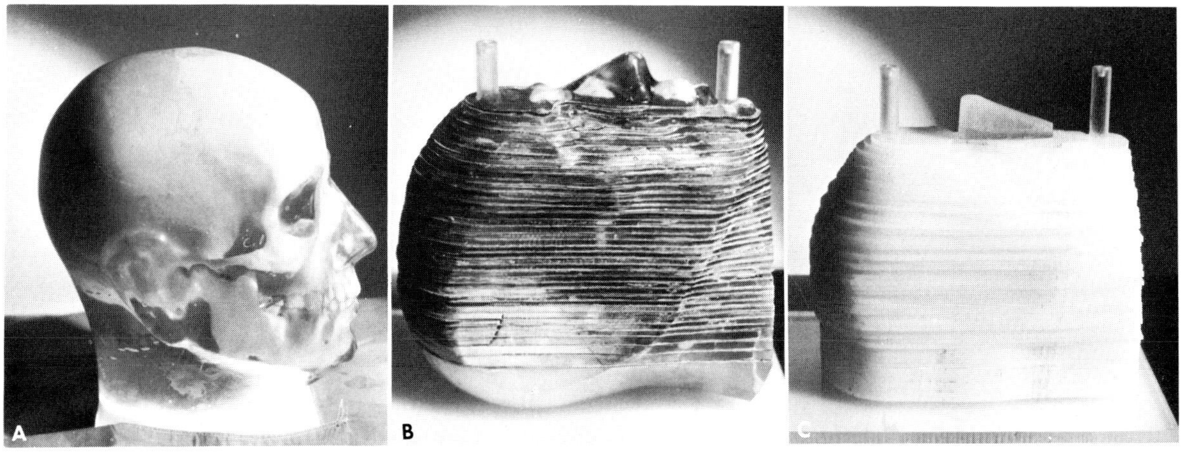

Fig. 6-8. Human skull embedded in human density plastic, **A,** was sectioned into 2 mm sections, **B,** and identical plastic models, **C,** of each section were made.

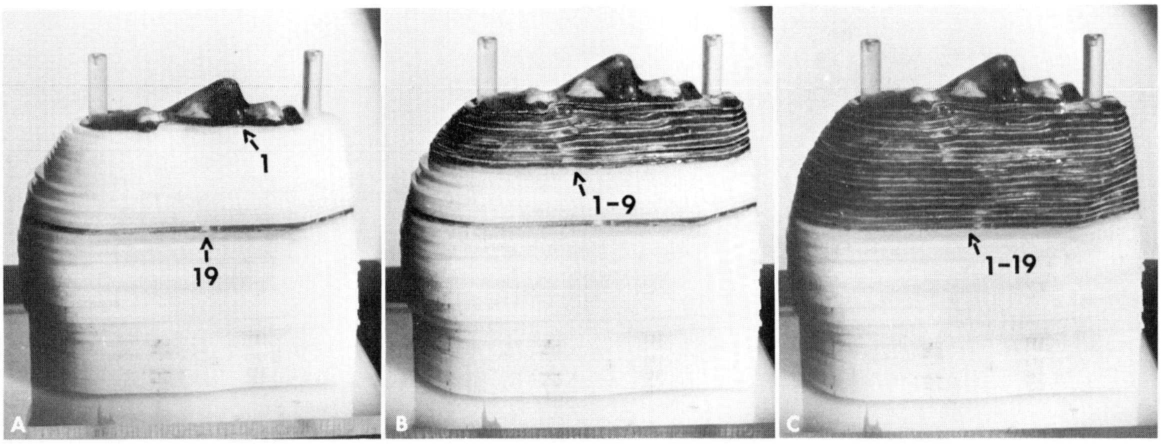

Fig. 6-9. By substituting plastic layers for layers of human skull, one may simulate influence of any predetermined layer or layers. For example, influence of layer *1* on layer *19* is depicted in **A**; of nine layers on focal plane *19* in **B**; and of eighteen layers on focal plane *19* in **C**.

blur pattern of any element section could be examined on the resulting tomogram. For example, in Fig. 6-9, *A,* only the anatomic section, number *19,* was chosen as the layer of focus. This section comprised approximately the posterior portion of the hard palate and the optic foramina. The first anatomic section containing the nasal bones and teeth was chosen as the layer to be blurred. Successive anatomic layers were added, one at a time, until this portion of the skull was completely reconstructed (Fig. 6-9, *B* and *C*). The original tomograms were then copied on 16 mm motion picture film. Projection of this film strip permitted visual examination of the development of the blur pattern of most of the structures of the skull. The influence of the summation of the element tomograms was then represented. Three films of each series were selected for photographic comparison. With a linear longitudinal movement the addition of the first layer showed the influence of the incisor teeth and nasal septum (Fig. 6-10, *A*), even though these structures were about 8 cm out of the focal plane. When half the element layers had been added (Fig. 6-10, *B*), the influence of these structures became more significant. When all the sections of this portion of the skull were reassembled, the linear effect was most striking because much of the detail in the midportion of the film was obscured and distorted (Fig. 6-10, *C*). By turning the tube movement 90° to a transverse direction, the linear effect was much less striking because the structures to be blurred were then perpendicular to the plane of section (Fig. 6-11). Those portions of the object parallel to the plane of section were still blurred incompletely, for example, the sphenoid ridges (Fig. 6-11, *B*). An elliptic tube movement showed a decided improvement in the residual blur. Again, however, even

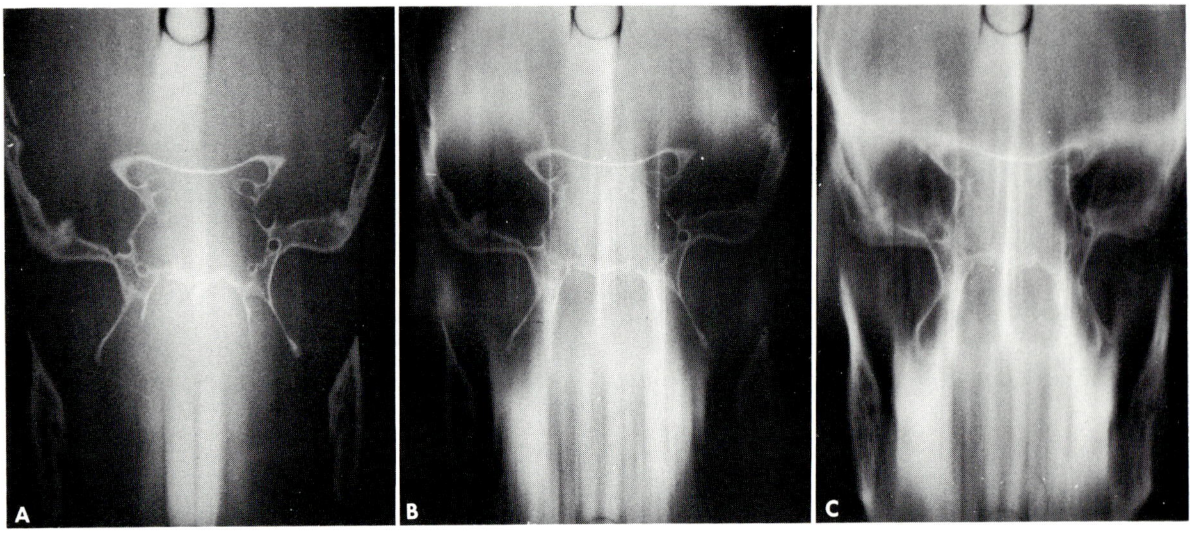

Fig. 6-10. Three tomograms of phantom skull shown in Fig. 6-9. **A,** Influence of even first element layer located 8 cm above focal plane is noted in tomogram. Teeth and nasal septum are incompletely blurred. This incomplete blur and the production of false images by linear movement are augmented when additional layers, **B** and **C,** are added.

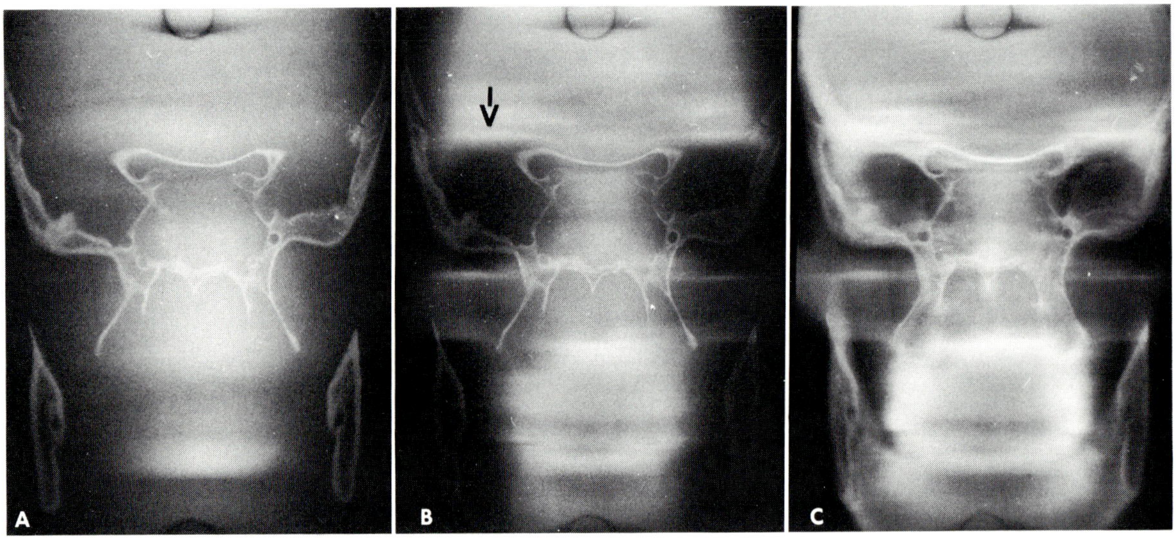

Fig. 6-11. Linear transverse obscuring movement demonstrates fewer extraneous shadows because bony elements to be obscured lie perpendicular to plane of section. Blurring of parallel bony elements is still incomplete, for example, in sphenoid ridges.

in the first film, the shadows of the teeth were still showing (Fig. 6-12, *A*). In the final tomogram (Fig. 6-12, *C*) the laminations of the phantom were clearly shown. These again represented false shadows that developed from the circular element of the ellipse.

A circular tube movement produced a better obscuring effect. As seen in the first film (Fig. 6-13, *A*), the teeth were only vaguely visualized and the roentgenogram was quite satisfactory when all the layers had been added (Fig. 6-13, *C*). False shadows were produced, however. For example, in Fig. 6-14 the shadows of the teeth recurred when circular movements employing different angles were used. Fig. 6-15 illustrates recurring false shadows of the supraorbital ridges that appear with circular movements of various angles. In addition, a circular blurring movement may produce an annulus of blur that may simulate soft tissues in the skull. An example is illustrated in Fig. 6-15, *B,* which shows a marginal blur pattern of the nares that suggests mucosal thickening. This pattern is another type of factitious

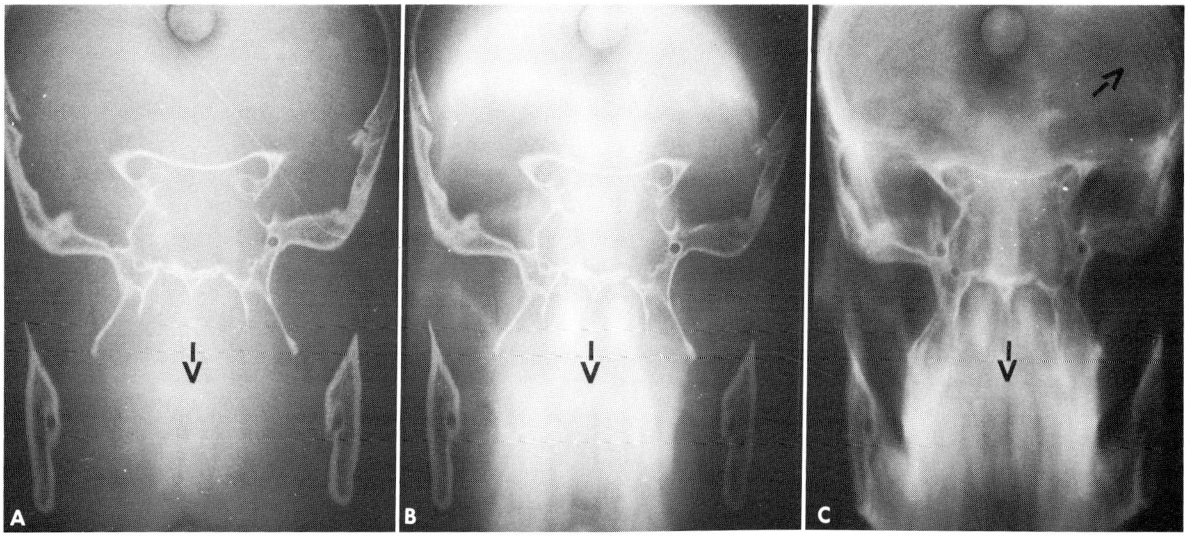

Fig. 6-12. Elliptic obscuring movement shows more nearly complete and uniform blur. Striated effect seen in **C** is probably summation effect arising from superimposition of shadows of laminations of the phantom skull. Also the linear element of this movement can be recognized by persistence of shadows of the teeth.

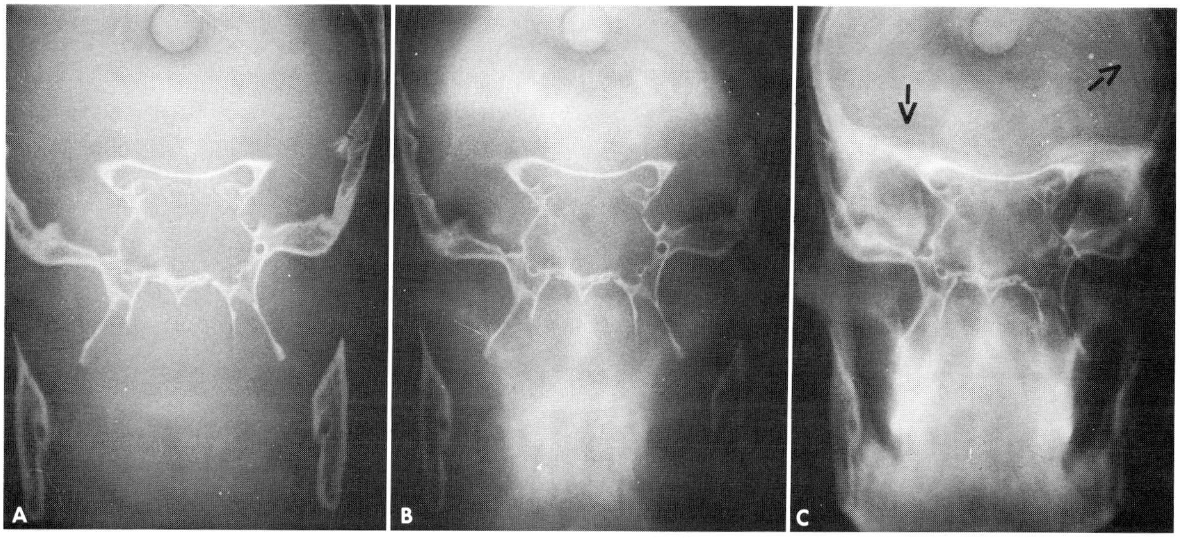

Fig. 6-13. Circular obscuring movement (36° circle) more completely effaces elements of adjacent layers. Shadows of teeth are completely blurred out in **A.** Laminations in **C** are prominent, as they were in elliptic movement, and a false shadow of supraorbital ridge has appeared.

shadow, which may occur with circular movements.

With a hypocycloidal movement the teeth are not recognized in any of the layers and the summation effect of the laminations of the phantom is somewhat less than it is with the circular movement (Fig. 6-16).

A clinical example is even more striking when accuracy of the image produced by linear tomographic movements is compared with that from a satisfactory pluridirectional motion. The tomogram of the base of the skull of a living patient, illustrated in Fig. 6-17, *A,* was obtained with hypocycloidal motion. Most of the basal structures were well defined, such as the posterior portion of the sphenoid sinus, the basiocciput, the jugular foramina, the hypoglossal canals, the foramen magnum, and portions of the petrous pyramid. A linear tomogram (Fig. 6-17, *B*) obtained with a 30° angle at the same level, at the same time, on the same patient showed significantly less detail. The posterior wall of the sphenoid sinus was not identified, and the lateral margins of the basiocciput were not seen. The foramina were

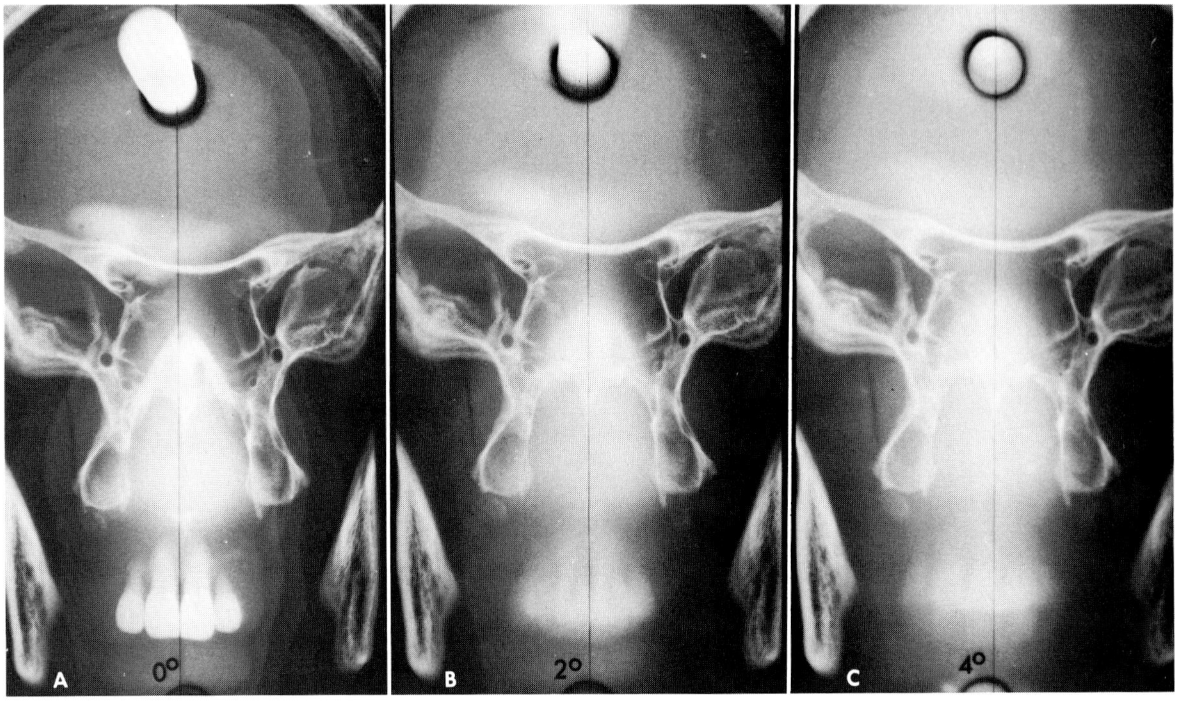

Fig. 6-14. Roentgenograms obtained at various angles to illustrate influence of blur patterns with circular movements. **A,** Layer *1* on focal plane *19* (Fig. 6-9). **B,** With 2° angle, shadows of teeth are fairly well effaced. **C,** At 4°, shadows of teeth have recurred at different location from that on original plain roentgenogram (**A**). These are false shadows occurring in circular blurring system.

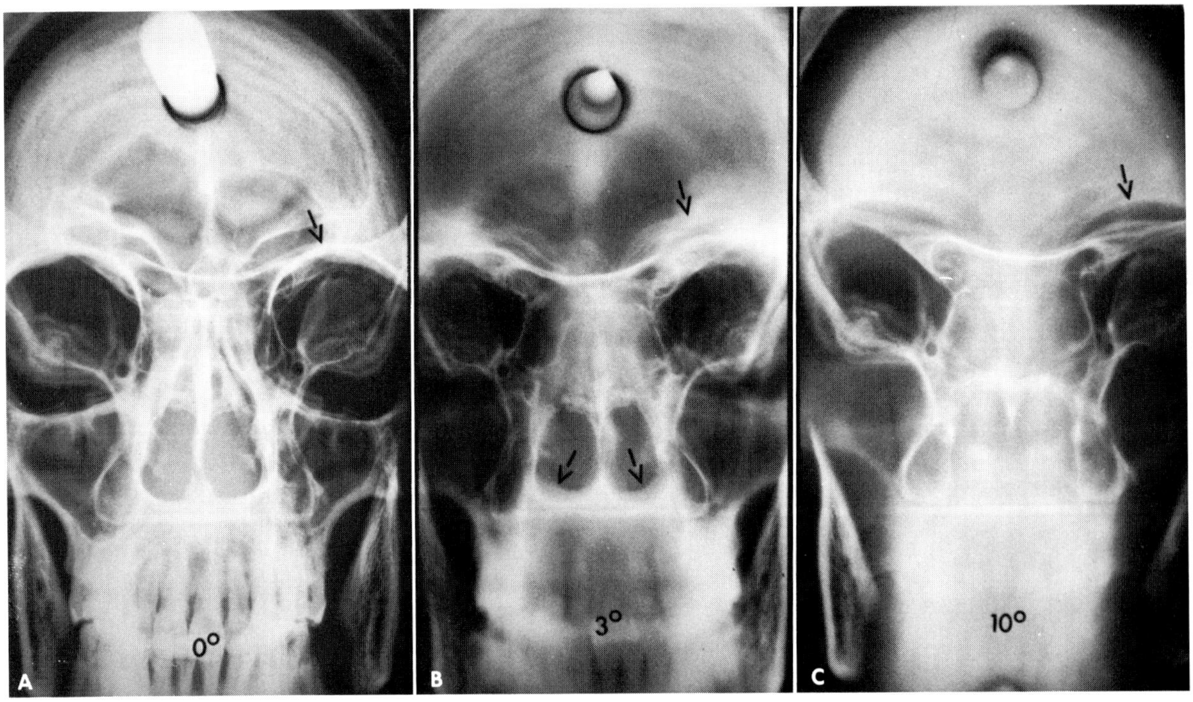

Fig. 6-15. Nine layers superimposed over focal plane as in Fig. 6-9, *B,* illustrate that at 10° circular movement, blur pattern of orbital margin is displaced to simulate shadow of supraorbital ridge. At 3°, annular pattern of nares suggests increase in soft tissue at this level. These are both factitious shadows that could cause confusion on interpretation.

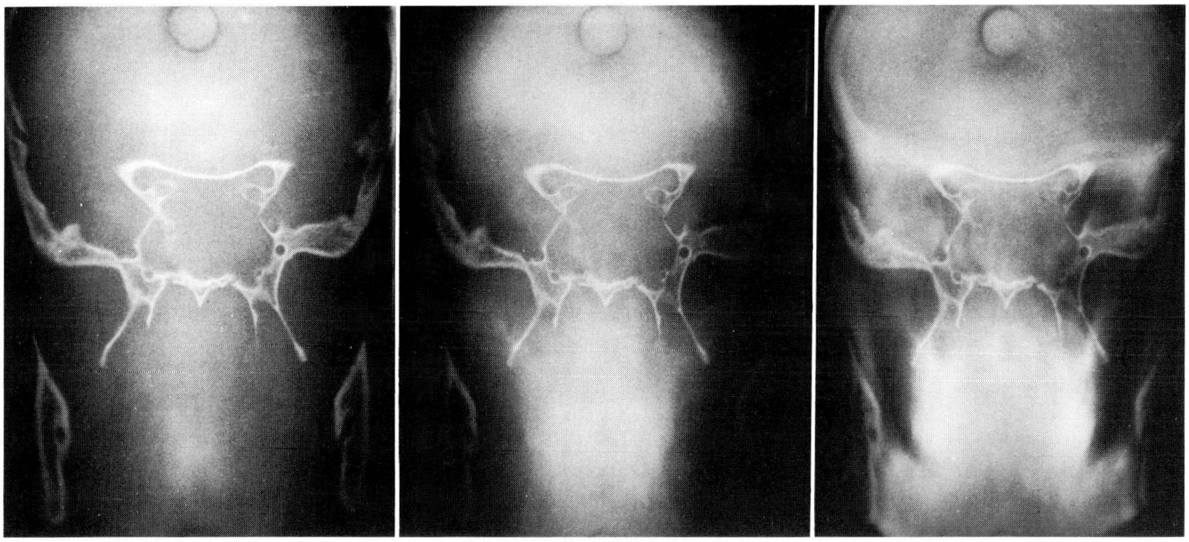

Fig. 6-16. Hypocycloidal obscuring movement shows complete blurring throughout with preservation of focal plane image and absence of false images.

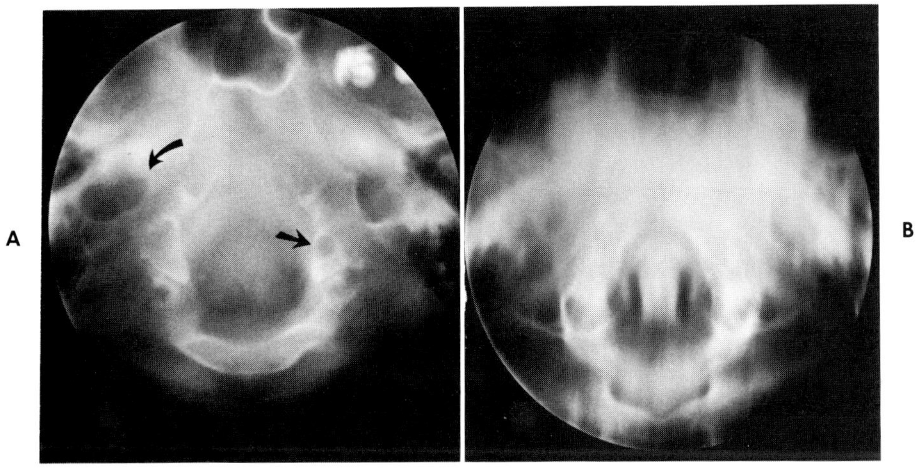

Fig. 6-17. A, Hypocycloidal tomogram of base of skull shows most of normal structures and foramina. **B,** Linear tomogram at same level. Note the incomplete image formation of the basal structures and the incomplete blurring of the odontoid.

poorly visualized, and the shadow of the odontoid, which is not at this level, was clearly visualized.

This evidence indicates clearly that *a good pluridirectional movement is essential for satisfactory tomograms of the skull.*

SECTION THICKNESS

The thickness of any tomographic section is a function of the angle subtended during the tube-film movement. (The thickness of a linear section cannot be measured since it varies with the relationship of the object to be blurred to the tomographic movement.) If the thickness of the section is plotted against the angle of the section with circular movements, a hyperbolic function results (Fig. 6-18). The change in section thickness is greatest with angles between 0° and 10° (decreasing from infinity at 0° to a section 5 mm thick at 10°), and there is only a 4 mm decrease in thickness with all angle changes from 10° to 48°.

In general, the choice of thickness of the tomographic section relates to the body organ of interest and its relation to the objects to be blurred. When objectionable shadows to be effaced are some distance from the plane of interest, a small blurring angle is employed (1° to 10°). In the skull, however, where an abundance of objectionable shadows is superimposed, the widest possi-

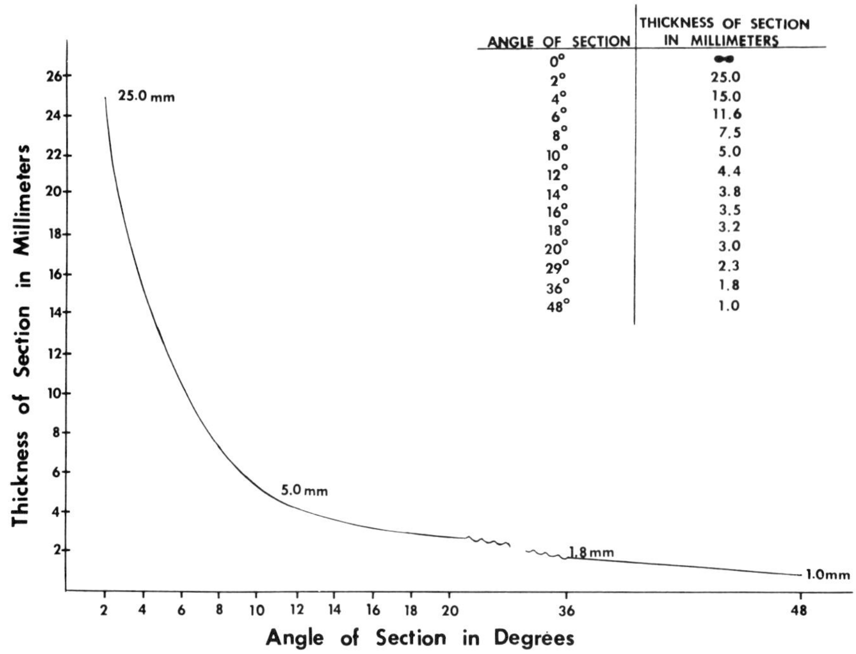

ANGLE OF SECTION	THICKNESS OF SECTION IN MILLIMETERS
0°	∞
2°	25.0
4°	15.0
6°	11.6
8°	7.5
10°	5.0
12°	4.4
14°	3.8
16°	3.5
18°	3.2
20°	3.0
29°	2.3
36°	1.8
48°	1.0

Fig. 6-18. Plotting angle of section against thickness of section in millimeters proves to be a hyperbolic function. Greatest influence of angular change appears between 0° and 10°.

ble angle is required to produce maximal effacement of objects in neighboring element layers. There is a geometric limit, however, for section angles greater than 60° produce geometric distortion in the focal plane image sufficient to negate the reduction in section thickness. A tomographic section about 1 mm thick provides satisfactory tomograms of the structures of the skull, including the middle ear. If a view is desired of the ventricular system outlined with air or of a segment of the curved calvarium or large calcified lesions within the cranial vault, then a thicker section may be employed.

OTHER FACTORS AFFECTING TOMOGRAM

In any tomographic system, blurring is progressive; hence some blur will always be inherent, which is characteristic of the obscuring movement and the pendular angle. The secret of a good tomogram is to keep the blur to a minimum. The difference between a high-quality tomogram and a poor one is slight; therefore attention to all those other factors that influence the focal plane image is extremely important. The addition of any unwanted blur makes the difference between a "blurogram" and a tomogram of highest diagnostic quality.

General factors that influence the tomogram are as follows:

1. *Tube-pivot/pivot-film distance* defines the geometry of the section, the magnification, and any distortion. Magnification is not undesirable, for it facilitates visualization of the smaller structures, particularly in areas such as the middle ear. The inherent blur is also magnified, but this does not appear to be objectionable.
2. *Mechanical properties of the device* must be such that no unwanted motion occurs during the obscuring movement. This quality can be easily checked by roentgen exposure through a pinhole in a lead diaphragm to provide a tracing of the obscuring movement. The tracing should contain no aberrant motion.
3. *Use of the proper film and screen thickness* is important. For areas of high contrast, single emulsion film may be an advantage and good screen contact is imperative.
4. *Wave form and beam quality* are important in that it is desirable to approximate a monochromatic beam as closely as possible. A three-phase generator provides a noticeable advantage and is more sparing of tube life than is a single-phase generator.
5. *Size of the focal spot* is extremely important. In every instance the focal spot should be the smallest obtainable. A 0.3 mm focal spot provides the most satisfactory tomograms of the middle ear, although a 0.6 mm focal spot is acceptable. Survey tomograms of coarser structures, such as the facial bones, may be obtained with a 1.2 mm focal spot. In general, however, it is desirable to use the smallest focal spot permissible.
6. *Control of secondary radiation* by means of suit-

Table 6-1. Modern pluridirectional tomographic devices

Apparatus	*Manufacturer*	*Domestic distributor*	*Pluridirectional movement*	*Range of section thickness with pluridirectional movement*
Polytome Universal Polytome Horizontal	Massiot Philips, Paris, France	Philips Medical Systems, Inc.	Elliptic, circular, hypocycloidal	Zonography to 1.0 mm
Multi-Planigraph	Siemens-Reiniger-Werke, Erlangen, Germany	Siemens Corp.	Elliptic, circular	1.1 mm (40° ellipse) 1.6 mm (30° circle) (measurement by author)
Pluristrator Eurostrator	Zuder, Genoa, Italy	Schick X-Ray Corp. All major domestic distributors	Circular Circular, spiral (2 spires)	Zonography to 1.6 mm 25 mm to 1.4 mm
Mimer	Elema-Schonander, Stockholm, Sweden	Elema-Schonander, Inc.	Semicircular (180°)	Not known
Radiotome	Massiot Philips, Paris, France	Philips Medical Systems, Inc.	Circular (axial transverse)	0.8 mm
Layergraph	Toshiba, Tokyo, Japan	Profexray Division, Litton Industries	Circular, hypocycloidal	Zonography to approx. 1.0 mm
Stratomatic	Compagnie Générale de Radiologie, Paris, France	CGR Medical Corp.	Circular, spiral (3 spires)	Zonography to approx. 1.0 mm
Maxitome	General Electric Medical, Liège, Belgium	General Electric Co.	Pseudosinusoidal	1.4 mm
Ultragraph	Isotopan, Rome, Italy	Picker Corp.	Circular	Approx. 2.0 mm
Plurigraph	Picker GmbH., Estelkamp, Germany	Picker Corp.	Elliptic, circular	Zonography to approx. 2.0 mm

able grids and maximum collimation is more important to tomography than it is to general roentgenography.

7. *Complete immobilization of the patient* is essential. A head box* is more desirable to immobilize the skull than are the various types of head clamps usually provided with most tomographic devices. The exposure times with the more complex movements are from 3 to 6 seconds, and control of the inherent motion of the patient's head during these long exposure times is essential.
8. *Shortest exposure time permissible* for any given tomographic device is important because it reduces the chance of patient motion. Unfortunately most of the present devices require fairly long exposure times, with the complex pluridirectional movements varying from 3 to 12 seconds.
9. *Developing procedure* should be kept constant. Automatic developing techniques have been entirely satisfactory.
10. *Contrast in a thick-section tomogram* is higher than in a thin-section. Therefore occasions may arise, for example in soft-tissue studies, when the differences of radiographic density of structures under examination are so slight that thick-section tomography will give more information than thin-section tomography even though the blurring effect is less satisfactory.

TOMOGRAPHIC DEVICES WITH MULTIDIRECTIONAL BLURRING

The employment of linear tomography has proved to be of limited use in any area, especially in the skull. Therefore, attention will be given only to those tomographic devices that provide pluridirectional movements. Approximately twelve new tomographic devices have come to my attention, and all but two of these have been described completely in a previous communication (Brünner et al., in press). Table 6-1 identifies the modern pluridirectional devices that are known to me. There may well be other units of which I have no knowledge. The tomographic devices commercially available are, with one exception, manufactured in Western Europe.

*Obtainable from Nosivol Specialty Co., Box 741, Temple City, Calif. 91780.

They are identified in Table 6-1 by their trade name, manufacturer, domestic distributor, tomographic movements, and section thickness when known.

Polytome

The Polytome is offered in two models, Universal and Horizontal. The former is constructed on a heavy base so that the entire unit can be raised to a 90° position, permitting tomography of erect patients. This feature is essential if air myelography of the spinal canal is desired and also when tomography is desirable during pneumoencephalography. Examinations of the lower cervical spine in the lateral projection are technically easier in the erect position, which permits better depression of the shoulders. The erect position is also used when fluid levels are sought and when there are small pulmonary lesions adjacent to the diaphragm. The occasional patient with orthopnea also must be examined in the erect position. All other tomographic procedures may be performed by means of horizontal tomography.

Both the Universal and the Horizontal units have the same tomographic system, namely, the x-ray tube and film tray situated at opposite ends of a jointed parallelogram. The tabletop moves through the plane of focus, a feature that is most desirable in providing a fixed tomographic system with a constant magnification factor at any tomographic level. Both Polytome models are provided with linear, elliptic, circular, and hypocycloidal blurring movements with a range of small circular movements in the area of zonography. The thinnest section, approximately 1 mm, is produced by the hypocycloidal movement with a pendular angle of 48°. Blurring above and below the intended plane of focus is complete. The Universal model can be used for conventional roentgenography to a limited degree when it is set for a 0° circle. The Horizontal model has provisions for complete general roentgenography. The layer height in both units is adjustable through a range of 23 cm, and on the newer units the layer height adjustments are motor driven at 1 mm increments.

Multi-Planigraph

The Multi-Planigraph is a multipurpose table for the examination of recumbent patients. It permits body-section roentgenography with linear, elliptic, and circular blurring. It also serves as a conventional Bucky table with vertical or oblique beams. The tube may be detached from the table and be used in combination with other examination units such as a Bucky wall stand, vertical cassette stand, or similar units. Three blurring movements are provided: linear, circular, and elliptic. Provisions are now available for zonography with circular movements. Two pluridirectional obscuring movements are available, each with a single, relatively wide angle (30° circular and 40° elliptic). These allow section thicknesses of about 1.6 mm and 1.1 mm respectively.

Pluristrator

The Pluristrator is designed specifically for tomography with circular and linear blurring. Adjunctive features include routine roentgenography with and without a Bucky diaphragm and magnification techniques. The objective plane is changed by moving the level of the fulcrum from 1 to 22 cm above the tabletop. Each change of focal plane level therefore alters the degree of magnification of the tomogram. The same is true of all units that change the layer of cut by adjusting the level of the focal plane. This fact must be accounted for when small structures, such as the internal auditory canal, are measured, particularly if the sections are obtained while the head is in the same lateral position for filming each internal auditory canal. The only pluridirectional movement on this device is circular blurring with a wide range of angles (0° to 40°). According to my measurements, section thicknesses for this unit vary from 1.8 to 8.4 mm at one focal plane level.

Eurostrator

The Zuder Company offers a second unit, basically similar in design to the Pluristrator, called the Eurostrator.* This unit is also equipped for standard roentgenography and tomography with linear and circular blurring. In addition, a spiral movement is available that progresses through approximately two spires. The focal plane level is also adjusted by moving the fulcrum from 2 to 24 cm above the tabletop. Exposure angles from 2° to 40° are provided; these permit section thicknesses of from 2.4 cm to 1.4 mm. The change from one technique to another may be done automatically, and interval sections can be preset to function automatically.

Mimer

The universal neuroradiologic unit manufactured by Elema-Schonander, the Mimer, is equipped for unidirectional and multidirectional tomography. For linear motion the patient must be in a sitting position, whereas circular movements may be executed with the patient horizontal. The circular movement provides an arc of only 180°, which compromises the image of the focal plane to some extent. The section level is moved by adjustment of the height of the table.

Radiotome

The Radiotome is adaptable only for axial transverse tomography. The patient rotates in one direction while

*Both units are imported by the Shick X-Ray Corporation and are distributed by all major domestic distributors.

the film, on a platform perpendicular to the long axis of the patient, rotates in the opposite direction. The tube is stationary on the wall. Adjustment of the unit is somewhat cumbersome, but a good horizontal axial tomogram approximately 0.8 mm thick can be obtained.

Layergraph

Many of the features described for the Polytome have been incorporated in the Layergraph. This unit was originally presented in two models, LGC-2, equipped only for circular blurring, and LGC-3, which provides both circular and hypocycloidal blurring movements. The two models are basically similar in design, differing only in the gear mechanism to provide the hypocycloidal movement. Conventional roentgenography is possible. The tube and Bucky tray are located at opposite ends of a jointed parallelogram and are attached to a gear box by a simple yoke. The focal plane is fixed, as in the Polytome, with an enlargement factor of 1.23×. This unit is being redesigned, and the new units have not yet come to the United States.

Stratomatic

The Stratomatic is a new device developed by the Compagnie Générale de Radiologie, in Paris, and is being distributed in the United States by the CGR Medical Corporation. It has provisions for tomography (in horizontal positions) with linear, circular, and trispiraled blurring movements. Circular movements in the area of zonography of from 0° to 20° are available with preset circles of 6°, 20°, 30°, and 45°. Exposure times vary from 25/100 to 6 seconds. The compound movement is trispiraled with an angular displacement beginning at 45° and decreasing to 12°. This tomographic movement will provide a thin section, about 1 mm thick. The Stratomatic provides for versatile conventional roentgenography, automatic sequences of multiple exposures on one film, and pushbutton mode selection.

Maxitome

Another new pluridirectional device is the Maxitome, manufactured by General Electric Medical, in Liège, Belgium. This new unit will be distributed by the parent company, General Electric, in the United States. It is somewhat similar in design to the Multi-Planigraph and provides for tomography only in horizontal positions. The blurring movements are linear in multiple directions and pseudosinusoidal. Only a prototype unit has been developed, and the device is being redesigned. Zonography is possible with a small-angle linear movement, and the pseudosinusoidal movement is estimated to provide a section about 1.4 mm thick. Preset indicators on this device allow layer change and automatic, sequential, multiple exposures on one film. Provisions for general roentgenography are also included.

Ultragraph

The Ultragraph is a universal x-ray unit designed for linear and circular tomography, neuroradiography, and special procedures. The unit also serves for routine and casualty roentgenography and for magnification techniques. It consists of an L-arm, a C-arm, a vertical stand, and a control console.

Linear tomography may be performed on any angle of the L-arm and C-arm for unlimited projections. A choice of four angles, 8°, 16°, 20°, and 40°, is available. Circular tomography is possible at any angle of the L-arm with the C-arm perpendicular to it. Only a single angle of 30° is available with exposure times of 3 or 4.7 seconds. The tomographic properties of this device are therefore somewhat limited, particularly in pluridirectional techniques confined to a single 30° circle.

Plurigraph

The Plurigraph is a second new device that is being imported by the Picker Corporation. I have not yet had a chance to examine the specifications of this device, and only fragmentary information is available. Its basic design is supposedly somewhat similar to that of the Siemens Multi-Planigraph, and the unit is equipped for linear, circular, and elliptic tomography. The circular movements are confined to a 10° movement for zonography and a 30° wide-angle circular movement. Elliptic movement is available at a 30° and a 40° angle. Additional information about the characteristics of this device are obtainable from the Picker Corporation.*

TECHNIQUES TO MONITOR QUALITY OF TOMOGRAPHIC DEVICES

In view of the increasing number of tomographic devices, some basis for comparison of different machines and some technique for periodic checking of their performance are important. The physical properties of a body-section device that affect the picture are mechanical stability, geometric form of the obscuring movement, formation of false images, and thickness of section. Most of these may be evaluated readily by two simple phantoms: a pinhole with a lead diaphragm and a composite phantom† (Fig. 6-19). This technique has been described more completely in a previous communication (Littleton, 1970). The tube-film obscuring movement may be traced with a lead diaphragm in whose center a 2 mm beveled pinhole has been located. The lead diaphragm is positioned about 12 cm outside the plane of focus. An exposure (120 ma at 65 kv) is made through the full cycle of the obscuring movement.

---

*Picker Corporation, 595 Miner Road, Cleveland, Ohio 44143.
†Obtainable from 3-M Company, 3M Center, St. Paul, Minn. 55101.

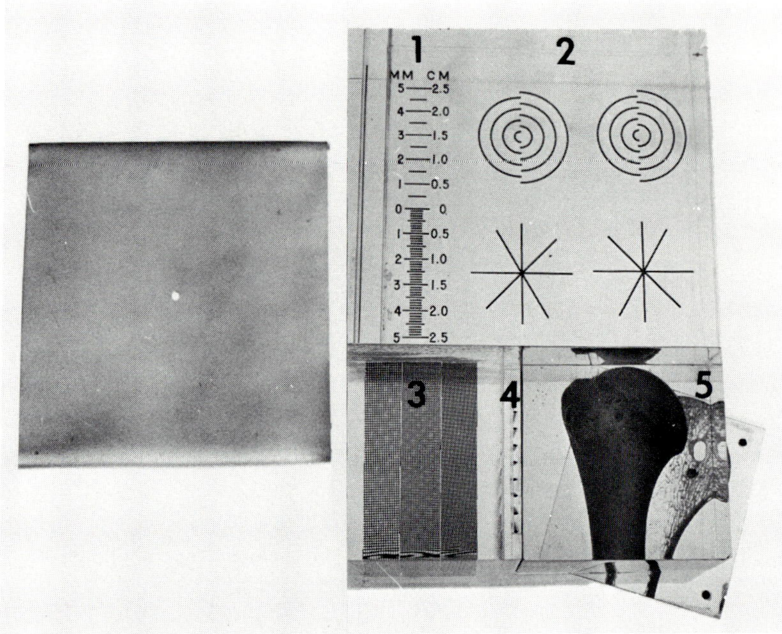

Fig. 6-19. Photograph of pinhole lead diaphragm and compound phantom containing five test patterns to evaluate following qualities of any tomographic system: *1,* thickness of focal plane, magnification, geometric distortion, interval thickness; *2,* focal plane image, blur characteristics; *3,* resolution; *4,* completeness of marginal occurrences of x-ray beam; *5,* quality and accuracy of image of simulated lesion in head of humerus.

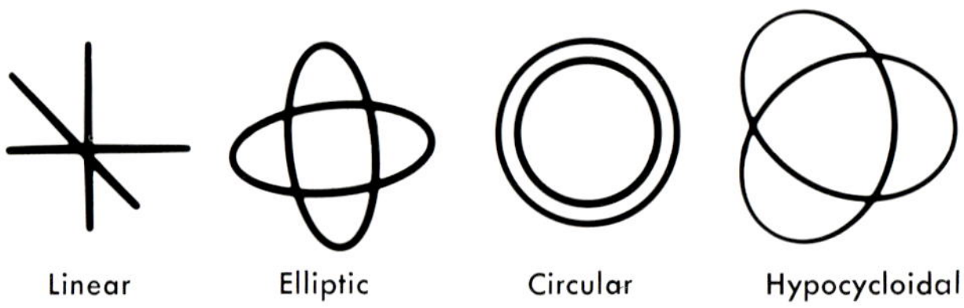

Fig. 6-20. Pinhole tracings of four basic tomographic movements.

The cassette is in the Bucky tray. The resultant patterns provide the following wealth of information:

1. *Geometric form of the movement* (ellipse, circle, hypocycloid, or other) is recorded. Fig. 6-20 is an example of four tracings from the same device all of which show satisfactory performance.
2. *Any mechanical instability in the apparatus* may be apparent in the pinhole tracings. Fig. 6-21, *C,* shows significant unwanted motion during an elliptic movement. This amount of unwanted motion adds additional blur to the tomogram.
3. *Completeness of the exposure* can be evaluated in the tracing. The open section of the elliptic tracing in Fig. 6-21, *B,* indicates that the exposure is not complete throughout the blurring movement. Skip areas of greater magnitude can adversely affect the focal plane image. Fig. 6-21, *E,* is a tracing of a device that should have provided a half circle. The tracing indicates that the tube is energized only during a small arc of the sweep. The effective blurring movement is therefore a small-angle linear sweep rather than a half circle.
4. *Variation in intensity of exposure,* which may be a factor of tube speed, will be noted as a change in the density of the pattern as seen in the spiral tracing in Fig. 6-21, *D.*
5. *Pendular angles* can be measured from the pinhole tracings. A spot exposure is made with the tube in zero position, and its relation to the entire tracing allows the half angles to be checked.
6. *Orientation of the movement* with reference to the long axis of the table is also apparent. Fig. 6-21, *B* and *C,* shows two elliptic patterns, neither of which is aligned with the long axis of the table.

A single exposure of the composite phantom (Fig. 6-19) brings into focus five test patterns on one film (or singly if desired by blocking out the other patterns with lead shields). The first test pattern has been described in detail previously (Littleton, 1965). This device permits the direct reading of section thickness, the accuracy of the section-level indicator, the exactitude of the section intervals, the magnification factor, and geometric distortion. The second pattern consists of two identical

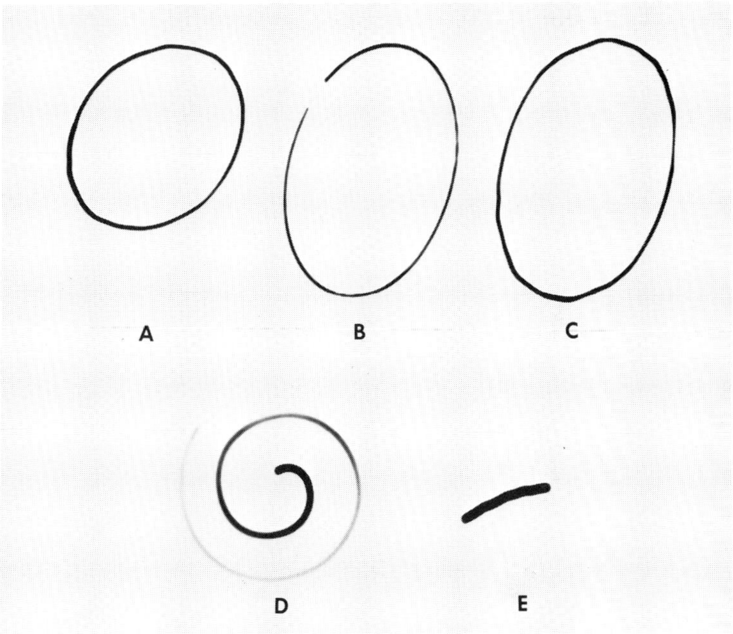

Fig. 6-21. Tracings of five unsatisfactory tomographic devices. **A,** Intended circle is actually describing ellipse oblique to long axis of table. **B,** Elliptic movement shows incomplete exposure. **C,** Elliptic movement oblique to long axis of table illustrates significant unwanted motion. **D,** Spiral movement shows effect of change in tube speed with increasing blackening during central portion of spire. **E,** Tracing from device designed to provide semicircular obscuring movement. Tube is energized only for 20°. Effect of obscuring movement therefore will be that of small-angle linear tracing rather than that of intended semicircle.

designs of 0.010-inch copper wire arranged in arcs and radii. One design is in the plane of focus, and the other 5 mm above the focal plane. The first of these two designs represents the image of the focal plane, and the other the blur from any element layer outside the focal plane. From this test pattern the quality of the blur can be examined and its effectiveness projected. The sharpness of the focal plane image also may be visualized. The third pattern consists of three strips of wire mesh (20, 30, and 50 lines per inch respectively). Each strip is inclined 7°. The focal plane image through the strips provides an evaluation of resolution in the tomogram. A good device should resolve 50 lines per inch. In addition, false-image formation is detected when screen patterns above and below the focal plane level recur.

The completeness of the marginal occurrences of the beam and therefore the accuracy of the roentgen record of the focal plane image may be assessed from the fourth test pattern. This pattern represents one radius of a phantom previously described by Stieve (1964).

The final evaluation of focal plane image can be made in the fifth test pattern in this phantom. The proximal one fourth of a human humerus is embedded in plastic of human density. A simulated lytic lesion, which is removable, is present in the center of the focal plane. A tomogram through the focal plane is then compared to a plain roentgenogram of the focal plane level, and the accuracy of the tomographic image is evaluated.

TOMOGRAPHIC TECHNIQUE

All technical problems of tomography cannot be reviewed completely in this chapter. The exposure time of most tomographic devices is fixed according to the technique selected. For example, a 6-second exposure is necessary for a hypocycloidal movement. For circular movements the exposure varies from 1 to 3 seconds on different devices, and a wide selection of times is possible with linear movements. With a fixed time therefore only the kilovoltage and the milliamperage may be varied. In general, an attempt is made to use the optimal kilovoltage for the part to be examined. The milliamperage, then, becomes the primary variable, and the extent to which it can be varied depends on the particular transformer and control supplying the unit. Optimal tomograms are obtained by minor variations of optimal kilovoltage and major variations of milliamperage. Table 6-2 indicates the suggested techniques for various tomographic studies of the skull. These factors were chosen primarily for the hypocycloidal movement of the Polytome. They are applicable in a general way, however, to most of the other modern pluridirectional devices.

Table 6-2. Sample technique chart

Examination	*Position*	*Movement*	*Interval separation*	*Factors*
Skull	AP, lateral, axial	Hypocycloidal	3-5 mm	AP—kv 65-75 ma 50 Lat—cut 25 ma Axial—add 75 ma Time—6 sec
Sinuses and facial bones	AP, lateral	Hypocycloidal	3-5 mm	AP—kv 60-70 ma 50 Lat—cut 25 ma Time—6 sec
Mandible	AP, lateral	Hypocycloidal	2 mm	AP—kv 60-70 ma 50 Lat—cut 25 ma Time—6 sec
Temporomandibular joints	Lateral, open and closed	Hypocycloidal	2 mm	Lat—kv 65-70 ma 25 Time—6 sec
Nasopharynx	AP, lateral (with Valsalva)	Hypocycloidal	2 mm	AP—kv 60-70 ma 50 Lat—cut 25 ma Time—6 sec
Middle ear	AP, lateral, 20° oblique	Hypocycloidal	AP and obl—1 mm Lat—2 mm	AP—kv 65-75 ma 40-60 Lat—cut 5 kv Obl—add 3 kv Time—6 sec Remove grid
Pneumoencephalogram	AP, lateral	Hypocycloidal, 10° circle	5 mm	AP—kv 65-75 ma 50 Lat—cut 25 ma Time—6 sec (hypocycloidal) 3.2 sec (10° circle)

These techniques have been employed with the following:
- High-speed screens
- Grid unless otherwise specified
- Three-phase generator
- Focal spot 0.3 and 1.2
- Maximum collimation
- Massiot Philips Polytome

REFERENCES

Brünner, S., Valvassori, G. E., and Barrett, A.: Modern thin-section tomography, Charles C Thomas, Publisher. (In press.)

Littleton, J. T.: A visual examination of laminagraphic systems, Amer. J. Roentgen. **91**:1153-1162, 1964.

Littleton, J. T.: A new test object to determine section thickness in any tomographic system, Guthrie Clinic Bull. **34**:166-171, 1965.

Littleton, J. T.: A phantom method to evaluate the clinical effectiveness of a tomographic device, Amer. J. Roentgen. **108**:847-856, 1970.

Littleton, J. T., and Winter, F. S.: Linear laminagraphy. A simple geometric interpretation of its clinical limitations, Amer. J. Roentgen. **95**:981-991, 1965.

Stieve, F. E.: Apparative Ausrustung zur mehr dimensionalen Tomographie, Roentgen-Bl. **17**:369-400, 1964.

Ziedses des Plantes, B. G.: Eine neue Methode zur Differenzierung in der Röntgenographie (Planigraphie), Acta Radiol. **13**:182-192, 1932.

PART II

Skull maturation

CHAPTER 7

Fetal skull

E. Leon Kier

Much information that pertains to the embryology of the skull has accumulated in the anatomic literature, but the fetal period has attracted little neuroradiologic interest (Berkvens, 1950; Theiler, 1963; Potts et al., 1969).

ROENTGEN EVALUATION

Roentgenographic studies of skull development demonstrate the progression of ossification and supplement conventional gross and histologic studies. The development of the fetal skull is critical, and the more we know about it the better will be our understanding of some of the anomalies and variations seen in clinical practice.

The material studied roentgenographically consisted of dry fetal skulls and fetuses preserved in 10% formalin. The fetal ages of the dry skulls were assessed by the occipitofrontal and biparietal diameters (Scammon and Calkins, 1929). The ages of the preserved fetuses were assessed by measurement of the crown-rump length (Patten, 1953) and the occipitofrontal and biparietal diameters and by estimation of the gestation age. The skulls of the preserved fetuses were separated from the cervical spine at the occipitoaxial junction. The intracranial contents were evacuated via the foramen magnum and an incision through the anterior fontanelle. The soft tissues covering the cranium were removed. Roentgenograms of the skulls were obtained in the lateral, anteroposterior, modified anteroposterior (Caldwell), half-axial, and basal projections.

The preserved skulls were then separated by dissection into the occipital, temporal, sphenoid, parietal, frontal, and mandibular components. The separated components were roentgenographed in various projections that simulate their position in the intact skull.

All the roentgenograms were obtained with a Siemens Biangulix rapid x-ray tube, using the 0.25 mm focal spot at a focal-film distance of 32 inches. Kodak type M film in a cardboard holder was used, and the skulls and specimens were placed directly on the cardboard holder.

DEVELOPMENTAL PATTERN

The complex developmental pattern of the skull is well summarized by Davies and Davies (1962).

The calvarial bones develop in the mesenchymal masses that surround the brain. The development of the skull can be classified into three overlapping stages: the membranous stage, the cartilaginous stage, and the ossification stage.

The bones of the mature skull likewise fit into three groups, depending on their origin (Henderson and Sherman, 1964): (1) cartilaginous origin—ethmoid; (2) membranous origin—parietal, frontal, nasal, lacrimal, and zygomatic; vomer, mandible, maxilla, and palate; and (3) mixed cartilaginous and membranous origin—occipital, sphenoid, and temporal.

Membranous stage

At the beginning of the second month of fetal life, thick masses of mesenchyme form around the brain. These first appear in the occipital region, where they surround the notochord and extend forward toward the hypophysis to outline the clivus and dorsum sellae. The mesenchymal masses further extend into the regions of the ethmoid, nasal septum, and greater sphenoid wing and enclose the optic and auditory centers. Plates of mesenchyme also form the future cranial vault. The mesenchyme surrounds the various cranial nerves forming the primitive cranial foramina.

I am grateful to E. S. Crelin, Jr., Ph.D., Professor of Anatomy, Yale University School of Medicine, for his advice and assistance in obtaining the material for dissection.

Cartilaginous stage

Chondrification of the skull begins during the second fetal month and is limited to the base of the skull. Chondrification takes place primarily in three regions: posteriorly around the notochord and the auditory centers, medially around the hypophysis, and anteriorly in the region of the nasal septum. The bones of the base of the skull are thus preformed in cartilage whereas the bones of the vault are ossified in membrane. The cartilaginous skull base—the chondrocranium—is continuous with the cranial vault. Thus the origin of some of the cranial bones is both cartilaginous and membranous. As ossification proceeds, the chondrocranium diminishes in size. At birth the chondrocranial remnants are still present in the nose, sphenoid, and occipital bones, the foramen lacerum, and the spheno-occipital and petro-occipital synchondroses.

Ossification stage

Frontal bones

The frontal bone ossifies from two centers that develop in the external layer of the membranous covering of the brain (Davies and Davies, 1962; Trotter and Peterson, 1966). The centers appear at about the eighth week of fetal life, one in the region of each superciliary arch. From these centers ossification extends upward and backward, to form the orbital plate, and downward, to form the nasal segment. At birth the bone consists of two halves separated by the frontal (metopic) suture.

Roentgenograms of the frontal bones demonstrate the radiating pattern of ossification. The configuration of the orbital plates changes with age so that the distance between the anterior and posterior margins of the orbital plates is increased (Fig. 7-1). This changing config-

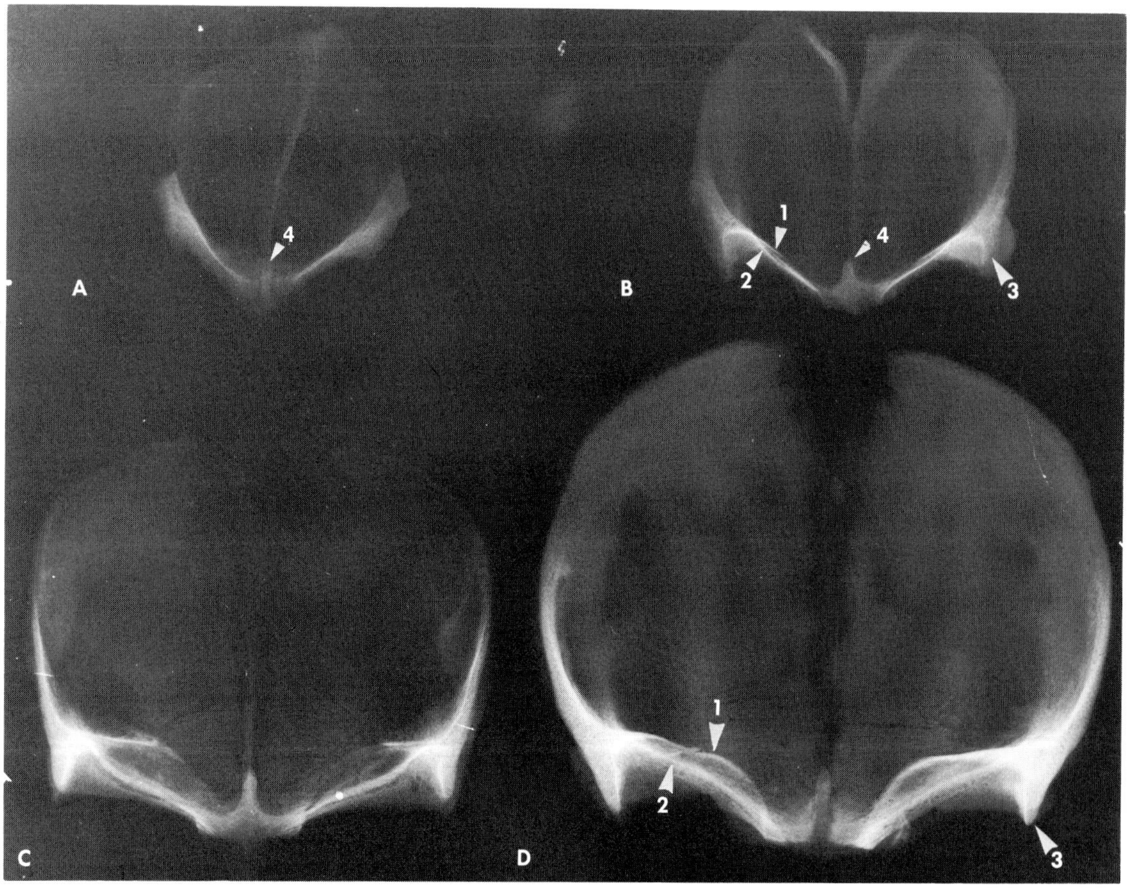

Fig. 7-1. Radiographs of dissected fetal frontal bones: **A,** 12 weeks; **B,** 20 weeks; **C,** 28 weeks; **D,** 36 weeks. Distance between anterior (*1*) and posterior (*2*) margins of orbital plate increases with fetal age. Zygomatic process (*3*) is progressively more caudal in relation to crista galli (*4*). These changes may result from growth of brain and eye. Note the ossifying crista galli at 12 weeks fetal age.

uration is probably the result of increase of ocular size. The zygomatic processes assume a lower position in relation to the crista galli (Fig. 7-1). The lower position of the zygomatic process is probably caused by an increase of brain size.

Ethmoid bone

The crista galli is ossified by the twelfth week of fetal life (Fig. 7-1). This finding contradicts the anatomic literature that describes ossification of the crista during the first year after birth.

Parietal bones

Ossification of the parietal bone begins during the seventh week of fetal life from two centers that form at the region of the parietal tuberosity (Davies and Davies, 1962). They unite early, and ossification extends gradually toward the margins of the bone in a radial manner. The angles of the bone are the last to ossify. Roentgenographic examination reveals the radial ossification and the grooves for the middle meningeal vessels (Fig. 7-2).

Mandible

In about the sixth week of fetal life, the mandible begins to ossify (Davies and Davies, 1962). Each half ossifies in dense membranous tissue from a center near the mental foramen. The condylar regions ossify from separate cartilaginous centers.

Calcification in the deciduous teeth begins during the fifth fetal month, and at birth the crowns are nearly completed (Blount and Lachman, 1966).

The mandibular ossification centers in the 12-week fetus (Fig. 7-3, *A*) and the onset of dental calcification

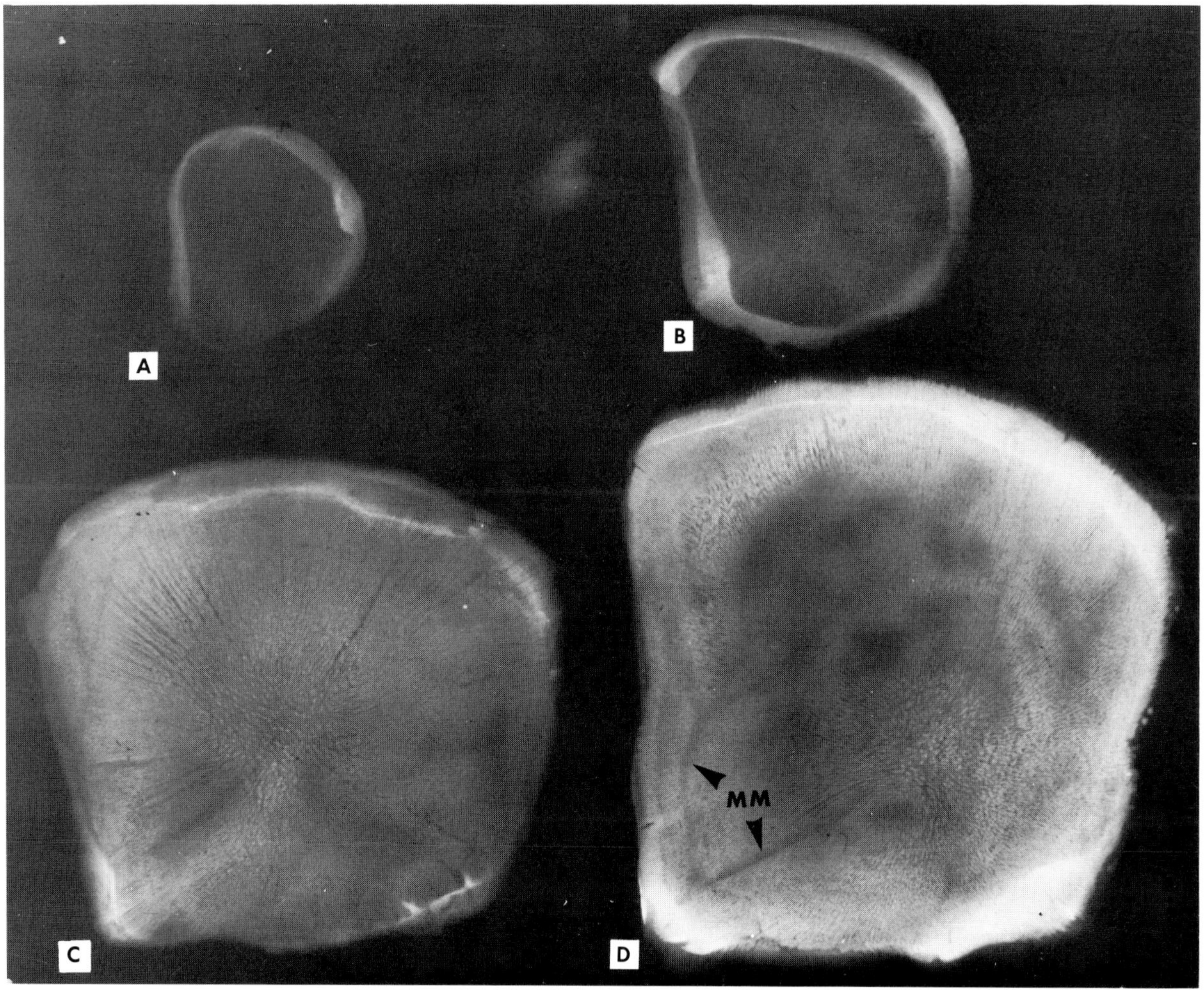

Fig. 7-2. Dissected fetal parietal bones: **A,** 12 weeks; **B,** 20 weeks; **C,** 28 weeks; **D,** 36 weeks. Note the central ossification process in the 20-week fetus. Middle meningeal vascular grooves (*MM*) are present in 36-week fetus.

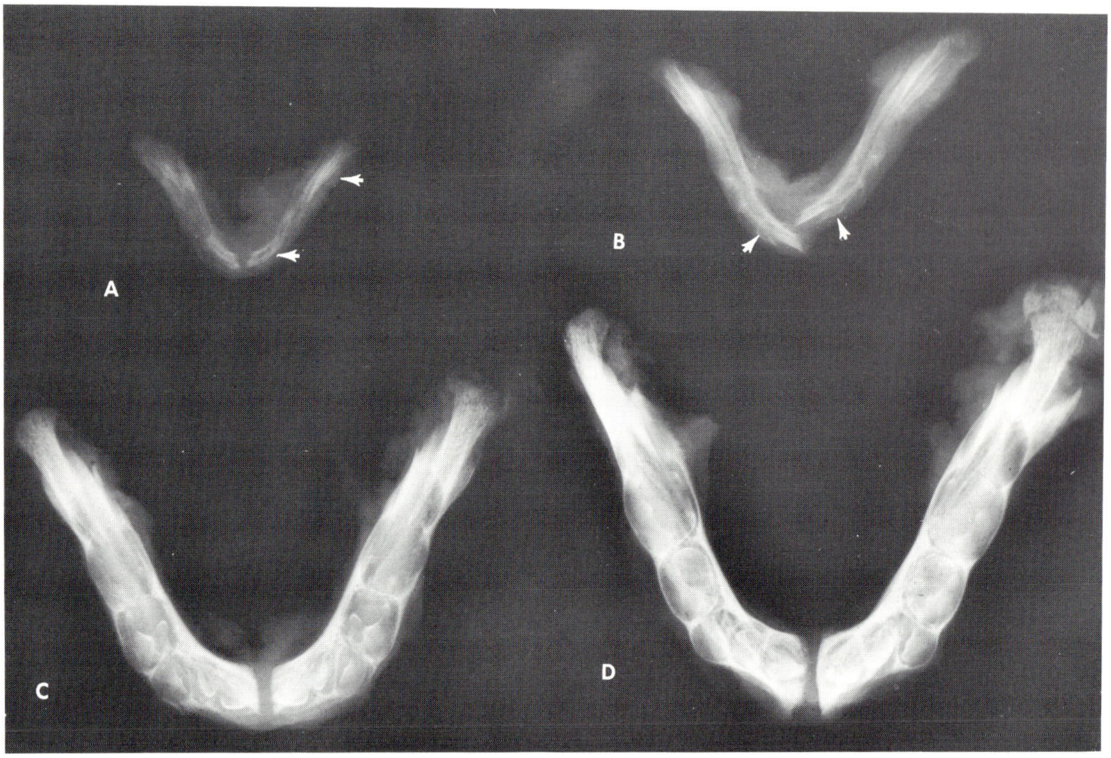

Fig. 7-3. Dissected fetal mandibles: **A,** 12 weeks; **B,** 20 weeks; **C,** 28 weeks; **D,** 36 weeks. Two ossification centers in each half of mandible are well seen in 12-week fetus. Early patterns of calcification of teeth (arrows) are seen in 20-week fetus. Pattern and sequence of calcification of cusp and crown can be followed in 28-week and 36-week fetuses.

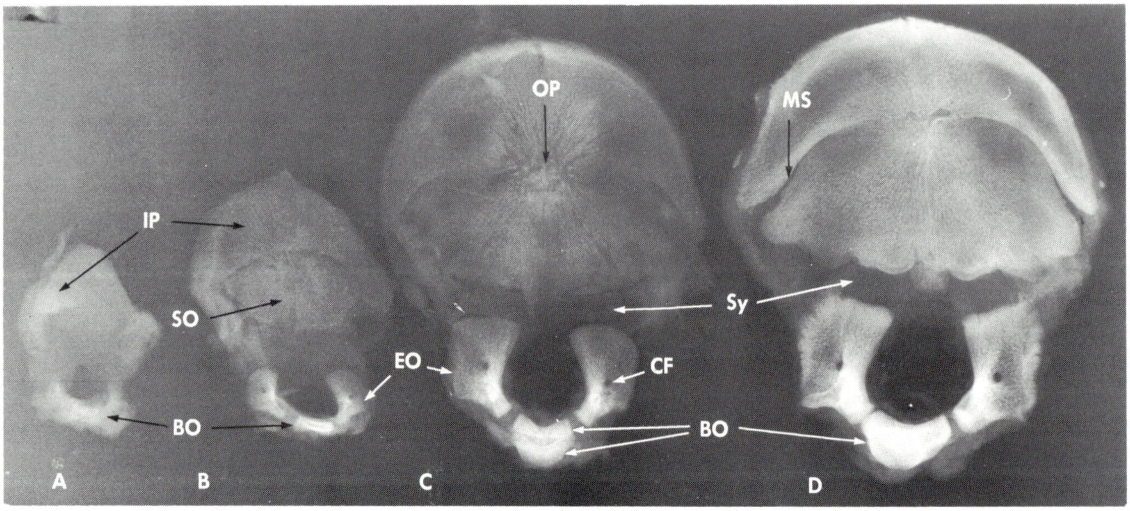

Fig. 7-4. Dissected occipital bones: **A,** 12 weeks; **B,** 20 weeks; **C,** 28 weeks; **D,** 36 weeks. At 12-week stage, basioccipital (*BO*) ossification center is well defined and interparietal (*IP*) center has appeared. Supraoccipital, *SO,* center does not appear until later age. Note that at the 20-week stage (**B**) the occipital squama is becoming a single structure with a central ossification center at the future occipital protuberance (*OP*). Condylar foramen (*CF*) and exoccipital ossification center (*EO*) are indistinct but present at 12-week stage. In later stages these structures are clearly visible. Variability in ossification of synchondrosis region (*Sy*) is demonstrated by greater amount of ossification in 28-week stage than in 36-week fetus. Mendosal suture (*MS*) is shown at 36 weeks.

in the 20-week fetus (Fig. 7-3, *B*) are well seen in roentgenograms.

Occipital bone

The fetal occipital bone consists of four segments that surround the foramen magnum. The basal segment (basioccipital) is anterior, the squamous segment is posterior and inferior, and the lateral segments (exoccipitals) lie on each side of the foramen magnum. These four parts are the result of the ossification pattern of the occipital bone.

At birth the basioccipital, the two exoccipitals, and the squama are separated by strips of cartilage. The squama is formed by the supraoccipital and interparietal ossification centers (Fig. 7-4). The anatomic literature is in agreement that the basal and the two lateral parts are ossified, each from a single center that appears in cartilage from the sixth to twelfth week of fetal life. There is also agreement that the inferior portion of the squama (supraoccipital) is formed in cartilage from two ossification centers and that the superior portion (interparietal) is formed in membrane. Disagreement

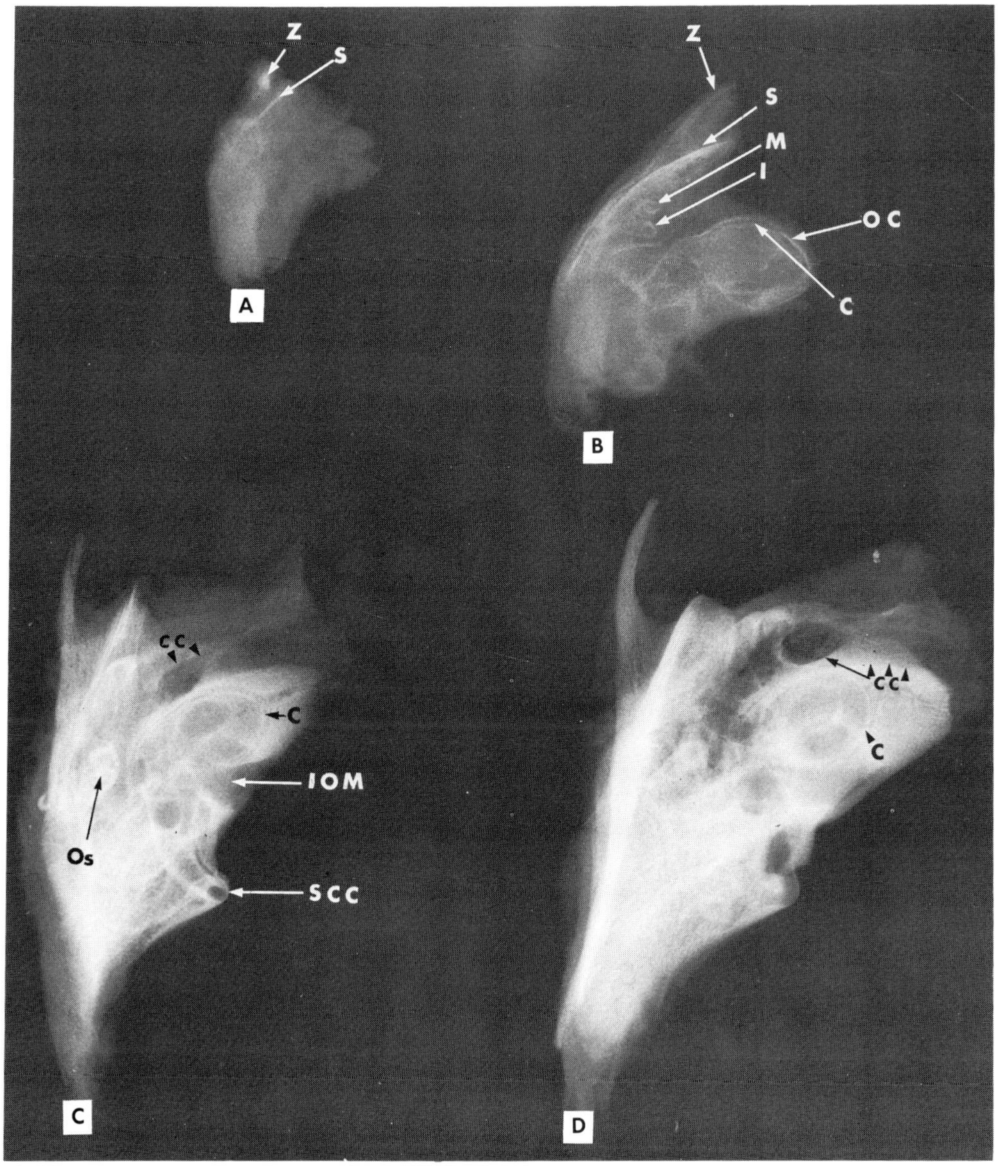

Fig. 7-5. Dissected fetal temporal bones: **A,** 12 weeks; **B,** 20 weeks; **C,** 28 weeks; **D,** 36 weeks. Simulated basal projection. At 20-week stage, malleus (*M*) and incus (*I*) can be seen. Otic capsule (*OC*) and cochlea (*C*) have begun to ossify. At 28-week stage, ossicles (*Os*), cochlea (*C*), carotid canal (*CC*), internal auditory meatus (*IOM*), and semicircular canals (*SCC*) can be seen.

exists, however, as to the number of ossification centers that form the inferior portion of the squama (supraoccipital). The importance of this question relates to the diagnosis of midline occipital fractures (Franken, 1969).

Roentgenographic examination of the occipital bone at various fetal ages reveals the following: (1) the basioccipital region is the site of the earliest well-defined ossification center (Fig. 7-4, *A*); (2) two ossification centers appear to participate in the formation of the definitive basiocciput (Fig. 7-4, *C*); (3) the interparietal region ossifies earlier than the supraoccipital region (Fig. 7-4, *A*); (4) the various segments of the occipital squama unite early, and a radial ossification pattern originates at the region of the future occipital protuberance (Fig. 7-4, *B* to *D*). Ossification of the posterior margin of the foramen magnum varies greatly. Caffey (1953) pointed out in detail the various accessory centers of ossification that may develop in this region.

Temporal bone

The complex anatomy and development of the temporal bone (Figs. 7-5 to 7-7) have been comprehensively investigated and presented by Bast and Anson (1949). Only the features that are relevant to the roentgenographic material will be described.

Of the three parts that constitute the temporal bone at birth, the squamous and tympanic parts develop in membrane and the petrous part in cartilage (Trotter and Peterson, 1966).

The squamous portion is formed from one center that appears as early as the eighth week of fetal development with the ossification .extending into the zygomatic process. The ossification center for the tympanic part appears from the ninth to the tenth fetal week. At birth it forms an incomplete ring, opening superiorly.

The cartilaginous petrous portion begins to ossify during the fifth fetal month. More than fourteen ossification centers appear, and ossification is almost com-

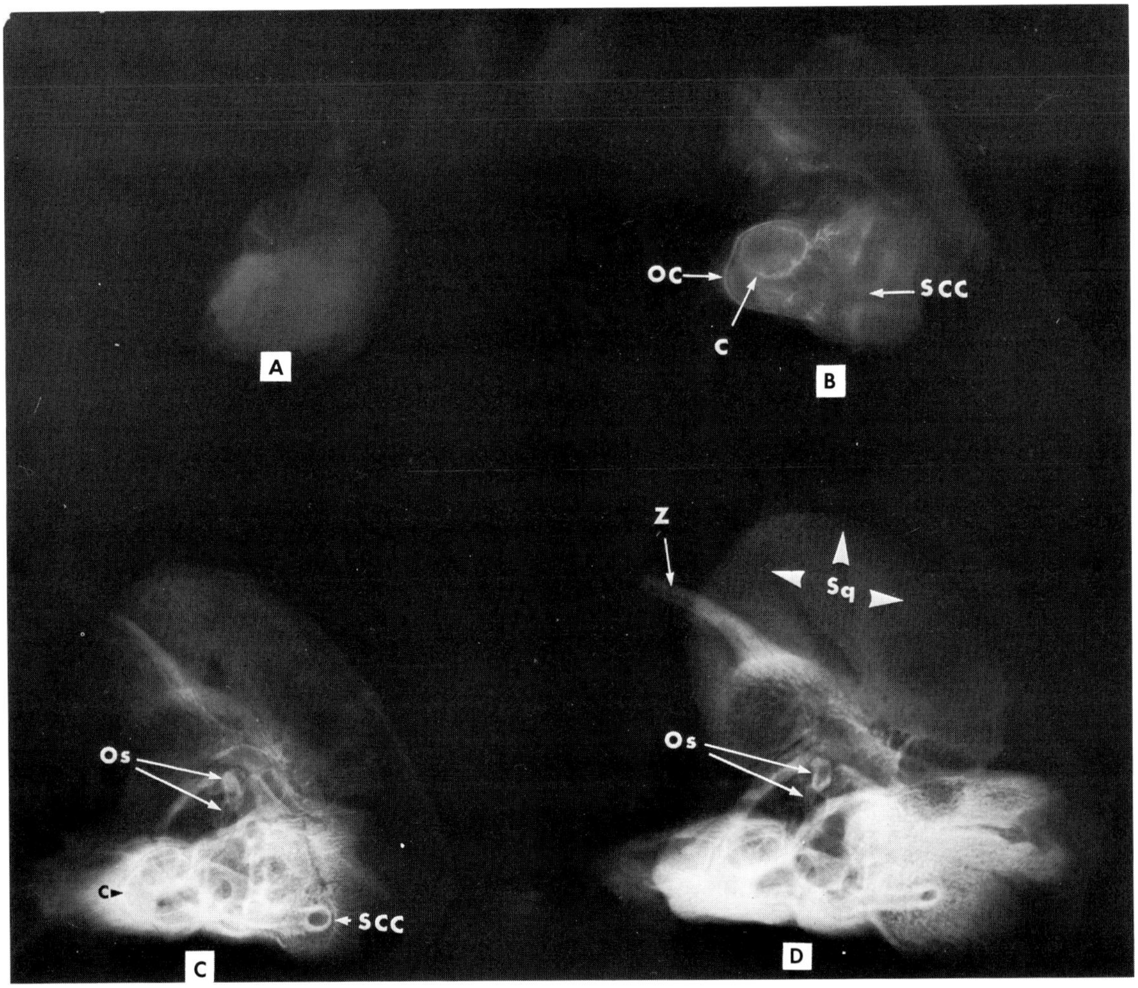

Fig. 7-6. Dissected fetal temporal bones: **A,** 12 weeks; **B,** 20 weeks; **C,** 28 weeks; **D,** 36 weeks. Simulated Stenvers projection shows that semicircular canals (*SCC*) ossify later than otic capsule (*OC*) and cochlea (*C*). Ossicles (*OS*), including manubrium, are extremely well seen. *Sq,* temporal squama; *Z,* zygomatic process.

plete by the end of the sixth month (Anson, 1966). Ossification proceeds from the cochlea backward to the semicircular canals. The ossicles begin to ossify during the fifth fetal month and attain almost full adult size at birth (Crelin, 1969).

Maxilla, vomer, and palatine bone

The maxilla, vomer, and palatine bone begin to ossify during the eighth week of fetal life (Davies and Davies, 1962). Roentgenograms show that the ossification of these structures in the region of the posterior choanae is prominent in the 12-week fetus and the 20-week fetus (Fig. 7-8).

Sphenoid bone

The ossification of the sphenoid is complex. Up to nineteen separate ossification centers may appear in the sphenoid anlage (Augier, 1931). These centers may be grouped into five major areas: the lesser wings—presphenoid, postsphenoid, basisphenoid—the greater wings, and the pterygoid plates.

Pterygoid plates and greater wings of sphenoid. The pterygoid plates ossify in membrane, whereas the greater wings of the sphenoid ossify in both cartilage and membrane (Fig. 7-8). About the eighth week an ossification center for the root of the greater wing appears near the foramen rotundum. The remainder of the greater wing

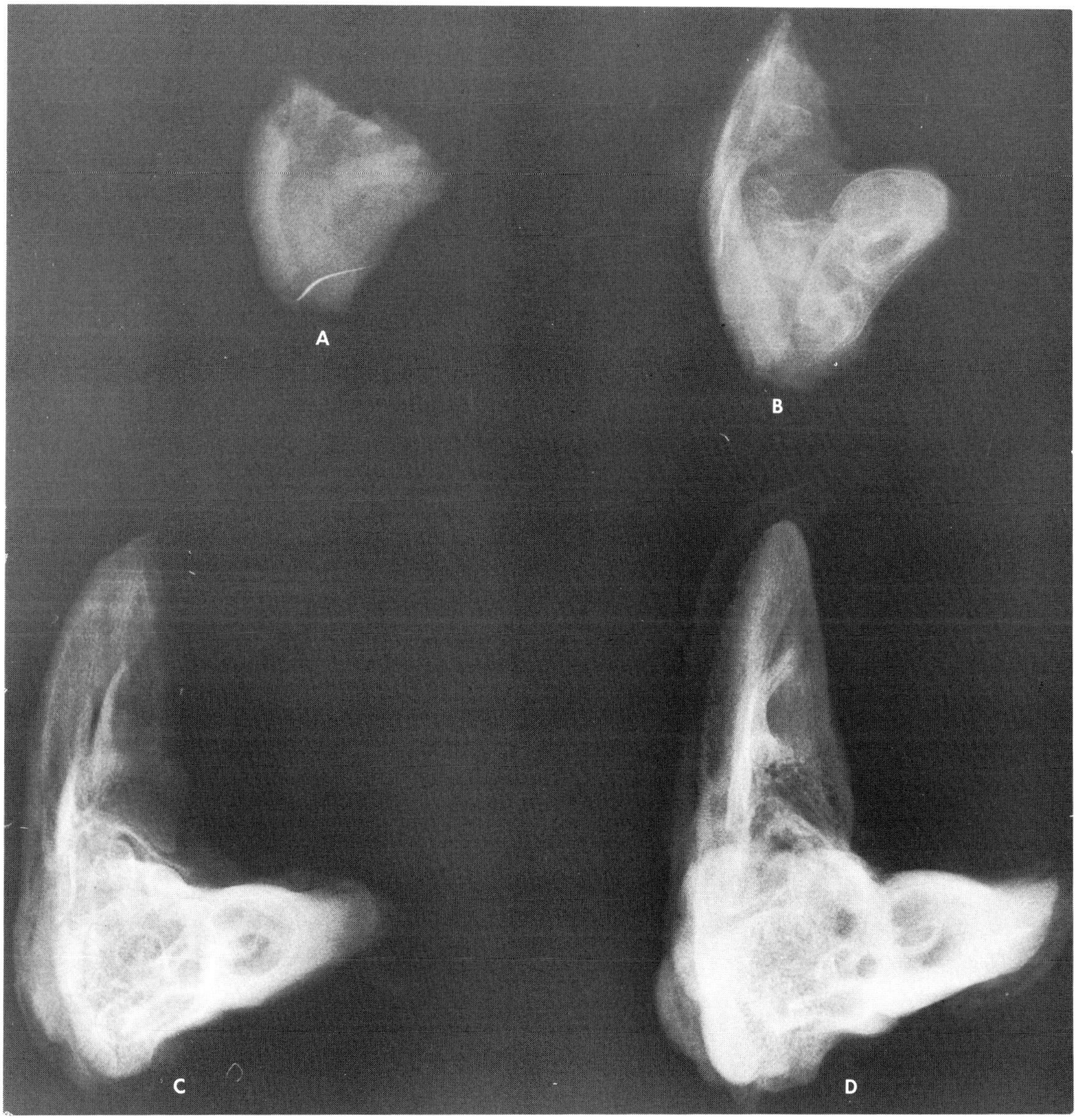

Fig. 7-7. Dissected fetal temporal bones: **A,** 12 weeks; **B,** 20 weeks; **C,** 28 weeks; **D,** 36 weeks. Simulated anteroposterior projection shows increasing angle between petrous and squamous portions as fetus gets older.

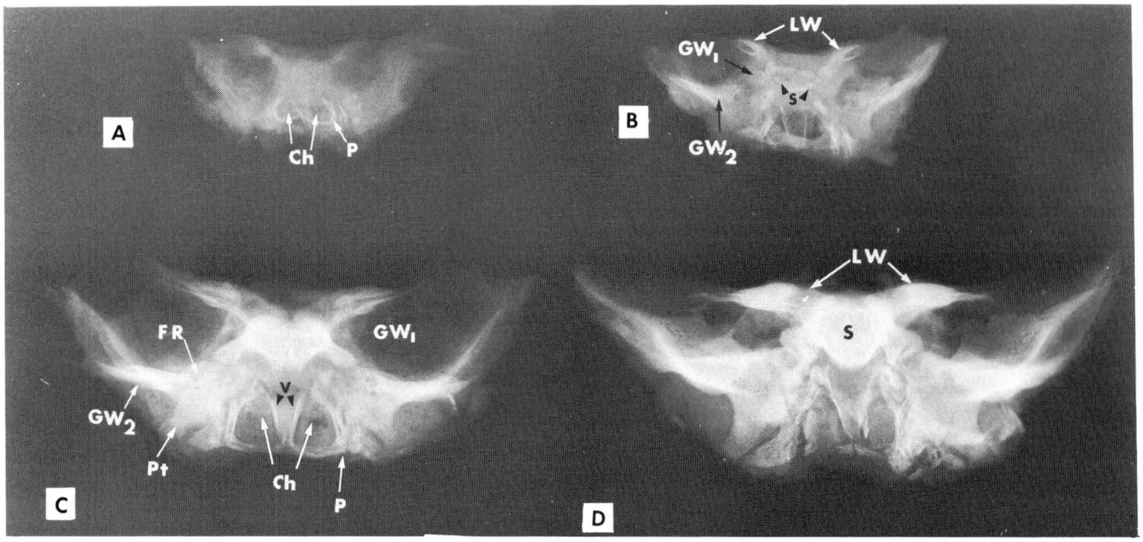

Fig. 7-8. Dissected fetal sphenoid bones in simulated anteroposterior projection. Note the prominent ossification of the palatine bone (*P*) that outlines the choanae (*Ch*) in 12-week fetus. **A,** Vomer (*V*) is faintly visualized. During 20-week, **B,** and 28-week, **C,** stages, the greater wing develops from two separate centers: one arises from sphenoid body (GW_1) and one arises in membrane (GW_2). The latter also gives rise to the pterygoid plates (*Pt*). In 36-week stage, **D,** note how the sphenoid body (*S*) arises from multiple centers, which eventually fuse. *LW,* Lesser wing of sphenoid; *FR,* foramen rotundum.

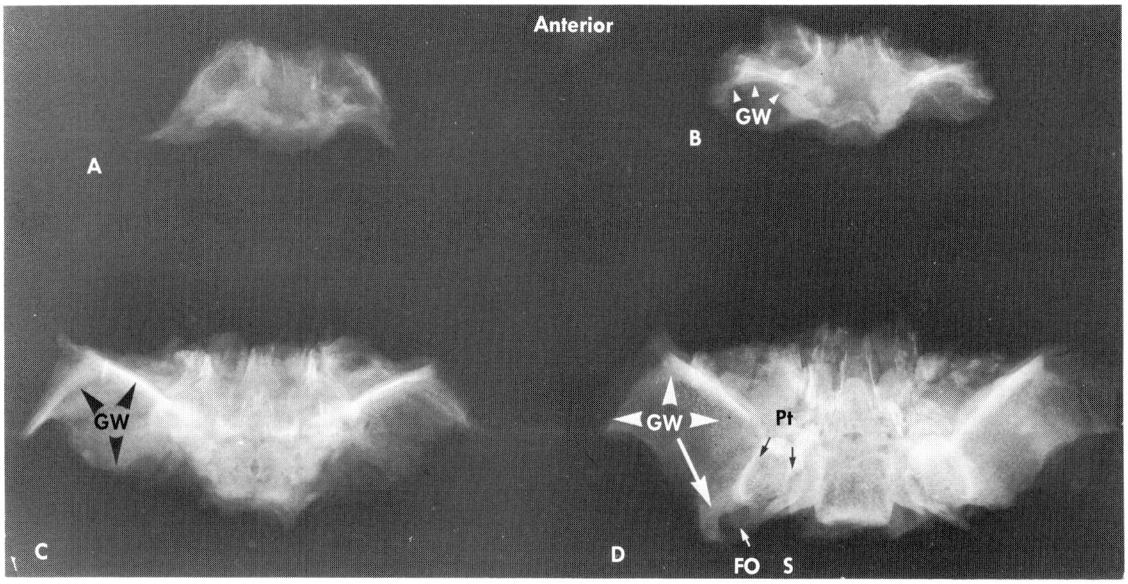

Fig. 7-9. Dissected fetal sphenoid bones: **A,** 12 weeks; **B,** 20 weeks; **C,** 28 weeks; **D,** 36 weeks. Simulated basal projection shows progressive backward growth of greater wing (*GW*). This growth may explain frequency of an incompletely outlined foramen ovale or spinosum (*FO S*) at birth. *Pt,* Pterygoid plates.

ossifies in the membrane and the ossification extends downward into the pterygoid plates (Davies and Davies, 1962). The hamulus, however, ossifies in cartilage. Of interest roentgenographically is the frequent lack of complete ossification of walls of the foramen ovale and foramen spinosum (Fig. 7-9). (See Chapter 16.)

Optic canal (Kier, 1966). The following description is necessary to understand the developmental transformation of the primitive calvarial opening (which surrounds the optic nerve and ophthalmic artery) from a shallow foramen to a canal with depth and two distinct openings. The optic strut is the inferior root of the lesser

A
B
C
D

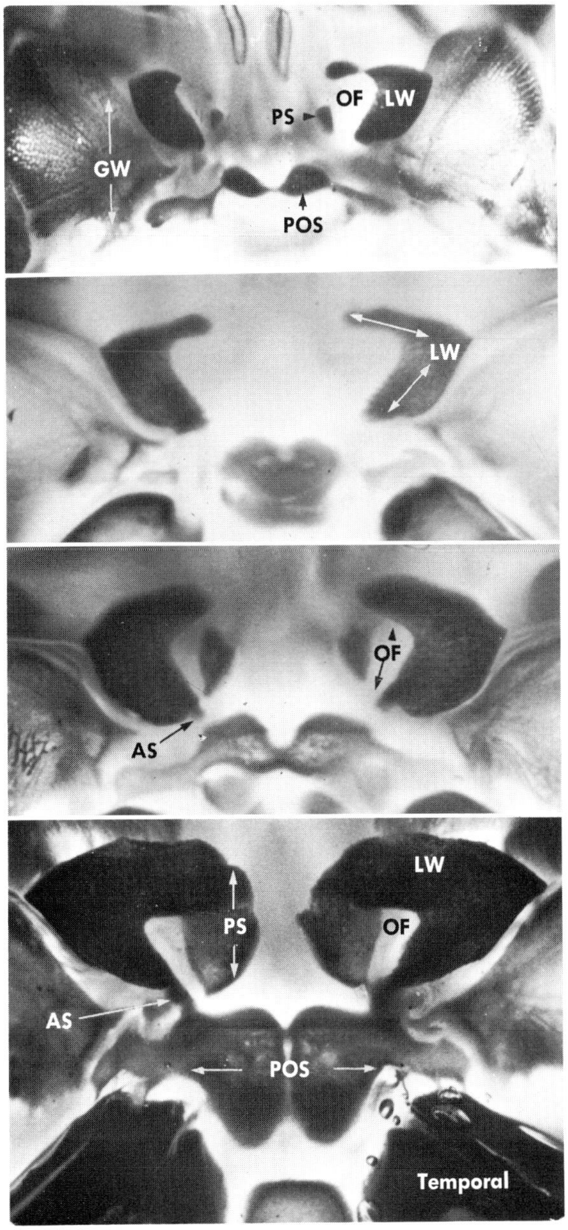

Fig. 7-10. Photographs of base of skull in cleared and alizarin-stained fetal specimens showing ossification of cartilaginous optic foramen (ossification centers appear in black). **A,** A 12-week fetus. Two ossification centers of lesser sphenoid wing (*LW*) outline anterosuperior and lateral margins of optic foramen (*OF*). Presphenoid (*PS*) center is beginning to ossify. **B,** A 14-week fetus with advanced ossification of lesser sphenoid wing. Presphenoid is not yet ossified. **C,** A 16-week fetus with further ossification around optic foramen. Anterior segment of optic strut (*AS*) extends from lesser wing toward postsphenoid ossification center (*POS*). **D,** A 17-week fetus. Anterior segment of optic strut is fused to postsphenoid. Note the keyhole-shaped optic foramen. *GW,* Greater sphenoid wing. (From Kier, E. L.: Invest. Radiol. **1**:346-362, 1966.)

wing of the sphenoid, separating the optic canal from the superior orbital fissure.

The development of the optic canal can be divided into three stages: (1) formation of the cartilaginous optic foramen, (2) ossification of the cartilaginous foramen, and (3) transformation of the bony foramen into a bony canal.

The cartilaginous optic foramen ossifies during the 12 to 17 weeks of fetal life (Fig. 7-10). The first ossification center outlines the lateral border of the future optic foramen. A separate center forms anterosuperiorly. These two centers join to form the bony lesser wing of the sphenoid, which outlines the lateral and superior border of the foramen. The presphenoid center appears medial to the foramen and gradually enlarges to form the medial border of the foramen. The lesser wing may be well ossified before the presphenoid center appears (Fig. 7-10, *B*).

A small linear ossification extends from the lesser wing toward the postsphenoid center and eventually joins the two centers. This linear ossification represents the first segment of the optic strut, which forms the inferolateral border of the optic foramen. The first segment of the optic strut joins the lesser wing only to the postsphenoid (Fig. 7-10, *D*). At the end of the ossification period, a bony foramen with a keyhole appearance is evident (Fig. 7-10, *D*).

The bony optic canal begins to form during the fifth month of fetal life. At the beginning of this stage, the bony optic foramen is relatively large, with a keyhole appearance (Figs. 7-11, *A,* and 7-12, *A*). The formation of the new posterior segment of the optic strut transforms the primitive optic foramen into a canal with two distinct openings.

The posterosuperior strut segment develops by new bone formation in two different forms. It may develop as an elongated bony ridge that extends from the lesser sphenoid wing medially to join the presphenoid center. It may also be formed by two bony ridges, one arising from the lesser wing, the other from the presphenoid center. These two ridges grow toward each other (Figs. 7-11, *B,* and Fig. 7-12, *B*). Therefore at this stage the optic strut consists of two separate segments: (1) an anteroinferior segment, extending from the lesser wing to the postsphenoid, and (2) a posterosuperior segment, extending from the lesser wing to the presphenoid.

A foramen is present at this time between the two strut segments (Figs. 7-11, *C,* and 7-12, *C*). It is not a functional foramen since no structures pass through it. The foramen is transitory and becomes obliterated by the fusion of the two segments into a single strut during the last 2 months of fetal life (Figs. 7-11, *D,* and 7-12, *D*).

The transformation of the optic foramen into a canal

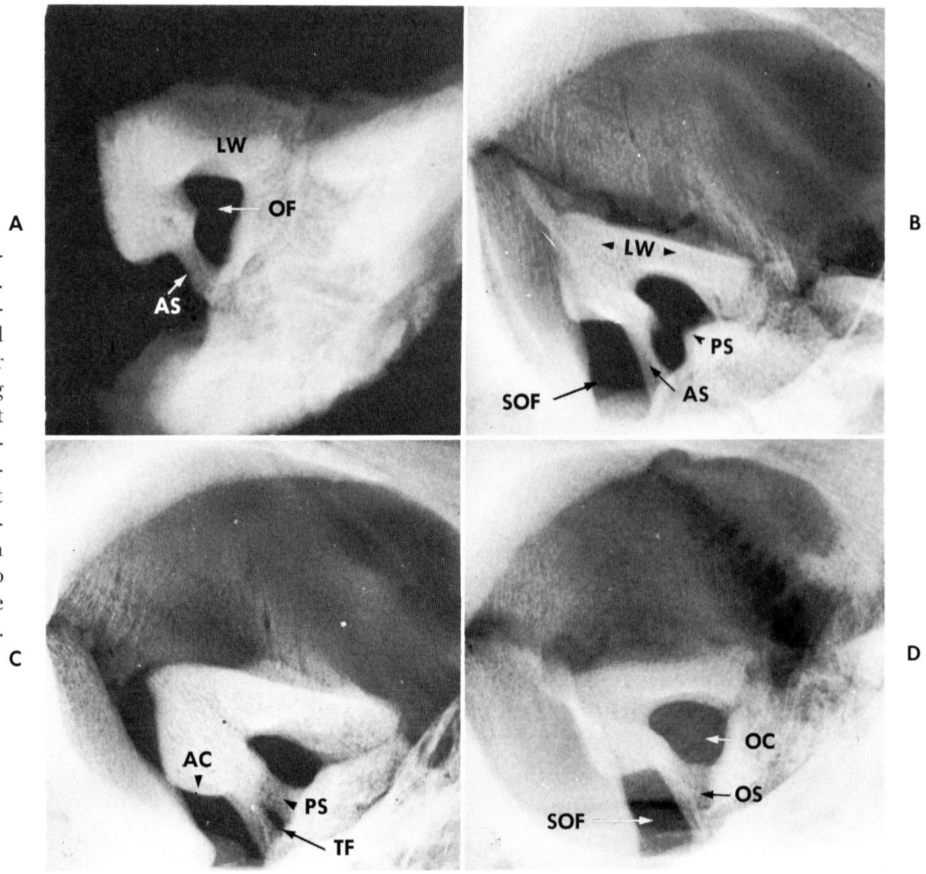

Fig. 7-11. Dissected and dry fetal specimens showing formation of optic canal. **A,** A 28-week fetus. Large keyhole-shaped optic foramen (*OF*) is still present. **B,** A 31-week fetus. Posterior optic strut segment (*PS*) is beginning to form. Anterior optic strut segment (*AS*) separates optic foramen from superior orbital fissure (*SOF*). **C,** A 35-week fetus. Segment of posterior strut is fully formed and separated from anterior segment by transitory foramen (*TF*). **D,** A 38-week fetus. The two strut segments are fused into a single optic strut. (From Kier, E. L.: Invest. Radiol. **1**:346-362, 1966.)

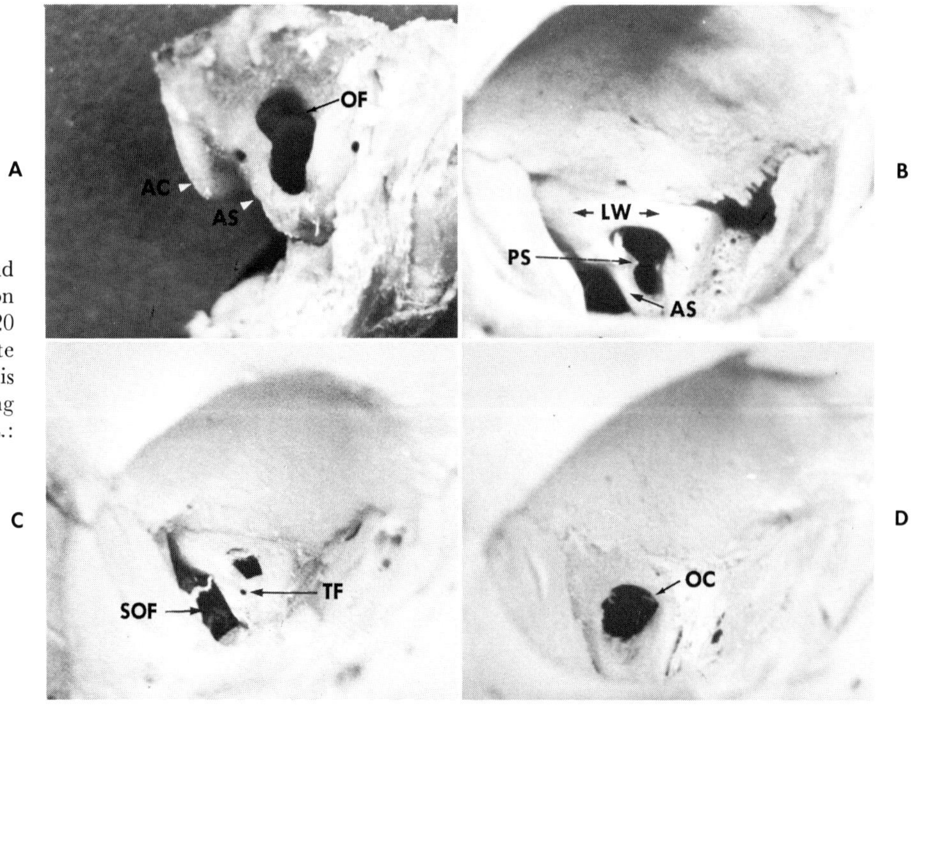

Fig. 7-12. Apex of orbit in dissected and dry fetal specimens showing formation of optic canal: **A,** 12 weeks; **B,** 20 weeks; **C,** 28 weeks; **D,** 36 weeks. Note the transitory foramen (*TF*), which is seen frequently in fetal skulls during the last trimester. (From Kier, E. L.: Invest. Radiol. **1**:346-362, 1966.)

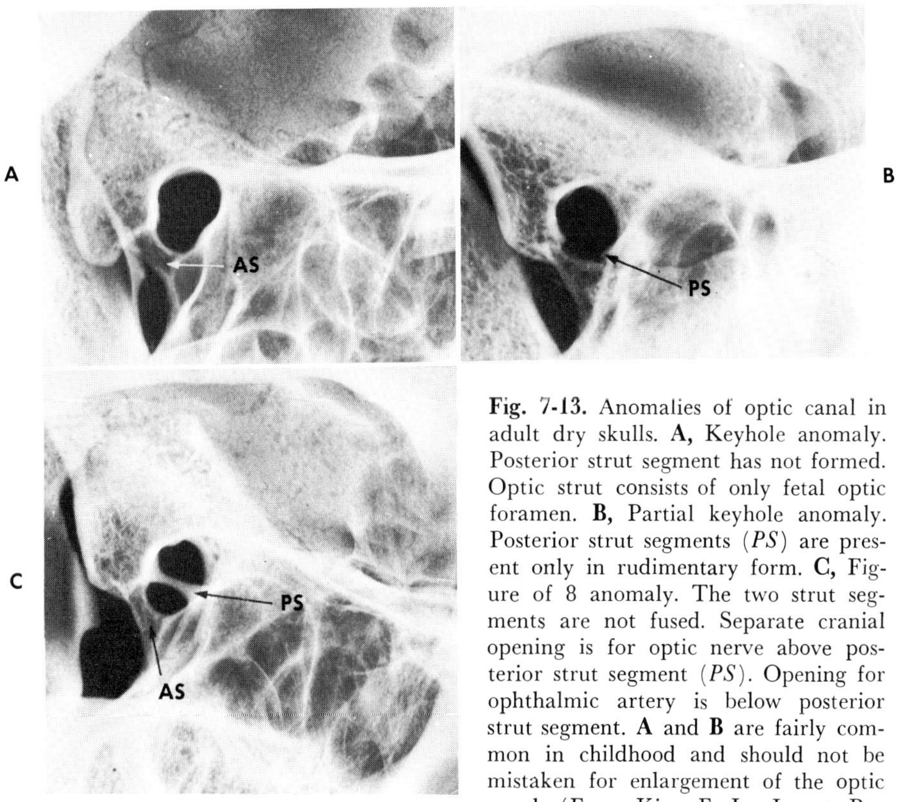

Fig. 7-13. Anomalies of optic canal in adult dry skulls. **A,** Keyhole anomaly. Posterior strut segment has not formed. Optic strut consists of only fetal optic foramen. **B,** Partial keyhole anomaly. Posterior strut segments (*PS*) are present only in rudimentary form. **C,** Figure of 8 anomaly. The two strut segments are not fused. Separate cranial opening is for optic nerve above posterior strut segment (*PS*). Opening for ophthalmic artery is below posterior strut segment. **A** and **B** are fairly common in childhood and should not be mistaken for enlargement of the optic canal. (From Kier, E. L.: Invest. Radiol. **1**:346-362, 1966.)

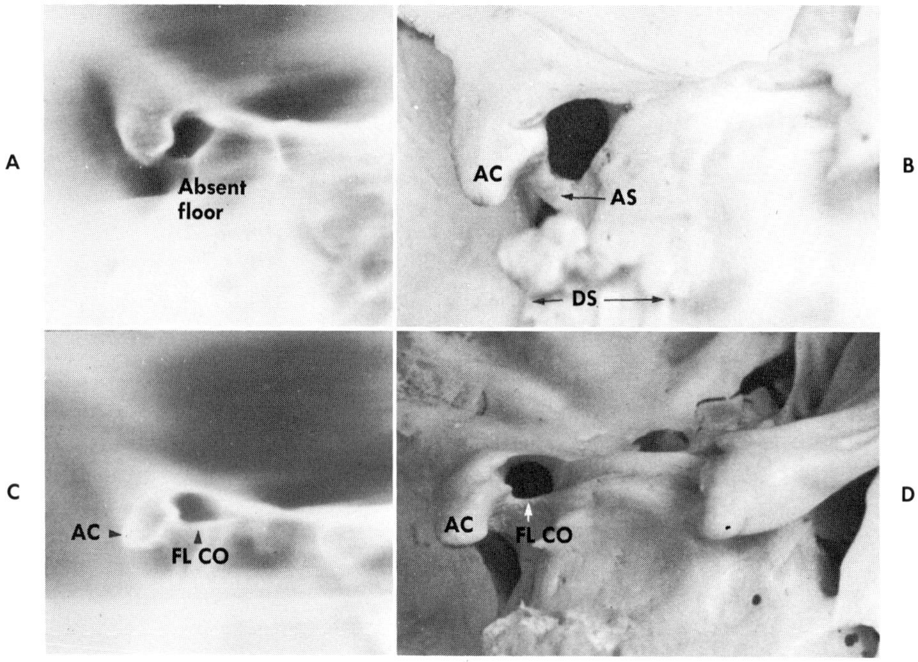

Fig. 7-14. Absent floor of cranial opening of optic canal. Tomogram obtained in plane perpendicular to long axis of canal shows that floor of cranial opening in keyhole anomaly is absent, **A.** This structure (*FL CO*) is clearly visible in tomogram of normal canal, **C.** Corresponding anatomic specimens demonstrate that posterior half of optic canal floor, which forms cranial opening in normal specimen, **D,** is absent in keyhole anomaly, **B.** Absence of this segment of the floor of the canal should not be mistaken for an erosion. (From Kier, E. L.: Invest. Radiol. **1**:346-362, 1966.)

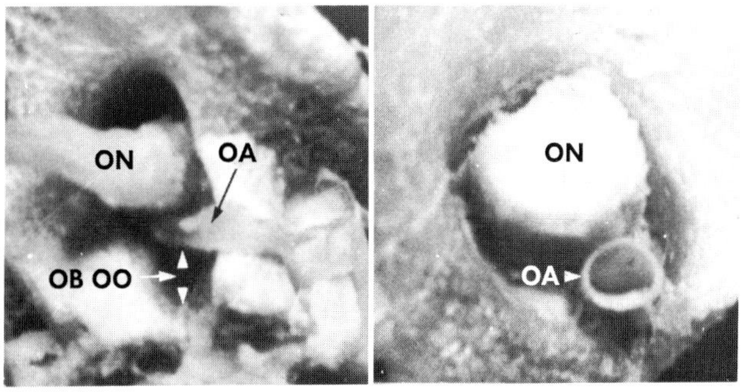

Fig. 7-15. Dissected orbital openings of optic canals showing changing relative size of orbital opening. Optic nerve (*ON*) and ophthalmic artery (*OA*) occupy only part of large orbital opening in 2-month-old infant. **A,** Lower segment of this opening (*OB OO*) is obliterated during childhood. **B,** In adulthood, orbital opening of optic canal tightly surrounds soft tissue within it.

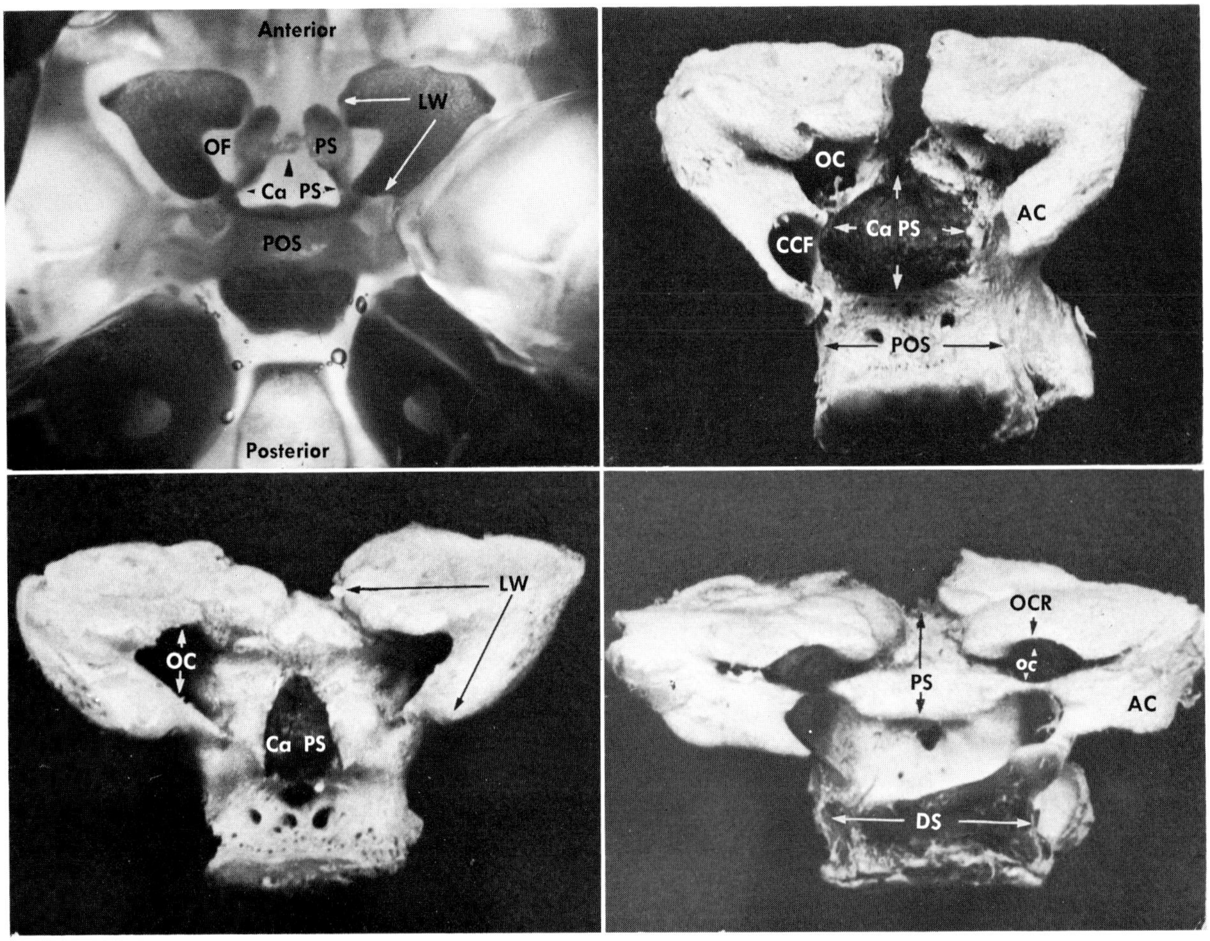

Fig. 7-16. Superior aspect of specimens of fetal sphenoid bone showing ossification of presphenoid. **A,** Cleared and alizarin-stained skull base of 16-week fetus (cartilage appears white, ossification centers appear black). Central presphenoid is still cartilaginous (*Ca PS*). *LW,* Lesser sphenoid wing; *OF,* optic foramen; *PS,* ossified presphenoid; *POS,* postsphenoid (floor of sella). **B,** Dissected sphenoid specimen of 20-week fetus. Note the large round (olivary) cartilaginous eminence of the presphenoid (*Ca PS*) anterior to the floor of the sella. *AC,* Anterior clinoid process; *CCF,* caroticoclinoid foramen; *OC,* optic canal. **C,** Dissected sphenoid specimen of 32-week fetus. Note the diminishing size of the cartilaginous presphenoid (*Ca PS*). **D,** Dissected sphenoid specimen of 4-day-old infant. Superior surface of presphenoid is completely ossified. Note the superior position of the optic canal roof (*OCR*) as compared with the presphenoid (*PS*). *DS,* Dorsum sellae. (From Kier, E. L.: Amer. J. Roentgen. **102:**747-767, 1968.)

may be a slow process continuing into childhood, may become arrested at an intermediate stage, or may not take place at all. These factors should be considered in the evaluation of the optic canal for possible enlargement or erosion (Figs. 7-13 and 7-14). (See Chapter 21.)

An optic canal with a large orbital opening is frequent in childhood. This feature should be considered in the evaluation of optic canals for possible enlargement (Fig. 7-15).

Sella (Kier, 1968). Certain aspects of the development of the superior surface of the body of the sphenoid are included in the discussion of the sella to complete the understanding of sphenoid development.

This development consists of four stages: (1) chondrification of the sphenoid body, (2) prenatal ossification, (3) postnatal development of the planum sphenoidale, and (4) variable posterior growth of the planum sphenoidale.

Stage 1. Chondrification of sphenoid body. According to Augier (1931) chondrification first takes place behind the pituitary gland. The cartilaginous plate extends forward, surrounding the stalk of Rathke's pouch, and forms the cartilaginous presphenoid anteriorly. Fawcett (1910) stated that the dorsum sellae chondrifies independently of the rest of the sphenoid.

Stage 2. Prenatal ossification. The last portion of the

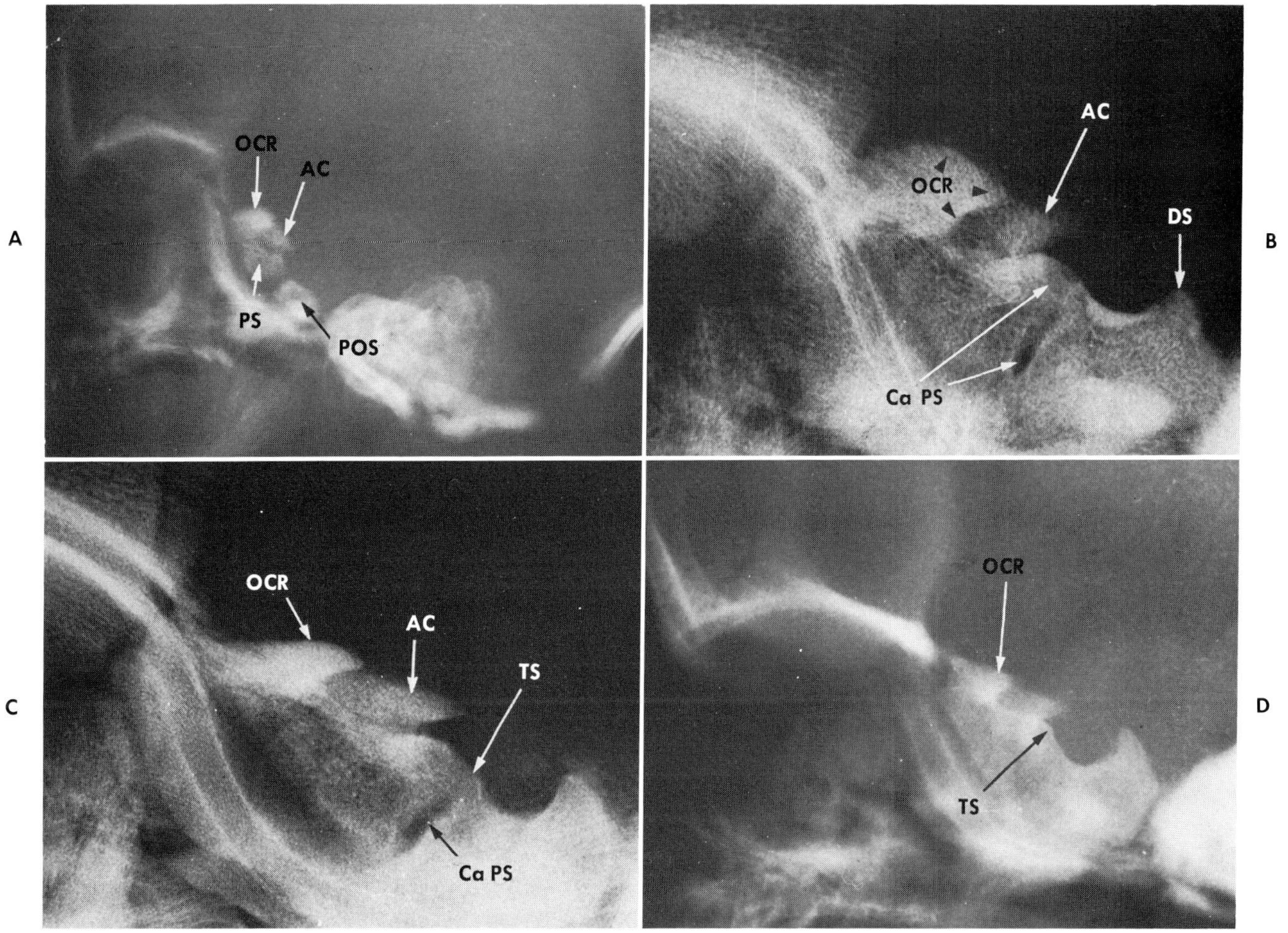

Fig. 7-17. Lateral roentgenograms of skull show ossification of presphenoid. **A,** A 28-week fetus. Region of future tuberculum sellae is not as yet ossified. Note the superior position of the optic canal roof (*OCR*). *AC,* Anterior clinoid process; *PS,* presphenoid; *POS,* postsphenoid (floor of sella). **B,** A 34-week fetus. Anterior sellar wall is partially ossified. Note the size and prominence of the optic canal roof (*OCR*). Intersphenoid synchondrosis is actually the centrally located remnant of the cartilaginous presphenoid (*Ca PS*). *DS,* Dorsum sellae. **C,** A 38-week fetus. Tuberculum sellae (*TS*) is further ossified. Note the flattening of the optic canal roof. **D,** Normal 2-week-old infant. Note the following features of the normal newborn sphenoid: planum sphenoidale is not present; anterosuperior margin of sellar fossa—tuberculum sellae (*TS*)—is ossified and well defined; roof of optic canal is prominent and is most superior sphenoid structure. (From Kier, E. L.: Amer. J. Roentgen. **102:**747-767, 1968.)

superior surface of the sphenoid body to ossify, except for the dorsum sellae, is the anterosuperior margin of the sella. At the 16-week stage of fetal development (Fig. 7-16, *A*), the floor of the sella has been formed by the ossified postsphenoid. The lesser sphenoid wings are well ossified. The lateral presphenoid center, which outlines the medial border of the optic foramen, and a small deep middle presphenoid center are both present. The region of the anterior wall of the sella is still cartilaginous, round, and superiorly convex. The term olivary eminence (Lawrence, 1894) is an appropriate description. This cartilaginous presphenoid olivary eminence is delimited posteriorly by the sharp anterior margin of the postsphenoid, laterally by the bony union of the presphenoid and postsphenoid at the level of the optic strut, and anteriorly by the paired lateral and single middle presphenoid centers (Thomson, 1902; Kodama, 1965).

The cartilaginous presphenoid eminence becomes gradually ossified, in the last trimester, by backward and medial growth of the presphenoid centers (Figs. 7-16 and 7-17) (Lawrence, 1894). A progressively smaller column of cartilage is found at the center of the ossifying presphenoid in the region of the anterior sellar wall—the future tuberculum sellae. This central cartilaginous column extends from the superior to the inferior surfaces of the sphenoid body. At birth the superior end of this column is ossified, although at times it is quite fragile. The intrasphenoid portion of this column may not be completely ossified until the end of the first year of postnatal life. The craniopharyngeal canal is not radiologically visible (Lowman et al., 1966).

Thus at birth (Fig. 7-16, *D*) the superior surface of the sphenoid body consists of: (1) the ossifying dorsum sellae, (2) the ossified postsphenoid (sellar floor), and (3) the ossified presphenoid, which forms the anterosuperior wall of the sella and extends anteriorly toward the cribriform plate. Of note is the superior position of the roof of the optic canals on each side of the presphenoid.

Stage 3. Postnatal development of planum sphenoidale. At birth the planum sphenoidale, the smooth superior surface of the anterior sphenoid that joins the two lesser sphenoid wings, has not yet formed (Fig. 7-16, *D*). During the first year of life, the medial center of the presphenoid continues to enlarge in height. Eventually this center fuses with the anterosuperior roots of the lesser sphenoid wings (Fig. 7-18, *A*). This fusion results in the formation of the planum sphenoidale. The two anterosuperior roots of the lesser sphenoid wings may enlarge and meet in the midline without the participation of the middle presphenoid center.

Stage 4. Variable posterior growth of planum sphenoidale. The planum sphenoidale may continue to enlarge

A

B

C

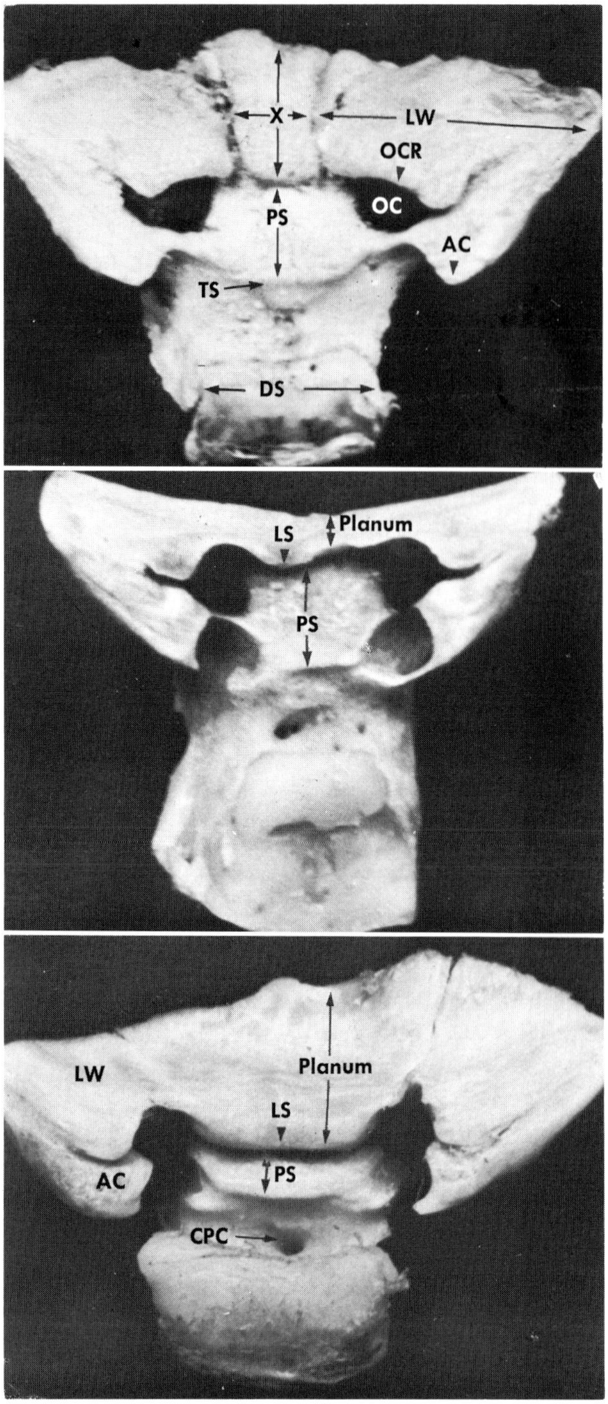

Fig. 7-18. Superior aspect of dissected specimens of sphenoid bone of infants showing formation of planum sphenoidale. **A,** A 3-month-old infant. Note the additional presphenoid center (*X*) between the superior roots of the lesser sphenoid wings (*LW*). *AC,* Anterior clinoid process; *OC,* optic canal; *OCR,* optic canal roof; *TS,* tuberculum sellae; *DS,* dorsum sellae; *PS,* presphenoid. **B,** A 14-month-old infant. Narrow planum sphenoidale is delimited posteriorly by thin limbus sphenoidalis (*LS*). Note the wide uncovered presphenoid (*PS*). **C,** A $2\frac{1}{2}$-year-old infant. Note the pronounced posterior growth of the planum sphenoidale resulting in almost total coverage of the presphenoid. Limbus sphenoidalis is still separate from underlying presphenoid. (See Fig. 7-6, *C.*) *CPC,* Craniopharyngeal canal. (From Kier, E. L.: Amer. J. Roentgen. **102**:747-767, 1968.)

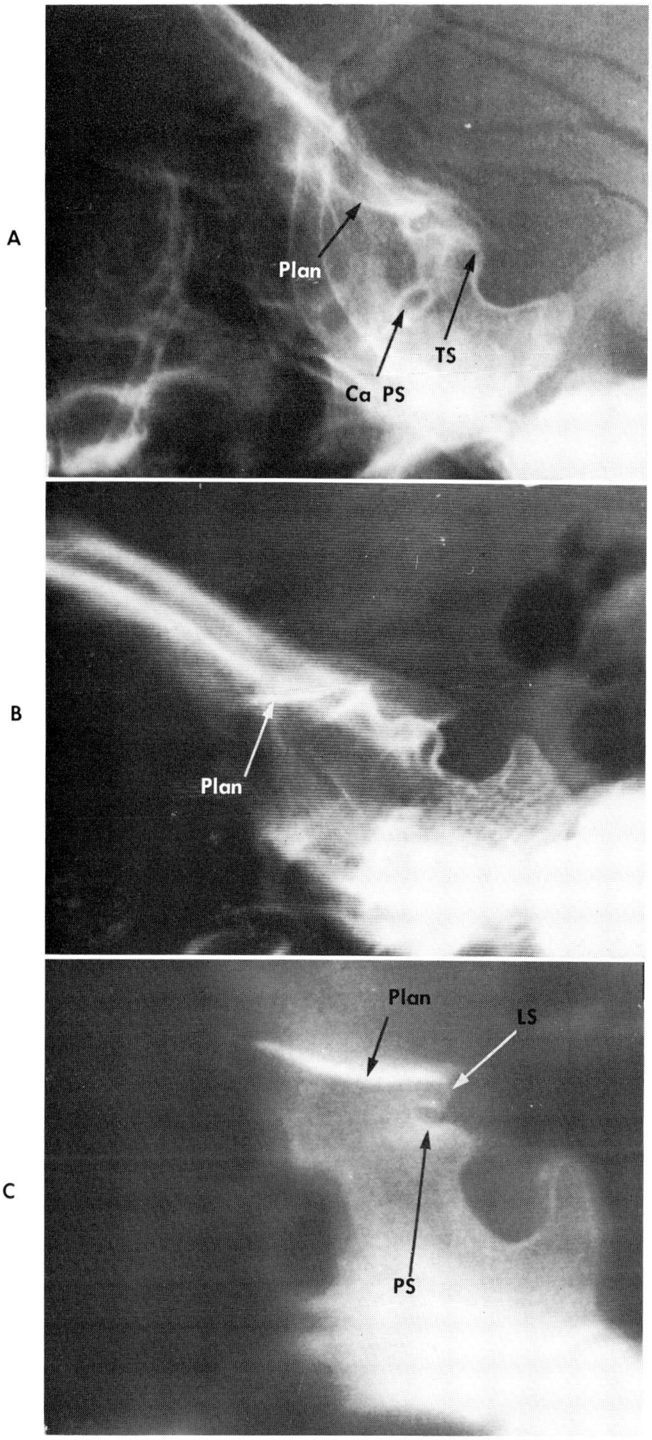

Fig. 7-19. Lateral roentgenograms of skull demonstrate various stages in development of planum sphenoidale. **A,** A 4-month-old infant. Planum sphenoidale (*Plan*) is beginning to form. Note the intrapresphenoid cartilage (*Ca PS*) and the well-defined tuberculum sellae (*TS*). **B,** Autotomogram of 12-month-old infant shows well-formed planum sphenoidale. **C,** Autotomogram of 2-year-old infant. Note the posterior extent of the planum sphenoidale. Thick limbus sphenoidalis (*LS*) is still distinct from underlying presphenoid (*PS*). (From Kier, E. L.: Amer. J. Roentgen. **102:**747-767, 1968.)

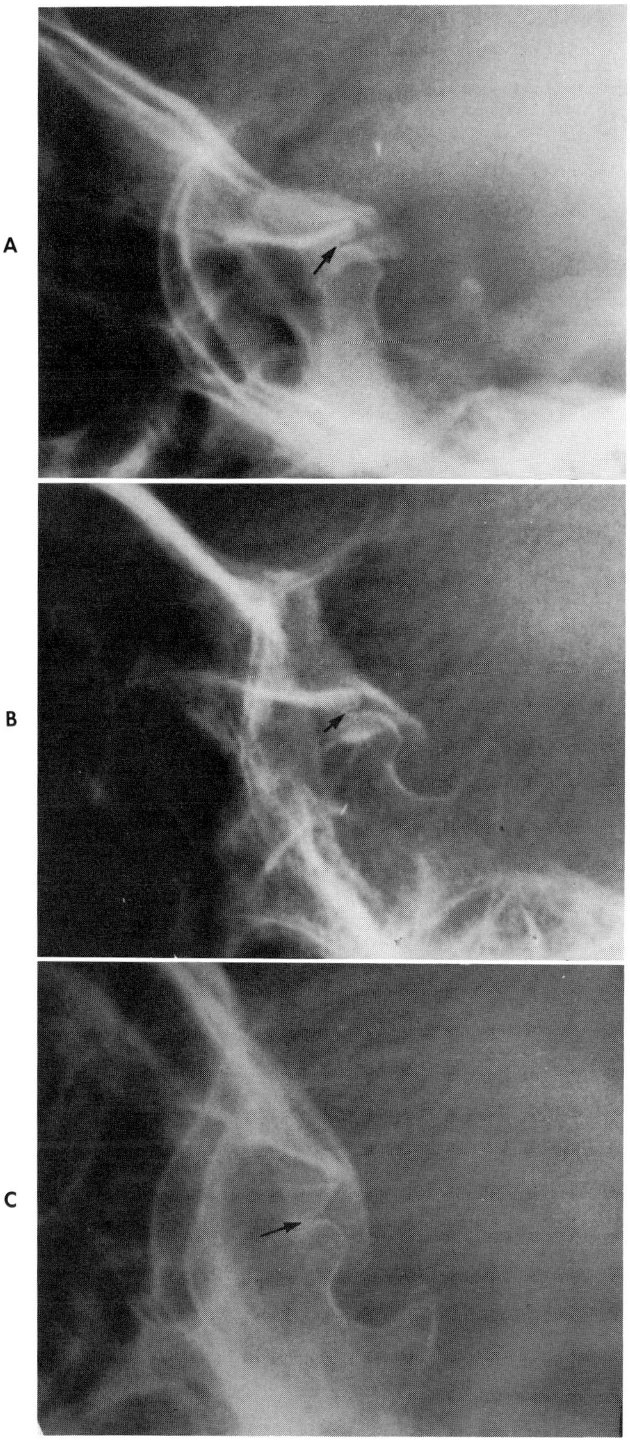

Fig. 7-20. Roentgenograms demonstrate a notch (arrow) present before fusion of limbus sphenoidalis to underlying presphenoid. This notch is frequent during childhood and should not be mistaken for persistent intersphenoid synchondrosis. **A,** 4 years; **B,** 5½ years; **C,** 6 years. (From Kier, E. L.: Amer. J. Roentgen. **102:**747-767, 1968.)

in width by variable posterior growth. This growth takes place mainly in the first year of life and overlaps the superior surface of the presphenoid. During this growth the posterior margin of the planum—the limbus sphenoidalis—is separate from the underlying presphenoid (Figs. 7-18 and 7-19). This separation may remain for a long period after the development of the planum (Fig. 7-20). In the adult the two structures are fused together.

The configuration of the superior surface of the definitive presellar sphenoid is governed by these variations in the posterior growth of the planum. The region of the presphenoid not overlapped by the planum remains as the definitive chiasmatic sulcus. Thus a narrow planum is associated with a wide chiasmatic sulcus (Fig. 7-21) (Schaeffer, 1924; Pendergrass et al., 1956) and a wide planum with a narrow chiasmatic sulcus.

This developmental information is of great importance in the evaluation of the sphenoid bone in lateral skull roentgenograms of young infants. An elongated *sulcus chiasmaticus* before the formation of the planum sphenoidale should not be mistaken for an abnormal feature; nor should the normally prominent roof of the optic canal during early infancy be mistaken for the planum sphenoidale. These errors account for many of the normal infants described in the literature, supposedly with a "J sella" or an "abnormal excavation" of the sulcus chiasmaticus. In effect, very few pathologic conditions present true abnormalities of the tuberculum sellae, sulcus chiasmaticus, planum sphenoidale, and optic canal roof.

The terms J and omega sellae, as currently used, are diagnostically meaningless and are adverse to the objective assessment of the sphenoid in infancy. A "normal J sella" or a "normal omega sella" is a radiologic myth and should be discarded.

A

B

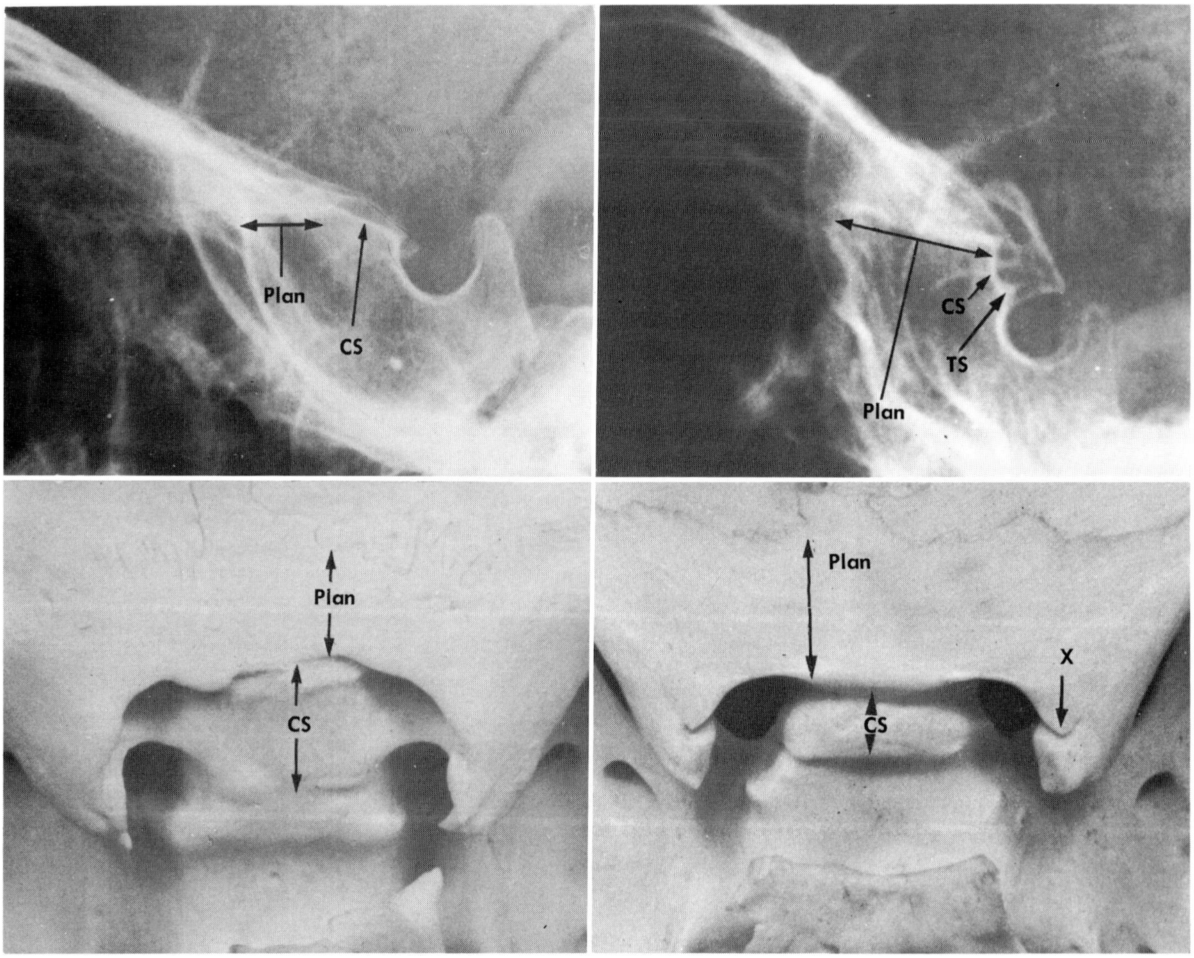

C

D

Fig. 7-21. Definitive presellar sphenoid. **A** and **B,** Roentgenograms of children. **C** and **D,** Views of superior surface of adult sphenoid specimens. Inverse relation between widths of planum sphenoidale (*Plan*) and chiasmatic sulcus (*CS*) is demonstrated. Note the vertical chiasmatic sulcus and the small tuberculum sellae (*TS*) in **B.** *X,* Overgrowth of anterior clinoid by optic canal roof. (From Kier, E. L.: Amer. J. Roentgen. **102**:747-767, 1968.)

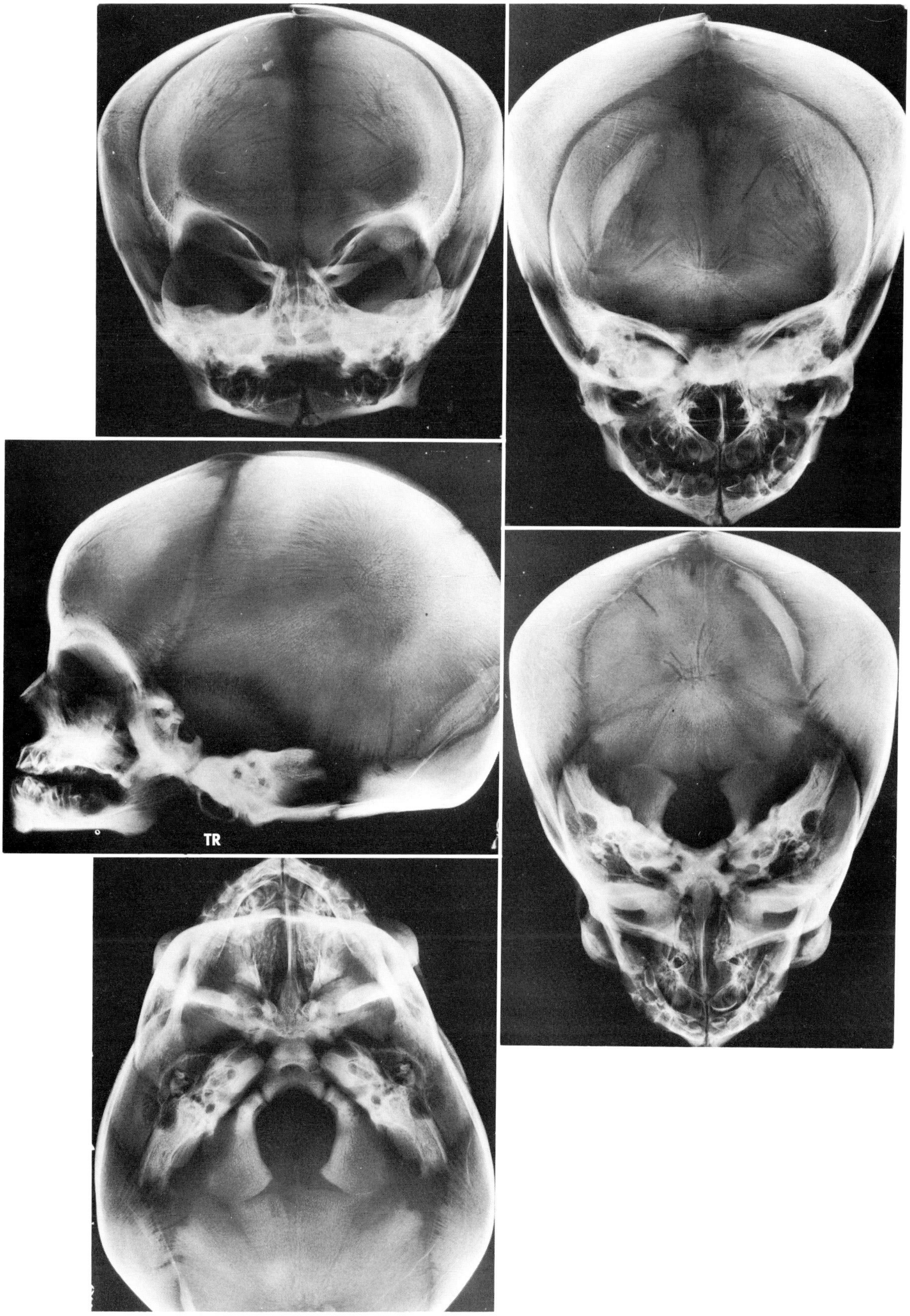

Fig. 7-22. A 28-week dry fetal skull in standard roentgenographic projections. Note the extremely fine detail that can be seen in the temporal bone. Both optic canals are visible in fetal period. Tympanic ring (*TR*) develops postnatally into external auditory meatus.

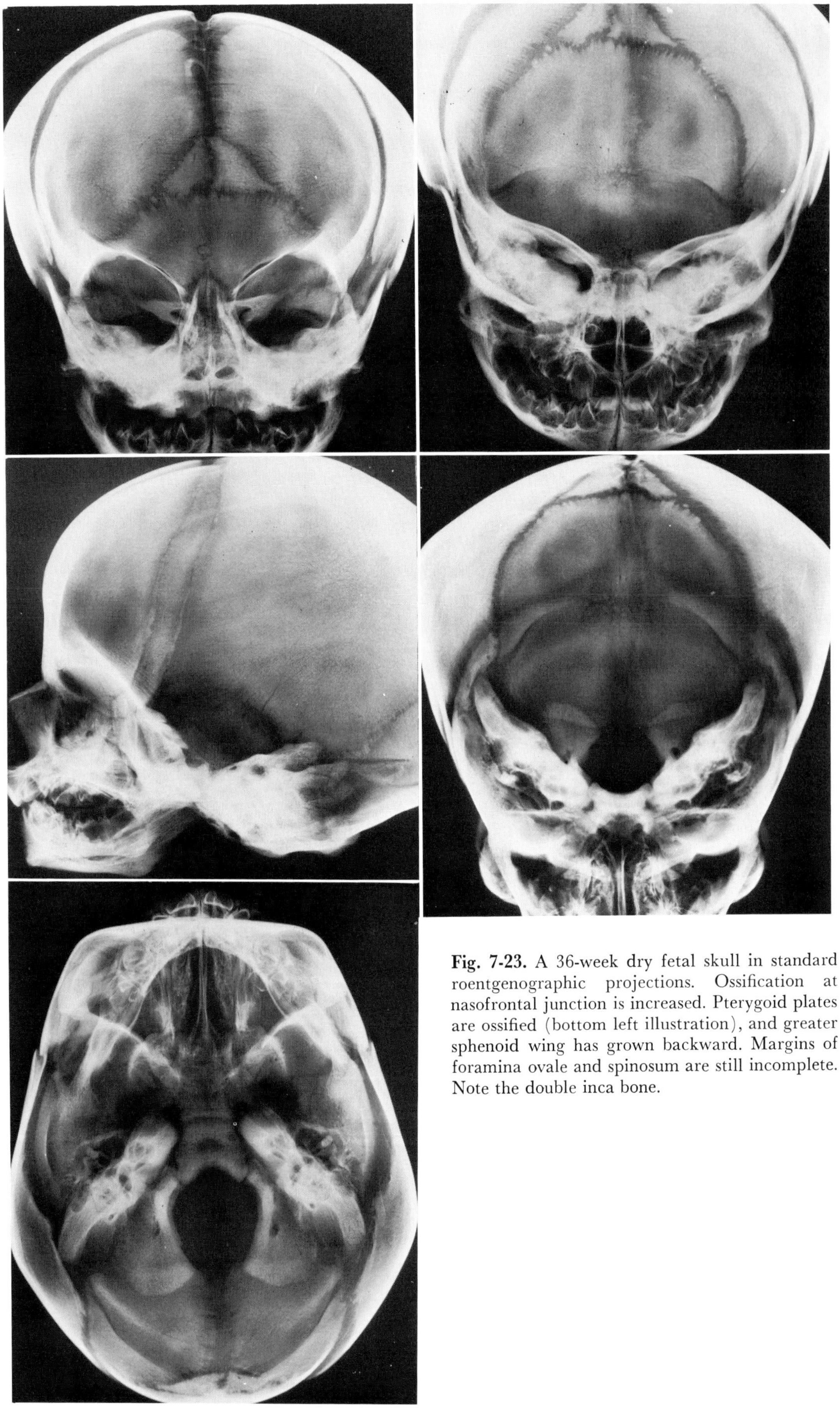

Fig. 7-23. A 36-week dry fetal skull in standard roentgenographic projections. Ossification at nasofrontal junction is increased. Pterygoid plates are ossified (bottom left illustration), and greater sphenoid wing has grown backward. Margins of foramina ovale and spinosum are still incomplete. Note the double inca bone.

Maturing fetal skull

The components of the fetal skull change relatively little during the last 2 months of fetal life (Figs. 7-22 and 7-23).

REFERENCES

Anson, B. J.: Organs of hearing and equilibrium. In Anson, B. J., editor: Morris' human anatomy, ed. 12, New York, 1966, McGraw-Hill Book Co.

Augier, M.: Squelette cephalique. In Poirier, P., and Charpy, A., editors: Traite d'anatomie humaine, ed. 4, Paris, 1931, Masson & Cie, vol. 1.

Bast, T. H., and Anson, B. J.: The temporal bone and the ear, Springfield, Ill., 1949, Charles C Thomas, Publisher.

Berkvens, T.: Radiography of the fetal skull, Acta Radiol. **34:** 250-252, 1950.

Blount, R. F., and Lachman, E.: Digestive system. In Anson, B. J., editor: Morris' human anatomy, ed. 12, New York, 1966, McGraw-Hill Book Co.

Caffey, J.: On the accessory ossicles of the supraoccipital bone: some newly recognized roentgen features of the normal infantile skull, Amer. J. Roentgen. **70:**401-412, 1953.

Crelin, E. S.: Anatomy of the newborn: an atlas, Philadelphia, 1969, Lea & Febiger.

Davies, D. V., and Davies, F., editors: Gray's anatomy, ed. 33, London, 1962, Longmans, Green & Co., Ltd.

Fawcett, E.: Notes on development of human sphenoid, J. Anat. **44:**207-222, 1910.

Franken, E. A.: The midline occipital fissure: diagnosis of fracture versus anatomic variants, Radiology **93:**1043-1046, 1969.

Henderson, S. G., and Sherman, L. S.: Roentgen anatomy of the skull in the newborn infant. In Etter, L., editor: Atlas of roentgen anatomy of the skull, Springfield, Ill., 1964, Charles C Thomas, Publisher.

Kier, E. L.: Embryology of the normal optic canal and its anomalies; an anatomic and roentgenographic study, Invest. Radiol. **1:**346-362, 1966.

Kier, E. L.: The infantile sella turcica; new radiologic and anatomic concepts based on a developmental study of the sphenoid bone, Amer. J. Roentgen. **102:**747-767, 1968.

Kodama, G.: Developmental studies on presphenoid in human sphenoid bone, Okajima Folia Anat. Jap. **41:**159-177, 1965.

Lawrence, T. W. P.: Position of the optic commissure, J. Anat. **28:**xviii-xx, 1894.

Lowman, R. M., Robinson, F., and McAllister, W. B.: Craniopharyngeal canal, Acta Radiol. [Diagn.] **5:**41-54, 1966.

Patten, B. M.: Human embryology, New York, 1953, The Blakiston Co.

Pendergrass, E. P., Schaeffer, J. P., and Hodes, P. J.: The head and neck in roentgen diagnosis, ed. 2, Springfield, Ill., 1956, Charles C Thomas, Publisher.

Potts, D. G., Svare, G. T., and Bergeron, R. T.: The developing brain—correlation between radiologic and anatomical findings, Acta Radiol. [Diagn.] **9:**430-439, 1969.

Scammon, R. E., and Calkins, L. A.: The development and growth of the external dimensions of the human body in the fetal period, Minneapolis, 1929, University of Minnesota Press.

Schaeffer, J. P.: Some points in regional anatomy of optic pathways with especial reference to tumors of hypophysis cerebri and resulting ocular changes, Anat. Rec. **28:**243-279, 1924.

Theiler, K.: Embryonale und postnatale Entwicklung des Schädels. In Olsson, O., editor: Handbuch der Medizinischen Radiologie, Berlin, 1963, Springer-Verlag, vol. 7/1.

Thomson, A.: Osteology. In Cunningham, D. J., editor: Textbook of anatomy, New York, 1902, The Macmillan Co.

Trotter, M., and Peterson, R. R.: Osteology. Arthrology. In Anson, B. J., editor: Morris' human anatomy, ed. 12, New York, 1966, McGraw-Hill Book Co.

CHAPTER 8

Changes of the skull during childhood

John P. Dorst

Abnormalities of the skull in infants and children cannot be appreciated without knowledge of the normal pattern of skull growth and development. This pattern results from the interaction of many forces. Abnormalities of one or more of these forces deform the developing skull. Some of the forces that contribute to normal growth of the skull and the consequences of compromise of these forces are here described and illustrated.

NORMAL GROWTH AND DEVELOPMENT OF SKULL

In the embryo the mesenchyme of the skull consists of three divisions. The first is the cerebral capsule, which covers the brain and leptomeninges and later develops into the dura mater, the skullcap (calvarium), and the scalp (Moss and Young, 1960). The second division forms the face. The third division provides a floor for the brain case (neurocranium) and a roof for the face.

Chondrification of the third division initiates skull development. Later, enchondral ossification converts this division into the bony chondrocranium—so named because it is the only part of the skull that is preformed in cartilage. In the face and cerebral capsule, portions of the mesenchyme are converted directly to bone without an intermediate cartilaginous stage (Arey, 1965). This process is termed intramembranous or dermal bone formation, and the resultant bone is called membrane bone.

Chondrocranium

The skull in primitive fishes of the shark type (elasmobranches) lacks a roof and consists of a cartilaginous base (chondrocranium) with capsules for the olfactory organs, eyes, and ears. The skull in the early human embryo is similar, and only later is membrane bone added in the skullcap and face. Thus the human chondrocranium is both phylogenetically and developmentally the most primitive part of the skull (Patten, 1968).

Since the chondrocranium forms both the floor of the brain case and the roof of the face, it is a critical region of skull development that coordinates the developing neural and facial skeletons (Moss and Greenberg, 1955). It also provides, in the occipital condyles, the only junction of the skull with the somatic skeleton.

Multiple enchondral ossification centers appear in the embryonic chondrocranium, and they enlarge and coalesce to form the seven bones of the adult chondrocranium. Three of these bones are unpaired—the ethmoid, sphenoid, and occipital bones. The other four are the paired temporal bones and the inferior turbinates (Patten, 1968). The ethmoid and the two turbinates develop completely from cartilage. The other four are only in part chondrocranial bones since they include contributions from the membranous skull. The contributions are small in the sphenoid, where they form the tips of the greater wings and parts of the medial pterygoid plates, and in the occipital bone, where they form the portion above the superior nuchal line. The membranous contributions are large in each temporal bone. Here only the petrous pyramid belongs to the chondrocranium, and the squamosa, zygomatic process, and annulus are formed of membrane bone.

In the adult skull the chondrocranium extends from the root of the nose to the superior nuchal line. The exact lateral margins are difficult to identify because the original intramembranous and enchondral ossification centers have coalesced into single bones. With minor exceptions, however, the chondrocranium forms the neurocranial floor. Membrane bone forms the face and the neurocranial vault or calvarium (Arey, 1965).

In the occipital bone of the infant, the mendosal suture divides the membranous interparietal portion of the squamosa from the larger chondrocranial portion. The medial portion of the mendosal suture nearly always is closed by the time of birth. When it remains open, the portion of the occipital bone above the mendosal suture is known as the interparietal bone. True interparietal bones are rare in the human skull, although at times large wormian bones have been misinterpreted as interparietal bones.

Progression from cartilage to bone is orderly in all chondrocranial bones, as it is in the ends of the growing long bones. Enchondral ossification occurs about the periphery of each chondrocranial bone, and the strips of unossified cartilage between the bones form the chondrocranial sutures. The age at which the chondrocranial sutures will close is as predictable as that for epiphyseal closure of the long bones. For example, the occipitosphenoid suture usually closes between 16 and 20 years of age (Irwin, 1960).

The brain and other soft tissues of the head influence development of the chondrocranium only slightly, but their effect on the calvarium and face is profound. In fact, the growth potential of all cartilage bone appears to be intrinsic in either the cartilage or, more likely, the precartilaginous mesenchyme. Murray and Huxley (1925) demonstrated this potential by grafting the basal piece of the left posterior limb bud of a 4-day chick embryo onto the chorioallantoic membrane of another chick embryo. At 4 days the limb bud was minute, merely an exaggeration of the wolffian ridge. Five days later it had developed into a well-formed, still cartilaginous, femur with only a trace of adjacent muscle and other soft tissue. Thus these workers demonstrated that precartilaginous tissues have a growth potential distinct from that of the surrounding soft tissues.

The chondrocranium has been proved to be the most stable and predictable portion of the skull. Indeed chondrocranial growth parallels general body growth much more closely than it does brain growth.

Calvarium

Before bone forms in the vault, condensations develop in the cerebral capsule that mature into fibrous bands within the outer layer of the dura mater. These bands attach to the high points of the chondrocranium—the crista galli, lesser wings of the sphenoid, and petrous apices. They underlie the future major calvarial sutures and divide the cerebral capsule into several *fields*.

Without the intervention of a cartilaginous stage, eight bone islands appear in the center of each of these fields just outside the dura, during the ninth and tenth fetal weeks. These islands are the single ossification centers for the two parietal bones and the two temporal squamosae, the paired centers for the frontal squamosa, and the two centers for the interparietal portion of the occipital bone (Moss and Young, 1960; Patten, 1968). By a process of appositional growth around the periphery, each island enlarges toward the fibrous tracts that define its field. There it almost meets the adjacent bones, forming the sutures. More bone is added to the periphery only when the cerebral capsule expands, and the capsule expands only in response to enlargement of the neural mass—the brain, leptomeninges, and cerebrospinal fluid. Growth of the calvarium therefore is purely passive, the bones literally floating outward in the expanding cerebral capsule. No active growth center exists in the periphery of a membrane bone of the calvarium that forces it to grow regardless of the development of the neural mass. Consequently the size and shape of the endocranial surface of the calvarium depend on the size and shape of the dura, which in turn are determined by the surface of the brain and the leptomeninges (Moss and Young, 1960; Enlow, 1968).

In the first 2 months of intrauterine life, the development of the central nervous system (CNS) exceeds the development of all other components of the body. The CNS forms 25% of the body mass at 8 weeks. Thereafter somatic growth outstrips neural growth so that the CNS forms only 10% of the body mass at birth. After birth, somatic growth continues to exceed neural growth, and at 5 years the CNS contributes only 5% to body mass, and in the adult but 2% (Watson and Lowery, 1967).

The brain of an average full-term newborn infant weighs approximately 335 gm, about 25% of its eventual adult weight. By 6 months the weight has increased to 660 gm, 50% of the adult weight, and by 2 years it has reached 80% of its adult weight (Coppoletta and Wolbach, 1933). Postnatal brain growth is almost 60% complete by the end of the first year, 80% complete by the end of the third year, and 95% complete by the end of the eighth year. The average weight of the brain at 10 years is almost as great as that in the adult. Minimal growth continues to at least 25 years and probably throughout life (Watson and Lowery, 1967).

Because of rapid brain growth during the first year, initial bone apposition is principally at the periphery of each calvarial bone. Bone is also added, however, to the exocranial and endocranial surfaces, which thickens the calvarium. The endocranial apposition would decrease the neurocranial volume except that the open sutures permit the calvarial bones to passively float outward within the expanding cerebral capsule. The size of the neural mass alone determines the neurocranial volume (Moss and Young, 1960; Enlow, 1968).

Bone resorption on the diploic surfaces of both the inner and the outer calvarial tables widens the diploe and prevents the calvarial bones from becoming excessively thick and heavy. Moreover, as the cerebral capsule expands, the arc of curvature of each calvarial bone decreases through a remodeling process. This process is similar to that in the metaphyses and diaphyses of the growing long bones. In the calvarium this remodeling is accomplished through combined apposition and resorption on the exocranial, diploic, and endocranial surfaces of both tables (Enlow, 1968).

That chondrocranial and calvarial sutures are different should be clear from the foregoing discussion. The periphery of each chondrocranial bone is an active growth center that pushes the adjacent bones away. Consequently the final size of the chondrocranium is influenced little by the brain and other adjacent soft tissues. Calvarial sutures, however, are passive growth sites where adjacent bones are never pushed apart. Instead bone is deposited only when the neural mass grows. This deposition maintains a relatively constant width for the calvarial sutures, which slowly narrow with advancing age (Moss and Young, 1960; Enlow, 1968).

In contrast to the chondrocranial sutures, closure of the calvarial suture is not predictable and varies greatly. McKern and Stewart (1957) found some portions of the sagittal suture closed in 9% of males 17 to 18 years old. In males 31 to 40 years old, it was closed in 72%. Comparable figures for the lambdoid suture were 3% and 39%, and for the coronal suture 1% and 25%. In the same skulls the basilar suture was closed in 78% of males 17 to 18 years old and in 100% of males 21 and older. These results were obtained by direct inspection of the ectocranial surface of each skull. Christensen and his co-workers (1960) showed that a suture may appear open on roentgenographic examination when inspection of both the ectocranial and endocranial surfaces suggests that it is closed.

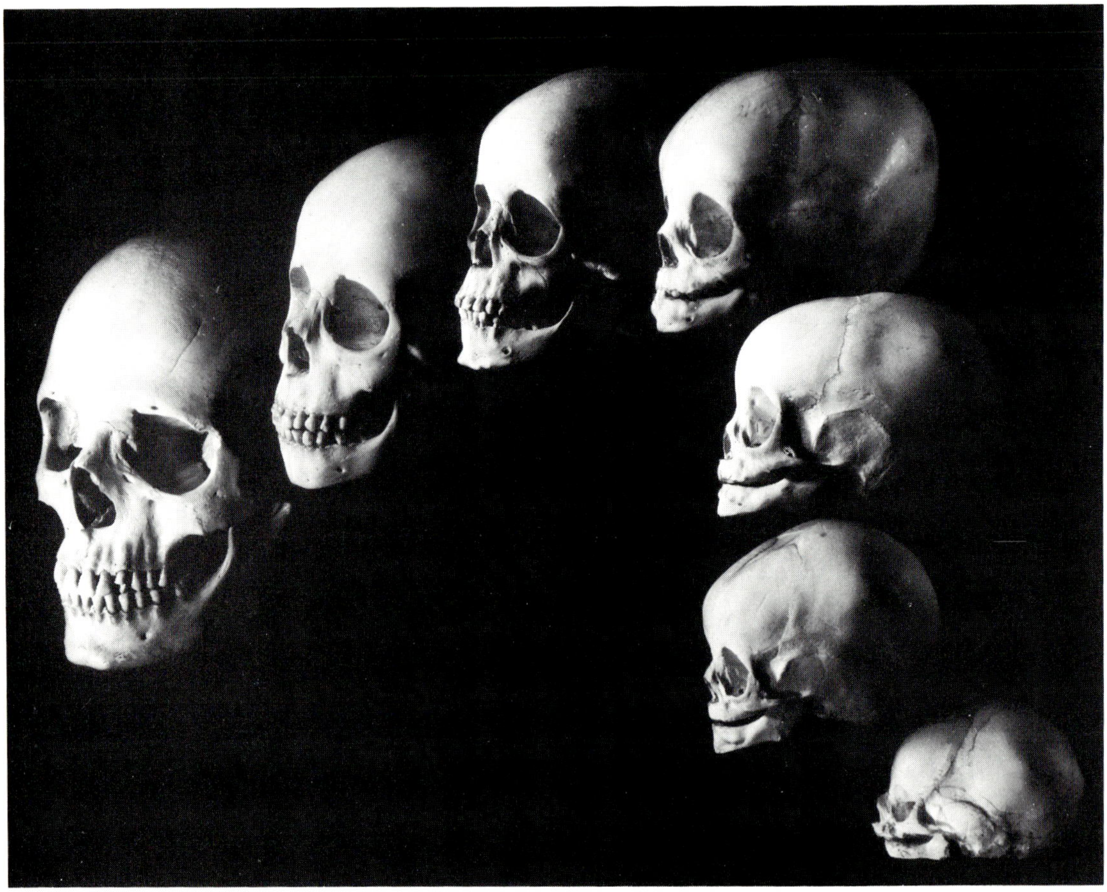

Fig. 8-1. Development of skull in first year of life (vertical column) and subsequently (horizontal row). Approximate ages of skulls are late prenatal (bottom right), 2 months, 5 months, 8 months (top right), 5 years, 7 years, and adult. (Courtesy L. M. Allison, Department of Medical Illustration, and D. H. Enlow, Professor of Anatomy, University of Michigan Medical School.)

Face

Facial growth is limited during fetal life, and at birth the face comprises 10% of total skull volume. During the first 6 months of postnatal life, neurocranial growth continues to exceed facial growth. Subsequently facial development exceeds neurocranial and begins to parallel general somatic development. By 10 years brain and neurocranial development are almost complete but facial growth is active. The face participates in the general adolescent growth spurt so that in the adult the face comprises 30% to 35% of the skull volume (Watson and Lowery, 1967).

Comparison of skull and body heights is informative. By the end of the eighth week of intrauterine life, the head comprises one half the length of the body; at birth it constitutes one fourth. As stated before, the CNS comprises 10% of the total body mass at birth and only 2% in the adult. Therefore a fivefold reduction in the portion of body height formed by the head might be anticipated between birth and full growth. Only a twofold reduction occurs, however; and in the adult the head forms one eighth of the total body height (Jackson, 1928). The difference is contributed by the face, and most facial growth occurs after birth (Fig. 8-1).

The chondrocranium forms the roof of the face. In the embryo, chondrocranial development precedes facial development and the face literally hangs from the chondrocranium. Consequently the width and protrusion of the face are largely determined by the width and length of the chondrocranium (Scott, 1953). Most abnormalities of the upper, central part of the face are probably caused by malformations of the chondrocranium. Malformations of the ears, mouth, and mandible are related to abnormal development of the first two branchial arches (Albers, 1963).

ROENTGENOGRAPHIC EVALUATION

Evaluation of the shape and size of the skull is best obtained by observation, palpation, and use of the tape measure. These methods reveal deformities and asymmetries as well as abnormalities in size that may be difficult or impossible to appreciate on roentgenograms. The measurement should be compared to appropriate standards for age, sex, and ethnic group (Nellhaus, 1968). Once an abnormality of shape or size is discovered, roentgen examination may establish the cause.

The radiologist should appreciate the relative proportions of the skull comprised by the neurocranium and face at various ages (Fig. 8-1). This knowledge is best gained by experience, but the excellent roentgenograms of normal skulls of infants and children reproduced by Shapiro and Janzen (1960) are useful guides.

At birth the *volume* of the neurocranium is eight to nine times as great as the *volume* of the face. At 2 years this ratio is 5:1, at 6 years 3:1, and in the adult 2:1 (Watson and Lowery, 1967). It is difficult for the radiologist to deal with volumes. A well-positioned lateral roentgenogram of the skull, however, shows clearly the relative *areas* in the midsagittal plane of the neurocranium and the face. At birth the midsagittal neurocranial area is four to four and a half times as large as the facial area, when the jaws are closed. (Roentgenograms usually show the mouth open, indicating that the infant was voicing resentment at being photographed; the radiologist must close the infant's jaws, either in his mind or by drawing a closed jaw on the film, before comparing neurocranial and facial areas.) In the child of 2 years, the midsagittal area of the neurocranium is about three to three and a half times as great as the area of the face; at 6 years the ratio is approximately 2.5:1; and in the adult 1.5:1 to 2:1.

Reliable measurements of the length, width, and height of the neurocranium may be derived from cephalometric roentgenograms of the skull, in which positioning and magnification are precisely controlled. When these measurements are derived from routine roentgenograms of the skull (Haas, 1952), however, they frequently are misleading.

The index provided by Cronqvist (1968) may be applied to measurements obtained from routine skull roentgenograms with moderate reliability. Cronqvist related the length, height, and width of the neurocranium to the width of the chondrocranium. He evaluated the width of the chondrocranium indirectly by measuring the distance between the two mandibular necks on the anteroposterior roentgenogram. Since chondrocranial growth reflects body growth, I have not been surprised that Cronqvist's indices proved useful in evaluating the skull when body growth was normal but misleading in some children with growth disturbances. Austin and Gooding (1971) have recently reevaluated the roentgenographic measurements of skull size in children. They agree that Cronqvist's index is a sensitive test of skull size. Unlike Cronqvist, they found the index to be age-dependent and suggested new values for infants and children under 5 years (Chapter 10).

Gordon (1966) devised a moderately complicated formula for estimating neurocranial volume from routine skull roentgenograms. Its extensive use seems unlikely except when clinical measurements are impossible. I have had no experience with it.

ABNORMAL SKULL GROWTH AND DEVELOPMENT

Effects of pressure

During vaginal delivery external pressure molds the neurocranium. With *molding,* the frontal and occipital bones fold toward each other and the parietal bones are displaced outward. The parietal bones overlap the margins of the frontal and occipital bones, and one parietal bone overlaps the margin of the other at the sagittal suture. After birth, normal intracranial pressure quickly re-expands the skull. Overlapping of the sutures usually disappears within 24 hours of delivery, but mild outward displacement of the parietal bones may persist several days.

The infant's calvarium is relatively soft and can be deformed by external pressure. The tower skull seen in certain African tribes who bind the heads of their infants and children is a striking example. A more common one is *postural flattening.*

When an infant habitually lies with his head in one position, the dependent portion of the calvarium is flattened and the remainder is secondarily deformed (Greene, 1931; Moss and Young, 1960). Postural flattening is most common when motor development is retarded. In a normal infant, however, postural flattening will develop if the child habitually holds the head in one position (e.g., as with wryneck). If a light or toy is the only source of stimulation near a crib, the infant may face that source most of the time and postural flattening may result. On occasions postural flattening is iatrogenic (Fig. 8-2).

Most often postural flattening involves the occiput, because the infant has been placed face upward. If he persistently faces sideways, the dependent side of the skull is flattened. Unusual calvarial deformities result when the infant faces obliquely, possibly with his chin elevated or depressed.

Intrinsic, as well as extrinsic, pressure molds the calvarium. The cerebral convolutions press on the inner table to cause the normal *digital markings.* Occasionally these markings can be identified in the neonate. They increase from 1 to 4 years of age, remain constant from 4 to 9 years, decline somewhat from 9 to 14 years, and then again increase slightly. They are usually most prominent in the period from 4 to 9 years (du Boulay, 1956).

Because the specific gravity of the brain exceeds that of the cerebrospinal fluid, the brain sinks in the fluid and rests against the dependent part of the neurocranium. Consequently the most prominent digital markings are noted along the neurocranial base in normal erect children and adults. When postural flattening has developed, digital markings are confined to the dependent half of the calvarium (Fig. 8-2).

Effects of abnormal brain growth

As explained in the first section of this chapter, brain growth has little effect on the development of the chondrocranium. It does not affect development of the face, but is the principal determinant of calvarial growth and form (Scott, 1953; Young, 1959). More precisely the entire neural mass—brain, cerebrospinal fluid, and meninges—rather than the brain alone, directs calvarial growth. When the neural mass is abnormally large, the chondrocranium forms an abnormally small portion of the neurocranium and the calvarium is enlarged. When the neural mass is abnormally small, the chondrocranium forms an abnormally large portion of the neurocranium and the calvarium is small.

With *hydrocephalus* the neural mass expands too quickly. The cerebral capsule keeps pace, and the contained islands of calvarial bone are rapidly separated. Appositional bone deposition increases at the periphery of each calvarial bone, possibly at the expense of surface apposition, since the bone tends to be unusually thin. When the hydrocephalus is mild, increased peripheral bone apposition maintains normal suture width; with severe hydrocephalus bone apposition cannot keep pace and the sutures widen (Fig. 8-3). Since the face and chondrocranium are not enlarged (Moss and Young, 1960), the large dermal neurocranium bulges out above

A

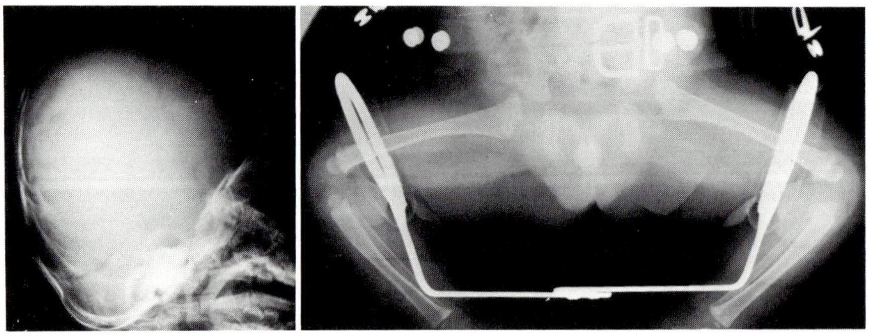

B

Fig. 8-2. A, Mentally normal 8-month-old infant with severe postural flattening of occiput. Because brain sinks in cerebrospinal fluid, digital markings are limited to posterior third of neurocranium. **B,** Brace that was intended to reduce congenitally dislocated hips maintained infant in supine position and was cause of occipital flattening. (From Dorst, J. P.: Radiol. Clin. N. Amer. **2**:347-366, 1964.)

its chondrocranial attachments. The bulge is particularly apparent anteriorly, where it forms the characteristic frontal bossing of hydrocephalus.

The neurocranium is also enlarged in two uncommon conditions: macrencephally and hydranencephaly. *Macrencephaly* (literally a large brain) is present in the occasional individual of normal or unusual intelligence. The term is usually reserved, however, for large and malformed brains, which often are diffusely overgrown with protoplasmic microglia. Clinically epilepsy or mental deficiency, or both, is present in these patients (Blackwood et al., 1963).

In *hydranencephaly* the lateral ventricles are enormous and the cerebral cortex is reduced to a virtual membrane that contains the cerebral vessels. The calvarial size usually is normal at birth and increases rapidly in the next few months (Blackwood et al., 1963).

A small neurocranium is almost always the result of a small brain. When the circumference of the head is more than 2 standard deviations below the mean for age and sex, intelligence is almost always subnormal (O'Connell et al., 1965). Microcrania is an adequate term, but *micrencephaly* better expresses the implications of a small neurocranium.

If the stature of the micrencephalic child is normal, the face and chondrocranium are of normal size but the vault of the cerebral capsule and the contained membranous neurocranium (calvarium) are small (Figs. 8-4 and 8-5). The forehead slopes—exactly the opposite of the bossing seen in hydrocephalus. The calvarial bones are carried apart abnormally slowly within the small cerebral capsule. Consequently they are small and close together. The sutures are narrow for the chronologic age and occasionally close prematurely. Moreover, each calvarial bone usually is abnormally thick, indicative of decreased peripheral and increased surface apposition of bone, as compared with the normal skull. Digital markings usually are reduced or absent. Occasionally, for unknown reasons, these markings are prominent in the skulls of patients with moderate micrencephaly (Fig. 8-6). The paranasal sinuses and mastoid air cells frequently are unusually large. The length and width of the chondrocranium are normal, but the cranial fossae are shallow (Scott, 1953; Young, 1959; Moss and Young, 1960).

When cerebral atrophy is caused by brain damage in the late intrauterine period, the size of the calvarium may be normal before birth. During vaginal delivery severe molding occurs, which persists because intracranial pressure is low. A few months later an abnormally thick calvarium and persistent molding will be found in such an infant (Fig. 8-7).

When severe micrencephaly results from factors early in intrauterine life, deformity of the skull may be so great that the skull resembles a monkey's (Fig. 8-8). Analysis shows that the chondrocranium and face are relatively normally formed and that the small neurocranium is what gives the entire skull its nonhuman appearance.

In micrencephalic patients the stature is frequently somewhat reduced and the size of the chondrocranium and face is correspondingly reduced. When stature and brain growth are reduced to the same extent, no disproportion results between the size of the calvarium and the size of the chondrocranium and face. Micrencephaly is then difficult to recognize roentgenographically unless measurements are employed. As explained previously, these measurements are frequently unreliable. Cronqvist's indices are not helpful since they compare the size of the entire neurocranium to the size of the chondrocranium. Clearly, direct measurement of the circumference of the head is the easiest and best method of diagnosis.

One might argue that when stature and brain size

A

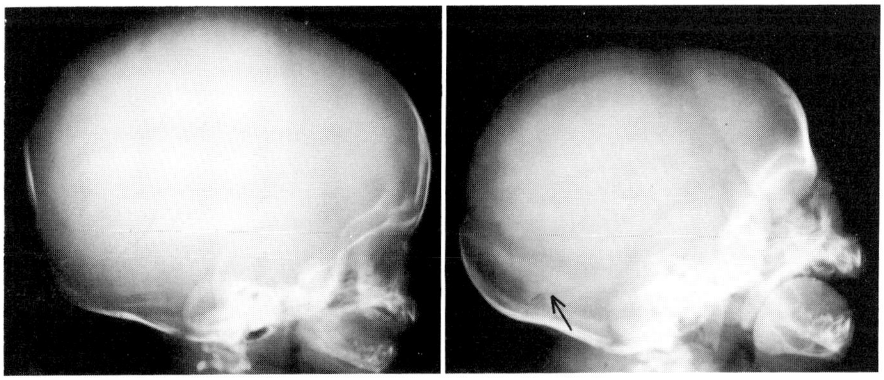

B

Fig. 8-3. A, Roentgenogram of skull of 10-day-old infant with hydrocephalus, large calvarium, and abnormally wide sutures. **B,** Roentgenogram of skull of normal 10-day-old infant, for comparison. Arrow points to mendosal suture. (From Dorst, J. P.: Radiol. Clin. N. Amer. **2**:347-366, 1964.)

A B C D

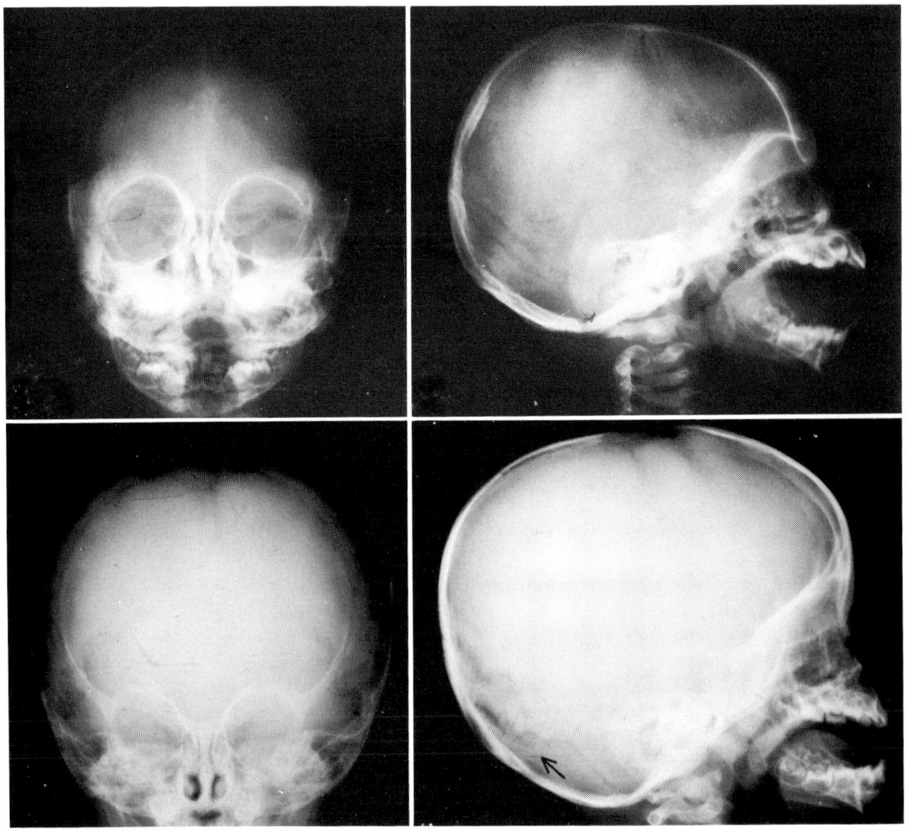

Fig. 8-4. A and **B,** Frontal and lateral roentgenograms of skull of 10-month-old girl with severe retardation of motor and mental development. Compared to the face, the calvarium is small. Rather than usual frontal bossing, the forehead slopes. Anterior fontanelle is prematurely closed. **C** and **D,** Roentgenograms of skull of normal 10-month-old boy, for comparison. Arrow points to mendosal suture. (From Dorst, J. P.: Radiol. Clin. N. Amer. **2:** 347-366, 1964.)

A B

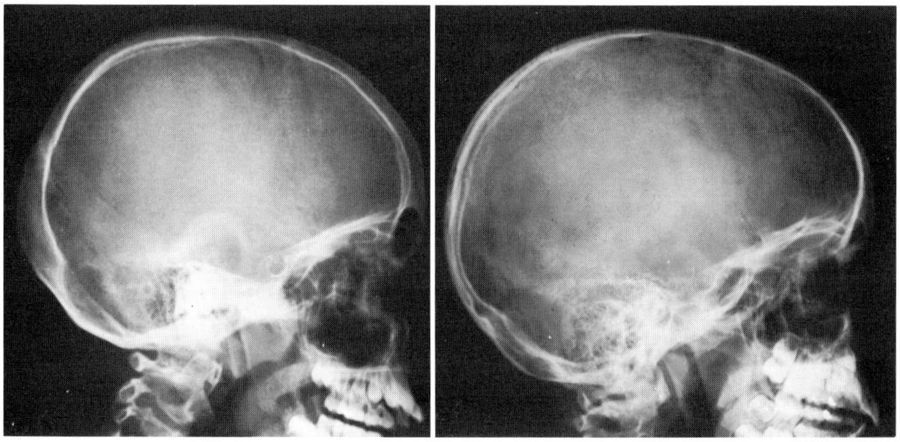

Fig. 8-5. A, Roentgenogram of 9½-year-old girl with severe retardation of mental and motor development after meningitis at 2 years. Size and thickness of calvarium, relative to face, would be normal in adult but are quite abnormal at age 9. Sinuses are large. **B,** Normal child, age 9½ years, for comparison. (From Dorst, J. P.: Radiol. Clin. N. Amer. **2:**347-366, 1964.)

A 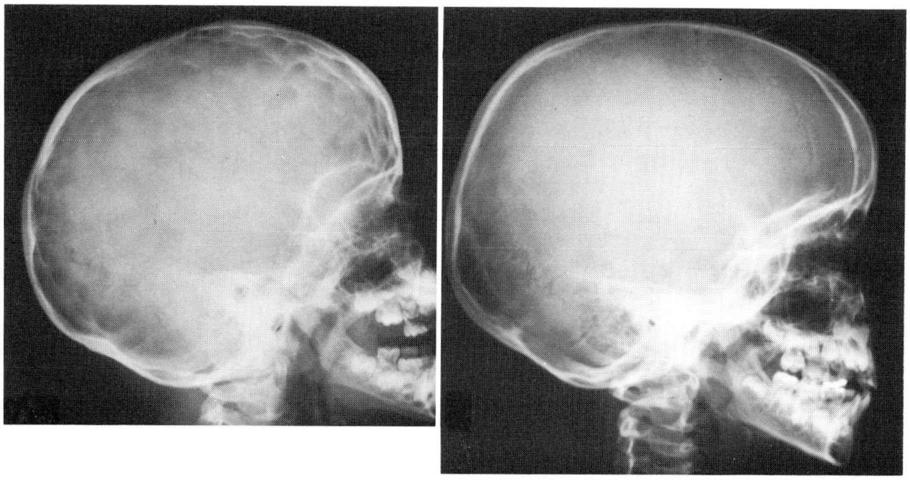 B

Fig. 8-6. A, Micrencephaly and delayed motor and mental development have been apparent since infancy in this 6-year-old girl. Despite small calvarium, diploe is not thickened and digital markings are unusually prominent. **B,** Skull of normal child, age 6½ years, for comparison. (From Dorst, J. P.: Radiol. Clin. N. Amer. **2**:347-366, 1964.)

A B C 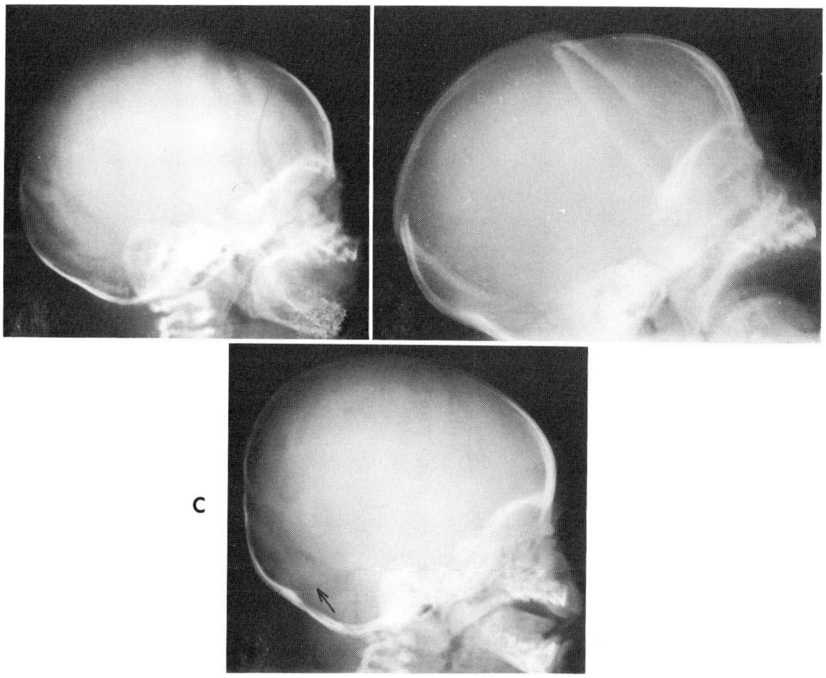

Fig. 8-7. A, Normal molding of calvarium in neonate. Occipital and frontal bones are slightly elevated. **B,** Residual molding and abnormally thick calvarium of 3½-month-old infant in whom size of skull did not increase since birth. Thick calvarium distinguishes this skull from normal neonatal skull. **C,** Normal 3¼-month-old infant. Arrow points to mendosal suture. (From Dorst, J. P.: Radiol. Clin. N. Amer. **2**:347-366, 1964.)

A

B

C

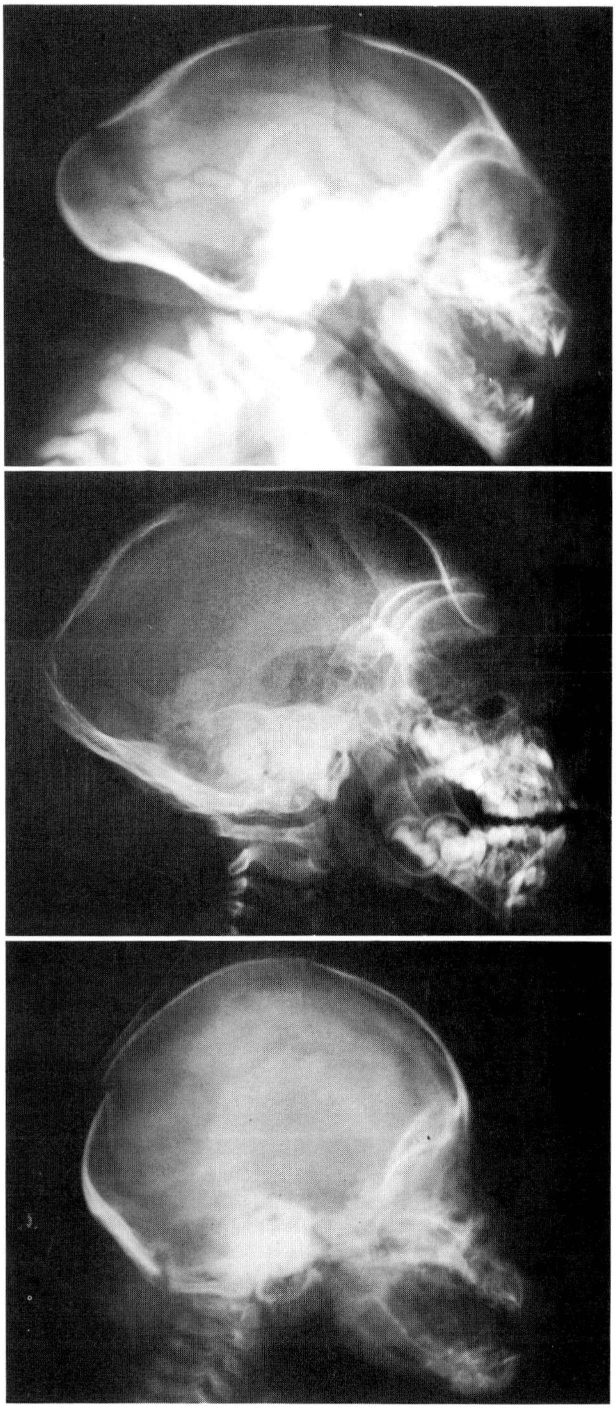

Fig. 8-8. A, Skull roentgenogram of 2-week-old human infant with intrauterine growth retardation and extreme micrencephaly. Calvarium is thick and forehead slopes. **B,** Severe micrencephaly in 20-month-old boy who apparently neither sees nor hears and responds to pain only with weak withdrawal. **C,** Skull of monkey. (**A** from Dorst, J. P.: Radiol. Clin. N. Amer. **2**:347-366, 1964; **C** courtesy Frederic N. Silverman, M.D., Cincinnati, Ohio.)

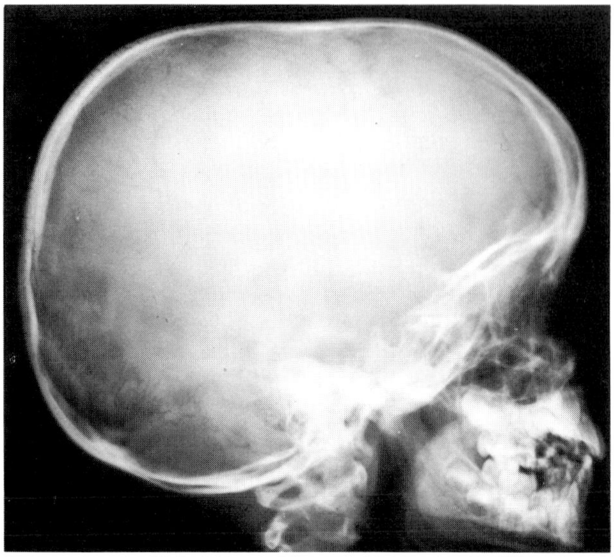

Fig. 8-9. Quite intelligent $8\frac{3}{4}$-year-old pituitary dwarf. Neurocranium is normal for his age and too large for face and chondrocranium, which are proportionate to his reduced stature. (From Dorst, J. P.: Radiol. Clin. N. Amer. **2**:347-366, 1964.)

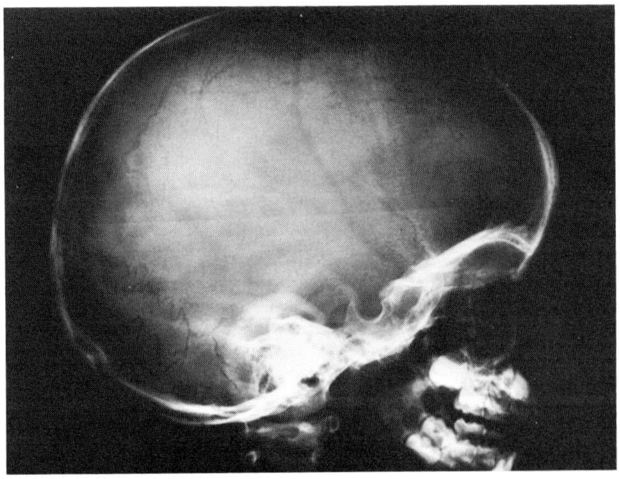

Fig. 8-10. A $3\frac{2}{3}$-year-old boy with mental retardation and even greater growth retardation. Circumference of the head is that of average 2-year-old boy, and height age is 10 months. Consequently growth of face and chondrocranium is more retarded than neurocranial growth, and findings on roentgenogram could easily be misinterpreted as arrested hydrocephalus.

A 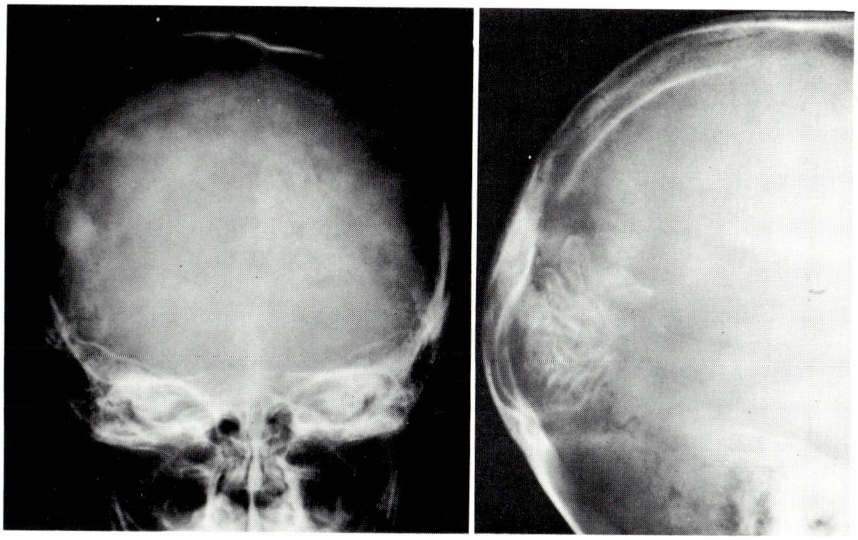 B

Fig. 8-11. A 6-year-old girl with typical clinical features of the Sturge-Weber syndrome. **A,** Left cerebral hemisphere is hypoplastic; consequently left side of calvarium is considerably smaller than right. **B,** Characteristic serpentine cortical calcifications within the left occipital cortex. (From Dorst, J. P.: Radiol. Clin. N. Amer. **2**:347-366, 1964.)

are similarly reduced the patient is not truly micrencephalic, for he has adequate brain for his height. This is incorrect, and such patients are nearly always mentally subnormal. The circumference of the skull of a mentally normal, short individual usually is normal for his chronologic age and increased for his height age (O'Connell et al., 1965; Cloutier and Stickler, 1968; Nellhaus, 1968). The size of the chondrocranium and face is proportionate to the reduced stature, but the size of the neurocranium is correct for the chronologic age. On roentgenograms the consequent disproportion between the face and the calvarium is difficult to differentiate from that seen with mild hydrocephalus or macrencephaly (Fig. 8-9).

Occasionally in a significantly micrencephalic child, stature is more reduced than brain growth. In this situation the roentgenogram of the skull is likely to be misinterpreted as showing hydrocephalus or macrencephaly (Fig. 8-10).

When growth of one cerebral hemisphere is impaired, the calvarium is smaller and thicker over the involved hemisphere than over the normal one. The central portion of the chondrocranium is usually unaffected. The lateral portion, particularly the petrous ridge, may be slightly elevated on the involved side. This change, however, is less common and usually less striking than the decreased circumference and increased thickness of the involved half of the calvarium (Fig. 8-11).

Effects of abnormal bone formation

In *achondroplasia* all cartilage bone is abnormal, including the chondrocranium. Membrane bone ossifies normally, but the calvarium and face are secondarily deformed because of their attachments to the short chondrocranium. Since the nasomaxillary component of the face hangs from the chondrocranium, the root of the nose and the midface are recessed. The jaws, particularly the mandible, which develops from the first branchial arch, are less affected.

The brain in achondroplasia is usually slightly large, as are the ventricles (Cohen et al., 1967). Since the chondrocranium forms a disproportionately small part of the covering of the brain, the membranous cranium is correspondingly enlarged. This disproportion gives the achondroplastic dwarf his characteristic facies. The calvarium is large, and there is frontal bossing (Fig. 8-12). The midface is recessed, the nose is flat, and the jaws are relatively prognathic.

Although the chondrocranial foramina, including the foramen magnum, are small in achondroplasia, compression of the cranial nerves and brainstem is rare. (Spinal nerve root compression, however, is not uncommon.) The incidence of hydrocephalus in achondroplasia is increased (Fig. 8-12, *B*), and some authors have related hydrocephalus to the small size of the foramen magnum; yet in some achondroplastic infants with hydrocephalus, the foramina of Luschka and Magendie have been demonstrated by pneumoencephalography to open *above* the foramen magnum. To implicate the small foramen magnum in the hydrocephalus therefore is difficult.

In most of the chondrodystrophies, not all cartilage bone is abnormal. In pseudoachondroplastic spondyloepiphyseal dysplasia, for example, body proportions are similar to those encountered in achondroplasia but the

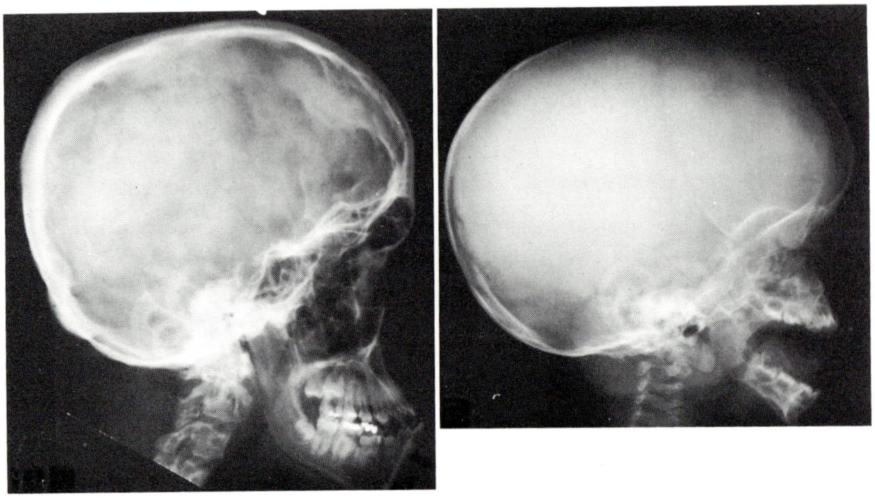

Fig. 8-12. A, A 15-year-old girl with achondroplasia. Small chondrocranium causes sunken midface and striking depression of root of nose. **B,** An 8-month-old girl with achondroplasia and hydrocephalus. (From Dorst, J. P.: Radiol. Clin. N. Amer. **2**:347-366, 1964.)

skull and face are normal (Ford et al., 1961). The primary abnormality in this condition apparently involves the epiphyses. Because the chondrocranial bones lack epiphyses, they are unaffected in pseudoachondroplastic spondyloepiphyseal dysplasia and the skull consequently is normal.

Abnormal membrane bone formation affects the calvarium in a number of conditions. These include cleidocranial dysostosis, pyknodysostosis, the otopalatodigital syndrome, the Hallerman-Streiff syndrome, osteogenesis imperfecta, progeria, frontonasal dysplasia, pachydermoperiostosis, and hypothyroidism. In these conditions each calvarial bone is small and the sutures are wide. An abnormally large number of wormian bones frequently accompany the wide sutures. Both membrane bone and cartilage bone are abnormal in conditions such as rickets and hypophosphatasia. These bones may also be abnormal in an infant born of a mother who had osteomalacia or hyperparathyroidism or who attempted abortion with aminopterin (Bretz et al., in press).

Effects of premature suture closure

When two or more calvarial bones unite before brain growth is complete, these bones are no longer free to float passively outward within the expanding cerebral capsule. To accommodate the growing brain, additional expansion occurs at the sutures that remain open.

When the sutures close prematurely after 3 to 5 years of age, postnatal brain growth is more than 80% complete. The remaining brain growth is not sufficient to significantly deform the neurocranium. When closure occurs earlier, the compensatory growth at the open sutures leads to a deformed calvarium.

This condition is often referred to as *craniosynostosis* or *craniostenosis*. The second term implies that brain growth is inhibited by the premature closure of the suture. Clearly this implication is wrong since only when brain growth continues does calvarial deformity develop (Weidenreich, 1941).

Craniosynostosis most commonly involves the sagittal suture (Fig. 8-13). Compensatory growth occurs in the coronal and lambdoid sutures, lengthening the calvarium. Moreover, at the time the sagittal suture fuses, the junction angle of the two parietal bones is consistent with the size of the brain case. Once fusion occurs, this angle cannot change and remodeling of the parietal surfaces is impeded so that in the older child the junction of the two parietal bones is abnormally acute. The term scaphocephaly (meaning boat head) is particularly descriptive of this condition since it encompasses both the long narrow shape of the skull and the keel-like deformity along the sagittal suture.

A more complex deformity occurs when one or more of the other sutures close prematurely. For example, when one half of the lambdoid suture fuses, the squamosa of the occipital bone is flattened on the involved side. The skull bulges laterally, behind the ear, because of compensatory growth in the occipitomastoid and parietomastoid sutures (Fig. 8-14). Even in the rare situation when all of the sutures close prematurely, brain growth is usually not affected. The skull is distinctive and not suggestive of micrencephaly (Fig. 8-15).

On occasions, premature closure of a suture is related to the abnormal calvarial bone that forms in such conditions as hypophosphatasia and healing rickets. Usually the cause of premature closure is unknown. One possible explanation derives from the great variability in the age when each calvarial suture closes. Premature closure of a suture may merely represent closure in the first part of that range.

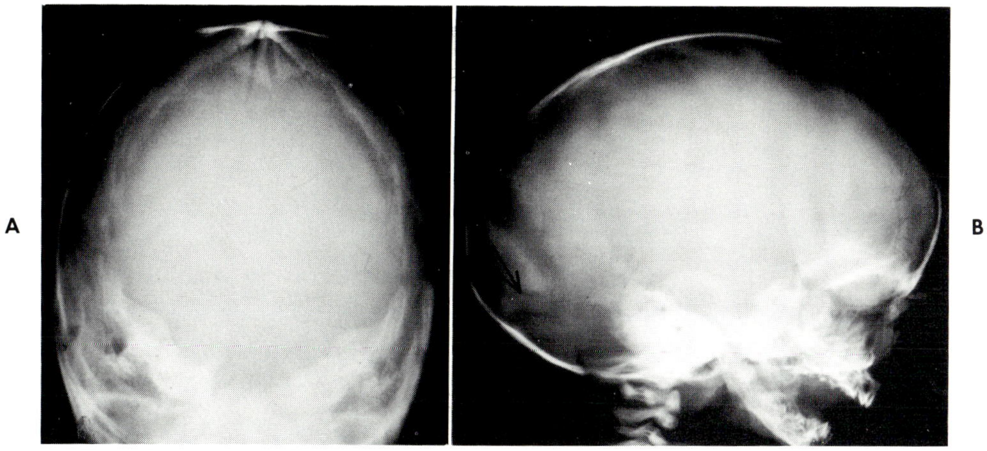

Fig. 8-13. A 1-month-old infant with premature closure of sagittal suture. **A,** The suture is functionally closed, and thick bony margins form a palpable ridge. **B,** Also seen are striking dolichocephaly, mild widening of coronal and lambdoid sutures, and relatively small face. Arrow points to mendosal suture. (From Dorst, J. P.: Radiol. Clin. N. Amer. **2:** 347-366, 1964.)

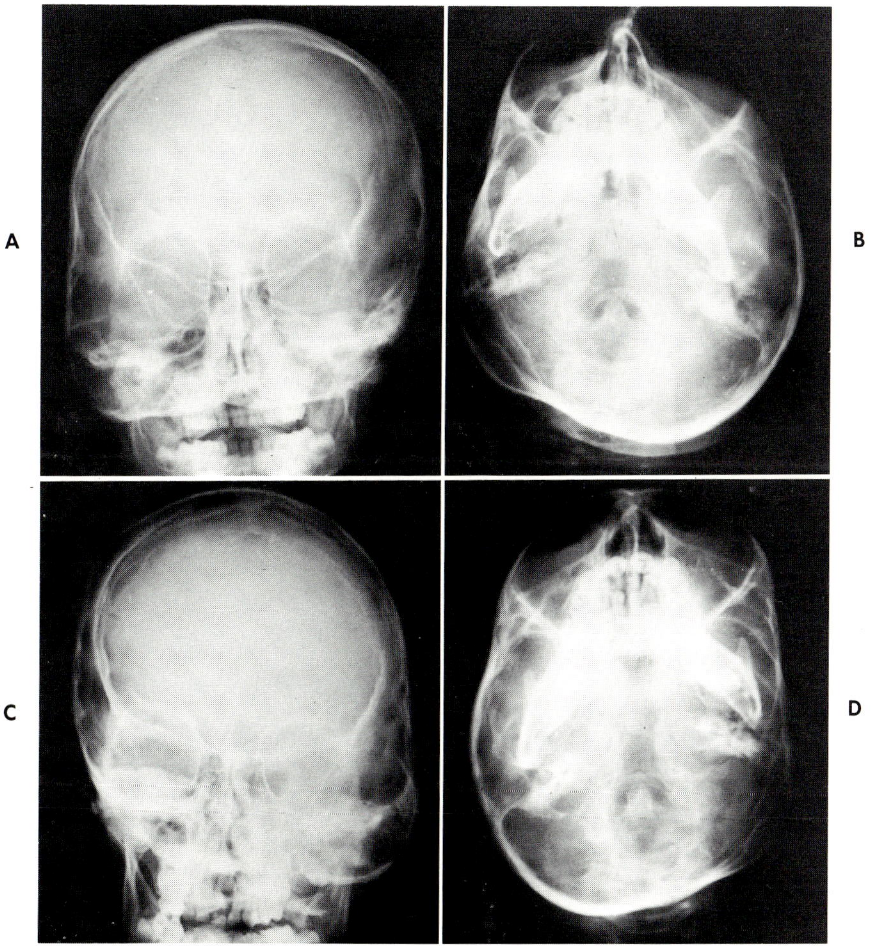

Fig. 8-14. Sisters with plagiocephaly, the result of premature closure of one limb of lambdoid suture. **A** and **B,** In younger sister, age 6 years, the right limb of lambdoid suture is prematurely closed. (**A,** Right half of posterior fossa is deeper than normal and, **B,** its posterolateral wall is flattened.) **C** and **D,** Older sister, age 7 years, with premature closure of left limb of lambdoid suture. (From Dorst, J. P.: Radiol. Clin. N. Amer. **2:**347-366, 1964.)

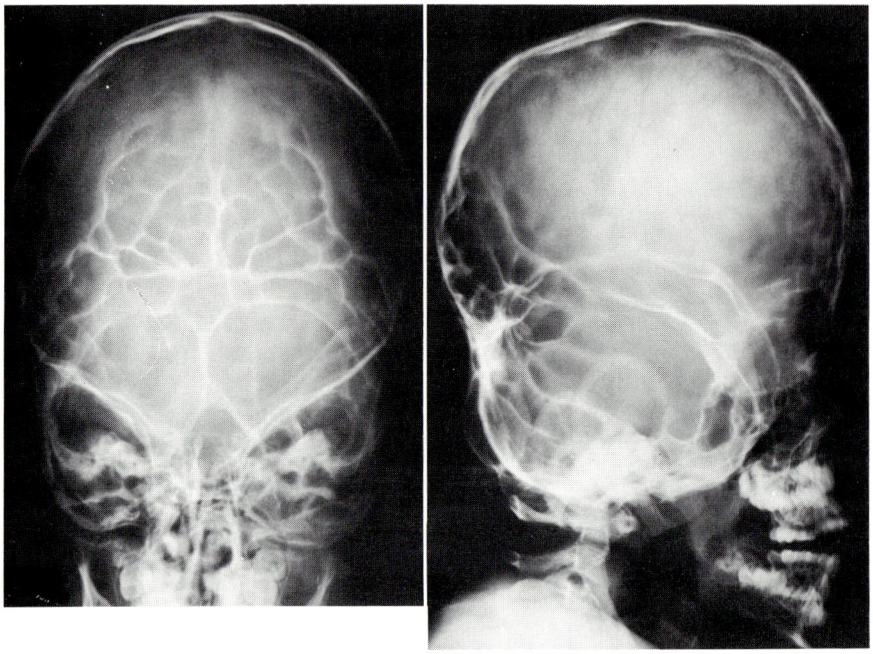

Fig. 8-15. A 5½-year-old girl with premature closure of all calvarial sutures. Presumably lambdoid suture closed first, then next in order sagittal, squamosal, and coronal sutures. Neurocranial volume is normal. (From Dorst, J. P.: Radiol. Clin. N. Amer. **2:**347-366, 1964.)

Moss and Young (1960) have suggested another explanation of craniosynostosis. Moss (1960) showed that section of the fibrous dural band beneath the metopic suture in the rat delayed closure of the suture. Similar dural bands underlie all of the major sutures and attach to the high points of the chondrocranium. Moss and Young (1960) expressed the belief that the common denominator in all cases of craniosynostosis is malformation of the chondrocranium. The malformation causes increased tensions within the cerebral capsule, particularly in one or more of the fibrous dural tracts. The increased tension in the dural tracts leads in turn to premature closure of the overlying sutures. The association of chondrocranial and facial malformations with premature suture closure is at times obvious, as in Crouzon's syndrome of craniofacial dysostosis.

Influence of function on form of skull

Studies in comparative anatomy suggest that the form of the skull in various animals is in large measure determined by the functions of the skull. As stated in the preceding discussion, the size and shape of the neurocranium are determined by three factors: (1) size of the neural mass, (2) form of the chondrocranium, and (3) state of the cerebral capsule. When the relative size of the neural mass is more appropriate to a monkey than to a man, the appearance of the skull is simian rather than human (Fig. 8-8).

The skull may be considered as being comprised of several functional components, each associated with specific soft parts. This concept has been expressed clearly by Moss (1964):

> The head consists of a number of relatively independent and yet coordinated functional cranial components. These components are related to the major functions of the head—sight, respiration, speech, swallowing, and so forth. Each cranial component includes all of the skeletal and related soft tissues necessary to carry out these separate functions effectively. . . . Each supposedly individual bone is, in reality, composed of a number of relatively independent functional components. . . . Each component is, in turn, related to its *functional matrix*—those soft tissues within which the individual osseous components exist and grow. *It is of the utmost importance that we realize that the growth of bone is dependent primarily upon the growth of its functional matrix.**

To give an example, the frontal bone forms portions of the brain case and the orbits and thus is related to the functions of thought and sight. In fact, independent functional components can be identified within such an apparently simple element as the parietal bone. They are the two calvarial tables and the diploe (Moss and Young, 1960). One diploic function is production of blood. When this function is increased in severe or prolonged anemia or in polycythemia, the diploe widens and the calvarium thickens (Fig. 8-16). The calvarial tables protect the brain, and the outer table also provides attachments for the intrinsic and extrinsic muscles of the scalp. This function accounts for the thick skull

---

*From Moss, M. L.: Vertical growth of the human face, Amer. J. Orthodont. **50:**359-376, 1964.

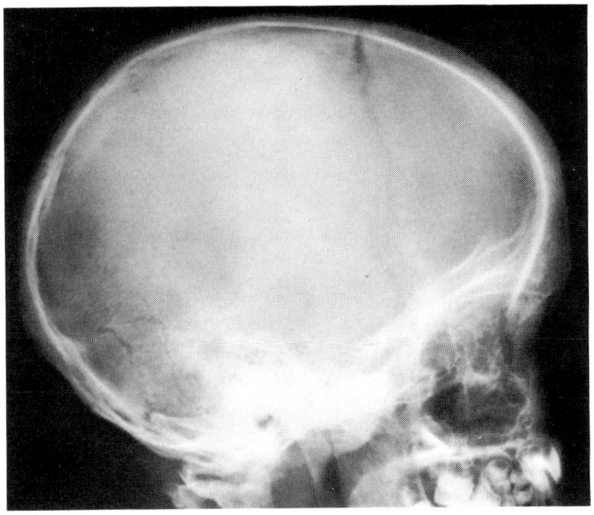

Fig. 8-16. Skull roentgenogram of 4⅔-year-old boy with polycythemia secondary to cyanotic congenital heart disease (tetralogy of Fallot). Hematocrit had varied from 51% to 71%. Diploe is unusually granular and thicker than normal, particularly in supraorbital region. (From Dorst, J. P.: Radiol. Clin. N. Amer. **2**:347-366, 1964.)

in many animals. It is not important in man, except possibly in the micrencephalic (Dorst, 1964).

SUMMARY

The pattern of normal growth of the skull results from the interaction of many forces, both extrinsic and intrinsic to the skull. Many of these forces are related to the functions of the skull, and the skull may be considered as a collection of functional cranial components. When during the period of active skull growth one or more of these forces are abnormal, the skull is deformed correspondingly.

REFERENCES

Arey, L. B.: Developmental anatomy, ed. 7, Philadelphia, 1965, W. B. Saunders Co.

Albers, G. D.: Branchial anomalies, J.A.M.A. **183**:399-409, 1963.

Austin, J. H. M., and Gooding, C. A.: Roentgenographic measurement of skull size in children, Radiology **99**:641-646, 1971.

Blackwood, W., McMenemey, W. H., Meyer, A., Norman, R. M., and Russell, D. S.: Greenfield's neuropathology, ed. 2, Baltimore, 1963, The Williams & Wilkins Co.

Bretz, G. W., Bowerman, J. W., and Dorst, J. P.: Differential diagnosis of delayed calvarial ossification. (In press.)

Christensen, J. B., Lachman, E., and Brues, A. M.: A study of the roentgen appearance of cranial vault sutures: correlation with their anatomy, Amer. J. Roentgen. **83**:615-627, 1960.

Cloutier, M. D., and Stickler, G. B.: (Letter to the editor) Head circumference in children with idiopathic hypopituitarism, Pediatrics **42**:209-210, 1968.

Cohen, M. E., Rosenthal, A. D., and Matson, D. D.: Neurological abnormalities in achondroplastic children, J. Pediat. **71**:367-376, 1967.

Coppoletta, J. M., and Wolbach, S. B.: Body length and organ weights of infants and children, Amer. J. Path. **9**:55-70, 1933.

Cronqvist, S.: Roentgenologic evaluation of cranial size in children, Acta Radiol. [Diagn.] **7**:97-111, 1968.

Dorst, J. P.: Functional craniology: an aid in interpreting roentgenograms of the skull, Radiol. Clin. N. Amer. **2**:347-366, 1964.

du Boulay, G.: The significance of digital impressions in children's skulls, Acta Radiol. **46**:112-122, 1956.

Enlow, D. H.: The human face. An account of the postnatal growth and development of the craniofacial skeleton, New York, 1968, Harper & Row, Publishers.

Ford, N., Silverman, F. N., and Kozlowski, K.: Spondyloepiphyseal dysplasia (pseudo-achondroplastic type), Amer. J. Roentgen. **86**:462-472, 1961.

Gordon, I. R. S.: Measurement of cranial capacity in children, Brit. J. Radiol. **39**:377-381, 1966.

Greene, D.: Asymmetry of the head and face in infants and children, Amer. J. Dis. Child. **41**:1317-1326, 1931.

Haas, L. L.: Roentgenological skull measurements and their diagnostic applications, Amer. J. Roentgen. **67**:197-209, 1952.

Irwin, G. L.: Roentgen determination of the time of closure of the spheno-occipital synchondrosis, Radiology **75**:450-452, 1960.

Jackson, C. M.: Some aspects of form and growth. In Robbins, W. J., and others, editors: Growth, New Haven, 1928, Yale University Press.

McKern, T. W., and Stewart, T. D.: Skeletal age changes in young American males, Technical report EP-45, Natick, Mass., 1957, Environmental Protection Research Division, Quartermaster Research and Engineering Command, U. S. Army.

Moss, M. L.: Inhibition and stimulation of sutural fusion in the rat calvaria, Anat. Rec. **136**:457-467, 1960.

Moss, M. L.: Vertical growth of the human face, Amer. J. Orthodont. **50**:359-376, 1964.

Moss, M. L., and Greenberg, S. N.: Postnatal growth of the human skull base, Angle Orthodont. **25**:77-84, 1955.

Moss, M. L., and Young, R. W.: A functional approach to craniology, Amer. J. Phys. Anthropol. **18**:281-292, 1960.

Murray, P. D. F., and Huxley, J. S.: Self differentiation in the grafted limb-bud of the chick, J. Anat. **59**:379-384, 1925.

Nellhaus, G.: Head circumference from birth to eighteen years: practical composite international and interracial graphs, Pediatrics **41**:106-114, 1968a.

Nellhaus, G.: Head circumference in children with idiopathic hypopituitarism, Pediatrics **42**:210-211, 1968b.

O'Connell, E. J., Feldt, R. H., and Stickler, G. B.: Head circumference, mental retardation and growth failure, Pediatrics **36**:62-66, 1965.

Patten, B. M.: Human embryology, ed. 3, New York, 1968, Blakiston Division, McGraw-Hill Book Co.

Scott, J. H.: The variability of cranial and facial dimensions in modern skulls, Brit. Dent. J. **94**:27-31, 1953.

Shapiro, R., and Janzen, A. H.: The normal skull, a roentgen study, New York, 1960, Paul B. Hoeber, Inc.

Watson, E. H., and Lowery, G. H.: Growth and development of children, ed. 5, Chicago, 1967, Year Book Medical Publishers, Inc.

Weidenreich, F.: The brain and its role in the phylogenetic transformation of the human skull, Trans. Amer. Philosoph. Soc. **31**:321-442, 1941.

Young, R. W.: The influence of cranial contents on postnatal growth of the skull in the rat, Amer. J. Anat. **105**: 383-410, 1959.

CHAPTER 9

Alterations in the skull with aging

Fred J. Hodges, III

Fundamental to all radiologic interpretation is an appreciation of normal roentgen anatomy; and since no human beings (except perhaps identical twins) are exactly alike, "normal" must include a considerable number of variations. In the early years of life, normal is obviously age dependent. The progressive development of the skull from birth to adulthood pursues a well-known and fairly regular pattern as recorded roentgenographically. A similar, regular, and reliable series of changes might be assumed between early adulthood through old age, but such a metamorphosis is not definite or predictable. After the second or third decade, conjecture as to age based on the roentgen appearance of the skull alone is unreliable. Variations from the normal adult appearance, seen in the aging skull, are rather loosely correlated with age. Although many features of the skull are statistically associated with older age, prediction of the age based on roentgen features is not easy in a given case nor is reliance on the known age in predicting the normal limits roentgenographically. Of course, many changes in the skull are frankly pathologic and not truly normal. Because these changes are anticipated or common in certain ages, they are considered within normal limits. When seen at other ages, the same features may be suggestive of prematurity or of a different pathologic origin and significance.

Yet the many alterations that do accompany aging, even though they are inconstant and do not fall into a regular schema, are worthy of consideration. Some are the result of diseases that are more common in, or unique to, advancing age, such as atherosclerosis and senile osteoporosis. Others are idiopathic and may occur at any age but are more common later in life. These are the so-called physiologic intracranial calcifications and benign hyperostosis. Still other changes, although truly senile, may be imperceptible or unrecognizable on standard roentgenograms (at least without benefit of earlier films for comparison). Examples are the subtle changes in bone architecture or minute changes in size and shape of the skull.

The great usefulness of earlier roentgenograms for comparison is obvious, but for various reasons these are seldom available. Satisfactory roentgenograms of the skull were not possible before the advent of the Potter-Bucky diaphragm, in 1917; hence the maximum period of observation is about 50 years. The hazards involved in storing the earlier, highly flammable, cellulose acetate films and the ever-increasing demand for space have resulted in the regular disposal of old films in most departments. Moreover, repeated or interval roentgenography of the skull of *normal persons* over a period of years is uncommon. The rare discovery of old roentgenograms is frequently disappointing because of differences in projection, technique, and quality, which interfere with or negate exact comparison. These circumstances account for the scarcity of satisfactory comparable roentgenograms of the same skull obtained during one or more decades between the ages of 25 and 100 years, and they explain the paucity of data. Instead we must rely heavily on studies of dried skulls of known ages and on roentgenographic findings in older persons for comparison with those in younger patients.

SUTURES

With advancing age the cranial sutures become progressively fused (Ashley-Montague, 1938). Whereas nearly all adult skulls when dried remain firmly in one piece, the sutures are not necessarily fused, only tightly interlocked. The sutures do fuse, however (i.e., solid bony union occurs with increasing age). Closure of the entire length of the suture is not simultaneous and does not necessarily involve the entire depth. Most reports concerning the sutures are based on visual inspection of dried skulls; hence they do not indicate whether the fusion is of the full depth of the suture or merely of the surface edges. Apparently the inner, endocranial aspects of sutures fuse in a more orderly fashion whereas the outer, ectocranial, serrated margin is subject to considerable variation (Todd and Lyon, 1924, 1925). Roentgenography may show either the endocranial, the ectocranial, or the internal aspect of the suture, and the findings may not correlate with those of direct inspection. Furthermore, if the projection is slightly oblique through a suture, roentgenography may fail to show the suture, suggesting closure even when not actually present. For these reasons, assessment of sutures on a dried skull is not strictly applicable to studies on routine skull roentgenograms. Even in dried specimens, inconsistencies and variations are present; consequently studies of these specimens are unreliable for judging age (Singer, 1953). For example, Brooks (1955) noted that in two different groups of dried skulls all of the vault sutures were frequently united, suggesting a minimum age of 46 years, whereas all the circummeatal sutures were open, indicating a maximum age of 37. Furthermore, closure of suture correlates less often with age in females than in males. The sutures in females tend to remain open longer or fail to fuse at all.

The major reports on this subject are those of Todd and Lyon (1924, 1925), who described the fundamental modal of closure in the vault as beginning in the sagittal suture at age 22 years. The coronal closure begins at age 24, and the lambdoid at 26. Complete fusion results by 35, 41, and 47 years respectively. These authors described a condition that they called lapsed union of the sagittal and lambdoid sutures, in which actual fusion does not take place, but growth ceases and a ridge of bone forms along the endocranial edge of the suture. They classified this state as fusion in formulating the modal of closures. Obviously roentgenograms in this condition would show the suture to be unfused. The sutures bordering the squamous portion of the temporal bone rarely close completely even in old age (Harris, 1933) but usually begin to close at about the age of 35 years. The closure pattern in a large series is quite irregular.

Roentgenographic examination of the skull shows the sagittal suture to be closed frequently after 35 to 40 years of age and usually after the age of 50. The lambdoid, and especially the coronal, sutures frequently are closed at least in part after the age of 50 years, whereas the others are frequently, if not uniformly, identifiable on some views even in the 90's. Variations in the pattern of closure are of no significance, except for obvious early closure before adulthood (synostosis) and strikingly delayed closure. The metopic suture, when present in adults, usually remains open indefinitely.

THICKNESS

Significant generalized increase or decrease in the thickness of the skull concomitant with advancing age is not borne out by measurements of dried skulls (O'Leary, 1952), but slight increased thickening has been shown roentgenographically (Israel, 1968; Kraft and Finby, 1969). Local increased thickening in the frontal region is the result of increased thickness primarily of the inner table of the skull. It is frequently seen in older skulls and is the so-called hyperostosis frontalis interna that occurs mainly in women. This thickening begins in middle age but does not regularly increase or decrease after that (Moore, 1955). It does not correlate with cerebral atrophy and must be regarded as an innocent abnormality, not a progressive function of aging (Fig. 9-1). Thickening of other cranial bones is also seen but is not typical (Fig. 9-2).

Thinning also has received attention in regard to aging, especially the so-called parietal thinning. Although thinning is more common with advancing age, it is not confined to later years. Camp and Nash (1944) noted it in ten of ninety-eight patients younger than 31 years. Its complete significance is not known, but

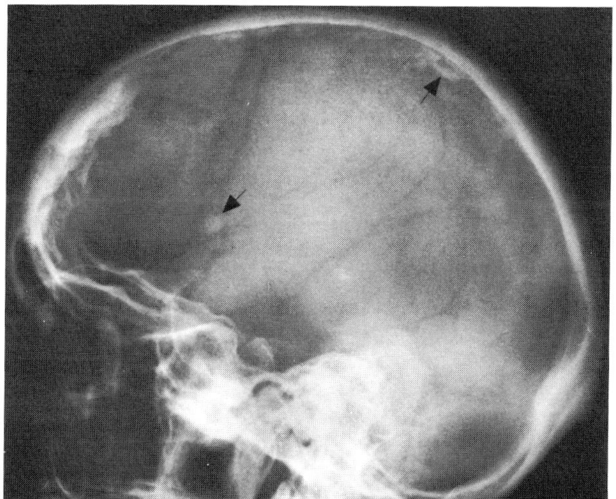

Fig. 9-1. A 42-year-old white woman. Several findings are common to old age but are also frequently seen in middle age: dense calcification in dura (arrows), calcified pineal and petroclinoid ligaments, well-developed hyperostosis of frontal bone, and fused major sutures. Note the absence of recognizable osteoporosis, perhaps the most reliable sign of advancing years. Vascular grooves are common to any adult age. Vascular diploic channels are frequently lacking but when present suggest young or middle adulthood since they are said to disappear in old age.

evidence suggests that this thinning is an inherited dysplasia and not a common function of aging (Gershon-Cohen et al., 1953). Steinbach and Obata (1957) reported observation of a patient over a 16-year period (from age 69 to 85 years) with roentgenographic proof of significant increase in thinning during that time. They thus confirmed the opinion of Schmidt (cited by Camp and Nash, 1944) that at least one form of parietal thinning is associated with osteoporosis and progresses with age. This single case report emphasizes the dearth of, but desire for, skull roentgenograms at intervals over a long period for evaluation of alterations from the normal.

Parietal thinning is shown on frontal roentgenograms as a flattening or depression of the outer table of the parietal bones at the expense of diploic bone while the inner table remains unaffected. The thinning is seen in the lateral view as a darkening along the upper edge of the parietal region. This darkening or radiolucency may be seen, however, without parietal thinning (Fig. 9-3), as pointed out by Gershon-Cohen and his co-workers (1953). A simple explanation is that the transverse thickness of the head, which is widest at the dense midparietal area, tapers toward the vertex, resulting in less density. If the tapering begins suddenly, it produces a fairly distinct edge of radiolucency. The edge-on view of the vertex bone across the midline provides the top limit to the radiolucency. This phenomenon is not restricted to old age but is seen more commonly in older persons, probably because of osteoporosis.

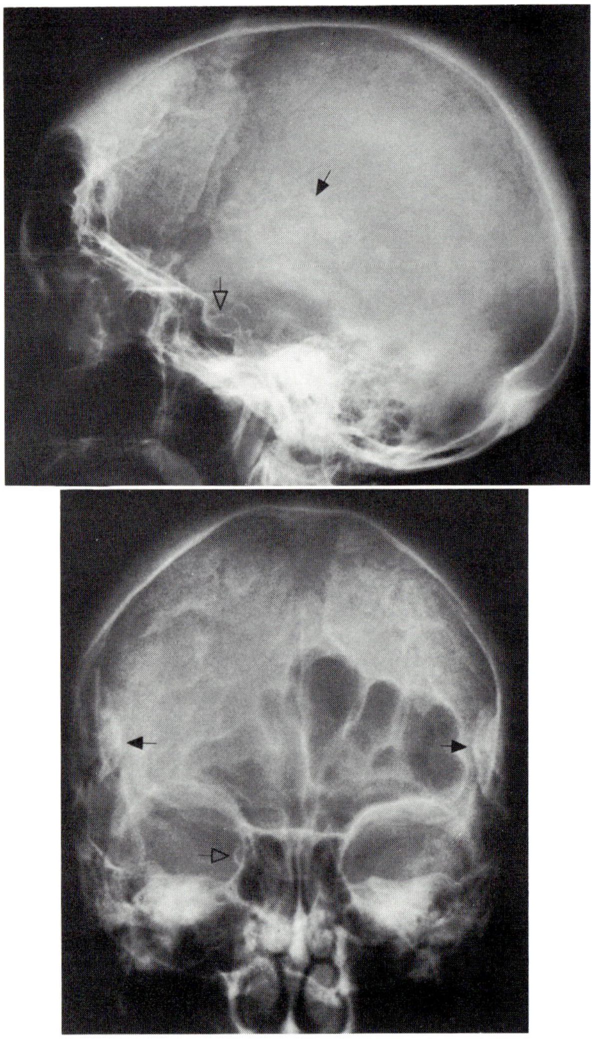

Fig. 9-2. Frontal and lateral roentgenograms of skull of 83-year-old white woman show typical benign idiopathic hyperostosis on inner table of frontal bone cordoned off by dural veins. Similar hyperostosis noted bilaterally on the frontoparietal bones (solid arrows) is presumably of the same etiology. Note the tubular carotid artery calcification (open arrow), the suture fusion, the osteoporosis of sella turcica, and the calcified pineal body.

A

B

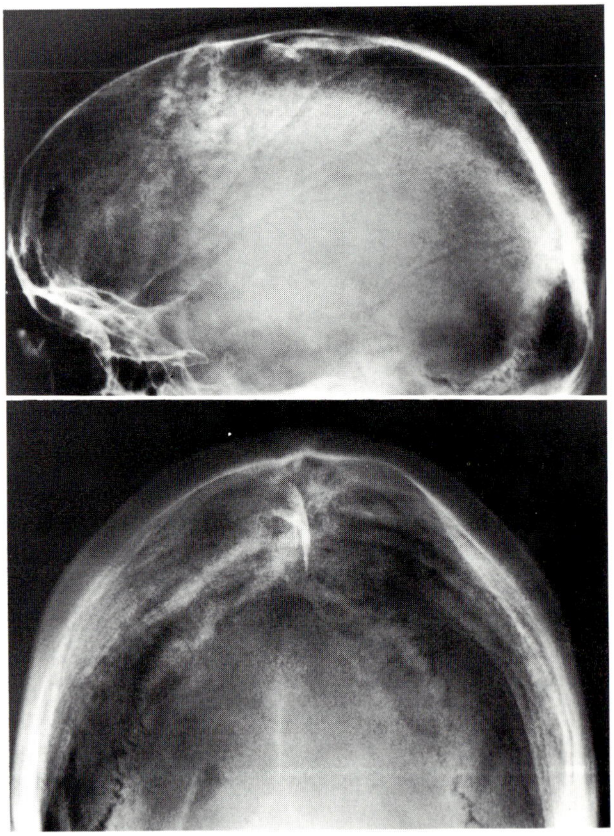

Fig. 9-3. A 44-year-old Negro man. **A,** Dark band or crescent is clearly visible along top of skull from coronal to lambdoid suture, typical of that seen with parietal thinning. In **B,** however, no thinning (or thickening) is apparent, but skull slopes fairly abruptly toward midline. Consequently, transverse diameter of head rapidly diminishes, absorbing less and less radiation. Note the physiologic calcification in the dura adjacent to the sagittal sinus. Upper coronal and total lambdoid sutures are clearly persistent, but sagittal suture is closed.

DENSITY

A generalized decrease in skeletal mass (and roentgenographic density) is universal with aging (Arnold et al., 1966). Decrease in radiodensity of the calvarium attributed to senile osteoporosis is apparently the rule in older individuals. It is not always evident on isolated examination (Gershon-Cohen et al., 1953) and is absent in about one third of persons over the age of 60 years. Osteoporosis (loss of bone mass) may be indistinguishable from osteomalacia (loss of calcium), especially in the skull. Skeletal osteoporosis affects women earlier and to a greater degree than it does men (Newton-John and Morgan, 1968). The diffuse form of benign hyperostosis may mask or offset the osteoporotic effect.

MARKINGS AND TEXTURE

In addition to the granular or honeycomb pattern of the diploe and the sutures, a number of markings in the cranial vault are shown on routine roentgenograms: (1) vascular grooves, channels, and foramina, (2) digital impressions, (3) bony ridges, and (4) pacchionian depressions.

Jones (1912) described a sharpening in delineation of meningeal veins with age. Harris (1933) described a prominence of grooves for the meningeal vessels up to the age of 35 years. After this age the diploic venous channels are more prominent from the age of 50 to 60 years, after which the meningeal vessel grooves again are more prominent. Heinrich (1941) stated that he had never seen a general increase in diploic venous channels but rather a decreased frequency of these channels in senility. Differentiation between diploic venous channels and meningeal grooves may be difficult. Without interval roentgenograms these changes may be difficult to prove, but vascular grooves, both arterial and venous, are regularly present in older skulls (Figs. 9-2, 9-4, and 9-5). The classic intradiploic channels are distinctly less common. Since osteoporosis diminishes the diploic bone pattern and density, it probably also diminishes the clarity of diploic channels. These channels would be affected to a much greater extent than would the grooves, which are outlined by compact inner table bone. A slight hyperostosis of the inner table, accentuating the grooves in some instances, is also hard to exclude.

Concerning the pacchionian depressions, reports in the literature are conflicting. Basmajian (1952) described a general enlargement of these structures with age. O'Leary (1952) also stated that the pacchionian granulations may be hypertrophied in old age. In the same text Cobb (1952) expressed the belief that the pacchionian depressions and granulations do not show any change with age. Heinrich (1941) reported that he had never seen a steady increase of the depressions in older age, and Bondareff (1959) stated that they may hypertrophy with age.

An interesting radiolucency, closely resembling pacchionian depressions, is not infrequent in the occipital bone. It is close to the midline just below the transverse sinuses or torcular Herophili and seems to be associated

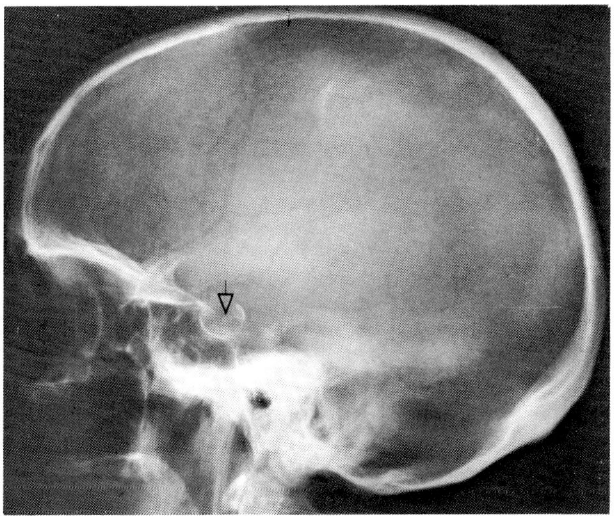

Fig. 9-4. A 97-year-old white woman. Calcification of carotid siphon (arrow) and fusion of sutures, except for the lower lambdoid and temporo-occipital, are characteristic of advanced age. Note the absence of both physiologic intracranial calcification and hyperostosis, two findings associated with older age but frequently lacking. Both meningeal grooves and diploic vascular markings can be identified on original roentgenograms; but bony architecture is diminished, suggesting generalized osteoporosis.

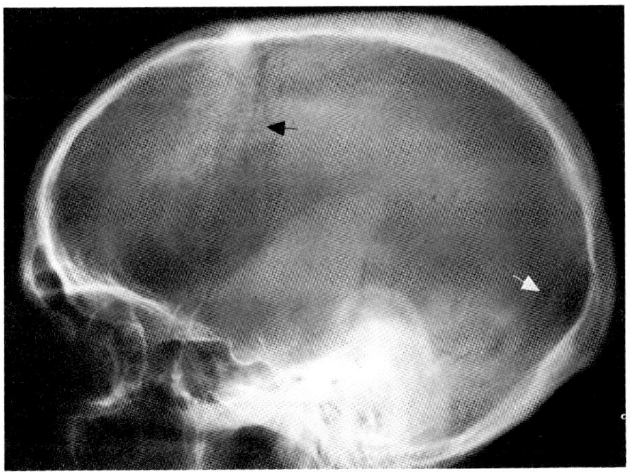

Fig. 9-5. A 105-year-old Negro man. Some osteoporosis of dorsum and clinoids is present, but none of the other signs associated with aging (e.g., vascular calcification, physiologic calcification, loss of bony architecture or markings, hyperostosis). Coronal suture is suggested by poorly demonstrated zigzag markings (black arrow); and lambdoid and temporo-occipital sutures (white arrow) and vascular grooves are clearly present.

with aging, since it has been found only in adults beyond middle age. So far, no patient has been followed long enough for investigators to know definitely that this radiolucency increases in size with further aging; but experience suggests that it does. Somewhat similar markings result from dilated emissary veins or from various other pathologic entities, but the location and appearance are quite characteristic. In only two instances has biopsy or postmortem examination been performed, and in both cases the nonossified tissue was brain, probably of cerebellar origin (Goldring et al., 1964).

Digital impressions seen in the young disappear slowly after maturity and are considered abnormal after middle age.

Bony ridges for the attachment of muscles or dura show no roentgen change during adult aging except to share in the general osteoporosis.

CALCIFICATION

Various intracranial calcifications are visible roentgenographically, but their cause and significance are unknown. These include the pineal, choroid plexus, falx, tentorium, and other portions of the dura, especially the petroclinoid ligament.

The general impression is that the incidence of these so-called physiologic calcifications increases in older age. In the pineal the incidence of calcification increases chiefly before adulthood, however, and is minimal with further aging. Heinrich (1941) reproduced a table from Lorenz that showed the incidence of pineal calcification to be about 70% at the age of 20 years. After the age of 60 years, it was present in only 79% of skulls (i.e., a 9% increase in incidence over a period of 40 or more years). No satisfactory statistical analysis of dural and choroid plexus calcification was found. As with the pineal, apparently the extent of calcification does not increase significantly with aging and only minimally so in early adulthood. All of these calcifications correlate better with developmental maturation than with postmaturity aging.

SELLA TURCICA AND PARASELLAR REGION

Changes with aging in and about the sella turcica are sufficiently common and detectable to warrant special consideration. Osteoporosis (loss of bone mass), as elsewhere, is common if not invariable in the sella turcica after the age of 50 or 60 years. It may not be obvious, however, and when present may be difficult to distinguish from the effects of increased intracranial pressure or of adjacent disease. A thin but nevertheless discrete rim of bone without sellar enlargement is characteristic of osteoporosis. In the absence of an aerated sphenoid sinus underlying the sella, this thin line of osteoporosis may be difficult to demonstrate. Another source of thinning is

A 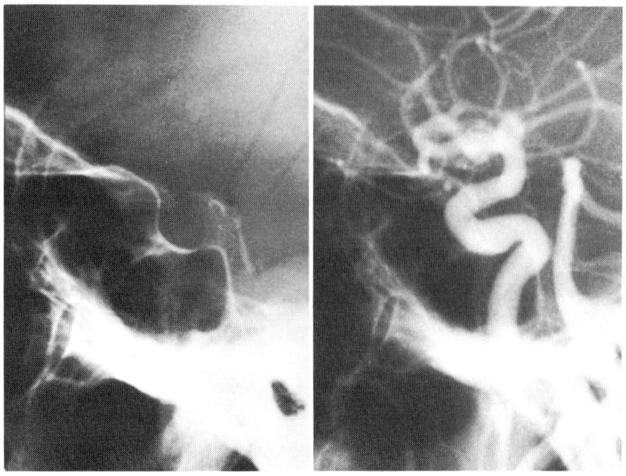 B

Fig. 9-6. A 49-year-old woman. **A,** Dorsum sellae between floor of sella and posterior clinoid is barely visible, suggesting osteoporosis. **B,** Angiography shows that thin zone exactly corresponds to lateral notch or groove in dorsum in which this posterior carotid siphon runs. It is probably a normal feature although perhaps accentuated by atherosclerotic dilatation (ectasia) of carotid artery. Note that the retrodorsum calcification in **A,** which might be mistaken for calcification of the basilar artery, does not conform to this artery and is actually a physiologic calcification in the petroclinoid ligament.

the narrowing of the dorsum sellae from side to side, apparently resulting from the carotid arteries. Ectasia of these vessels, which may accompany advancing age with or without calcification, probably accentuates these grooves or notches. It therefore decreases the transverse thickness of bone in the dorsum, simulating osteoporosis or pressure atrophy. In the lateral view this decrease may result in apparent discontinuity between the top of the dorsum and its base (Fig. 9-6). In the same manner the carotid sulcus, including the undersurface of the anterior clinoid, may be deepened, adding to the appearance of osteoporosis. These changes are not normal features of adult age. Like elongation and dilatation of the aorta, they are accepted as a common though pathologic accompaniment of aging. At any age these same changes may be associated with pathologic enlargement of the carotid arteries, such as occurs with large arteriovenous shunts or cavernous internal carotid aneurysms.

Probably no significant change in shape of the sella turcica or increase in its size is attributable to aging after adulthood. A slight increase in size, at least through the age of 50 years, was described by Schinz and co-workers (1952), however.

As mentioned earlier, calcification in the carotid vessels and in the petroclinoid ligaments is frequently seen adjacent to the sella turcica (Figs. 9-2 and 9-4). Carotid calcification, signifying atherosclerosis, is to some extent correlated with aging, but petroclinoid ligament calcification is not. Except for thinning secondary to carotid ectasia and the loss in density accompanying generalized osteoporosis, changes in the clinoids as the result of aging are not noted regularly.

MISCELLANEOUS

Whether various features of the skull are the result of aging may be questioned. These features either show no significant variation with aging or have not been investigated in relation to aging.

Shape of skull. A number of linear measurements and angles investigated by Zuckerman (1955) showed a statistical increase with aging. The differences were so slight as to be of no practical concern from the roentgenologic point of view.

Base of skull. The complex features of the base of the skull, excluding the sella turcica, apparently have not been studied specifically in regard to age. I have observed no distinct changes. Heinrich did state that the petrous apices have a more "ground glass" appearance in the aged. Probably this change is just another manifestation of osteoporosis.

Soft tissues. Obvious outward changes of aging are, of course, baldness and wrinkling as well as sagging and atrophy of the skin. Loss of subcutaneous fat and resultant folding and wrinkling of the skin may be visible on roentgenograms, much as they appear on chest roentgenograms of infants (Fig. 9-7). The nasopharyngeal shadow caused by prominent adenoid tissue in the young may persist into adulthood but usually not beyond the ages of 30 to 40 years. A nasopharyngeal shadow after that age demands direct examination to rule out neoplasm.

A

B

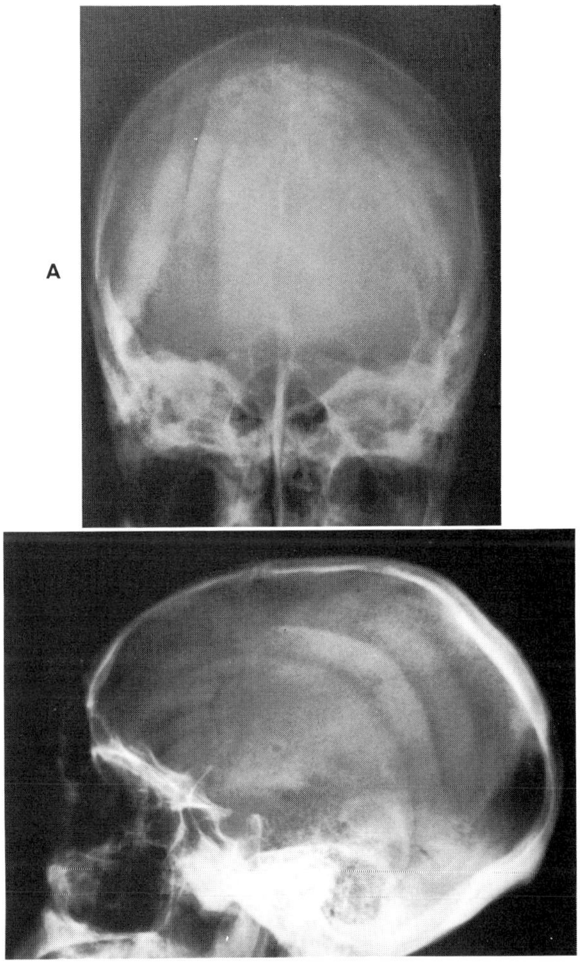

Fig. 9-7. An 82-year-old Negro man. **A,** Prominent folds of loose skin cast vertical shadows over right side. This view was exposed with patient supine. Folds are caused by head resting on a sponge, sliding redundant skin laterally. **B,** Skull of 64-year-old Negro man with similar prominent folds of loose skin.

SUMMARY

The effects of aging on the roentgen appearance of the skull from early adulthood through senility are surprisingly slight and disappointingly inconstant. Although a gradual fusion of the cranial sutures of the vault is noted, wide variations exist. The appearance of calcified dural structures, pineal body, and choroid plexus is not age specific or significantly progressive. Thickening of the bone is so slight as to be appreciated only by comparing many roentgenograms over a long period of time or by comparing many dried skulls. The same may be stated about the changes in the shape of the skull. Parietal thinning affects only a small percentage of skulls, and progression has been documented in only one case. Osteoporosis is probably the most constant change with age; but it may or may not be evident, depending on the previous degree of bone thickness and denseness. Calcification in the carotid siphon is a common finding in skulls of persons more than 50 years of age but is in reality a pathologic finding. Changes in the various markings and bony patterns of the skull are probably the result of osteoporosis or hyperostosis. Benign hyperostosis indicates middle age or older.

Hyperostosis, pineal calcification, and various dural calcifications in the presence of closed sutures do not necessarily indicate old age. Furthermore, most of the features associated with aging may be lacking or minimal in advanced age. Apparently the skull has been developed to outlast the individual it serves.

REFERENCES

Arnold, J. S., Bartley, M. H., Tont, S. A., and others: Skeletal changes in aging and disease, Clin. Orthop. **49:**17-38, 1966.

Ashley-Montague, M. F.: Aging of the skull, Amer. J. Phys. Anthrop. **23:**355-375, 1938.

Basmajian, J. V.: The depressions for arachnoid granulation as criterion of age, Anat. Rec. **112:**843-846, 1952.

Bondareff, W.: Morphology of the aging nervous system. In Birren, J. E., editor: Handbook of aging and the individual, Chicago, 1959, University of Chicago Press.

Brooks, S. T.: Skeletal age at death: the reliability of cranial and pubic age indicators, Amer. J. Phys. Anthrop. **13**:567-590, 1955.

Camp, J. D., and Nash, L. A.: Developmental thinness of the parietal bones, Radiology **42**:42-47, 1944.

Cobb, W. M.: Skeleton. In Lansing, A. I., editor: Problems of aging, ed. 3, Baltimore, 1952, The Williams & Wilkins Co.

Gershon-Cohen, J., Schraer, H., and Blumberg, N.: Flat heads among the aged due to thin parietal bones, Geriatrics **8**: 596-598, 1953.

Goldring, S., Hodges, F. H., and Luse, S. A.: Ectopic neural tissue of occipital bone, J. Neurosurg. **21**:479-484, 1964.

Harris, H. A.: Bone growth in health and disease, London, 1933, Oxford University Press.

Heinrich, A.: Alternsvorgänge in Röntgenbild, Leipzig, 1941, George Thieme.

Israel, H.: Continuing growth in the human cranial skeleton, Arch. Oral Biol. **13**:133-137, 1968.

Jones, F. W.: On the grooves upon the ossa parietalia commonly said to be caused by the arteria meningea media, J. Anat. Physiol. **46**:228-238, 1912.

Kraft, E., and Finby, N.: The aging skull—comparative interval study of 25 years. Presented at the XIIth International Congress of Radiology, Tokyo, October, 1969.

Moore, S.: Hyperostosis cranii, Springfield, Ill., 1955, Charles C Thomas, Publisher.

Newton-John, H. F., and Morgan, D. B.: Osteoporosis: disease or senescence? Lancet **1**:232-233, 1968.

O'Leary, J. L.: Aging in the nervous system. In Lansing, A. I., editor: Problems of aging, ed. 3, Baltimore, 1952, The Williams & Wilkins Co.

Schinz, H. R., Baensch, W. E., Friedl, E., and Uehlinger, E.: Roentgen diagnostics, New York, 1952, Grune & Stratton, Inc., vol. 11.

Singer, R.: Estimation of age from cranial suture closure. A report on its unreliability, J. Forensic Med. **1**:52-59, 1953.

Steinbach, H. L., and Obata, W. G.: The significance of thinning of the parietal bones, Amer. J. Roentgen. **78**:39-45, 1957.

Todd, T. W., and Lyon, D. W.: Endocranial suture closure, Amer. J. Phys. Anthrop. **7**:325-384, 1924.

Todd, T. W., and Lyon, D. W.: Cranial suture closure, Amer. J. Phys. Anthrop. **8**:23-71, 149-168, 1925.

Zuckerman, S.: Age changes in the basicranial axis of the human skull, Amer. J. Phys. Anthrop. **13**:521-539, 1955.

PART III

Skull vault

CHAPTER 10

Size and Shape

Charles A. Gooding

Comprehensive analysis of skull roentgenograms of infants or children may be difficult for one unaccustomed to dealing with young patients. Full understanding of the pathophysiologic alterations that have produced the current morphologic situation requires knowledge of normal growth and development patterns of children and knowledge of the embryologic basis of these patterns. Pathologic representation of congenital and acquired disease entities must also be known (Jackson, 1956; Dorst, 1964; Campbell, 1966).

NORMAL PROPORTIONS

The size and shape of the vault of the skull are determined to a large extent by the size of the brain and its rate of growth (Caffey, 1967). When the skull is obviously excessively large (Fig. 10-1) or inordinately small (Fig. 10-2), exact criteria for estimation of cranial size are superfluous, aside from assessing serial studies for progression or regression of the process. Alternatively, when the changes are slight, less subjective techniques must be used.

Craniofacial proportion concept

A basic concept in evaluation of the pediatric skull is that the size of the face usually parallels the gen-

I herewith gratefully acknowledge the review of this material and the suggestions offered by Dr. Richard D. Hoare, Hospital for Sick Children, Great Ormond Street, London, England.

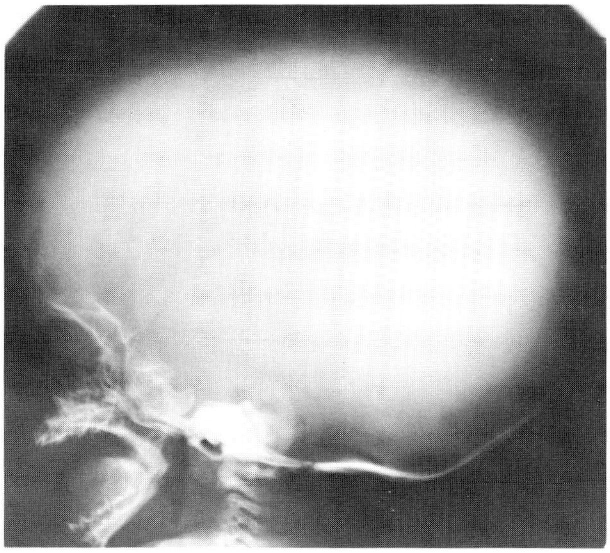

Fig. 10-1. A 6-week-old child with severe communicating hydrocephalus producing enlargement of vault and extreme craniofacial disproportion.

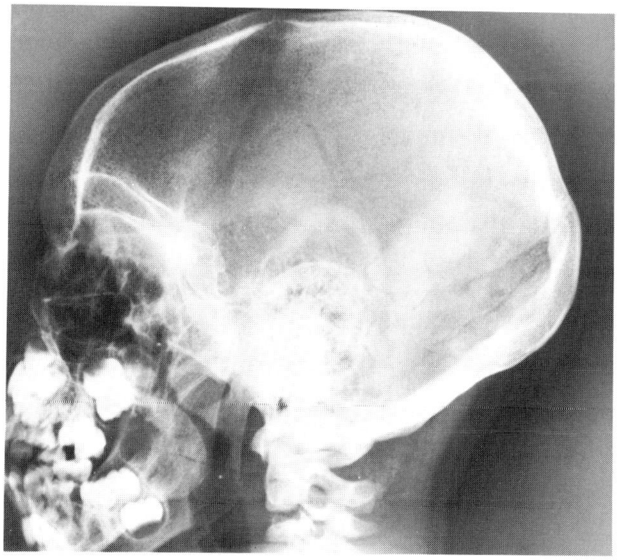

Fig. 10-2. Micrencephaly. Craniofacial disproportion with cranial vault too small relative to size of facial bones and mandible. Diploic structure of vault is thickened, and sutures are not as wide as would be expected in child of this age.

eral somatic growth and is independent of the growth of the brain. With experience the normal craniofacial proportions at the different age levels are appreciated, and deviation (i.e., craniofacial disproportion) is recognized as an indication of intracranial abnormality. What is the necessity for craniofacial proportions, and why will absolute measurements not suffice? Haas, in 1952, collected data on length, width, and height of the skull in various age groups. The range of normal was so broad, however, that generally evaluation of craniofacial interrelationship proved to be of more value. Gordon (1966) similarly collected data on calvarial measurements at different ages, but the volumetric formula he derived is cumbersome for frequent use.

Volume ratio

A second basic concept in the evaluation of the pediatric skull is that the size of the calvarium is merely a representation of the volume of its contents. The rate of brain growth is known to be greater than the rate of growth of the remainder of the body in early fetal life. By the second fetal month the brain comprises 25% of the total body weight. This decreases to 10% at birth, to 5% at 5 years, and to 2% by adulthood. By the end of the first year of life, postnatal brain growth has been 50% completed; by the end of the second year, 75%; and by the end of the sixth year, 90%. The growth stops at the age of 10 to 12 years.

Thus at birth the cranial volume is approximately

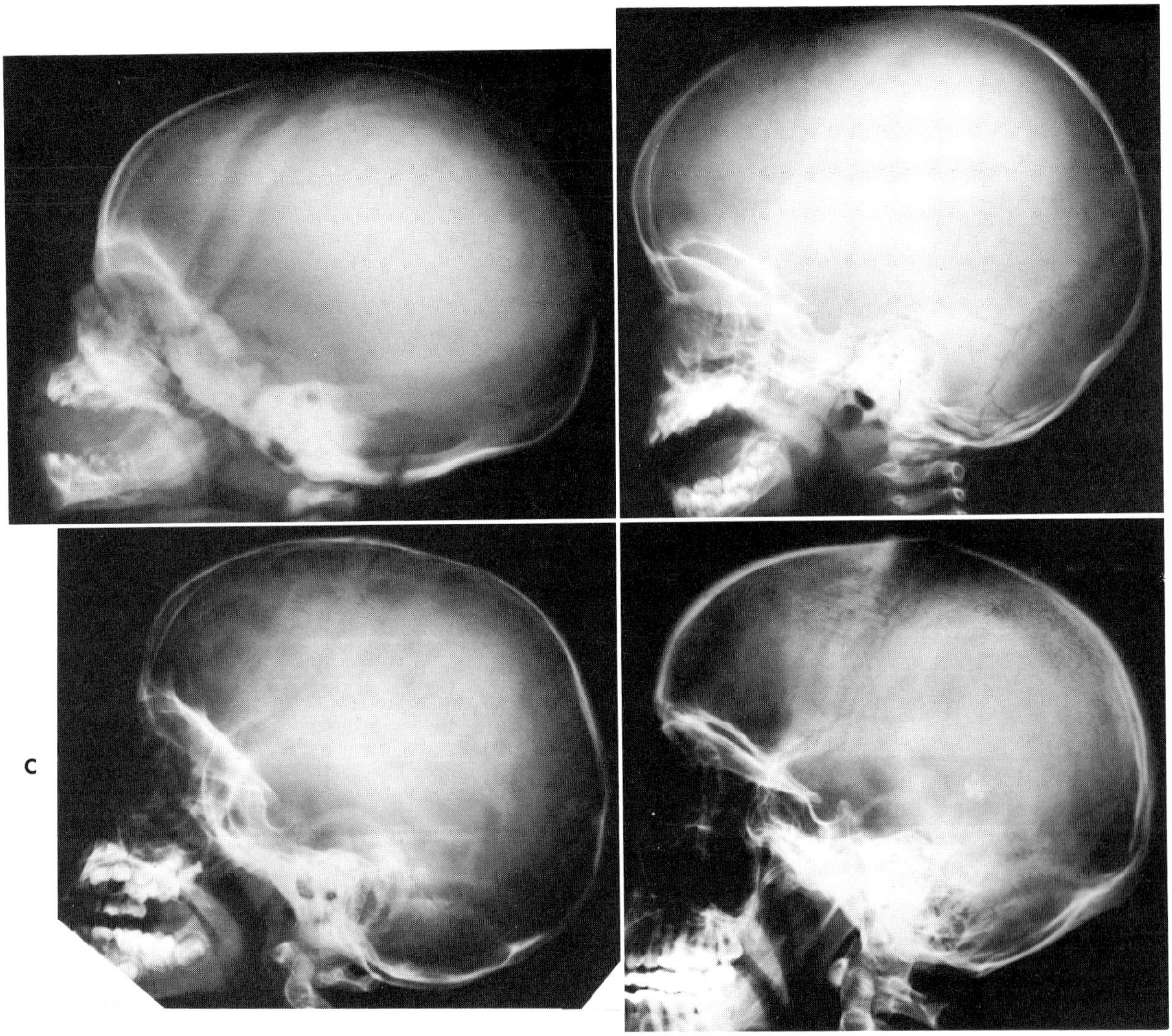

Fig. 10-3. Change in craniofacial midsagittal area with age. Anteroposterior diameter of all cases illustrated has been equalized to emphasize this feature. **A,** Newborn. **B,** Age 18 months. **C,** Age 6 years. **D,** Adult.

eight times as great as the volume of the face (Fig. 12-11). In the 2-year-old child the ratio of cranial volume to facial volume is 5:1; in the 6-year-old 3:1; and at 12 years 2.5:1 (Watson and Lowery, 1967). At 18 years of age, the craniofacial volume ratio is 2:1, which represents adult proportions.

Midsagittal area ratio

Craniofacial proportions are more easily estimated, although perhaps less accurately, on a lateral area basis than on a volume basis. At birth the area of the cranium on a lateral view of the skull (which, in fact, is a midsagittal area) is four times the facial area; by 2 years this ratio is 3:1; by 6 years 2.5:1; and by adulthood approximately 1.5:1 (Fig. 10-3).

Cronqvist cranial index

The increased need for more reliable and objective criteria to assess the size of the cranial vault prompted Cronqvist (1968) to construct new cranial indices. His technique utilized the two concepts just described. Only lateral and anteroposterior views were necessary to ascertain his index (Fig. 10-4). The measurements included the greatest length *(L)*, greatest width *(W)*, and greatest height *(H)* between the inner tables of the skull. The last measurement is the maximum perpendicular distance between the vault of the skull and a line drawn from the nasion to the posterior margin of the foramen magnum. The summation of the measurements is divided by the maximum distance between the inner margins of the two necks of the mandible as measured in the anteroposterior view *(M)*. The quotient is then multiplied by the factor of 10.

$$\text{Cronqvist cranial index} = \frac{H + L + W}{M} \times 10$$

The normal range (i.e., ± 2 standard deviations) is 51 to 56. The advantage of having the intermandibular distance as a denominator is that this measurement reflects growth of the cranial base and is generally not affected by change in intracranial content. The wide range of the normal spectrum is thereby narrowed. Cronqvist's technique is useful for charting head size progression or regression during therapy.

Austin and Gooding (1971) applied Cronqvist's index to a North American population and found many false-positive measurements, particularly in children less than 2 years of age. Because the Cronqvist index indiscrimi-

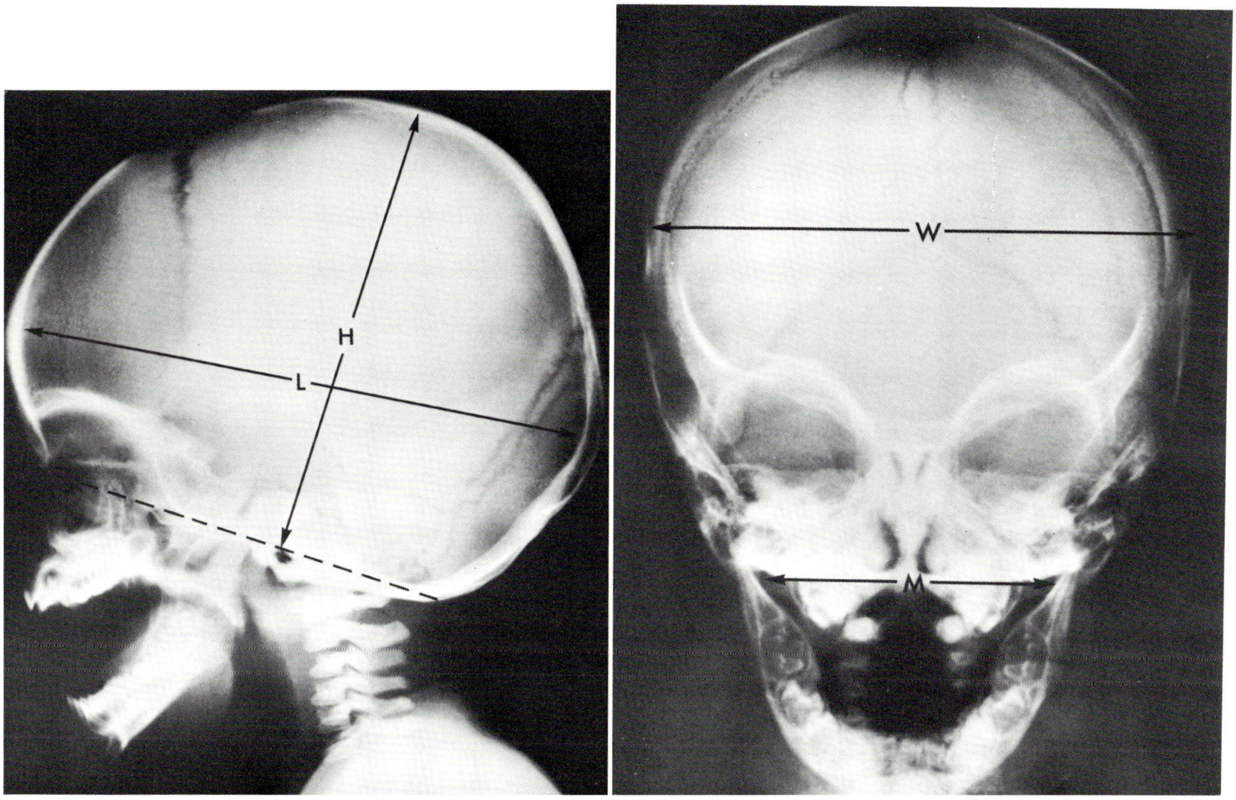

Fig. 10-4. Anteroposterior and lateral views of normal skull indicate sites of measurement for determination of Cronqvist index. *H,* Height; *L,* length; *W,* width; *M,* distance between mandibular necks. (From Austin, J. H. M., and Gooding, C. A.: Radiology **99:**641-646, 1971.)

Table 10-1. Roentgenologic indices of cranial size of children: normal mean values*

Age	*L + H + W* (± 2 *SD*)	*Cranial index of Cronqvist* (± 2 *SD*) $\frac{L+H+W}{M} \times 10$
1 mo	327 ± 26 mm	57 ± 5
2-3 mo	355 ± 43	58 ± 4
4-6 mo	391 ± 30	57 ± 4
7-9 mo	421 ± 42	57 ± 5
10-12 mo	421 ± 36	56 ± 6
1 yr	441 ± 45	56 ± 6
2 yr	456 ± 32	56 ± 7
3 yr	470 ± 45	55 ± 5
4 yr	464 ± 34	52 ± 6
5 yr	465 ± 37	53 ± 5

*From Austin, J. H. M., and Gooding, C. A.: Roentgenographic measurement of skull size in children, Radiology 99:641-646, 1971.

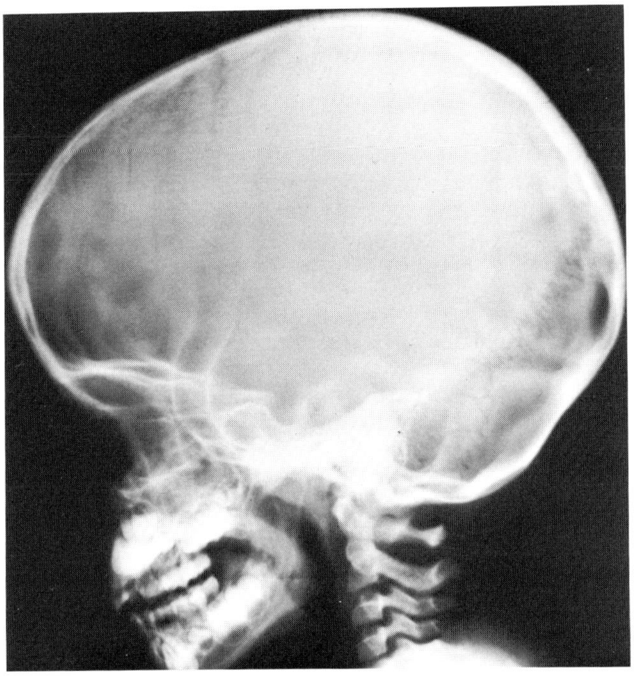

Fig. 10-5. A 5-year-old boy with hypopituitarism. Note the apparent craniofacial disproportion resulting from delayed somatic growth of the facial structures and the concomitant normal growth of the brain.

nately included data from children all younger than 7 years, without specification of age, Austin and Gooding hypothesized that the index may vary with age. In their analysis of skull roentgenograms of 262 American children, they found the Cronqvist cranial index to be a function of age, decreasing in value as age increases (Table 10-1). For seventy-one normal newborn infants the mean cranial index was 57 ± 5 (± 2 standard deviations). For twenty-four normal 5-year-old children the mean cranial index was 53 ± 5 (± 2 standard deviations). The difference between the cranial index for these two age groups is statistically significant ($p < 0.001$).

A single measure of the sensitivity of any index is the coefficient of variation, which is the percentage of the mean comprised by one standard deviation. The cranial index of Cronqvist appeared most sensitive in infants from birth through 9 months of age. This index should be used routinely in any assessment of the skull in this age group. From 9 months through 5 years, however, a single summation index of length plus height plus width has proved slightly more sensitive than the Cronqvist index. In this age group the summation index should be used first; and if it is borderline or abnormal, the Cronqvist cranial index should be applied. These two indices for the first 5 years of life are provided in Table 10-1.

One of the entities that limit the value of determination of craniofacial proportion is hypopituitarism (Fig. 10-5). The somatic growth of the pituitary dwarf is retarded and the face underdeveloped, but neural growth is normal; this gives an illusion of a large calvarium (Nellhaus, 1968b). The lack of other stigmata of increased intracranial pressure and the crowded teeth and small sella turcica that are seen sometimes point to the correct diagnosis. Assessment of retardation of skeletal maturation corroborates the impression.

Clinical correlation

Clinical correlation should be utilized in all instances that represent roentgenographic craniofacial disproportion. Measurement of head circumference is one of the clinical parameters widely used as an index of brain growth and development. Studies of normal head circumference for North American infants have been reported by Silver and Deamer (1948); for American-born Caucasian children by Pryor (1966); and for Negro, Japanese, Alaskan, Eskimo, and Russian children by Nellhaus (1968a). The definition of microcrania used by Pryor and Thelander (1968) is a head circumference 2 or more standard deviations below the mean for age and sex. Similarly macrocrania may be assumed to mean a head circumference greater than 2 standard deviations above the mean.

In addition to determination of head circumference, a complete neurologic examination, including transillumination of the vault, should be performed on all infants and children with roentgenographic evidence of macrocrania.

MACROCRANIA

A greater than normal volume of the calvarium indicates macrocrania. Macrocrania may be symmetric or asymmetric.

Symmetric macrocrania

Diploic space enlargement

Symmetric macrocrania secondary to enlargement of the diploic space, as in thalassemia (Powell et al., 1965; Hirata and Gooding, 1970) (Fig. 10-6) or Cooley's anemia, sickle-cell disease, or congenital spherocytosis shall be mentioned only *en passant*. This type of macrocrania results in increased measurements of head circumference, but inner table–to–inner table diameters, or the intracranial volume, are not increased.

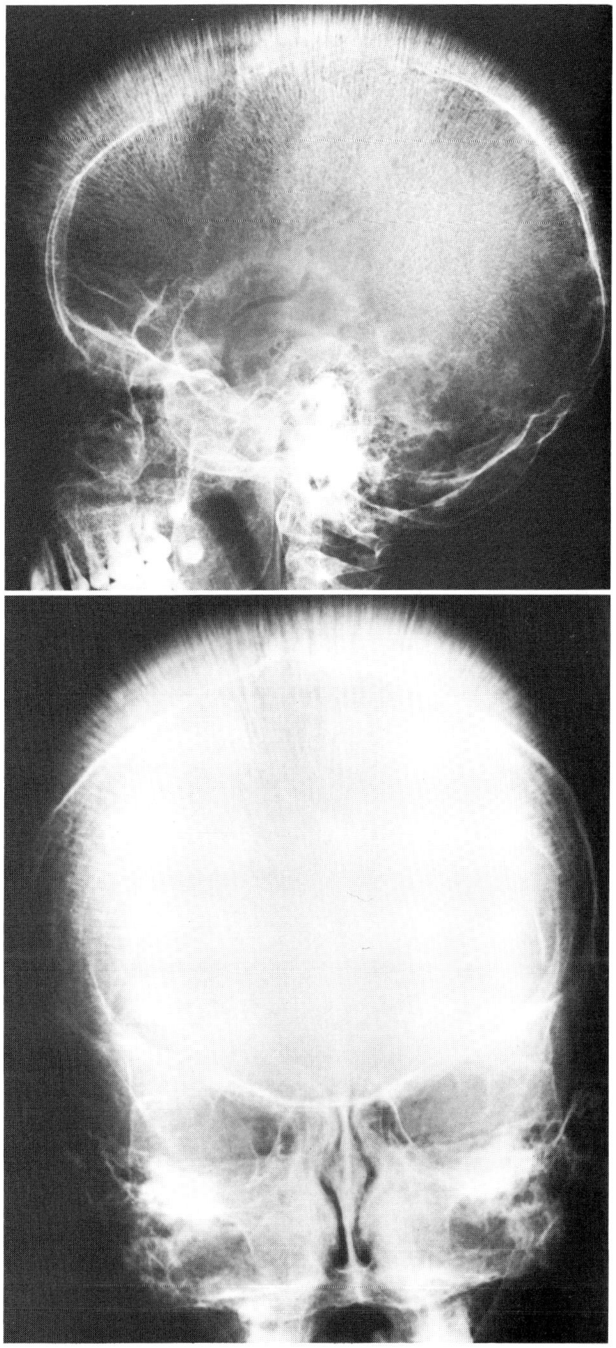

Fig. 10-6. Anteroposterior and lateral views of skull in thalassemia in 17-year-old boy show vault increased in size because of increased calvarial thickening. Head circumference is increased, but intracranial volume is not. Hair-on-end appearance by vertical striations is characteristic, as is obliteration of paranasal sinuses. (From Hirata, T., and Gooding, C. A.: Amer. J. Dis. Child. **119**:505-506, 1970.)

A

B

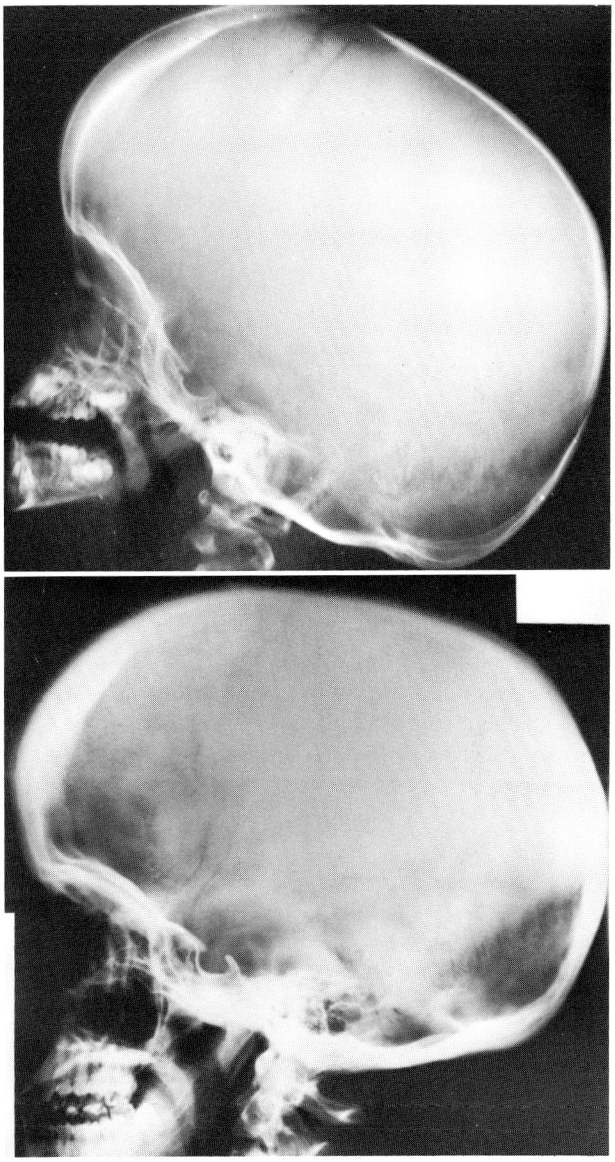

Fig. 10-7. Arrested hydrocephalus. **A,** Age 2 years. Craniofacial disproportion with macrocrania and open anterior fontanelle is present. The vault is thickened. **B,** At age 18 years, thickness of vault has increased but size of calvarium has changed little.

Hydrocephalus

The most common cause of symmetric macrocrania is increased intracranial pressure, secondary to hydrocephalus. In infants and children the sutures respond to increased intracranial pressure by becoming diastatic, and membranous new bone forms at their margins. When the increase in pressure is indolent and develops over a prolonged interval, such as occurs with communicating hydrocephalus, bone has an opportunity to grow at the margins. Although the interdigitations of the sutures may be elongated, suture separation may not be seen (Fig. 10-1). Conversely, with most cases of obstructive hydrocephalus in children, the sudden increase in intracranial pressure causes the bones at the sutures to separate.

Arrested hydrocephalus, either spontaneous or postoperative, refers to hydrocephalic children in whom is manifested a sudden halt of skull growth. Resumption of this growth at a normal rate takes place after a normal relation of head and body size is restored (Fig. 10-7) (Schick and Matson, 1961). A late complication of arrested hydrocephalus has been the development of remarkable calvarial thickening and premature fusion of the cranial sutures (Moseley et al., 1966; Anderson et al., 1970). The thickening of the vault in children who had had ventricular shunts was at the expense of the intracranial volume and was termed the *contracting skull* by Griscom and Oh (1970).

Subdural hematoma

Subdural hematomas in infants are most frequently caused by trauma, but the injury may be most inconspicuous. Purulent meningitis produces subdural effusions, which on examination of plain roentgenograms are indistinguishable from traumatic or idiopathic varieties. Subdural hematomas may follow pneumoencephalography, probably because of rupture of veins that cross the subdural space. In severe subdural hematoma, macrocrania may be present, the sutures may widen, and the anterior fontanelle may bulge. The cranial enlargement may be asymmetric. Generally, cranial enlargement with subdural hematoma is not as great as with hydrocephalus, particularly of the obstructive type. In long-standing subdural hematomas focal thinning of bone and focal expansion of the cortex may be observed.

Ingraham and Matson (1944) found fractures of the cranial vault in fewer than 15% of their large series of subdural hematomas. The fracture may be situated on the side contralateral to the hematoma. Caffey (1946) found fractures frequently in other bones in infants with chronic subdural hematoma. In every infant with an unexplained subdural hematoma, the skeleton should be surveyed to exclude trauma elsewhere.

Familial macrencephaly

Sometimes macrocrania is normal when it is present on an inherited basis. Bakwin and his co-workers (1964) described a familial condition that consisted of macrocrania, generalized osteoporosis of the long bones, and multiple fractures. In patients with epilepsy or mental deficiency, large malformed brains have also been described (Blackwood et al., 1963). The shape of these enlarged calvaria is not unusual.

Cerebral gigantism (Sotos' syndrome)

Cerebral gigantism, or Sotos' syndrome, was described in 1964 and refers to hypothalamic acceleration of growth associated with cerebral atrophy and mental retardation. The ventricles are slightly dilated and the pituitary fossae are normal (Abraham and Snodgrass, 1969). The skull vault is enlarged but not unusual in shape.

Hydranencephaly

Infantile hydranencephaly, another cause of macrocrania, manifests agenesis of the cerebral mantle, perhaps secondary to compression of the carotid arteries by the umbilical cord or amniotic strands. The lateral ventricles are dilated tremendously and are surrounded by cerebral cortex that has been reduced to a membrane. The ventricles fill practically the entire cranial cavity, whereas a small mass of malformed cerebral tissue occupies the skull base (Hamby et al., 1950; Olive and DuShane, 1953). The lateral ventricles do *not* communicate with the third ventricle. This lack of communication is of diagnostic significance in differentiating hydranencephaly from severe hydrocephalus. The size of the hydranencephalic vault is usually normal at birth and increases rapidly in the first few months of life. The shape is not specific.

Gargoylism

Gargoylism, also called dysostosis multiplex and lipochondrodystrophy, was described in 1917 by Hunter and amplified in 1919 by Hurler. Children with this syndrome are dwarfs and are infantile, with mental retardation, large skulls, puffy myxedematous skin, hepatosplenomegaly, and corneal clouding. The skulls of patients with the Hurler-Hunter syndrome are most impressive because of the thickness of the bones of the calvarium and the complete absence of normal convolutional impressions (Fig. 10-8). Hypertelorism and heavy supraorbital ridges are seen (Horrigan and Baker, 1961). According to Russell (1949) the hydrocephalus in these patients is the result of fibrous thickening of the dura and leptomeninges. She stated that this thickening was secondary to meningeal accumulation of lipoid particles that obstructed the subarachnoid space. The particles

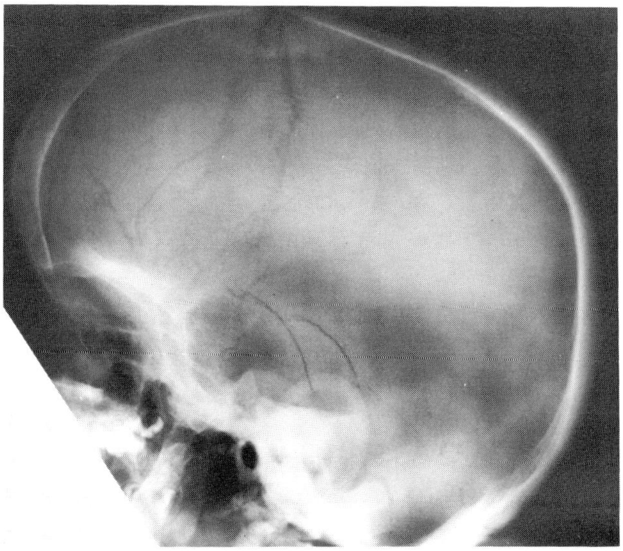

Fig. 10-8. Hurler-Hunter syndrome. Note the thickening of the vault, particularly in the frontal bone, and the concave chiasmatic sulcus.

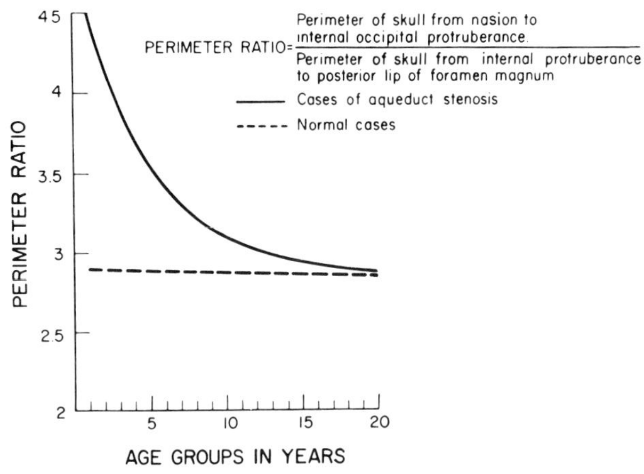

Fig. 10-10. Perimeter ratio for normal children and children with aqueduct stenosis. (From Schechter, M. M., and Zingesser, L. H.: Radiology **88**:905-916, 1967.)

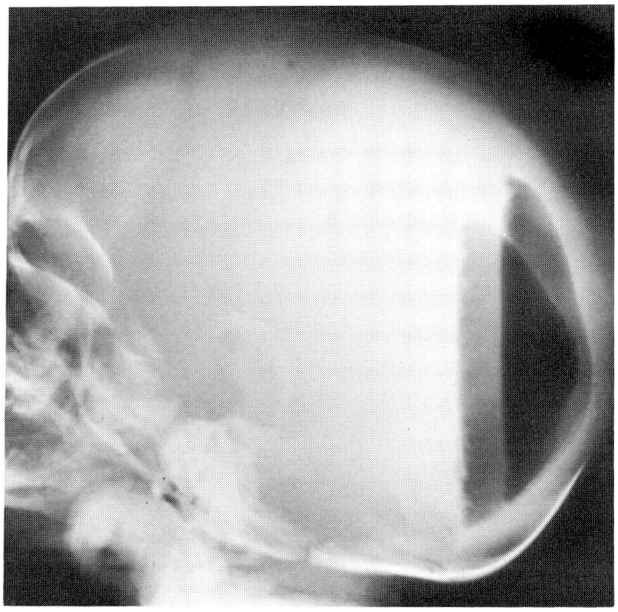

Fig. 10-9. Aqueduct stenosis in newborn infant. Note the craniofacial disproportion, the small squamous portion of the occipital bone, and the increased perimeter ratio. Ventricles are dilated.

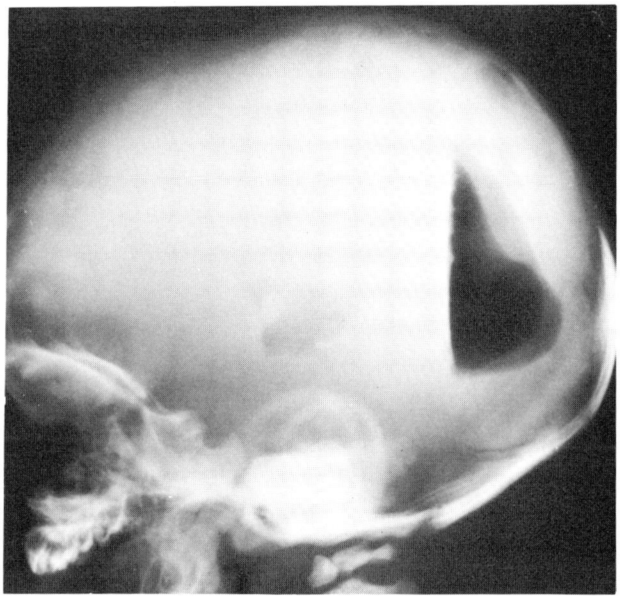

Fig. 10-11. A 2-month-old boy with aqueduct stenosis. Note the very small squamous portion of the occipital bone. Craniofacial disproportion is present with perimeter ratio increased. Aqueduct stenosis is evident on this ventriculogram.

now are believed to be not lipid but a complex macromolecular mucopolysaccharide.

Asymmetric macrocrania

Aqueduct stenosis

The term aqueduct stenosis describes a group of lesions that obstruct the aqueduct of Sylvius. Periaqueductal gliosis and miscellaneous inflammatory lesions, such as tuberculosis, toxoplasmosis, and histoplasmosis, may produce narrowing of the aqueduct. Congenital aqueduct stenosis, however, is a maldevelopment of the aqueduct and, according to Russell (1949), comprises various types. These include aqueducts that (1) are histologically normal but abnormally small, (2) are forked and branched and then become atretic, and (3) have a septum or membrane.

When congenital aqueduct stenosis exists, hydrocephalus may be present at birth as macrocrania or the head may increase in size rapidly in infancy. Separation of the cranial suture in patients with aqueduct stenosis is seen in infancy, in childhood, and even in adolescence. Other roentgenographic signs are (1) enlargement of the occipital channel of the emissary vein and (2) demineralization of the dorsum sellae in children more than 7 years of age. Two of the most characteristic findings on plain roentgenograms in patients with aqueduct stenosis are a relatively small posterior fossa and a low inion (Fig. 10-9). Unfortunately these signs are not uniformly present.

A numerical value has been applied to the preceding described findings by Schechter and Zingesser (1967), who devised what they termed a perimeter ratio. This ratio refers to the perimeter of the skull from the nasion to the internal occipital protuberance. It is divided, by the perimeter of the skull, from the internal protuberance to the posterior lip of the foramen magnum (Fig. 10-10). Normally this ratio is stable at about 2.9:1 for all ages. Because of dilated lateral ventricles and the resultant capacious calvarium relative to the diminutive posterior fossa, the ratio in aqueduct stenosis is increased. It is particularly increased in the first 5 years of life, up to 4.5:1.

Ventriculography (Fig. 10-11), necessary to confirm the diagnosis, is sometimes supplemented by pneumoencephalography and cerebral arteriography.

Dandy-Walker syndrome

The Dandy-Walker syndrome is a name coined by Benda in 1954 to describe the congenital occlusion of the foramina of Magendi and Luschka. The cerebellum is often underdeveloped because of the enormous dilatation of the fourth ventricle, but the brainstem remains normal. This entity, which produces hydrocephalus, was initially described in 1914 by Dandy and Blackfan, was amplified in 1921 by Dandy, and further elucidated in 1942 by Taggart and Walker.

Most patients with the Dandy-Walker syndrome present symptoms by the age of 2 years, although the range in the eighty-five cases reviewed by Juhl and Wesenberg (1966) was from newborn to 59 years. The etiology is unknown, and there is no genetic component. Various congenital anomalies associated with the Dandy-Walker syndrome include agenesis of the corpus callosum, encephaloceles, tracheoesophageal fistulae, polycystic kidneys, and many others.

In contrast to the relatively small posterior fossa seen with aqueduct stenosis, that seen with the Dandy-Walker syndrome is greatly expanded (Fig. 10-12). This expansion is most evident on the lateral view of the skull. A tremendous dilatation of the fourth ventricle, the result of atresia of its foramina, causes flattening of the supraoccipital portion of the occipital squama and thin-

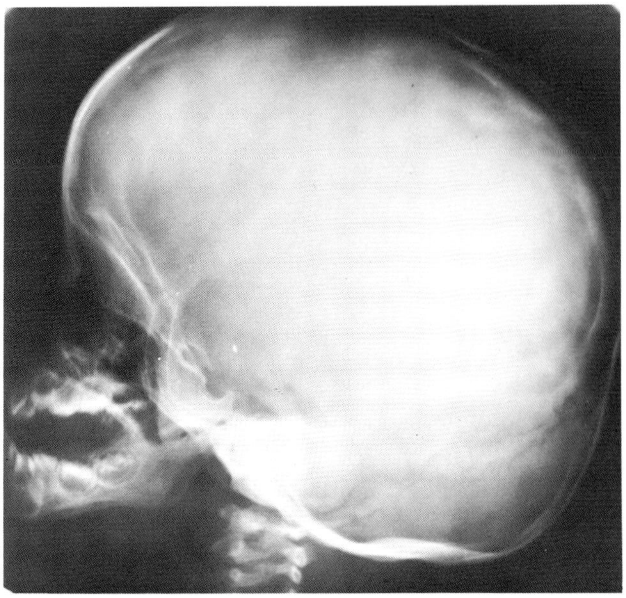

Fig. 10-12. An 11-month-old girl with Dandy-Walker malformation. Craniofacial disproportion is present, the head being too large relative to the size of the facial structures. Chiasmatic sulcus is concave, and area of squamous portion of occipital bone is increased. Note that the inferior portion of the occipital bone is horizontal and that it thins as it turns superiorly.

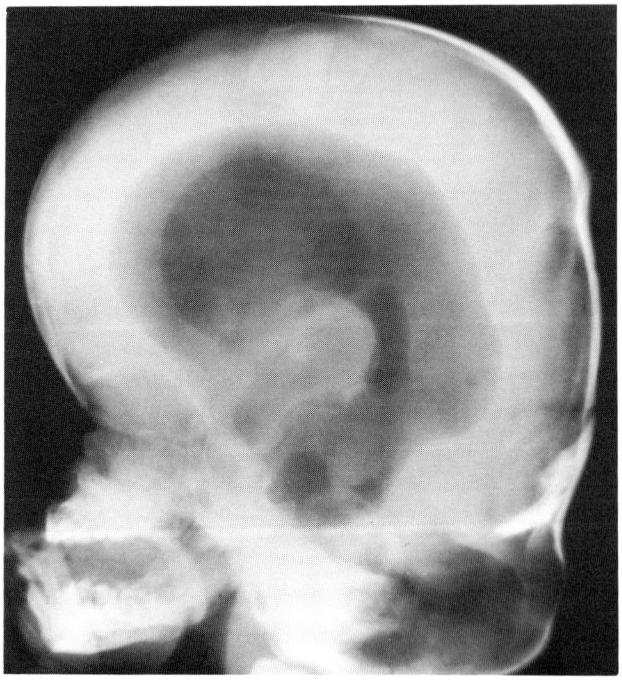

Fig. 10-13. Craniostenosis in 6-week-old girl, in association with Dandy-Walker malformation. Ballooning of posterior fossa is secondary to tremendous dilatation of fourth ventricle as a result of atresia of foramina of Magendie and Luschka. The craniostenosis has accentuated this abnormality.

ning of the interparietal portion just superior to it (Fig. 10-13). The grooves of the lateral sinus and the torcular Herophili are positioned inordinately high, and this is now considered a pathognomonic sign. A line constructed on the lateral roentgenogram of the skull, from the floor of the orbit through the external auditory canal to a point below the inion, is called the Bucy line. Normally the lateral sinus grooves are quite close to this line, but in the Dandy-Walker malformation the lateral sinus grooves are far above it. These grooves are never seen in the first year of life, and identification is constant only after the second year. Even then they are seen in only half the patients. To evaluate children less than the age of 2 years, Juhl and Wesenberg (1966) described what they termed a lambdoinnominate line. The line was drawn on a lateral roentgenogram of the skull. It started at the lambda or midpoint of the posterior fontanelle and extended to the innominate synchondrosis. The synchondrosis was seen on the lateral view 1 or 2 cm posterior to the posterior margin of the foramen magnum. The area posterior and inferior to the lambdoinnominate line corresponded roughly to the squamous portion of the occipital bone. In the Dandy-Walker syndrome, because of the cystic expansion of the fourth ventricle, this area is markedly increased. The magnitude of the increase is directly proportionate to the degree of dilatation of the fourth ventricle.

Achondroplasia

Achondroplasia is a disease of enchondral bone formation that is inherited as an autosomal dominant trait but that also occurs sporadically. Usually the head is enlarged, but intellectual development is within a normal range.

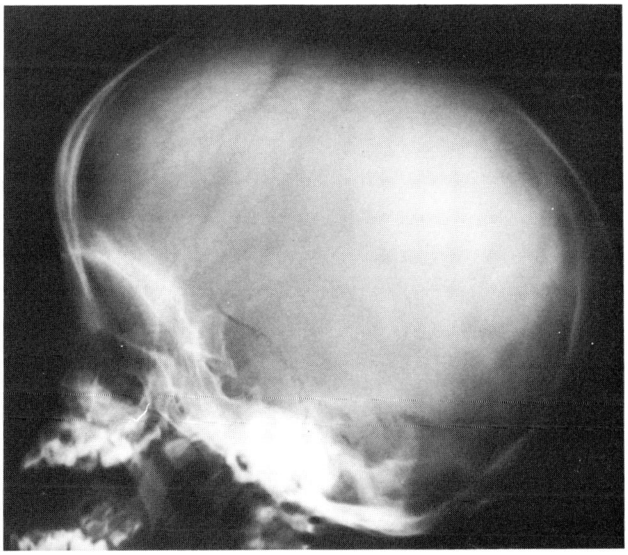

Fig. 10-14. Achondroplasia in 11-month-old boy. Note that the nasion is depressed and the frontal bone bulges anteriorly. Craniofacial disproportion is present, with skull vault too large for size of facial bones. Chiasmatic sulcus is concave.

The skull of these children manifests increased vertical diameter. The base of the skull is relatively short as a result of premature fusion of spheno-occipital synchondrosis. The basilar synostosis results in a brachycephalic appearance (Fig. 10-14). Because the nasion is anchored to the base of the vault and because of delayed enchondral bone growth at the base, the nasion is depressed and the frontal bone bulges anteriorly above it.

Air encephalograms in eight of fifteen achondroplastic children were reported by Cohen and co-workers (1967). All showed some degree of ventricular dilatation, but in only two were cerebrospinal fluid shunting procedures indicated. The cortical mantle remained thick in all patients.

Subdural hematomas

Focal subdural hematomas can cause asymmetric macrocrania and also focal asymmetry without macrocrania. In the neonatal period, subdural hematomas in the posterior fossa may be more frequent than has previously been recognized (Gilles and Shillito, 1970). In this instance separation of the lambdoid sutures often is not prominent.

Expanded middle fossa

The anterior wall of the middle fossa, formed by the greater wing of the sphenoid, may be evaluated in the lateral position (preferably by tomography) or in the submentovertical position. The middle fossae are sometimes asymmetric in normal individuals (Taveras and Wood, 1964). The curve of the anterior margin of the middle fossa may increase when the middle fossa enlarges. This increased curve may result from middle fossa subdural hygromas, chronic subdural hematomas, and subarachnoid cysts (Fig. 10-15), and occasionally it will occur in cases of slowly growing temporal lobe tumors. Porencephalic dilatation of the temporal horn may also cause asymmetric enlargement (Fig. 10-16). The size of the temporal fossa may decrease, as is seen in patients with temporal lobe atrophy or cerebral hemiatrophy. In the latter instance the temporal fossa may be small without concomitant cranial hemihypertrophy.

Craniosynostosis

Asymmetric macrocrania may be seen in instances of craniosynostosis. For example, when the sagittal suture closes prematurely, the cranial vault is elongated in a sagittal plane. With unilateral closure of a cranial suture, brain growth will occur parallel to that suture and asymmetry results. Some of the most extreme examples of this (fortunately seldom seen today) are instances of

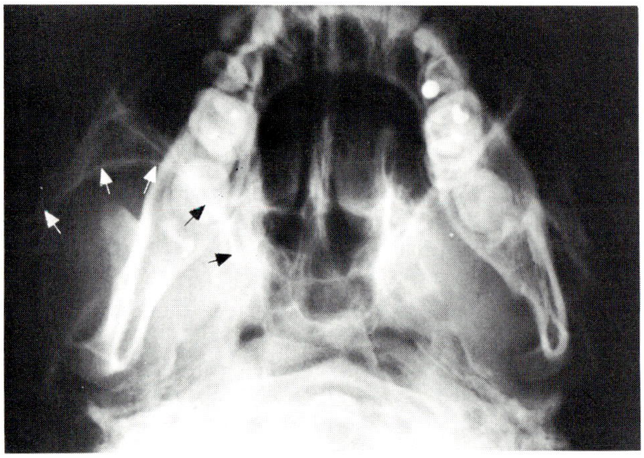

Fig. 10-15. Subarachnoid cyst of right middle fossa, basal view. Note the asymmetry with increased convexity of that portion of the sphenoid bone that forms the anterior margin of the right middle fossa (arrows). (Courtesy Leslie M. Zatz, M.D., Palo Alto, Calif.)

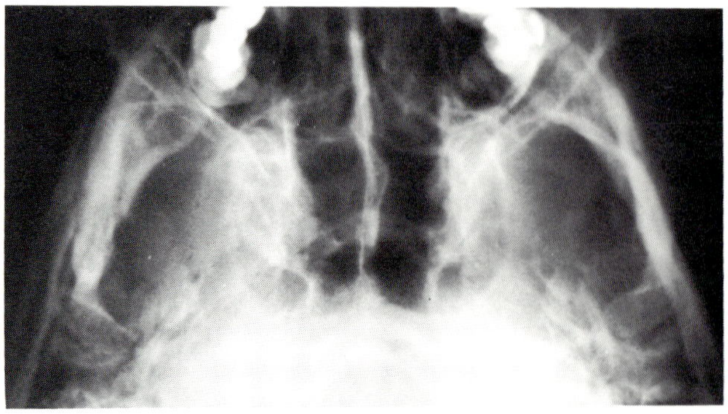

Fig. 10-16. Basal view of skull. Note the asymmetric anterior margins of the middle fossa with the right side enlarged because of porencephalic dilatation of the right temporal horn.

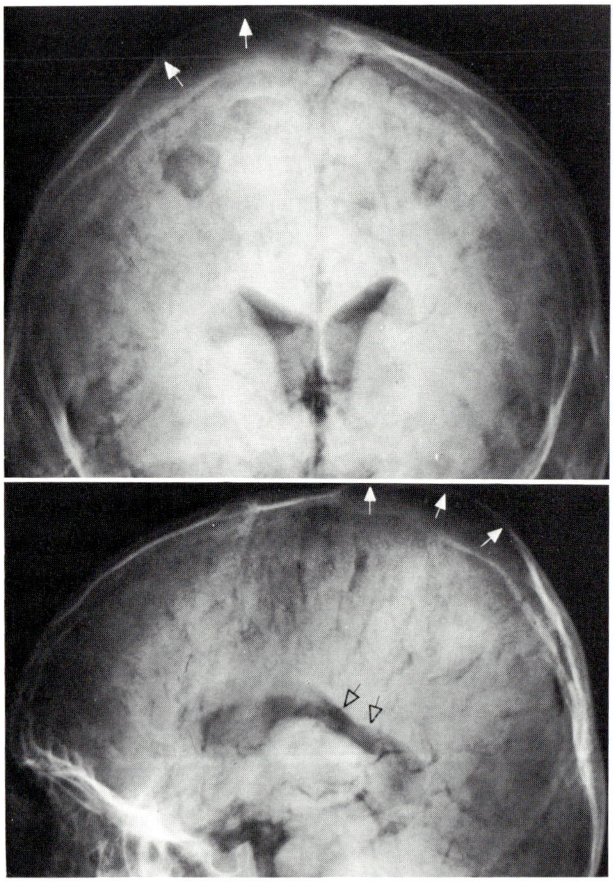

Fig. 10-17. A 10-year-old boy with parietal convexity oligodendroglioma. Anteroposterior and lateral views of skull with air in ventricular system show focal skull asymmetry with thinning of cortex and focal bone expansion of right parietal region (solid arrows). Note the depression of the roof of the lateral ventricle (open arrows).

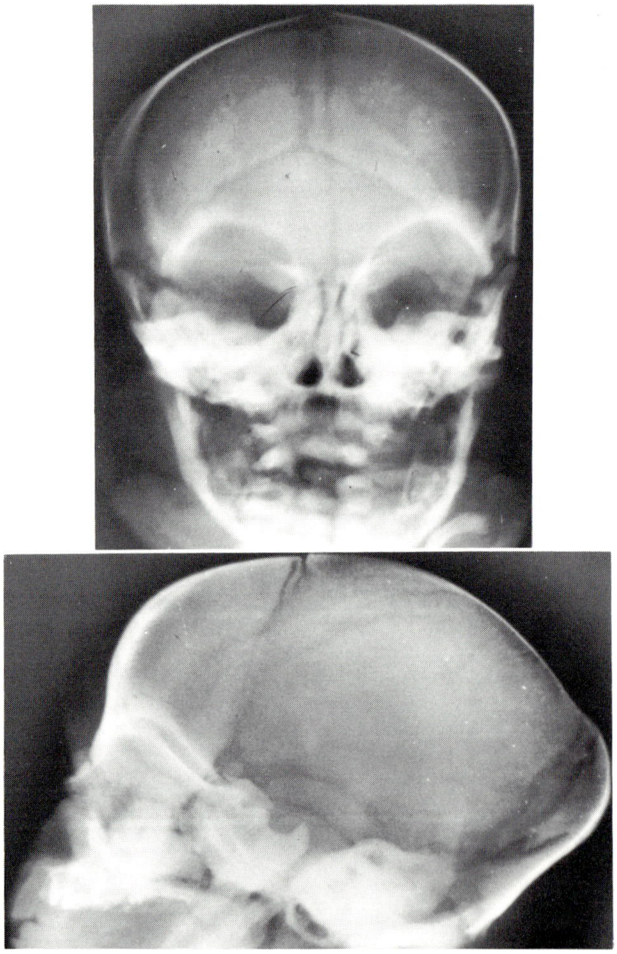

Fig. 10-18. Micrencephaly. Calvarium is much too small relative to size of facial structures and mandible. Sutures are open. Vault is small because brain has not grown normally.

neglected premature closure of the lambdoid and coronal sutures, giving a grotesque tower skull (Chapter 12).

Tumors and subarachnoid cysts

Tumors and subarachnoid cysts situated adjacent to the skull vault may cause focal calvarial asymmetry and enlargement (Fig. 10-17). Generally asymmetry indicates that the process is not of recent onset.

Cephalhematoma

As cephalhematoma becomes ossified and incorporated into the skull vault, focal asymmetry may be observed. The characteristic ossification processes of this entity consist of initial ossification at the periphery, followed by central ossification.

Postural flattening

In mentally retarded children who are left in the supine position for long intervals, flattening of the posterior parietal bone and squamous portion of the occipital bone develops.

Bathrocephaly

Bathrocephaly refers to focal bulging asymmetry of the occipital bone, either above or below the mendosal suture in the neonate. It is of no clinical significance and becomes less prominent with age (Fig. 12-6).

MICROCRANIA

Microcrania results from failure of the normal growth rate of the brain (Fig. 10-18). Most frequently a small vault is the result, not of total premature craniostenosis but of a small brain, and this situation is more accurately described as micrencephaly. Intelligence is almost always subnormal when the circumference of the head is more than 2 standard deviations below normal for the age (Pryor and Thelander, 1968). In a child of normal mentality with short stature, the circumference of the skull is normal for the chronologic age, and increased for the height age (O'Connell et al., 1965; Cloutier and Stickler, 1968; Nellhaus, 1968b).

Symmetric microcrania

The causes of symmetric microcrania are many, and the following classification is modified after that in Farmer's *Pediatric Neurology* (1964):

1. Genetic—recessive micrencephaly, phenylketonuria, aminoaciduria
2. Chromosomal—Down's syndrome, trisomy 13-15
3. Intrauterine injury—radiation, rubella (Cooper et al., 1969), toxoplasmosis (Holden and Whitehead, 1951)
4. Perinatal—cortical atrophy, cytomegalic inclusion disease (Allen and Riley, 1958)
5. Craniosynostosis (Andersson and Gomes, 1968) (See Chapter 12.)

The skull of the child with micrencephaly reflects diminished brain growth not only by reduced size but also by specific characteristic stigmata (Gordon, 1970). The forehead slopes backward because of diminished intracranial content. The width of the suture is diminished for the chronologic age, and occasionally the su-

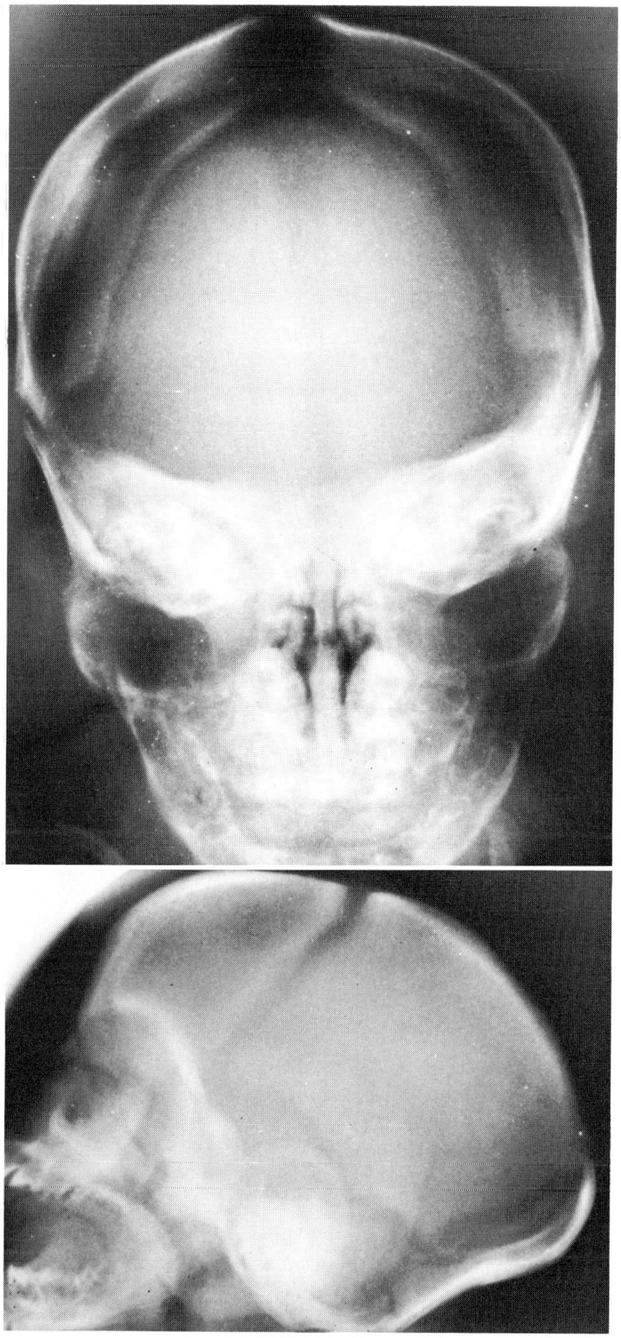

Fig. 10-19. Newborn infant with micrencephaly. Vault is much too small for size of face, and sutures are open. Cause of microcrania in this infant is failure of brain growth.

tures are closed prematurely. Convolutional impressions are usually reduced or absent. The diploic width is thickened compared with the width of the normal skull (Fig. 10-19).

Radiation to the fetus in utero has been documented as a cause of microcrania both experimentally and in clinical studies. In a study from Hiroshima, seven of eleven pregnant women within 1,200 meters of the atomic blast gave birth to micrencephalic children; beyond 1,200 meters 194 had no micrencephalic progeny (Farmer, 1964).

Arhinencephaly

Micrencephaly, in association with marked orbital hypotelorism and absence or hypoplasia of the median facial bones, is seen in holoprosencephaly (arhinencephaly) (Kurlander et al., 1966).

Defective development of the median facial structures differentiates patients with holoprosencephaly from micrencephalic patients. Chromosomal studies suggest that two groups of holoprosencephalies exist, both with identical craniofacial malformation. One group has multiple severe extracephalic anomalies such as malformations of the ear and gastrointestinal tract; the other group has no extracephalic anomalies.

Arhinencephaly has been produced experimentally by feeding pregnant sheep the plant *Veratrum californicum* and by feeding mice vitamin A, rabbits alloxan, and rats vincristine (Bligh and Lawrence, 1967). In man arhinencephaly is associated with maternal diabetes and trisomy 13-15.

Asymmetric microcrania

Occipital encephaloceles

An asymmetric form of micrencephaly is present in patients with encephaloceles. When neural contents herniate outside of the calvarium, the diminished volume of intracranial content is reflected by the vault. In instances of occipital encephalocele, the anterior fossa is decreased in volume and thus the frontal bone slopes posteriorly rather than has the normal anterior convexity. The size of the soft-tissue sac at the occiput is not an indication of the sac's contents. The diminished capacity of the anterior fossa therefore assumes importance in the differential diagnosis of encephalocele and myelomeningocele.

Down's syndrome

A brachycephalic type of micrencephaly is seen in patients with mongolism, or Down's syndrome. The calvarial deformity is not evident at birth but becomes manifest by the age of 3 months because of retarded growth, particularly at the spheno-occipital synchondrosis. Associated skull findings include hypotelorism because of marked hypoplasia of the paranasal sinuses, nasal bones, maxilla, and sphenoid. The calvarium is often thin and lacking in diploic structure (Spitzer et al., 1961; Roche et al., 1961; Gerald and Silverman, 1965; Roche, 1966).

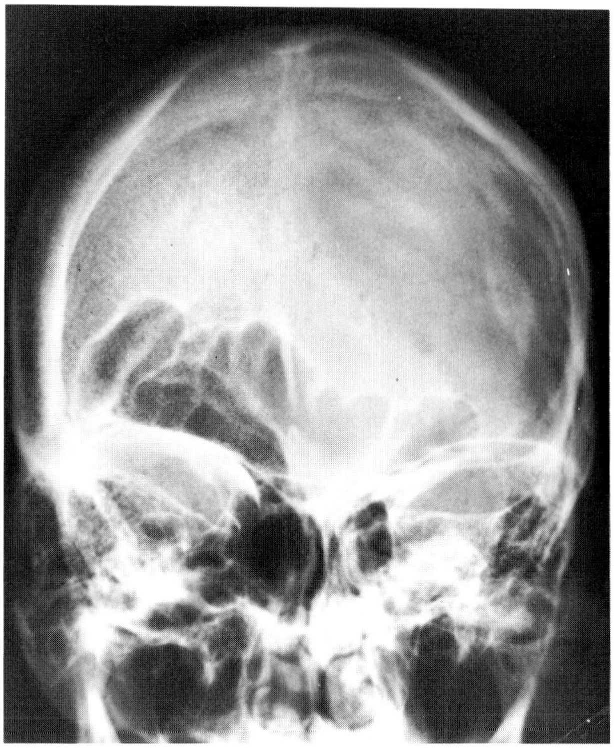

Fig. 10-20. Young adult woman with right-sided cerebral hemiatrophy. Cranial vault is thickened on right side. Ipsilateral enlargement of frontal sinus, elevation of right petrous pyramid, tilting of crista galli to the right, and asymmetry of mastoid and sphenoid sinus are visible.

Unilateral cerebral atrophy

A most characteristic form of microcrania is produced by unilateral cerebral atrophy. Generally the degree of microcrania is slight. The stigmata on the skull roentgenogram include thickening of the diploic space of the vault on the affected side, enlargement of the ipsilateral orbit, elevation of the ipsilateral petrous pyramid, tilting of the crista galli to the affected side, and displacement of the superior sagittal sinus to the affected side (Fig. 10-20) (Dyke et al., 1933).

REFERENCES

Abraham, J. M., and Snodgrass, G. J. A. I.: Sotos' syndrome of cerebral gigantism, Arch. Dis. Child. **44**:203-210, 1969.

Allen, J. H., and Riley, H. D.: Generalized cytomegalic inclusion disease with emphasis on roentgen diagnosis, Radiology **71**:257-262, 1958.

Anderson, R., Kieffer, S. A., Wolfson, J. J., and others: Thickening of the skull in surgically treated hydrocephalus, Amer. J. Roentgen. **110**:96-101, 1970.

Andersson, H., and Gomes, S. P.: Craniosynostosis. Review of the literature and indications for surgery, Acta Paediat. Scand. **57**:47-54, 1968.

Austin, J. H. M., and Gooding, C. A.: Roentgenographic measurement of skull size in children, Radiology **99**:641-646, 1971.

Bakwin, H., Golden, A., and Fox, S.: Familial osteoectasia with macrocranium, Amer. J. Roentgen. **91**:609-617, 1964.

Benda, C. E.: The Dandy-Walker syndrome or the so-called atresia of the foramen Magendie, J. Neuropath. Exp. Neurol. **13**:14-29, 1954.

Blackwood, W., McMenemey, W. H., Meyer, A., and others: Greenfield's neuropathology, ed. 2, Baltimore, 1963, The Williams & Wilkins Co.

Bligh, A. S., and Lawrence, K. M.: The radiological appearances in arhinencephaly, Clin. Radiol. **18**:383-393, 1967.

Caffey, J.: Multiple fractures in the long bones of infants suffering from chronic subdural hematoma, Amer. J. Roentgen. **56**:163-173, 1946.

Caffey, J.: Pediatric x-ray diagnosis, ed. 5, Chicago, 1967, Year Book Medical Publishers, Inc.

Campbell, J A.: Roentgen aspect of cranial configuration, Radiol. Clin. N. Amer. **4**:11-31, 1966.

Cloutier, M. D., and Stickler, G. B.: Head circumference in children with idiopathic hypopituitarism, Pediatrics **42**:209-210, 1968.

Cohen, M. E., Rosenthal, A. D., and Matson, D. D.: Neurological abnormalities in achondroplastic children, J. Pediat. **71**:367-376, 1967.

Cooper, L. Z., Ziring, P. R., Ockerse, A. B., and others: Rubella. Clinical manifestations and management, Amer. J. Dis. Child. **118**:18-29, 1969.

Cronqvist, S.: Roentgenologic evaluation of cranial size in children, Acta Radiol. [Diagn.] **7**:97-111, 1968.

Dandy W. E.: Diagnosis and treatment of hydrocephalus due to occlusions of the foramina of Magendie and Luschka, Surg. Gynec. Obstet. **32**:112-124, 1921.

Dandy, W. E., and Blackfan, K. D.: Internal hydrocephalus; an experimental, clinical and pathological study, Amer. J. Dis. Child. **8**:406-482, 1914.

Dorst, J. P.: Functional craniology: an aid in interpreting roentgenograms of the skull, Radiol. Clin. N. Amer. **2**:347-366, 1964.

Dyke, C. G., Davidoff, L. M., and Masson, C. G.: Cerebral hemiatrophy with homolateral hypertrophy of the skull and sinuses, Surg. Gynec. Obstet. **57**:588-600, 1933.

Farmer, T. W.: Pediatric neurology, New York, 1964, Harper & Row, Publishers.

Gerald, B. E., and Silverman, F. N.: Normal and abnormal interorbital distances with special reference to mongolism, Amer. J. Roentgen. **95**:154-161, 1965.

Gilles, F. N., and Shillito, J.: Infantile hydrocephalus: retrocerebellar subdural hematoma, J. Pediat. **76**:529-537, 1970.

Gordon, I. R. S.: Measurement of cranial capacity in children, Brit. J. Radiol. **39**:377-381, 1966.

Gordon, I. R. S.: Microcephaly and craniostenosis, Clin. Radiol. **21**:19-31, 1970.

Griscom, N. T., and Oh, K. S.: The contracting skull, Amer. J. Roentgen. **110**:106-110, 1970.

Haas, L. L.: Roentgenological skull measurements and their diagnostic applications, Amer. J. Roentgen **67**:197-209, 1952.

Hamby, W. B., Krauss, R. F., and Beswick, W. F.: Hydranencephaly: clinical diagnosis, Pediatrics **6**:371-383, 1950.

Hirata, T., and Gooding, C. A.: Thalassemia major, Amer. J. Dis. Child. **119**:505-506, 1970.

Holden, W. S., and Whitehead, A. S.: The radiological appearances in congenital toxoplasmosis, Brit. J. Radiol. **24**:38-40, 1951.

Horrigan, W. D., and Baker, D. H.: Gargoylism: a review of the roentgen skull changes with a description of a new finding, Amer. J. Roentgen. **86**:473-477, 1961.

Ingraham, F. D., and Matson, D. D.: Subdural hematoma in infancy, J. Pediat. **24**:1-37, 1944.

Jackson, H.: Asymmetry and growth of the skull, Brit. J. Radiol. **29**:521-535, 1956.

Juhl, J., and Wesenberg, R.: Radiological findings in congenital and acquired occlusion of foramina of Magendie and Luschka, Radiology **86**:801-813, 1966.

Kurlander, G., DeMyer, W., Campbell, J. A., and others: Roentgenology of holoprosencephaly, Acta Radiol. [Diagn.] **5**:25-40, 1966.

Moseley, J. E., Rabinowitz, J. G., and Dziadiw, R.: Hyperostosis cranii ex vacuo, Radiology **87**:1105-1107, 1966.

Nellhaus, G.: Head circumference from birth to eighteen years; practical composite international and interracial graphs, Pediatrics **41**:106-114, 1968a.

Nellhaus, G.: Head circumference in children with idiopathic hypopituitarism, Pediatrics **42**:210-211, 1968b.

O'Connell, E. J., Feldt, R. H., and Stickler, G. B.: Head circumference, mental retardation, and growth failure, Pediatrics **36**:62-66, 1965.

Olive, J. T., and DuShane, J. W.: Hydranencephaly, Amer. J. Dis. Child. **85**:43-46, 1953.

Powell, J. W., Weens, H. S., and Wenger, N. K.: The skull roentgenogram in iron deficiency anemia and in secondary polycythemia, Amer. J. Roentgen. **95**:143-147, 1965.

Pryor, H. B.: Charts of normal body measurements and revised width-weight tables in graphic form, J. Pediat. **68**:615-631, 1966.

Pryor, H. B., and Thelander, H.: Abnormally small head size and intellect in chidren, J. Pediat. **73**:593-598, 1968.

Roche, A. F.: The cranium in mongolism; a critical review, Acta Neurol. Scand. **42**:62-78, 1966.

Roche, A. F., Seward, F. S., and Sunderland, S.: Nonmetrical observations on cranial roentgenograms in mongolism, Amer. J. Roentgen. **85**:659-662, 1961.

Russell, D. S.: Observations on the pathology of hydrocephalus, Great Britain Medical Research Council Special Report Series 265, London, 1949, Her Majesty's Stationery Office.

Schechter, M. M., and Zingesser, L. H.: The radiology of aqueductal stenosis, Radiology **88**:905-916, 1967.

Schick, R. W., and Matson, D. D.: What is arrested hydrocephalus? J. Pediat. **58**:791-799, 1961.

Silver, H. K., and Deamer, W. C.: Graphs of the head circumference of the normal infant, J. Pediat. **33**:167-171, 1948.

Spitzer, R., Rabinowitch, J. Y., and Wybar, K. C.: A study of the abnormalities of the skull, teeth and lenses in mongolism, Canad. Med. Ass. J. **84**:567-572, 1961.

Taggart, J. K., and Walker, A. E.: Congenital atresia of the foramens of Luschka and Magendie, Arch. Neurol. Psychiat. **48**:583-612, 1942.

Taveras, J. M., and Wood, E. H.: Diagnostic neuroradiology, Baltimore, 1964, The Williams & Wilkins Co.

Watson, E. H., and Lowery, G. H.: Growth and development of children, ed. 5, Chicago, 1967, Year Book Medical Publishers, Inc.

CHAPTER 11

Thickness and texture

Romeo Ethier

NORMAL FEATURES

The cranial vault should be regarded as the mirror of the underlying brain and not as simply a part of the bony skeleton. Growth of the cranial vault is directly related to brain growth; this is a basic principle in neuroradiology (Fig. 11-1).

Bone grows along the sutures and also along the tables through a constant remodeling process as the bones of the vault are pushed away by the expanding brain (Ham and Leeson, 1961). Along the tables a slow but continuous erosion and reconstruction occurs, by combined osteoclastic and osteoblastic mechanisms, until the bones reach their final shape and thickness around the fully grown brain. Along the sutures new bone is formed, which increases the capacity of the calvarium to accommodate the growing brain. Although the brain is

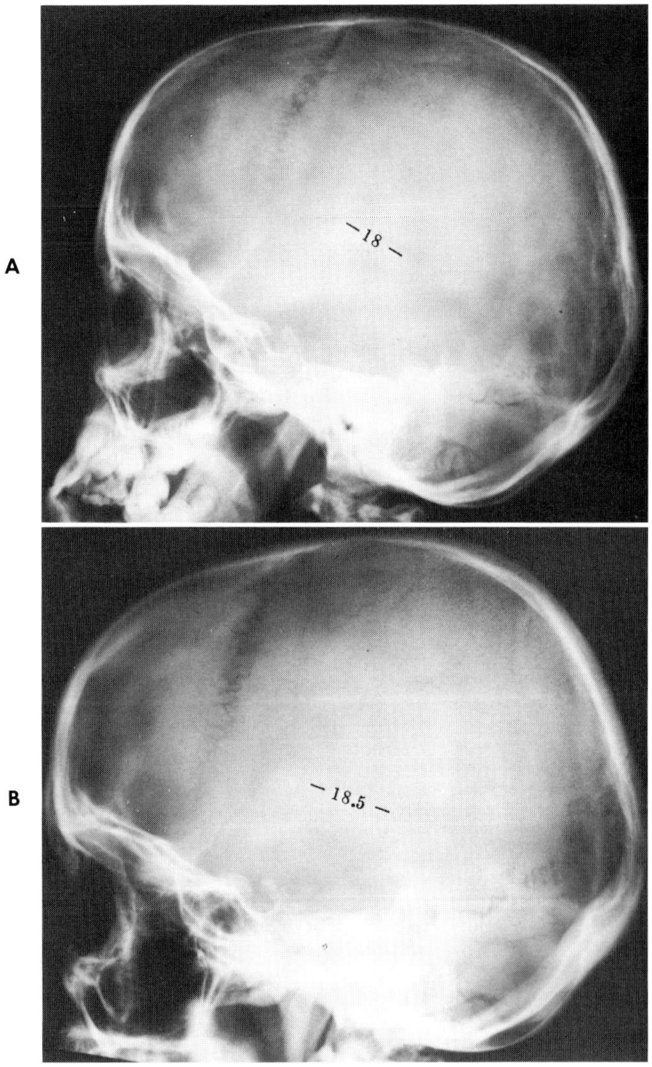

Fig. 11-1. Normal brain and skull growth. **A,** Thin vault with numerous brain markings in 9-year-old child. **B,** Same individual at age 21 years. Vault is thicker and brain markings have faded. Internal diameters indicate some cerebral growth in the interval.

I would like to express my most sincere gratitude to my associates, Dr. J. L. Vézina and Dr. D. Melançon for their magnificent support and encouragement.

My deepest gratitude also goes to Mr. C. Hodge for his skillful photographic work and to Miss M. Siegmann for her intelligent cooperation in writing this chapter.

I would like further to thank Dr. M. Molot, Dr. E. B. Karateew, Dr. R. Wee, and Dr. D'Arcy D. Lawrence for their constructive criticisms.

fully developed by the age of 14 years, thickening of the calvarial bones continues until the general somatic growth ends. In adults with a well-developed brain, the skull is large but relatively thin, whereas in adults with cerebral hypoplasia, it is small but relatively thick (Fig. 11-2).

The calvarial thickness varies widely in different individuals. The thickest part of a normal vault should not exceed 1 cm. If it measures more, some degree of cerebral underdevelopment, or a systemic disease, whether active or healed, should be suspected. The skull of adult epileptic patients afflicted with cerebral hypoplasia since early age tends to be thicker than the skull of normal individuals (Fig. 11-3). Some authors have pointed out that the size and thickness of the skull vary with sex. According to them the skulls of women are thicker and smaller than those of men (Pendergrass et al., 1956). The skulls of Negroes also are said to be thicker and larger than those of Caucasians. The first statement appears true, but I have not verified the latter.

In the analysis of roentgenograms of the skull, the cranial vault should be studied systematically. First the overall thickness and the general texture of the calvarium should be estimated. Then a critical study of the various tables and associated features should be made.

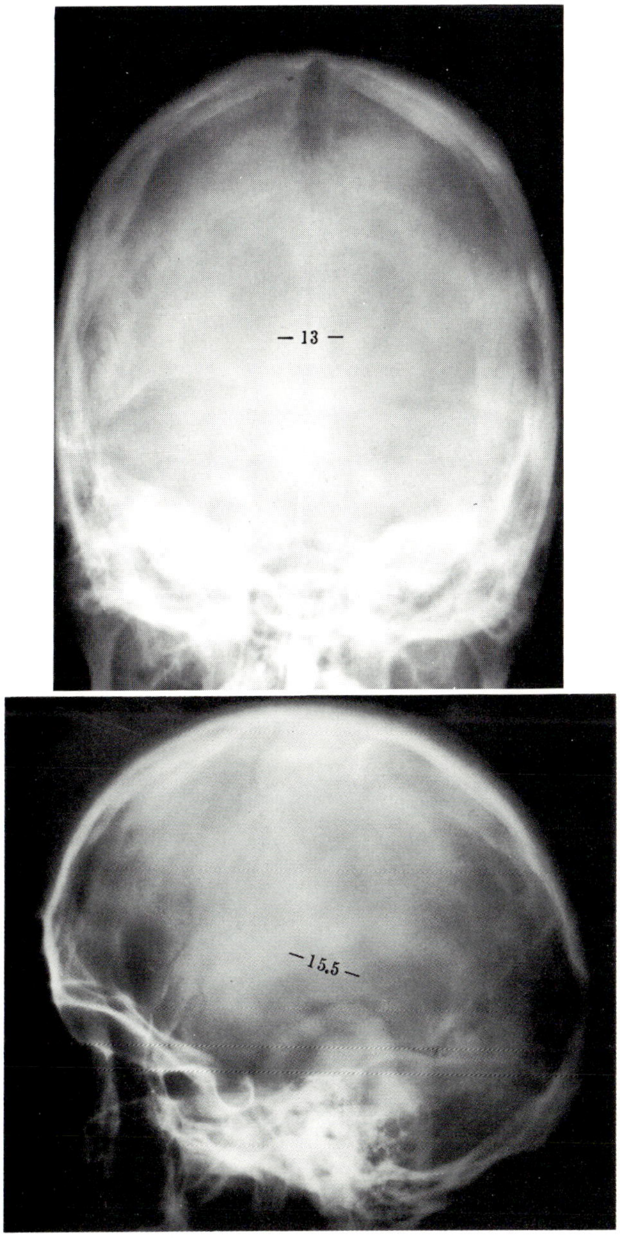

Fig. 11-2. Microcrania and micrencephaly. Small thick skull in 20-year-old epileptic female with I.Q. of 60. Note the small internal (or cerebral) diameters and the thick vault.

Tables

The calvarium, along the convexity, is well differentiated into three layers: the inner, the middle, and the outer tables. The inner and outer tables are composed of compact bone, the middle of cancellous bone.

The thickness of the normal skull is proportionate to the width of the middle table. Skulls with a prominent middle table are thick and are referred to as diploic skulls (Fig. 11-4). Those with little or no diploe are thin and are called compact skulls since they are composed essentially of compact bone (Fig. 11-5). In areas where the middle table is abundant, as in the parietal eminences, the skull is thick. It is thin where the middle table is less developed or absent, as in the supraorbital portions of the frontal squama or in the superior quadrants of the occipital squama. Parts of the cranial vault that are well protected by muscles are often very thin.

The *inner table* varies little in thickness, except in

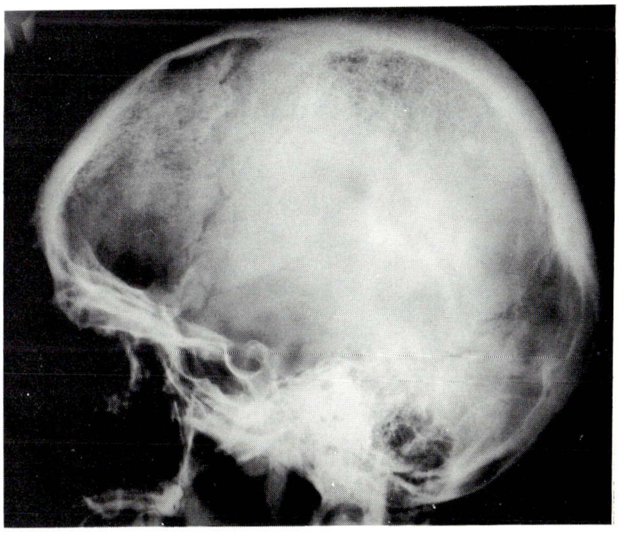

Fig. 11-3. Cerebral hypoplasia. Abnormally thick cranial vault indicating some degree of cerebral hypoplasia in 17-year-old patient with idiopathic epilepsy.

places where it is eroded by vascular structures and brain markings. It is usually thinner than the outer table, although the reverse is not infrequent in a normal skull. It is generally more fragile than the outer table. It is perforated by many minute channels containing the communicating veins that exist between the diploic veins and the meningeal veins or sinuses (Fig. 11-6). Not uncommonly these fine perforating channels are seen on roentgenograms of good quality. Occasionally, larger perforations, the *parietal foramina,* can be observed in the posteromesial aspect of the parietal bones. These foramina not only involve the inner table but also extend through the middle and outer tables (Fig. 11-7). They appear as small, radiolucent, round structures sur-

A

B

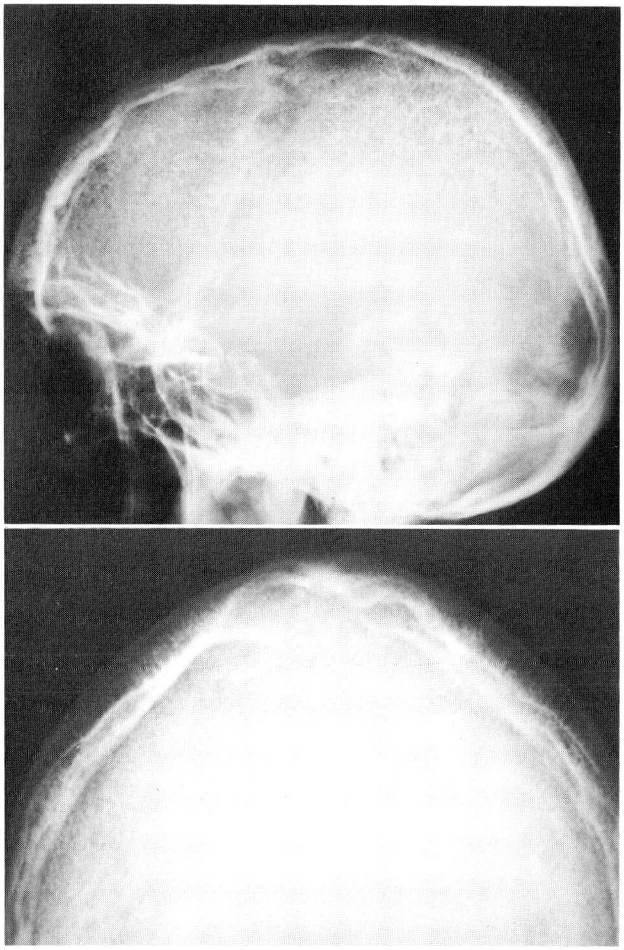

Fig. 11-4. Diploic skull. Striking mosaic-like appearance of skull with well-developed diploe.

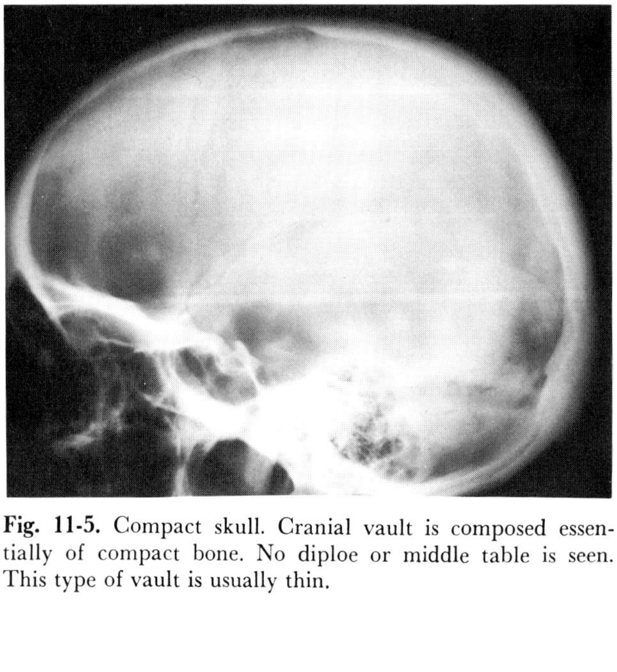

Fig. 11-5. Compact skull. Cranial vault is composed essentially of compact bone. No diploe or middle table is seen. This type of vault is usually thin.

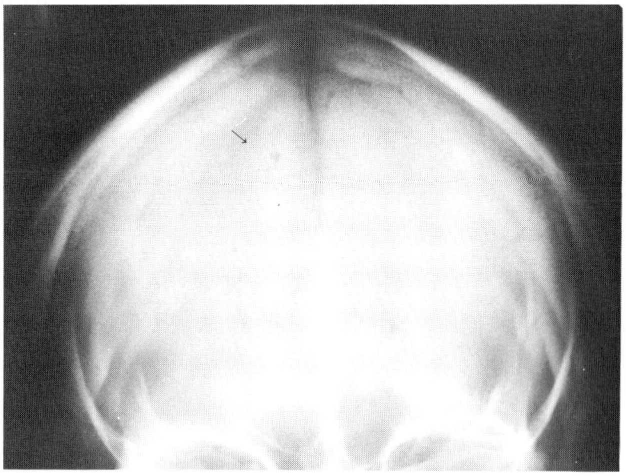

Fig. 11-6. Fine perforating emissary vessels (arrow) are numerous, mainly in frontal bone. Most of them run through minute foramina, which are hidden by the other tables.

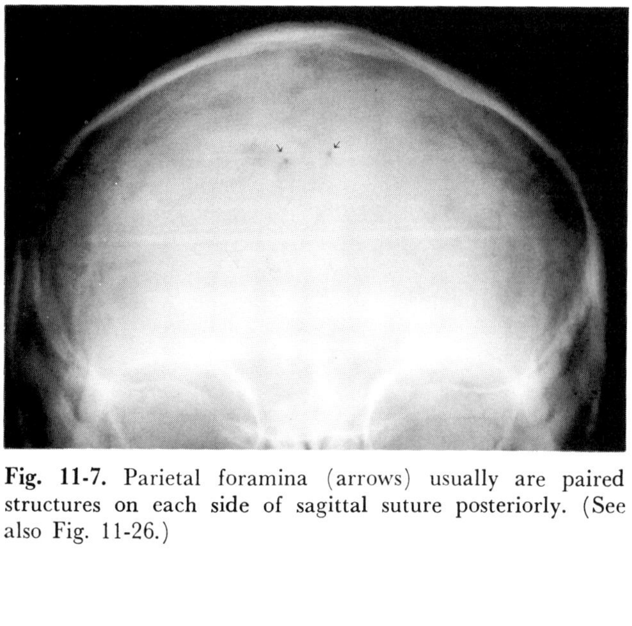

Fig. 11-7. Parietal foramina (arrows) usually are paired structures on each side of sagittal suture posteriorly. (See also Fig. 11-26.)

rounded by a halo of dense compact bone. Their margins are lined with periosteum, formed by the union of the endocranium and the pericranium (Gray, 1967).

The *middle table* or diploe is composed of an irregular network of bony trabeculae and vascular spaces. The bony trabeculae unite the outer and inner tables in such a way that maximum protection is achieved in case of injury. Probably also the blood within the diploe further acts as a fluid cushion to absorb traumatic forces. On roentgenograms of the skull, these trabeculations form a mosaic-like pattern, which vascular channels modify according to their number and configuration.

The *outer table* varies even less in thickness than does the inner table and appears rather smooth on roentgenograms. It tends to be thicker anteriorly when the frontal sinuses are not well developed. Often it is thinner along the parietal eminences, just above the temporal lines. Like the inner table it is perforated by many minuscule connecting veins, but these fine bony channels are rarely seen. Frequently, on lateral projections, fine serrations are seen on either side of the vertex between the bregma and the lambda. They do not represent vascular channels but are produced by the sagittal suture (Fig. 11-8).

Convolutional markings

The inner table of the skull is normally molded by the convolutions of the brain, resulting in digital mark-

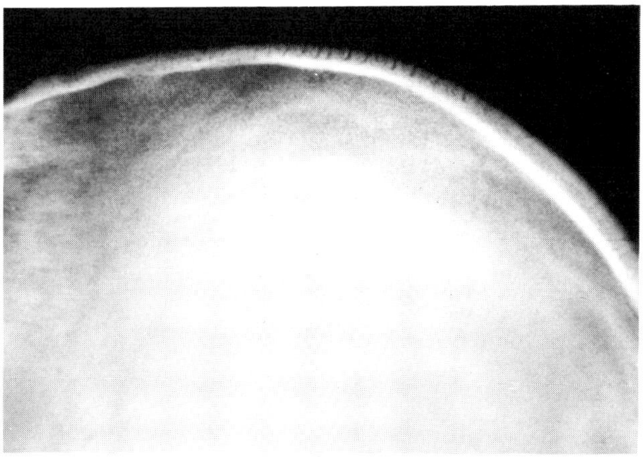

Fig. 11-8. Sagittal suture. Closeup lateral view of vertex shows serrations of sagittal suture that unite outer and middle tables of parietal bones.

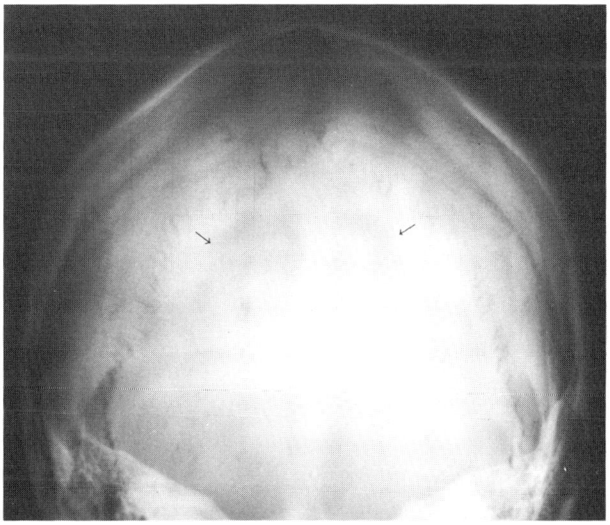

Fig. 11-9. Occipital brain markings. Arrows point to grossly oval, well-demarcated, radiolucent zones between lambdoid suture and grooves for transverse sinuses. Their edges are curved, as with other brain markings. They are best observed in patients with thin cranial vaults.

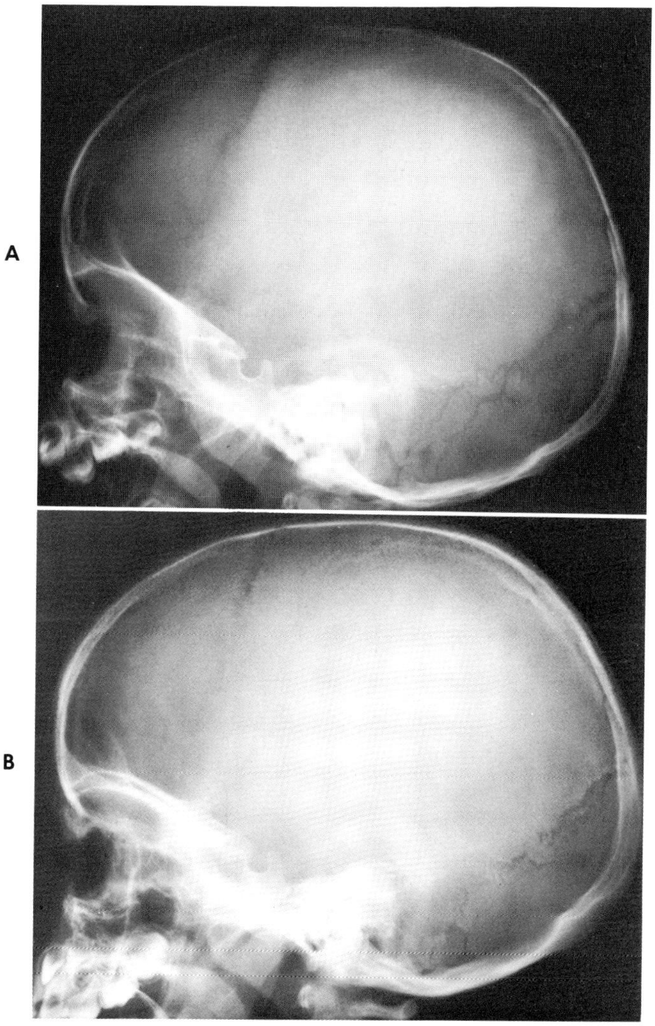

Fig. 11-10. Micrencephaly. **A,** Onset of seizures at age 14 months during febrile episode, possibly encephalitis. At that time brain markings were present. **B,** Thick featureless cranial vault 15 months later. Note the disappearance of brain markings and the remarkable increase in thickness of the vault in the interval. Skull has remained small because of brain damage and impaired cerebral development.

A

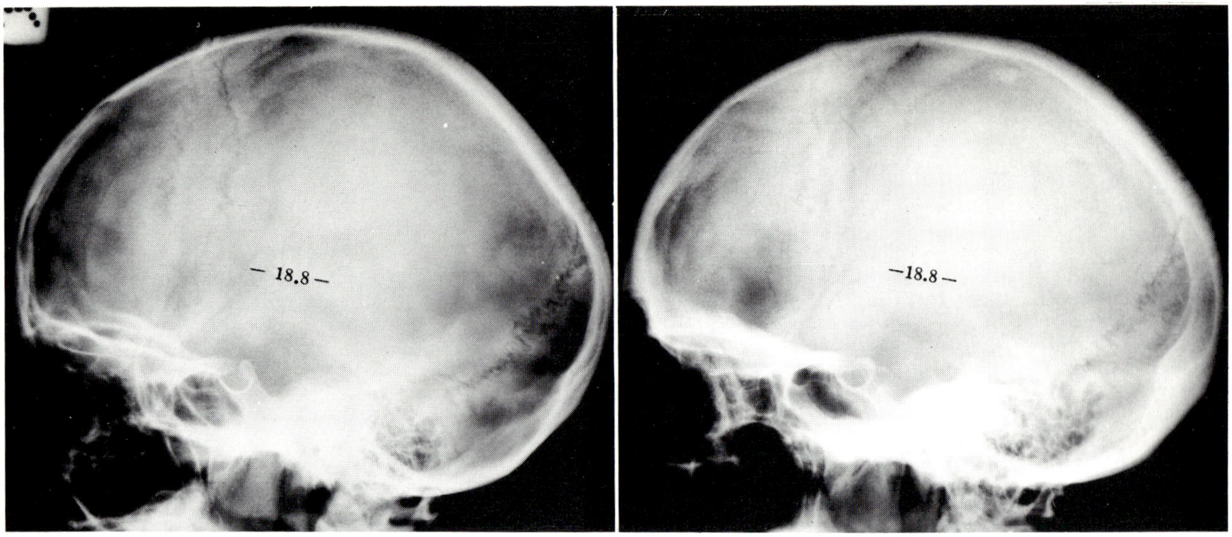

B

Figs. 11-11. Arrest of brain growth. **A,** At age 8 years, development of brain ceased. **B,** By 16 years, internal diameters had remained the same, brain markings had disappeared, and vault had doubled in thickness.

A

B

C

D

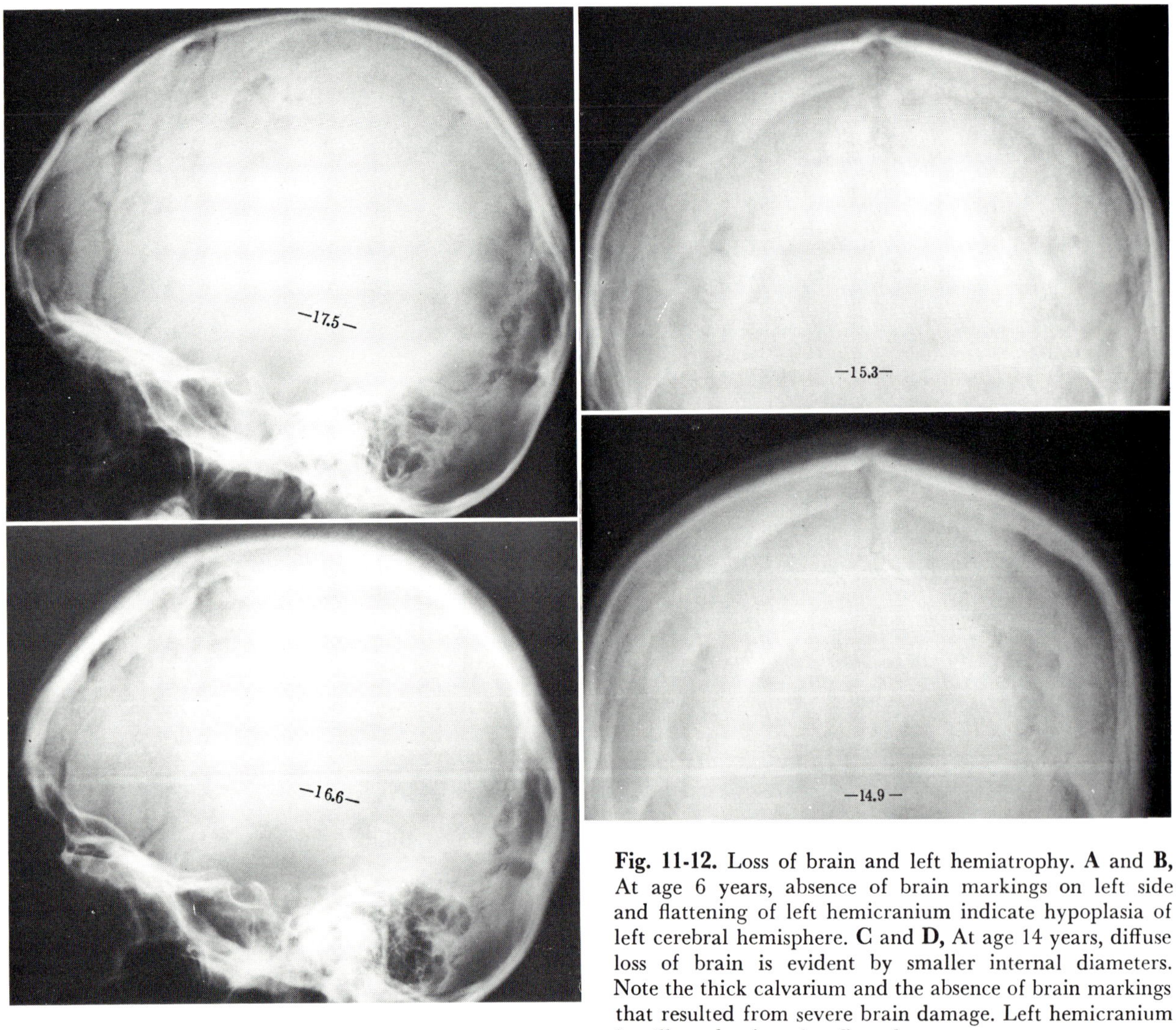

Fig. 11-12. Loss of brain and left hemiatrophy. **A** and **B,** At age 6 years, absence of brain markings on left side and flattening of left hemicranium indicate hypoplasia of left cerebral hemisphere. **C** and **D,** At age 14 years, diffuse loss of brain is evident by smaller internal diameters. Note the thick calvarium and the absence of brain markings that resulted from severe brain damage. Left hemicranium is still predominantly affected.

ings. These markings may be compared to the finger impressions formed on the surface of a wet ball of clay when grasped by the hand. They usually do not exceed the diameter of a medium-sized finger, which diameter could serve as a guide in the gross evaluation of brain markings in chronic intracranial hypertension (Fig. 11-13).

In childhood, convolutional markings are numerous and are as prominent along the cranial vault as along the base. During adolescence, growth of the brain decelerates, resulting in less prominent convolutional markings. In time, with the cessation of normal brain growth, these markings actually disappear. This phenomenon is aided by a concomitant thickening of the dura. Occasionally, in the normal skull, brain markings may be seen only opposite the occipital poles and not be apparent elsewhere. On frontal projections they appear as two symmetric areas of radiolucency in the superior occipital quadrants. These areas should not be confused with other conditions (Fig. 11-9).

In young patients the recognition that brain markings are absent is extremely important. If such convolutions are totally absent, arrest of cerebral growth must be suspected (Fig. 11-10). This cessation of brain growth is documented best when the internal diameters of the skull are measured on serial examinations. When the diameters remain the same or decrease, arrest of brain growth (Fig. 11-11) or an actual loss of brain tissue can be affirmed (Fig. 11-12). Absence of cerebral markings on one side of the cranial vault indicates either that the brain is not growing on this side or that a collec-

A

B

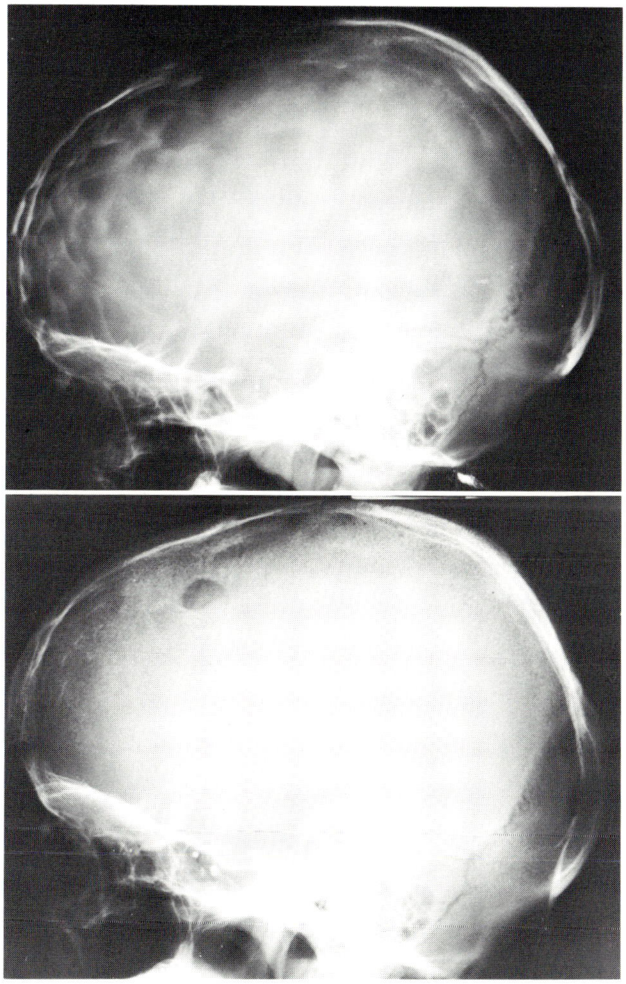

Fig. 11-13. Pressure changes. **A,** Abnormally large brain markings in child recently operated on for medulloblastoma. **B,** Three years after irradiation and surgery, brain markings had disappeared and thickness of vault increased.

A

B

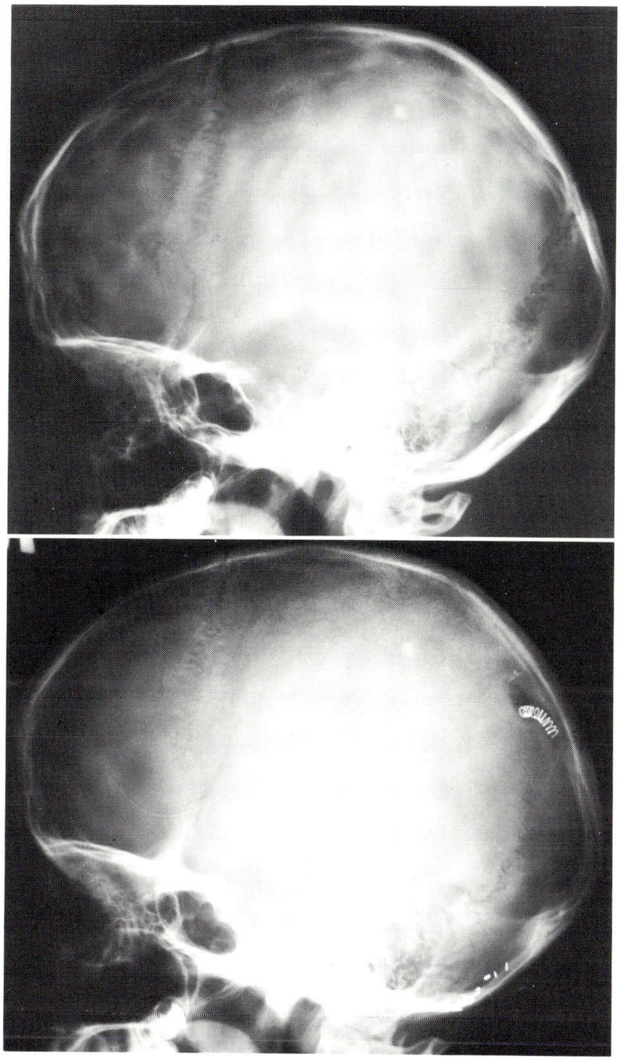

Fig. 11-14. Reduction of intracranial pressure after Torkilsen shunt. **A,** Thin vault, slightly widened sutures, prominent brain markings, and pressure changes about sella in 10-year-old patient with toxoplasmosis. **B,** Twelve months later, complete disappearance of pressure changes after shunt operation. Cranial vault increased in thickness, since it was no longer subjected to high intracranial pressure. Note how rapidly these changes took place.

tion of fluid is interposed between the brain and the vault. In the latter case some bulging and thinning of the cranial vault may be seen (Fig. 11-43). Fewer markings on one side of the vault than on the other may be the only definite sign of hypoplasia of a cerebral hemisphere. Stereoscopic views show this asymmetry rather strikingly.

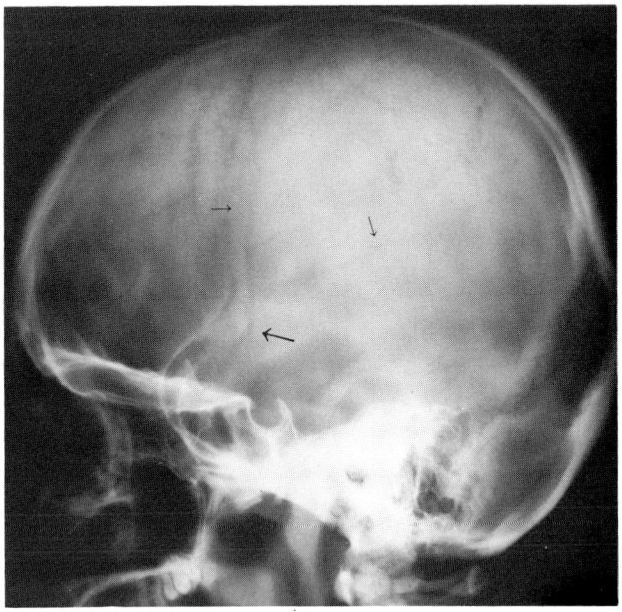

Fig. 11-15. Arterial meningeal grooves. Normal appearance of the grooves for middle meningeal artery and branches (arrows). Note how they taper gradually.

After a severe head injury the eventual disappearance of brain markings indicates that the brain has been damaged extensively. In contrast, the fading of accentuated brain markings after surgery or radiotherapy means that the cerebral hypertension has been relieved (Fig. 11-13). Proper interpretation of these variations is of great interest also in postoperative evaluation of ventricular shunts (Fig. 11-14).

Vascular grooves and channels

Inner table. Vascular structures that indent the inner table are the branches of the middle meningeal arteries and veins and the dural sinuses.

The main trunk of the meningeal artery bifurcates along the anterolateral wall of the middle fossa into anterior and posterior branches. The anterior branch may become embedded in bone, for a variable distance, shortly after its origin. Above the pterion it parallels the coronal suture on its parietal side and gives off frontal and parietal twigs. The posterior branch curves posteriorly along the superior aspect of the temporal squama and divides into parietal and occipital branches (Fig. 11-15). Many normal variations exist, however. As a rule the meningeal grooves seen along the inner table on both sides of the skull are symmetric in size and number. The grooves containing the meningeal arteries taper progressively as they ascend toward the superior aspect

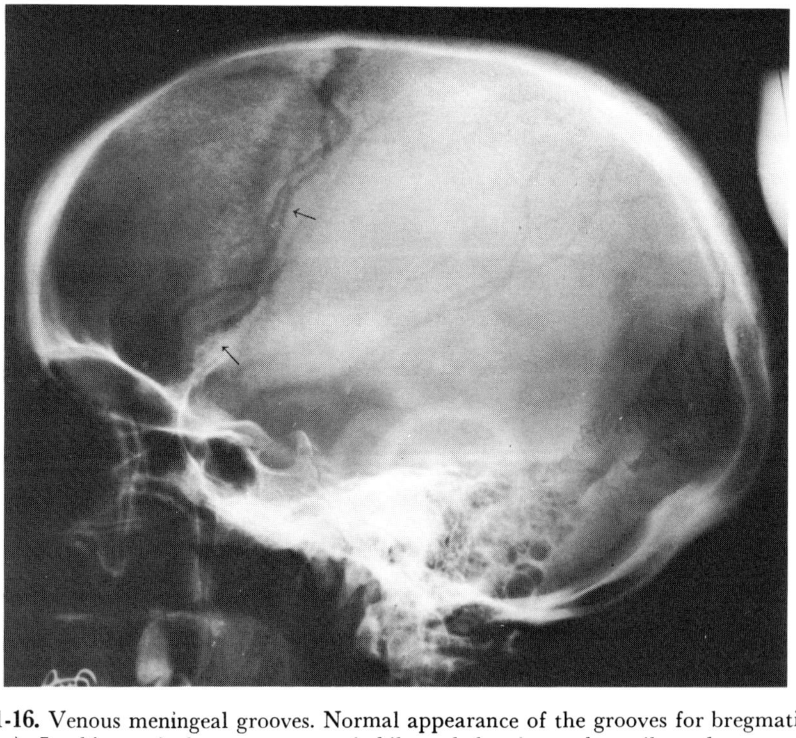

Fig. 11-16. Venous meningeal grooves. Normal appearance of the grooves for bregmatic vein (arrows). In this particular case, groove is bilateral; but it can be unilateral.

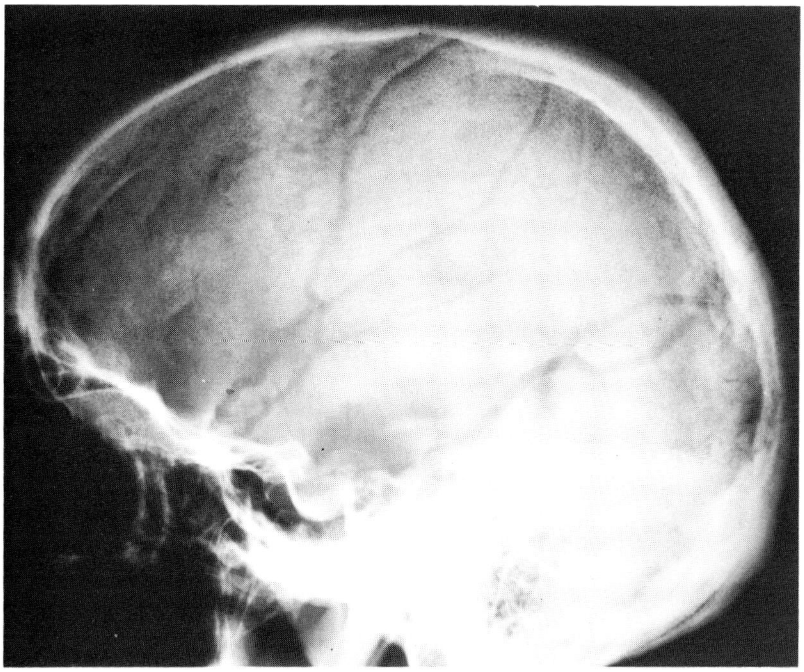

Fig. 11-17. Cerebral arteriovenous fistula. Enlarged arterial and venous meningeal grooves bilaterally. When observed on an otherwise normal skull, they are suggestive of arteriovenous fistula, either meningeal or cerebral in location.

of the skull. They are often referred to as arterial grooves, but this designation is not absolutely correct since meningeal arteries are usually accompanied by two veins. In contrast, venous grooves change little in caliber throughout their course.

The most common venous groove is the so-called bregmatic groove, which runs along the coronal suture (Fig. 11-16). It contains a large meningeal vein, which empties into the sphenoparietal or the superior longitudinal sinus, either directly or through venous lakes. Because the blood can flow in either direction, the groove remains fairly uniform in width throughout its entire course. The meningeal veins represent important collateral channels in cases of thrombosis of the superior longitudinal sinus.

Increase in size, number, and tortuosity of the arterial grooves on one side of the skull is indicative of a lesion. These features are frequently observed in meningiomas, fibrous dysplasia, and tumors of the cranial vault. The grooves are enlarged strikingly on both sides of the skull when the meningeal circulation contributes to the blood supply of either a cerebral or a meningeal arteriovenous malformation (Fig. 11-17). They may be rather prominent bilaterally in Paget's disease, even in the absence of sarcomatous degeneration. Enlargement has also been reported in progressive intracranial arterial occlusions (Taveras, 1969). The meningeal arteries in this condition become the main collateral system through which the brain receives its blood supply.

The grooves for the large intradural sinuses are deeper and wider than those for the meningeal vessels. The main sinus groove of the cranial vault is the sagittal sulcus, in which runs the superior longitudinal sinus. On frontal projections it appears as a smooth curved elevation of the inner table along the midline (Fig. 11-

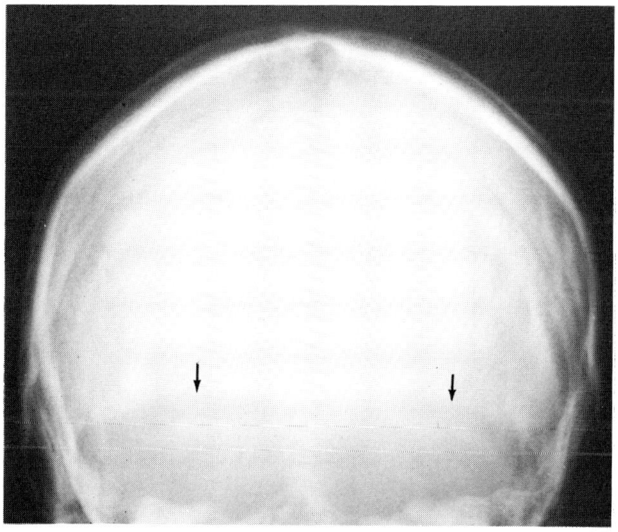

Fig. 11-18. Sinus grooves. Smooth elevation and erosion of inner table along midline superiorly caused by the superior longitudinal sinus. Similar grooving of occiput, but seen *en face* due to transverse sinuses. Note that the groove of the right transverse sinus is wider than that of the left (arrows).

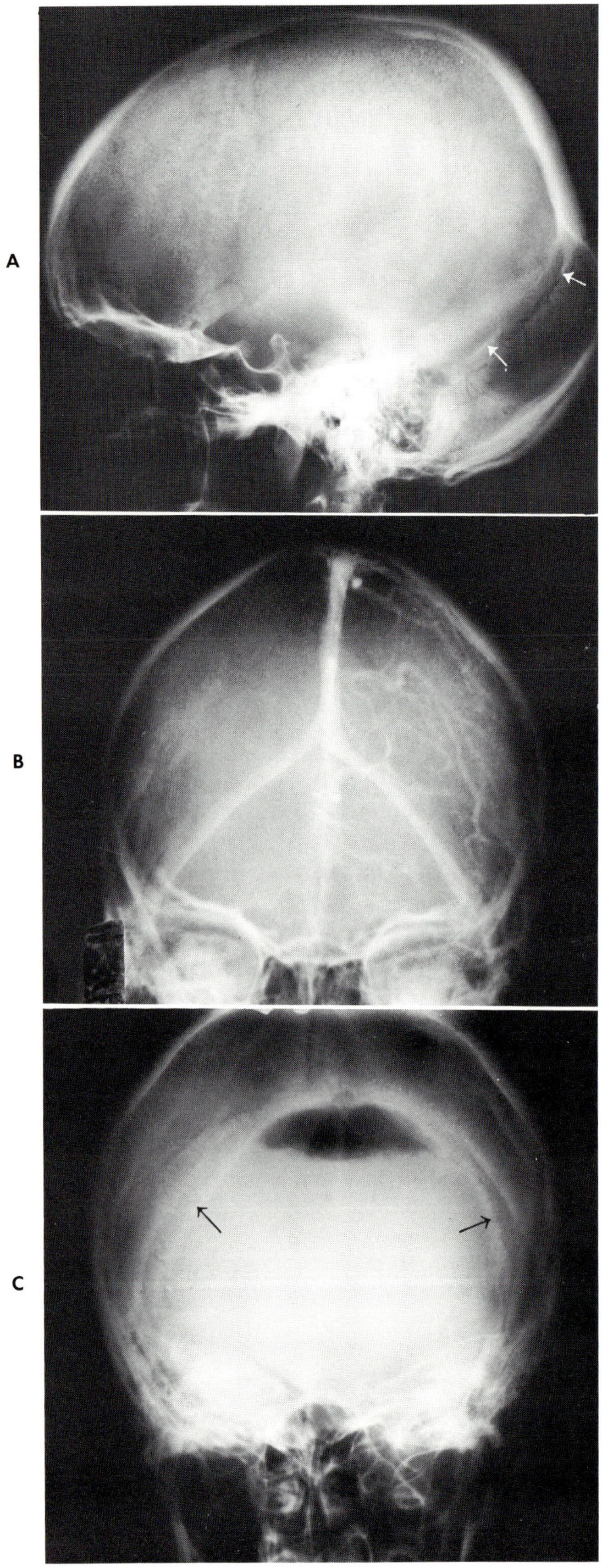

18). Immediately underneath, a V-shaped dural calcification on both sides of the sinus is common (Fig. 11-102). The longitudinal sinus runs from the crista galli to the internal occipital protuberance. At this point it either joins the straight sinus to form the torcular Herophili or continues into one of the transverse sinuses. The transverse sinuses travel along the periphery of the tentorium and lie in grooves that run horizontally across the occipital squama (Fig. 11-18). They divide the occipital squama into two halves: the supratentorial or occipital and the infratentorial or cerebellar. Since the occipital bone is relatively thin, the grooves for the transverse sinuses are more apparent than the sagittal sulcus, the right usually more so than the left. With high insertion of the tentorium, the grooves run along the lambdoid sutures (Fig. 11-19).

Middle table. As already mentioned, the diploe of the skull contains numerous veins (Fig. 11-20). In some skulls a rather well-organized diploic circulation is shown and veins are recognizable in the frontal, parietal, and occipital regions. These veins are sometimes referred to as the diploic channels of Breschet (Fig. 11-21). This topographic distribution is rare (Testut and Latarjet, 1949). More commonly the diploic channels are scattered at random. In the parietal eminence, where the diploe is usually thickest, the channels frequently appear stellate (Fig. 11-22). The channels vary so much in shape and size that no significant diagnostic criterion can be attributed to them.

Besides diploic veins, there are diploic lakes, which appear as irregular grossly oval or round areas of radiolucency. They rarely exceed 2 cm in their longest diameter and are most common in the parietal bones. Another location is on either side of the grooves for the transverse sinuses, where clusters of diploic lakes are seen occasionally (Fig. 11-23). Although the diploic lakes are frequently irregular in contour, they are well demarcated and the bone around them is intact. Occasionally their identification, as such, may be difficult. Appropriate tangential views or tomographic sections, however, show them quite clearly within the diploe with intact outer and inner tables. When the diploic lakes are small and numerous, they may resemble multiple metastases; and only by serial studies is proper identification possible (Fig. 11-24).

Fig. 11-19. High transverse sinus grooves and bulging occipital squama. **A,** Grooves for transverse sinuses run along lambdoid sutures whenever insertion of tentorium is high. **B,** High position of transverse sinuses at carotid angiography. **C,** Large cisterna magna extends up to lambda. Note the high position of the transverse sinus grooves (arrows). These features are commonly associated and represent a normal variant.

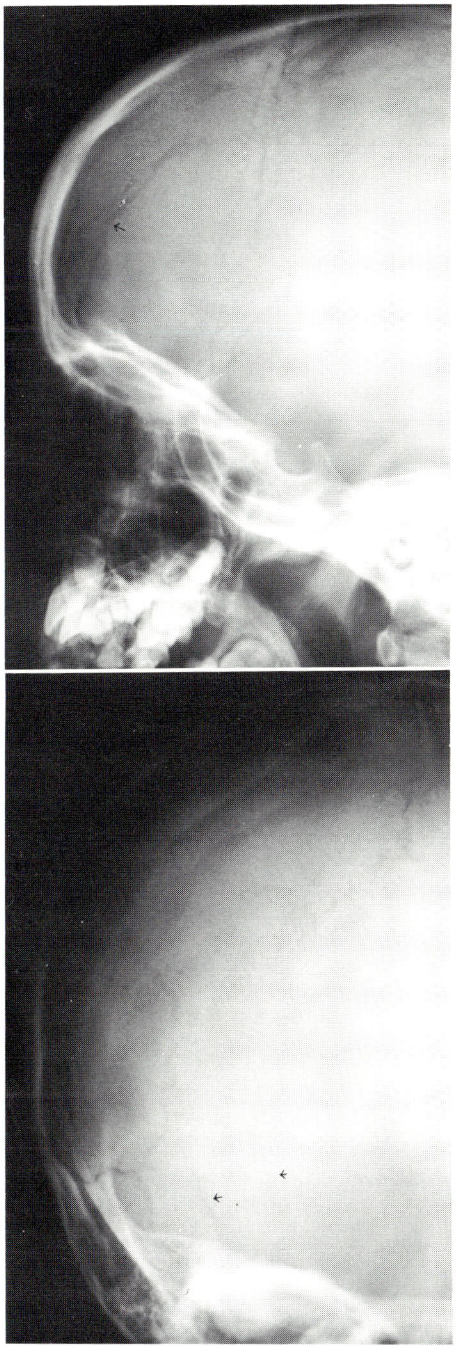

Fig. 11-20. Diploic veins. Frequently these veins pursue an angular course and are usually lined with faint parallel bony walls (arrows), which differentiate them from fracture lines. They are not as radiolucent as a fracture of similar width.

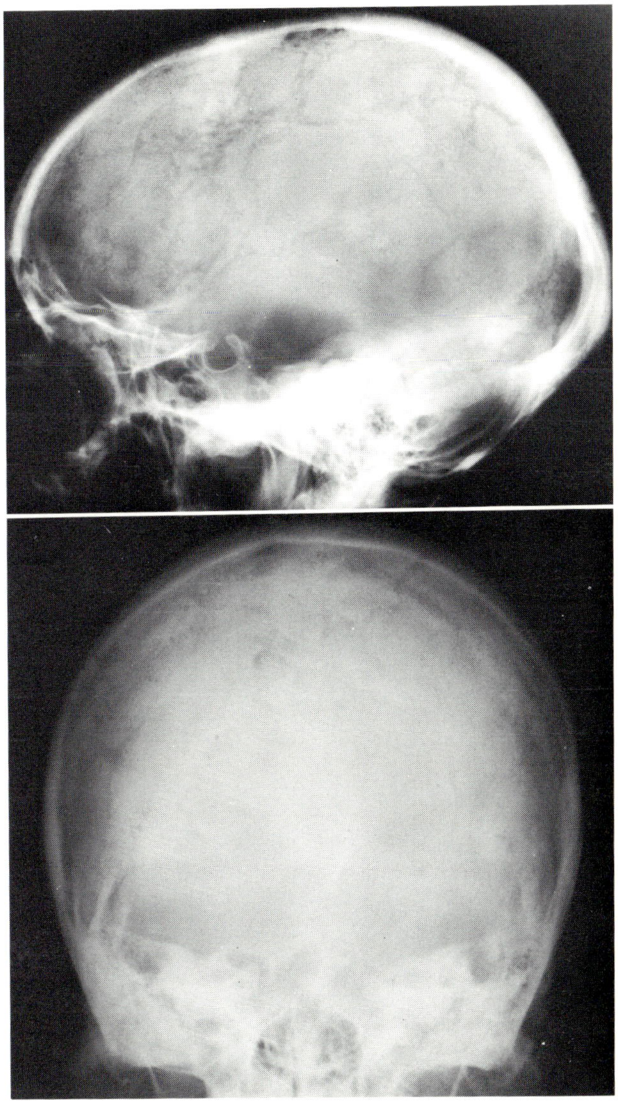

Fig. 11-21. Diploic channels of Breschet. Numerous venous channels in diploe of frontal and parietal bones fairly symmetrically distributed on both sides of vault.

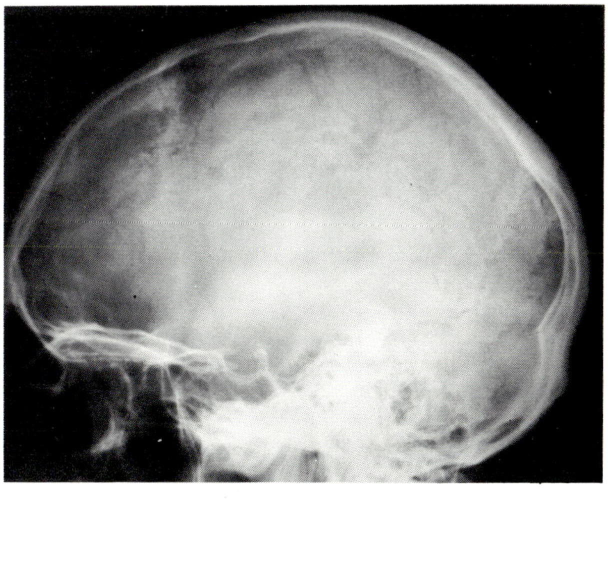

Fig. 11-22. Parietal diploic veins. Frequently in the parietal area, diploic veins follow a stellate course as they radiate from venous lakes. They are usually symmetric on each side of vault.

Outer table. Two vascular grooves have been described along the outer table of the cranial vault (Schunk and Maruyama, 1960). One is supraorbital in location and is said to be due to the supraorbital artery. The other runs along the outer table of the temporal squama and parietal bone above the external auditory meatus. It is produced by the middle temporal branch of the superficial temporal artery (Fig. 11-25). Close analysis reveals that these grooves taper and branch as do other arterial grooves.

The many vascular grooves and channels just described should be recognized as such and not be mistaken for fractures. An old fracture through a diploic part of the skull, however, may appear exactly like a diploic vein and probably becomes a vascular channel with healing. The arterial grooves along the inner and outer tables of the skull are less radiolucent in general than fracture lines. In addition, the elevated bony edges along the grooves appear as faint parallel dense lines. Their exact location along the inner and outer tables is greatly facilitated by stereoroentgenography.

Transosseous emissary veins. In the cranial vault, emissary veins are most frequent in the region of the occipital protuberance and in the parasagittal and posterior aspects of the parietal bones. These veins represent an anastomotic system between the intracranial and extracranial venous systems.

In the occipital region the emissary veins run a sinuous course in bony channels between the torcular Herophili and the occipital scalp veins. In the superior parietal

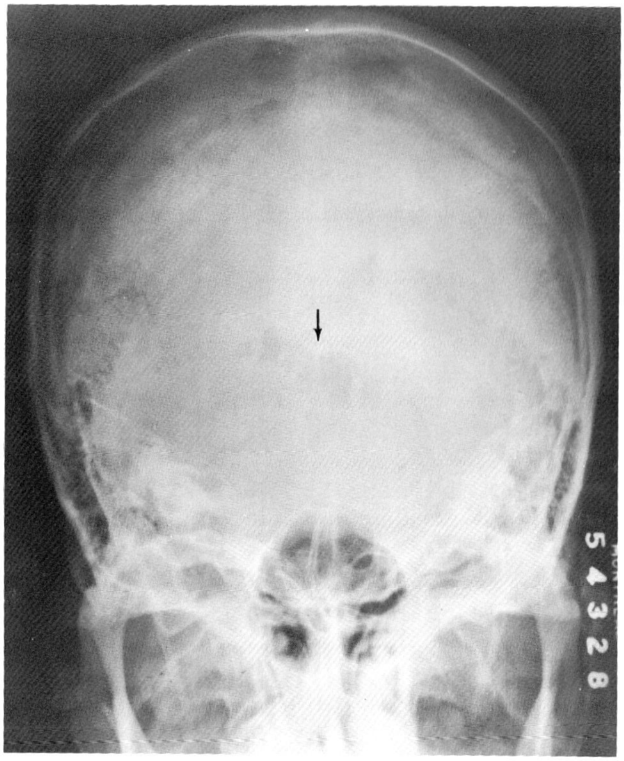

Fig. 11-23. Occipital diploic lakes. Numerous cavities within diploe of occipital bone are lined with thin walls of compact bone (arrow). They are usually seen in region of the torcular Herophili. Lateral views in such cases show that the position of the inner table remains normal; or the table may bulge slightly intracranially, which differentiates these cavities from pacchionian granulations.

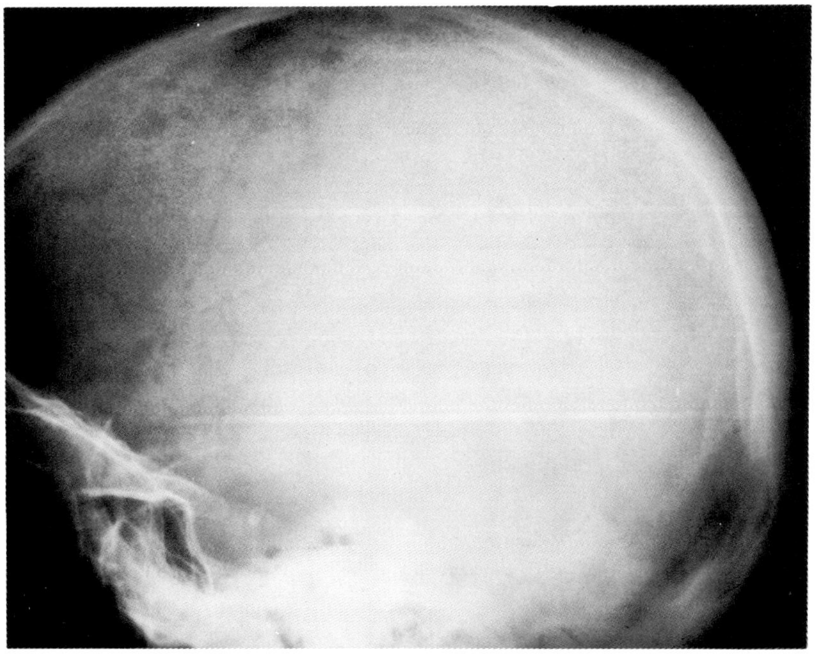

Fig. 11-24. Diploic venous lakes. Numerous small radiolucent zones resemble multiple osteolytic lesions.

regions the emissary veins of Santorini join the longitudinal sinus with the parietal scalp veins. They pass through the parietal foramina, which are seen in the superior part of the parietal bones, approximately 3.5 cm above the lambdoid suture (Fig. 11-26). Along with the emissary veins there is frequently a branch of the occiptal artery.

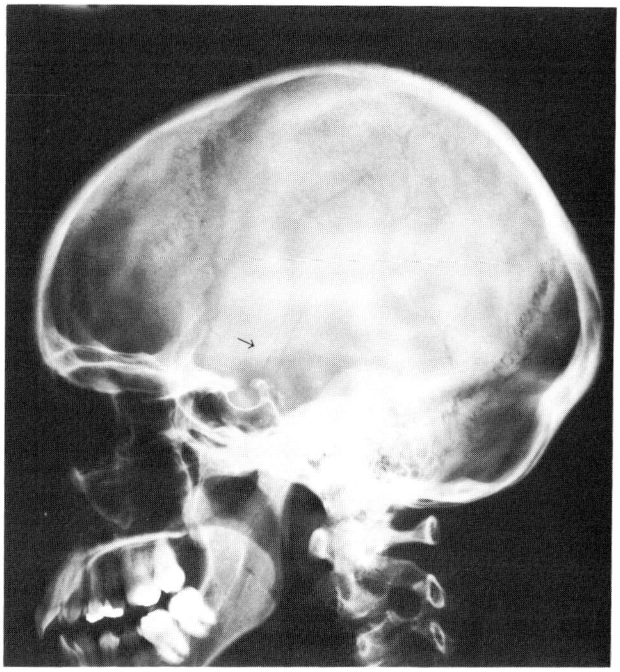

Fig. 11-25. Middle temporal artery grooves. Linear grooves (arrow) run vertically on each side of vault. They extend across temporal squama and fade out rapidly along inferior part of parietal bone. (From McRae, D. L.: In Caveness, W. F., and Walker, A. E., editors: Head Injury Conference Proceedings, Philadelphia, 1966, J. B. Lippincott Co.)

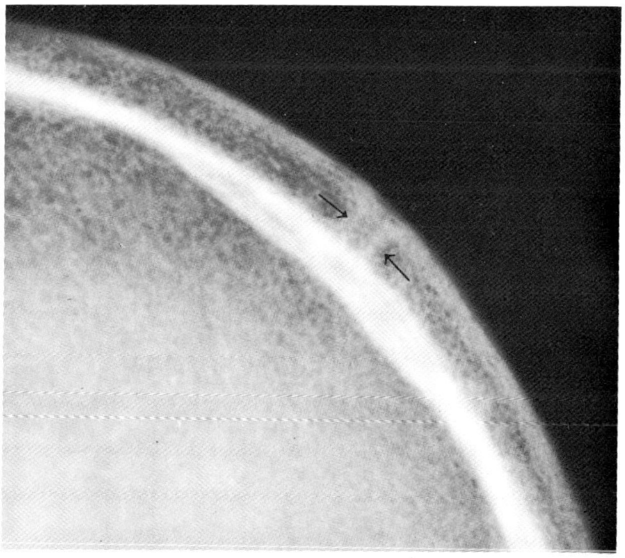

Fig. 11-26. Normal parietal foramen. Closeup lateral view of the foramen, through which passes the emissary vein of Santorini, shows walls parallel and lined with compact bone (arrows).

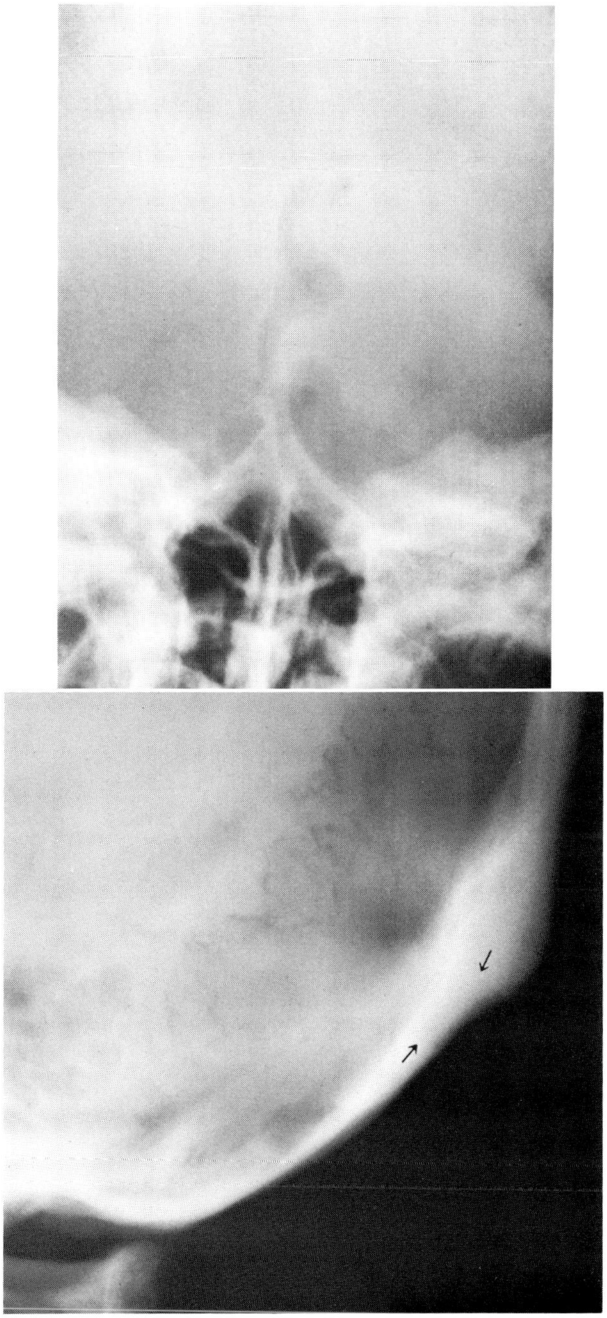

Fig. 11-27. Enlarged occipital emissary veins. Large intraosseous and transosseous channels (arrows) result from hypertrophied tortuous emissary veins in patient with increased intracranial pressure of long duration.

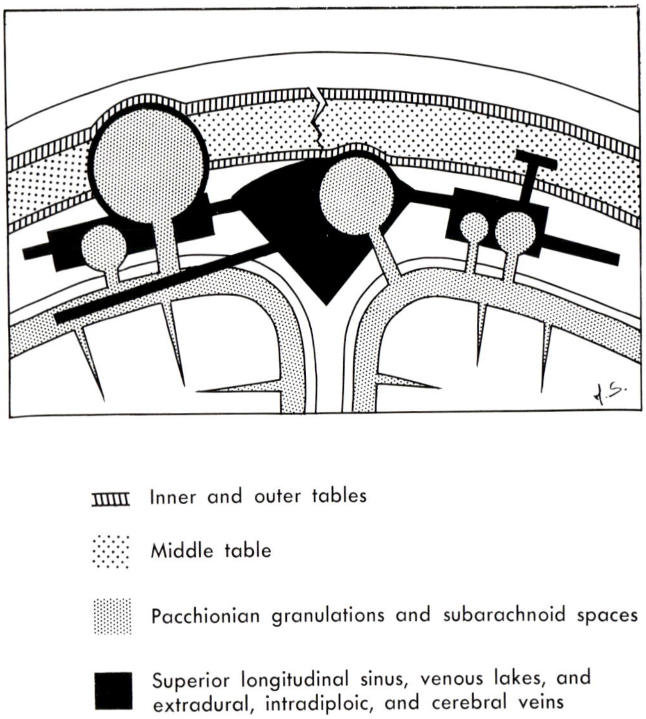

Fig. 11-28. Pacchionian granulations. Schematic representation of some of many possible locations of these granulations.

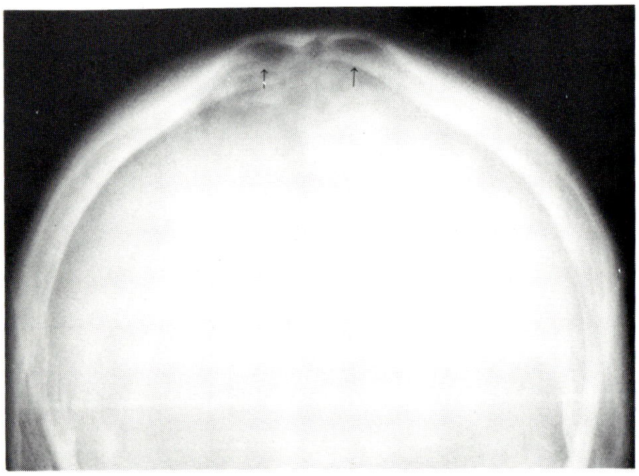

Fig. 11-29. Pacchionian granulations. Smooth curved erosions of inner and middle tables (arrows) on both sides of midline. They are more frequently seen just behind the bregma in the anterior half of the parietal bones.

In long-standing increased intracranial pressure these anastomotic vessels assume an important role (Fig. 11-27). More cerebral venous blood passes through them, and they become enlarged. According to Lindblom (1936), if the bony channels for the occipital emissary veins measure more than 2 mm, raised intracranial pressure is indicated. This interpretation has been challenged recently (Yuhl and Schmitz, 1969). Because of insufficient data, however, the conclusions reached by these authors are far from convincing.

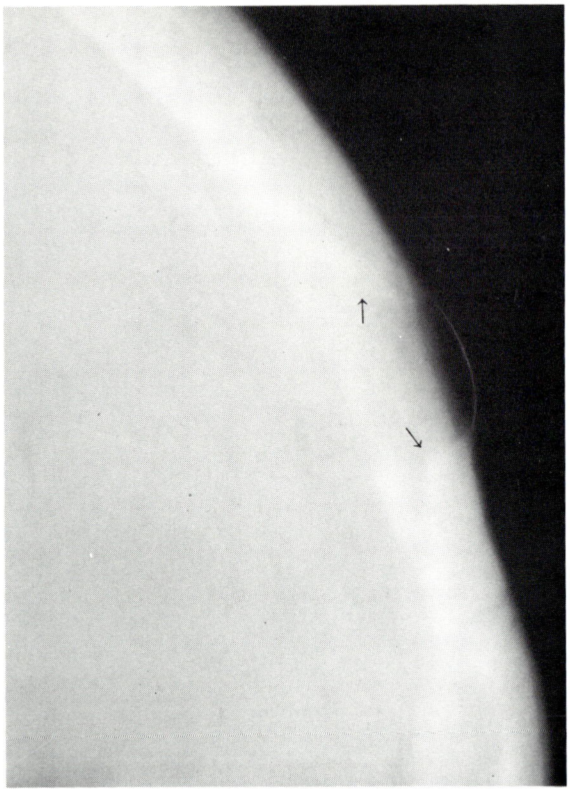

Fig. 11-30. Pacchionian granulations. Funnel-shaped erosion of inner and middle tables (arrows), caused by this type of granulation. Note the erosion and bulge of the outer table (retouched).

Pacchionian granulations. These arachnoid extensions are intradural in location. They project into the lumen of the main sinuses or the venous lacunae that are located immediately lateral to the sinuses (Fig. 11-28). Large granulations reach the inner table and produce smooth local elevations and erosions. They are common in the parasagittal region (Fig. 11-29). Occasionally they erode into the diploe and into the outer table, which may become very thin and even bulge externally. If diagnosis is difficult, tangential views of the area demonstrate smooth and funneled edges of the erosion. These edges are farther apart at the inner table level than at the outer. This characteristic indicates quite clearly that the process originates inside the skull and is of a benign nature (Fig. 11-30). If there is any doubt, follow-up studies may be carried out. At times pacchionian granulations are situated in unusual sites along meningeal or diploic veins (Fig. 11-31), and their identification may present a problem. Careful analysis with the aid of stereoscopic tangential views, however, will reveal the true nature of the erosions in most cases.

A

B

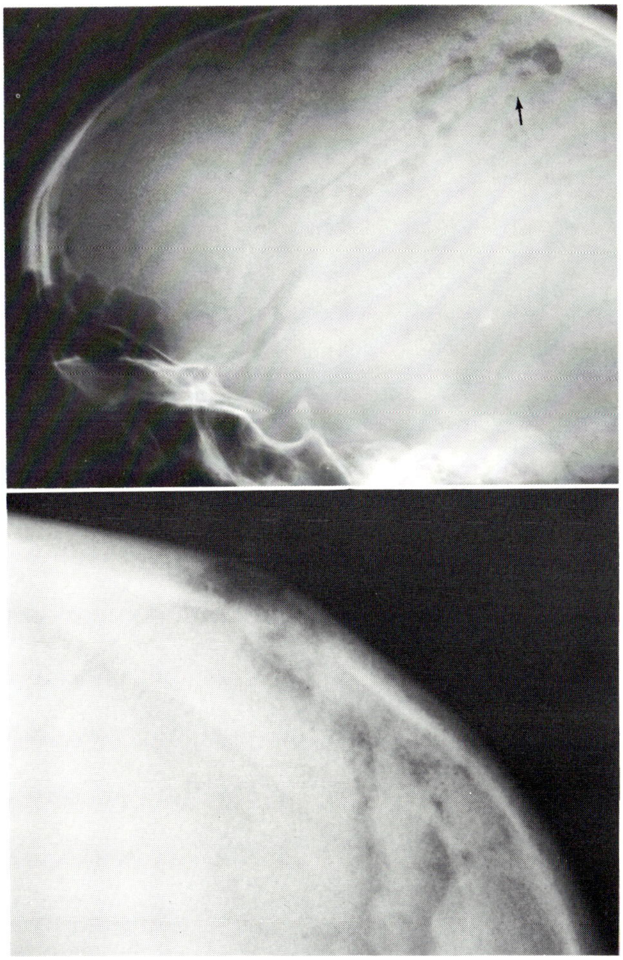

Fig. 11-31. Unusual pacchionian granulations. **A,** Cluster of small and medium-sized arachnoid granulations (arrow) along meningeal vein. **B,** Tangential view shows outer table bulging but intact; inner and middle tables have been eroded by the granulations.

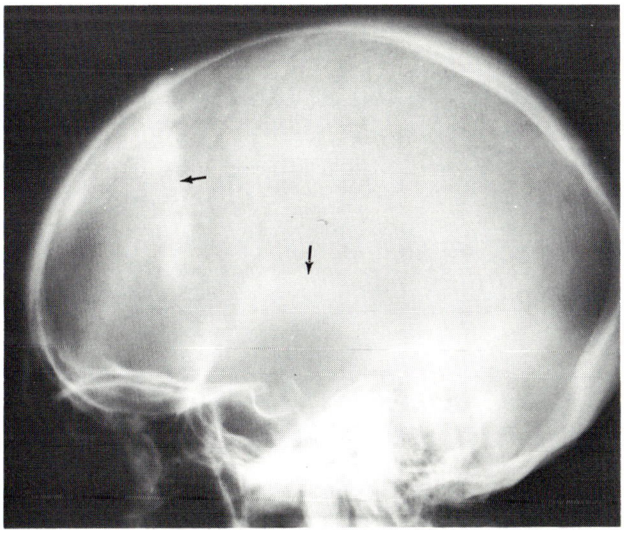

Fig. 11-32. Sutural sclerosis. Wide dense bony bands (arrows) along coronal and squamosal sutures. They are common in elderly people and also in micrencephalic patients.

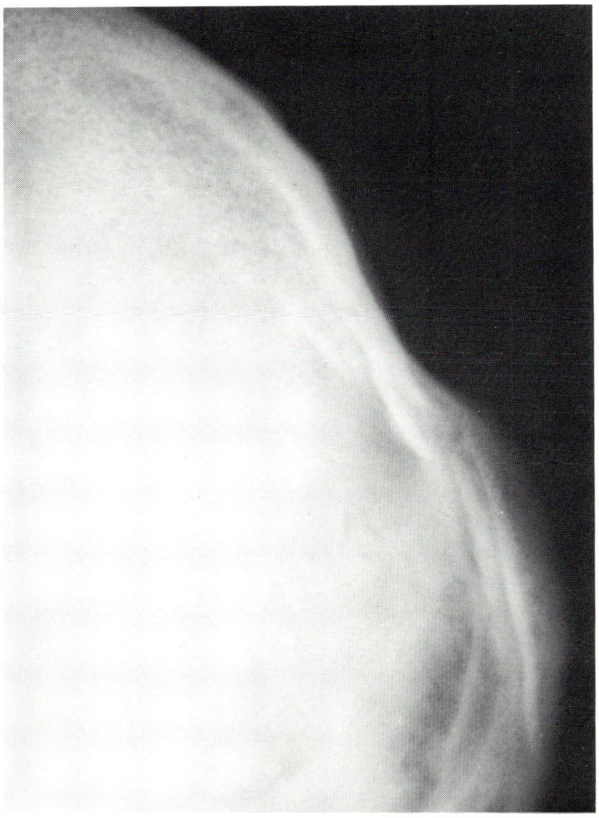

Fig. 11-33. Bathrocephaly. Developmental steplike deformity of the posterior aspect of cranial vault. Occipital bone overrides parietal bone. In traumatic cases this condition must be differentiated from depressed fracture.

Sutural sclerosis and bony ridges

Not uncommonly a dense band is seen along the sutures, the result of the continuous bridging process that takes place (Fig. 11-32). These bands vary in width and may be quite wide at times, measuring up to 15 mm. This sutural sclerosis does not reflect a pathologic entity. It is a physiologic condition that becomes more apparent with advancing age. The progressive deposition of bone is mainly in the diploe and along the inner table.

In bathrocephaly the edges of the lambdoid suture appear dense. The increase in density is caused by the overriding of the parietal bone by the occipital squama and does not represent sutural sclerosis. The lateral projection in this particular variant is most informative (Fig. 11-33).

Grossly triangular zones of increased density may be seen along the superior and lateral aspects of the grooves for the transverse sinuses. They are usually seen when the grooves are deep and are the result of relatively thick bony edges. Most of the time they are bilateral and symmetric so that they are rarely mistaken for pathologic hyperostoses (Fig. 11-34).

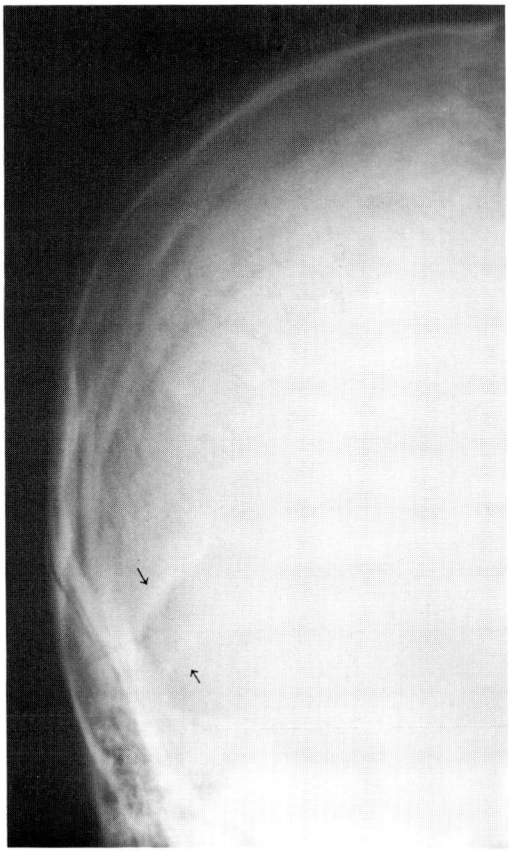

Fig. 11-34. Bony ridges. Frequently these are seen along lateral portions of deep transverse sinus grooves. They result from thick, raised, bony margins on each side of the groove (arrows).

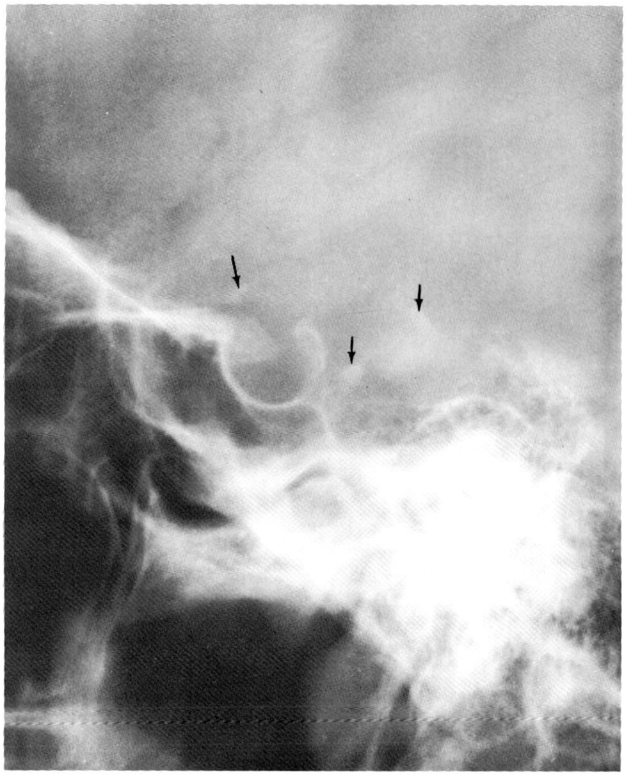

Fig. 11-35. Temporal enostoses. Small bony crests (arrows) on inner table of temporal squama project between brain markings. They are frequently seen along inferior half of temporal squama and are usually triangular in shape. Because they project over sellar region, they are misinterpreted occasionally for parasellar or suprasellar calcifications.

The opposite is true, however, of the small bony ridges on the inner surface of the temporal squama. These are frequently misinterpreted as parasellar or suprasellar calcifications on single lateral projections. These ridges, or enostoses, are small curvilinear or triangular elevations of the inner table around and in between brain markings (Fig. 11-35). They are easily recognized as such on stereoscopic views.

ABNORMAL FEATURES

In the investigation of neurologic diseases, the discovery of a lesion or an anomaly of the cranial vault is not uncommon. The accurate diagnosis of every lesion seen on roentgenograms of the skull is not possible. A definite diagnosis can be achieved, however, in most cases if two simple rules are followed: first, the location of the pathologic process must be determined accurately (i.e., determine which table of the vault is affected); second, the type of bony changes that are produced at the site of the lesion must be appreciated.

Location of bone changes

Generally speaking, a variety of pathologic entities is specific to each table. For example, meningiomas are known to affect the inner table first, whereas metastatic lesions are usually seen in the diploe. Because of the close relation between the brain, the meninges, and the skull, bony alterations of the inner table are generally indicative of underlying cerebral or meningeal abnormalities. Intramedullary or diploic changes indicate a completely different group of diseases, such as lymphomas, metastatic lesions, and metabolic disorders that have their origin or extension in cancellous bone. The outer table, which is composed of compact bone, can be the site of lesions common to other similar bones. Since it is closely related to the scalp, however, it reflects soft-tissue lesions as well.

Involvement of all tables may indicate only an extension of a process that started primarily in one table; but it may also reflect a specific group of neurologic disorders.

Because of the oval shape of the skull, tangential views

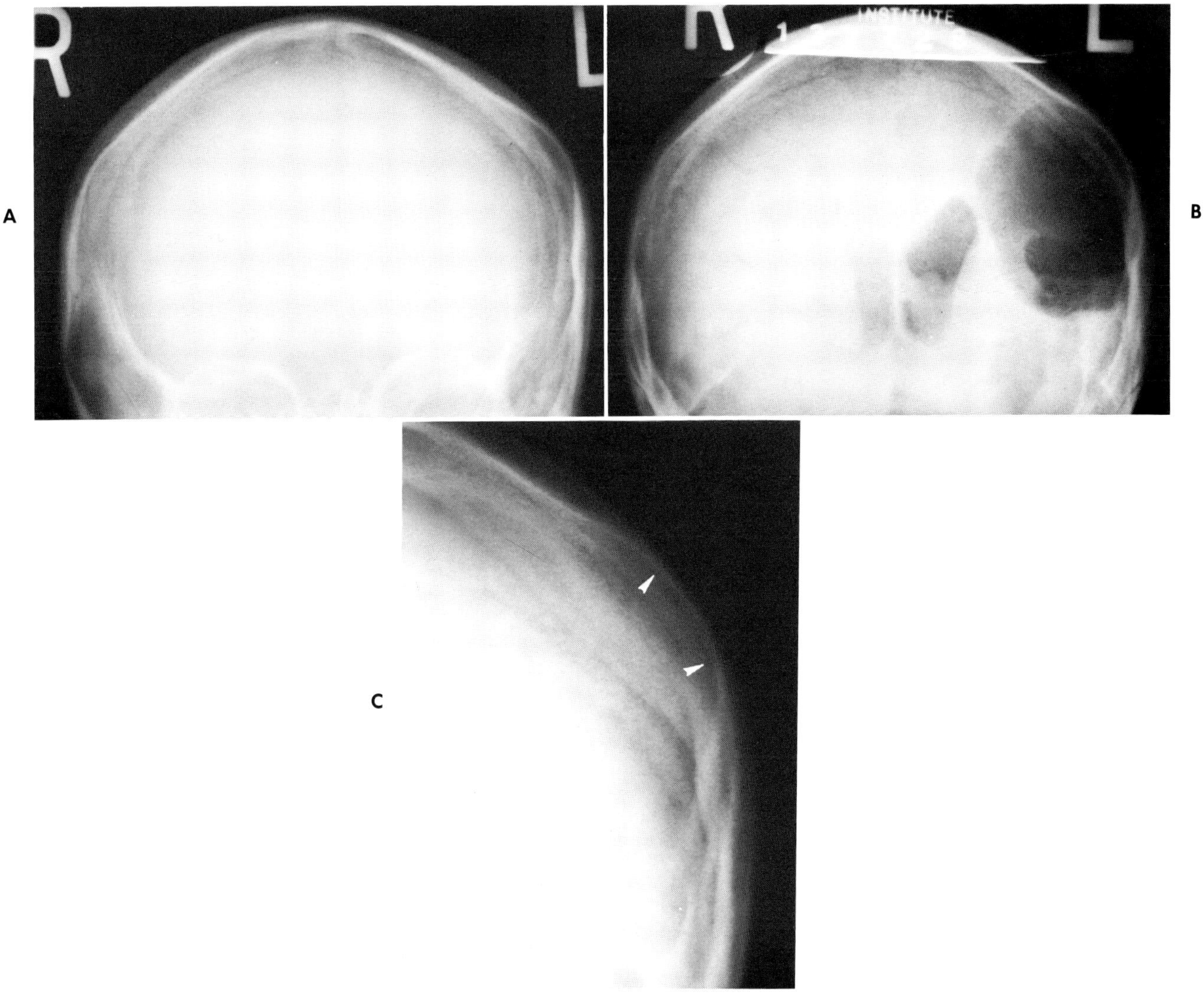

Fig. 11-36. Left frontal erosion and left-sided atrophy (porencephalic cyst). **A,** Note the smooth elevation and thinning of the inner and middle tables on the left compared with the right. **B,** Erosion is caused by superficial cyst beating against inner aspect of cranial vault at each cardiac pulsation. **C,** Closeup view of the erosion showing alteration of cranial contour (arrowheads).

are required to demonstrate a lesion of the vault adequately. Whether a lesion originates in the inner, middle, or outer table is relatively easy to determine with high-quality tangential views. In some cases local changes will be seen; in others, two of the tables, or even all three tables, will be affected. The tangential views also provide additional information regarding the nature of the bone changes. The roentgenographic technique applied varies with the thickness of the vault, the type of lesion, and the presence or absence of involvement of the scalp. True frontal views of the lesion are also necessary whenever the conventional projections do not provide sufficient information. Stereoscopic views are preferred since the lesion can be studied in depth without disturbing superimpositions. Similar information is obtainable with multiple fine tomographic sections.

Classification of bone changes

The character and the nature of a lesion in the vault are revealed by the type of bone changes. To analyze the changes fully, the bony texture in the center and at the periphery of the lesion must be compared carefully with the texture of normal bone. When the margins of a lesion are sharply demarcated from normal bone, the lesion is usually benign. An area of destruction with peripheral invasion indicates the presence of an aggres-

A

B

C

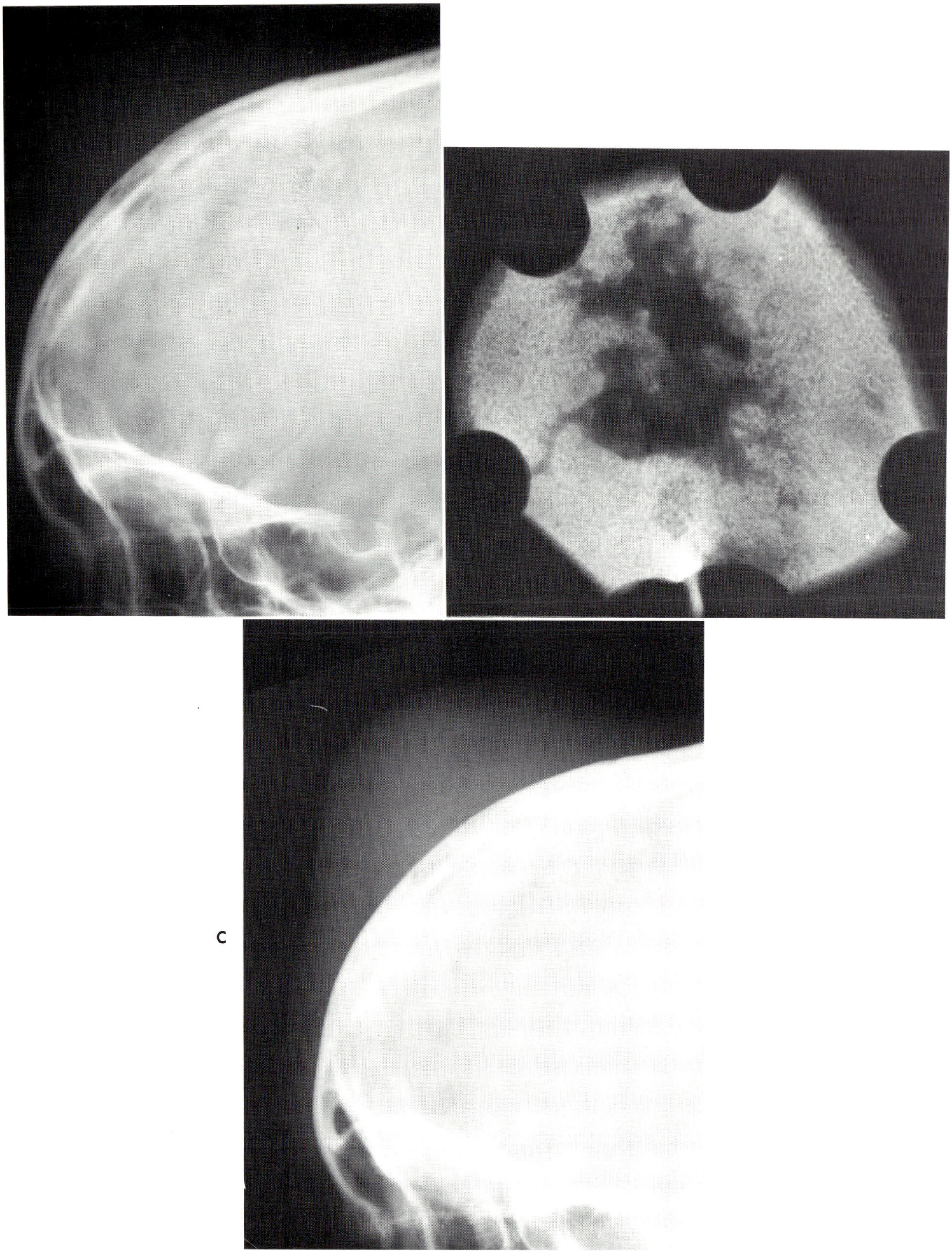

Fig. 11-37. Osteolytic process. Moderately extensive destruction of frontal bone secondary to osteomyelitis. **A** and **B,** Margins of lesion are rather indistinct. This indistinctness is better appreciated on roentgenogram of specimen where area of bone destruction appears separated from normal bone by poorly demarcated zone of invaded bone. **C,** Marked swelling of scalp, indicating permeation of outer table by infection.

sive lesion, such as neoplasm or acute infection. Conversely, sclerosis around an osteolytic zone denotes a more benign or more chronic process.

For practical purposes the focal or diffuse osseous changes observed on skull roentgenograms may be classified into six main categories: (1) erosive, (2) osteolytic, (3) osteoblastic, (4) atrophic, (5) hypertrophic, and (6) mixed.

Erosive changes

The word *erosion* as here used means progressive thinning of bone from pressure exerted by an adjacent mass. For this reason the surface of an erosion is always curved and frequently smooth. Erosions are always well demarcated by bone of normal texture (Fig. 11-36). Thinning of bone is progressive, from the periphery of the erosion to the center. At times the bone may be completely eroded in the center. Frequently the sloping borders, composed of normal compact bone, appear very dense when seen tangentially.

Erosion along the inner table of the skull always reflects an intracranial anomaly, whereas an erosion of the outer table indicates a scalp lesion. Erosive lesions of the middle table are expansile in nature and eventually displace the inner and outer tables.

Osteolytic changes

The osteolytic type of change is seen in more aggressive processes such as infections and malignant growths. With these processes the bone is destroyed and replaced by abnormal tissue, extensively altering the bony texture. The changes are more marked in the center of the lesion, where bony trabeculae may have completely disappeared. They are less pronounced at the periphery, where trabeculae may still be identified but are less numerous. At times bony debris or sequestra can be seen in the center of the lesion. The edges of such a process are irregular and poorly demarcated, indicating the invasive nature of the lesion. Infiltration and swelling of the scalp may be prominent features (Fig. 11-37).

Osteoblastic changes

Bone-forming processes are chronic in nature and consequently are either benign conditions or low-grade neoplasms (Fig. 11-38). The degree of sclerosis or hyperostosis, which are the two main types of osteoblastic changes, depends on the nature and duration of the lesion.

In hyperostotic lesions the cranial vault becomes locally thicker and denser. Benign lesions are usually uniformly dense, and their contours smooth and sharply demarcated. In low-grade neoplasms the margins of the hyperostosis are ill defined and irregular and the surfaces of such neoplasms are frequently rugose and

A

B

C

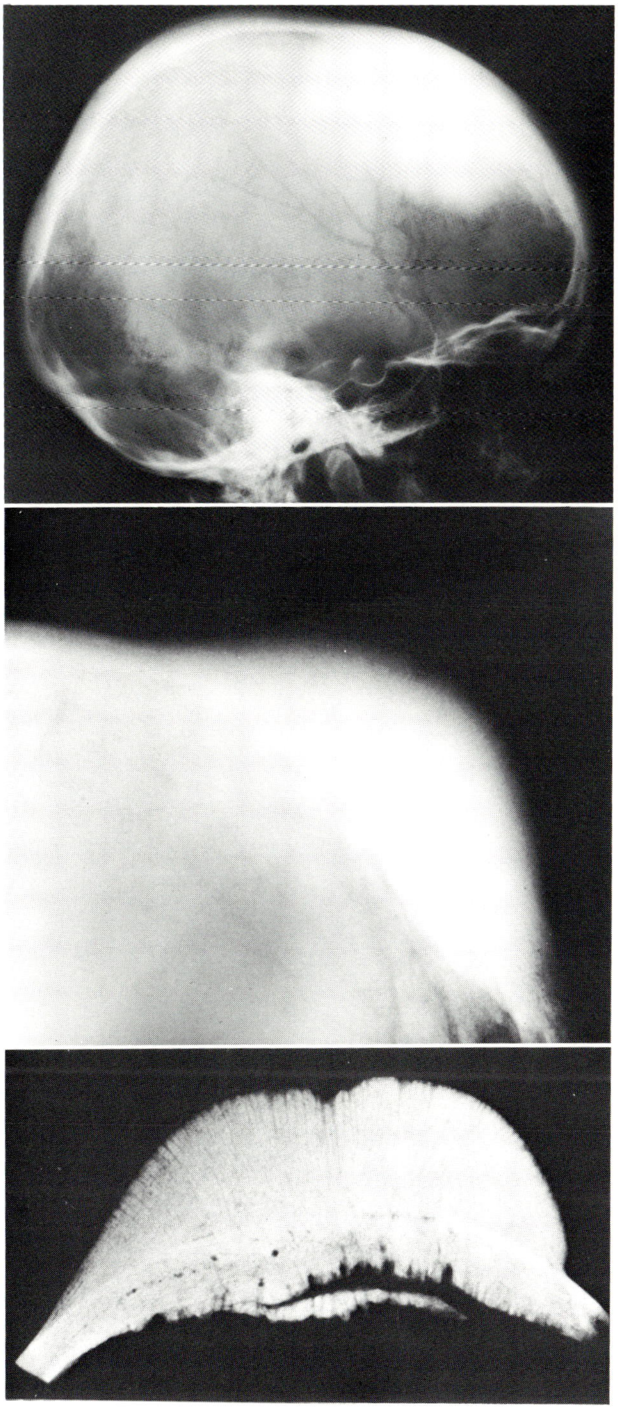

Fig. 11-38. Meningioma. **A,** Large sclerotic lesion of left frontal squama is associated with numerous enlarged meningeal grooves. **B,** Tangential view shows that the bony mass is growing extensively on external surface of skull. Recognition of an abnormal inner table, however, warrants diagnosis of meningioma. **C,** Roentgenogram of specimen shows various features of the lesion (i.e., radial ossification, permeation of middle and outer tables by tumor, and grossly abnormal inner table).

uneven. Bony spicules or lamellae are frequent in hyperostotic lesions and may be seen in benign lesions. A hyperostosis that results from a slow-growing tumor may be associated with prominent vascular grooves caused by enlarged meningeal vessels that supply this area. Changes resulting from perforating vessels of extracranial origin should also be sought.

In reactive sclerosis the cranial vault is denser, but not necessarily thicker, than normal. The increased density is the result of diffuse deposition of bone along or between preexisting trabeculae or lamellae. This protective reaction tends to limit the extension of diseases. Other sclerotic reactions, caused by different mechanisms, may be observed in devitalized fragments of bone and also in the healing phase of a disease process.

Atrophic (or hypoplastic) changes

Thinning of bone without any other alteration, or absence of bone, is a feature of many developmental, congenital, and posttraumatic conditions. The thinned-out areas in the cranial vault have no specific configuration; however, the bony edges are frequently beveled and smooth.

Since roentgenographically the difference between hypoplasia and atrophy is only a matter of degree, these two changes are discussed under the same heading.

Hypertrophic changes

In the group of hypertrophic changes, the cranial vault is increased in thickness. This increase may be the result of an unusually thick but otherwise normal inner table, as in hyperostosis frontalis interna, or all three tables may be uniformly thick. The bone itself in all cases is of normal texture and density.

Mixed changes

The most common category of bone changes is the mixed group. These changes are present in many lesions. They are the most difficult to assess since many combinations are possible. Their critical analysis is always rewarding. Such changes may consist of areas of bone rarefaction, associated with hyperostosis or sclerosis (Fig. 11-39), or be a mixture of bone atrophy and hypertrophy. In neoplastic and infectious diseases, bone is ordinarily destroyed and replaced by neoplastic or inflammatory tissues; occasionally it is eroded instead of destroyed. In developmental or dysplastic diseases, bone is sometimes replaced by fibrous tissue or cartilage.

The areas of sclerosis or hyperostosis are also related to the underlying disease process. Reactive sclerosis is common to certain invasive lesions, such as low-grade neoplasms and infections. In bone dysplasias formation of dense islands of erratic bone is frequent. In some bone tumors hyperostosis is the prominent feature.

This analytic approach and a general knowledge of the possible entities are of great help in the diagnosis and management of cranial vault abnormalities. In many cases a definite diagnosis is possible from the roentgenographic examination alone. In other instances, in which the diagnosis is not absolute but the process has been

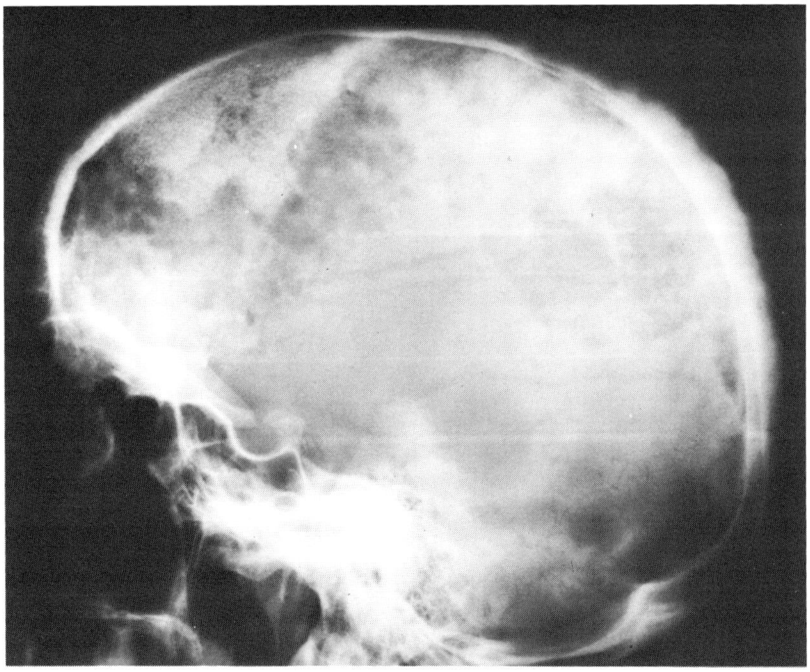

Fig. 11-39. Mixed changes. Multiple areas of bone destruction surrounded by and associated with areas of sclerosis in fibrous dysplasia.

established as benign, simple serial examinations prevent unnecessary investigations and explorations.

This combined topographic and qualitative method is applied to various anomalies and lesions of the skull that are discussed in the following paragraphs.

Inner table

Erosive changes

Along the inner table erosive change is always seen with superficial lesions of the brain or meninges. The deformity is the result of the combined effects of the underlying abnormality and cerebral pulsations. Remodeling of the inner table takes place to accommodate the local increase in intracranial pressure. Bulging of the other tables over the eroded inner table is not uncommon (Fig. 11-40). A process that produces an erosion indicates that it has been present for a long time and is either inert or growing very slowly. Focal erosive changes may be observed in different acquired patho-

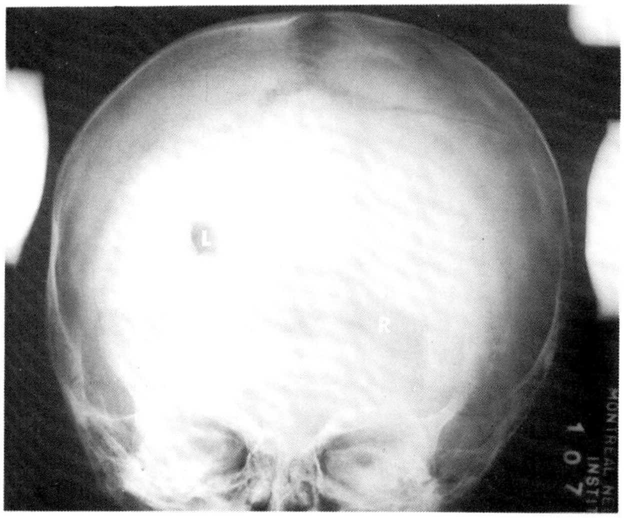

Fig. 11-40. Erosion and bulging of cranial vault. Brow down view shows extensive erosion of inner aspect of right hemicranium associated with focal bulging. Massive displacement of ventricular system by a large mass, which was found to be an old intracerebral hemorrhagic cyst at operation.

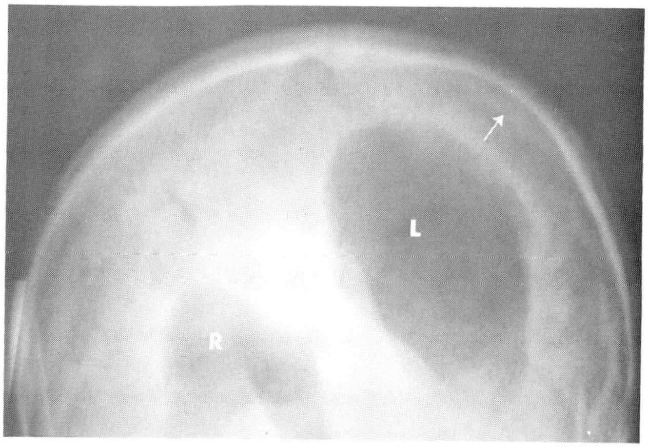

Fig. 11-41. Left parietal erosion. Smooth elevation and thinning of inner table (arrow) caused by pulsations of greatly enlarged posterior horn on the left side.

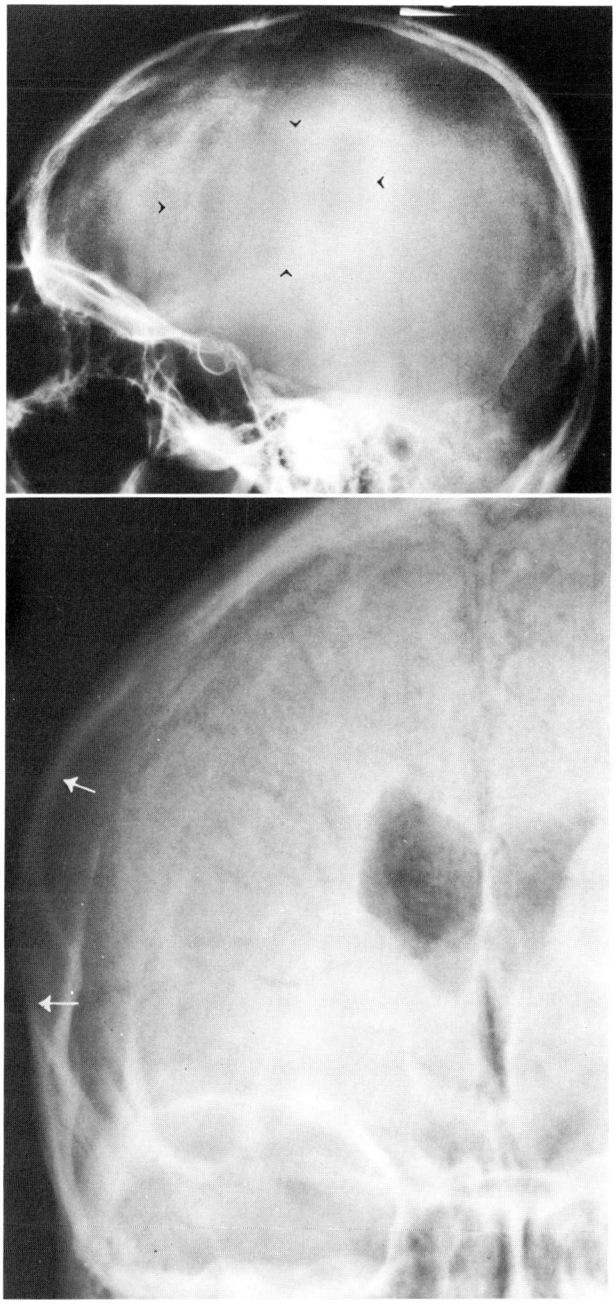

Fig. 11-42. Superficial cerebral cyst. Extensive erosion of inner table (denoted by arrowheads) associated with thinning and bulging of middle and outer tables (white arrows) in the right midfrontal and posterior frontal regions. When associated with signs of atrophy of ipsilateral hemisphere, these erosive changes are usually indicative of superficially situated cerebral cysts.

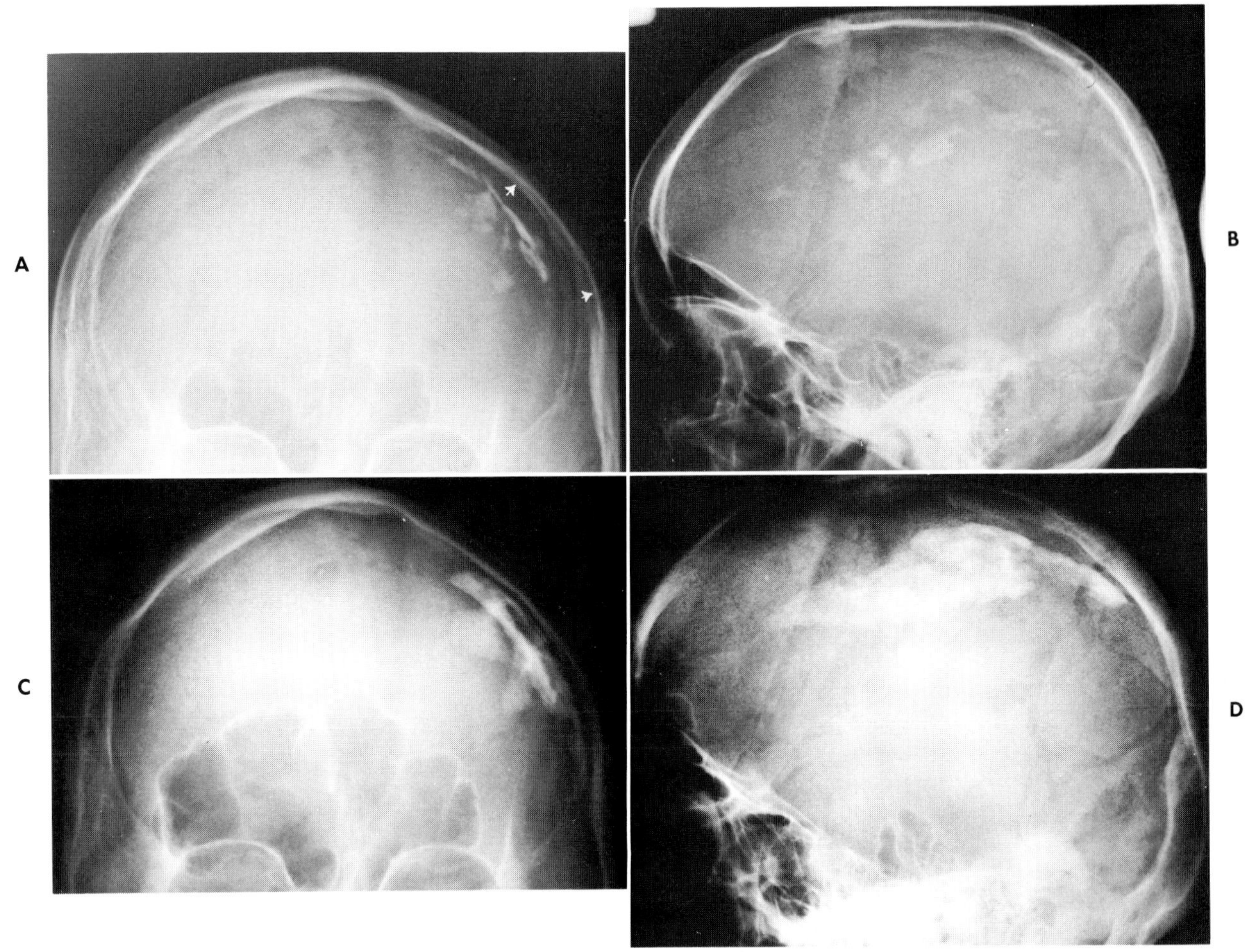

Fig. 11-43. Calcified chronic subdural hematoma. **A** and **B,** Slight but definite elevation and erosion of inner table (arrows) opposite flat inert calcifications, typical of this condition. Note the relatively thin left hemicranium. **C** and **D,** Ossified chronic subdural hematoma in the same patient 22 years later. Note the diffuse irregular ossification of the old fluid collection.

logic conditions, such as degenerative, posttraumatic, and neoplastic processes.

With *focal damage to the cerebrum,* a focal enlargement of the lateral ventricles may compensate for the loss of brain substance. In some patients the pulsations of that ventricular diverticulum eventually cause a smooth erosion and bulging of the inner table and occasionally some bulging of the other tables (Fig. 11-41). In other patients the damaged part of the brain eventually becomes a fluid-filled cyst and identical changes are seen along the inner table (Fig. 11-42). Frequently the classic signs of hemiatrophy of the ipsilateral hemisphere are obvious, thus facilitating the diagnosis (Dyke et al., 1933). When superficial cysts communicate with the cerebrospinal fluid pathways, they fill with gas during pneumoencephalography (Fig. 11-36, *B*).

Chronic juvenile subdural hematoma may cause erosion and thinning of the cranial vault. Flat plaquelike calcifications, frequently present in the membrane around the collection of fluid, are of great diagnostic value (Fig. 11-43, *A* and *B*). Ossification of hematomas is rare but may take place in the subdural spaces (Fig. 11-43, *C* and *D*).

In *craniocerebral erosion*—a term introduced by Penfield—the erosive process affects not only the inner table but all three tables as well. This term is more appropriate than *leptomeningeal cyst* or *growing fracture,* other designations applied to this entity (Penfield and Jasper, 1954). It is included in the present discussion because the changes develop first along the inner table. The shape of the erosion is related to the type of fracture caused by the initial trauma. Long erosions are usually the result of linear fractures (Fig. 11-44). More complex forms may be seen after a comminuted fracture (Fig. 11-45). The eroded edges are frequently scalloped as well as beveled from inside. This interesting posttraumat-

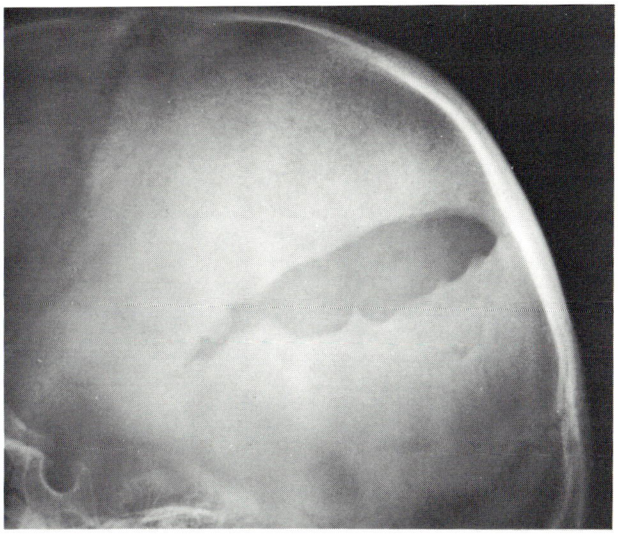

Fig. 11-44. Craniocerebral erosion. Long erosion of parietal bone with scalloped beveled edges is result of a dural tear at time of previous linear fracture. (From McRae, D. L.: In Caveness, W. F., and Walker, A. E., editors: Head Injury Conference Proceedings, Philadelphia, 1966, J. B. Lippincott Co.)

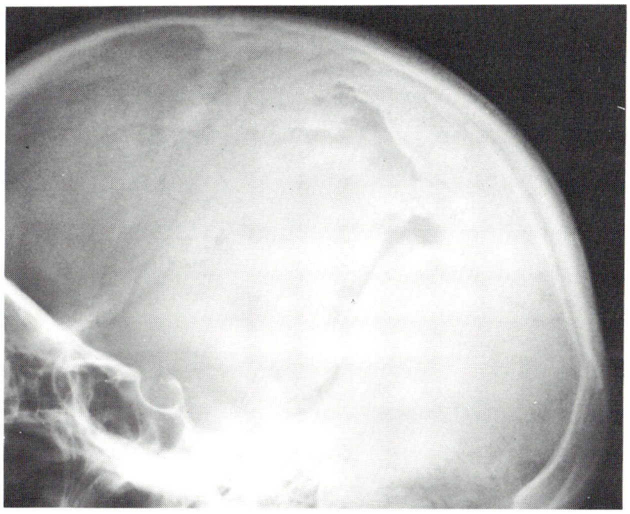

Fig. 11-45. Craniocerebral erosion. Linear and circular erosions scattered in right parietal and temporal bones result from an old severe comminuted fracture. (From McRae, D. L.: In Caveness, W. F., and Walker, A. E., editors: Head Injury Conference Proceedings, Philadelphia, 1966, J. B. Lippincott Co.)

ic complication results from a dural tear at the fracture site. Fractures wider than 3 mm are usually associated with dural tears through which the brain and the leptomeninges herniate. The edges of the fracture may then become eroded by the pulsating brain or meninges or by both (McRae, 1966b).

Slowly growing superficial gliomas can erode the inner

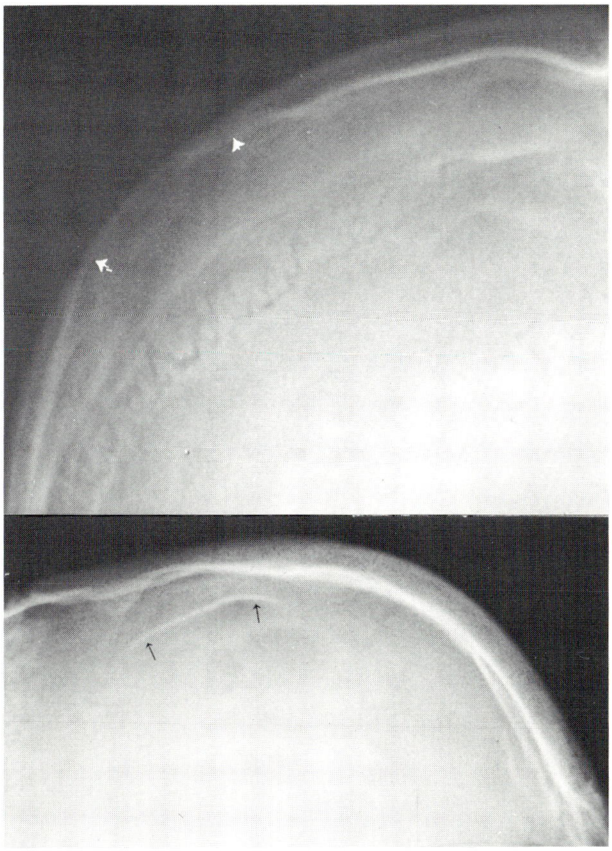

Fig. 11-46. Right parietal astrocytoma. Arrows point to erosion of inner and middle tables of right parietal bone in a 15-year-old patient with focal epilepsy since age of 2 years.

table (Fig. 11-46). In the absence of calcification within the lesion, a specific diagnosis may be possible only with cerebral angiography or pneumoencephalography. Meningiomas rarely cause a simple erosion, and therefore this possibility should not be strongly entertained when such an erosion of the inner table is seen.

Focal erosive changes are also seen in *developmental anomalies*. An abnormally distended sinus or superficial cerebral vein that drains an arteriovenous malformation may erode the inner table and even the middle table. When an erosion is seen along the midline, a distended superior longitudinal sinus must be suspected; but a definitive answer will be obtained only by arteriography (Fig. 11-47). The detection of an extensive midline erosion along the inner aspect of the occipital squama, resulting from an unusually large cisterna magna, is not uncommon (Fig. 11-48). Usually, associated anomalies permit immediate recognition of this entity, which has no clinical significance. Because the tentorium in this condition has a high position, the grooves for the transverse sinuses course more obliquely than normal. For the same reason the internal occipital protuberance is not present. Bulging of the superior half of the occipital

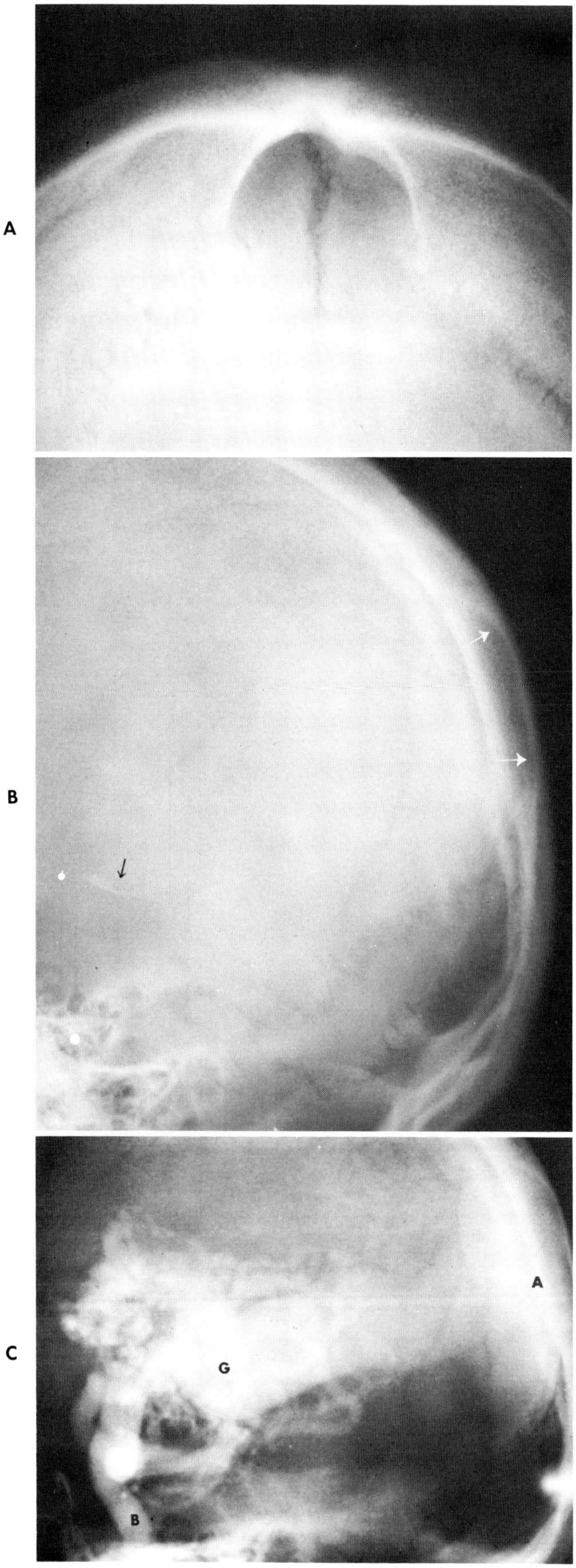

squama is a frequent feature. At pneumoencephalography this large cisterna magna should not be confused with an atrophic process of the occipital lobes. The occipital lobes are elevated and are situated above the large cisterna magna.

Osteolytic changes

Osteolytic change along the inner table is rarely the first manifestation of a disease. *Dural metastasis* may destroy the inner table; but, in addition, other lesions are usually seen in the diploe. *Meningiomas* rarely cause destruction of the inner table without producing other changes.

Osteoblastic changes

The most common acquired lesion, which causes a localized hyperostosis of the inner table, is *meningioma*. Since the inner table is always affected first, it must be studied with great care, and usually tangential views are indicated. The hyperostosis alters the inner table, which becomes gradually thicker. At the same time the cerebral and diploic surfaces of the inner table lose their crisp margins and become more irregular and indistinct. The slightest increase in thickness of the inner table must be regarded with suspicion, especially in patients who present focal neurologic signs.

In meningioma *en plaque* the hyperostosis along the inner table may be extremely minimal and therefore difficult to recognize (Fig. 11-49). In more advanced cases the middle table becomes involved by the hyperostosis and the changes are seen more readily (Fig. 11-50). Slowly growing meningiomas may be clinically silent for a long time. The hyperostosis, in those circumstances, may evolve into a large bony mass that affects the three tables and even elevates the scalp. Although the diagnosis of meningioma seems obvious, it cannot be confirmed unless appropriate tangential views demonstrate an unequivocal hyperostotic inner table (Fig. 11-51). When the diagnosis of meningioma is considered, the vascular grooves in the vicinity of the suspected area must be scrutinized thoroughly. The reason for this scrutiny is that meningiomas receive a large portion of their blood supply from the meningeal circu-

Fig. 11-47. Aneurysm of superior longitudinal sinus. Midline erosion results from focal distention of superior longitudinal sinus. **A** and **B,** Extensive erosion of inner and middle tables of both parietal bones posteriorly (white arrows). Note the sharp demarcated margins lined with compact bone and the aneurysmal calcifications in region of the vein of Galen (black arrow). **C,** Extensive arteriovenous malformation drains into elevated and distended straight sinus and empties into greatly enlarged longitudinal sinus. *A,* Aneurysm; *B,* basilar artery; *G,* vein of Galen. (Courtesy D. Levy, M.D., and R. J. Tuttle, M.D., St. Joseph's Hospital, Hamilton, Ontario.)

A 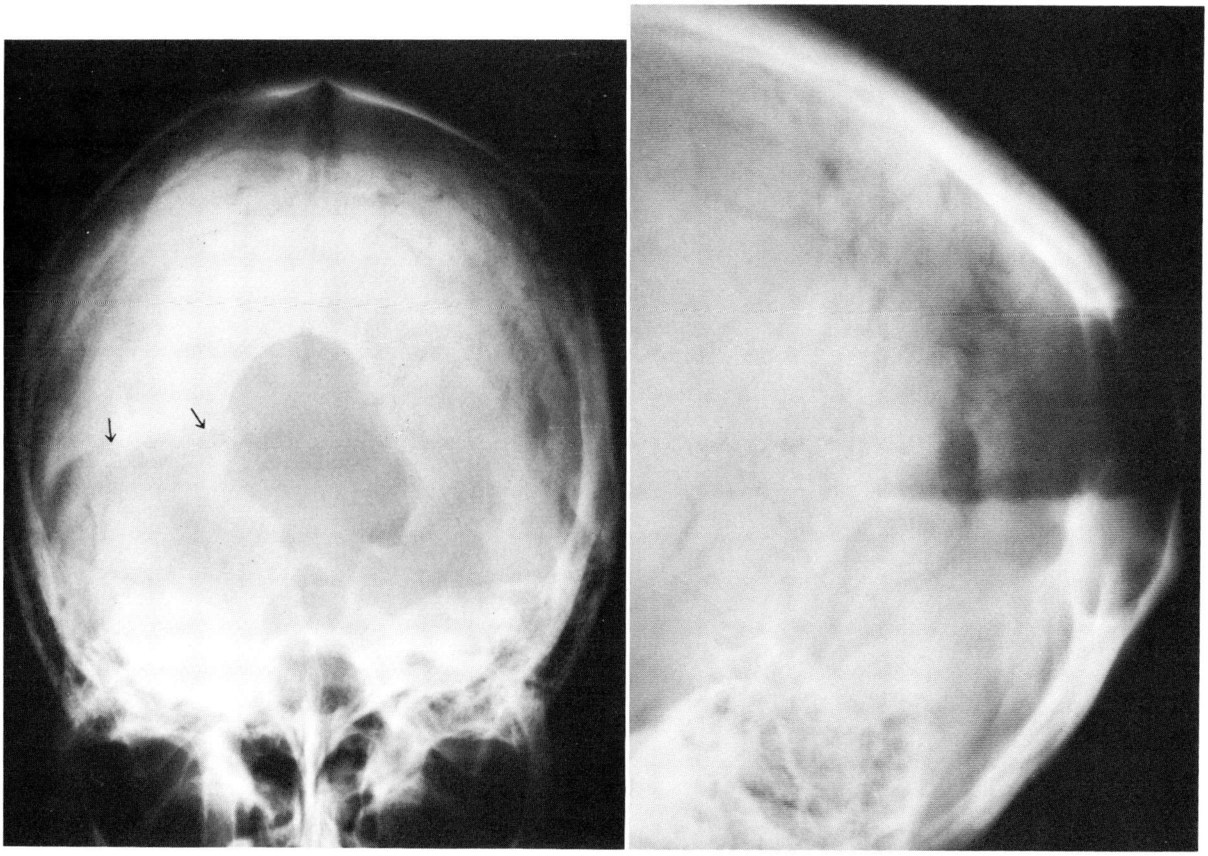 B

Fig. 11-48. Large cisterna magna. **A,** Large central erosion of occiput. Note the upward sweep of the right transverse sinus (arrows) near the erosion. **B,** Anomalous cisterna magna partly filled with gas at pneumoencephalography. Note the bulging of the superior portion of the occipital squama and the absence of internal occipital protuberance.

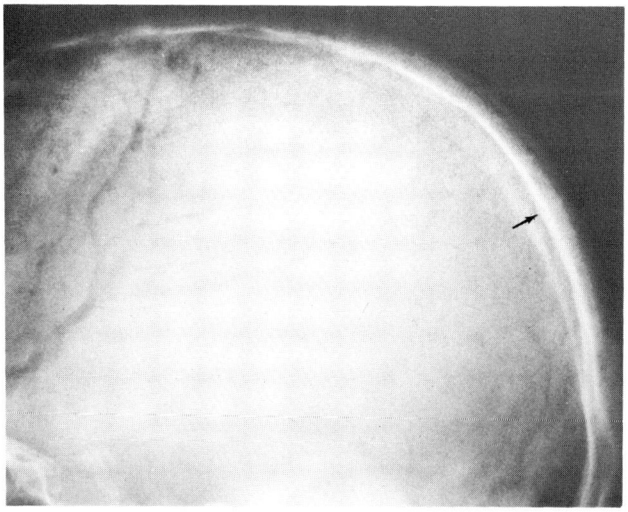

Fig. 11-49. Meningioma *en plaque.* Slight increase in thickness of inner table along posterior third of left parietal bone (arrow). With extension of hyperostosis in the diploe, the sharp interface between middle and inner tables disappears. Note the increase in the number of meningeal grooves.

lation. The identification of prominent vascular grooves running toward an area of hyperostosis is extremely valuable in establishing the diagnosis. Equally important is the search for perforations due to enlarged branches of the scalp arteries that penetrate the skull to supply the tumor (Fig. 11-52). On basal views an enlarged foramen spinosum on the side of the hyperostosis is a clear indication of an enlarged middle meningeal artery (Traub, 1961). Such an enlargement, however, is uncommon.

Frontal hyperostosis that results from a meningioma may be mistaken for a localized form of hyperostosis frontalis interna. Hyperostosis frontalis does not develop along the course of either the longitudinal sinus or the superficial cerebral veins. Prominent grooves are seen therefore to encroach on the areas of hyperostosis frontalis. In meningiomas such grooves are absent since the brain and its vessels are dislocated away from the cranial vault by the growing tumor.

Occasionally a calcified superficial cerebral lesion is mistaken for a meningioma. Adequate tangential views,

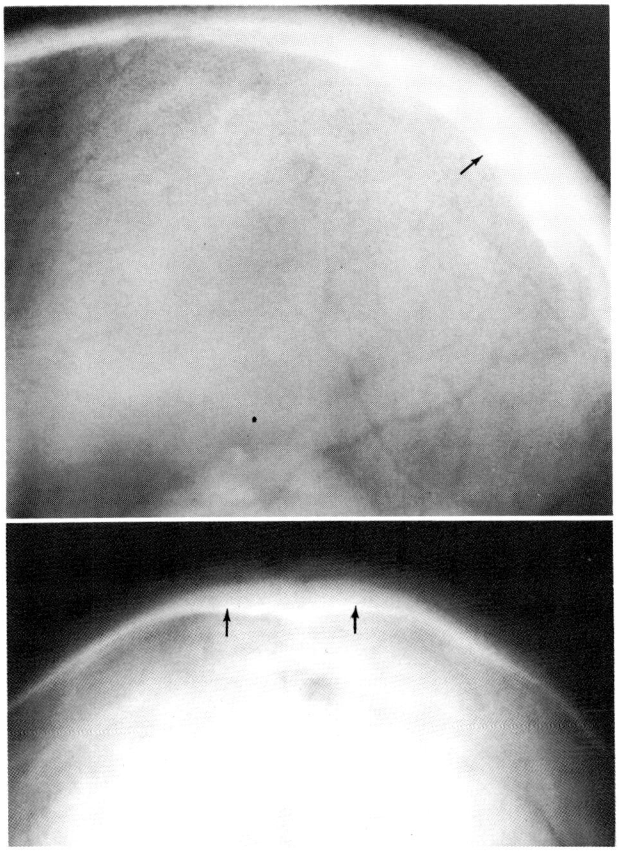

Fig. 11-50. Meningioma *en plaque*. **A,** Indistinct inner table (arrow) along superior and posterior aspects of parietal bones on lateral view. Some hypertrophy of posterior meningeal grooves exists. **B,** Anteroposterior tangential view shows hyperostosis involving the inner table, which becomes progressively thicker near midline (arrows).

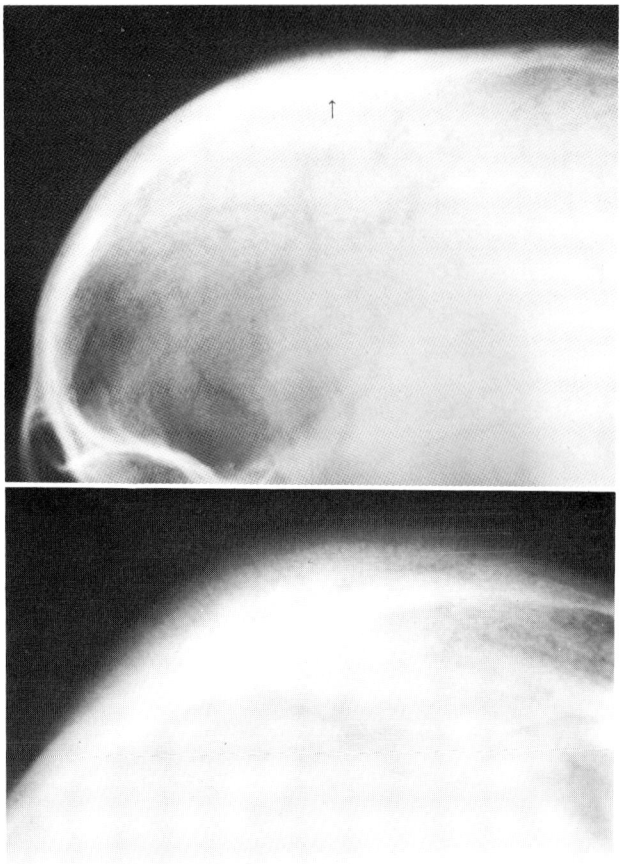

Fig. 11-51. Meningioma. **A,** Diffuse hyperostosis of superior and posterior parts of left frontal squama (arrow). Different tables cannot be identified clearly through the hyperostosis. **B,** Tangential view shows extent of tumor but more specifically the hyperostosis of the inner table, which is of prime interest in the diagnosis of this condition.

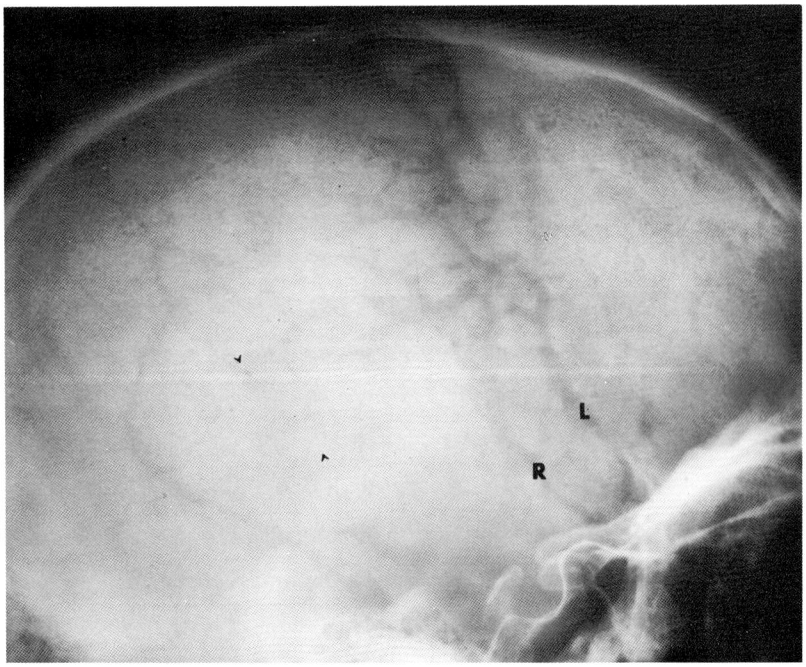

Fig. 11-52. Meningioma, vascular supply. Minimal diffuse hyperostosis in anterolateral part of left parietal bone. Marked increase in size and number of left meningeal grooves. Note the multiple small foramina in the center due to perforating vessels (arrowheads). Lateralization of abnormal vessels is greatly facilitated by stereoscopy.

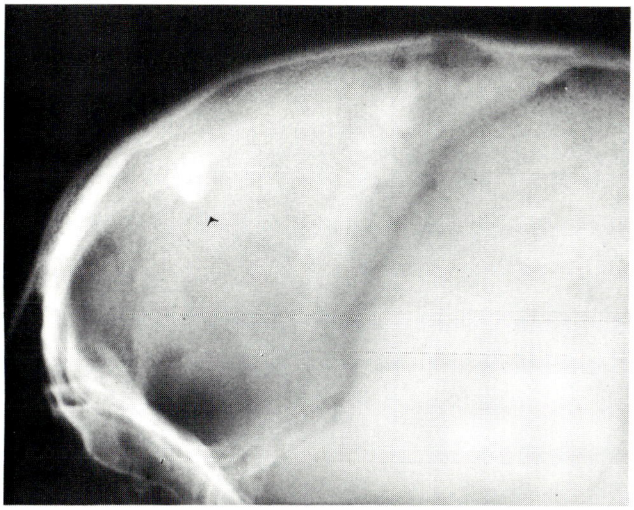

Fig. 11-53. Osteoma, inner table. Well-demarcated nodule with density and texture of normal compact bone is indicated by arrowhead.

however, always show a space between the inner table and the calcified cerebral mass.

Another rare osteoblastic lesion along the inner table is *osteoma.* This lesion is mainly seen along the inner table of the frontal squama (Fig. 11-53). It may be sessile or nodular. Sessile osteomas may resemble meningiomas; however, their cerebral surface is always smooth and sharply demarcated as opposed to that of a meningioma. No hypertrophied meningeal grooves or perforating vessels are associated with osteoma. A firm diagnosis of osteoma of the inner table on the basis of a single examination would be hazardous. Serial examinations are necessary every 6 months or every year. Osteomas are fairly stable lesions and expand only minimally over the years. Only then should the diagnosis be definite.

Atrophic or hypoplastic changes

Craniolacunia falls into the hypoplastic category, although the cranial vault is not differentiated into three layers when this condition is observed. The multiple thin zones are almost surely the result of hypoplasia of the inner aspect of the vault, secondary to maldeveloped immature meninges. Such hypoplasia is strongly suggested by the presence of other meningeal abnormalitics seen in this condition. For example, in our experience, nearly every case of craniolacunia is associated with various degrees of communicating hydrocephalus, which indicates some malfunction of the meninges. In addition, the incidence of meningocele and myelomeningocele is high with craniolacunia (McRae, 1966a). Against the fact that the lacunae are the result of brain markings is the disappearance of the lacunae with time, even during the course of progressive low-grade hydrocephalus (Fig. 11-54). (See Chapter 28.)

A

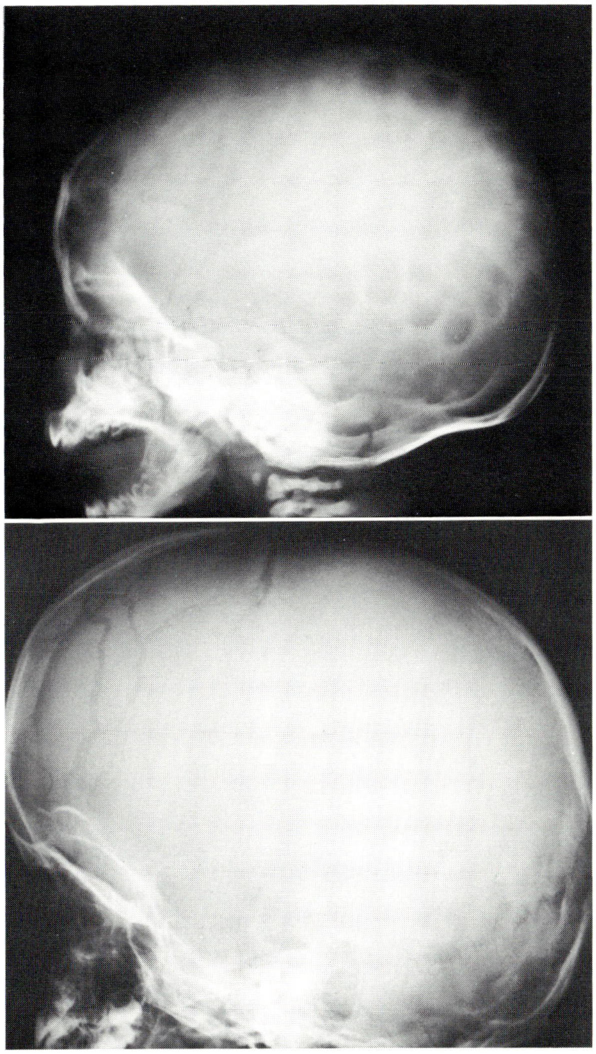

B

Fig. 11-54. Fading craniolacunae. **A,** Multiple round thin areas of hypoplastic bone surrounded by normal bone in a neonate. **B,** Same patient, untreated, 4 years later. Note the thin but normally ossified vault and the disappearance of lacunar markings even in the presence of obvious chronic and subacute raised intracranial pressure.

Hypertrophic changes

Hypertrophy of the inner table is seen in *hyperostosis frontalis interna.* This type of hyperostosis is characterized by thickening of the inner table of the frontal squama. The cerebral surface of the thickened inner table remains smooth and sharply demarcated, although occasionally it may be very uneven. The texture of the hypertrophied inner table retains the normal appearance of compact bone. Hyperostosis of the skull has been studied and reported by many authors (Morel, 1929;

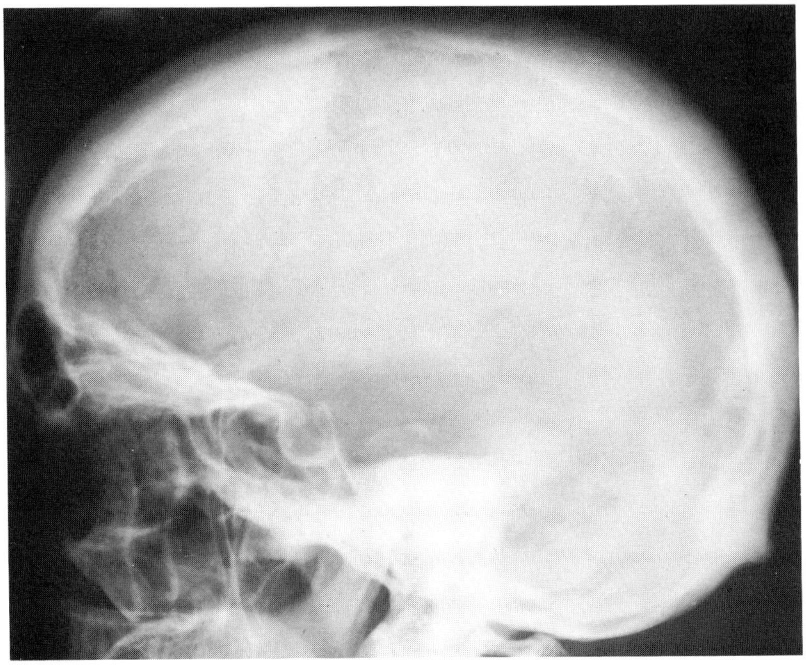

Fig. 11-55. Hyperostosis frontalis interna. Diffuse thickening of inner table of frontal and parietal bones in a 22-year-old mentally retarded patient. Cranial vault is generally thick, as would be expected in such patients. Of interest is the combination of cerebral hypoplasia and hyperostosis interna.

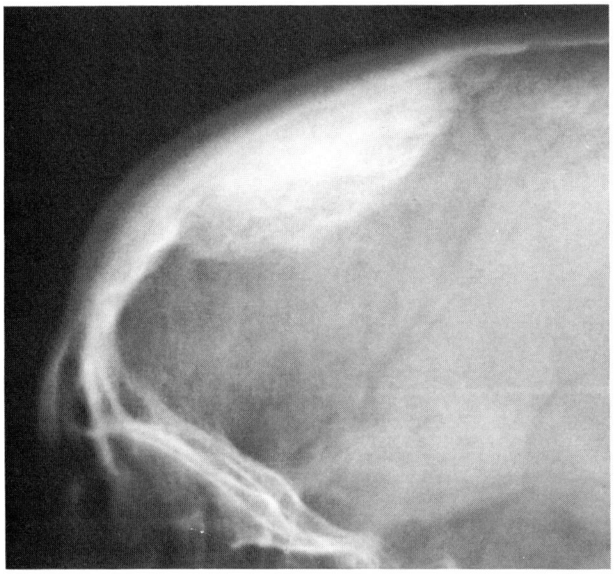

Fig. 11-56. Hyperostosis frontalis. Mixed sessile and nodular forms. Bilateral thickening of inner table of frontal squama appears as corrugated dome on three-dimensional studies.

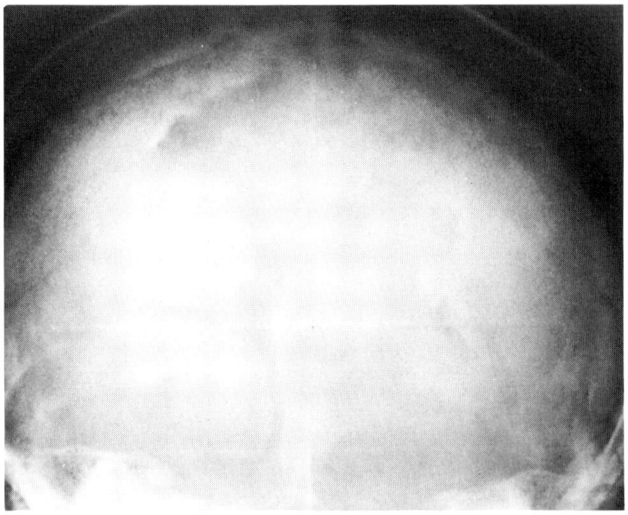

Fig. 11-57. Vascular grooves in hyperostosis frontalis. This form of hyperostosis does not develop over prominent superficial cerebral veins, a striking feature of the condition.

Moore, 1955; Salmi et al., 1962). It is more common in females than in males. Although it is more frequent in patients older than 40 years, it may be seen in younger individuals also (Fig. 11-55). The clinical and experimental studies conducted since this entity was recognized have not yet yielded satisfactory explanations for its formation. Perhaps this physiologic bony thickening is indicative of brain loss in adults (Stewart, 1941; Dorst, 1964).

In the fully developed form of hyperostosis frontalis interna, a moderate thickening of the inner table is associated with sessile and nodular formations (Fig. 11-

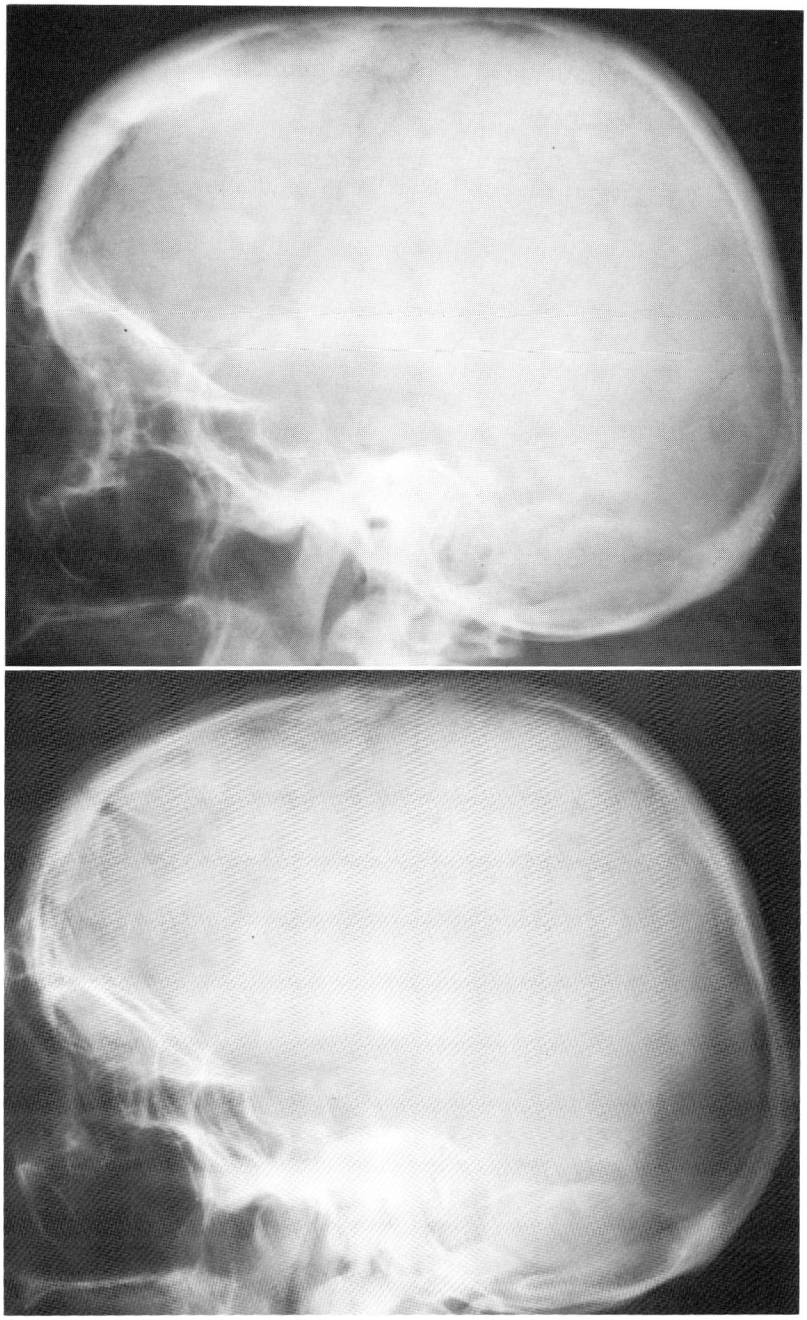

Fig. 11-58. Changes with time in hyperostosis frontalis. **A,** Mild degree of hyperostosis in 56-year-old patient. **B,** Some, but little, progression 9 years later.

56). The appearance varies widely from single to multiple nodules, or from a single patch of hyperostosis to diffuse thickening. The hyperostosis does not alter the position of either longitudinal sinus or superficial veins, which appear strikingly delineated (Fig. 11-57). Follow-up studies demonstrate that the hyperostosis progresses over the years but that it does so at a very slow pace (Fig. 11-58).

Roentgenographically this condition usually offers no diagnostic difficulty. At first glance localized forms may resemble meningiomas, but tangential views should bring out the benign character of the process.

Mixed changes

Osteoblastic and osteolytic. This type of alteration of the inner table is probably the most common early presentation of *meningioma* and for practical purposes is pathognomonic of this condition. As the tumor grows in

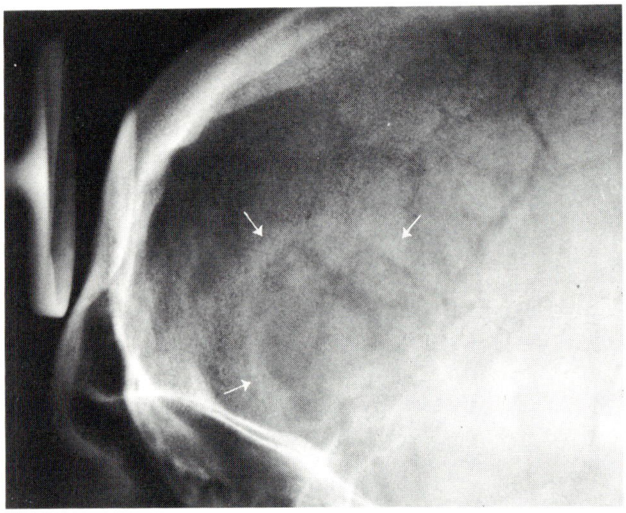

Fig. 11-59. Meningioma. Mixed changes include destruction of inner table in center of lesion (arrows) with sclerosis of inner table at periphery.

the inner table, it tends to destroy bone opposite its center and to induce reactive bone formation at the periphery. The destruction of bone is partly the result of tumor invasion and partly of increased vascularity (Fig. 11-59). Identification of these changes may be extremely difficult in the early stages, and even with arteriography the lesion may be missed. This difficulty stresses the importance of high-quality plain roentgenograms, especially stereoscopic views.

More advanced forms are seen readily and are essentially diagnostic of meningioma (Fig. 11-60). In those instances the inner table is destroyed, and signs of invasion are seen in the middle table. In more severe cases the outer table is also involved. Patches of sclerosis are usually seen at the periphery of the lesion. In meningioma the inner table is always affected first, which must be remembered when such a diagnosis comes to mind.

The pattern of dural metastasis from *neuroblastoma* may be mixed, but the changes usually appear first along the base then along the cranial vault.

Erosive and osteoblastic. In *craniocerebral erosion* (leptomeningeal cyst) the brain may be in apposition to the vault where the dura has been torn. Bone reaction in such cases may be of two different types. In some areas the bone is eroded by the pulsating brain, either directly or by interposed encysted fluid. In other areas the bone reacts by forming spicules, which grow into the cortical surface of the brain, causing the cerebrum to hanging from the inner aspect of the vault. This reactive become extremely adherent to the cranial vault (Fig. 11-61). On stereoscopic views the spicules of bone may be identified. They appear like small dense stalactites

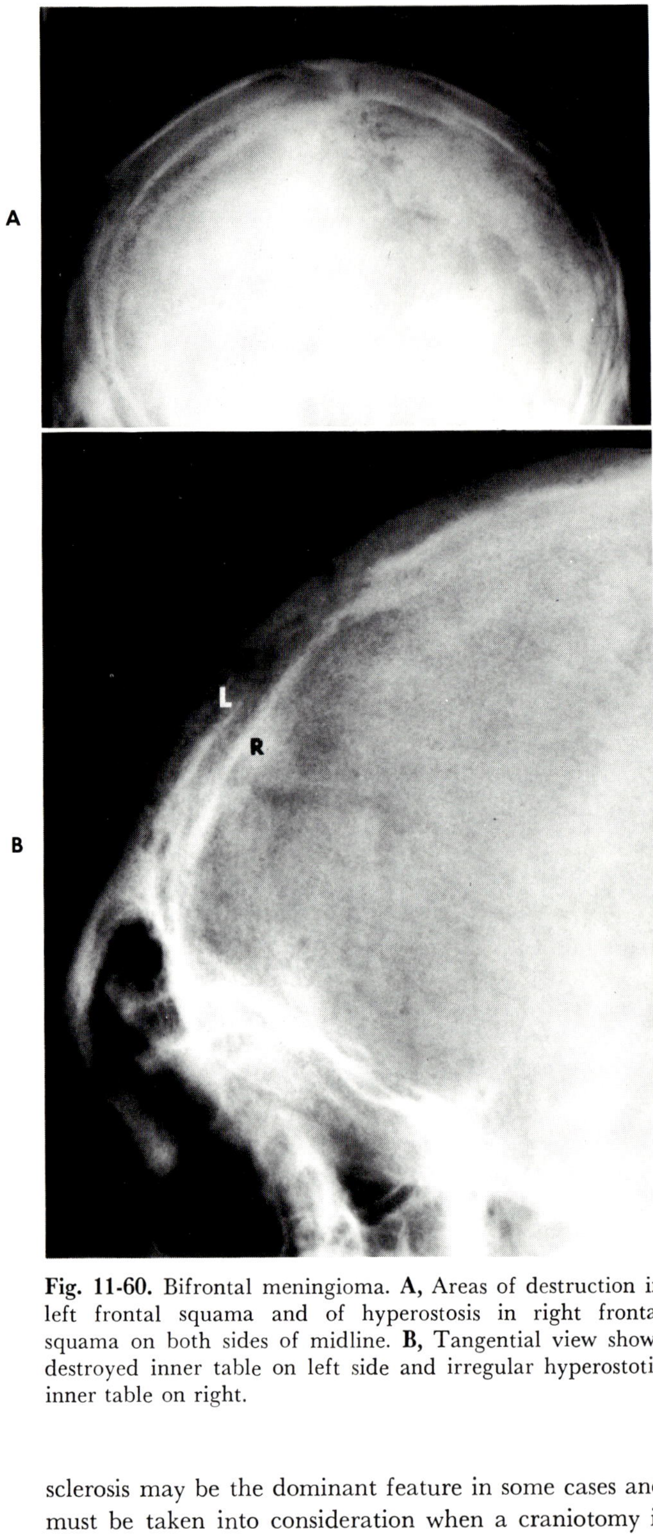

Fig. 11-60. Bifrontal meningioma. **A,** Areas of destruction in left frontal squama and of hyperostosis in right frontal squama on both sides of midline. **B,** Tangential view shows destroyed inner table on left side and irregular hyperostotic inner table on right.

sclerosis may be the dominant feature in some cases and must be taken into consideration when a craniotomy is contemplated (Fig. 11-62).

Erosions and sclerosis are also seen in *chronic epidural abscesses.* In this condition the erosions result from encapsulated pus. The diffuse peripheral sclerosis represents either a form of reactive sclerosis or a low-grade osteitis (Fig. 11-63).

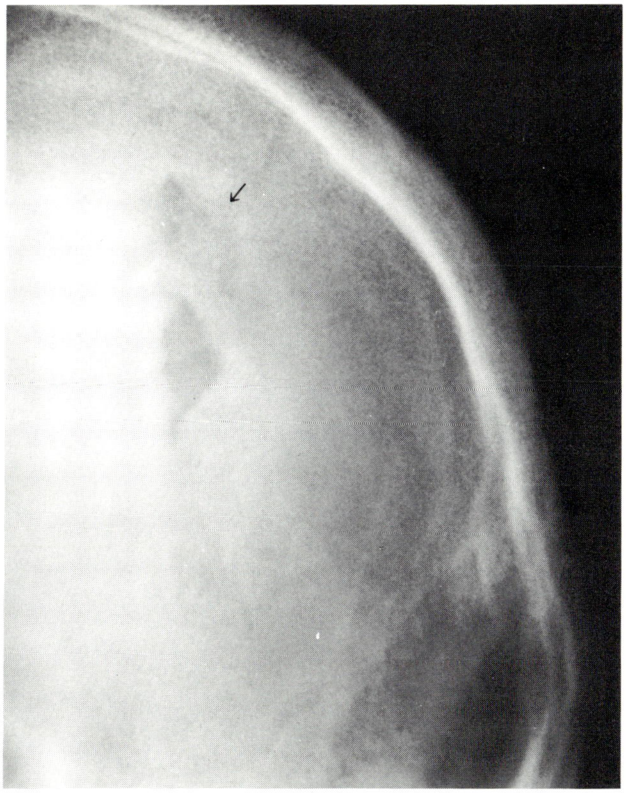

Fig. 11-61. Craniocerebral erosion. Grossly oval erosion, with scalloped edges, the result of an old linear fracture. Immediately above are seen residual small erosions and bony spicules of inner table (arrow).

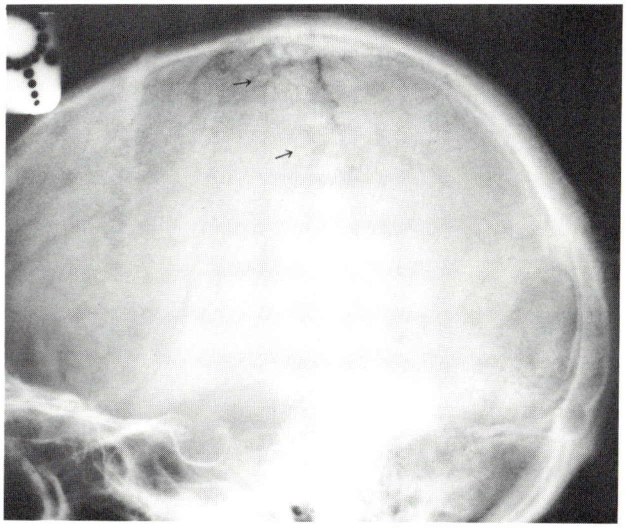

Fig. 11-62. Chronic craniocerebral erosion. Old partially healed fracture associated with small erosions along and on each side of fracture. Striking feature is the multitude of small, closely packed, bony spicules arising from inner table and growing into adjacent brain in middle and upper central regions (arrows).

Fig. 11-63. Chronic epidural empyema. Multilobulated erosive process of left frontal squama (arrows). Extensive sclerosis of inner table is seen at periphery of erosions, which indicates presence of low-grade inflammatory process. Combination of inner table erosions and sclerosis is pathognomonic of this condition.

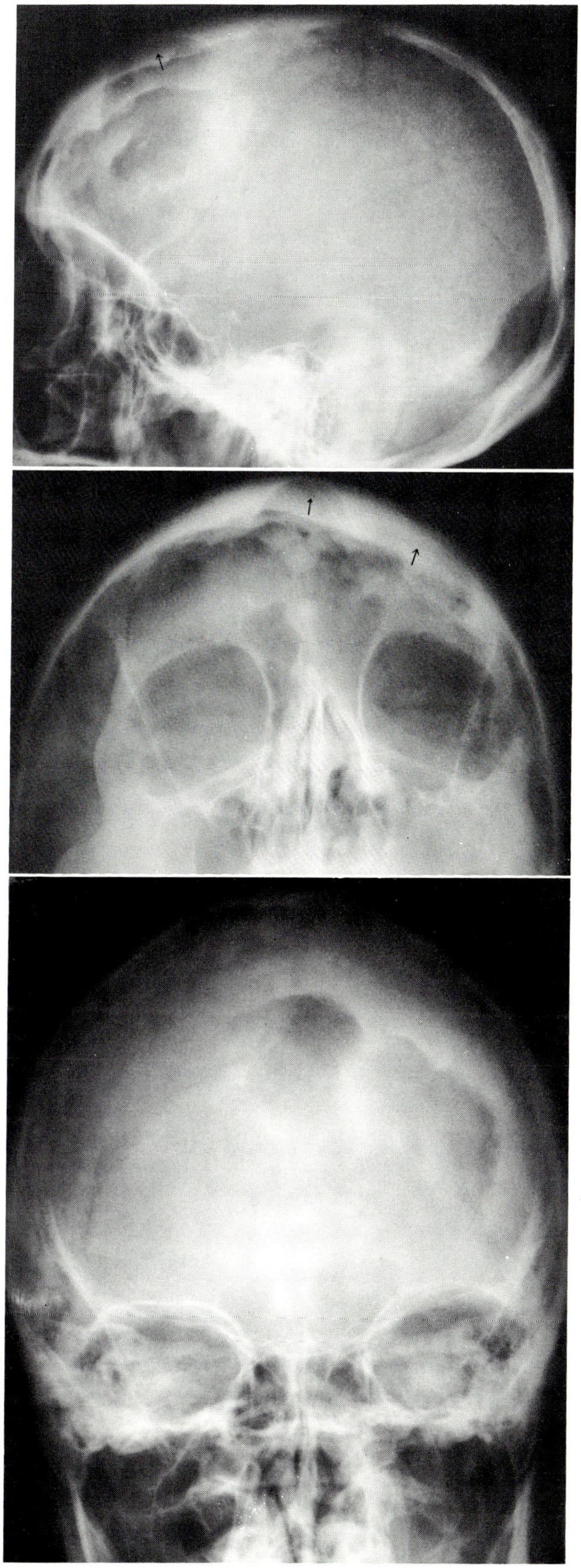

11-63

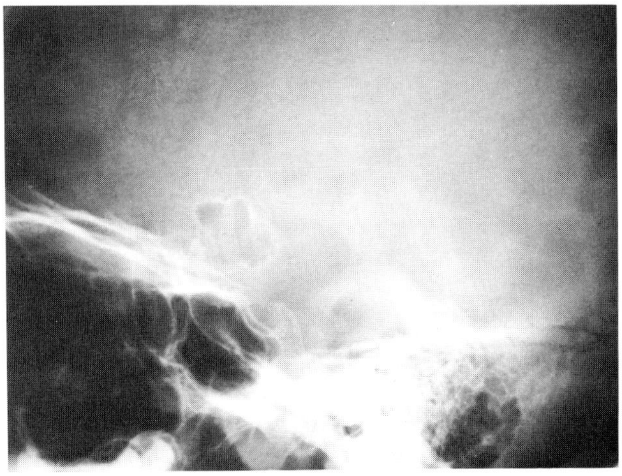

Fig. 11-64. Epidermoid. Typical blown-glass appearance of an intraosseous epidermoid. Margins are quite sharp and consist of compact bone, whereas remainder of lesion is mainly radiolucent keratin.

Middle table

Erosive changes

Intramedullary epidermoid tumors are tumors of ectodermal origin, lined with stratified squamous epithelium and filled with a mass of keratin (Patriquin et al., 1969). As they grow in the diploe, they gradually erode the bony trabeculae by pressure. At the same time new compact bone forms at the periphery, producing well-corticated margins to these lesions (Fig. 11-64). If the tumors grow over a long period, they will erode into the inner and outer tables, which then become displaced in opposite directions in a curvilinear manner (Fig. 11-65). The appearance of the intramedullary epidermoid tumor is essentially the same as that of an ordinary bone cyst. The lesion itself, inside the dense margins, appears radiolucent since it contains nonradiopaque material.

The *brown tumors of hyperparathyroidism, neurofibromas,* and *dermoids* may have a similar appearance, but they are extremely rare.

Osteolytic changes

Osteolytic changes may be focal, multiple, or diffuse.

Focal. These destructive changes with signs of peripheral invasion are seen exclusively with aggressive processes, such as malignant neoplasms and subacute and acute infections. The middle table is involved first. As the lesion progresses, the adjacent parts of the inner and outer tables become involved and eventually are completely destroyed. The margins of the destroyed zone are always poorly demarcated and grossly circular.

Focal changes are seen in different types of *intramedullary tumor.* The roentgenographic signs indicate a malignant lesion, but no specific diagnosis can be of-

A

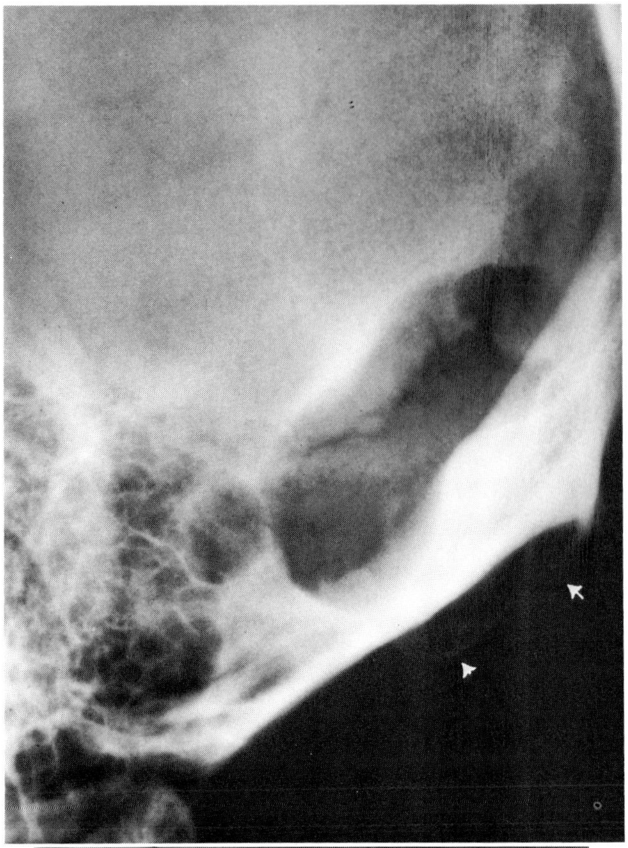

B

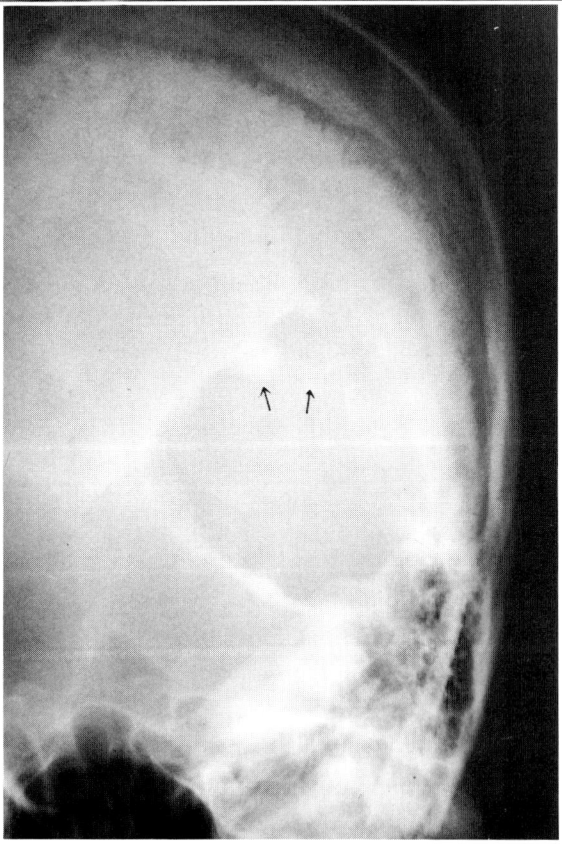

Fig. 11-65. Epidermoid. Eroding and expanding process of left occipital squama. **A,** Marked thinning and bulging of outer table (arrows). **B,** Residual thin fragments of inner table (arrows). Note the sharp corticated margins.

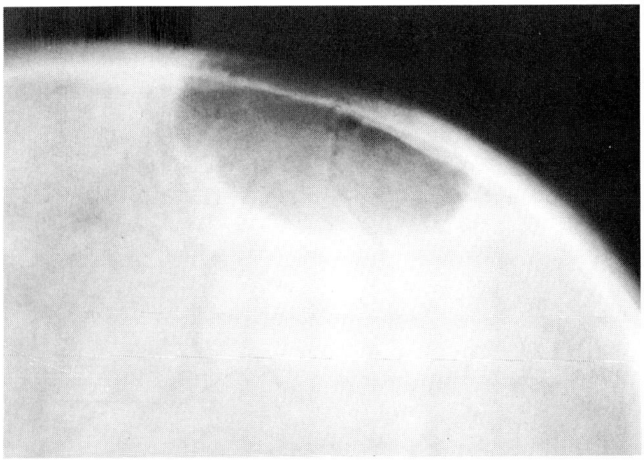

Fig. 11-66. Metastatic carcinoma. This case illustrates complete osteolysis in the center of the lesion and peripheral invasive changes. Destructive changes affect mainly the diploe, indicating that lesion is essentially intramedullary in origin.

A

B

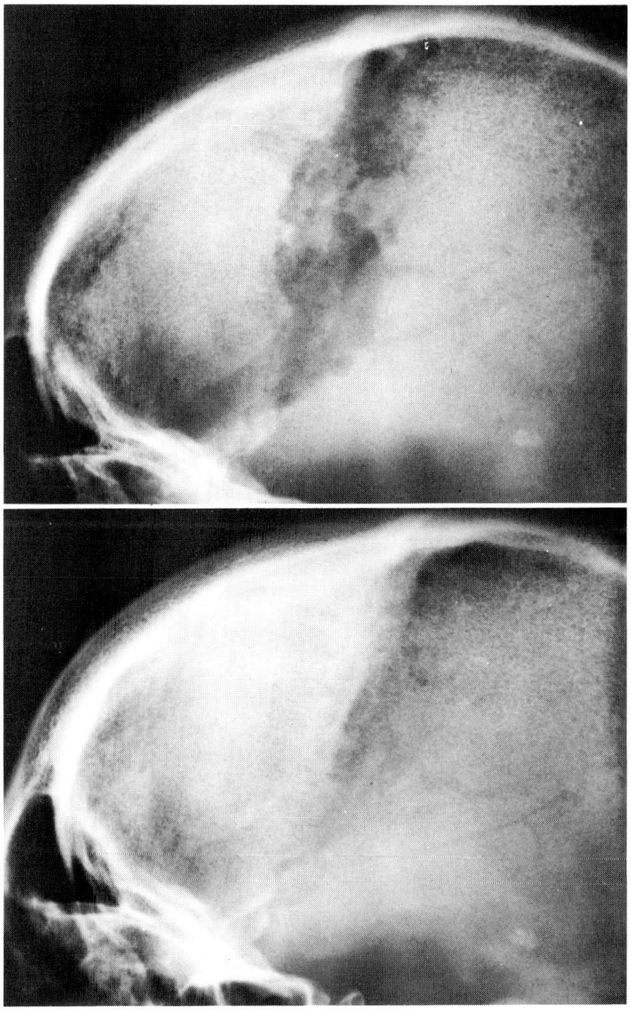

Fig. 11-67. Osteomyelitis. **A,** Irregular zone of destruction on both sides of right coronal suture with numerous typical fistulous tracts along some vascular channels. **B,** Normal skull 3 months before.

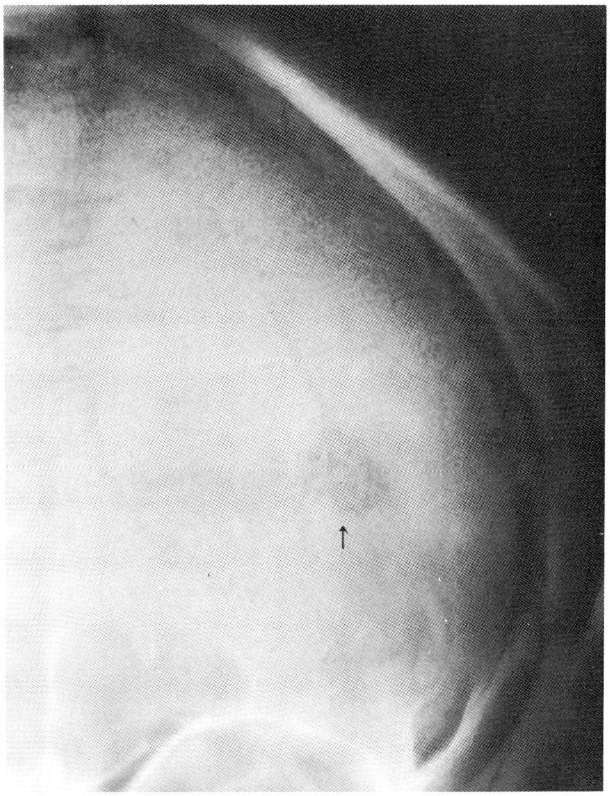

Fig. 11-68. Osteomyelitis. Early phase of development of the disease in the diploe. Multiple minute perforations are slightly larger than normal diploic spaces (arrow).

fered. Solitary myelomas, reticulum cell sarcomas, fibrosarcomas, osteolytic sarcomas, melanosarcomas, and single metastatic osteolytic lesions may all appear identical (Fig. 11-66).

Bone destruction was frequently extensive in *osteomyelitis* before the advent of antibiotics (the bone changes requiring 3 or 4 weeks to appear); but now, when the diagnosis is suspected clinically, active antibiotic therapy is started immediately. Because of this early treatment, osteomyelitis of the cranial vault has become a rare entity. The disease may develop, however, after successful control of the acute phase and discontinuance of treatment. Six to twelve weeks after the initial episode the acute signs may reappear, and examination of the skull may then reveal extensive changes (Fig. 11-67). Since osteomyelitis develops in the diploe, the first modifications to appear are slightly enlarged diploic spaces. These are the result of focal destruction of bony trabeculae (Fig. 11-68). Usually the edges of the destroyed zone are much more irregular than in neoplastic diseases. Numerous fistulous tracts are seen to extend into the diploe from the area of destruction. The infection spreads rapidly along the intradiploic vascular channels (Fig. 11-69). Small islands of incompletely destroyed bone are seen, mainly between confluent tracts.

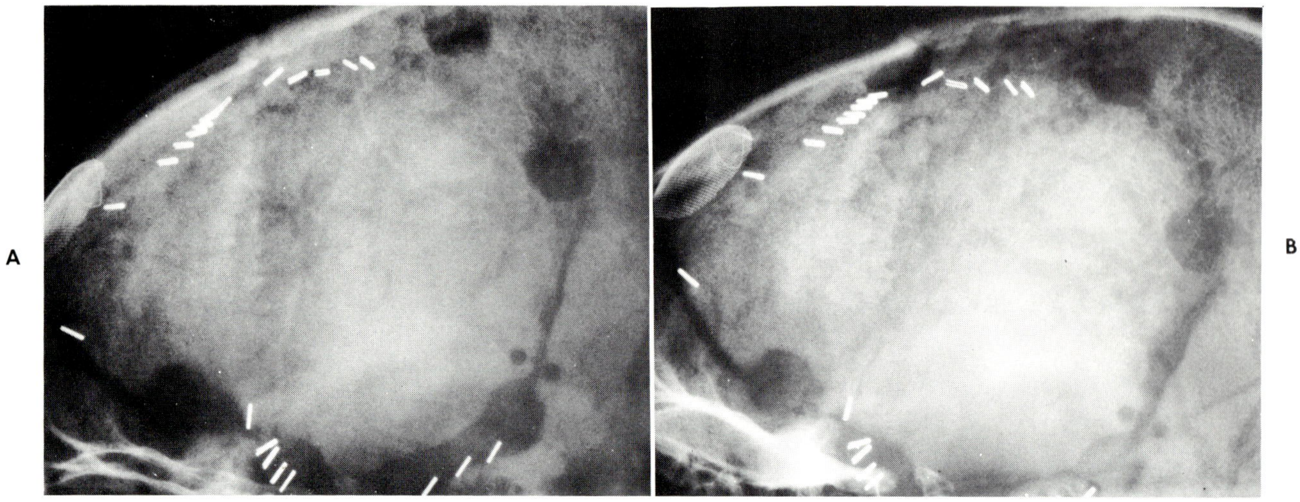

Fig. 11-69. Osteomyelitis of bone flap. **A,** Normal appearance of bone flap 2 months after operation. **B,** Osteomyelitis 5 weeks later. Note the propagation of the disease along pre-existing diploic vascular channels.

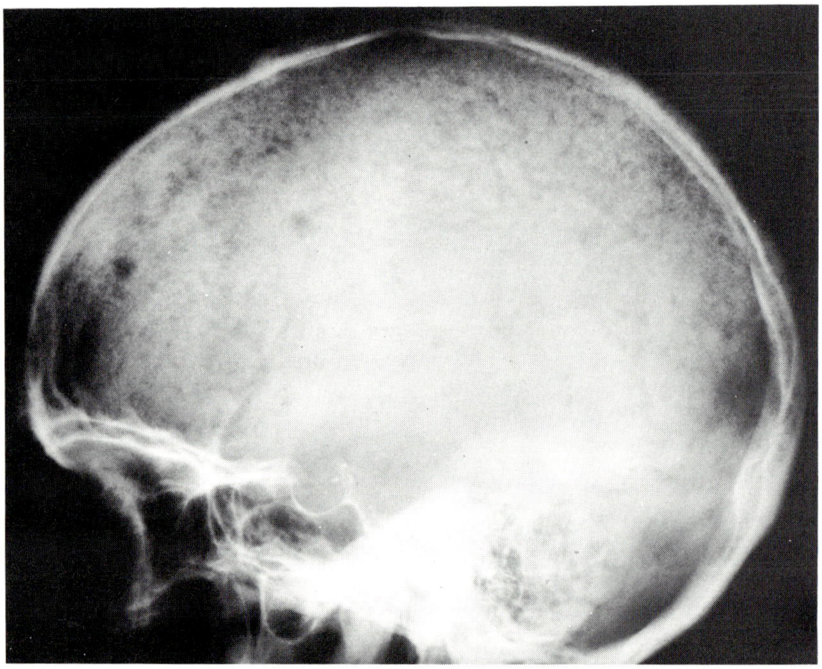

Fig. 11-70. Multiple myeloma. Multiple small irregular zones of bone destruction scattered throughout diploe. In the cranial vault, differentiation of these lesions from metastatic lesions is almost impossible.

Multiple. This type of destruction is commonly seen in *multiple myeloma* and *metastatic tumors* (Fig. 11-70). In addition to the central area of total destruction, a halo of invaded bone surrounds the lesion (Fig. 11-71). This peripheral zone of invasion is better seen around the larger lesions. The adjoining bone is of normal texture. Similar changes may be seen in other intramedullary neoplastic diseases, such as *leukemia* and *lymphoma.*

Radiation necrosis presents the same appearance. If irradiation has been focal, multiple small areas of bone destruction are localized to the area treated (Fig. 11-72). If the entire head has been treated, the lesions are diffuse (Fig. 11-73). These changes may appear years after the initial treatment, as revealed by annual follow-up studies (Figs. 11-72 and 11-73).

In children multiple large areas of bone destruction are a common manifestation of *Hand-Schüller-Christian*

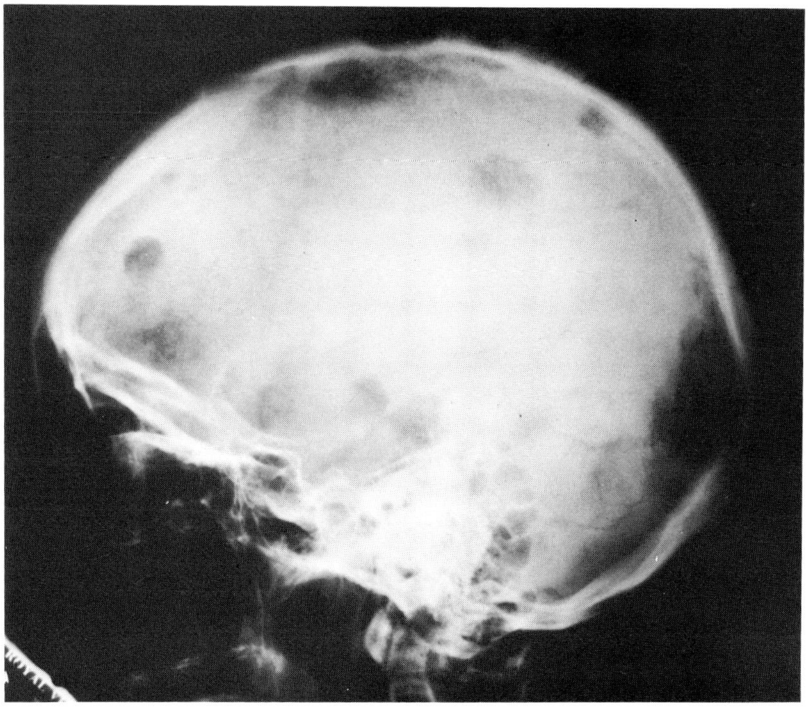

Fig. 11-71. Osteolytic metastasis. Edges of multiple lytic lesions are irregular because of uneven destruction and invasion. (Courtesy R. G. Fraser, M.D., Royal Victoria Hospital, Montreal, Quebec.)

A

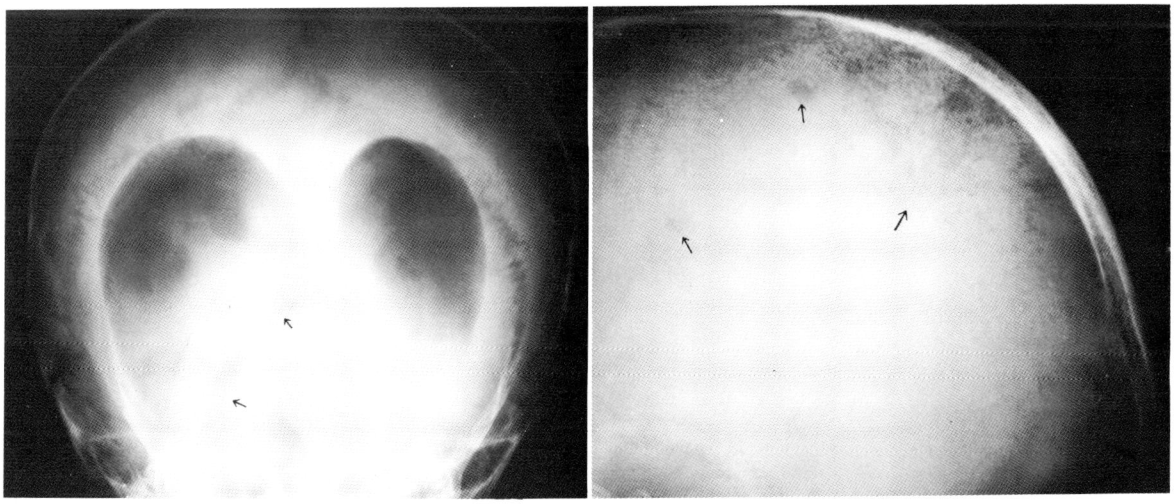

B

Fig. 11-72. Radiation necrosis. **A,** Preoperative ventriculogram in 14-month-old child. Presumptive diagnosis of fourth ventricle medulloblastoma (arrows) was confirmed by microscopy. **B,** Patient had annual follow-up studies, but not until 9 years after irradiation were small irregular areas of bony rarefaction (arrows) seen scattered in both parietal bones.

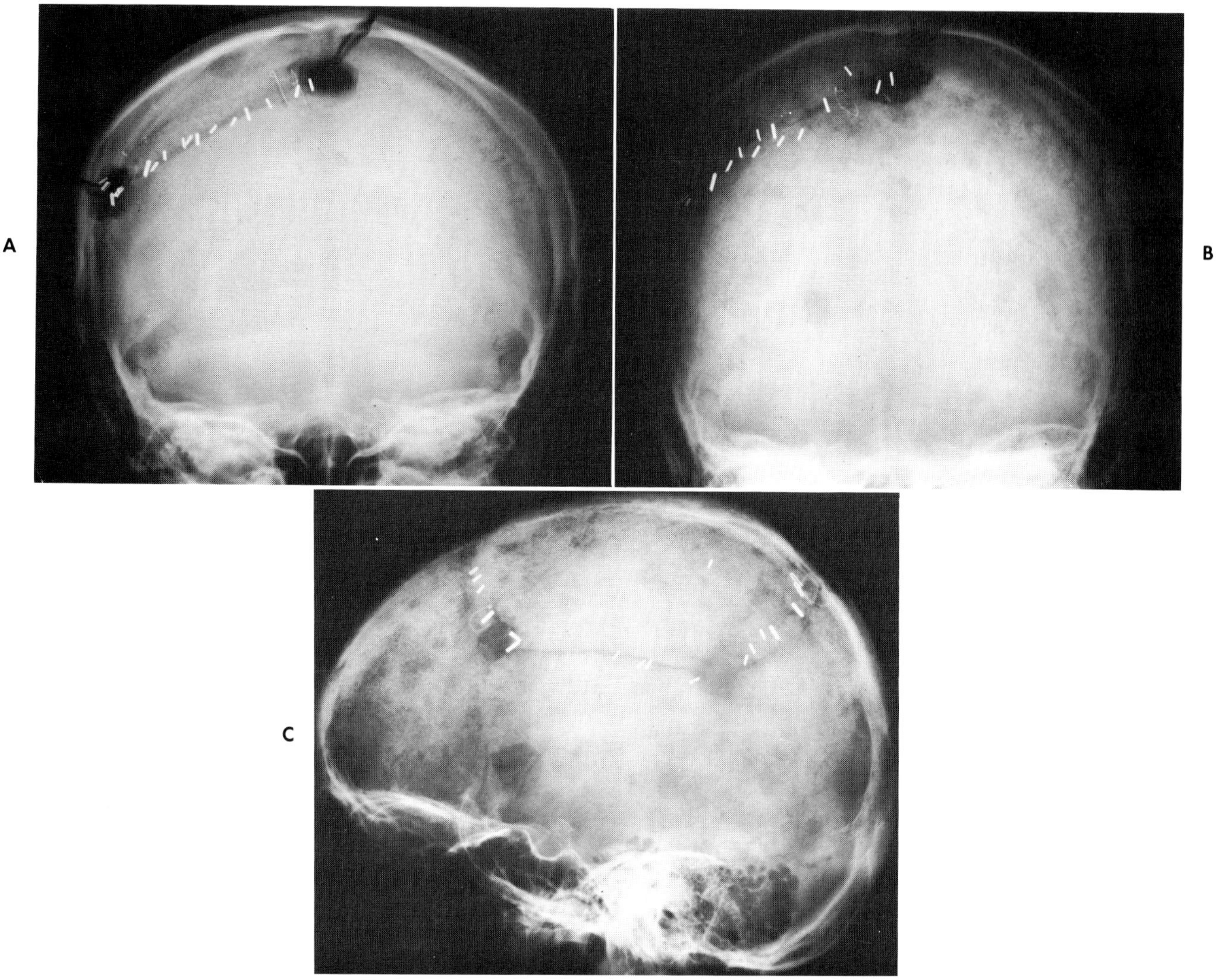

Fig. 11-73. Radiation necrosis. **A,** Normal appearance of skull after recent craniotomy for right parietal astrocytoma. **B** and **C,** After annual follow-up examinations, numerous intradiploic lesions were seen 10 years after radiation therapy.

disease (Fig. 11-74). The bony edges are irregular and frequently serrated, as in eosinophilic granuloma, but without marginal sclerosis. The absence of sclerosis seems to differentiate these two related conditions. Eosinophilic granuloma is believed to represent the benign form of Hand-Schüller-Christian disease.

Diffuse. This type of lysis of cancellous bone is a less common initial manifestation of disease and is difficult to recognize on a single examination. This change is observed mainly in metabolic and idiopathic diseases. *Hyperparathyroidism* initially produces a diffuse loss of cancellous bone. The diagnosis is usually not established at that stage but only when the three tables are affected (Fig. 11-112).

Bone destruction is rare in idiopathic diseases. Among these, *osteoporosis circumscripta* (Paget's disease) is probably the most common; it is considered idiopathic for lack of better classification. The disease is discovered incidentally in most cases; but when it is symptomatic, a dull ache over the area is the usual complaint. The edges of the lesion are usually well demarcated and frequently irregular rather than circular as in acquired conditions. Osteoporosis circumscripta is nearly always progressive, and the classic form of Paget's disease develops eventually. Rarely, however, it may regress (Fig. 11-75). (See Chapter 38.)

Osteoblastic changes

Focal and multiple osteoblastic changes are mainly seen in tumorous and developmental processes.

In *osteogenic sarcoma,* areas of neoplastic bone are closely packed and the lesion appears dense. As the

A

B

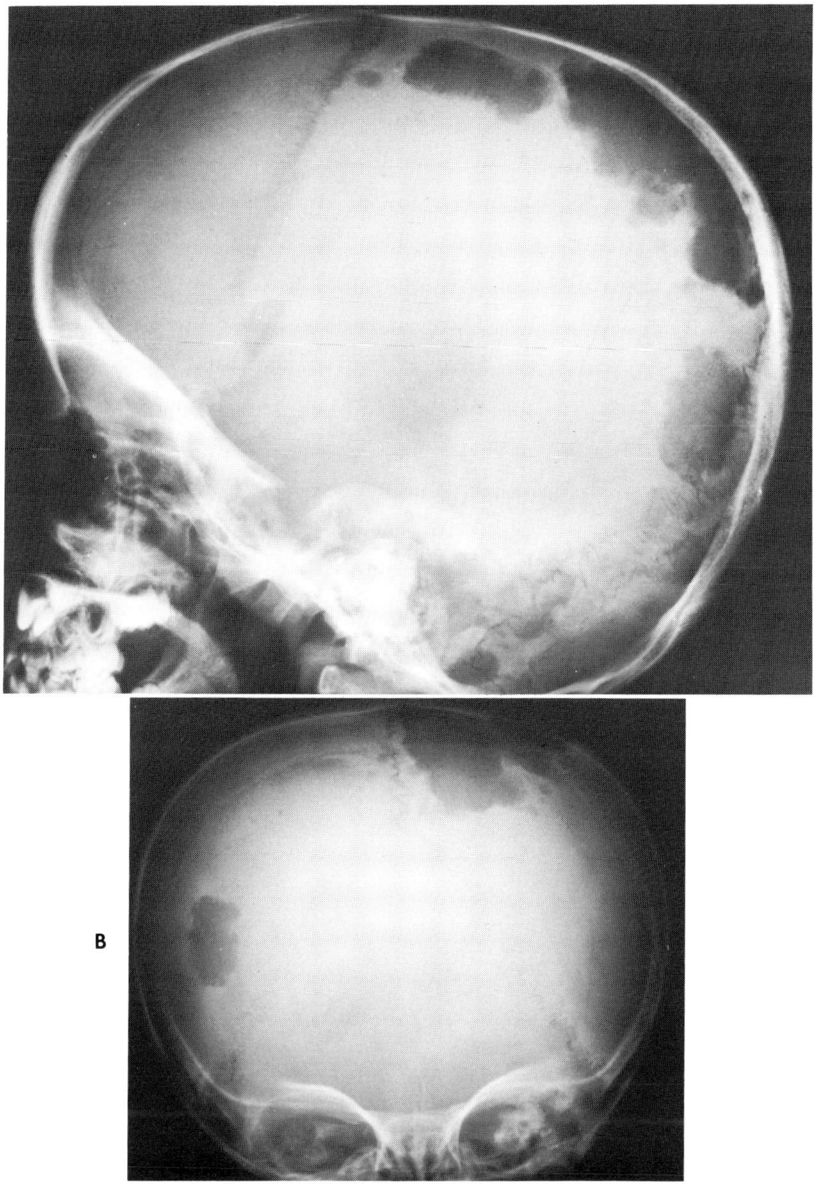

Fig. 11-74. Hand-Schüller-Christian disease. Multiple large areas of destruction of cranial vault. Margins are irregular and indicate an invasive process. Numerous similar lesions also affect base of skull. Lesions appear to be purely lytic.

tumor grows within the middle table, it pushes the inner and outer tables apart. These tables finally are invaded and incorporated within the tumor. The bony trabeculae are usually well formed, but their spatial distribution is quite erratic. As with osteosarcoma elsewhere, spicules may be seen to radiate from the tumor into the soft tissues.

Osteoblastic metastatic lesions from carcinoma are found in the cranial vault, where their features are the same as in other bones. They are round with ill-defined margins. Their bony texture is abnormal, for the bone is formed in a haphazard manner. Their density is fairly uniform, and they resemble the dense nodules that are seen in Paget's disease. The site of the primary tumor is commonly the prostate.

Bone islands may develop in the middle table. They are usually small, dense, well-demarcated structures, of an essentially benign appearance. Histologically they are composed of normal bone. The pattern of the diploe surrounding these islands is also normal.

In *tuberous sclerosis* multiple sclerotic nodules are occasionally seen within the middle table. They are of uniform density and are usually poorly demarcated (Fig. 11-76). They are close to the inner table, which may be

A 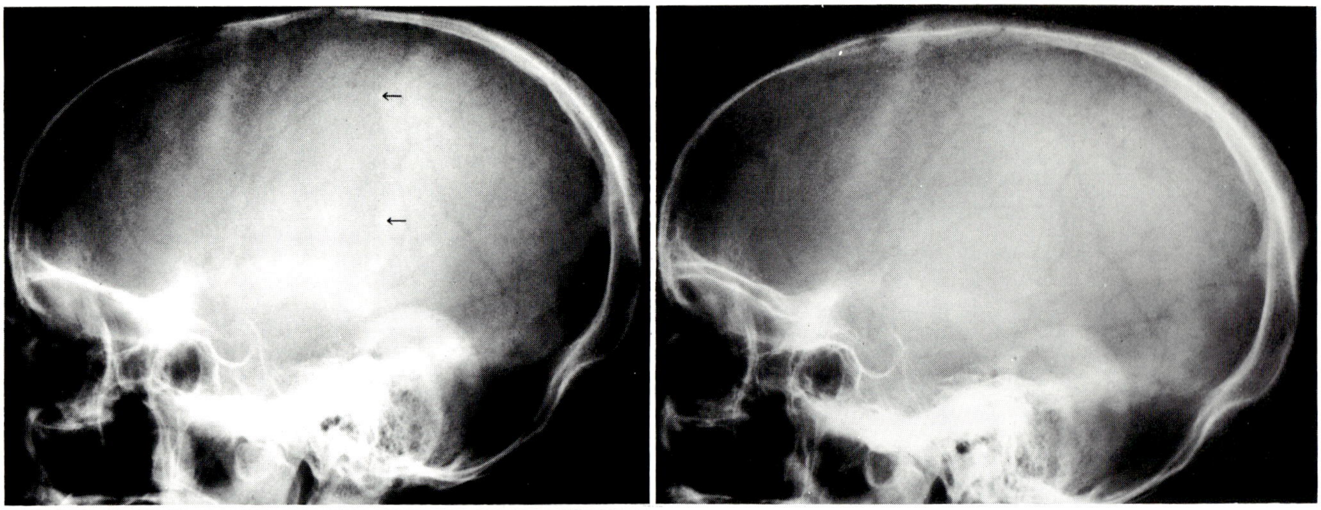 C

B 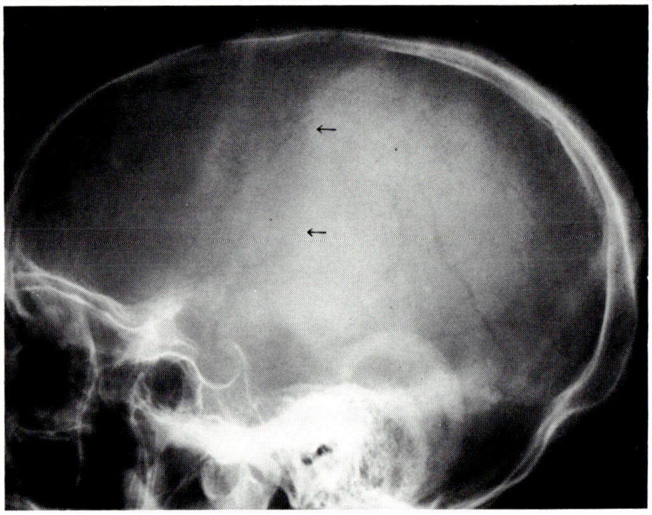

Fig. 11-75. Osteoporosis circumscripta. **A,** Extensive destruction of right frontal and parietal middle tables. Note the sharp linear demarcation between normal and abnormal bone in the midparietal area (arrows). **B,** Three years later, disease has regressed (arrows). **C,** Five years later, further regression. Skull would be reported as normal if not compared with previous examinations.

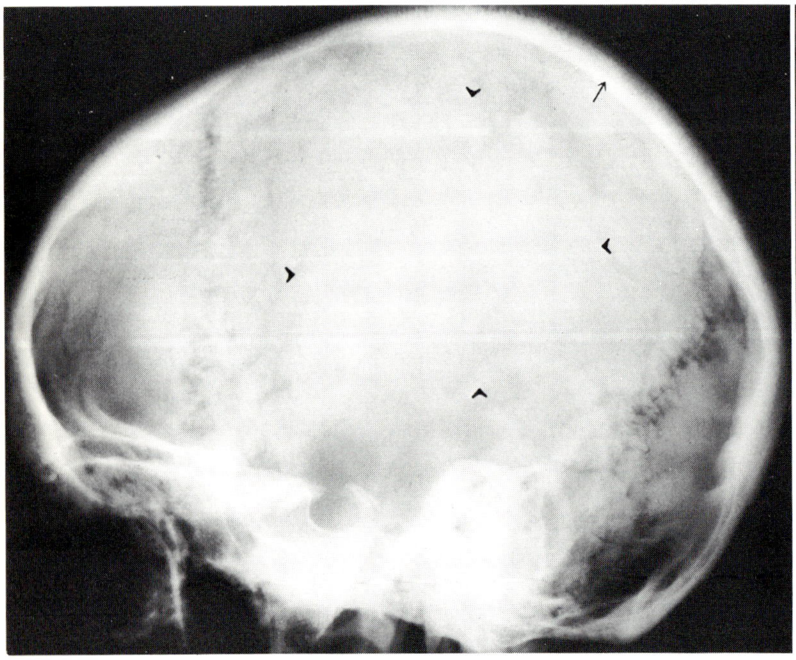

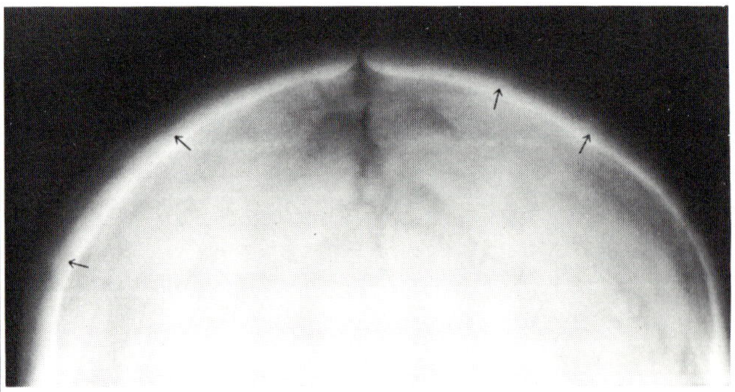 B

Fig. 11-76. Tuberous sclerosis. **A,** Numerous small ill-defined sclerotic nodules are scattered in parietal bones (arrowheads). **B,** They appear to be grouped along inner half of middle table (arrows).

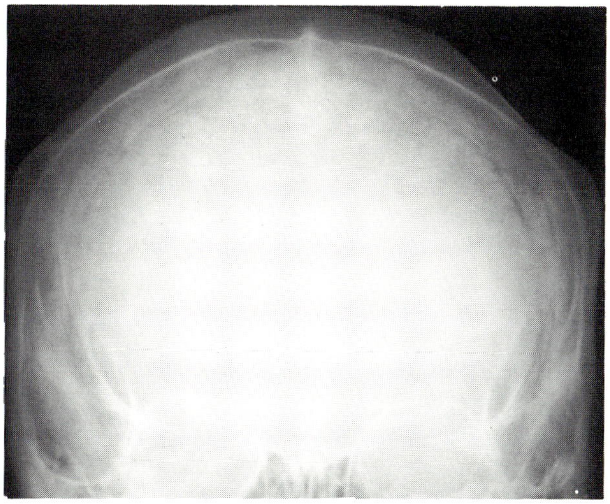

Fig. 11-77. Biparietal thinning, grooved type. Moderate atrophy of outer table on both sides over parietal depressions. On the right, atrophy of middle table is moderate; on the left, severe. Inner table is intact.

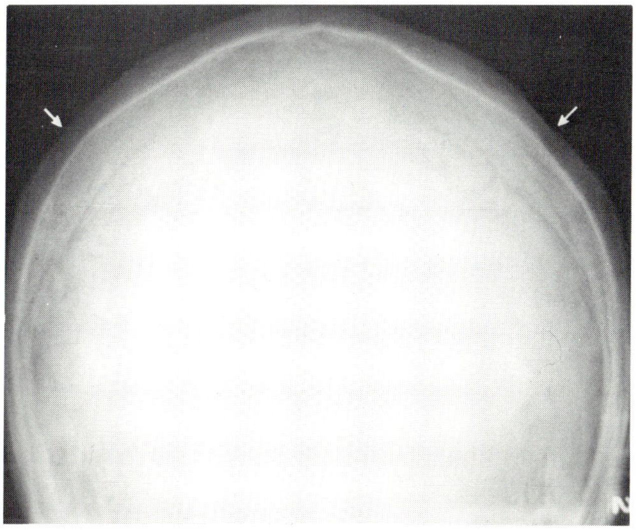

Fig. 11-78. Biparietal thinning. Arrows point to flat type on the right, grooved type on the left.

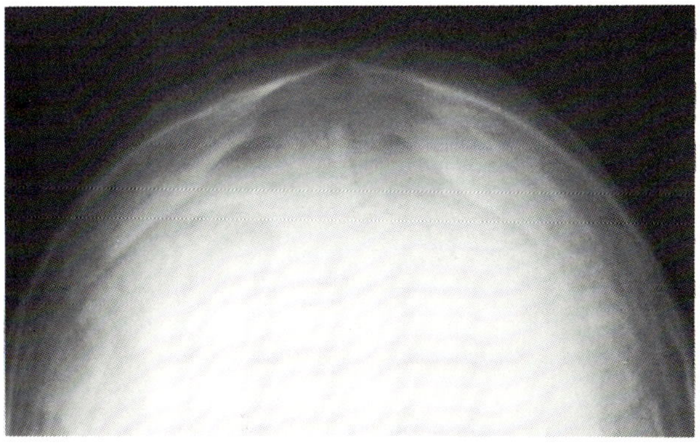

Fig. 11-79. Biparietal thinning in 17-year-old male with severe thinning of both parietal bones.

somewhat increased in thickness. These nodules do not differ from those seen in the medullary cavity of other affected bones (Lagos et al., 1968).

Diffuse sclerotic or hyperostotic changes of the middle table are usually manifestations of *metabolic* or *developmental diseases.* The classic appearance of the middle table in anemias, particularly the brushlike pattern in Cooley's anemia, is well known. Equally recognized is the extensive sclerosis of the middle table in osteopetrosis. Various types of anemias and bone dysplasias are associated with marked sclerosis of the middle table. These entities are usually diagnosed before they are brought to the attention of the neuroradiologist.

Atrophic (hypoplastic) changes

Atrophy or hypoplasia of the middle table appears to be the dominant feature in moderately advanced *biparietal thinning* (Figs. 11-77 and 11-78). Camp and Nash (1944) described flat and grooved types and called this condition developmental thinness of the parietal bones. They observed the condition more commonly in males than in females, and they noted that the flat type is more frequent than the grooved type. Parietal thinning is mainly seen during the fourth and fifth decades of life, but it is also found in younger individuals (Fig. 11-79). Follow-up studies show that the process progresses slowly over the years. Cursory studies of well-developed forms of this condition suggest that the process started in the diploe. In patients in whom we are able to see this condition develop over the years, the outer table thins out first and then the diploe (Fig. 11-102).

Some loss of diploe is frequently observed in postoperative *bone flaps* of adult skulls. Tangential views show that with time the bone flap becomes thinner,

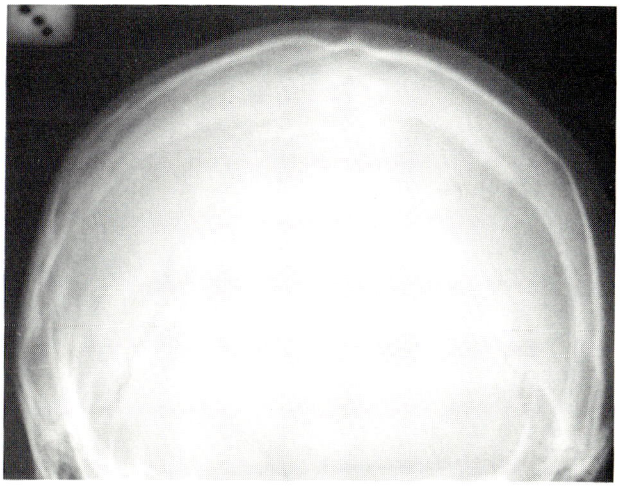

Fig. 11-80. Left cerebral hemiatrophy. Flattening and increase in thickness of left hemicranium in 20-year-old epileptic with history of meningoencephalitis at age 7 months. Note the overgrowth of the middle table.

mainly at the expense of the middle table. Under these circumstances bony fusion between the flap and the surrounding skull is always delayed and may never develop. The scalp overlying the flap is also thinner than elsewhere.

In *unilateral cerebral hypoplasia* the cranial vault may be thinner on the affected side than on the normal side. The middle table, which is usually quite thick in such cases, may be hypoplastic, accounting for the relative thinning of the vault on the affected side. The reasons for this finding are not clear, but the change emphasizes the intricate relation between the brain and the skull.

Hypertrophic changes

Diffuse overgrowth of the middle table is a common feature of the cranial vault in *cerebral atrophy* in early life. This overgrowth is the result of retarded growth

A

B

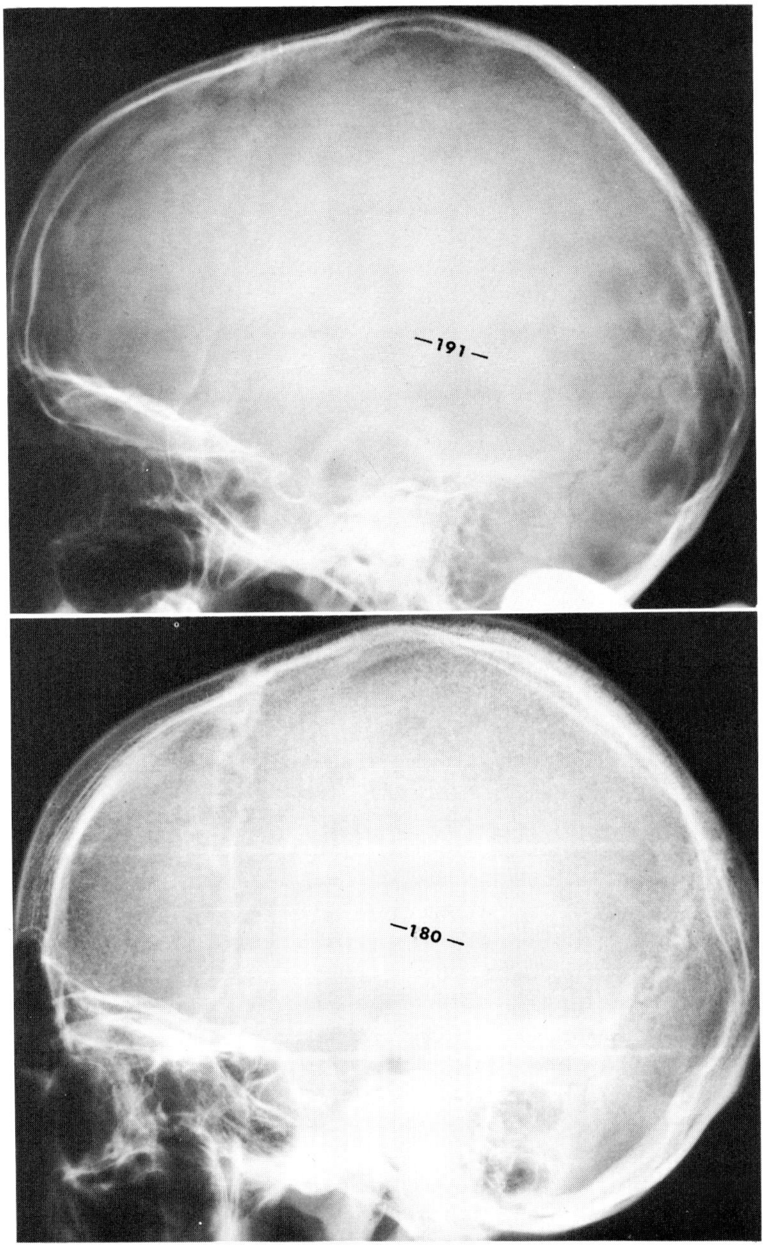

Fig. 11-81. Remodeling of cranial vault during progressive brain loss. **A,** Normal skull at age 7 years, at the time of measles encephalitis. **B,** At age 15 years, same external diameters of skull but much shorter internal diameters. Note in the frontal squama the superimposition of several old inner tables that are slowly incorporated into the middle table.

of the brain. The hypoplastic brain does not exert as much erosive pressure on the vault as would a normal growing brain. Consequently the bone proliferates more freely and increases in thickness. The middle table appears sooner than usual and continues to expand until late adolescence. During this time the inner and outer tables remain relatively normal in thickness (Fig. 11-80). If growth of the brain becomes retarded midway or late in childhood, the bone changes are less pronounced. Even in that age group, however, the changes can be striking if brain growth is arrested suddenly and an actual loss of brain follows. Remarkable remodeling of the cranial vault takes place. As the brain decreases in size, new inner tables are formed and absorbed and the middle table becomes thicker (Fig. 11-81). This loss of brain is appreciated best when the inner diameters of the skull are measured, since clinically the skull size remains normal.

A rare manifestation of *hyperostosis frontalis* is a focal eccentric expansion of the middle table, with inward bulging of the inner table (Perou, 1964). The inner table at that point is usually thicker than elsewhere.

Mixed changes

The appearance of mixed changes, observed in numerous lesions, is caused partly by productive osseous

A

B

C

D

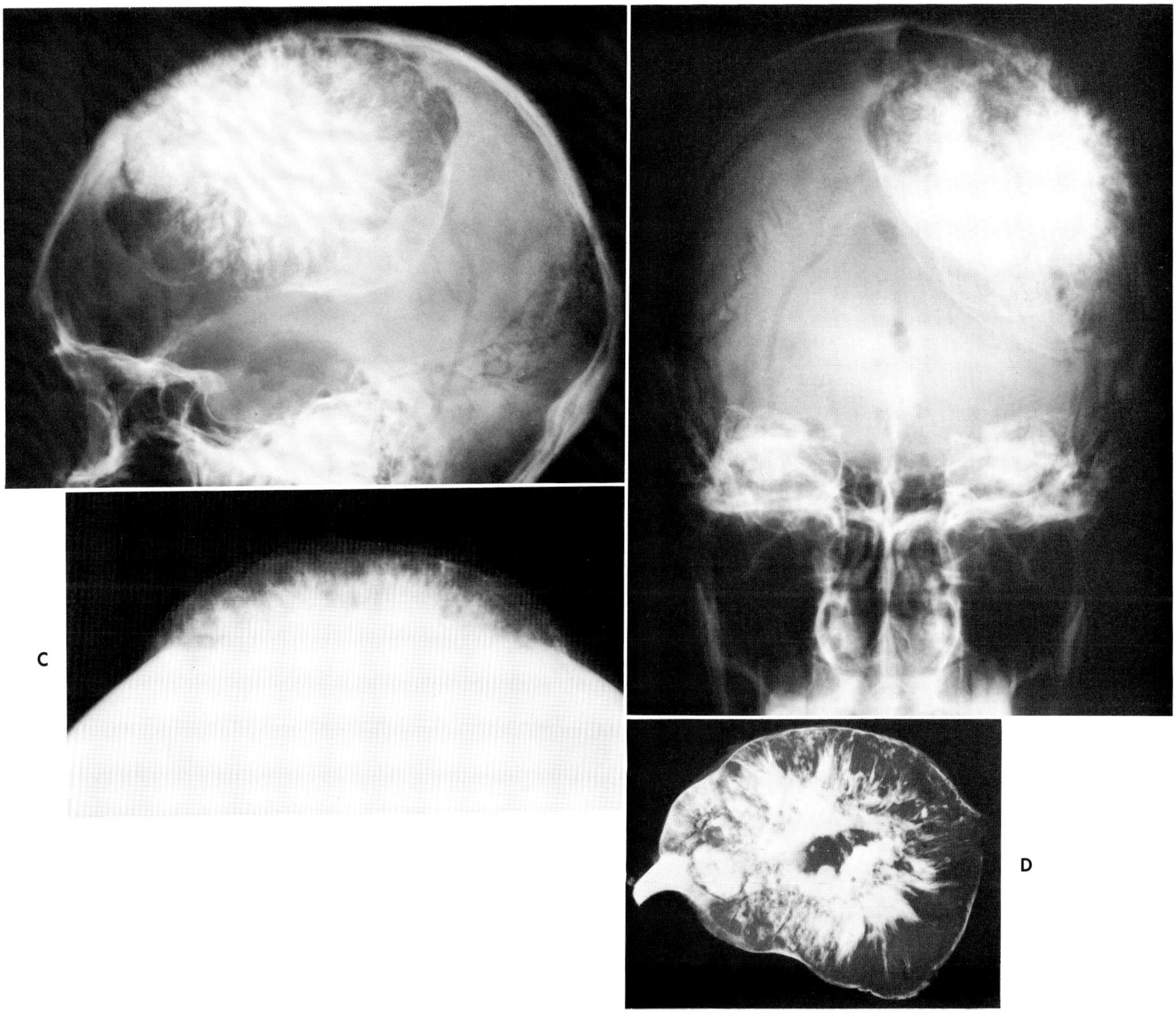

Fig. 11-82. Osteosarcoma. **A** to **C,** Large intracranial and extracranial mass whose bulk is composed of bony nodules and spicules. Periphery of lesion consists mainly of nonossified matrix. Tumor is still lined by thin but intact inner and outer tables that have been spread apart markedly. **D,** Roentgenogram of specimen shows those particular features well.

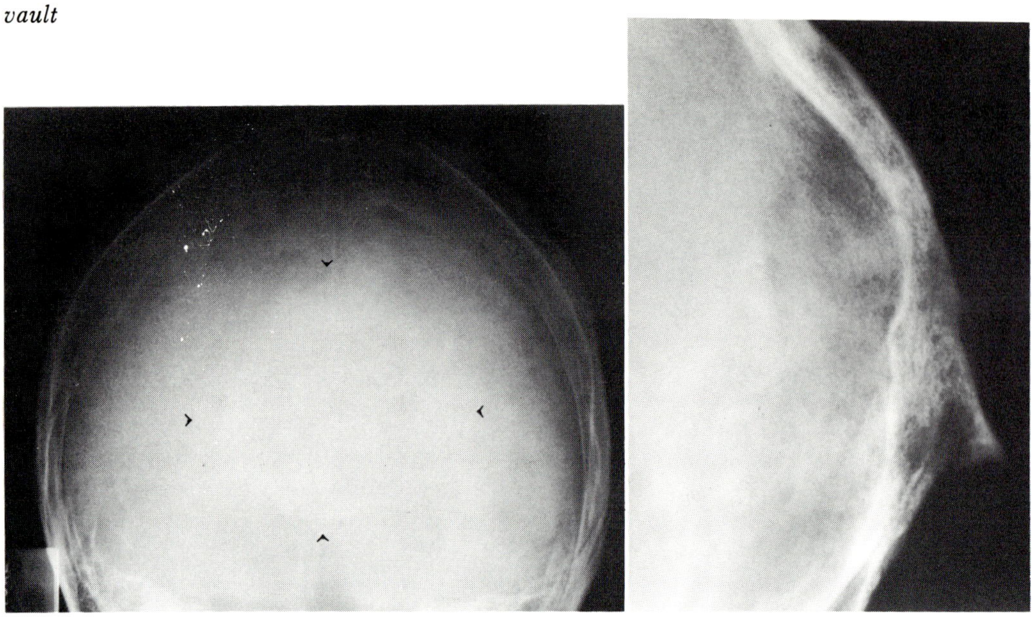

Fig. 11-83. Primary melanosarcoma. Rapidly growing malignant lesion has invaded and destroyed bone. It extends through inner and outer tables, which have been replaced rather than displaced by the tumor. Some marginal sclerosis (arrowheads) probably represents reactive new bone formation.

A 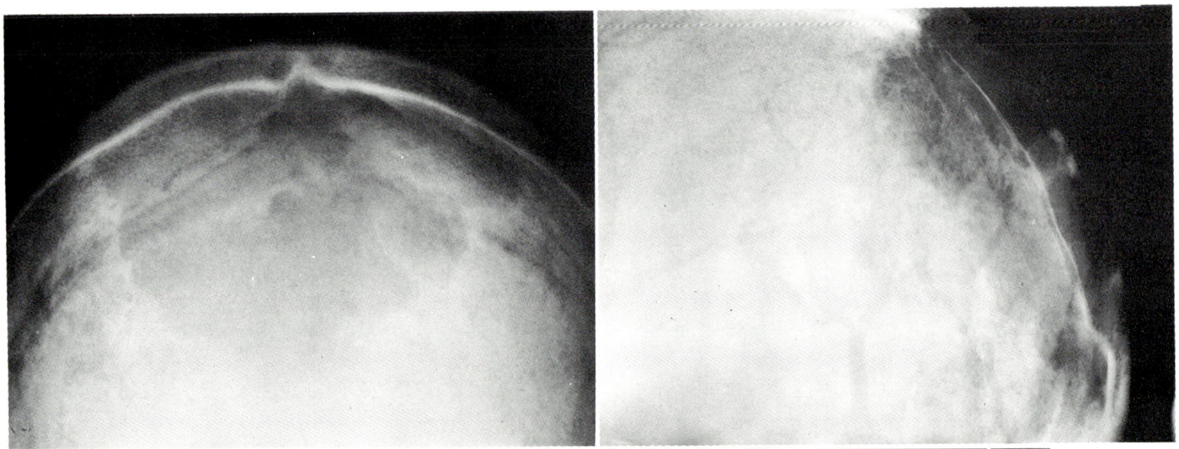 B

Fig. 11-84. Solitary myeloma. **A** and **B,** Large irregular parieto-occipital destructive lesion with minimal peripheral sclerosis. **C,** Mixed character of lesion is brought out by tangential view, which shows that the process has extended from diploe into scalp, where numerous bony spicules can be seen.

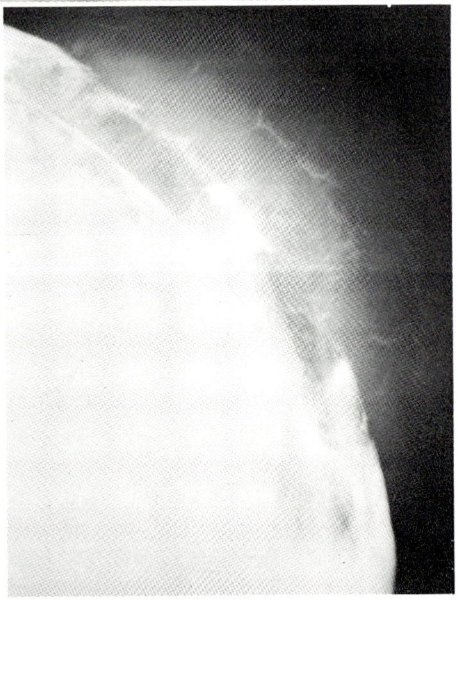

C

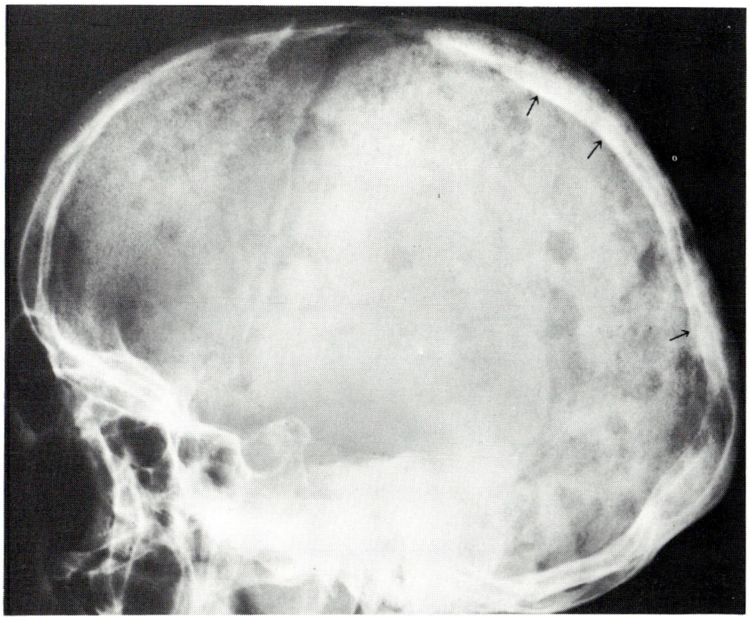

Fig. 11-85. Osteolytic and osteoblastic metastases. Numerous osteolytic lesions (arrows) are associated with osteoblastic lesions distributed mainly along superior parts of parietal bones in patient with prostatic carcinoma.

A

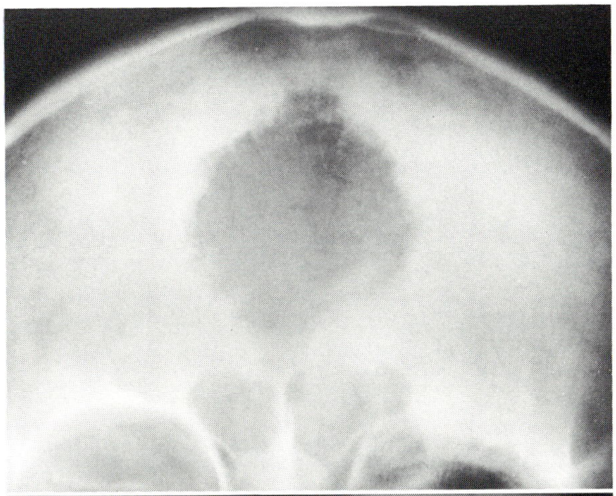

B

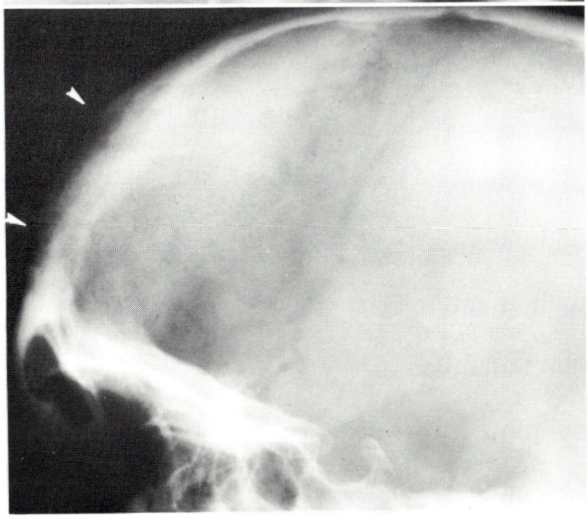

Fig. 11-86. Metastatic melanosarcoma. **A,** Midfrontal destructive process with irregular edges. Moderate degree of peripheral sclerosis is present. Similar changes are seen in left orbit secondary to direct spread from melanosarcoma of the eye. **B,** Tangential view shows that maximal changes are in middle table (arrowheads).

changes and partly by abnormal or destroyed bone. It is the most common manifestation of diseases of the middle table. Attempts to recognize whether the bony texture in the lucent areas is modified or destroyed are important in the establishment of a diagnosis. When the bone is actually destroyed, infectious and neoplastic lesions must be considered. If the bony texture is modified (or dysplastic), in other words, replaced by fibrous tissue or noncalcified cartilage, developmental conditions are more likely. For practical purposes lesions can be classed as osteolytic and osteoblastic or as dysplastic and osteoblastic.

Osteolytic and osteoblastic. Mixed osteolytic and osteoblastic changes may be seen in *sarcoma.* Low-grade tumors behave as other intramedullary lesions and displace the inner and outer tables apart through a constant remodeling process (Fig. 11-82). In rapidly expanding malignant tumors, such as melanosarcoma, the peripheral tables are destroyed rather than displaced (Fig. 11-83).

In lymphomatous lesions, such as *Hodgkin's disease,* the bony trabeculae that are formed are poorly defined and the osteoblastic lesions poorly outlined. The areas of bone destruction are also poorly demarcated. These lesions rarely expand the middle table. They can destroy the inner and outer tables, however, and grow intracranially or in the scalp. In solitary *myelomas* the extracranial part of the tumor may be quite large (Fig. 11-84).

Mixed osteolytic and osteoblastic *metastatic neoplasms* are well known to develop in the cranial vault; usually they present no diagnostic difficulty (Fig. 11-85). They may cause areas of destruction, surrounded by sclerosis, when they grow slowly (Fig. 11-86). If solitary, such lesions are difficult to diagnose.

In rare instances *meningiomas* may produce changes identical to those of an intramedullary tumor (Fig. 11-87). Meningiomas can, of course, develop around the margins of an erosion produced by a pacchionian gran-

A

B

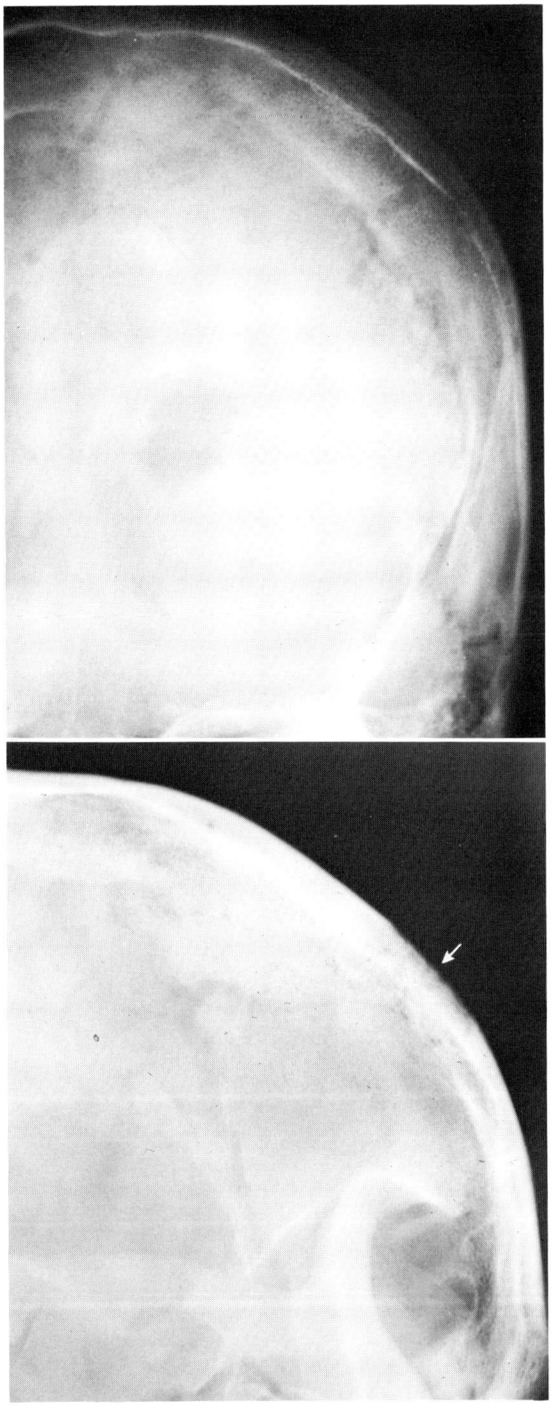

Fig. 11-87. Left frontal meningioma. **A,** Osteolytic lesion surrounded by sclerotic margins. **B,** Tangential view shows extensive destruction of middle table as well as of inner and outer tables, suggesting a lesion of intradiploic origin (arrow). These changes are atypical for meningioma, except perhaps for those that arise around a pacchionian granulation embedded in bone. Note the widened vascular grooves.

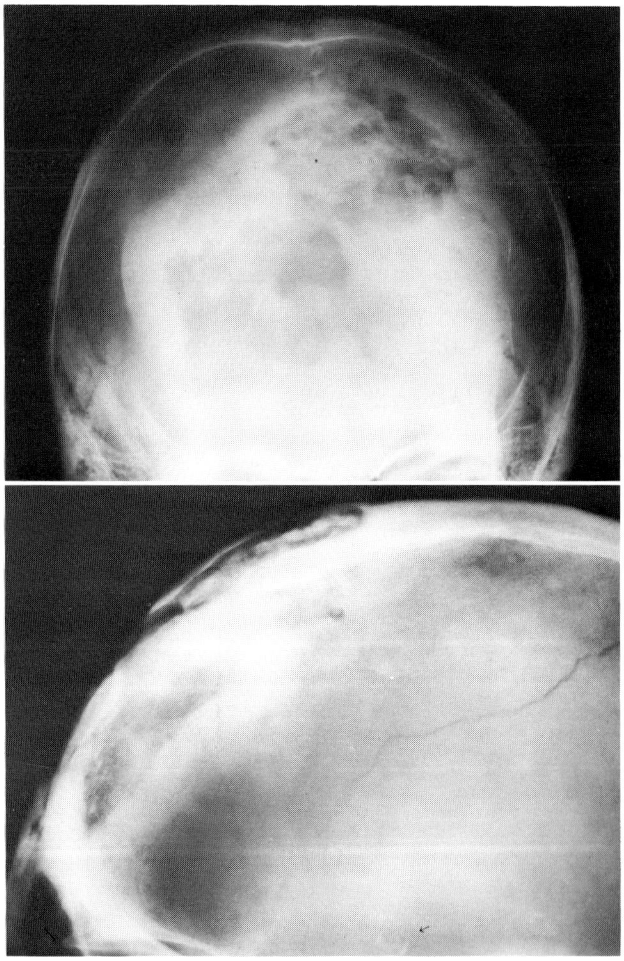

Fig. 11-88. Syphilitic osteomyelitis. Large areas of bone destruction surrounded by extensive marginal sclerosis. Note the large sequestra in the superior frontal region. These changes, as well as a berry aneurysm, were discovered incidentally after a head injury in which patient sustained a skull fracture.

ulation and grow mainly in the middle table. Everytime an unusual lesion is seen, meningioma must be considered as a diagnostic possibility, particularly when vascular grooves are widened.

A mixed pattern is the rule in *chronic inflammatory processes*. Among these, chronic osteomyelitis produces the most diverse appearance. Areas of reactive sclerosis are shown as dense irregular patches, and sequestra appear as dense isolated fragments. Areas of destruction appear as poorly demarcated lucent zones (Fig. 11-88). The inner and outer tables are always involved to some degree. They are partially destroyed and thin in some places and are sclerosed and thick in others.

In infancy, before the development of a medullary cavity, *chronic osteitis* of the skull has a polymorphous appearance (Fig. 11-89).

Eosinophilic granuloma destroys the middle table and at the same time produces various degrees of marginal sclerosis (Fig. 11-90). The lytic part of the lesion is so striking that the sclerosis around it may be missed. The edges of the osteolytic area are irregular and frequently serrated. The peripheral sclerosis varies in intensity and

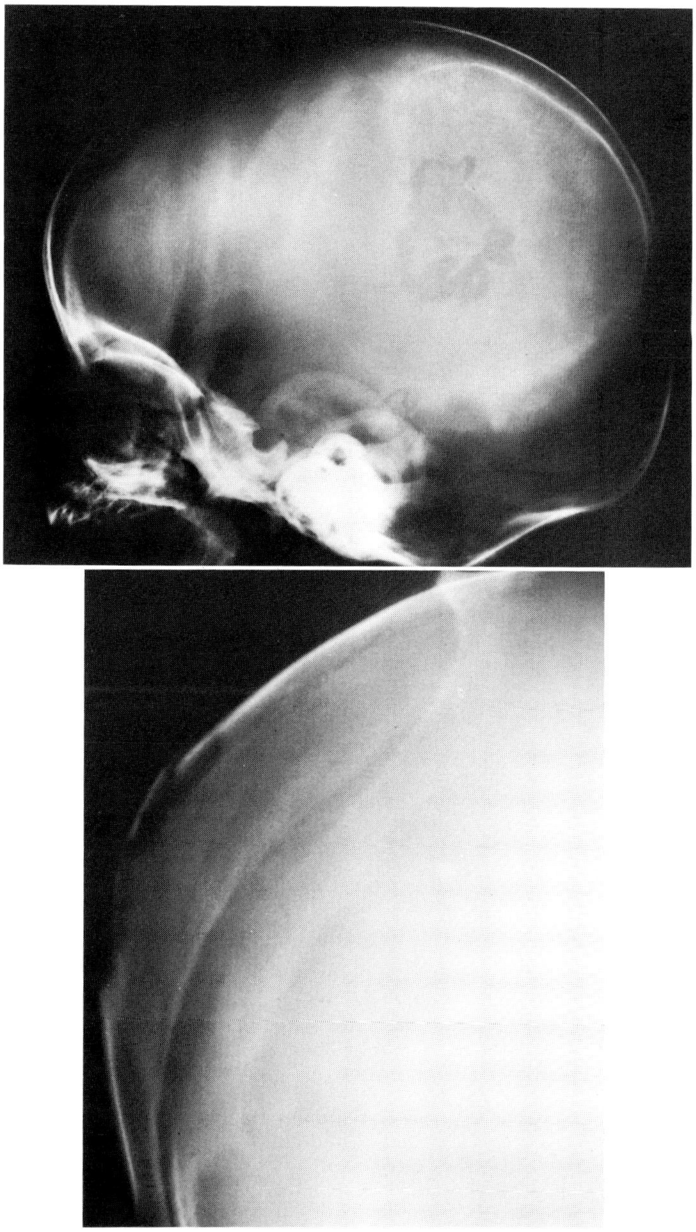

Fig. 11-89. Osteomyelitis and cephalhematoma in 1-month-old baby. Irregular zone of bone destruction contains large sequestra over the right parietal eminence.

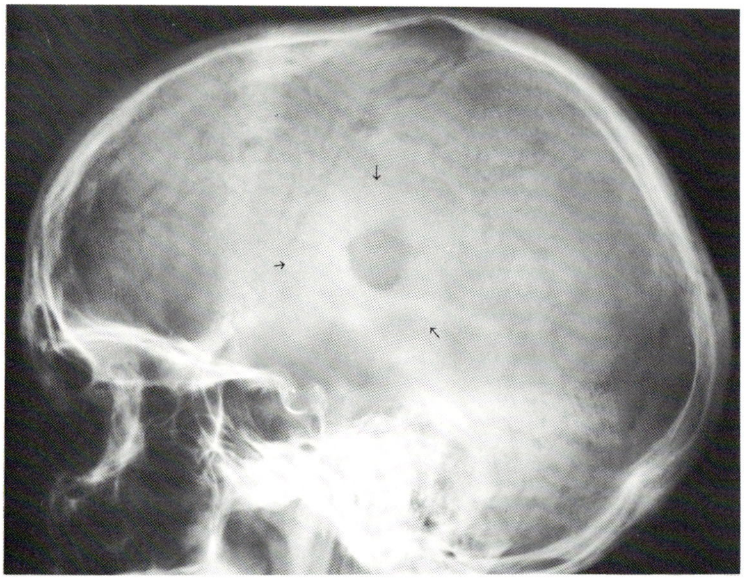

Fig. 11-90. Eosinophilic granuloma. Focal destruction of left parietal bone with irregular margins. Note the relatively wide halo of sclerosis (arrows) around the lesion.

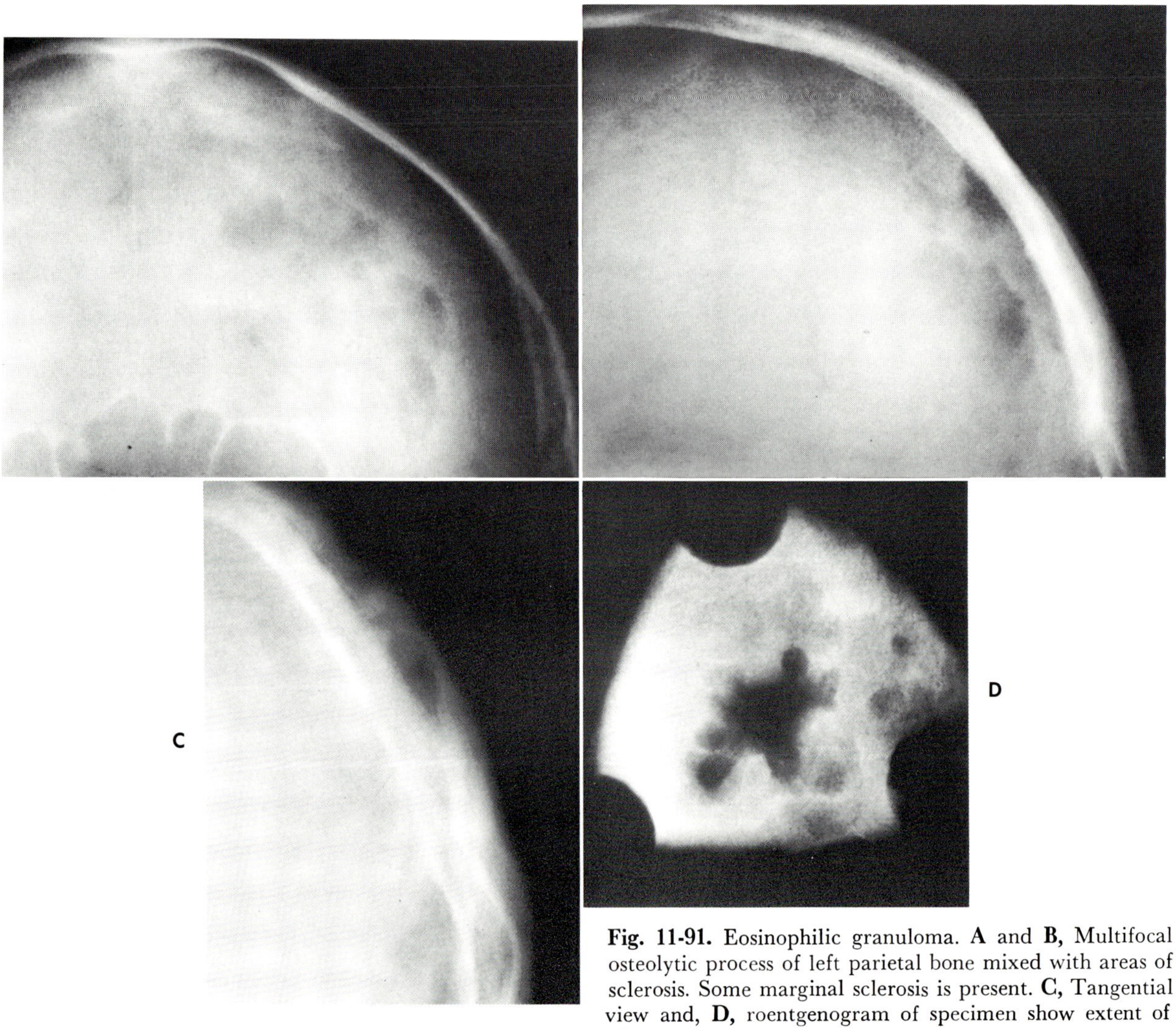

Fig. 11-91. Eosinophilic granuloma. **A** and **B,** Multifocal osteolytic process of left parietal bone mixed with areas of sclerosis. Some marginal sclerosis is present. **C,** Tangential view and, **D,** roentgenogram of specimen show extent of changes.

gradually merges with normal bone. Multiple lesions in one area tend to coalesce (Fig. 11-91). Eosinophilic granuloma is observed mostly in children and in young adults and becomes symptomatic when it breaks through the inner or outer table.

Dysplastic and osteoblastic. A rather poorly understood entity named *doughnut lesion* has a characteristic appearance (Keats and Holt, 1969). As its name implies, it is a circular lesion, usually not exceeding 2 cm in diameter. The center of the lesion is mainly fibrous, whereas the periphery consists of dense closely packed bony trabeculae (Fig. 11-92). The exact nature of this entity is not known, but the lesion is believed to be a benign reparative process of some sort that is asymptomatic. We have seen this type associated with osteoma and also with fibrous dysplasia (Fig. 11-93). Some of the so-called doughnut lesions are endosteomas; others probably represent the early, and possibly the only, manifestation of many bone diseases.

A

B

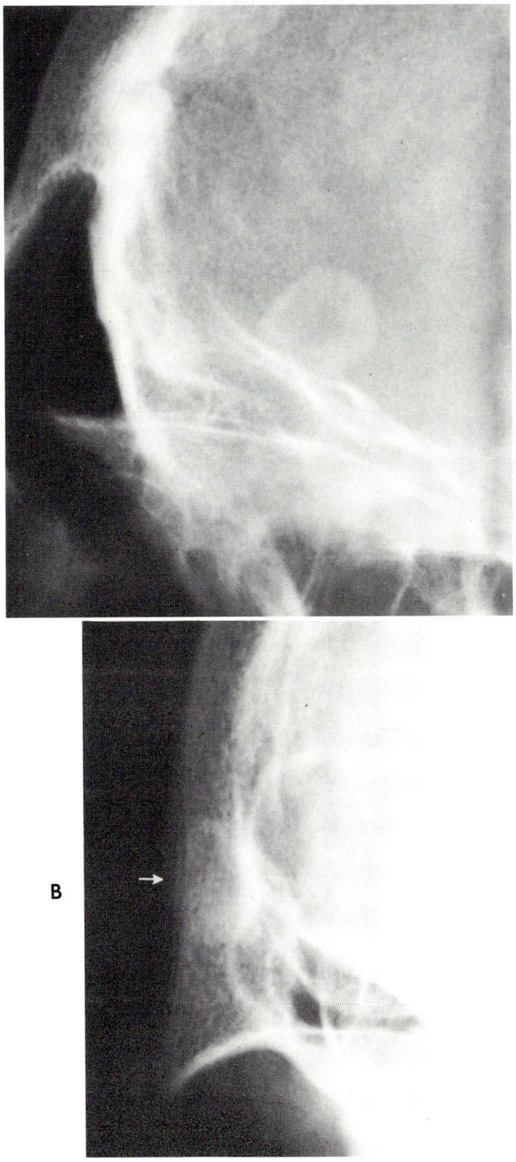

Fig. 11-92. Doughnut lesion. **A,** Lateral view shows well-demarcated circular lesion with sclerotic margin and radiolucent center. **B,** Intradiploic location is marked by arrow on tangential view.

A mixed pattern is the most common finding in *fibrous dysplasia* of the vault. The overall appearance varies with the relative amounts of fibrous cartilaginous and osseous tissues within the lesion. Cysts may also form. Tangential views nearly always show some degree of expansion of the middle table, which resembles a blister (Fig. 11-93). The outer table bulges while the normal curvature of the inner table is maintained (Leeds and Seaman, 1962). Sclerosis in this condition consists of two main forms: (1) a marginal sclerosis that is more or less distinct and (2) poorly defined dense round nodules of various size within the lesion itself. The bulk of the lesion is mainly radiolucent but has a ground-glass appearance due to the presence of immature bone. Roentgenograms of surgical specimens show a striking difference between the normal and the dysplastic middle table. The diploe is highly modified. The trabeculae are closely packed, numerous, and small with minute vascular spaces between them (Fig. 11-93, *C*).

Fibrous dysplasia is a well-vascularized lesion, and stereoscopic examinations usually reveal widening of the meningeal grooves on the side of the lesion. The meningeal arteries on selective external carotid angiograms frequently appear somewhat enlarged. Many fine twigs radiate into the lesion from the meningeal branches (Fig. 11-94). In addition, associated dilatation and even aneurysmal distentions of the extracranial arteries may be seen (Lin et al., 1969).

Another developmental anomaly that may resemble fibrous dysplasia is *cavernous hemangioma.* It too expands the middle table by displacing the outer table. The inner table may remain in normal position. The main difference lies in the size of the medullary spaces, which are larger than normal, so that the lesion appears honeycombed. Radiating bony spicules are commonly seen in the superficial part of the lesion and are usually at right angles to the external surface. Some marginal sclerosis also is usually present (Fig. 11-95). This classic appearance is not often seen. Atypical forms of the condition resemble other focal intramedullary lesions, such as epidermoid, or eosinophilic granuloma. Selective external carotid arteriography is helpful in establishing the diagnosis in these cases (Rosenbaum et al., 1969).

A mixed pattern is also seen in the classic form of *Paget's disease.* Since the outer and inner tables are usually involved, this condition will be discussed later.

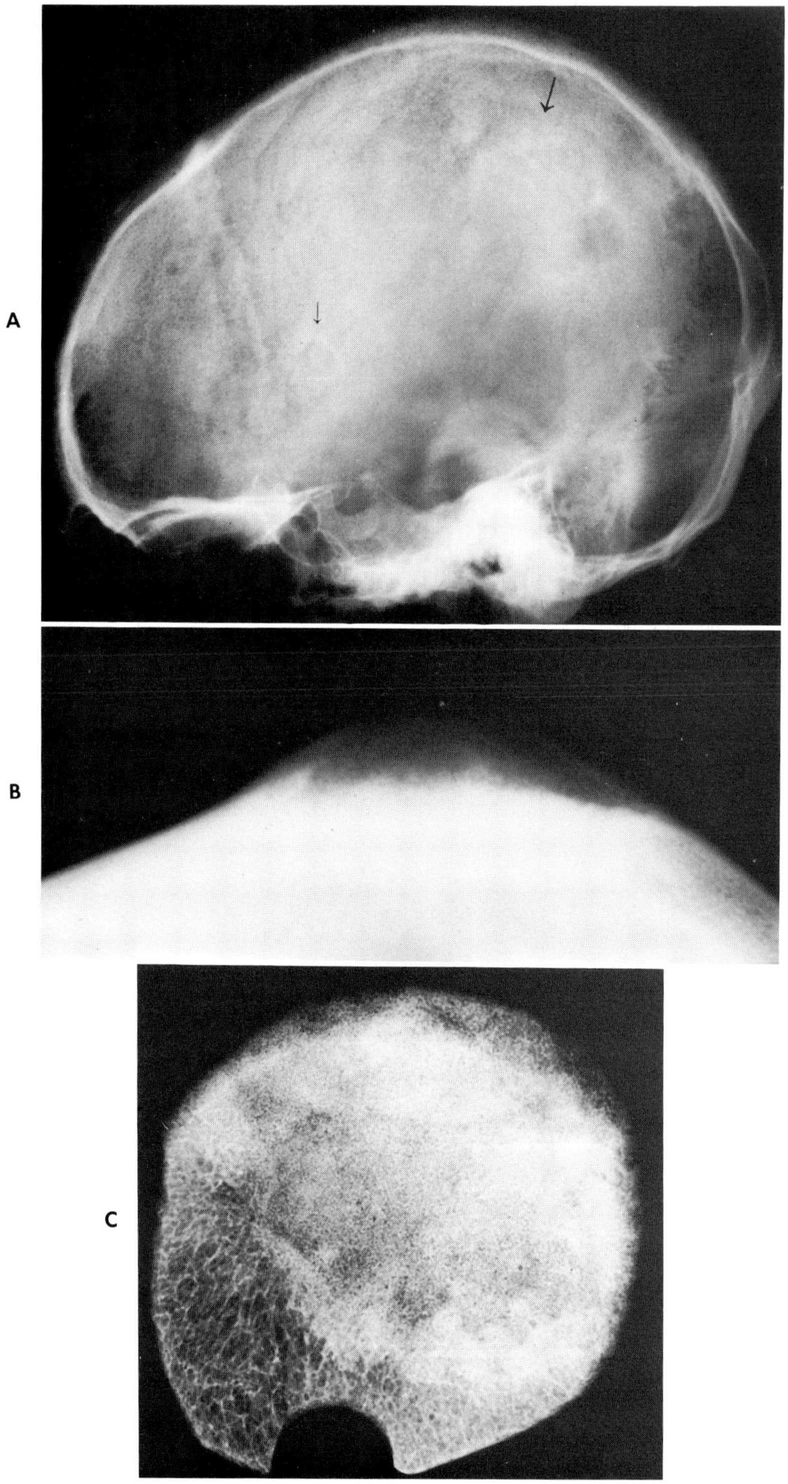

Fig. 11-93. Fibrous dysplasia. **A,** Two zones of bone rarefaction (arrows) surrounded by and mixed with areas of sclerosis in right parietal bone. Note the doughnut-like appearance of the smaller one. **B,** Tangential view shows poorly formed bony trabeculae in expanded middle table. Note the curvilinear elevation of the outer table and the normal position of the inner table. **C,** Specimen brings out difference between normal diploe (bottom left) and erratic bone formation in center and at periphery of lesion.

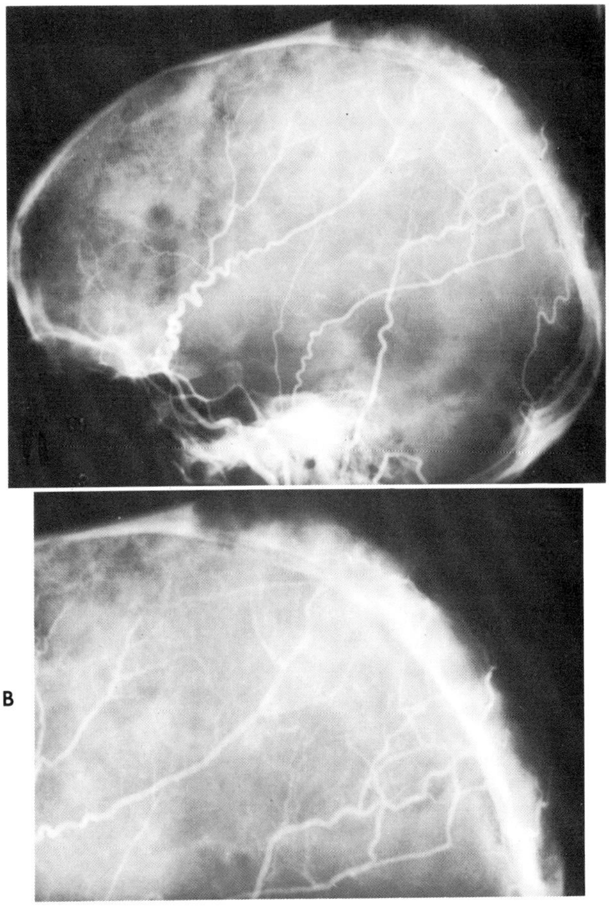

Fig. 11-94. Meningeal arterial supply in fibrous dysplasia. **A,** Selective external carotid angiogram shows remarkable enlargement and tortuosity of the main branches of the middle meningeal artery and of the meningeal branch of the occipital artery. **B,** Note the rich vascular supply in the right parietal region.

Outer table

Erosive changes

An erosion of the outer table is indicative of a mass in the scalp of long duration.

The most common scalp lesion is a *sebaceous cyst.* It causes a smooth depression of the outer table and, if allowed to grow for several years, an atrophy of the middle table. Other relatively benign masses, such as *neurofibromas* or *dermoid cysts,* may produce similar changes. The curvilinear depression of the outer table is usually best demonstrated by tangential views (Fig. 11-96).

Osteolytic changes

Focal destructive changes that affect primarily the outer table are rare and, again, are the result of scalp lesions. Demonstration on the same roentgenogram of both the abnormality of the scalp and the bone alteration is difficult. Most of the time one set of films is

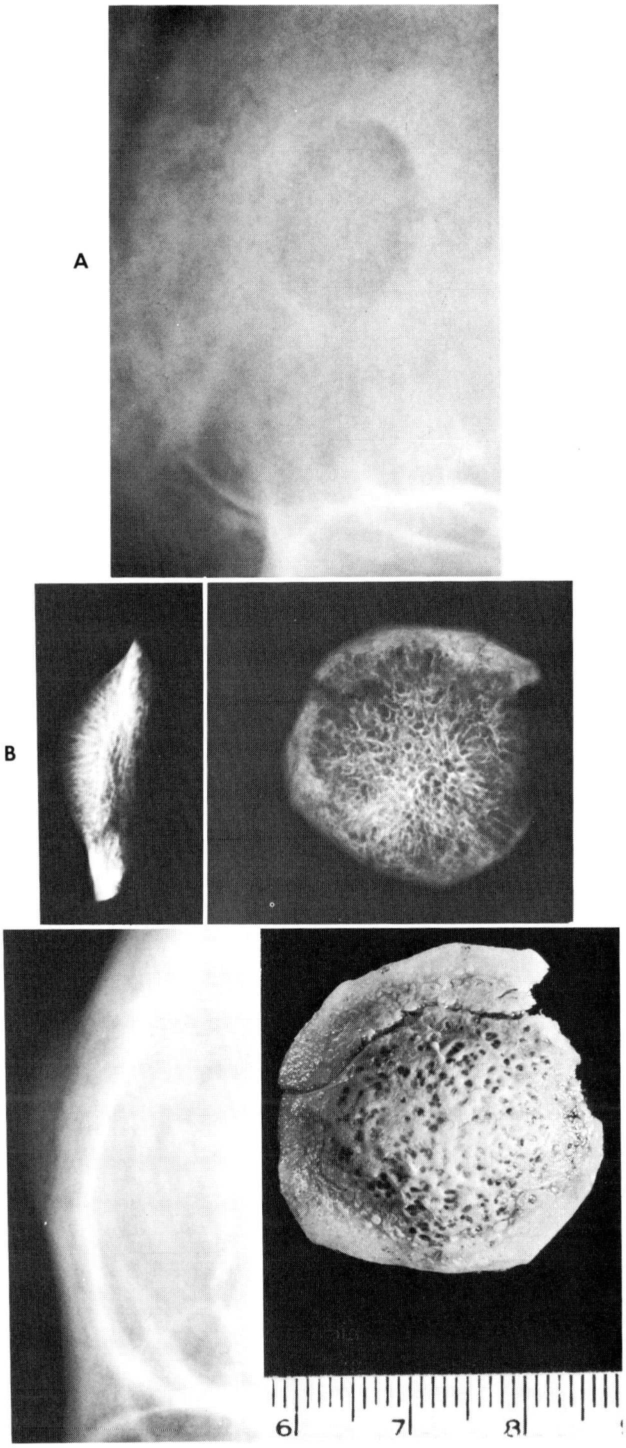

Fig. 11-95. Hemangioma of bone. **A,** Large vascular spaces contained within osseous channels resemble magnified diploe. There is slight but definite sclerosis around the lesion. **B,** Roentgenogram of specimen shows quite well the vertical arrangement of vascular channels. **C,** Tangential view shows expansion of the middle table, the elevated outer table, and the thin but undisplaced inner table. **D,** Note the multiple perforations of the bulging outer table on the photograph of the specimen.

A

B

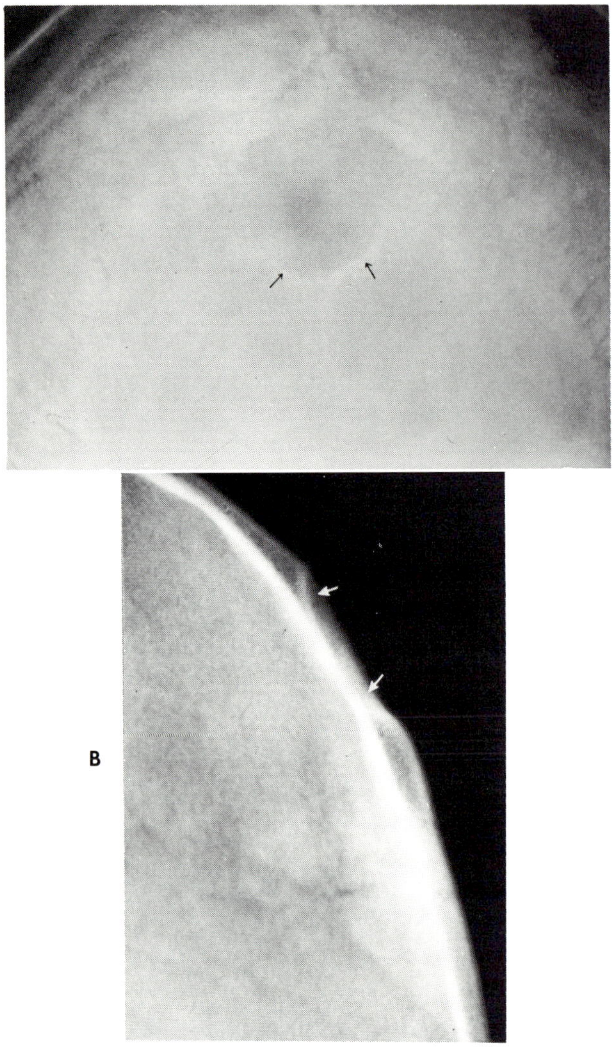

Fig. 11-96. Dermoid cyst of scalp. Erosion primarily of outer aspect of skull, as indicated by smooth depression and thinning of outer table (arrows), and secondarily of middle table. Although the nature of the process can be surmised on frontal view, **A,** tangential view, **B,** demonstrates the process best.

necessary for the vault and another set for the scalp.

Most of the osteolytic lesions of the outer table result from *scalp metastases* (Fig. 11-97). The changes are usually minimal; and unless the involved area is carefully evaluated, the lesion may be missed completely on routine skull examinations. The roentgenographic study of bone specimens provides additional information as to the extent of the lesion (Fig. 11-98).

Destruction of the outer table may be secondary to *scalp infections,* but ordinarily the disease spreads rapidly to the middle table.

Osteoblastic changes

Focal hyperostotic lesions of the outer table are mainly related to bone tumors; and among these, benign *oste-*

A

B

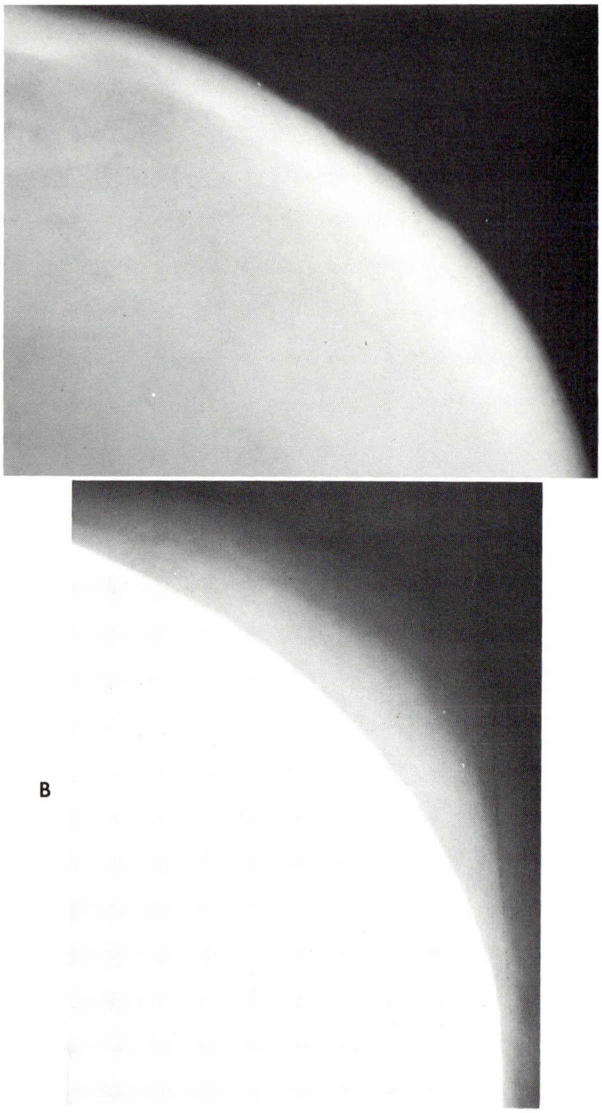

Fig. 11-97. Metastatic breast carcinoma. **A,** Normal technique. Tangential view shows irregular areas of bone destruction that involve outer table of left parietal bone. **B,** Soft-tissue technique of same area demonstrates swelling of scalp.

A

B

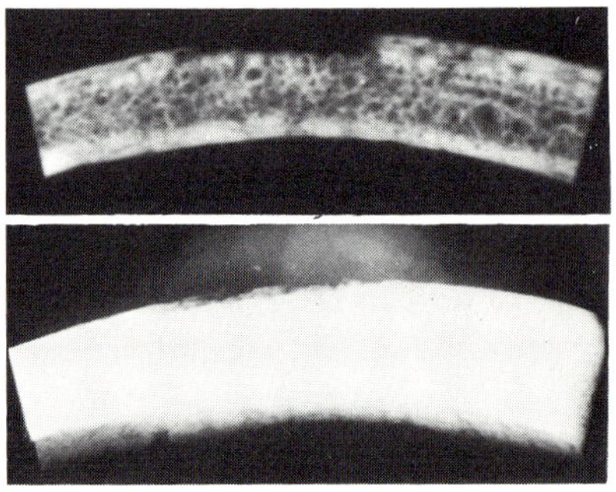

Fig. 11-98. Metastasis to outer table. **A,** Roentgenogram of surgical specimen shows destroyed outer table. Note the permeation of remaining segments of that table and of part of the middle table. **B,** Infiltrated and swollen scalp.

A

B

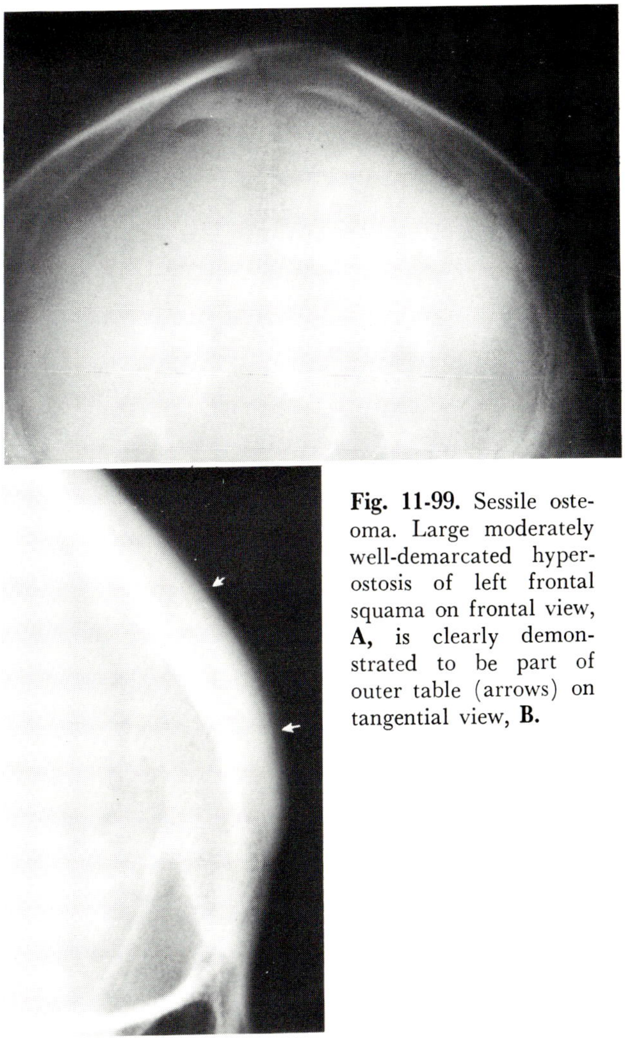

Fig. 11-99. Sessile osteoma. Large moderately well-demarcated hyperostosis of left frontal squama on frontal view, **A,** is clearly demonstrated to be part of outer table (arrows) on tangential view, **B.**

A

B

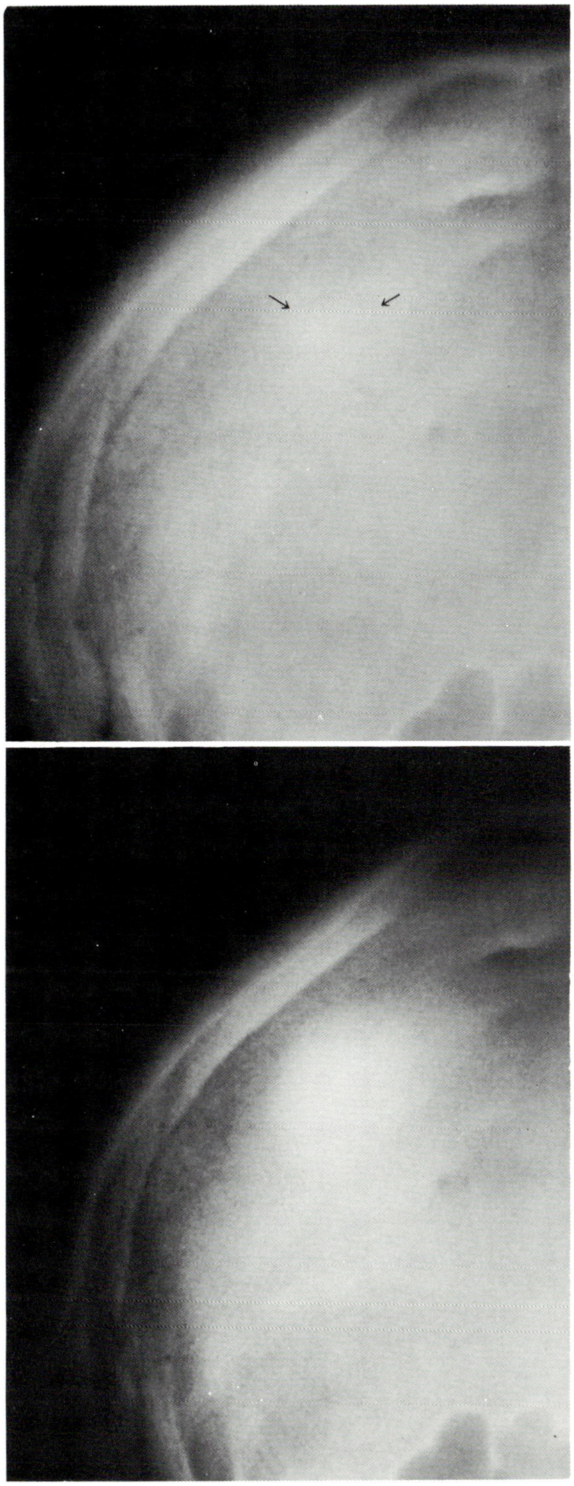

C

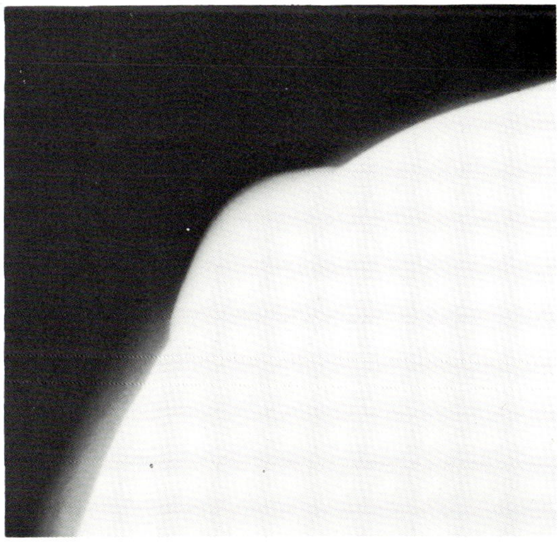

Fig. 11-100. Osteoma (growing). **A,** Small osteoma (arrows) of outer table in 35-year-old woman. **B,** Same patient 11 years later. Lesion has grown to fair size but remains well delineated. **C,** Osteoma is best seen on tangential view.

omas are the most frequent. They are usually sessile (Fig. 11-99). Comparison with previous examinations is of great value in establishing the rate of growth. On tangential views these osteomas appear as smooth curved elevations (Fig. 11-100).

Periosteal osteogenic sarcoma also appears as a dense bony mass. Both the density and the surface of the mass are very irregular, however, which differentiates this lesion from osteoma (Fig. 11-109).

Atrophic changes

Progressive thinning of the outer aspect of the vault is the main feature of *biparietal thinning,* occurring in compact skulls (Fig. 11-101). In diploic skulls, atrophy of the outer table is probably the first manifestation of this condition. It takes place before the development of any atrophy of the middle table. Slight thinning of the outer table is likely to be disregarded or missed on skull examinations. Whenever comparative studies are available over a period of 10 or more years, the fact becomes evident that thinning of the outer table takes place before thinning of the middle table (Fig. 11-102). For this reason we believe that parietal thinning is initiated in the outer rather than in the middle table.

Interparietal thinning refers to a midline depression of the vault along the posterior half of the sagittal suture

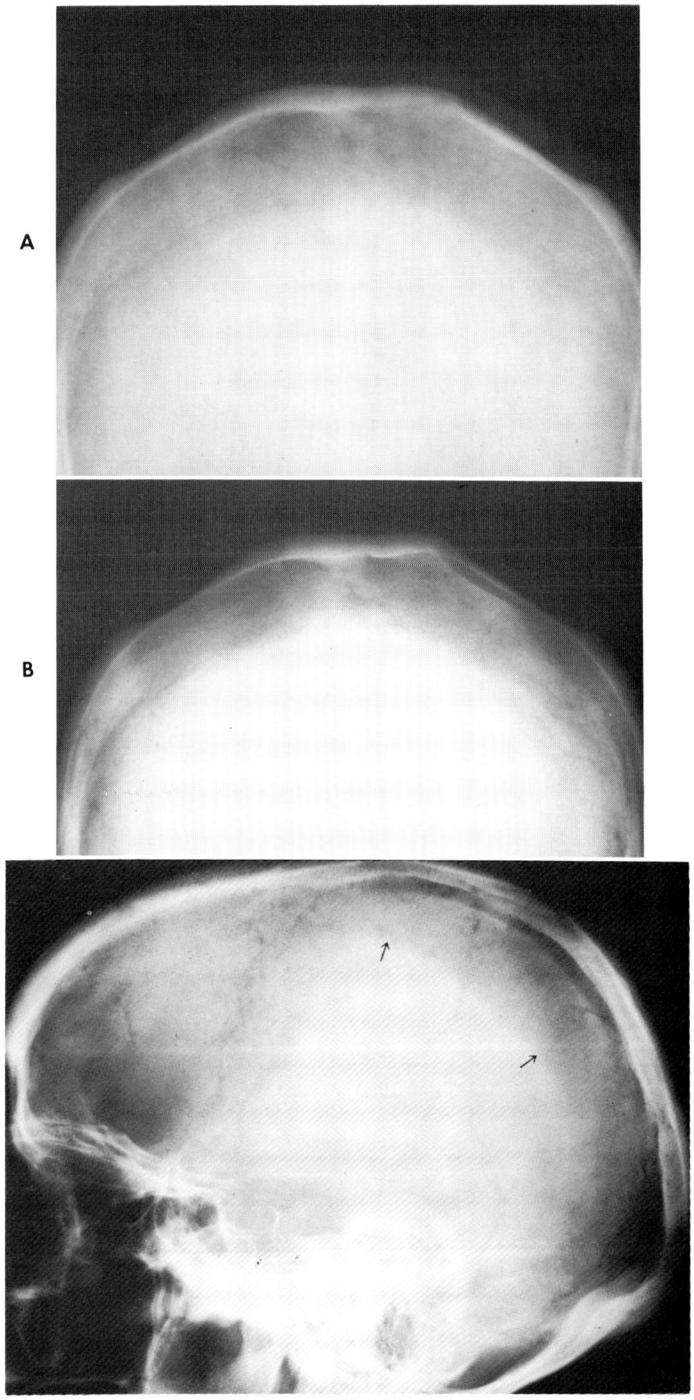

Fig. 11-101. Biparietal thinning. **A,** Thinning of outer aspect of vault in 58-year-old patient whose skull is composed essentially of compact bone. **B,** Same patient 73 years of age with further loss of bone. **C,** Lateral view shows that entire length of parietal bone (arrows) is involved.

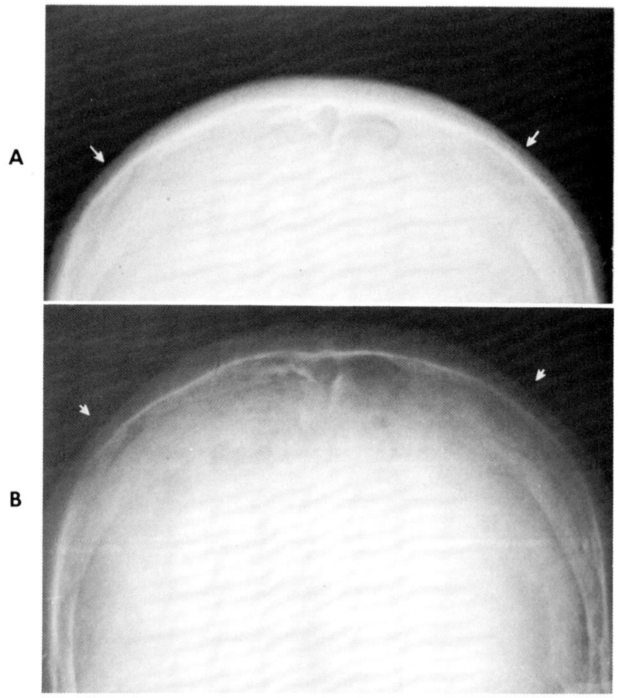

Fig. 11-102. Biparietal thinning. **A,** Minimal but definite thinning of outer table (arrows) along convexity of both parietal bones in 42-year-old woman with diploic skull. Middle table is intact. **B,** Same patient 18 years later with classic biparietal thinning.

(Fig. 11-103). This condition has not yet been surveyed but seems to be a moderately frequent entity in any age group. Sporadic and familial instances have been observed (Figs. 11-104 and 11-105). As in biparietal thinning, flat or groovelike depressions are noted. In this condition the outer table is also primarily affected and

A

B

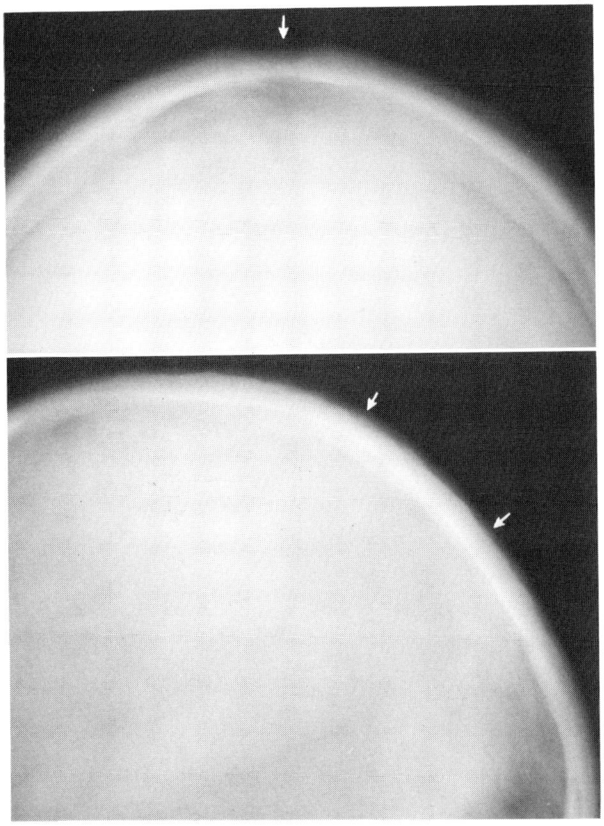

Fig. 11-103. Interparietal thinning. **A,** Smooth depression of superior aspect of cranial vault in 33-year-old woman. Either hypoplasia or atrophy of outer table is seen along midline (arrow). **B,** Superior and posterior aspects appear corrugated on lateral projection.

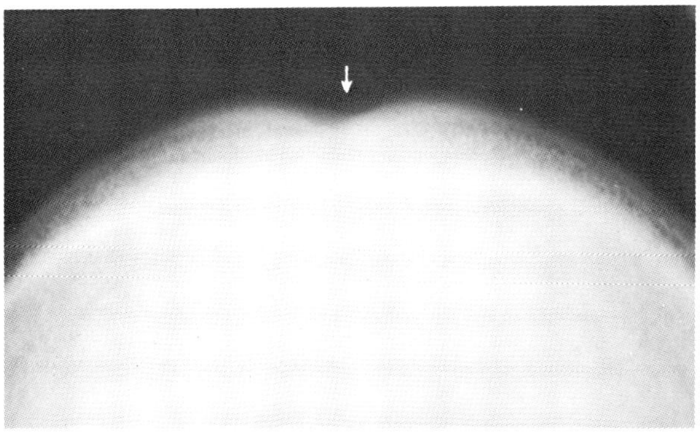

Fig. 11-104. Interparietal thinning. Deep midline groove (arrow) of outer table along sagittal suture in 29-year-old woman whose sister showed similar anomaly. Note that the outer table is rather thick on each side of the depression.

is thin or hypoplastic. With advancing age, atrophic changes appear in the diploe.

Whenever the local blood supply has been modified by *trauma* or surgery, the outer table atrophies. The outer table can disappear over a considerable distance adjacent to a craniectomy or in a bone flap (Fig. 11-106). This atrophy should not be mistaken for craniocerebral erosion.

Hypertrophic changes

Hypertrophy of the outer table alone is a rare phenomenon and is mainly observed in *old healed fractures* of the skull. The callus is usually linear and appears as a bony ridge, which differentiates this condition from osteoma.

Mixed changes

Mixed changes are most uncommon along the outer table. They are observed in *fibrosing osteitis,* a rare complication of skull fractures. The changes probably result

A

B

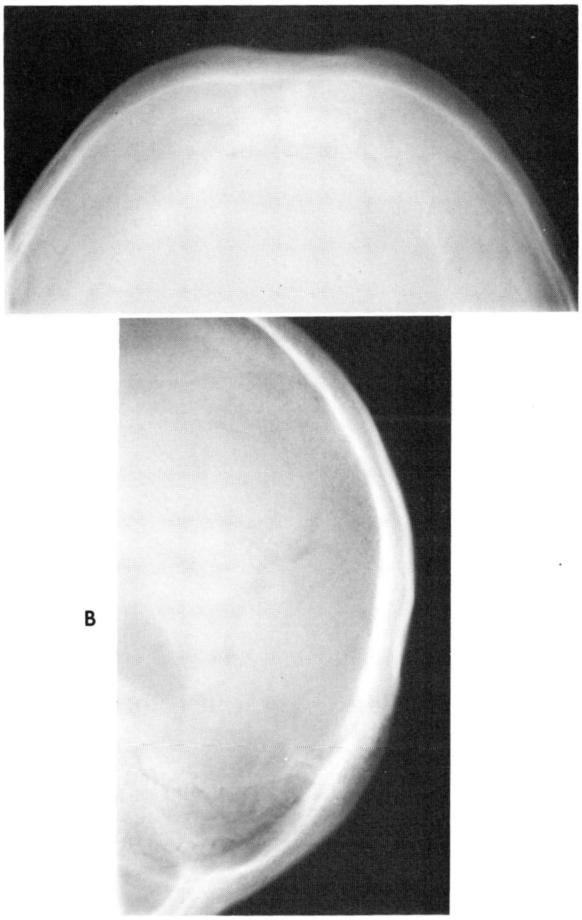

Fig. 11-105. Interparietal thinning and neurofibromatosis. **A,** Flat depression of superior aspect of skull in 13-year-old patient. **B,** Notched appearance of skull on lateral view.

A 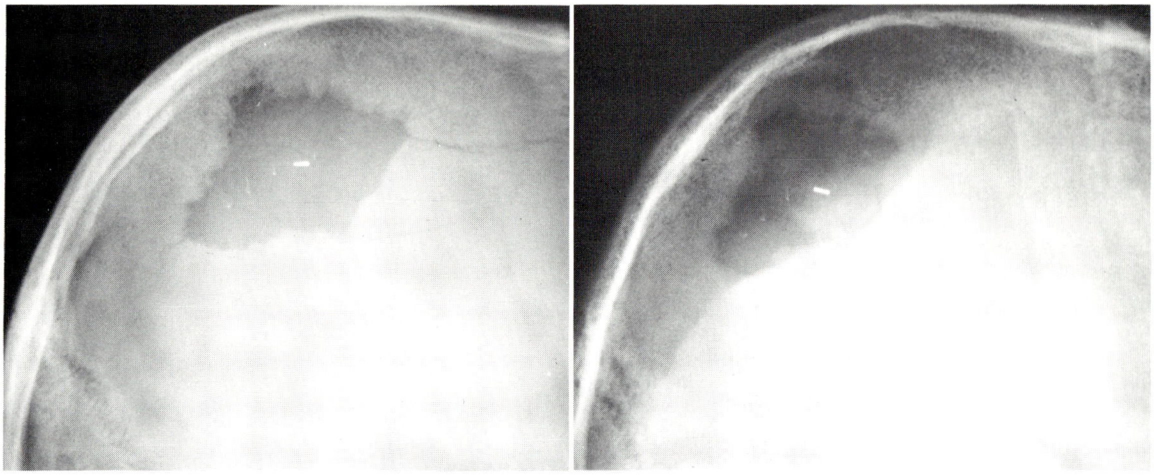 B

Fig. 11-106. Old craniectomy, posttraumatic atrophy. **A,** Depressed fracture and craniectomy at age 7 years. **B,** Partial healing of craniectomy at age 30 years; but in front of and behind operative site, the outer table is atrophied. This atrophy must be differentiated from craniocerebral erosion, which affects primarily the inner table.

A B C 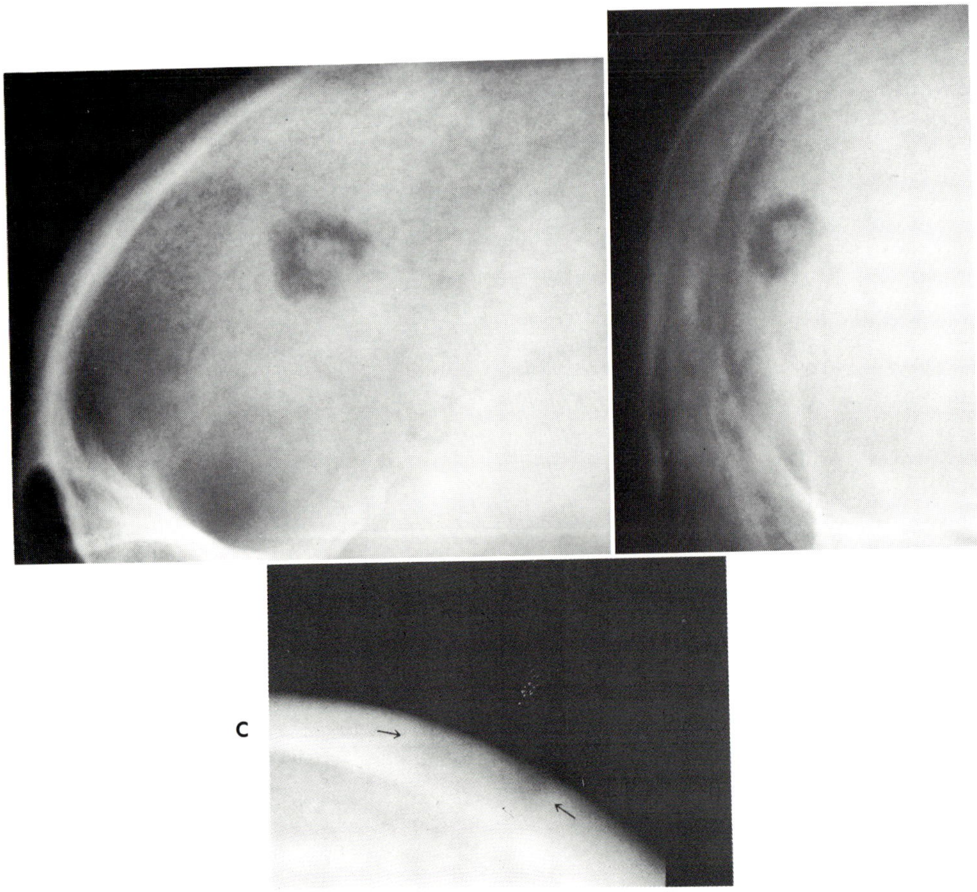

Fig. 11-107. Fibrosing osteitis. **A** and **B,** Standard views show well-localized destructive lesion associated with minimal marginal sclerosis and a pedunculated fragment of bone. **C,** Tangential view shows that destructive or reparative process is affecting primarily the outer table, but is also extending into the diploe (arrows). Bony fragment is a partially isolated segment of outer table.

A

B

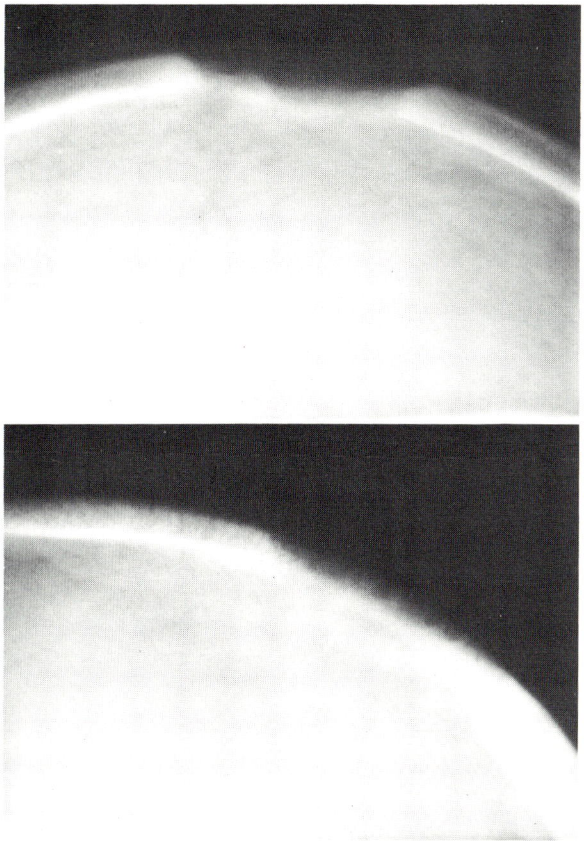

Fig. 11-108. Osteitis fibrosa. **A,** Frontal and, **B,** lateral views show extensive destruction of medial aspect of left parietal bone, with outer table showing maximal destruction. Note the sclerotic edges.

A

B

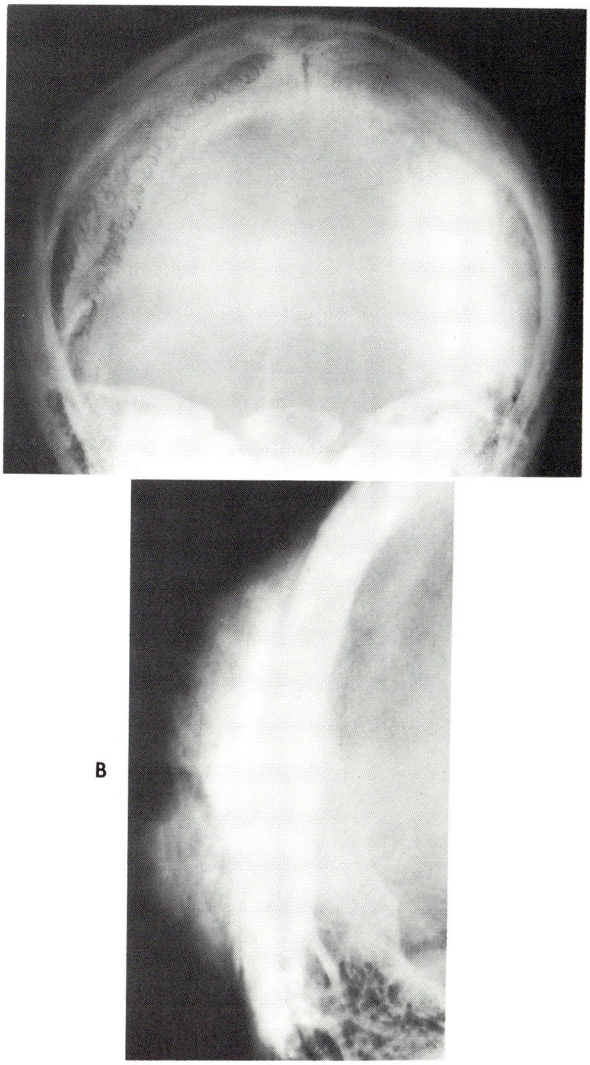

Fig. 11-109. Periosteal osteogenic sarcoma. **A,** Extensive hyperostosis of left occipital squama. **B,** Tangential view localizes the hyperostosis to outer table but, in addition, shows it to be uneven in both density and shape. Possibly the initial lesion was a benign osteoma that underwent sarcomatous changes.

from vascular necrosis, with secondary degeneration of bone into fibrous tissue. Usually some swelling of the scalp at the site of the previous injury is associated with destruction of the outer table. Minimal sclerosis exists around the edges, and a sequestrum may be seen in the center (Fig. 11-107). The bone alterations may be extensive, and all three tables may be destroyed. Destruction is maximal, however, along the outer table, and consequently the edges of the lesion are beveled in a characteristic manner from outside in (Fig. 11-108). Mixed changes may also be seen in tumors such as *periosteal osteosarcomas.* These lesions, although mainly osteoblastic, usually show poorly calcified zones of neoplastic tissue along their surface (Fig. 11-109).

All three tables

Extensive changes in the three tables of the cranial vault are common in infectious and tumorous processes. The diagnostic problem with these lesions is not so much their size or extension as their site of origin. This problem has been stressed in the preceding pages and will not be repeated under this heading.

Other specific conditions exist, however, in which the three tables are involved simultaneously and characteristic changes are usually seen on initial skull examinations.

Erosive changes

Total erosion in one area of the cranial vault is the result either of extrusion of intracranial contents or of intrusion of an extracranial process. Along the midsagittal plane, erosions of this type are mainly caused by meningoceles, meningoencephaloceles, or dermoids. In *meningoceles* and in *meningoencephaloceles* the margins of the eroded area are frequently raised and beveled. The edges may be lined with compact bone (Fig. 11-

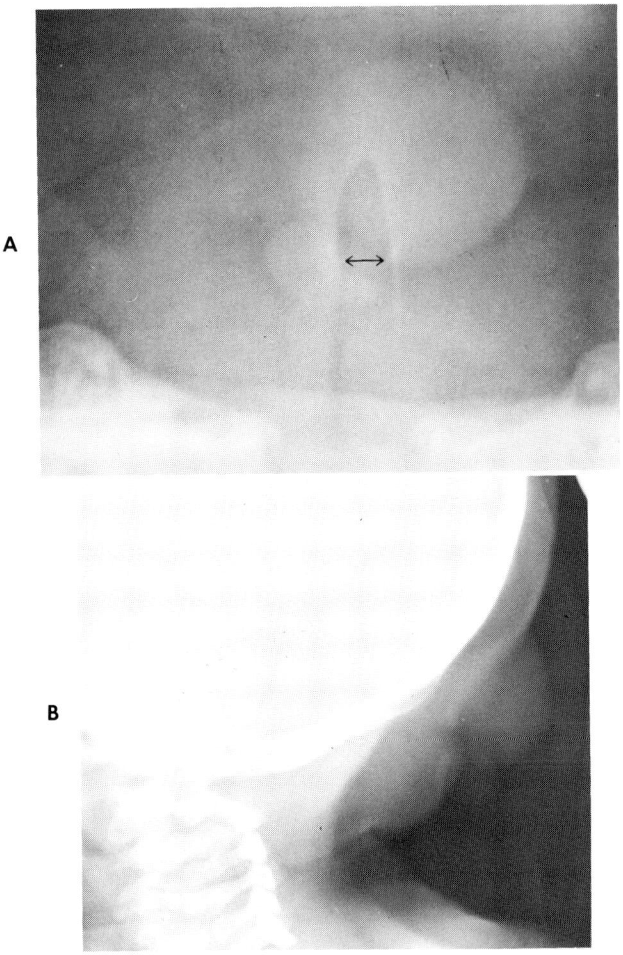

Fig. 11-110. Occipital meningocele. **A,** Midline triangular opening in occipital bone (double arrow) with well-corticated edges. Superimposed lobulated mass is extracranial in location, **B.**

110). An extracranial mass is readily seen in these cases.

Similar osseous changes are observed in intracranial *dermoids* except that the erosion is well demarcated with compact bone. It is usually funnel shaped, and the opening in the outer table is wider than in the inner table. When the cranial vault is thin, the erosion has parallel borders instead of being funnel shaped (Fig. 11-111).

Osteolytic changes

Diffuse destruction of the vault tables is occasionally seen in *hyperparathyroidism* (Fig. 11-112). The appearance is that of severe osteoporosis, more striking in diploic than in compact skulls. Early in the disease the cranial vault changes are more difficult to evaluate than those in the fingers or mandible. Consequently they are not usually looked for; but their recognition in unsuspected hyperparathyroidism is important.

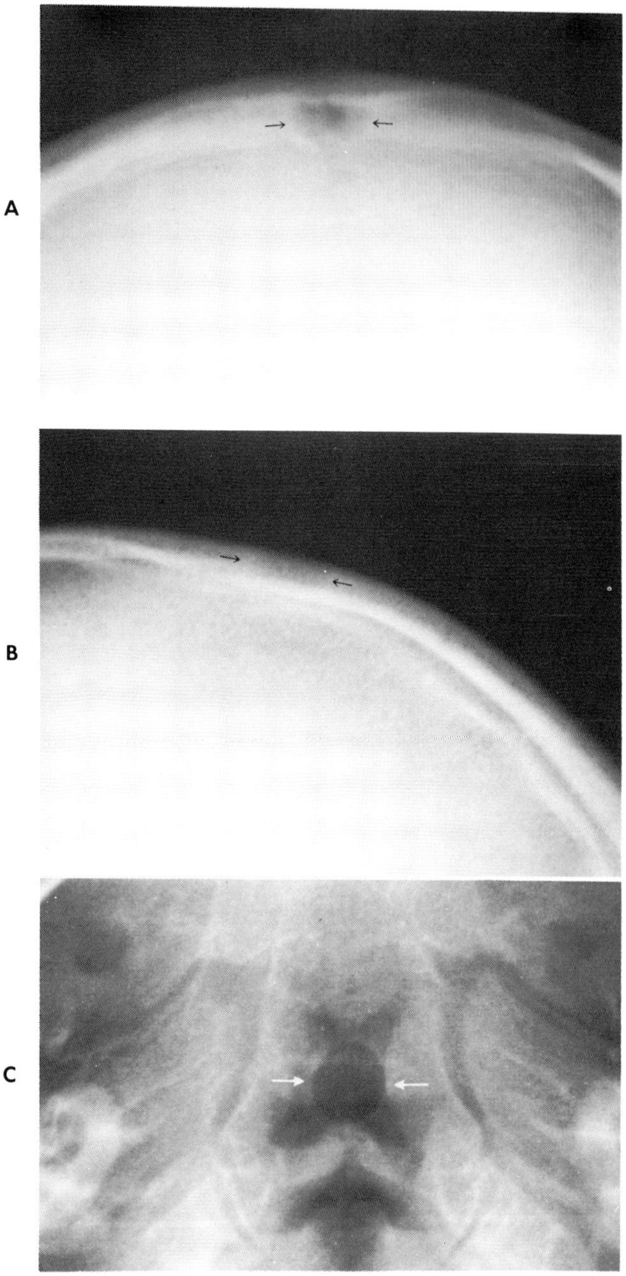

Fig. 11-111. Intracranial dermoid. **A** and **B,** Midline round well-demarcated opening through entire thickness of cranial vault at vertex. **C,** This is best seen on basal projection, which provides a frontal view of the anomaly (arrows).

Osteoblastic changes

Diffuse sclerosis and thickening of the cranial vault tables are usually manifestations of generalized forms of dysostoses such as advanced *tuberous sclerosis.*

Atrophic (hypoplastic) changes

Of the changes that affect the three tables simultaneously, atrophic changes are the most common and, of course, the most readily appreciated.

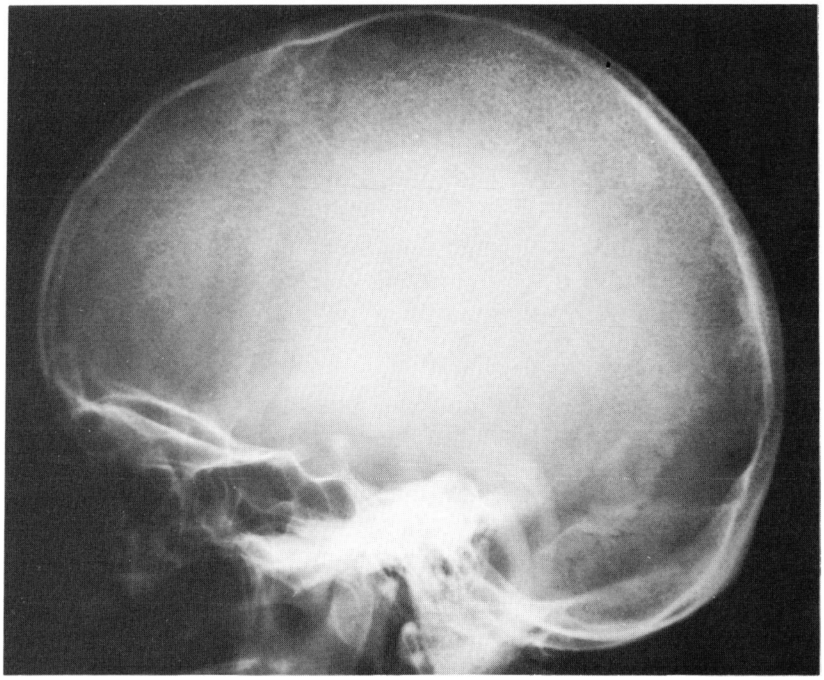

Fig. 11-112. Hyperparathyroidism. Mild diffuse osteoporotic changes of entire vault. Consequently the diploe stands out rather strikingly.

One of the most interesting diagnostic features of *neurofibromatosis* is the absence of bone formation along the sutures. These zones of bone deficiency are of various sizes and have irregular contour and thin beveled edges (Fig. 11-113). The sutural edges of the lesion are characteristically serrated, and the bone around the lesions is of normal texture. Palpation of the skull reveals soft areas that can be depressed where bone is missing. These calvarial lesions are similar in nature to the dysplasia of the greater wing of the sphenoid, which is also another feature of neurofibromatosis. Both seem to be related to a mesenchymal defect, which prevents the formation of bone in specific areas. Microscopic evidence of neurofibromatosis may be shown along the bony edges of the vault lesions (Saha et al., 1969). Previous reports indicate quite clearly, however, that neither the orbit nor the vault lesions result from overlying neurofibromas (Hunt and Pugh, 1961; Burrows, 1963).

Absence of bone is also a feature of *enlarged parietal foramina.* The foramina are secondary to a faulty ossification of the parietal fontanelle. Early in life the parietal fontanelle forms a single opening along the sagittal suture that later divides into two parts as the cranial vault grows and ossifies. The parietal fontanelles are situated on both sides of the sagittal suture at the junction of the posterior and middle thirds of the parietal bone. The site is the same in which parietal foramina are observed (Fig. 11-114). This developmental abnormality may be associated with deficient ossification of the lateral portions of the clavicles (Eckstein et al., 1963).

Similar perforations, the result of old *burr holes,* may be seen in the parietal bones. Usually, however, these are more lateral and posterior in location than are enlarged parietal foramina (Fig. 11-115). Their edges are usually beveled and smooth, but they may become irregular when the burr hole is partially filled with new bone formation. Changes along the bony margins of old craniectomies are identical (Fig. 11-116).

With *chronic intracranial hypertension* the cranial vault becomes diffusely atrophied (Fig. 11-117). As the vault enlarges, it becomes progressively thinner. This thinning is commonly observed early in life in such conditions as aqueduct stenosis and communicating hydrocephalus.

Hypertrophic changes

Remarkable but still poorly understood changes take place in the skull of *acromegalics.* A diffuse increase in thickness of the cranial vault of these patients seems to be produced by a relative hypertrophy of each table (Fig. 11-118). Which table will be affected most is impossible to predict since the thickness varies in different patients. The increase appears to be greatest in the outer table, less in the inner table, and least in the diploe. Hypertrophy of the cranial vault may continue even after complete surgical removal of the pituitary tumor. This progressive thickening appears then to result from a massive overgrowth of the middle table, partly at the expense of the outer and inner tables.

Generalized increase in thickness of the vault is also

A

B

C

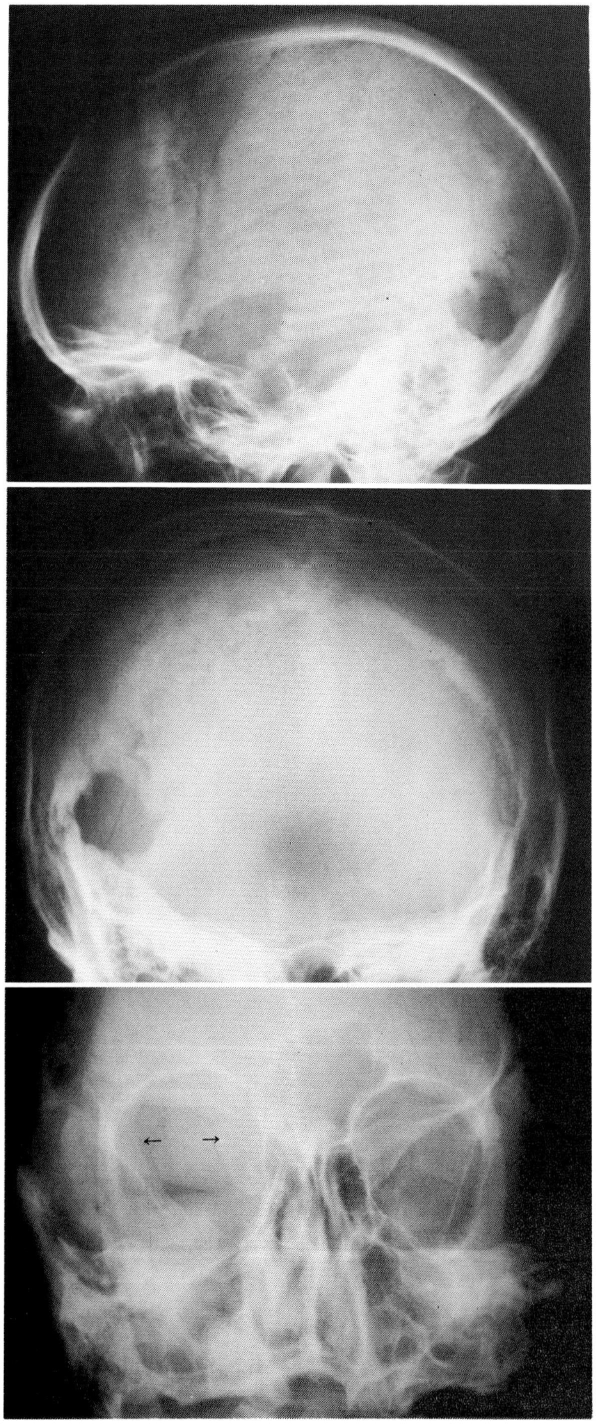

Fig. 11-113. Neurofibromatosis. Congenital areas of bone aplasia along right occipital and squamosal sutures, **A** and **B**, associated with hypoplasia of right greater wing, **C**. These findings are characteristic.

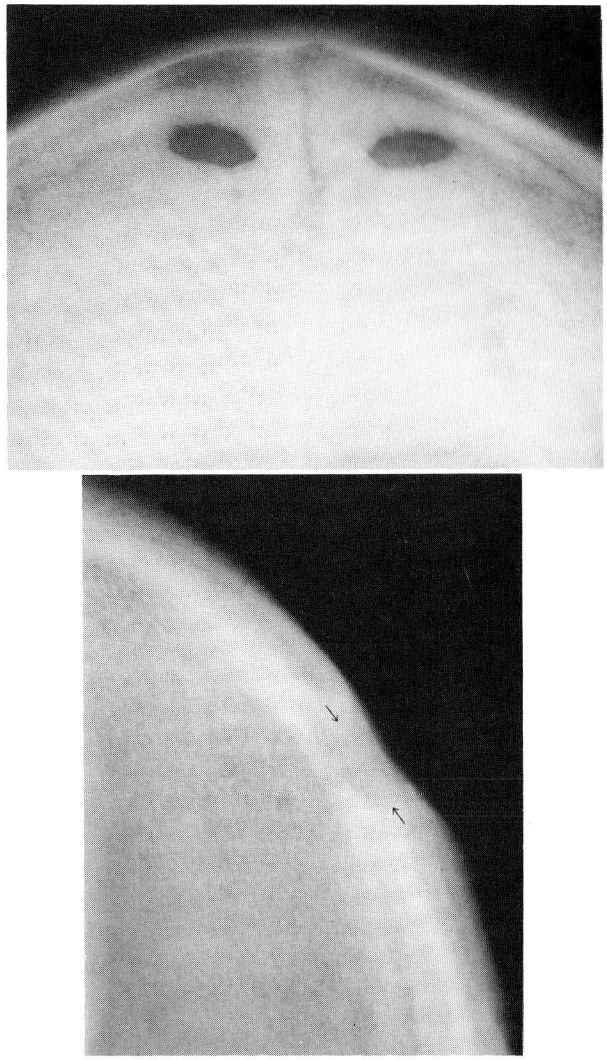

Fig. 11-114. Parietal fontanelles. Symmetric openings near midline in posteromesial aspects of parietal bones (arrows).

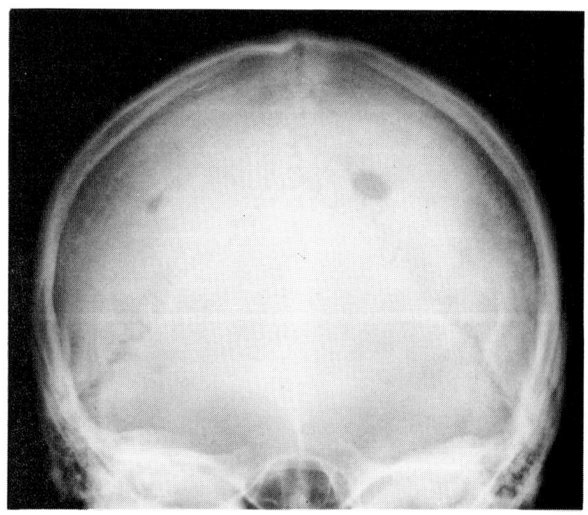

Fig. 11-115. Burr holes. Asymmetric openings of parietal bones, too posterior and too lateral to correspond to enlarged parietal foramina (parietal fontanelles).

A 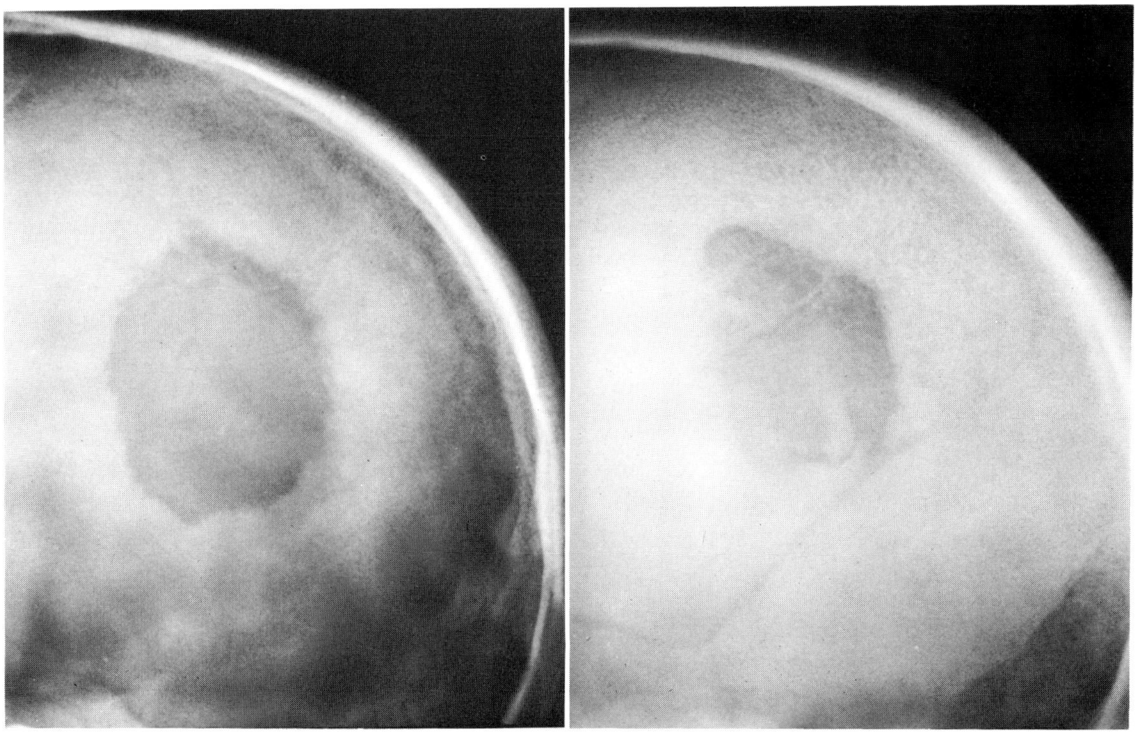 B

Fig. 11-116. Old craniectomy. **A,** Area of surgically removed bone in right parietal bone is partially filled in with new bone 14 years later, **B.**

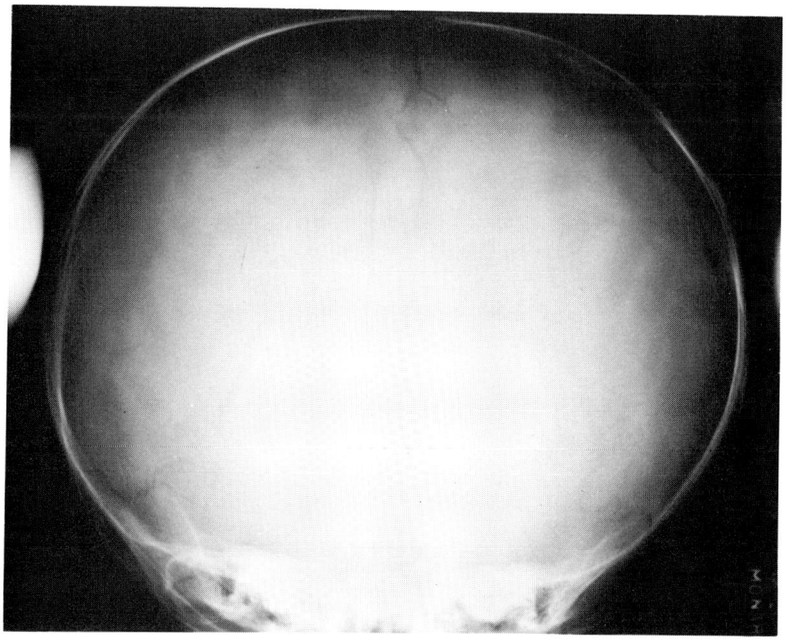

Fig. 11-117. Aqueduct stenosis. Thin enlarged vault in low-grade chronic intracranial hypertension.

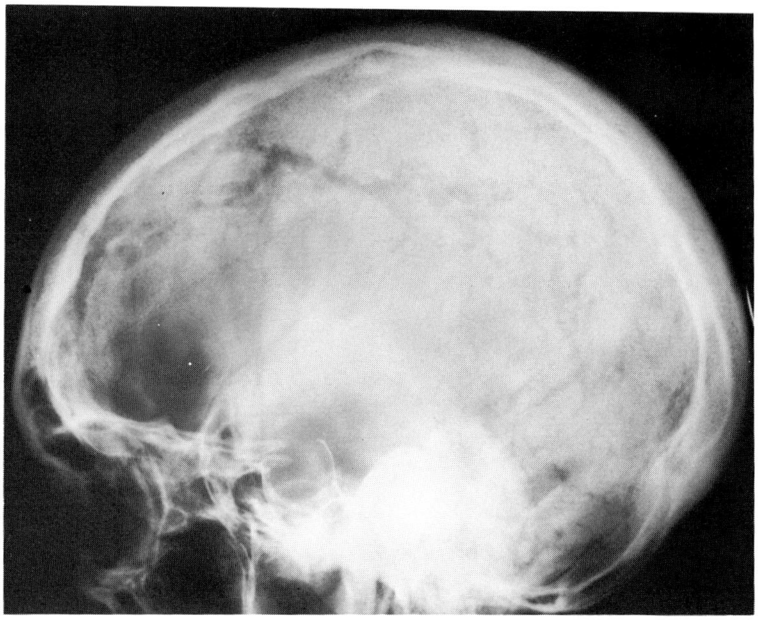

Fig. 11-118. Acromegaly. Moderately thick cranial vault is result of hypertrophy of all tables.

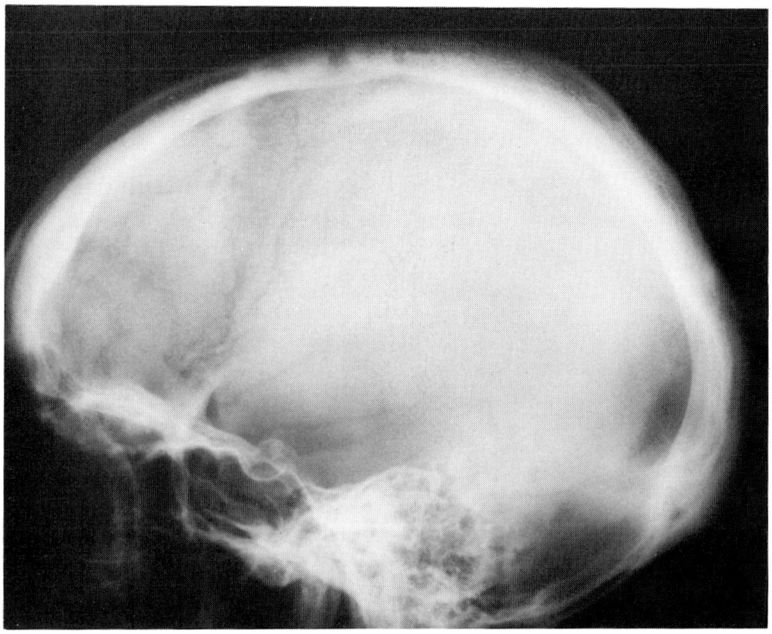

Fig. 11-119. Dystrophia myotonica. Generalized increase in thickness of cranial vault as well as marked hypertrophy of inner table.

seen in *dystrophia myotonica* (Di Chiro and Caughey, 1960). In this condition the thickness of the outer and middle tables is not increased as much as that of the predominantly affected inner table (Fig. 11-119). Hyperostosis frontalis interna may also be present, but this is considered a coincidental association.

Progressive increase in thickness of the cranial vault is expected after the *relief of raised intracranial pressure* (Figs. 11-13 and 11-14). The changes, which are fairly rapid, appear first along the inner table, which becomes thicker. Then the middle table grows, mainly at the expense of the thickened inner table. After an interval of between 8 and 12 months, the vault regains a normal thickness. The degree of cerebral damage caused by the intracranial hypertension determines whether the vault may remain normal or continue to thicken. The cranial vault thickens also in the *healing phase of rickets,* but the hypertrophic changes are most marked along the

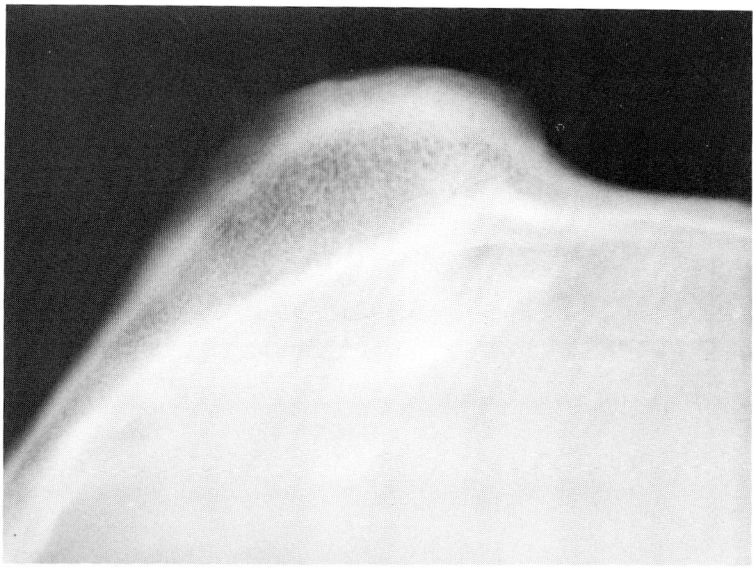

Fig. 11-120. Juvenile subgaleal hematoma. Superior frontal exostosis has developed over period of 20 years after scalp laceration and hematoma. Note the focal expansion of the diploe and the thick outer and inner tables.

outer table. The frontal squama or the parietal bones are usually affected.

Rather striking hypertrophic changes of the cranial vault can be seen in the rare persistent *cephalhematomas* or in *juvenile subgaleal hematomas* (Fig. 11-120). First, the fluid collection is organized; later it is completely incorporated within the vault by the induced bone reaction. Remodeling takes place, and the tables, predominantly the middle one, become thicker.

Mixed changes

Diffuse mixed changes are best observed in *Paget's disease*. Analysis of the changes in the vault in this condition reveals a specific involvement of each table in most cases. The changes are initiated in the middle table, which is thicker than normal and in which extensive reorganization has taken place. As the normal bony trabeculae disappear, the diploe is replaced progressively by areas of bone destruction and bony nodules. These nodules are poorly ossified and ill defined. They are seen mainly along the inner aspect of the middle table, where they pile up on the inner table. The changes in the outer layer of the middle table are mainly destructive. The inner table, on the diploic side, becomes hyperostotic, whereas the outer table becomes atrophic. Consequently the inner half of the vault in this disease is much more dense than the outer half (Fig. 11-121). When sarcomatous changes develop, they usually disrupt this pattern. As in fibrous dysplasia, increased tortuosity and size of the meningeal grooves is a frequent observation in Paget's disease.

Localized mixed changes may be found in *intracranial dermoids*. These changes consist of small irregular areas of bone destruction associated with pitted areas of sclerosis (Fig. 11-122). They result partly from the intraosseous portion of the lesion and partly from low-grade inflammation. Best appreciated on stereoscopic views, these curious osseous changes are usually associated with minute linear or curvilinear intracranial calcifications, indicating a cystic underlying lesion. The changes are characteristic of this condition, although not pathognomonic.

CONCLUSION

In conclusion, detailed thoughtful analysis of the radiologic changes caused by cranial lesions or anomalies is most informative. Time should not be lost trying to guess the nature of the lesion on the basis of incomplete examinations. Instead adequate information should be obtained by means of tangential views or other necessary projections. Optimum results are achieved when the radiologist himself positions the patient and at the same time examines the patient. The table from which the lesions arise must be determined since this knowledge will greatly influence the choice of the final diagnosis. Descriptive terms such as calvarial defects or areas of increased density do not reflect any specific pathology. They are used too freely to designate a wide variety of lesions and most of the time are used in too elusive a manner. As much information as possible should be obtained from the roentgenograms, and the changes thereon should be defined precisely by adequate scientific terminology.

Three-dimensional examinations are helpful, since

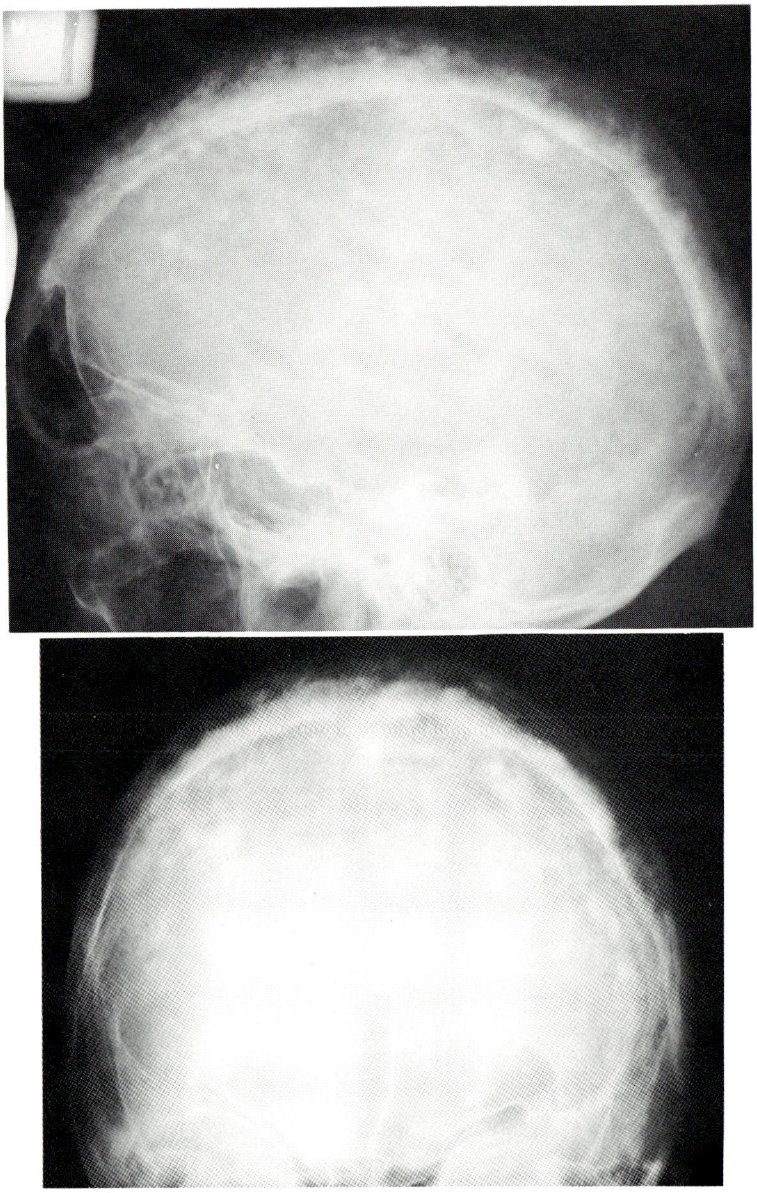

Fig. 11-121. Paget's disease. Classic appearance of skull in this condition. Note the accumulation of the bony nodules along the inner aspect of middle table and the marked osteoporotic changes in the outer aspect of that table. Inner table becomes hyperostotic, whereas outer table becomes atrophic.

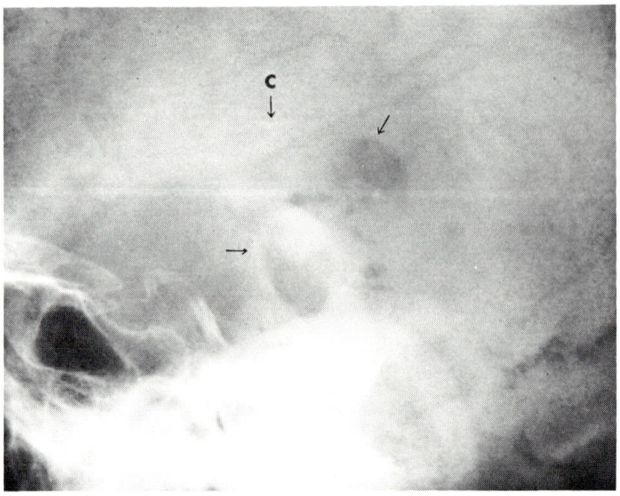

Fig. 11-122. Intraosseous and intracerebral dermoid. Partially osteolytic and osteoblastic changes in right temporal squama associated with extremely fine, linear, intracranial calcification (arrows). These findings, when observed, are quite typical of the lesion. *C,* Calcification.

direct observation of the lesion is achieved and comparison with other areas facilitated.

In dealing with cranial vault lesions, the close relation that exists between the skull, the meninges, and the brain should always be in mind. Intracranial diseases may be reflected by specific osseous changes, and in that respect the cranial vault differs from other bones and offers a greater diagnostic challenge.

REFERENCES

Burrows, E. H.: Bone changes in orbital neurofibromatosis, Brit. J. Radiol. **36**:549-561, 1963.

Camp, J. D., and Nash, L. A.: Developmental thinness of the parietal bones, Radiology **42**:42-47, 1944.

Di Chiro, G., and Caughey, J. E.: Skull changes in eighteen cases of dystrophia myotonica, Acta Radiol. **54**:22-28, 1960.

Dorst, J. P.: Functional craniology: an aid in interpreting roentgenograms of the skull, Radiol. Clin. N. Amer. **2**:347-366, 1964.

Dyke, C. G., Davidoff, L. M., and Masson, C. B.: Cerebral hemiatrophy with homolateral hypertrophy of the skull and sinuses, Surg. Gynec. Obstet. **57**:588-600, 1933.

Eckstein, H. B., Chir, M., and Hoare, R. D.: Congenital parietal "foramina" associated with faulty ossification of the clavicles, Brit. J. Radiol. **36**:220-221, 1963.

Gray, H.: Anatomy, descriptive and applied, ed. 34, London, 1967, Longmans, Green & Co., Ltd.

Ham, A. W., and Leeson, T. S.: Histology, ed. 4, Philadelphia, 1961, J. B. Lippincott Co.

Hunt, J. C., and Pugh, D. G.: Skeletal lesions in neurofibromatosis, Radiology **76**:1-20, 1961.

Keats, T. E., and Holt, J. F.: The calvarial "doughnut lesion": a previously undescribed entity, Amer. J. Roentgen. **105**:314-318, 1969.

Lagos, J. C., Holman, C. B., and Gomez, M. R.: Tuberous sclerosis: neuroroentgenologic observations, Amer. J. Roentgen. **104**:171-176, 1968.

Leeds, N., and Seaman, W. B.: Fibrous dysplasia of the skull and its differential diagnosis: clinical and roentgenographic study of 46 cases, Radiology **78**:570-582, 1962.

Lin, J. P., Goodkin, R., Chase, N. E., and Kricheff, I. I.: The angiographic features of fibrous dysplasia of the skull, Radiology **92**:1275-1280, 1969.

Lindblom, K.: A roentgenographic study of the vascular channels of the skull with special reference to intracranial tumors and arterio-venous aneurysms, Acta Radiol., supp. 30, pp. 1-146, 1936.

Moore, S.: Hyperostosis cranii, Springfield, Ill., 1955, Charles C Thomas, Publisher.

Morel, F.: L'hyperostose frontale interne. Syndrome de l'hyperostose frontale interne avec adipose et troubles cérébraux, Geneva, 1929, Chapalay & Mottier.

McRae, D. L.: Observations on craniolacunia, Acta Radiol. **5**:55-64, 1966a.

McRae, D. L.: The role of radiology in the management of the head-injured patient. In Caveness, W. F., and Walker, A. E., editors: Head Injury Conference Proceedings, Philadelphia, 1966b, J. B. Lippincott Co.

Patriquin, H., Melancon, D., Bertrand, G., and Ethier, R.: Epidermoids of the fourth ventricle, J. Canad. Ass. Radiol. **20**:37-43, 1969.

Pendergrass, E. P., Schaeffer, J. P., and Hodes, P. J.: The head and neck in roentgen diagnosis, Springfield, Ill., 1956, Charles C Thomas, Publisher.

Penfield, W., and Jasper, H.: Epilepsy and the functional anatomy of the human brain, Boston, 1954, Little, Brown & Co.

Perou, M. L.: Cranial hyperostosis, Springfield, Ill., 1964, Charles C Thomas, Publisher.

Rosenbaum, A. E., Rossi, P., Schechter, M. M., and Sheehan, J. P.: Angiography of haemangiomata of the calvarium, Brit. J. Radiol. **42**:682-687, 1969.

Saha, M. M., Agarwal, K. N., and Bhardwaj, O. P.: Calvarial bone defects in neurofibromatosis, Amer. J. Roentgen. **105**:319-321, 1969.

Salmi, A., Voutilainen, A., Holsti, L. R., and Unnerus, C. E.: Hyperostosis cranii in a normal population, Amer. J. Roentgen. **87**:1032-1040, 1962.

Schunk, H., and Maruyama, Y.: Two vascular grooves of the external table of the skull which simulate fractures, Acta Radiol. **54**:186-194, 1960.

Stewart, R.: Hyperostosis frontalis interna: its relation to cerebral atrophy, J. Ment. Sci. **87**:600-607, 1941.

Taveras, J. M.: Multiple progressive intracranial arterial occlusions: a syndrome of children and young adults, Amer. J. Roentgen. **106**:235-268, 1969.

Testut, J. L., and Latarjet, A.: Traité d'anatomie humaine, Paris, 1949, Gaston Doin & Cie, vol. 2.

Traub, S. P.: Roentgenology of intracranial meningiomas, Springfield, Ill., 1961, Charles C Thomas, Publisher.

Yuhl, E. T., and Schmitz, A. L.: The occipital emissary channel and increased intracranial pressure, Acta Radiol. **9**:124-127, 1969.

CHAPTER 12

Cranial sutures and fontanelles

Charles A. Gooding

NORMAL SUTURES AND FONTANELLES

Appearance in neonate

The soft membranous bones of the neonatal calvarium lie in an incompletely mineralized capsule. Each is separated by strips of connective tissue—sutures (Latin *sutura,* seam)—and more broad and irregular patches of connective tissue—fontanelles (French *fontanelle,* little fountain). The connective tissue of the sutures and fontanelles is continuous with the pericranium on the outer surface of the skull. On the inner surface it is continuous with the dura mater. Because of these elastic pliable intervals, the skull may be molded as necessary during the birth of the child (Fig. 12-1).

The suture that unites the frontal bone with the two

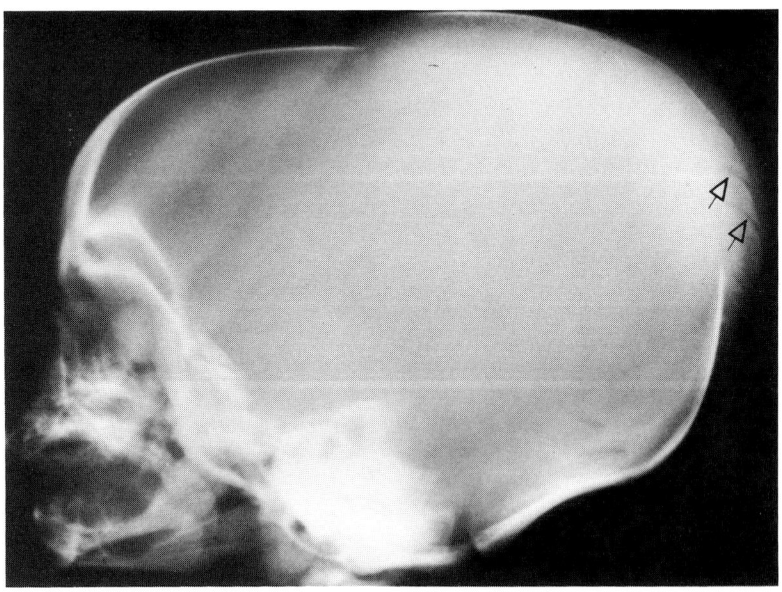

Fig. 12-1. Overriding parietal bone in normal newborn skull. This transient phenomenon is secondary to molding process that occurs during normal deliveries. Incidental note is made of small fissures in parietal bone (arrows), which are another variant of normal.

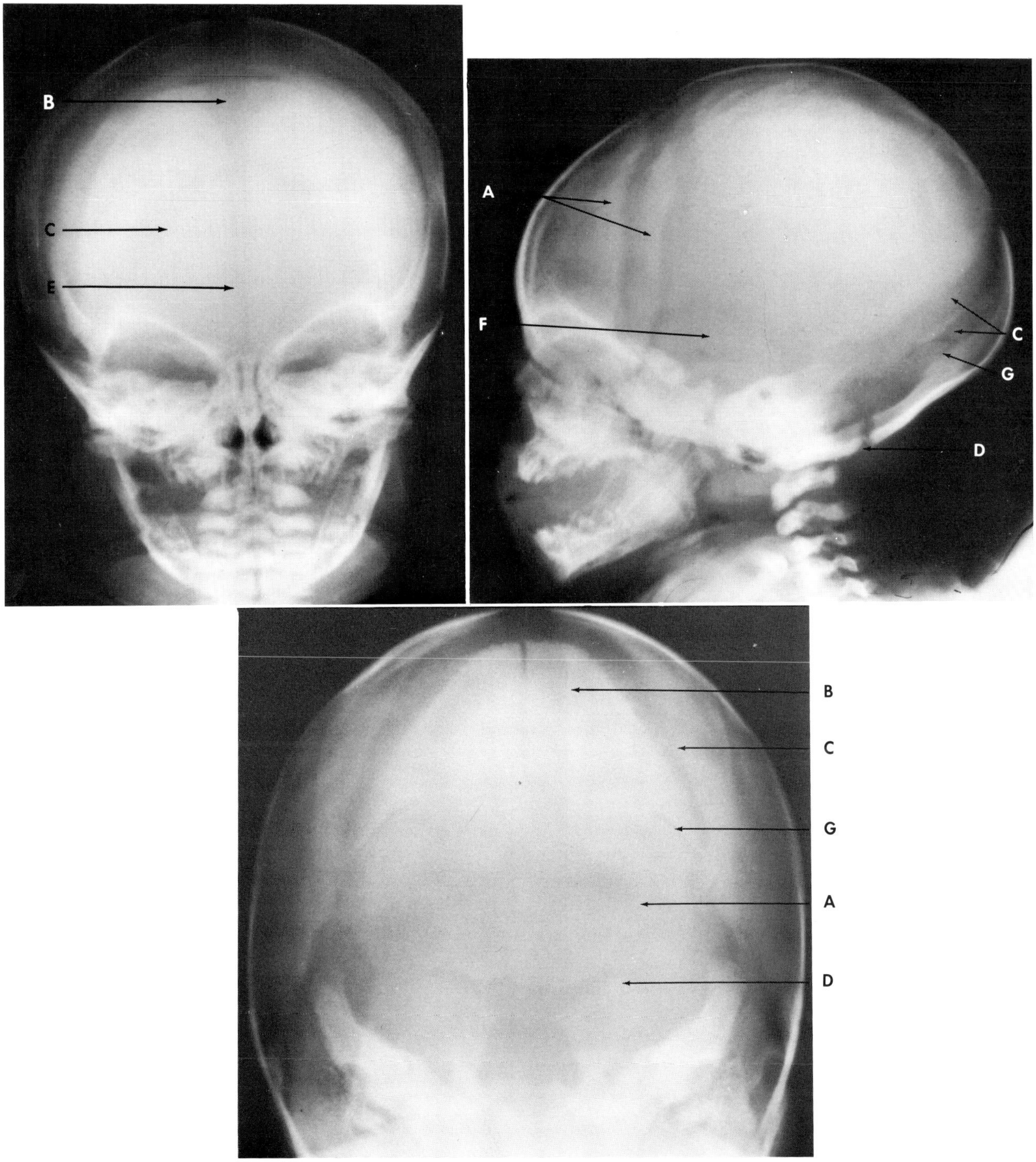

Fig. 12-2. Normal newborn skull, anteroposterior, lateral, and half-axial projections. *A,* Coronal suture; *B,* sagittal suture; *C,* lambdoid suture; *D,* innominate synchondrosis; *E,* metopic suture; *F,* squamosal suture; *G,* mendosal suture.

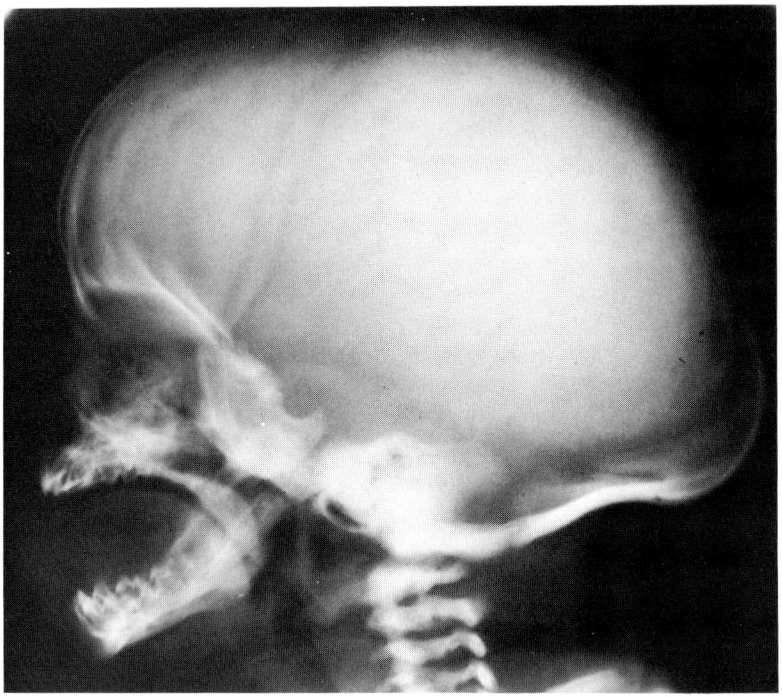

Fig. 12-3. Bathrocephaly in 2-week-old girl. Occipital bone bulges in posterior direction between mendosal suture and lambda. This bulging is a variant of normal and is of no clinical significance.

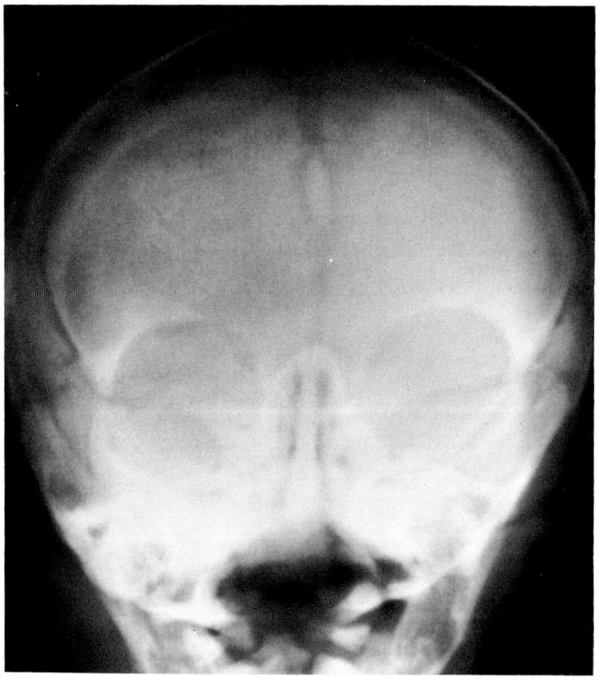

Fig. 12-4. Metopic sutural bone in newborn girl. Note the solitary ossification center in the metopic suture inferior to the anterior fontanelle.

parietal bones and arches across the skull from one side to the other is the coronal (Latin *corona,* crown or garland) (Fig. 12-2). The suture that unites the occipital bone to the two parietal bones is called the lambdoid suture. (It was so named because it looks like the Greek *lambda,* eleventh letter of the Greek alphabet.) The two parietal bones are separated by the sagittal suture (Latin *sagitta,* arrow). In a newborn skull the lambdoid suture, sagittal suture, and unossified anterior fontanelle resemble an arrow. The frontal bone is divided equally by a vertically oriented suture, called the frontal or metopic suture. The word is derived from the Greek *metōpon,* forehead (Torgerson, 1950).

The occipital bone of the neonate is comprised of four disjoined masses of bone that surround the foramen magnum. One of these masses is the *basiocciput,* which forms the clivus and the anterior margin of the foramen magnum. Another pair of masses consists of lateral or *exoccipital* bones separated from the basiocciput by a synchondrosis. The large *squamous* portion of the occipital bone forms the posterior margin of the foramen magnum and continues superiorly to the lambdoid suture (Fig. 12-5). This squamous portion is separated from the exoccipital bones by an innominate synchondrosis (Greek *syn,* together + *chondros,* cartilage). It is also semidivided in a transverse plane by the mendosal suture, which divides the occipital bone into a supraoccipital and an interparietal portion. The occipital bone occasionally manifests focal bulging asymmetry adjacent to the mendosal suture. This is referred to as bathro-

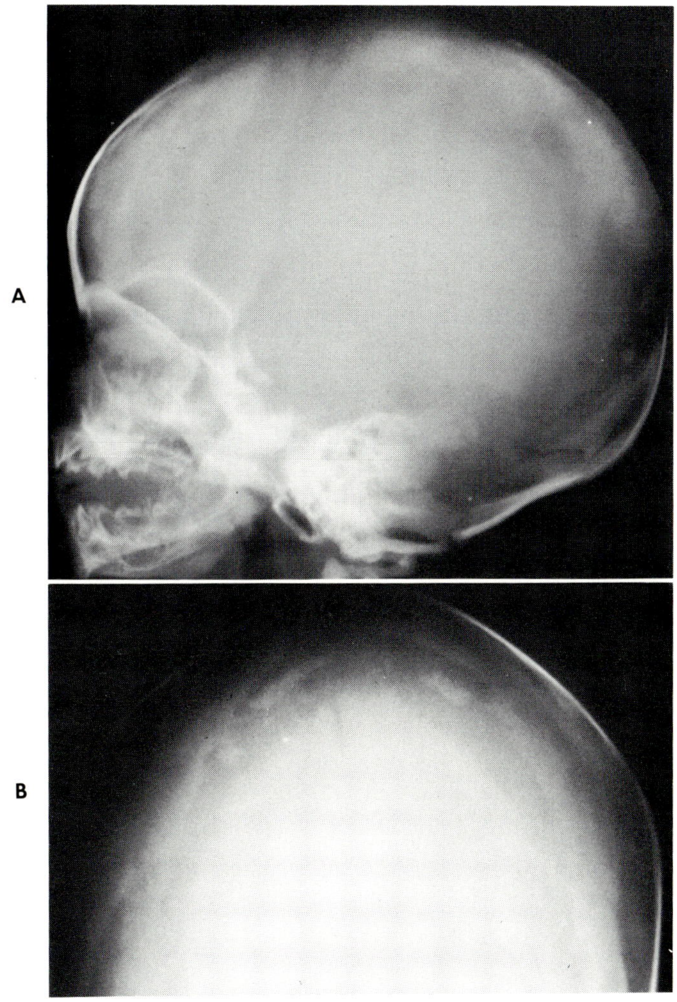

Fig. 12-5. Normal newborn boy. Several sutural bones or irregular foci of mineralization are present in lambdoid suture; this is a variant of normal.

cephaly (Greek *bathron,* step + *kephalē,* head) (Fig. 12-3). An occasional normal variant in the newborn skull is a persistent strip of connective tissue that forms a suture extending into the parietal bone, dividing the bone into a superior and an inferior portion. It is of no clinical significance and should not be mistaken for a fracture.

Below the parietal bone and extending into the base of the skull is the temporal bone. It is separated from the parietal bone by the squamosal suture (Latin *squama,* scale).

At birth, portions of the frontal and parietal bones at the bregma (i.e., where the sagittal suture meets the coronal suture) are not fully ossified and a diamond-shaped membranous area 3 cm in diameter, the anterior fontanelle, is present. An ossicle, called the anterior fontanelle bone, is occasionally seen within this fontanelle. It should not be mistaken for premature closure

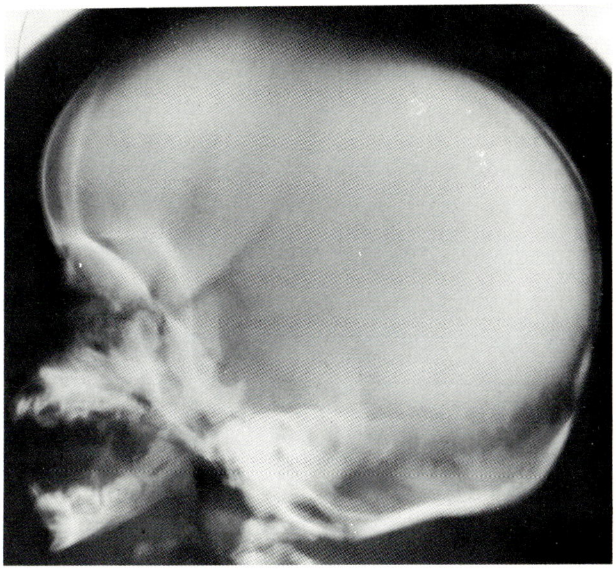

Fig. 12-6. Pyknodysostosis in 5-month-old boy. Solitary large interparietal bone is present at the lambda. Calvarium is inordinately dense.

of the fontanelle or fracture (Brown, 1961). Girdany and Blank (1965) found only five examples of such an entity recorded in the literature and described thirty-one examples. Nearly all of the children were boys, and in some this ossicle was not present at birth but developed later. Although usually single, the ossicles may be multiple. Sometimes a solitary bone is identified in the metopic suture (Fig. 12-4).

Early observers claimed that the anterior fontanelle increased in size from time of birth until about 9 months of age and then gradually closed. These observations have been challenged on the basis that the children studied were European children of the poorer classes, many with rickets (Acheson and Jefferson, 1954).

Fontanelles smaller than the anterior fontanelle sometimes are present along the midsagittal plane anterior and posterior to the diamond-shaped membranous area. A metopic fontanelle is seen sometimes anteroinferior to the anterior fontanelle, and the glabellar fontanelle occasionally is present inferior to this. Posterior to the anterior fontanelle, midway along the sagittal suture, is the parietal (sagittal) fontanelle, and at the lambda is the triangular shaped posterior fontanelle. Frequently, small irregularly shaped bones are seen in the lambda and along the lambdoid suture (Fig. 12-5). Some sutural bones persist within the suture and are not incorporated into the adjacent bone during mineralization and maturation. These are called wormian bones (after the Danish anatomist Oläus Worm). The largest of the sutural bones is the interparietal bone, which is triangularly shaped (Fig. 12-6). It merely represents the previously described interparietal portion of the occipital bone above the mendosal suture. A multitude of wormian bones are found in conditions associated with abnormal ossification, such as cleidocranial dysostosis, osteogenesis imperfecta, hypothyroidism, and hypophosphatasia.

A fetal wormian bone, which usually disappears by birth by completely fusing with the supraoccipital bone at the posterior margin of the foramen magnum, is called Kerckring's bone (Caffey, 1953). When seen at birth, it usually appears as an elongated process attached to the edge of the supraoccipital bone at the foramen magnum near the midsagittal plane. Several such cases, representing variants of midline sutural remnants, have been discussed by Franken (1969).

On each side of the neonatal skull may be seen the paired anterior lateral and posterior lateral fontanelles and the parietomastoid and temporosquamosal sutures, which join them.

Sutural width and closure

The membranous bone of the cranial vault is less dense than the cartilaginous bone of the skull base, and the thickness of its edges is gradually tapered. Because of thinness of the margins of bonc at the sutures, the sutural margins in neonates are often ill defined and difficult to see. When the bone edge is unusually well defined, follow-up examinations are indicated if the diagnosis of craniosynostosis in early infancy is to be established.

The width of the sutures in the neonate varies tremendously. In the lateral view the coronal and lambdoid sutures may be between 1.5 and 10 or 11 mm in diameter. In the half-axial view the sagittal and lambdoid sutures range from 3 mm in diameter to 17 and 11 mm respectively.

For evaluation of the width of sutures in children, Taveras and Wood (1964) expressed the belief that the most reliable measurement site is the top of the coronal sutures, as seen in the lateral view. In children older than 3 years, the width at the vertex should be less than 2 mm. In children between 2 and 12 months of age, it should not be more than 3 mm.

With increasing age, ossification of the skull causes the sutures and fontanelles to become narrower and smaller, until finally the latter are obliterated (Fig. 12-7). The velocity of this process varies in different individuals and may vary from side to side in the same individual's skull. The fontanelles are the first to close. The posterior, anterolateral, anterior, and posterolateral fontanelles are closed by 8 weeks, 3 months, 15 to 18 months, and 2 years respectively. Closure of the anterior fontanelle marks the disappearance of the last remnant of the membranous calvarium. After closure the skulls of the child and the adult are similar in most respects.

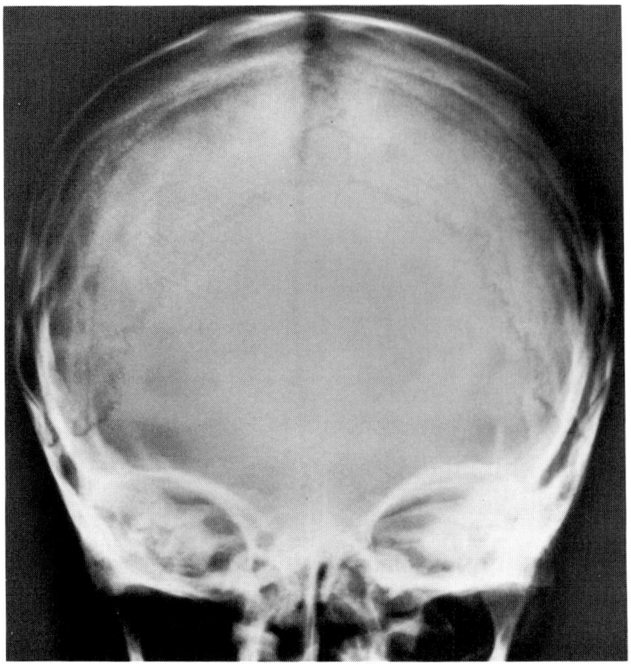

Fig. 12-7. Normal skull in 4-year-old child. Compare with Fig. 12-2 and note that the sutures are much more narrow and the fontanelles are closed.

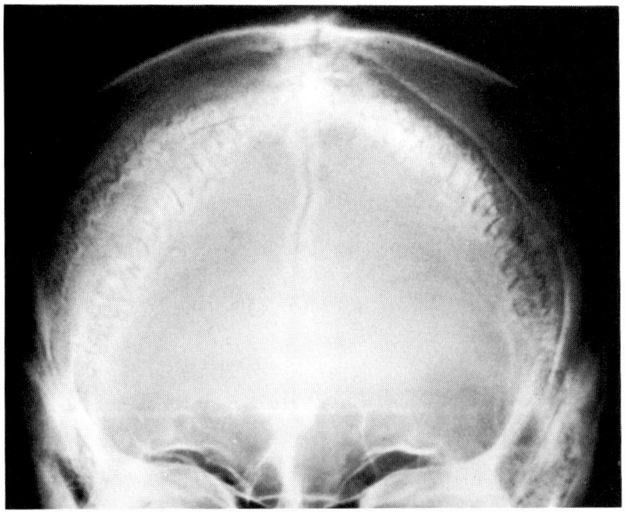

Fig. 12-8. Normal skull in 25-year-old patient. Note the perisutural sclerosis, which is a normal variant at this age.

The first suture to close is the mendosal suture, which closes several weeks after birth. The metopic suture begins to close in the second year and is usually completely obliterated during the third year; in about 10% of cases, it persists throughout life. When the metopic suture persists, either partially or completely, it may be distinguished from a fracture by its slight interdigitations. Sometimes there is a perisutural density of condensed bone (Fig. 12-8). When this suture continues inferiorly to the lower portion of the frontal bone, the frontal sinuses do not develop as usual.

The fissure between the exoccipital and the supraoccipital portions of the occipital bone (innominate synchondrosis) disappears during the second or third year. The coronal, lambdoid, and sagittal sutures all persist throughout infancy, childhood, adolescence, and early adulthood. They do not close until about the age of 30 years.

The term *double suture line* refers to the roentgenographically demonstrated superimposition in the adult skull of the normal interdigitating external portion of any suture and its corresponding straight portion of the inner table (Fig. 12-9). This appearance may be interpreted erroneously as a fracture. The difference between the sutures of the outer and the inner table is greatest in the sagittal suture and in the medial portions of the coronal and lambdoid sutures (Fig. 12-10).

The serrated nature of the lambdoid suture can best be appreciated by examination of a disarticulated specimen of the occipital bone (Fig. 12-11). Multiple inter-

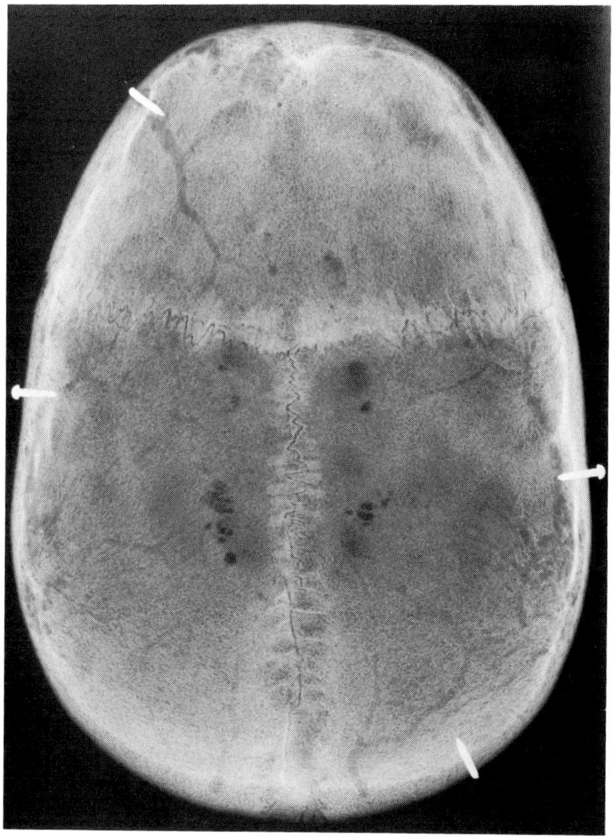

Fig. 12-9. Roentgenogram of skull vault specimen illustrates double suture line. Note that traversing the serpiginous suture, which represents sutural course on the outer portion of the vault, is a somewhat eratic linear lucency, which represents the suture on the inner aspect of vault.

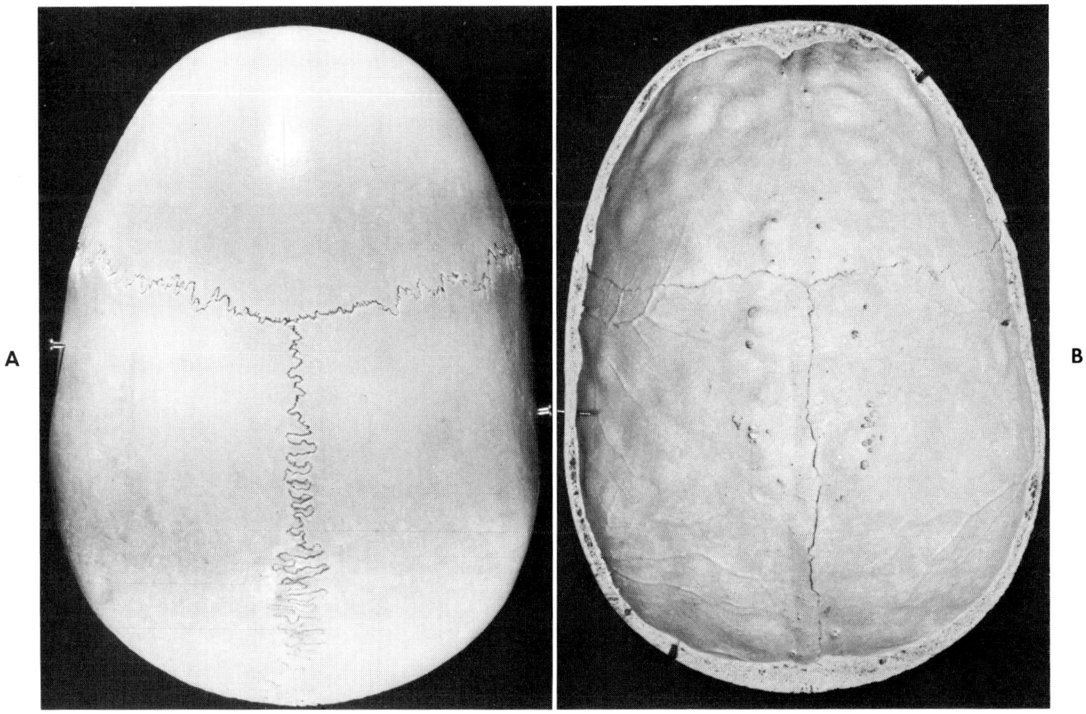

Fig. 12-10. A, Specimen of calvarium, outer surface. Note the serpiginous erratic course of the coronal and sagittal suture. **B,** Same specimen, inner surface. Sagittal and coronal sutures are less tortuous.

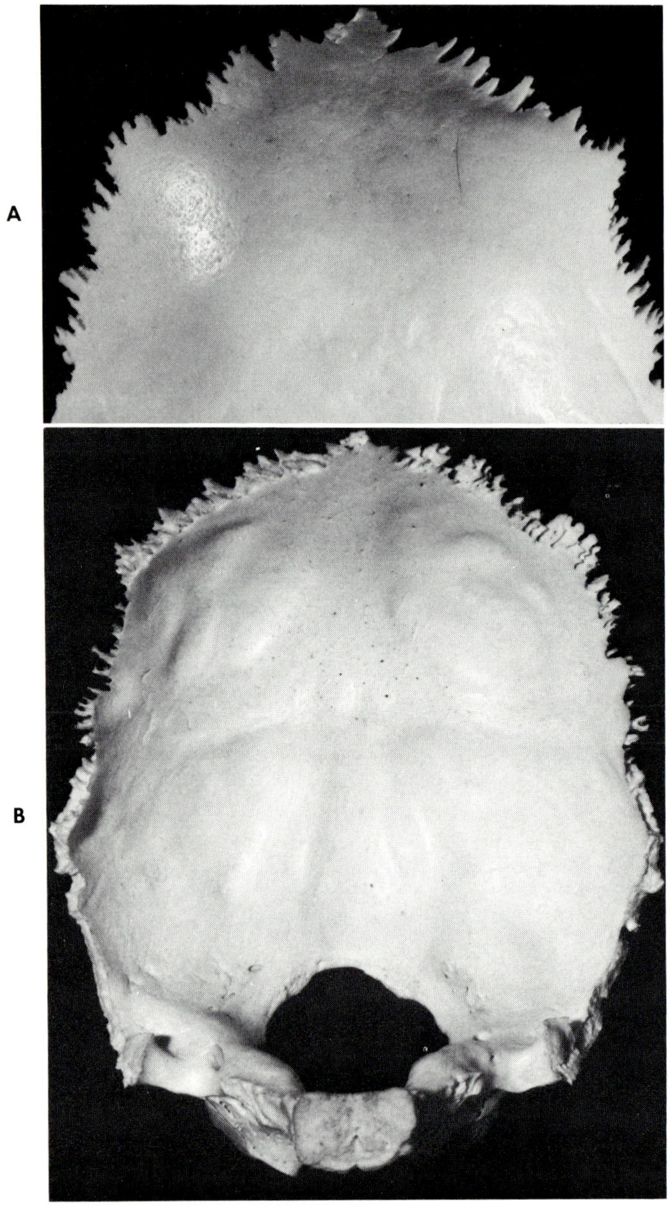

Fig. 12-11. Disarticulated specimen of occipital bone. A, External surface. B, Internal surface. Note the serpiginous irregular nature of the occipital bone at the lambdoid suture.

digitations with focal bony excrescenses serve to unite the occipital bone with the parietal bones at the lambdoid suture.

ABNORMAL SUTURE CLOSURE

Premature craniosynostosis

Premature craniosynostosis refers to fusion across the suture line, which appears in utero, in infancy, or in childhood (Andersson and Gomes, 1968). It results in obliteration of the involved suture and synostosis (Greek *syn,* together + *osteon,* bone) of the juxtaposed bone segments.

Historically, premature closure of the cranial sutures was described by Hippocrates; but the first important publication on the condition was that of Virchow in 1852. He ascertained that growth of the skull perpendicular to the suture that had been fused was impaired and that growth took place parallel to that suture. This phenomenon became known as Virchow's law (Freeman and Barkowf, 1962).

Primary premature craniosynostosis

Premature craniosynostosis has been classified by Duggan and co-workers (1970) according to the outline below.

*Classification of premature craniosynostosis (PCS)**

I. Primary (simple, idiopathic, isolated, true) PCS
  A. Brachycephaly (short head)—premature bilateral closure of the coronal and/or the lambdoid sutures
  B. Scaphocephaly (boat head), dolichocephaly (long head)—premature closure of the sagittal suture
  C. Plagiocephaly (oblique head)—unilateral premature closure of the coronal and/or lambdoid sutures
  D. Trigonocephaly (triangular head)—premature closure of the metopic suture
  E. Oxycephaly, acrocephaly, turricephaly (pointed head)—premature closure of all sutures
II. Secondary PCS
  A. PCS as a part of other known syndromes
    1. Crouzon's disease (craniofacial dysostosis)
    2. Apert's syndrome (acrocephalosyndactyly)
    3. Carpenter's syndrome (acrocephalopolysyndactyly)
    4. Treacher-Collins syndrome (mandibulofacial dysostosis)
    5. Craniotelencephalic dysplasia
    6. Orbital hypotelorism, arhinencephaly, trigonocephaly
    7. Kleeblattschädel—deformity syndrome (cloverleaf skull)
  B. PCS in association with other conditions
    1. Metabolic diseases
      a. Rickets
      b. Idiopathic hypercalcemia
      c. Gargoylism
      d. Hyperthyroidism
    2. Bone dysplasias and dysostoses
      a. Hypophosphatasia
      b. Achondroplasia
      c. Metaphyseal dysostosis
      d. Rubinstein-Taybi syndrome
      e. Mongolism
      f. Dysplasia of bone associated with hyperostosis
    3. PCS after ventriculovenous shunts
    4. PCS in association with microcephaly
    5. Hematologic disorders
      a. Congenital hemolytic icterus
      b. Polycythemia vera
      c. Sickle cell disease
      d. Thalassemia major
    6. Miscellaneous associated malformations

*From Duggan, C. A., Keever, E. B., and Gay, B. B.: Secondary craniosynostosis, Amer. J. Roentgen. 109:277-293, 1970.

The primary type of this process is the most common and is considered a disorder of the membranous bones of the skull or their anlage. Advanced stenosis of the cranium, with increased intracranial pressure and exophthalmos, has been seen to develop when the sutures were still open. Actual synostosis did not take place until many months later. These changes suggest that the synostosis is a result of a primary resistance to stretching of the preosseous membranous sutures.

Carefully designed animal experiments led Moss (1959) to conclude that the primary morphologic event in premature synostosis is malformation of the skull base. He expressed the opinion that positional disarrangement of the points of basal attachment of the dura prevented normal responses of the neural capsule to the forces of the growing brain. The same dural alteration predisposes to premature fusion of the suture. Therefore the fusion is a result, and not a cause, of the cranial malformation. Subsequent calvarial changes postnatally are obligatory changes, secondary to redirection of forces of brain growth.

The possibility exists that the primary disease in craniostenosis is not limited to the cranial mesenchyme but is widespread in the body. This possibility is based on the descriptions of associated defects, such as syndactylism (Park and Powers, 1920), biliary atresia, and congenital heart disease in these patients. Shillito and Matson (1968) in a review of 519 patients with craniosynostosis found multiple abnormalities in 13%. Most frequently these abnormalities were in patients with multiple synostosis, particularly when both coronal sutures were involved.

Primary premature craniosynostosis is more common in the male, and the ratio of males to females has been stated to be as high as 5:1. In the Boston series (Shillito and Matson, 1968) only sixty-three of 289 patients with sagittal synostosis were girls. By contrast, seventy-six of the 127 patients with synostosis of one or both coronal sutures were girls. In this entire series there were only three Negroes; all others were Caucasian. There is a familial tendency to premature synostosis, but the mode of inheritance is not known. Sagittal synostosis was seen approximately five times as frequently as the next common category of suture closure. Single coronal and bilateral coronal closures were almost equal in incidence, and many other much less frequent combinations were noted.

The radiologic recognition of premature craniosynostosis is based on the alteration in shape of the skull vault and also on the intrinsic appearance of the sutures. The prematurely closed suture may have just a small focal segment where fusion has occurred and the remainder of the suture may otherwise appear open. Therefore the entire extent of all sutures must be adequately visualized when roentgenograms of the skull are examined for premature craniostenosis.

Continued bone growth adjacent to the suture line in instances of premature craniostenosis alters the normal tapered appearance at this site to a squared or heaped up configuration that may be recognized in the neonate. This overgrowth sometimes can be clinically palpable as a hard ridge of bone along the suture. When the suture is finally closed, this ridge often disappears.

In contradistinction to the often asymmetric head shape of premature craniostenosis, the infant with microcephaly as a result of failure of normal brain growth manifests a normal shape to the head. Although the su-

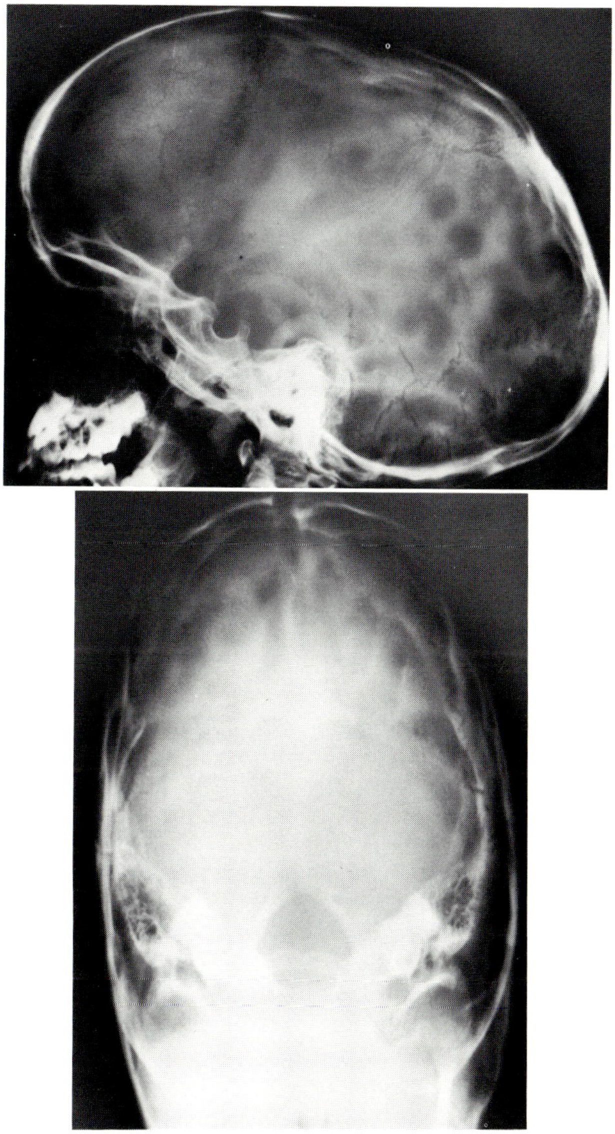

Fig. 12-12. Sagittal craniosynostosis in 9-year-old boy. Calvarium is markedly dolichocephalic because of premature closure of sagittal suture. Coronal, lambdoid, and squamosal sutures are normal.

tures may not taper, generally they are not fused. In some cases of microcephaly, however, the sutures may actually fuse. Focal thickening of the vault at the suture margins, as is seen in premature craniostenosis, is not seen in instances of microcephaly.

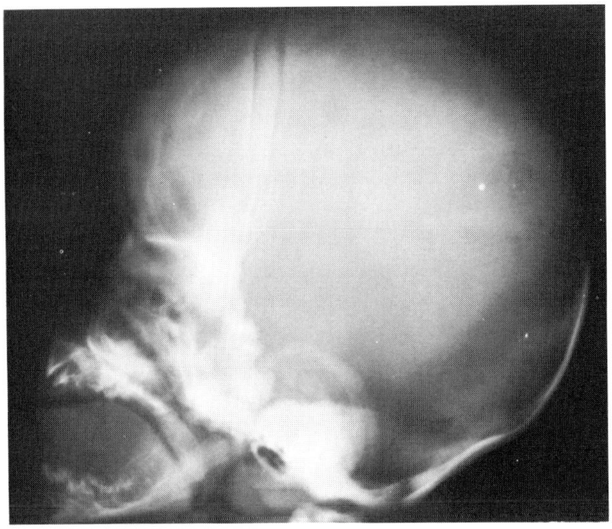

Fig. 12-13. Bilateral coronal craniosynostosis in 3-week-old girl. Note the narrowed coronal sutures with sclerosis at their margins; compare this appearance with the more normal-appearing lambdoid suture. Calvarium is brachycephalic.

Any description of craniosynostosis should include precise details regarding the suture or sutures involved and the quantitation of the degree of closure. General terms describing premature craniosynostosis, however, have been used for classic descriptive purposes.

When only the sagittal suture is involved (Fig. 12-12), the head is elongated and narrow and is termed dolichocephalic (Greek *dolichos,* long + *kephalē,* head) or scaphocephalic (Greek *skaphē,* skiff) because it resembles the upturned keel of a boat. A short segment of synostosis in the sagittal suture may produce the same degree of craniosynostosis as does involvement of the entire suture.

A brachycephalic (Greek *brachys,* short) type of craniosynostosis is produced by premature closure of the coronal or lambdoid sutures. With bilateral coronal synostosis the frontal fossa is markedly foreshortened and both orbits are oblique (Hope et al., 1955) (Fig. 12-13). Not to be confused with brachycephalic craniosynostosis is postural flattening of the posterior aspect of the skull. This flattening is acquired in early infancy from prolonged recumbency in the supine position and is a longstanding pressure phenomenon. It is most likely in infants neglected in cribs, or in defective infants with little head movement. Infants with inordinately soft skulls, as in osteogenesis imperfecta or rickets, also acquire such flattening.

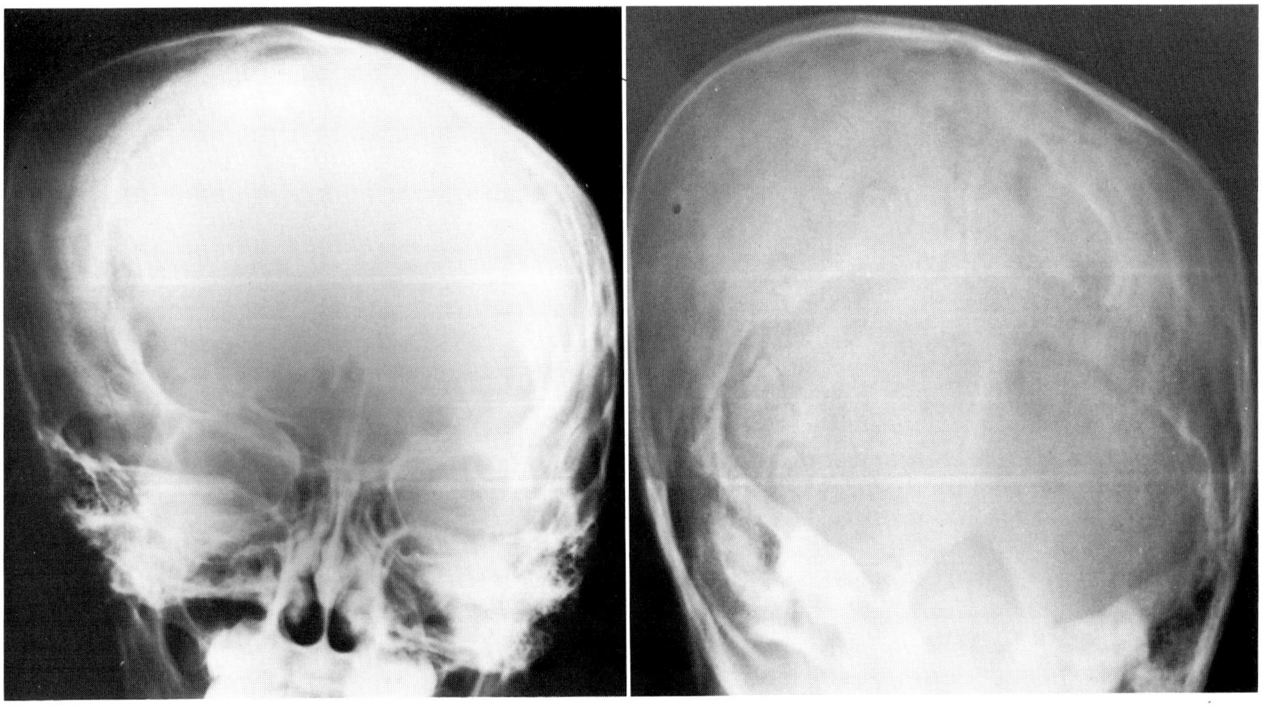

Fig. 12-14. Left coronal craniosynostosis in 2-year-old girl. There is harlequin appearance to left orbit, and superior orbital fissue on the left is elevated. Flattening of left parietal bone is caused by redirected brain growth.

Plagiocephaly (Greek *plagios,* oblique) is an irregularly shaped skull and results from unilateral coronal or lambdoid craniosynostosis (Fig. 12-14). It also occurs with generalized craniosynostosis when the sutures close at different times. Synostosis of one coronal suture prevents forward migration of the frontal bone on that side. Consequently a flattening is produced on the affected side and an apparent exaggeration of the frontal boss on the normal side. The flattened forehead is usually accompanied by a more prominent eye because of the associated orbital involvement. The involved orbit is shallow and oblique. In older children plagiocephaly must be differentiated from other conditions associated with focal calvarial expansion such as large subdural hematomas or hygromas.

Fauré and his co-workers (1967) reported nine cases of unilateral coronal craniosynostosis in which the clinical and radiologic features were described. In the frontal projection the orbit on the affected side was enlarged and elliptic and the lesser wing of the sphenoid was elevated. In addition, the innominate line of the greater wing of the sphenoid was displaced outward, and the nasal septum was inclined obliquely to the involved side (Figs. 12-15 and 12-16).

A grotesque trilobed skull results from hydrocephalus that is associated with intrauterine combined synostosis of the coronal and lambdoid sutures. The increased intracranial pressure produces bulging at the sagittal suture and squamosal sutures and has been called cloverleaf skull or Kleeblattschädel (Angle et al., 1967; Feingold et al., 1969). In these infants the ears are displaced downward, proptosis or exophthalmos is severe, and facial deformities are similar to those of craniofacial dysostosis. Deformities of the long bones, which resemble achondroplasia, have been described in many of the patients.

When the sagittal and coronal sutures are obliterated, the skull elongates vertically, a condition termed oxycephaly or acrocephaly. Because of the shallow orbits, it is often associated with marked exophthalmos. Syndactylism and polydactylism of the hands and feet frequently accompany this form (Table 12-1) (Cooper, 1953; Pfeiffer, 1964; Palacios and Schimke, 1969).

When the metopic suture fuses prematurely, trigonocephaly (Greek *trigonos,* triangular) results (Fig. 12-17). A sharp bony ridge runs down the center of the frontal bone along the metopic suture. The suture is well defined in profile on a submentovertical view of the skull. Trigonocephaly may be associated with hypotelorism and hypoplasia of the frontal lobes; but this is not always true. Some patients with trigonocephaly have normal brains (Currarino and Silverman, 1960). Furthermore, in milder cases, the trigonocephaly may regress.

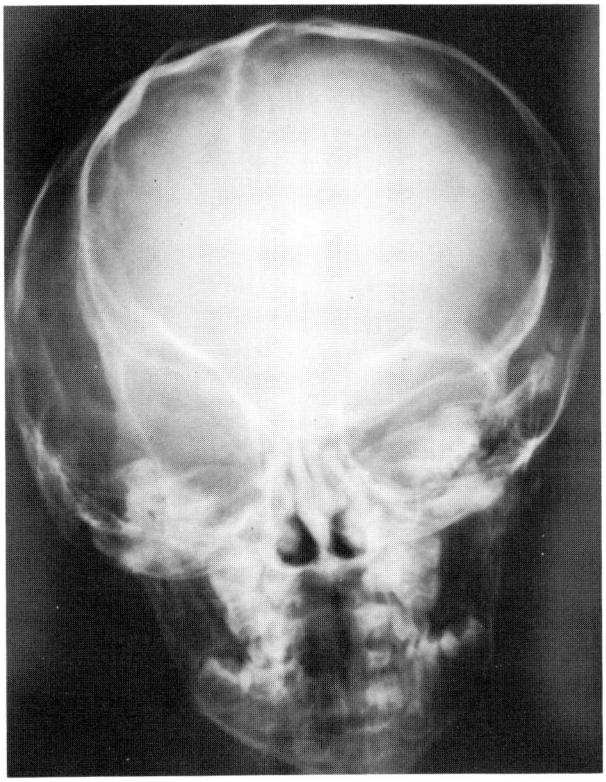

Fig. 12-15. Premature unilateral closure of right coronal suture. Note the harlequin appearance of the right orbit and the dense right coronal suture compared to the more normal left coronal suture. In addition, nasal septum and crista galli are tilted toward affected side.

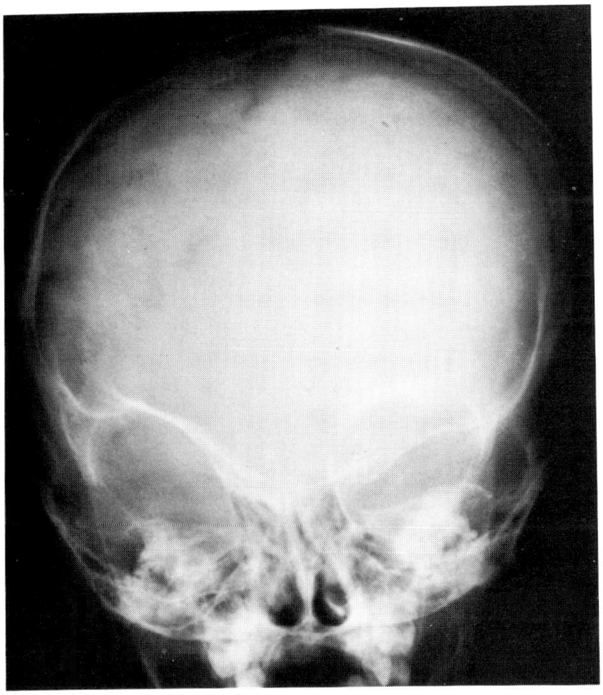

Fig. 12-16. Craniosynostosis of right coronal suture. Asymmetry of skull results from redirection of brain growth to the left and produces this form of plagiocephaly.

Table 12-1. Craniosynostosis associated with hand and foot deformities*

		Inheritance	*Features*
Acrocephalosyndactyly	A. Type I—Apert's syndrome	Autosomal dominant	Acrocephaly; hands and feet show *extreme* degree of syndactyly with synostosis of middle digits; most patients are mentally defective
	B. Type II—Crouzon's disease	Autosomal dominant	Acrocephaly; hypoplasia of facial bones, hypertelorism, exophthalmos
Acrocephalopolysyndactyly	A. Type I—Carpenter's syndrome, Noack's syndrome	Autosomal recessive probable; but genetic heterogeneity cannot be excluded	Peculiar facies, polydactyly, brachymesophalangy, mild soft tissue syndactyly, obesity, hypogenitalism, and mental retardation, skull changes not as severe as Apert's or Crouzon's syndrome
	B. Type II—Laurence-Moon-Biedl-Bardet syndrome	Autosomal recessive	Obesity, hypogonadism, mental retardation, postaxial polydactyly, and retinitis pigmentosa

*Modified from Palacios, E., and Schimke, N.: Craniosynostosis-syndactylism, Amer. J. Roentgen. 106:144-155, 1969.

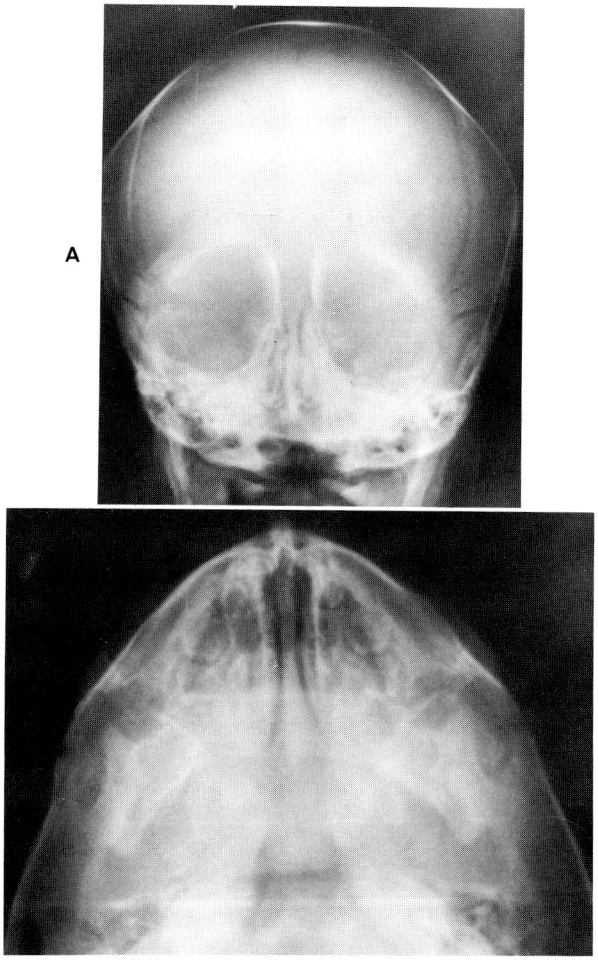

Fig. 12-17. Trigonocephaly. Interorbital distance is diminished, which produces hypotelorism, **A**, and frontal bone is sharply pointed at metopic suture, as seen on basal view, **B**. (Courtesy Dr. Richard D. Hoare, London, England.)

Delayed premature craniosynostosis

Delayed premature synostosis is of no clinical significance. It consists merely of variations in the shape of the skull, which may be a familial or racial trait. Taveras and Wood (1964) reported a tendency to premature synostosis of the lambdoid suture in late childhood, which allegedly is frequent among inhabitants of the Middle East. We have seen many roentgenograms of the skull from the Middle East that almost invariably showed brachycephaly but never closed lambdoid sutures.

Treatment of craniosynostosis

After the diagnosis has been established, surgical treatment is sometimes warranted to prevent exophthalmos, retardation, and injury of the cranial nerves. Surgery may also be indicated for cosmetic purposes. Current surgical technique (Matson, 1969) is similar to that described by Ingraham and Matson (1944) and has changed little in more than 25 years. It consists of removing a strip of bone 1 cm wide at the normal site of the involved suture. The pericranium is excised widely to retard formation of new bone, and polyethylene film strips are placed around the edges of the bone. Arbitrarily, Shillito and Matson (1968) chose the age of 4 to 6 weeks as most ideal for the operation in infants with single suture closure. In patients with multiple suture involvement or total synostosis, the operation has been performed during the first week of life. The surgical mortality rate of these authors was 0.39%, and the overall morbidity rate 14%; but permanent undesirable sequelae followed in only 0.58%.

The controversy regarding the need and value of surgery was emphasized in the long-term study of thirty-four children by Freeman and Borkowf (1962). They found no difference in cosmetic results in untreated and in surgically treated patients. In those treated, surgery

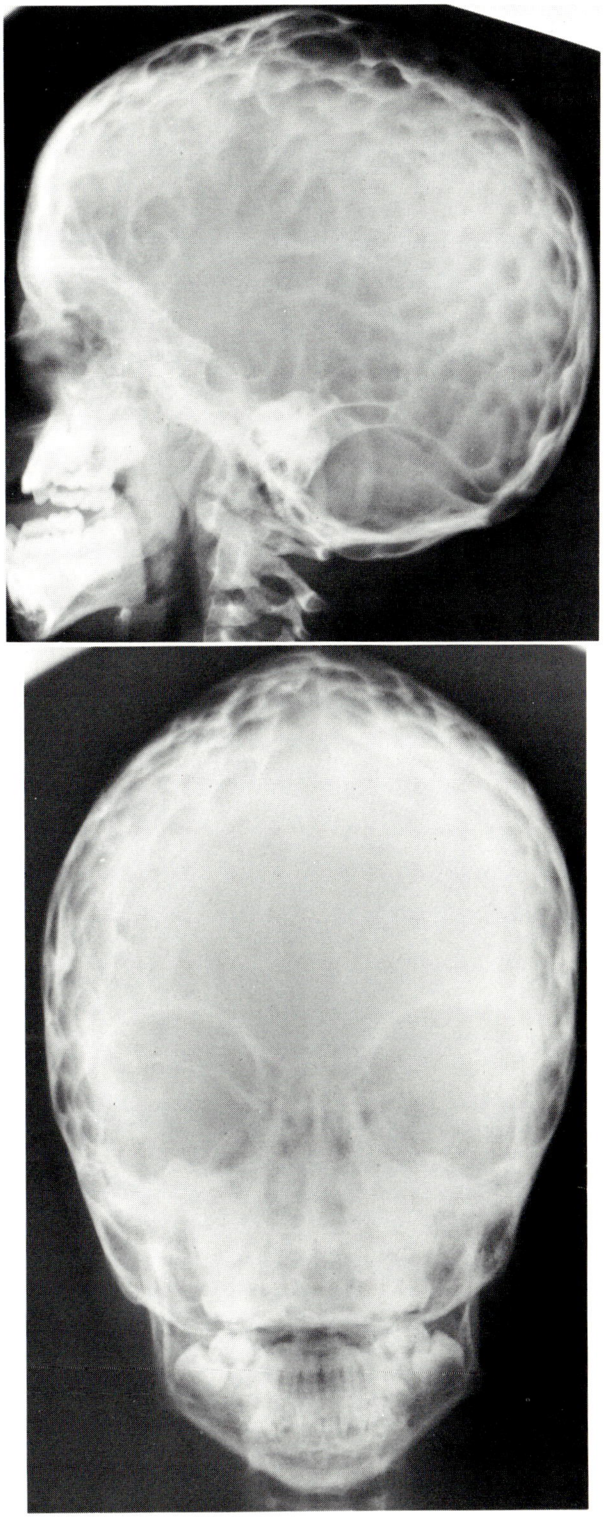

Fig. 12-18. Craniofacial dysostosis (Crouzon's disease) in 3-year-old girl. All the cranial sutures have closed prematurely; thus the convolutional impressions are exaggerated. Calvarium is somewhat brachycephalic; maxilla is hypoplastic.

did not prevent mental retardation. The authors advocated surgery only when papilledema or severe deformity was present.

We believe that if treatment is carried out early improvement in the shape of the head will result. Surgical treatment is essential as soon as the diagnosis is established in cases of bilateral coronal craniosynostosis and total craniosynostosis.

Secondary premature craniosynostosis

Secondary synostosis may exist when the brain fails to grow; hence, all sutures are simultaneously involved. As seen from the outline on p. 222, a variety of dysplasias, metabolic diseases, and hematologic disorders are incriminated as causes of this secondary form of craniostenosis.

In cases of generalized premature closure of the sutures, growth is limited in all directions and a microcephalic (Greek *mikros,* small) craniosynostosis is produced. This type of microcrania is associated with prominent convolutional impressions. It may be distinguished from microcephaly, produced by failure of brain growth, since the sutures in microcephaly are open.

Crouzon's disease (hereditary craniofacial dysostosis) is one form of generalized craniosynostosis associated with hypoplasia of the facial bones (Dodge et al., 1969) (Fig. 12-18).

Craniotelencephalic dysplasia, described by Jabbour and Taybi (1964), includes mental retardation and premature synostosis of the metopic, frontal, and sagittal sutures. The frontal squama is protuberant, and lacunar rarefaction of the frontal bone is seen. A similar case but with an encephalocele was described by Daum and his co-workers (1958).

Reilly and his group (1964) found premature craniosynostosis in about a third of all types of rickets and hypophosphatasia. The severity of the craniosynostosis correlated directly with that of rickets. Coleman and Foote (1954) described craniosynostosis in a 6-year-old boy with familial vitamin D–resistant rickets. The osseous deformities in vitamin D–resistant rickets are similar to those of classic nutritional rickets; however, in the familial resistant type, craniosynostosis develops only occasionally. Coleman and Foote's case allegedly was only the second reported of this condition. In the patients with hypophosphatasia reported by Currarino and his group (1957), craniosynostosis developed in all infants during the second year of life but led to symptoms in only a few.

Robinson and co-workers (1969) reported premature closure of the sutures of the skull in a boy with hyperthyroidism (Graves' disease). The roentgenogram of the skull demonstrated virtually total premature fusion of sagittal, coronal, and lambdoid sutures. Papilledema developed and a ventriculogram demonstrated normal-sized ventricles. When linear craniectomies were performed, the sutures were found to be closed.

We have seen secondary premature craniosynostosis in patients with idiopathic hypercalcemia and Caffey's disease (infantile cortical hyperostosis).

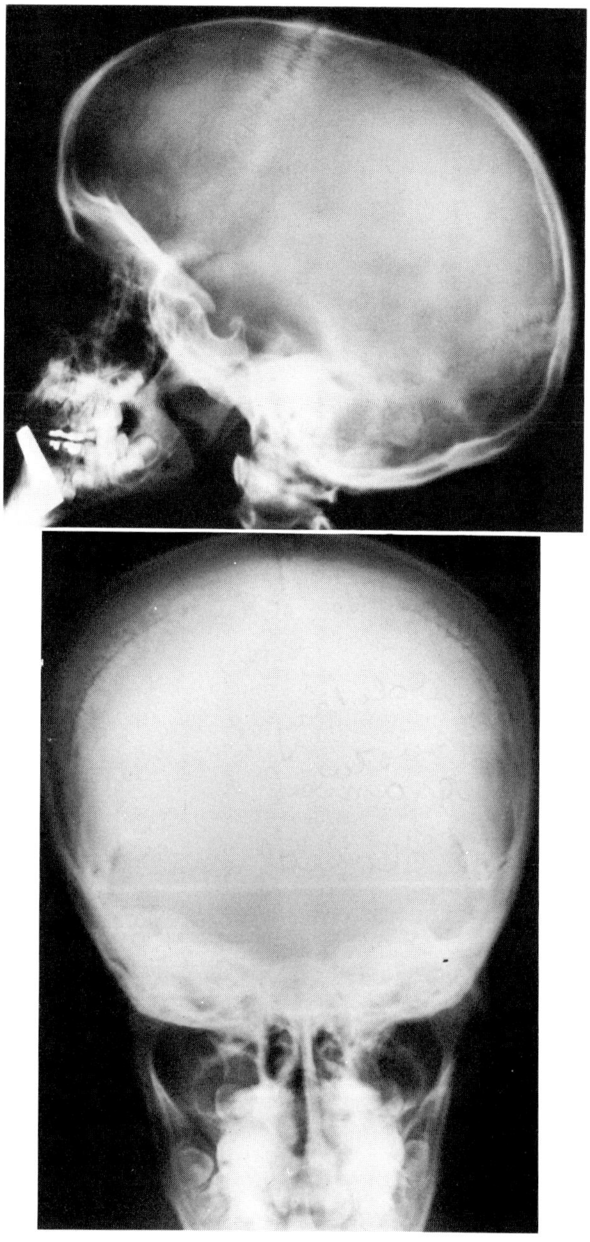

Fig. 12-19. Spurious widening of coronal suture in 7-year-old boy. Note that on the lateral view the superimposed coronal sutures give the illusion of elongation of the interdigitations; but, in fact, anteroposterior view shows that the sutures are normal.

Delayed suture closure

Retardation of maturation of skulls is seen in untreated cretins. Closure of sutures in untreated cretins may be markedly delayed. In congenital hypothyroidism the number of wormian bones is increased, and differentiation of the outer and inner tables of the vault is delayed. Delayed pneumatization of the mastoids and paranasal sinuses, delayed tooth development, macroglossia, and commonly an enlarged pituitary fossa are other changes in the hypothyroid skull (Bellini and Neves, 1956).

SUTURAL WIDENING

Sutural widening exists when the width of a suture is greater than normal for that age. Sutural widening

A 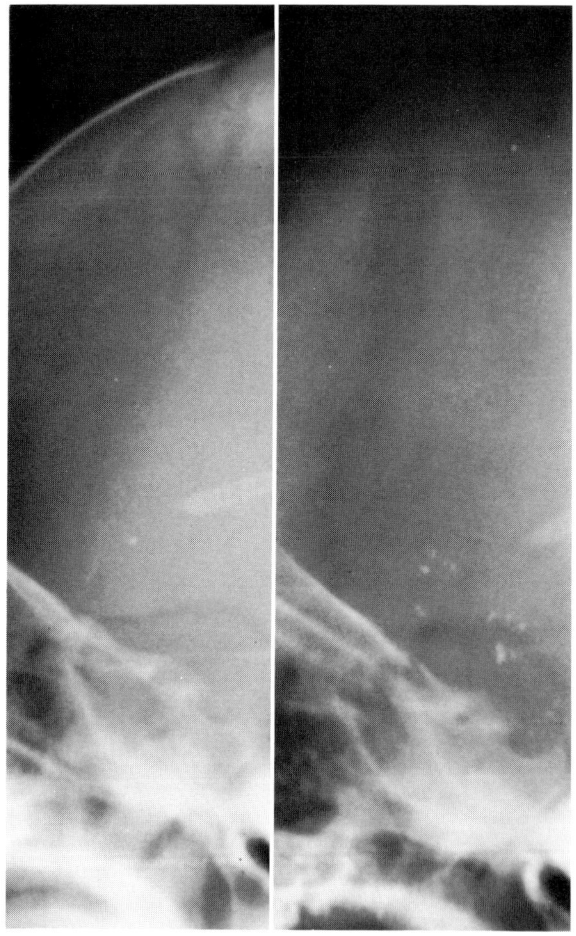 B

Fig. 12-20. A 3-month-old girl with suture diastasis development within 8 days. Ventriculoatrial shunt for treatment of aqueduct stenosis. **A,** Coned-down lateral view of coronal suture shows normal appearance of sutures and position of catheter tip in lateral ventricle. **B,** Eight days later, coronal suture bilaterally is diastatic because of blocked shunt catheter. In infants of this age, rapid sutural diastasis in response to increase in intracranial pressure is not unusual.

may result from increased intracranial pressure or from destruction of bone at suture margins. In the first instance the margins of the diastatic sutures are well delineated although the interdigitations may be of increased length. With destructive lesions, such as neuroblastoma or leukemia, the permeative nature of these entities produces a rarefied appearance at the suture margin.

Spurious widening of the coronal sutures may be seen on lateral views of the skull obtained with the head slightly oblique, so that the two sutures lie side by side (Fig. 12-19). If this artifact of positioning is suspected, it may be accurately assessed on roentgenograms obtained with more obliquity or on other views of the skull.

Increased intracranial pressure

The response of the cranial sutures to raised intracranial pressure depends on the age at which the increased pressure becomes manifest, the rapidity of its onset, and its duration.

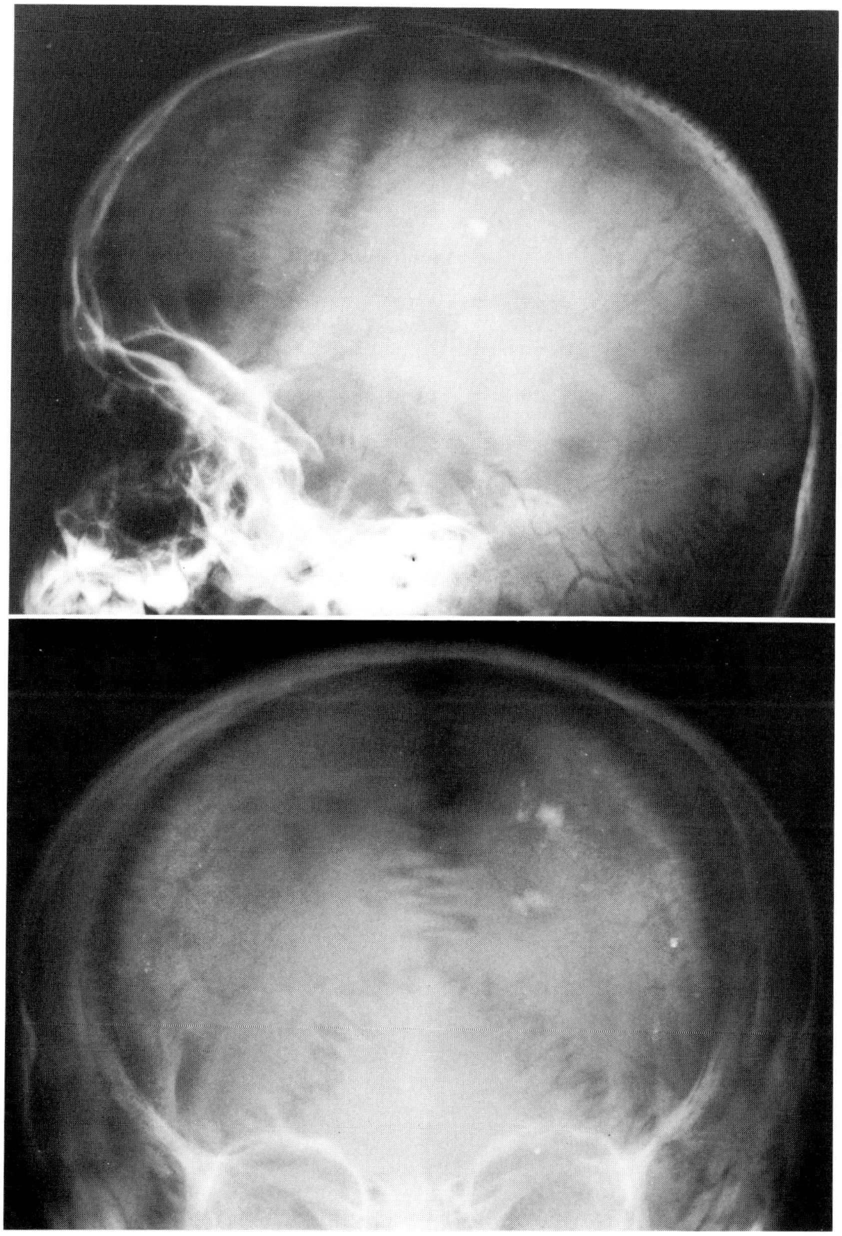

Fig. 12-21. Increased intracranial pressure secondary to meningioma in 6-year-old boy. Coronal suture is markedly diastatic, and sagittal suture less so. Note the elongated interdigitations.

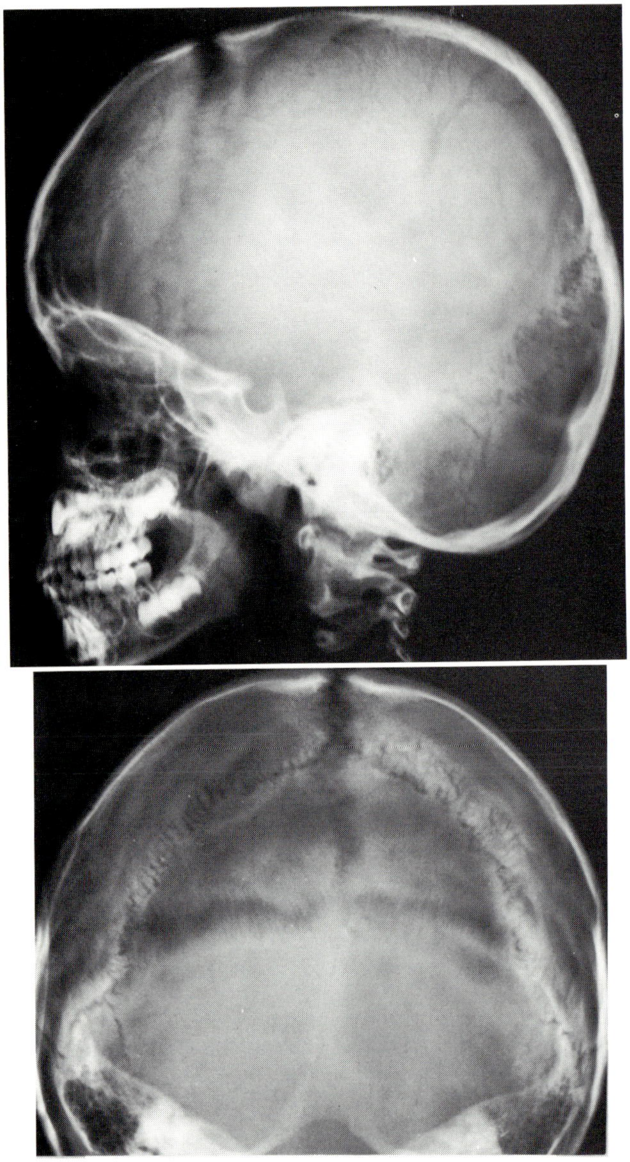

Fig. 12-22. Suture diastasis secondary to increased intracranial pressure in 3-year-old boy. Note that the coronal suture and, to a lesser degree, the sagittal suture are diastatic yet the lambdoid suture has not been affected.

In the neonatal period the calvarial mineralization is such that discernment of bone margins is difficult. Therefore identification of diastasis is made difficult. Furthermore, what are normal sutures in one infant may be diastatic in another because of the broad spectrum of normal variation. Detection of bulging of the soft tissues at the anterior fontanelle provides supportive evidence in the equivocal case of elevated pressure at this age. Reevaluation of the patient by serial clinical measurements of head circumference or resort to a more sophisticated diagnostic radiologic technique, such as pneumoencephalography, is necessary in some cases.

In children up to 8 or 9 years of age, sutural diastasis may occur within a few days of the development of acutely increased intracranial pressure (Fig. 12-20). du Boulay (1957, 1965) reported that diastatic sutures had been seen to develop 10 days after the onset of illness at 3 years of age, within 3 weeks at 5 years of age, and within 2 weeks at 8 years. Suture diastasis may also be the only evidence of raised intracranial pressure that is present. After 10 years of age, sutural diastasis is uncommon, except when the onset of long-standing raised intracranial pressure was at an earlier age. After this age it is seldom the only sign of raised pressure, and usually sellar changes and abnormal convolutional impressions are also noted.

In children with long-standing increased intracranial pressure, sharply pointed sutures and elongated interdigitations are manifested (Fig. 12-21). Although bone growth tends to close this diastasis, the closure is rarely complete until the increased intracranial pressure has been relieved.

The coronal and sagittal sutures are the earliest to become diastatic (Fig. 12-22). If one is in doubt about the sutures, the submentovertical view may settle the problem.

Hydrocephalus

The commonest cause of increased intracranial pressure in infancy is hydrocephalus. It is either of the communicating type, with defective resorption of cerebrospinal fluid, or of the noncommunicating or obstructive type. The latter frequently results from a congenital block at some point within the ventricular system (e.g., an aqueduct stenosis or atresia of the foramina of Magendie and Luschka).

In communicating hydrocephalus the sutures are normal, or slightly widened, since in this instance intracranial volume increases only gradually and the bone has time to grow at the sutures (Fig. 12-23). In noncommunicating hydrocephalus, however, dilatation of the lateral ventricles may be more rapid and the sutures are likely to be wide (Fig. 12-24). In most instances this generalization is correct. If in infants and young children the increased intracranial pressure is relieved suddenly, as may be achieved with an appropriate shunt, premature closure of the sutures may supervene. This closure is likely only if brain damage is present in addition to the hydrocephalus, as in severe meningitis or hemorrhage. If the head has already grown to adult size, this closure may be of little significance. In other children the changes that were described for premature craniosynostosis may develop. After surgical reduction of elevated intracranial pressure, the roentgenographic changes of increased intracranial pressure disappear within a few months.

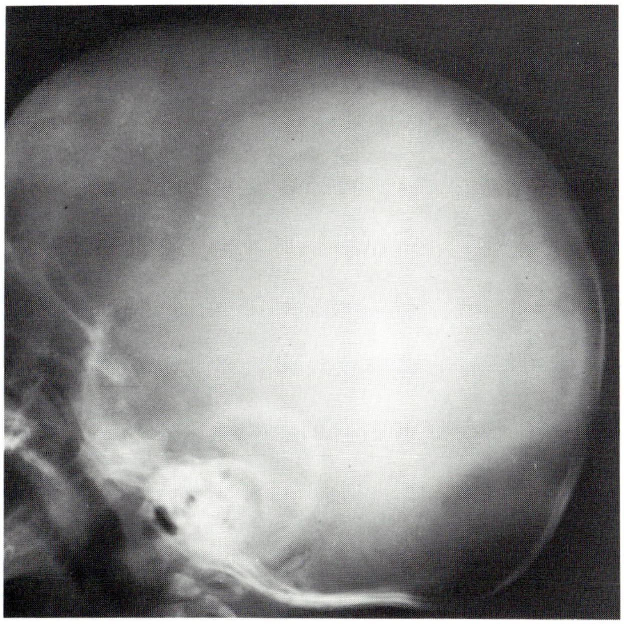

Fig. 12-23. Communicating hydrocephalus. Note the craniofacial disproportion; the vault is inordinately large. Sutures are not markedly diastatic because enlargement of vault has taken place over a long time and bone has grown at suture margin.

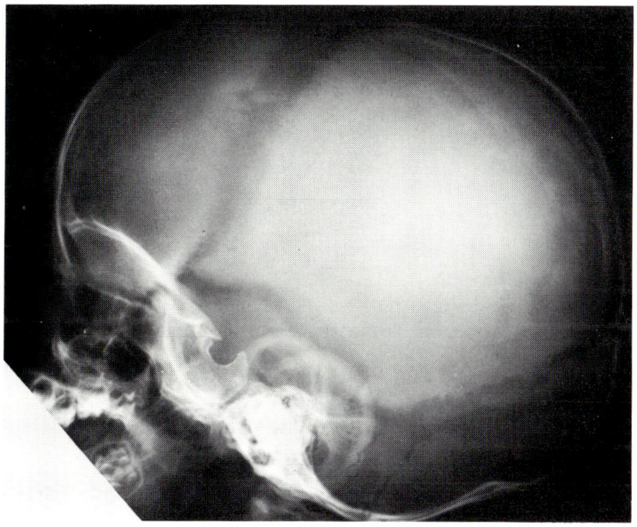

Fig. 12-24. Increased intracranial pressure with suture diastasis in infant girl. Note that all the sutures are widened. Because in infancy the skull can expand to accommodate intracranial pressure, increased digital impressions or sellar changes are usually not seen.

Vitamin A toxicity and deficiency

Acute and chronic poisonings resulting from vitamin A and also vitamin A deficiency have produced increased intracranial pressure (Marie and See, 1954; Bass and Caplan, 1955). With hypervitaminosis A an associated benign hydrocephalus with bulging fontanelle has been described. The hydrocephalus is transient and harmless, and it disappears rapidly when the intake of vitamin A is reduced. Experimentally this phenomenon has been produced in puppies. The probable mechanism of the hydrocephalus in this instance is an increased cellular activity of the choroid plexus, which produces excess cerebrospinal fluid (Knudson and Rothman, 1953).

In a patient with vitamin A deficiency, signs of increased intracranial pressure have disappeared 2 days after vitamin A was administered. Experimentally, increased cerebrospinal fluid pressure has also been reported in calves maintained on a diet deficient in vitamin A. Papilledema, syncope, and incoordination developed in these animals. When vitamin A was added, these signs disappeared (Moore and Sykes, 1940).

Pseudotumor cerebri

Pseudotumor cerebri associated with prolonged corticosteroid therapy was discussed by Walker and Adamkiewicz (1964), who reviewed twenty-four cases from the literature. Four of the patients had had diastatic sutures. The clinical manifestations included headache, nausea, vomiting, and papilledema, which tended to occur during the reduction or withdrawal phase of therapy. The serum electrolyte levels were normal, but urinary excretion of steroids tended to be low. The cerebrospinal fluid pressure was elevated, and the ventricles were small. The underlying mechanism may have been a transient hypophyseal adrenal suppression. The condition is usually self-limiting with appropriate management.

Tetracycline therapy

Fields (1961) described elevated intracranial pressure as early as 12 hours after tetracycline therapy was begun. In one of his patients with a bulging fontanelle, the roentgenograms of the skull demonstrated questionable spreading of the sutures. No skull roentgenograms were obtained on the other patient.

Therapy for deprivation syndrome

Capitanio and Kirkpatrick (1969) described three children with deprivation dwarfism who responded to emotional support and proper nutrition. This response was manifested by marked acceleration in growth and widening of the cranial sutures. At no time were signs or symptoms of increased intracranial pressure evident in any of these patients. The etiology of the increased sutural width is unknown in this circumstance. The increase was accompanied by an increase in head circumference and was presumed to represent rapid growth of the brain. This same phenomenon in five children was described by De Levie and Nogrady (1970), and in four additional patients by Sondheimer and his colleagues (1970).

Hypoparathyroidism

Steinberg and Waldron (1952) described increased intracranial pressure in about 15% of patients with idiopathic hypoparathyroidism. This association of increased intracranial pressure with idiopathic hypoparathyroidism and resultant diastatic sutures was illustrated by Caffey in a 3-year-old boy.

Brain tumors

The degree of suture widening varies greatly in patients with brain tumors. The generalizations given earlier in the discussion of increased intracranial pressure are most applicable here. To reiterate, the response of the sutures to a brain tumor depends on the age of the patient, the rate of growth of the tumor, and whether the tumor obstructs the flow of cerebrospinal fluid through the ventricular pathway. In young children, for example, with a medulloblastoma filling the posterior fossa and obstructing the foramina of the fourth ventricle, marked suture diastasis may be seen. At the other end of the spectrum is the elderly patient with a slowly growing glioma present for several years and producing absolutely no sutural abnormality. After the first decade of life, sphenoid bone changes, such as erosion of cortical bone along the anterior aspect of the dorsum sellae, assume more importance than does the status of the sutures in the diagnosis of increased intracranial pressure secondary to brain tumors.

Other causes of diastatic sutures

Increased intracranial pressure with widened sutures has also been attributed to other important causes. These include lead intoxication, nephritic encephalopathy, tuberculous and other types of meningitis, toxoplasmic encephalomyelitis, torula meningoencephalitis, and hydatid disease (McAfee, 1958).

In an analysis of 116 infants with subdural hematomas and effusions, Till (1968) found that the cranial sutures in half the patients were separated.

Bone destruction at sutural margin

Leukemia and neuroblastoma

Leukemia of the meninges and of the central nervous system, and infiltrates from neuroblastoma, are other causes of elevated pressure and suture widening (Fig. 12-25). The mechanism of split sutures in metastatic neuroblastoma was described recently by Carter and his group (1968). These authors noted that metastatic lesions of the skull were continuous with a similar tumor plaque in the epidural space. The tumor appeared to separate the dura from the inner table of the skull. These authors concluded that the diastatic sutures represented an accommodation to the bulky extradural metastatic growth. In addition, tumor infiltration, which caused destruction of marginal bone along the sutures, also produced a widening (Fig. 12-26).

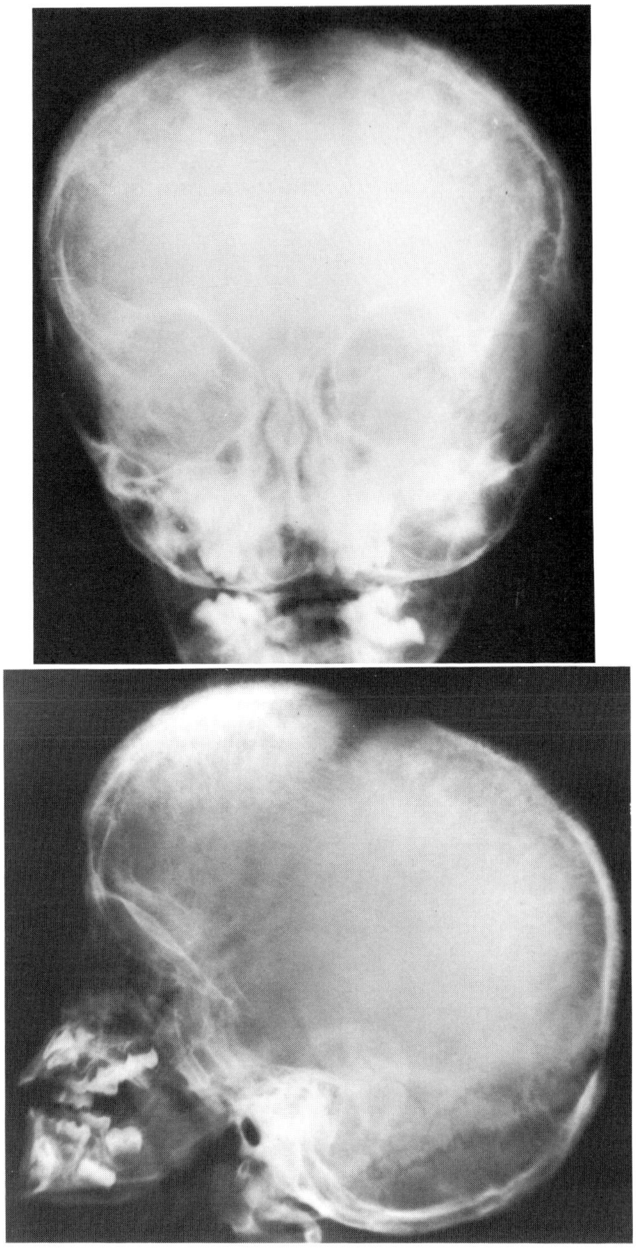

Fig. 12-25. Neuroblastoma in 3-year-old girl. Note the advanced diffuse metastatic neuroblastoma. Sutures are diastatic because of bulky extradural deposits.

ABNORMAL OSSIFICATION AT SUTURES

There are several entities that are characterized by defective mineralization at the skull sutures. Some of these have specific stigmata, which lead to an unequivocal roentgenographic diagnosis.

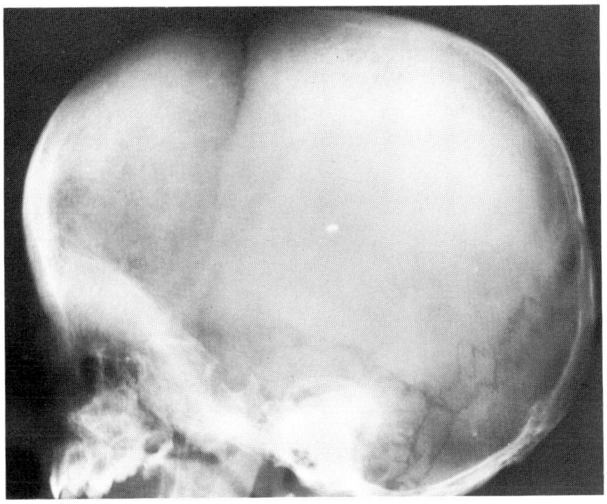

Cleidocranial dysostosis

Cleidocranial dysostosis involves delayed and defective ossification of the calvarium with associated hypoplasia of the clavicles. Also reported is defective ossification of the spine, pelvis, and long bones, and defective dention. A familial component is involved in this disease, but the disease also occurs sporadically (Keats, 1967).

Fig. 12-26. Metastatic neuroblastoma in 10-month-old boy. Note the irregularly decreased demineralization about the coronal suture and the diastasis of the suture.

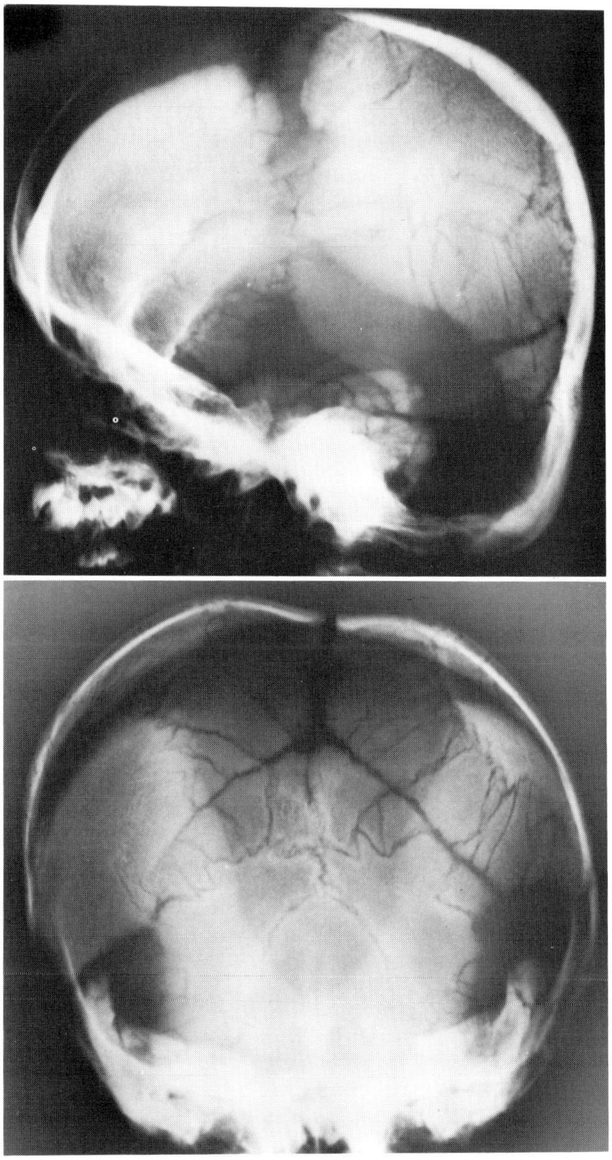

Fig. 12-27. Pyknodysostosis. Vault is dense. Defective mineralization is present, extending anteriorly from anterior fontanelle almost to nasion.

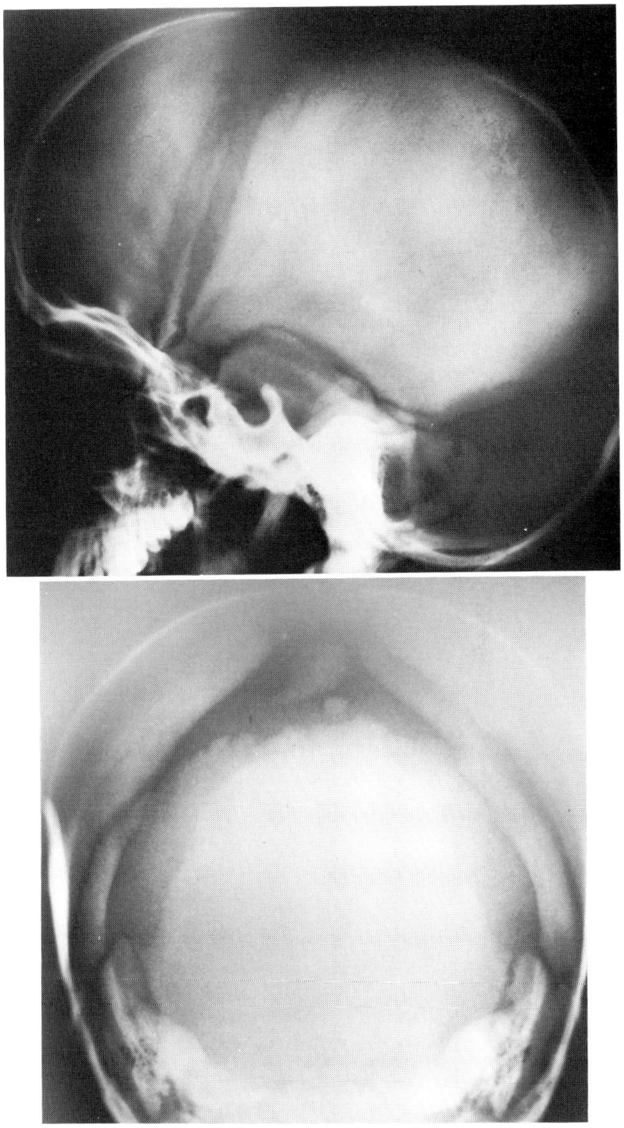

Fig. 12-28. Pyknodysostosis. Defective mineralization is seen at lambda and at bregma. Sutures do not have elongated digitations that characterize increased intracranial pressure. Widening is result of defective mineralization.

In early infancy most of the calvarium of patients with cleidocranial dysostosis is membranous with small foci of ossification. In childhood the calvarial mineralization increases, and a mosaic rarefaction develops. In later childhood midline defects persist along the sagittal suture, and particularly on the borders of the anterior fontanelle and metopic suture. The sutures are much wider than normal, and many accessory sutures and innumerable sutural bones are seen.

Pyknodysostosis

Pyknodysostosis is a term coined by Maroteaux and Lamy (1962) to describe a disease complex that combines some of the features of cleidocranial dysostosis with osteopetrosis (Figs. 12-27 and 12-28). It is characterized by short stature, separated cranial sutures, open fontanelles, and loss of mandibular angle. Dysplasia of the bones of the skull, partial aplasia of the terminal phalanges, dense bones, and frequent fractures are additional

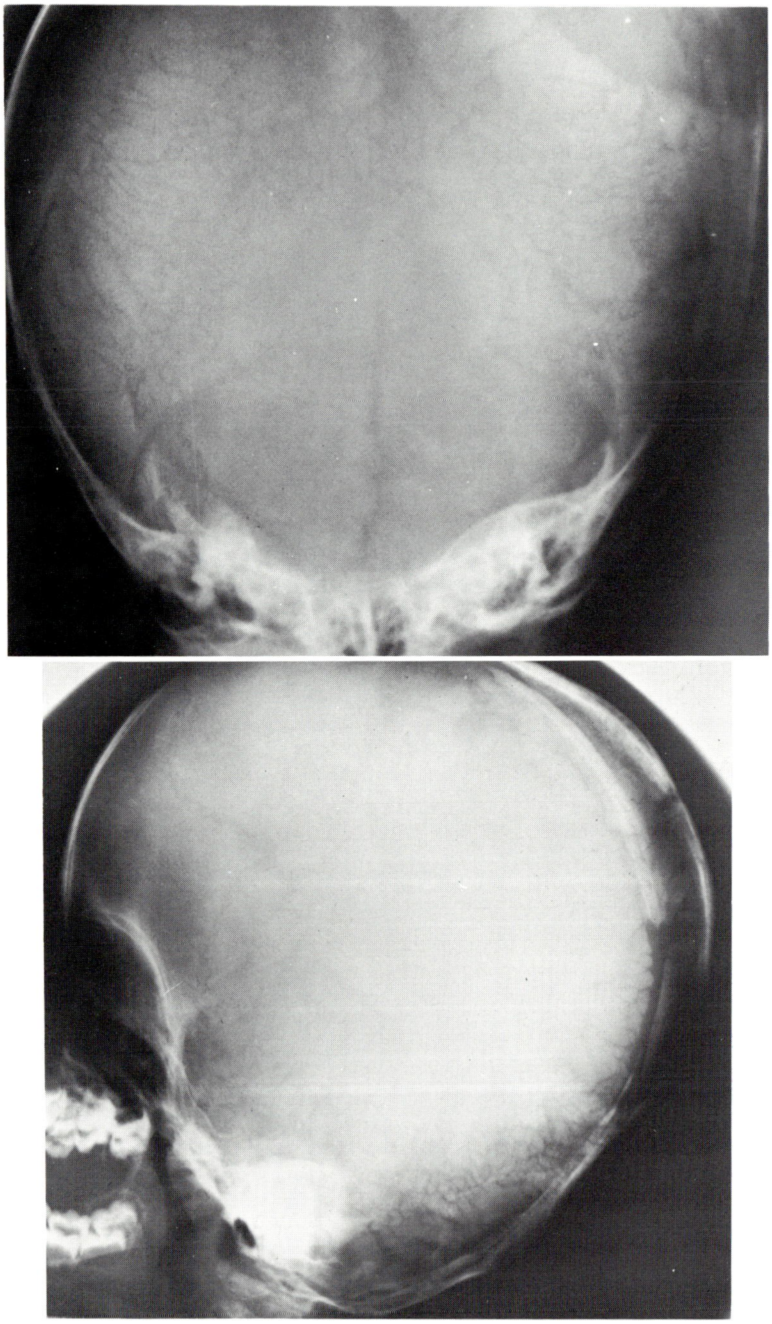

Fig. 12-29. Osteogenesis imperfecta in 2-year-old girl. Multiple wormian bones are evident throughout vault, with diffuse and focal areas of defective mineralization also manifested.

characteristics. The base of the skull may be strikingly flat (Shuler, 1963; Dusenberry and Kane, 1967).

Progeria

In progeria the fontanelles persist and the clavicles are often thin and short. This combination suggests that progeria and cleidocranial dysostosis may share some common causal factors (Margolin and Steinbach, 1968).

Osteogenesis imperfecta

Osteogenesis imperfecta is characterized by delayed and defective mineralization of membranous bones. In the neonate the calvarium may consist of a membranous sac with only a few small foci of isolated centers of ossification discernible. Numerous ossification centers appear as age increases in patients who survive, and the calvarium is gradually converted from membrane to bone. So many wormian bones are present that a mosaic rarefaction develops in the vault of the skull (Fig. 12-29). This severe rarefaction is seen usually in only three diseases: osteogenesis imperfecta, cleidocranial dysostosis, and hypophosphatasia (Currarino et al., 1957; Schwarz, 1963).

In later infancy and childhood the width of the sutures becomes normal and the fontanelles are not enlarged. The skull often becomes brachycephalic, probably because of pressure on the occipital bone in these infants, who frequently appear hypotonic.

Cranium bifidum

A midline round or shield-shaped defect near the anterior fontanelle may be seen and may persist into adult life. Sometimes the adjacent neural tissue also is defective and may bulge through the bony defect as a meningocele. When the defect is small without herniation, the term cranium bifidum occultum is used. The lesion may close spontaneously (TerraFranca and Zellis, 1953). It appears in patients with cleidocranial dysostosis but may also be present as an isolated finding without other manifestations.

Aminopterin poisoning

Several years ago, aminopterin was employed occasionally for therapeutic abortion. The drug was dis-

A

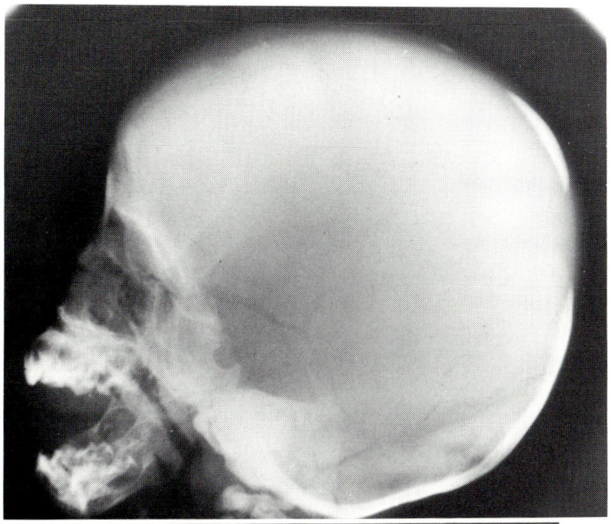

B

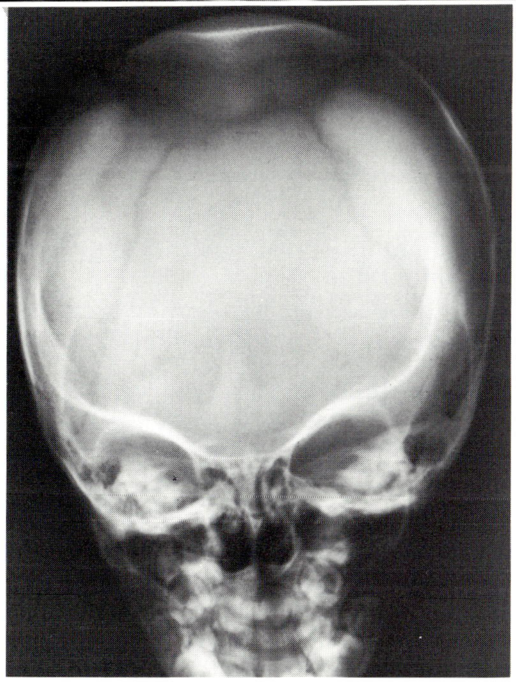

Fig. 12-30. Aminopterin poisoning. **A,** Three months. **B,** Eighteen months. Defective mineralization is evident initially. Parasagittal sutures are later evident.

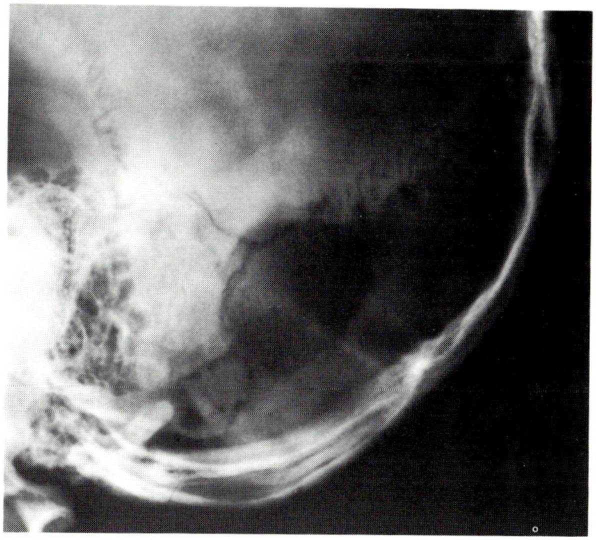

Fig. 12-31. Neurofibromatosis. Characteristic focal area of defective ossification in lambdoid suture is evident. This is a mesenchymal abnormality, and no underlying neurofibroma is present.

covered to cause multiple serious fetal anomalies, however, as seen in infants who did not succumb. Reports of children who survived such an attempted abortion described defective mineralization of the skull with ossification limited to the lower part of the skull (Fig. 12-30). In the infant described by Shaw and Steinbach (1968), two large ossified centers were seen within the posterior part of the sagittal suture. Subsequent roentgenographic examination showed progressive ossification of the membranous bones. The anterior ossification center within the sagittal suture became progressively larger and extended laterally. It produced a large midline bone and two sutures, one on each side. In the parietal region no central sagittal suture was present.

Neurofibromatosis

The skeletal lesions of neurofibromatosis have been completely discussed by Hunt and Pugh (1961). In three of the six patients with neurofibromatosis reported by Davidson (1966), an oval well-defined cranial defect (Fig. 12-31) appeared in the left lambdoid suture. Necropsy in one case showed progressive thinning of bone toward the center of the defect. No overlying or underlying cyst or tumor was evident. This solitary lambdoid lesion would appear to be a rather specific sign of neurofibromatosis.

Saha and his co-workers (1969) reported a case of neurofibromatosis with multiple osteolytic defects that spared the left lambdoid suture but involved the right lambdoid suture. On a review of the literature, these authors found that involvement of the right lambdoid suture is most rare.

REFERENCES

Acheson, R. M., and Jefferson, E.: Some observations of the closure of the anterior fontanelle, Arch. Dis. Child. **29**:196-198, 1954.

Andersson, H., and Gomes, S. P.: Craniosynostosis. Review of the literature and indications for surgery, Acta Paediat. Scand. **57**:47-54, 1968.

Angle, C. R., McIntire, M. S., and Moore, R. C.: Cloverleaf skull: kleeblattschädel-deformity syndrome, Amer. J. Dis. Child. **114**:198-202, 1967.

Bass, M. H., and Caplan, J.: Vitamin A deficiency in infancy, J. Pediat. **47**:690-695, 1955.

Bellini, M. A., and Neves, I.: The skull in childhood myxedema; its roentgen appearance, Amer. J. Roentgen. **76**:495-498, 1956.

Brown, W. H.: Anterior fontanel bone, J. Pediat. **58**:800-802, 1961.

Caffey, J.: On the accessory ossicles of the supraoccipital bone, Amer. J. Roentgen. **70**:401-412, 1953.

Capitanio, M. A., and Kirkpatrick, J. A.: Widening of the cranial sutures, Radiology **92**:53-59, 1969.

Carter, T. L., Gabrielsen, T. O., and Abell, M. R.: Mechanism of split cranial sutures in metastatic neuroblastoma, Radiology **91**:467-470, 1968.

Coleman, E. N., and Foote, J. B.: Craniostenosis with familial vitamin-D resistant rickets, Brit. Med. J. **1**:561-562, 1954.

Cooper, R.: Acrocephalosyndactyly; with report of a case, Brit. J. Radiol. **26**:533-538, 1953.

Currarino, G., Neuhauser, E. B. D., Reyerbach, G. C., and others: Hypophosphatasia, Amer. J. Roentgen. **78**:392-419, 1957.

Currarino, G., and Silverman, F. N.: Orbital hypotelorism, arhinencephaly and trigonocephaly, Radiology **74**:206-217, 1960.

Daum, S., Le Beau, J., and Minuit, P.: Dysplasie telencéphalique avec excroissance de l'os frontal, Sem. Hop. Paris **34**:1893-1896, 1958.

Davidson, K. C.: Cranial and intracranial lesions in neurofibromatosis, Amer. J. Roentgen. **98**:550-556, 1966.

De Levie, M., and Nogrady, M. B.: Rapid brain growth upon restoration of adequate nutrition causing false radiologic evidence of increased intracranial pressure, J. Pediat. **76**: 523-528, 1970.

Dodge, H. W., Jr., Wood, M. W., and Kennedy, R. L. J.: Craniofacial dysostosis; Crouzon's disease, Pediatrics **23**:98-106, 1959.

du Boulay, G.: The radiological evidence of raised intracranial pressure in children, Brit. J. Radiol. **30**:375-377, 1957.

du Boulay, G.: Principles of x-ray diagnosis of the skull, London, 1965, Butterworth & Co., Ltd.

Duggan, C. A., Keever, E. B., and Gay, B. B.: Secondary craniosynostosis, Amer. J. Roentgen. **109**:277-293, 1970.

Dusenberry, J. F., Jr., and Kane, J. J.: Pyknodysostosis, Amer. J. Roentgen. **99**:717-723, 1967.

Fauré, C., Bonamy, P., and Rambert-Misset, C.: Craniostenosis from premature unilateral fusion of the coronal suture, Ann. Radiol. **10**:32-42, 1967.

Feingold, M., O'Connor, J. F., Berkman, M., and others: Kleeblattschädel syndrome, Amer. J. Dis. Child. **118**:589-594, 1969.

Fields, J. P.: Bulging fontanel: a complication of tetracycline therapy in infants, J. Pediat. **58**:74-76, 1961.

Franken, E. A.: The midline occipital fissure; diagnosis of fracture versus anatomic variants, Radiology **93**:1043-1046, 1969.

Freeman, J. M., and Borkowf, S.: Craniosynostosis; review of the literature and report of 34 cases, Pediatrics **30**:57-70, 1962.

Girdany, B. R., and Blank, E.: Anterior fontanel bones, Amer. J. Roentgen. **95**:148-153, 1965.

Hope, J. W., Spitz, E. B., and Slade, H. W.: Early recognition of premature cranial synostosis, Radiology **65**:183-193, 1955.

Hunt, J. C., and Pugh, D. G.: Skeletal lesions in neurofibromatosis, Radiology **76**:1-20, 1961.

Ingraham, F. D., and Matson, D. D.: Subdural hematoma in infancy, J. Pediat. **24**:1-37, 1944.

Jabbour, J. T., and Taybi, H.: Craniotelencephalic dysplasia, Amer. J. Dis. Child. **108**:627-632, 1964.

Keats, T. E.: Cleidocranial dysostosis, Amer. J. Roentgen. **100**:71-74, 1967.

Knudson, A. G., and Rothman, P. E.: Hypervitaminosis A, Amer. J. Dis. Child. **85**:316-334, 1953.

Margolin, F. R., and Steinbach, H. L.: Progeria, Amer. J. Roentgen. **103**:173-178, 1968.

Marie, J., and See, G.: Acute hypervitaminosis A of the infant, Amer. J. Dis. Child. **87**:731-736, 1954.

Maroteaux, P., and Lamy, M.: Deux observations d'une affection osseuse condensante: la pycnodysostose, Arch. Franc. Pediat. **19**:267-274, 1962.

Matson, D. D.: Neurosurgery of infancy and childhood, ed. 2, Springfield, Ill., 1969, Charles C Thomas, Publisher.

McAfee, J. G.: The roentgen signs of systemic disease in the skull, Amer. J. Med. Sci. **236**:634-660, 1958.

Moore, L. A., and Sykes, J. F.: Cerebrospinal pressure and vitamin-A deficiency, Amer. J. Physiol. **130**:684-689, 1940.

Moss, M. L.: The pathogenesis of premature cranial synostosis in man, Acta Anat. **37**:351-370, 1959.

Palacios, E., and Schimke, N.: Craniosynostosis-syndactylism, Amer. J. Roentgen. **106**:144-155, 1969.

Park, E. A., and Powers, G. F.: Acrocephaly and scaphocephaly with symmetrically distributed malformations of the extremities, Amer. J. Dis. Child. **20**:235-315, 1920.

Pfeiffer, R. A.: Dominant erbliche Akrocephalosyndaktylie, Z. Kinderheilk. **90**:301-320, 1964.

Reilly, B. J., Leeming, J. M., and Fraser, D.: Craniosynostosis in the rachitic spectrum, J. Pediat. **64**:396-405, 1964.

Robinson, D. C., Hall, R., and Munro, D. S.: Graves' disease, an unusual complication: raised intracranial pressure due to premature fusion of skull sutures, Arch. Dis. Child. **44**:252-257, 1969.

Saha, M. M., Agarwal, K. N., and Bhardwaj, O. P.: Calvarial bone defects in neurofibromatosis, Amer. J. Roentgen. **105**: 319-321, 1969.

Schwarz, E.: The skull in skeletal dysplasia, Amer. J. Roentgen. **89**:928-937, 1963.

Shaw, E. B., and Steinbach, H. L.: Aminopterin-induced fetal malformation, Amer. J. Dis. Child. **115**:477-482, 1968.

Shillito, J., Jr., and Matson, D. D.: Craniosynostosis, a review of 519 surgical patients, Pediatrics **41**:829-853, 1968.

Shuler, S. E.: Pyknodysostosis, Arch. Dis. Child. **38**:620-625, 1963.

Sondheimer, F. K., Grossman, H., and Winchester, P.: Suture diastasis following rapid weight gain, Arch. Neurol. **23**:314-318, 1970.

Steinberg, H., and Waldron, B. R.: Idiopathic hypoparathyroidism: an analysis of 52 cases, including the report of a new case, Medicine **31**:133-154, 1952.

Taveras, J. M., and Wood, E. H.: Diagnostic neuroradiology, Baltimore, 1964, The Williams & Wilkins Co.

TerraFranca, R. J., and Zellis, A.: Congenital hereditary cranium bifidum occultum frontalis, Radiology **61**:60-65, 1953.

Till, K.: Subdural haematoma and effusion in infancy, Brit. Med. J. **2**:400-402, 1968.

Torgerson, J.: A roentgenological study of the metopic suture, Acta Radiol. **33**:1-11, 1950.

Walker, A. E., and Adamkiewicz, J. J.: Pseudotumor cerebri associated with prolonged corticosteroid therapy, J.A.M.A. **188**:779-784, 1964.

PART IV

Skull base

CHAPTER 13

Nasopharynx

Richard J. Rizzuti and Joseph P. Whalen

Radiographic study of the nasopharynx plays an important role in the diagnosis of disease in this region. It is particularly valuable in the diagnosis of malignant tumors of the nasopharynx. Many of these present late clinically, often after nodal metastasis has occurred (Lenz, 1942; Ackerman and del Regato, 1962). Once the clinical diagnosis is made, radiography is of value in localizing and determining the extent of the lesion. Radiographic demonstration of the lesion may also help the surgeon plan his biopsy. The roentgen diagnosis of nasopharyngeal abnormalities is dependent on a detailed knowledge of the radiographic anatomy of the nasopharynx and the manner in which this anatomy is altered by disease.

GROSS ANATOMY

Boundaries

The nasopharynx is a six-walled space, roughly cuboidal in shape with anterior and posterior walls, a roof and floor, and two lateral walls. It is situated at the base of the skull and is continuous with the nasal cavity anteriorly, the oropharynx inferiorly, and the middle ears laterally (via the eustachian tubes). It measures 2 to 3 cm from front to back, and approximately 4 cm in width and height. Its *anterior* boundary is formed by the vomer, the choanae, and the posterior aspects of the middle and inferior turbinates (Fig. 13-1). Its *posterior* wall is formed by the superior constrictor muscle. The nasopharynx here is separated from the atlas and the axis by the retropharyngeal space. The basiocciput and sphenoid bones comprise its *roof* (Fig. 13-2, *D*), from which projects the pharyngeal tonsil (of Luschka). The soft palate forms its floor, which separates the nasopharynx inferiorly from the oropharynx (Fig. 13-2, *A* to *C*). The lateral extension of the posterior wall is the pharyngeal recess (fossa of Rosenmüller), which, with the more anterior torus tubarius, forms each *lateral* wall

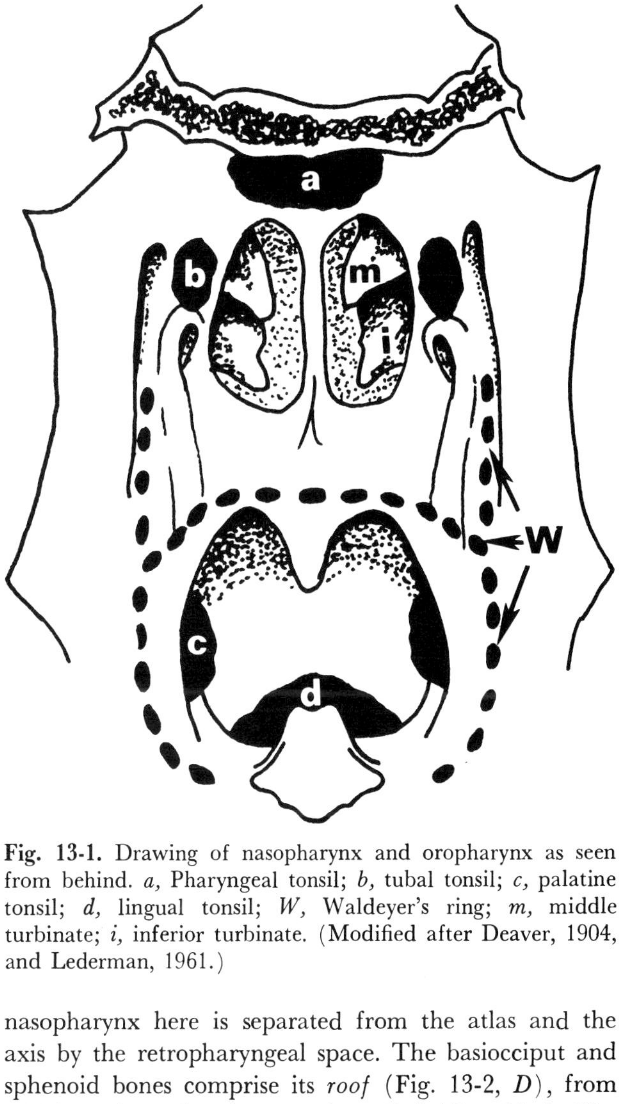

Fig. 13-1. Drawing of nasopharynx and oropharynx as seen from behind. *a,* Pharyngeal tonsil; *b,* tubal tonsil; *c,* palatine tonsil; *d,* lingual tonsil; *W,* Waldeyer's ring; *m,* middle turbinate; *i,* inferior turbinate. (Modified after Deaver, 1904, and Lederman, 1961.)

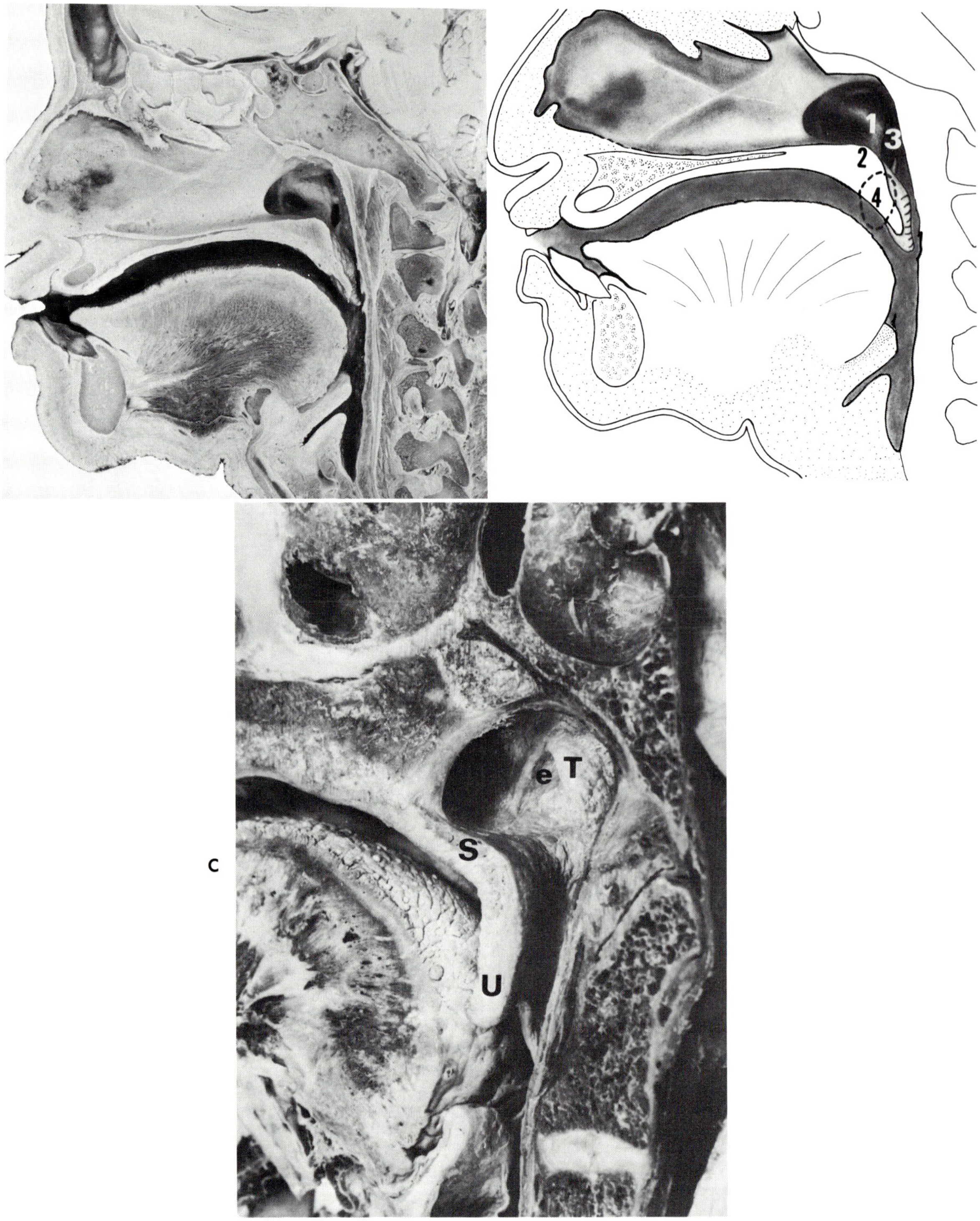

Fig. 13-2. Nasopharynx in lateral view. **A,** Anatomic sagittal section through nasopharynx. **B,** Diagram of **A.** *1,* Torus tubarius; *2,* soft palate; *3,* pharyngeal recess (fossa of Rosenmüller); *4,* plane of palatine tonsil, which lies laterally. **C,** Anatomic section, magnified view. *T,* Torus tubarius; *e,* eustachian orifice; *S,* soft palate; *U,* uvula. **D,** Roentgenogram of sagittal section of specimen at level of nasopharynx demonstrates bony landmarks. Relation of nasopharynx to sphenoid sinus, basisphenoid, basioccipital bones, and first and second cervical vertebrae is clearly demonstrated. Note the proximity of the nasopharynx to the neural structures. **E,** Roentgenogram in lateral projection shows soft tissue and bony structures in an adult. *t,* Torus tubarius; *e,* eustachian orifice; *i,* inferior turbinate. Black and white horizontal arrows indicate posterior walls of maxillary antra. **F,** Roentgenogram in lateral projection in a child shows normal nasopharyngeal soft tissues.

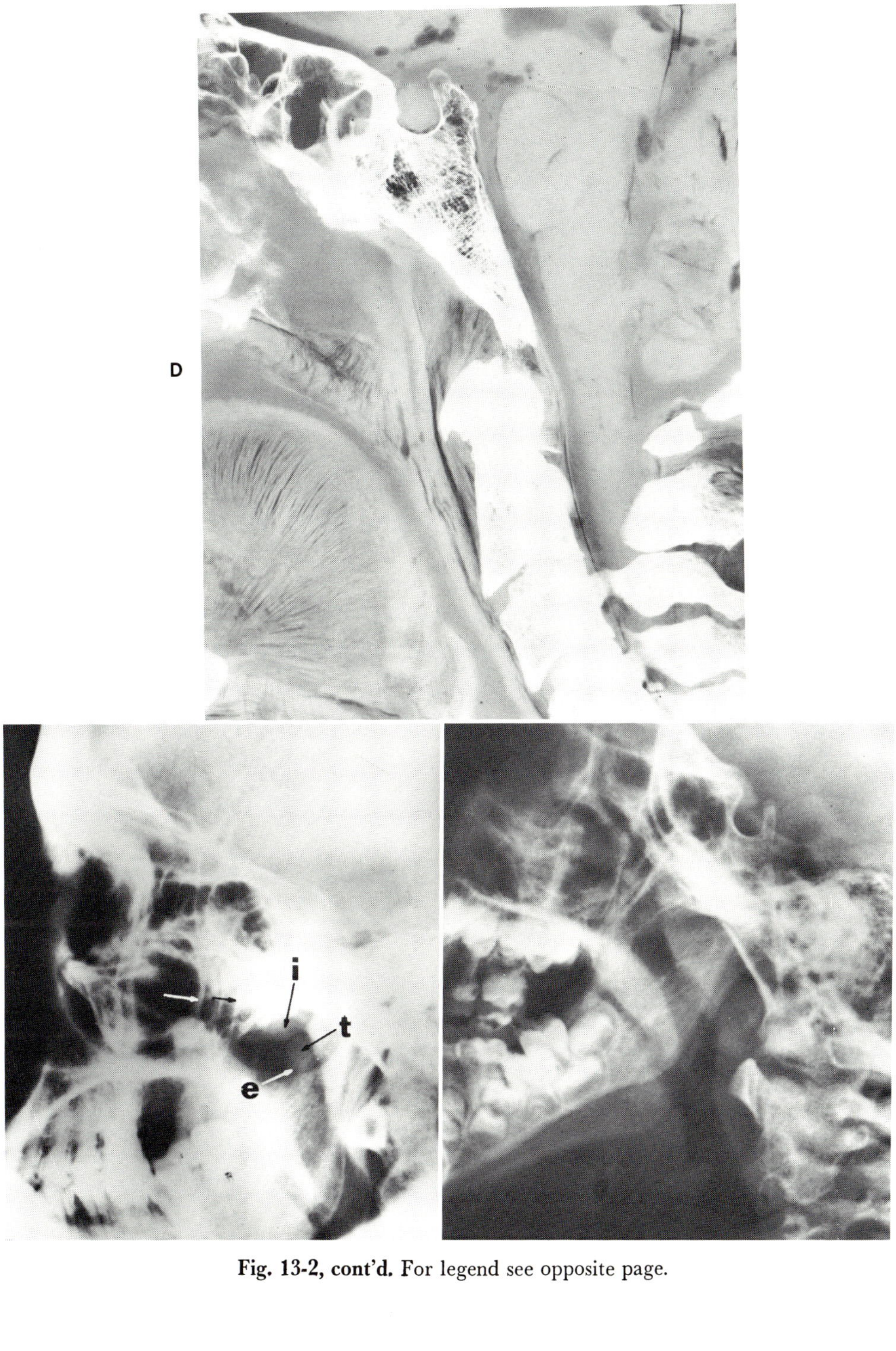

Fig. 13-2, cont'd. For legend see opposite page.

A
B
C

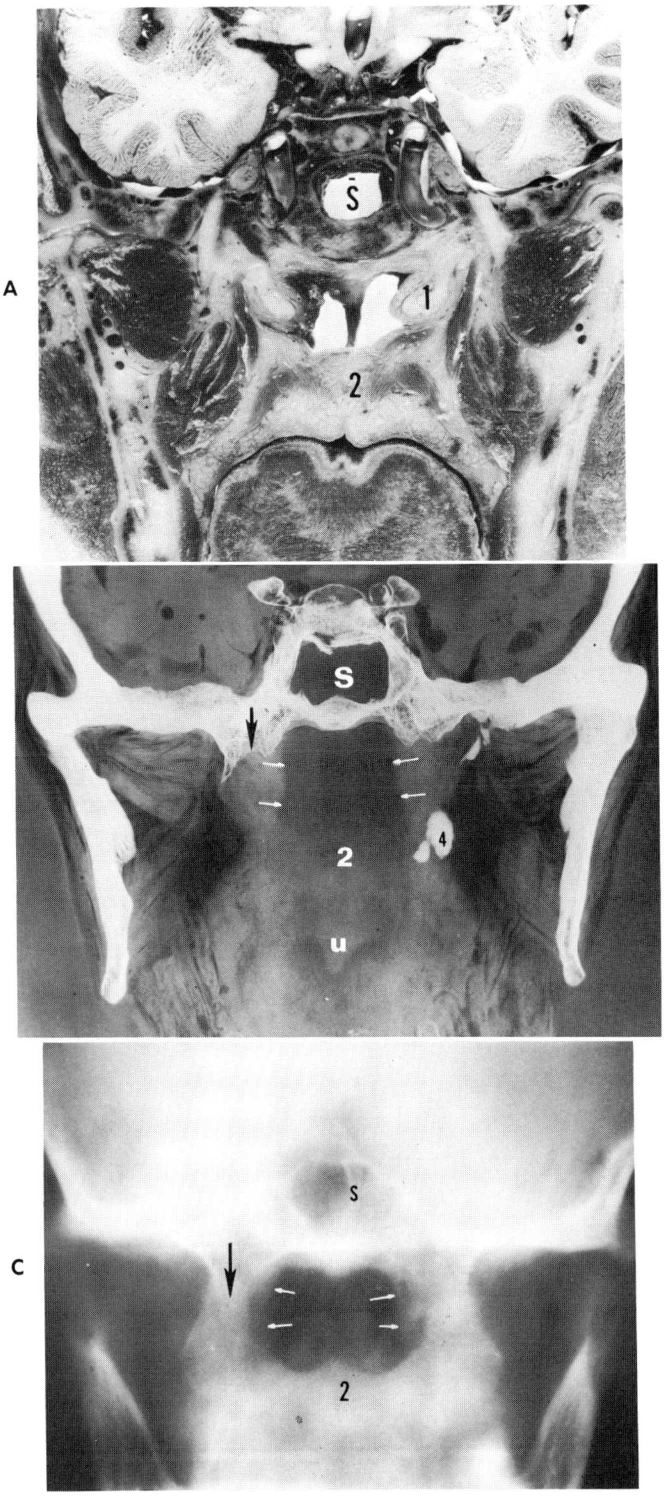

Fig. 13-3. Nasopharynx in frontal view. **A,** Anatomic coronal section through nasopharynx. *S,* Sphenoid sinus; *1,* torus tubarius; *2,* soft palate. **B,** Roentgenogram of coronal section of specimen at level of nasopharynx. *S,* Sphenoid sinus; *2,* soft palate; *4,* palatine tonsil calculus; *u,* uvula; white arrows indicate lateral pharyngeal wall; black arrow, pterygoid process. **C,** Clinical tomogram in AP projection. *S,* Sphenoid sinus; *2,* soft palate; white arrows indicate lateral nasopharyngeal wall; black arrow, pterygoid process.

(Figs. 13-2 to 13-4). The torus tubarius is cartilaginous above and behind and is perforated by the trumpet-shaped opening of the eustachian tube (Fig. 13-2, *C*). Two longitudinal folds delimit each torus, the salpingopalatine fold anteriorly and the salpingopharyngeal fold posteriorly.

Layers

The nasopharynx has four layers: mucosa, aponeurosis, muscle, and fascia (MacComb and Fletcher, 1967). The inner layer is the *mucosa,* which contains abundant lymphoid tissue. The superior wall, and to a degree the posterior wall, is thrown into numerous folds by this tissue to form the pharyngeal tonsil or adenoids (Weitz, 1946). This structure may be particularly prominent in children. Rich lymphoid accumulations are present at the eustachian orifices (the tubal tonsils) and longitudinally along the lateral walls. The two sides are bridged anteroinferiorly across the soft palate by lymphoid extensions that contribute to form the upper arch of Waldeyer's ring (Lederman, 1961; Ackerman and del Regato, 1962) (Fig. 13-1). The second layer, the *pharyngeal aponeurosis,* inserts at the pharyngeal tubercles of the basiocciput posteriorly, passes laterally just anterior to the carotid canal of each side, and extends anteriorly past the petrous tip to attach at the medial pterygoid plate (Fig. 13-4, *D*). The space thus described encloses the foramina lacera. The *muscular layer* is formed by the superior constrictor muscle, having cranial attachments anteriorly and posteriorly (MacComb and Fletcher, 1967). Laterally is the sinus of Morgagni, through which the eustachian tube enters. The fourth and outermost layer is the *buccopharyngeal fascia,* which is loosely connected posteriorly to the prevertebral

---

Fig. 13-4. Nasopharynx in axial view. **A,** Anatomic horizontal cross section through nasopharynx. **B,** Diagram of **A.** *M,* Maxillary sinuses; *1,* torus tubarius; *2,* soft palate; *3,* pharyngeal recess (fossa of Rosenmüller); *4,* plane of palatine tonsil, which lies more inferiorly; *5,* internal carotid artery. **C,** Roentgenogram of horizontal cross section of specimen at level of nasopharynx demonstrates soft tissue and bony landmarks. Arrow marks lateral pterygoid plate. *1,* Torus tubarius. **D,** Roentgenogram of dried skull in axial projection shows sphenoid bone, which contains foramen ovale (long arrow) and foramen spinosum (short arrow). White line, enclosing the foramen lacerum, depicts aponeurotic attachment to base of skull. **E,** Clinical roentgenogram in axial projection shows soft-tissue structures demonstrated in **A** and **B** and bony landmarks of **C** and **D.** White arrows outline posterior nasopharyngeal wall; small black arrows outline lateral aspects of oropharynx, not to be mistaken for lateral nasopharyngeal wall; large black arrow denotes lateral pterygoid plate. *1,* Tori tubarii with pharyngeal recess behind.

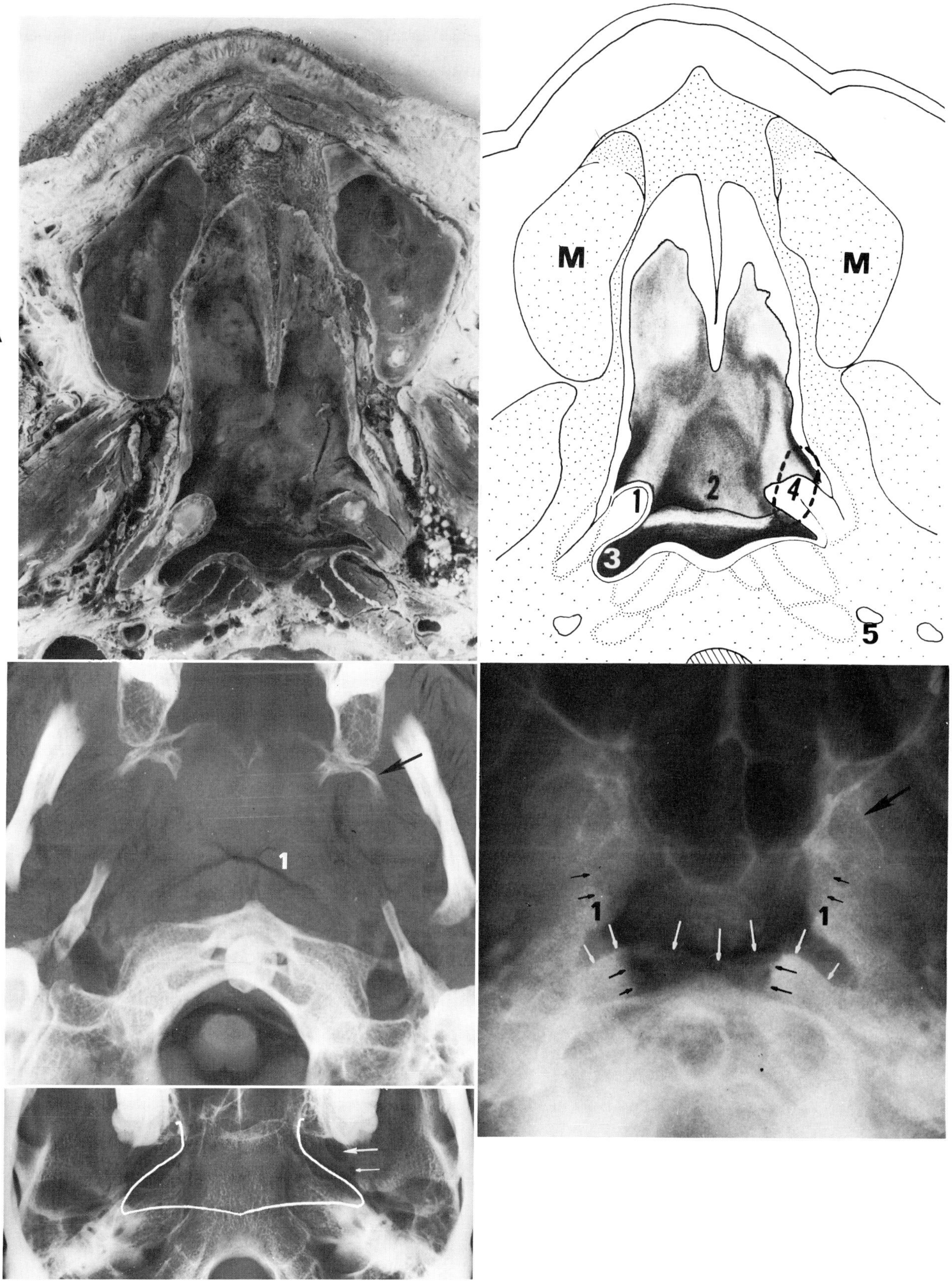

Fig. 13-4. For legend see opposite page.

layer of the deep cervical fascia. A potential space is thus formed that is continuous into the mediastinum (MacComb and Fletcher, 1967).

More distant relationships

Anterior to the nasopharynx are the nasal fossae, which in turn are related to the maxillary sinuses, the ethmoid sinuses, and the medial pterygoid plate. Posteriorly are the first two cervical vertebrae. Superiorly are the sphenoid sinuses and the middle cranial fossae; inferiorly is the oropharynx. The middle cranial fossa is separated from the lateral nasopharynx by the foramen lacerum, which contains mucosa and fibrocartilage only. The carotid canal is posterolateral to the foramen lacerum. The third, fourth, and sixth cranial nerves, together with the first and second divisions of the fifth cranial nerve, are close to the point where the carotid artery enters the skull. Lateral and slightly anterior to the foramen lacerum is the foramen ovale and the third division of the fifth cranial nerve.

Posterolaterally the fossa of Rosenmüller is related to the retroparotid space, or poststyloid portion of the lateral pharyngeal space. This space encloses several important structures: the superior cervical sympathetic ganglion, the last four cranial nerves, the internal carotid artery, and the internal jugular vein.

ROENTGENOGRAPHIC TECHNIQUE

Plain roentgenograms for the assessment of the nasopharynx should include axial and lateral projections, which usually give the most information. These views may be supplemented by stereoscopic axial and lateral films, paranasal sinus views, and Waters, Towne, straight posteroanterior, and Stenvers views, where indicated.

When an abnormality is suspected on the plain films, tomography should be performed. Anteroposterior and axial or subaxial tomograms are most helpful. Hypocycloidal motion is superior to linear tomography because it eliminates parasite shadows. A relative disadvantage is that the sections are so thin that a bony structure moving out of the plane of focus may be interpreted as being eroded. Also some contrast is lost (Potter and Seaman, 1966).

Positive contrast examination of the nasopharynx (with barium or oily contrast media) has been described and is advocated by some authors (Bloch and Quantrill, 1968). More recently cinefluorography has been used during positive contrast examination to study the mobility of the nasopharynx (Khoo et al., 1967). Other authors believe positive contrast studies to be contraindicated because the dense material may obscure bony abnormalities (Ho, 1967b). Generally this type of study is not necessary when hypocycloidal tomography has been performed.

Carotid and vertebral angiography is useful to demonstrate the extent of vascular lesions and their effect on adjacent vessels (Melot et al., 1958; Rosen et al., 1966). Furthermore, angiography may be helpful in predicting tumor pathology (Wilson and Hanafee, 1969).

ROENTGENOGRAPHIC ANATOMY

Air in the nasopharynx offers a natural contrast medium for identification of the soft-tissue structures. After these have been studied carefully, the normal bony landmarks should be identified. As in other anatomic regions, the nasopharyngeal structures best detailed are those seen in tangent, where there is significant interface between tissues of different densities. The lateral projection therefore is used to delineate anterior, posterior, superior, and inferior structures; and the frontal projection (tomogram) to delineate superior, inferior, and lateral landmarks. The axial projection is best for nasopharyngeal structures that are anterior, posterior, or lateral.

Lateral view

In the lateral view the structures most readily identified are the soft palate and the soft tissues comprising the roof and posterior walls. The soft palate is convex backward. Alteration of this appearance may be abnormal.

Although laterally placed and seen *en face,* the torus tubarius may be identified since it projects medially, thus creating a significant air–soft-tissue interface (Fig. 13-2, *E*). The lymphoid tissue of the roof (pharyngeal tonsil) is prominent in childhood (Fig. 13-2, *F*) and decreases with age. Indeed, prominence of nasopharyngeal lymphoid tissue in adulthood is abnormal. Many studies have been performed in an attempt to establish normal measurements for the soft tissues of the roof of the nasopharynx (Weitz, 1946; Oon, 1964; Ho, 1967b; Jóhannesson, 1968; Capitanio and Kirkpatrick, 1970). An absolute normal measurement is difficult to establish since, among the various studies, differences exist in the focus-film and patient-film distances. In one study (Ho, 1967b) the average adult thickness of the anterior roof of the nasopharynx, measured where the posterior edge of the nasal septum joins the skull base, was 8 mm (range 2 to 12.5 mm). The average thickness of the posterior roof of the nasopharynx was 17.8 mm (range 12 to 33 mm) in males and 15.7 mm (range 12 to 20 mm) in females. The posterior roof thickness was measured from the anterior lip of the foramen magnum to the point where the posterior wall of the nasopharynx meets the roof. The average thickness in children of 2 to 15 years was 13.4 mm (range 10 to 18 mm). This was the greatest width of the soft tissues measured anterior to the pharyngeal tubercule and perpendicular to the bony roof. Ho (1967b) emphasized that variations are wide and that a normal measurement does not preclude abnormality. A local thickening, however, should arouse suspicion even if the measurement is normal.

Adenoid hyperplasia is frequent in children. In their study of 257 children, Capitanio and Kirkpatrick (1970) found no measurable lymphoid tissue under age 1 month. After that age thickening of lymphoid tissue occurred up to age 2 years, after which time it leveled off at about 13.5 mm. Involution to the normal adult thickness has been variously reported from ages 10 to 25 years (Jóhannesson, 1968). The contour of the pharyngeal tonsil in childhood is convex from the roof into the nasopharyngeal lumen. Posteriorly the soft tissues describe a straight line (Groth, 1933).

A second convexity may be found in this region when a lateral skull is taken with the neck obliqued (Fig. 13-2, *F*). In children a full expiration may produce thickening of the posterior soft tissues (Grunebaum and Moskowitz, 1970). In the identification of the soft tissues, one must be careful to distinguish the inferior nasal turbinate (Hill, 1940) (Fig. 13-2, *E*) from the earlobe. These two structures may cause considerable confusion.

The bony structures to be identified on the lateral projection are the posterior walls of the maxillary sinuses and the pterygoid processes, which delimit the pterygopalatine fossae and canals (Fig. 13-2, *E*). These are seen to best advantage when the head is obliqued approximately 10° (Potter, 1969). The basisphenoid and basioccipital bones and the upper cervical vertebrae form the superior and posterior bony nasopharyngeal boundaries (Fig. 13-2, *D* to *F*). It is especially important to identify the sphenoid sinus since intracranial extension of nasopharyngeal malignancy may involve this structure. The hard palate should also be examined.

Anteroposterior view

The anteroposterior projection is more useful in evaluating the bony landmarks than the soft tissues since the bones of the nasal fossa obscure the soft-tissue structures on the plain film. Frontal tomography, however, is valuable in assessing soft-tissue as well as bony structures (Fig. 13-3, *C*).

Axial view

The air shadows seen in the axial projection are those of the oropharynx and the piriform sinuses, which are superimposed. The latter are capable of great variation in size and shape in different phases of respiration, as can be well shown on laryngography. The nasopharyngeal portion of the pharyngeal air column is more constant in appearance. These structures (the oropharynx and piriform sinuses) should not be confused with the nasopharynx (Fig. 13-4, *E*).

The torus tubarius protrudes into the lateral aspect of the nasopharyngeal air shadow. The pharyngeal recess (fossa of Rosenmüller), which in some individuals is 1 cm deep, lies behind the torus tubarius (Lederman, 1961) (Fig. 13-4, *E*). Malignancy in this region is common. Therefore it is important to compare the recesses on each side since the only finding with neoplasm may be partial obliteration of this space.

In assessing the posterior nasopharyngeal wall in the axial projection, one should observe the thickness of the soft tissues in front of the anterior arch of the atlas. If the x-ray beam is tangential to the air–soft-tissue interface, there will always be a soft-tissue shadow in front of the anterior arch of the first cervical vertebra (Fig. 13-4, *E*). Indeed, if air is seen behind the anterior arch of the first cervical vertebra, one is most likely looking at the piriform sinuses or the oropharynx since to cast the nasopharyngeal air shadow behind this vertebra would take extreme dorsiflexion of the neck.

Anteriorly the nasopharyngeal air shadow is continuous with that of the nasal fossa. Although the uvula is often identified, the soft palate is not usually seen in tangent. The base of the tongue may also be seen superimposed on the nasopharyngeal air column (Fig. 13-5, *A*).

After the soft-tissue structures have been identified, the bony landmarks should be studied. The sphenoid sinus plates as well as the clivus and posterior clinoid processes should be examined for their integrity. Three lines may superimpose in the axial view (Whalen and Berne, 1964). These are (1) the anterior wall of the middle fossa, which is concave posteriorly, (2) the posterior wall of the orbit, which follows a straight course, oblique outward, from posterior to anterior, and (3) the posterior wall of the maxillary sinus, which follows a similar course but is sigmoid in shape. The relationship of the latter to the pterygoid process should be noted since certain tumors may grow between the two, causing them to become separated.

The foramina of the skull base are often involved in nasopharyngeal cancer (Chapter 16). Most important are the foramina lacerum, ovale, and spinosum and the carotid canal (Fig. 13-4, *D*). The eustachian tubes extend medially in an oblique manner from posterior to anterior. Their proximal bony portions are seen in the region of the middle ear; and if this line is extended anteriorly, just medial to the foramina spinosum and ovale, the torus tubarius can be identified.

PATHOLOGY

Roentgenographic features

Soft-tissue abnormalities

The soft tissues may be altered by a mass that arises within the nasopharynx and projects into its air column

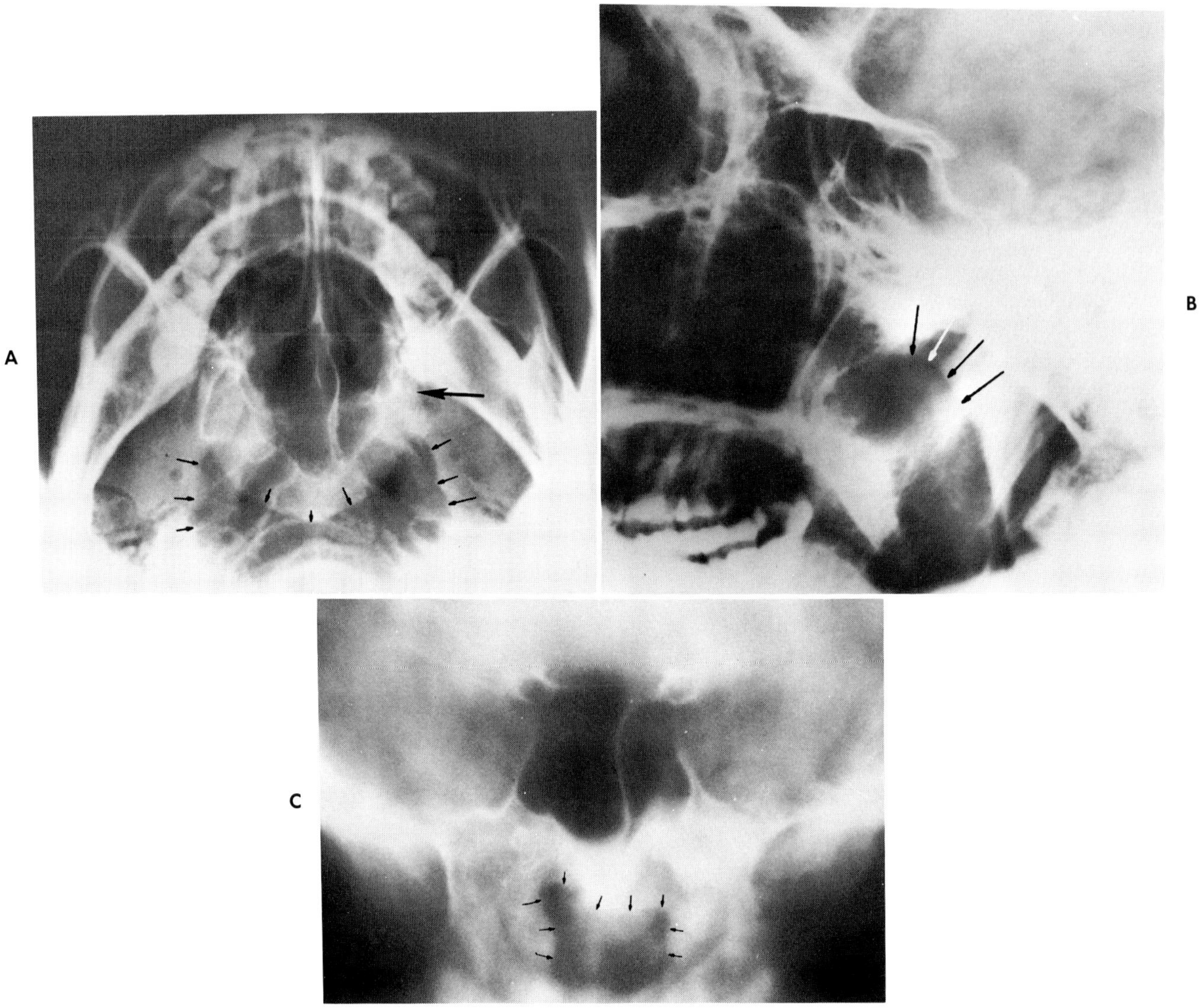

Fig. 13-5. Epidermoid carcinoma. **A,** Subaxial view demonstrates bone destruction of pterygoid bone (large arrow). Soft-tissue shadow of tumor is not visualized in this projection. Note the lateral aspects of the air-distended oropharynx (horizontal arrows), not to be mistaken for lateral nasopharyngeal walls. Base of tongue (vertical arrows) casts prominent shadow, outlined by oropharyngeal air (horizontal arrows), below nasopharynx. **B,** Lateral roentgenogram of skull demonstrates soft-tissue mass in roof of nasopharynx that encroaches on nasopharyngeal air shadow from above (arrows). **C,** Anteroposterior roentgenogram (tomographic section) demonstrates eccentric mass involving primarily the roof on the left side. Arrows outline the distorted nasopharyngeal air shadow. Note the evidence of bone involvement with reactive sclerosis of the left pterygoid process.

(Figs. 13-5 and 13-6); or the mass may arise outside the nasopharynx, which it may displace away from the side of the lesion. As a general rule the more intraluminal the mass in proportion to the displacement it causes, the more likely the lesion is to be primary in the nasopharynx. The greater the displacement in proportion to the size of the intraluminal mass, the more likely is the tumor to be extranasopharyngeal.

A soft-tissue mass that is intraluminal is visible on the routine plain roentgenogram; but it may require extra views or special procedures, such as tomography and rarely nasopharyngography, for more complete evaluation.

When the mass itself cannot be appreciated, specific indirect signs should be sought. Normally the lateral roentgenogram shows the soft palate to be convex backward. When a posterior mass reaches sufficient size, it causes downward flattening or even a posterior concavity

A

B

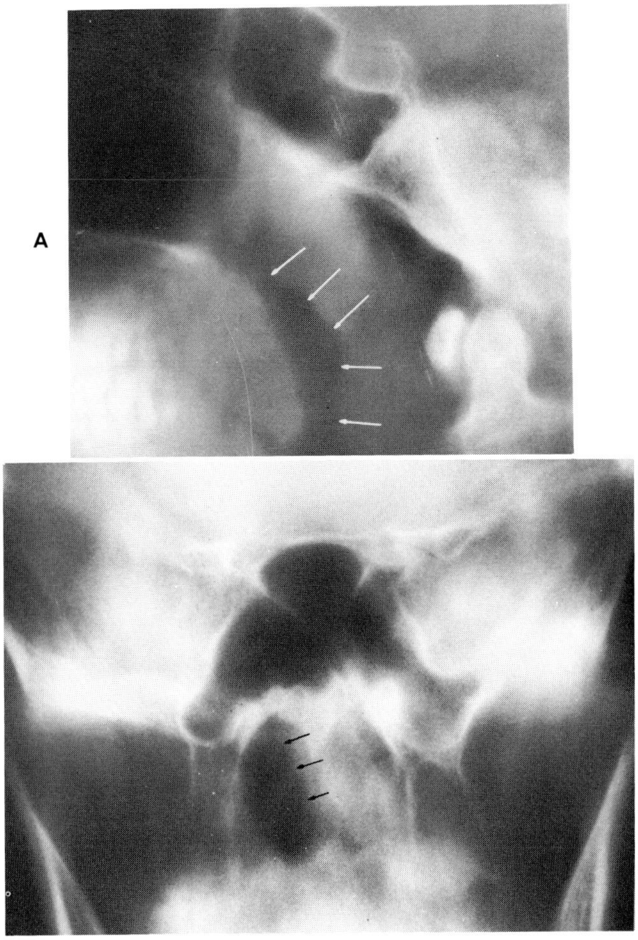

Fig. 13-6. Epidermoid carcinoma of nasopharynx. **A,** Lateral tomographic section shows posterior nasopharyngeal mass encroaching on nasopharyngeal air shadow (arrows). **B,** Anteroposterior tomographic section shows left lateral component of tumor that intrudes on lateral air shadow of nasopharynx (arrows).

A

B

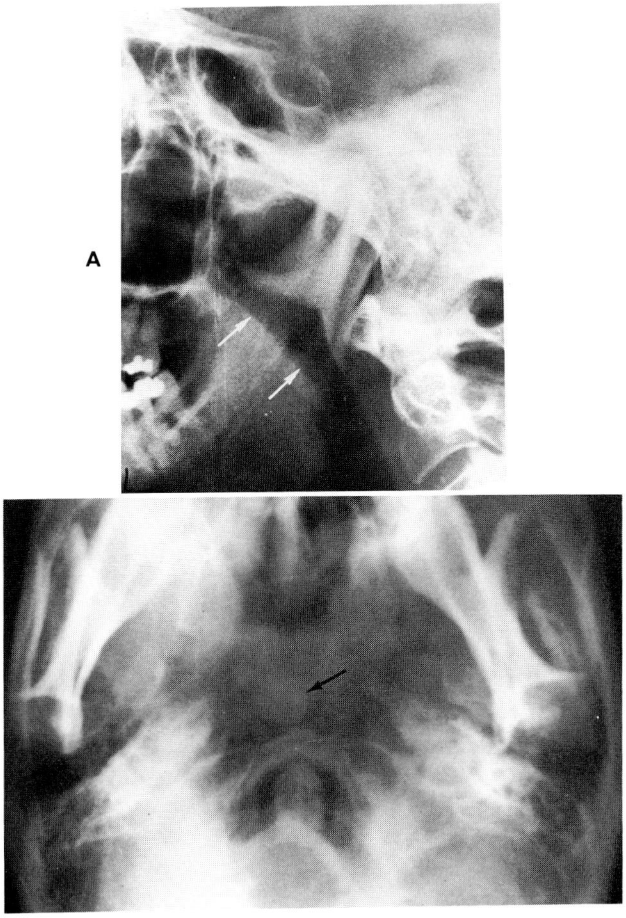

Fig. 13-7. Lymphosarcoma of nasopharynx. **A,** Soft-tissue shadow of tumor is seen to encroach on nasopharyngeal shadow from behind. Soft palate is flattened (arrows), suggesting more inferior and anterior extension by posterior mass. **B,** Roentgenogram in basal projection shows contralateral displacement of uvula (arrow), which verifies the more anterior and inferior extension of the tumor that is directly visualized in the lateral projection. (Courtesy F. W. Van Buskirk, M.D., University of Vermont, College of Medicine, Burlington, Vt.)

of the soft palate (Jönsson, 1941; Epstein, 1951) (Figs. 13-7, *A,* and 13-8, *B*). A laterally placed mass seen *en face* may not be appreciated directly when it does not produce a significant air–soft-tissue interface. It may cause depression of the soft palate, however. Even when a posterior mass is detected and a column of air is seen between it and the soft palate, flattening of the latter implies that the mass is lobulated and that an inapparent component causes this effect (Fig. 13-7, *A*). Thus the abnormality may be more extensive than suspected initially, and further investigation is warranted.

Related to depression of the soft palate is stretching of the posterior palatine arch (Jönsson, 1941). As the palate is displaced, tension on the posterior palatine arch causes it to stand out against nasopharyngeal air.

In the axial projection the uvula is often seen and may be displaced by an eccentric mass. A lateral mass is usually appreciated directly by its interface with nasopharyngeal air in this view. A superiorly placed or bulky mass can obscure the upper nasopharyngeal air column. With a lateral component the uvula may be displaced, leading to the suspicion of more extensive disease (Fig. 13-7, *B*).

Paranasal sinusitis may be a feature of nasopharyngeal neoplasm (Belanger and Dyke, 1943) and may result from obstruction or bone invasion by tumor. Mayer, in 1928, proposed that extension of masses into the cavernous sinus can cause vascular congestion, which clouds the paranasal sinus. Ipsilateral clouding of the mastoid, which is indistinguishable from acute and subacute mastoiditis, has been described (Miller et al., 1969).

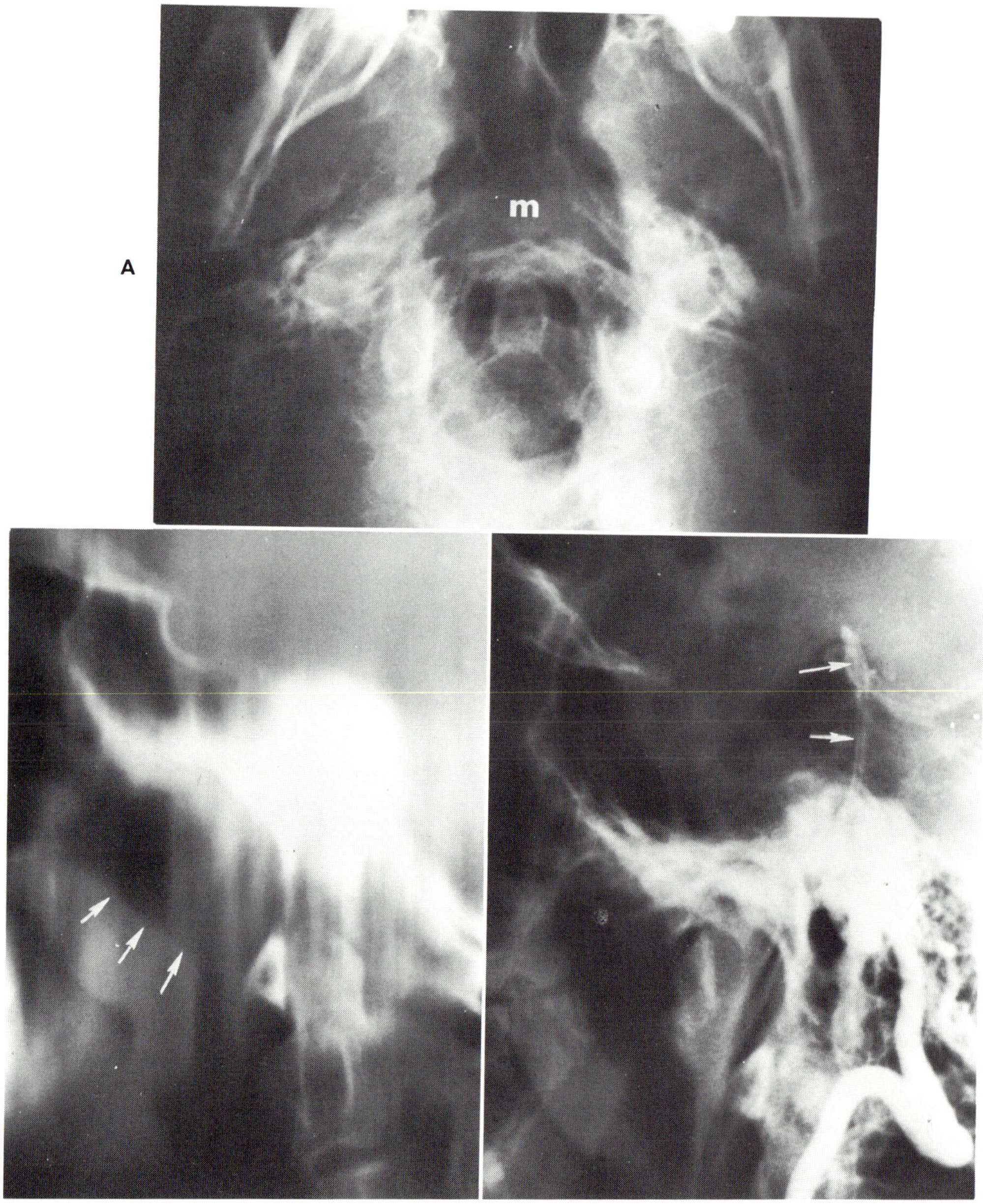

Fig. 13-8. Chordoma of clivus. **A,** Axial view of skull demonstrates ill-defined mass (*m*) intruding on air shadow of nasopharynx from behind. Destruction of clivus is also demonstrated. **B,** Lateral tomogram demonstrates displacement of soft palate with reversal of normal posterior convexity of nasopharyngeal surface to a posterior concavity (arrows), an indirect sign of nasopharyngeal mass. **C,** Lateral projection of vertebral artery arteriogram demonstrates posterior displacement of basilar artery (arrows), which establishes an intracranial component.

Bony abnormalities

A primary nasopharyngeal mass may cause destruction, sclerosis (or both), or displacement of the contiguous bony structures. Primary diseases of the bone, such as chondrosarcoma (Fig. 13-9) and osteogenic sarcoma, may also affect the nasopharynx secondarily. Careful examination of the bony structures is essential; and when abnormality is uncertain, tomography should be performed.

Bone may be destroyed in two ways: by *pressure erosion* or by actual *osseous invasion.* In both instances a margin of reactive sclerosis is usually seen. When pressure erosion causes bone destruction, an area of rarefaction with a thin well-circumscribed margin of reactive

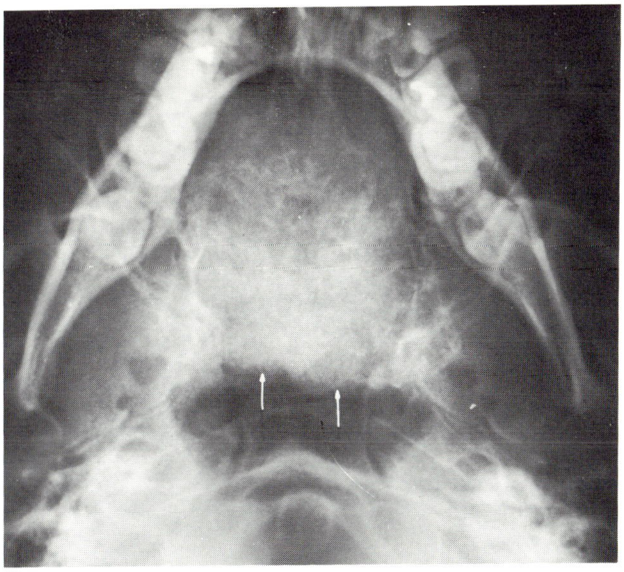

Fig. 13-9. Chondrosarcoma of hard palate. Tumor is seen to extend posteriorly into anterior nasopharynx (arrows).

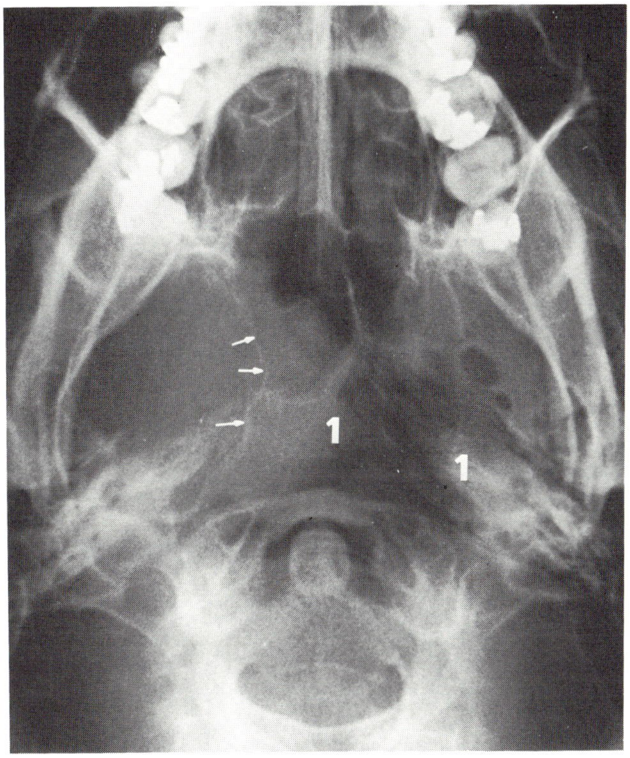

Fig. 13-10. Neurilemmoma of trigeminal nerve. Axial view of skull demonstrates large soft-tissue mass on the right. Mass extends into lateral aspect of nasopharynx but mainly displaces nasopharynx to the left, which suggests extranasopharyngeal origin. Displacement is appreciated when tori tubarii (*1*) on the two sides are compared. Pressure erosion of right sphenoid bone has resulted in loss of usual landmarks (foramina ovale and spinosum). Benign character of erosion is illustrated by well-circumscribed sclerosis (arrows). (Courtesy Fred Hodges, III, M.D., Johns Hopkins Hospital, Baltimore, Md.)

sclerosis is present. This type of bone involvement is seen in the benign tumors that grow slowly (Fig. 13-10). With bone invasion the area of destruction generally is more irregular, and a dense ill-defined margin of sclerosis may be present (Ho, 1967b) (Fig. 13-5, *A*). Such destruction is more characteristic of malignant tumor.

In evaluation of the base of the skull, the foramina, as well as the other bony landmarks, should be identified. (See Chapter 16.) A difference between the foraminal size of each side is not sufficient to be considered abnormal. Size can be influenced by projection and by normal variations. The diagnosis of foraminal involvement depends on (1) disappearance of the white bony cortex of the foramen, (2) a surrounding area of reactive sclerosis, and (3) irregularity of the foramen (Ho, 1967b).

Occasionally bone involvement is purely sclerotic. Sclerosis may be midline, eccentric, or bilateral, and it can extend posteriorly to include the anterior arch of the atlas and odontoid process (Potter, 1970). This type of bone reaction has been described in malignant nasopharyngeal tumors (Belanger and Dyke, 1943; Epstein, 1951); but it is also seen in inflammatory disease. The differential diagnosis includes fibrous dysplasia, meningioma, metastatic neoplasm, lethal midline granuloma, and some other lesions (Potter, 1970).

Specific disease processes

Malignant tumors

Primary nasopharyngeal tumors. By far the most important lesions of the nasopharynx are the malignant tumors. Of these, the most common are carcinomas and sarcomas (Schmidt, 1962).

Incidence (Martin and Blady, 1940; Scanlon et al., 1958; Lederman, 1961; Ackerman and del Regato, 1962; Bailar, 1967; Miyaji, 1967; Muir and Shanmugaratnam, 1967; Quisenberry and Heimann-Jasinski, 1967)

The incidence of cancer in the region of the nasopharynx has been variously reported as 0.3% to 2% of all malignant neoplasms in man. Although the Chinese are more often affected than any other ethnic group, some authors have expressed the belief that these are the China-born Chinese. Others have stated that the predisposing factor is more racial than environmental. Except in the Japanese, an increased relative frequency of nasopharyngeal cancers has also been noted in other Orientals. White populations are less commonly affected, especially in the United States.

Age and sex (Martin and Blady, 1940; Godtfredsen, 1944; Martin, 1957; Scanlon et al., 1958; Lederman, 1961; Ho, 1967a; Quisenberry and Heimann-Jasinski, 1967; Yeh, 1967)

In all groups males are more frequently affected than

females, in a ratio of from 2:1 to 4:1. The average age at the time of onset is about 45 years, and the peak is between 40 and 60 years. Among the Chinese these tumors develop at an earlier age. Nasopharyngeal tumors are not rare in youth, and some surveys include children as young as 3 and 4 years of age. Most such tumors in children are anaplastic carcinomas (lymphoepithelioma or transitional cell carcinoma).

Histology. Great discrepancies appear in the literature concerning the relative incidence of carcinoma and sarcoma and of the various histologic subtypes. These discrepancies may be more apparent than real and might result from differences in classification. Particular confusion exists in regard to lymphoepithelioma and transitional cell carcinoma. Yeh (1967) preferred to consider lymphoepithelioma as a form of transitional cell carcinoma and included both forms as varieties of epidermoid carcinoma. In his study of 1,437 malignant nasopharyngeal neoplasms in Taiwan, 99% were carcinomas (including epidermoid, adenocarcinoma, and undifferentiated forms). Sarcomas (reticulum cell sarcoma, lymphosarcoma, and acute lymphatic leukemia) comprised only 1%. In 1944, Godtfredsen reviewed 768 cases and added 454 of his own. In both groups he found identical relative frequencies, 56% and 44% for carcinoma and sarcoma respectively. Lymphoepithelioma and transitional cell carcinoma were included as forms of sarcoma, however, and the two combined constituted approximately 11%. Generally carcinoma appears more frequent than sarcoma. Among the carcinomas, epidermoids (of various degrees of differentiation) are the most common in many series, especially if lymphoepithelioma and transitional cell carcinoma are considered as subgroups (Miller, 1951; Fletcher and Million, 1965; Yeh, 1967). Adenocarcinoma is relatively rare, and unclassified carcinoma is of intermediate frequency. Of the sarcomas, lymphosarcoma and reticulum cell sarcoma are the types reported frequently. A simplified classification (modified after that of Yeh, 1967) is summarized in the outline that follows:

Common primary malignancies of the nasopharynx

I. Carcinoma
   A. Epidermoid (including transitional cell carcinoma and lymphoepithelioma)
   B. Adenocarcinoma
   C. Unclassified
II. Sarcoma
   A. Reticulum cell sarcoma
   B. Lymphosarcoma

Gross pathology. Malignant tumors of the nasopharynx are likely to appear as ulcerated, lobular, or exophytic masses.

In 1962 Ackerman and del Regato observed the following correlations between the histologic and gross pathologic changes:

The *ulcerated* lesion is usually situated posteriorly or posterolaterally in the fossa of Rosenmüller. Such a lesion is likely in the uncommon well-differentiated epidermoid carcinoma.

Most commonly the site of the *lobular* form is lateral and near the torus tubarius. This form is of the usual morphologic type seen in undifferentiated epidermoid carcinoma.

The *exophytic* tumor is a smooth, round, often large mass, which may be on a stalk. This form usually arises from the roof of the nasopharynx and usually is a lymphosarcoma of the pharyngeal tonsil. Lymphosarcomas may also arise from the lateral wall or posterolaterally in the fossa of Rosenmüller. In these latter sites the mass tends less to become large and project into the nasopharynx, as is the tendency of roof lesions.

The soft palate (floor) and anterior wall are rare sites of malignant nasopharyngeal tumor (Martin and Blady, 1940).

Clinical signs. The clinical manifestations in a patient with malignant disease of the nasopharynx depend on the route of spread as well as on the local effects.

Anterior extension into the nasal fossa, or a large mass in the nasopharynx, may cause obstruction of the upper air passages quite late in the disease (Martin and Blady, 1940). Anterior extension may also involve the maxillary sinus, the ethmoid sinus, or the medial pterygoid plate. Complaints of nasal symptoms were the most common presentation in the patients of Lederman's series (1961).

Posterior extension involves the first and second cervical vertebrae, whereas growth superiorly may extend into the base of the skull, the sphenoid sinuses, or the middle cranial fossa on one or both sides. Large masses may extend inferiorly into the oropharynx. Lateral extension often involves the foramen lacerum, which is separated from the nasopharynx only by mucosa and fibrocartilage. Some authors have stated that the foramen lacerum is the main route of malignant extension into the middle cranial fossa (Baylin et al., 1949). Others, however, argue that the fibrocartilage resists invasion and that the primary pathway is through the floor of the carotid canal (Lederman, 1961). When the foramen lacerum is involved, the tumor may encase the carotid artery and reach the cavernous sinus. Disturbance in function of the third, fourth, and sixth cranial nerves and the first and second divisions of the fifth cranial nerve may result (Lenz, 1942). The third division of the fifth cranial nerve is involved, with lateral extension of tumor to the foramen ovale. Invasion of the petrous bone may allow extension to the ear, but only at a stage when destruction has been extensive. The routes of spread are summarized in Fig. 13-11. At times the

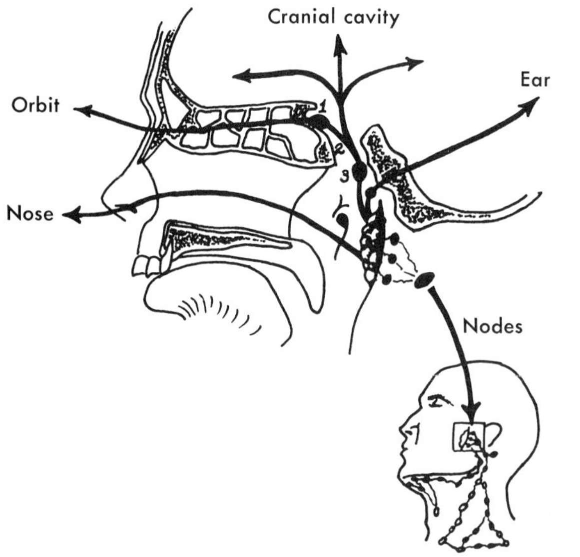

Fig. 13-11. Schematic drawing of routes of spread of primary neoplasms of nasopharynx. *1,* Sphenoid fissure; 2, foramen lacerum; *3,* carotid canal. (Modified from Baylin, G. J., Reeves, R. J., and Kerman, H. D.: Southern Med. J. **42:** 467-476, 1949.)

eustachian tube becomes occluded early (Baylin et al., 1949), which causes hypoacusis. Extension through the eustachian tube is unusual since the cartilage of the torus is resistant to malignant invasion. Extension into the orbit, with consequent proptosis, is relatively uncommon (Lederman, 1961, 1964).

Posterolaterally a tumor may extend into the retroparotid space or poststyloid portion of the lateral pharyngeal space. Here it may involve the superior cervical sympathetic ganglia, the last four cranial nerves, the internal carotid artery, and the internal jugular vein. The more medial structures are usually involved first.

Metastatic spread. Signs of metastasis are extremely important in the clinical manifestation of nasopharyngeal cancer. Lymph node metastasis is the rule in all histologic types, especially in tumors of the roof and of the posterior and lateral walls (Godtfredsen, 1944; Ackerman and del Regato, 1962; Teoh, 1967). On the patient's admission to the hospital, metastatic lymph nodes may be present in as many as 80% to 90% of the cases of nasopharyngeal cancer (Martin and Blady, 1940; Fletcher and Million, 1965; Pantangco et al., 1967). In 20%, cervical adenopathy may be the chief complaint (Lederman, 1961). Contralateral lymph node involvement is present in more than 50% of patients with metastasis (Lederman, 1961). Involvement of cranial nerves may be by direct extension of the tumor itself or by compression of the nerve by metastatic nodes. Facial nerve involvement is usually the result of contiguous nodal metastasis (Miller, 1951).

Metastasis to distant sites is most commonly associated with lymphoepithelioma, less often with lymphoma, and rarely with well-differentiated epidermoid carcinoma (Ackerman and del Regato, 1962). Metastasis may involve bone, distant lymph nodes, liver, lungs, spleen, skin, adrenals, and testes (Martin and Blady, 1940; Godtfredsen, 1944; Miller, 1951; Teoh, 1967). With lymphoepithelioma, metastasis to bone is most common and tends to involve mainly the axial skeleton. The bony lesions are most commonly lytic, although sclerotic or mixed metastasis is not unusual (Tan and Oon, 1967).

Prognosis. The 5-year survival rate averages about 25%. When the base of the skull is eroded, the 5-year survival rate is reduced to 12.5% (Godtfredsen, 1944). Lymphoma appears to afford the most favorable prognosis, and well-differentiated carcinoma the worst. Patients with lymphoepithelioma have an intermediate chance of survival (Lederman, 1961; Ackerman and del Regato, 1962).

Death is nearly always the result of intracranial spread or diffuse dissemination (Martin and Blady, 1940).

Radiologic features. The two characteristic features of nasopharyngeal cancer are a soft-tissue mass and destruction of the base of the skull (Jönsson, 1934).

In nearly all cancers of the nasopharynx, a *soft-tissue mass* is identified in the lateral or axial views (Baylin et al., 1949; Miller et al., 1969). Miller and his coworkers (1969) studied 102 malignant tumors, and in most instances a soft-tissue mass could be detected on both the lateral and the axial views. Those masses not visible were mostly flat or, when large, were usually situated laterally or in the fossa of Rosenmüller. Any mass seen in the axial view, regardless of its size, should be considered abnormal (Miller et al., 1969). When the posterosuperior nasopharyngeal soft tissue measures more than 1.8 cm in the lateral projection, abnormality must be suspected. Ho (1967b) stated that a normal measurement does not necessarily exclude disease since wide variations exist. A localized swelling, however, should cause suspicion of abnormality.

In roentgenograms, tumors of the nasopharynx may appear in two general forms: *infiltrative* (Figs. 13-5 and 13-6) or *lobulated* (Fig. 13-7). Prediction of the nature of a nasopharyngeal tumor is difficult by assessment of the soft-tissue morphology (Baclesse and Dulac, 1948). Certain features of the various tumors are suggestive, however. Larger masses are more likely to be malignant than benign (Jönsson, 1941); exceptions are angiofibromas that may attain tremendous size. Sarcomas, particularly, are often bulky, whereas epidermoid carcinomas are generally smaller and more prone to ulcerate (Godtfredsen, 1944; Scanlon et al., 1958). Ulceration is especially true of well-differentiated epidermoid carcinoma; it may also be a feature of tuberculosis of the nasopharynx (Jönsson, 1941).

Cancer of the nasopharynx is usually eccentric in location (Jönsson, 1941; Godtfredsen, 1944; Lederman, 1961). The fossa of Rosenmüller (and remaining lateral wall) and roof are the most common sites of origin of malignant lesions (about 75% together) (Jönsson, 1941; Scanlon et al., 1958; Lederman, 1961). Next in frequency is the posterior wall. The least common sites are the anterior wall and floor (nasopharyngeal surface of the soft palate), which account for only 5% to 10%. When the tumor is large, determination of its point of origin may be impossible (Scanlon et al., 1958). The location of a mass is not reliable in predicting malignancy versus benignity. Generally an eccentrically situated soft-tissue mass is more likely malignant than benign (Jönsson, 1941), except angiofibroma, to be described later. Midline masses may be of either variety. Malignant tumors of the lateral wall (including the fossa of Rosenmüller) may be of any histologic type. A large exophytic midline mass suggests lymphosarcoma of the pharyngeal tonsil (Ackerman and del Regato, 1962).

Erosion of the base of the skull has been reported in from 13% to 63% of patients with nasopharyngeal cancer. Most authors agree that epidermoid carcinoma causes bone destruction more frequently than does lymphoma (Jönsson, 1941; Godtfredsen, 1944; Baclesse and Dulac, 1948; Lederman, 1961). Since many malignant neoplasms are eccentric, the usual unilateral bone destruction is not surprising (Ho, 1967b), but bilateral and midline involvement may also occur (Miller et al., 1969).

The relative frequency of involvement of the various bones of the skull base depends on the location of the tumor. Anterior masses may involve the medial pterygoid plate and extend into the sphenoid sinus, posterior ethmoid cells, and maxillary sinus (Jönsson, 1941). When extension proceeds more anteriorly, the orbit and nasal fossa may be involved (Lederman, 1961, 1964). Whether the tumor originated in the nasopharynx or the nasal fossa cannot be stated when the nasal fossa is involved (Ho, 1967b). In tumors of the fossa of Rosenmüller, usually the foramen lacerum is involved, first at its posterolateral aspect (that portion formed by the petrous apex). In these instances the carotid canal is often also involved (Ho, 1967b). Lateral extension can lead to destruction of the foramina ovale and spinosum. Tumors growing superiorly may invade the sphenoid body. Extension to the sphenoid sinus not infrequently leads to sellar destruction (Baylin et al., 1949). Posterolateral extension into the petro-occipital fissure leads to involvement of the basiocciput (Ho, 1967b). A posterior tumor may involve the basiocciput directly. When invasion is extensive, many of the structures may be affected.

In general the osseous structures most commonly affected are the sphenoid and petrous bones. Of the foramina, the foramina lacerum and ovale (alone or together with the spinosum) are most frequently destroyed (Ho, 1967b). The sphenoid, ethmoid, maxillary, and frontal sinuses are affected in that order (Baylin et al., 1949). The middle cranial fossa is more commonly involved than the posterior fossa, and the anterior fossa the least often (Teoh, 1967).

Chordoma. A tumor of notochordal origin, chordoma is usually slow growing and of relatively low-grade malignancy. The fetal notochord is a midline structure that extends from the dorsum sellae to the coccyx. Occasionally, notochordal remnants are found dorsal to the clivus or in the soft tissues of the nasopharynx at the junction of the roof and the posterior wall. Chordomas develop anywhere in the axial skeleton, in order of decreasing frequency, in the sacrococcygeal, cranial, and vertebral regions (Wood and Himadi, 1950). They arise more often in the cervical spine than in the thoracic or lumbar spine (Dahlin and MacCarty, 1952). Grossly these tumors appear as gelatinous lobular masses with cystic areas of necrosis. They may contain degenerative calcification; or if bone has been invaded, it may be sequestered or fragmented (Wood and Himadi, 1950). Cranial chordomas are most common in the third and fourth decades of life although they may occur in children (Wood and Himadi, 1950). In most series the ratio of males to females is 2:1 (Windeyer, 1959).

Radiologic features. Chordoma may be primary nasopharyngeal or, depending on its primary site, may affect the nasopharynx secondarily after breaking through the clivus or upper cervical spine. In any of these locations, a soft-tissue mass may be present. Occasionally calcification is roentgenographically detectable within the tumor (Wood and Himadi, 1950; Dahlin and MacCarty, 1952; Windeyer, 1959); or when osseous destruction has occurred, fragmented or sequestered bone may be seen (Wood and Himadi, 1950; Windeyer, 1959). These tumors cause irregular osseous destruction of the basisphenoid and basioccipital bones (Fig. 13-8, *A*). Similar changes may involve the middle cranial fossa, foramen magnum, and occipital bone (Wood and Himadi, 1950). The sella is enlarged but not ballooned as is the case of intrasellar tumors, and the sphenoid sinus is frequently involved (Dahlin and MacCarty, 1952) (Fig. 13-8, *B* and *C*). Vertebral arteriogram will reveal posterior displacement of the basilar artery but no neovascularity (Windeyer, 1959) (Fig. 13-8, *C*).

Other malignant neoplasms. *Plasmocytomas* are occasionally reported in the nasopharynx (Godtfredsen, 1944; Greenfield, 1948; Fletcher and Million, 1965). They may be present at as early as 18 years of age (Greenfield, 1948) but are unusual before age 40 (Godtfredsen, 1944). Most often the nasopharyngeal plasmocytoma develops in the presence of generalized disease (Godtfredsen, 1944).

Other primary malignant tumors of the nasopharynx are rare. *Rhabdomyosarcoma* is a tumor of children and young adults (Lederman, 1961; Mani and Smith, 1968); and a predilection for the nasopharynx has been noted (Mani and Smith, 1968). Rhabdomyosarcoma may be vascular and may displace the posterior antral wall forward, thus simulating angiofibroma (Mani and Smith, 1968). *Malignant teratomas* (and the benign dermoid cysts) are present at birth or neonatally. This is an important diagnostic feature (Miller, 1951). These and other tumors of the neonate should be distinguished from adenoids before the age of 1 month. According to Capitanio and Kirkpatrick (1970), no adenoid tissue is roentgenographically measurable before that age.

Cases of *sarcoma botryoides* (Prior and Stoner, 1957) and *leiomyosarcoma* of the nasopharynx (Dobben, 1958) have been reported. Sarcoma may develop in any of the connective tissue elements, and metastatic spread from this tumor is not unknown (Lederman, 1961). (A more complete list of the uncommon tumors of the nasopharynx appeared in an article by Stout, 1941.)

Benign lesions of the nasopharynx

Juvenile angiofibroma. The most common benign tumor of the nasopharynx (Rosen et al., 1966), angiofibroma is also known as fibroma, juvenile basal fibroma, fibroid of the nasopharynx, and myxofibroma. It is a highly vascular neoplasm typically found in pubescent males, but it has been reported in patients of up to 50 years of age (Rosen et al., 1966). Occasionally it has been found in females (Holman and Miller, 1965; Fitzpatrick, 1967).

Grossly this tumor consists of a smooth shiny mass, which arises eccentrically from the roof of the anterior nasopharynx or from the posterior nasal fossa (Ackerman and del Regato, 1962). The tumor may reach considerable size, but it does not infiltrate locally. Its growth is by expansion and pressure erosion (Holman and Miller, 1965); and extension tends to be polydirectional along natural foramina and fissures (Wilson and Hanafee, 1969). A large tumor may fill the nasopharynx and extend anteriorly through the nares. Anterolaterally the orbit, maxillary antrum, zygoma, and mandible may be expanded (Massoud and Awwad, 1960). The tumor may extend superiorly into the sphenoid sinus and sella turcica, or it may involve the middle cranial fossa by extradural spread (Wilson and Hanafee, 1969).

Histologically the angiofibroma is a benign tumor composed of connective tissue, with prominent vascular components (Ackerman and del Regato, 1962). Lymph node metastasis (Massoud and Awwad, 1960) and sarcomatous change (Rosen et al., 1966) are rare, but not unknown. Bleeding, at times massive, may be a prominent feature; and biopsy is particularly hazardous. As the patient reaches adulthood, the tumor may regress spontaneously. Commonly after surgical treatment the tumor recurs. Irradiation or hormonal therapy may arrest the process until spontaneous involution begins (Ackerman and del Regato, 1962).

The tumor may appear as a well-circumscribed soft-tissue mass surrounded by air over a large portion of its circumference (Figs. 13-12 and 13-13). In their study of forty-six cases of juvenile angiofibroma, Holman and Miller (1965) stressed three characteristic roentgenographic features: (1) anterior bowing of the posterior maxillary wall in front of the expanding mass, (2) an area of lucency in the sphenoid bone with a well-marginated rim of sclerosis, characteristic of benign growth, and (3) occasional enlargement of the outer lower margin of the superior orbital fissure.

Potter (1969) described a posterior bowing sign in which the pterygoid process is displaced backward. Anterior bowing of the posterior maxillary wall and posterior bowing of the pterygoid process take place as the tumor insinuates itself between the posterior maxillary wall and the pterygoid process. This bony displacement signifies that the tumor has extended beyond the confines of the nasopharynx (Potter, 1969). Anterior bowing of the posterior maxillary wall has rarely been reported in other tumors (Holman and Miller, 1965; Mani and Smith, 1968; Potter, 1969). In such instances tomography may demonstrate destruction of the posterior wall of the pterygopalatine fossa (Potter, 1969).

The external carotid artery (ascending pharyngeal and internal maxillary branches) supplies the juvenile angiofibroma. Meningeal branches of the internal carotid artery, and the ophthalmic artery, may contribute to its blood supply when it grows intracranially. The tumor is therefore well shown by selective internal and external carotid arteriography. In the early arterial phase there is rapid filling of reticulated vessels, which are irregular in diameter but are of approximately equal size (Rosen et al., 1966). In the capillary phase a homogeneous blush appears, but no early venous filling (Wilson and Hanafee, 1969). The internal maxillary artery is usually displaced laterally. (See Chapter 58.)

Adenoid hyperplasia. Adenoid hyperplasia of the pharyngeal tonsil is common in childhood. According to Jóhannesson (1968) the normal pharyngeal tonsil enlarges rapidly in the first 2 years of life, after which its growth tapers off. Spontaneous involution has been reported variously from ages 10 to 25 years (Weitz, 1946; Jóhannesson, 1968). In childhood, adenoid hyperplasia may accompany upper respiratory tract infections; or its appearance may be unexplained.

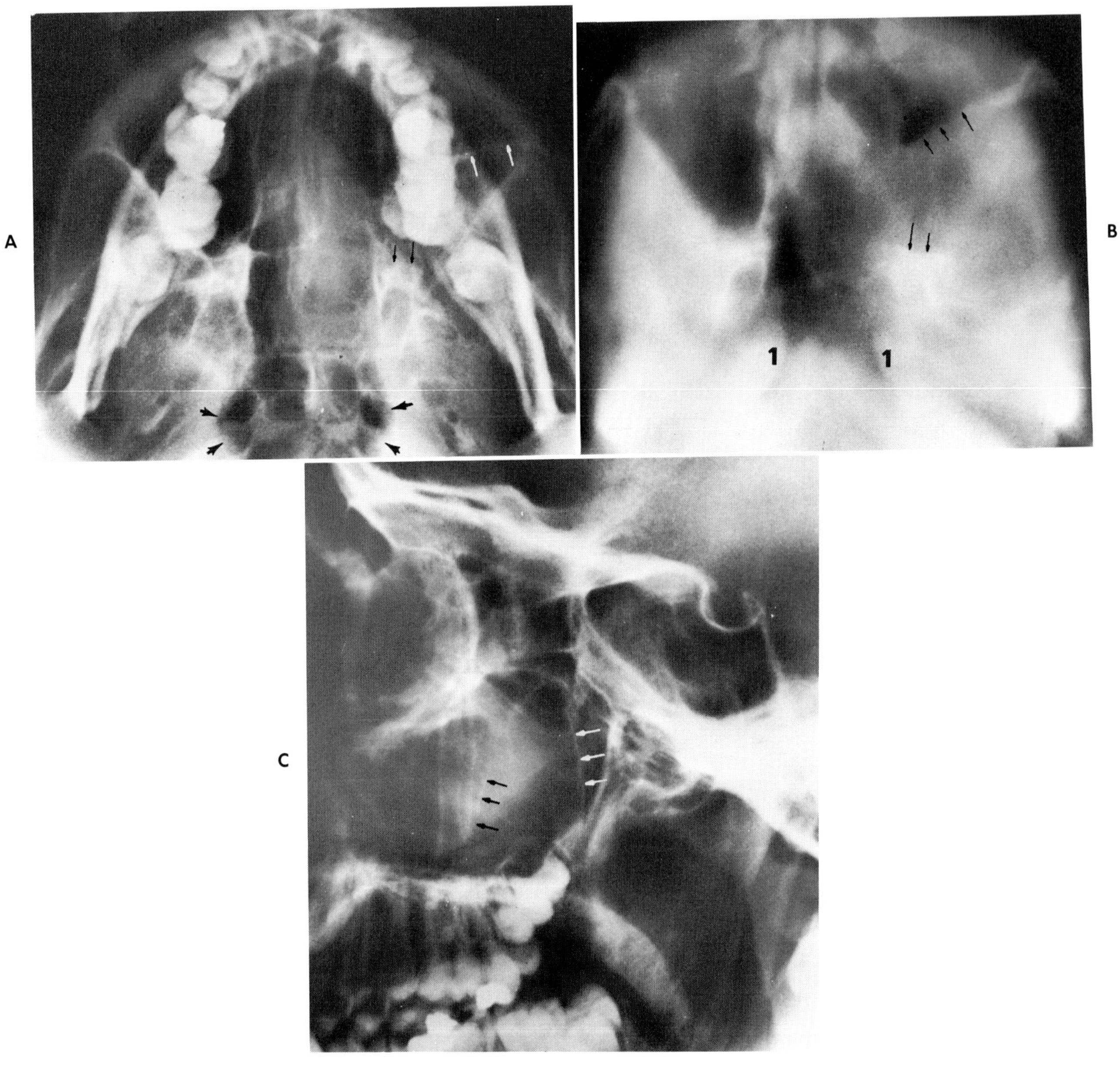

Fig. 13-12. Juvenile angiofibroma. **A,** Axial view of skull demonstrates soft-tissue mass in nasopharynx and nasal fossa. Posterior maxillary wall is displaced anteriorly (white arrows). Left pterygoid process is displaced slightly posteriorly (black arrows). Normal piriform sinuses are outlined by large arrows. **B,** Tomographic section in axial view verifies anterior position of posterior maxillary wall and slight posterior displacement of left pterygoid process. Sclerotic reactive change is seen in this pterygoid process. Note the normal posterior pharyngeal shadows with the tori tubarii (*1*) well outlined. This shadow does not correspond to air shadow in more inferiorly placed piriform sinuses demonstrated on plain roentgenogram. **C,** Lateral roentgenogram of skull demonstrates normal position of right posterior maxillary wall (white arrows) contrasted with anterior displacement of posterior wall of left maxillary antrum (black arrows). (Compare with Fig. 13-2, *E*.)

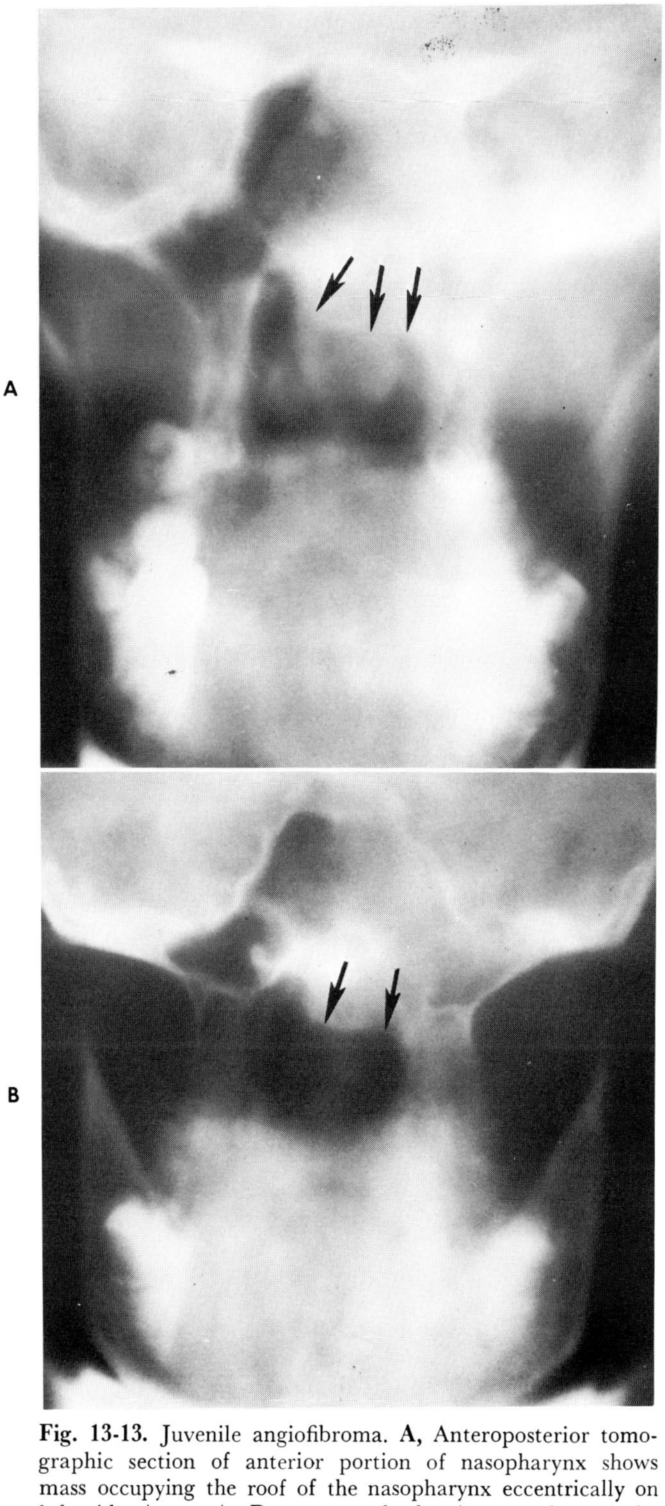

Fig. 13-13. Juvenile angiofibroma. **A,** Anteroposterior tomographic section of anterior portion of nasopharynx shows mass occupying the roof of the nasopharynx eccentrically on left side (arrows). Demonstrated also is extension of the mass into sphenoid sinus. **B,** Anteroposterior tomographic section of more posterior portion of nasopharynx demonstrates mass in the roof of the nasopharynx on left side (arrows) to a lesser degree than does section through the more anterior portion.

Adenoid hyperplasia is characterized roentgenographically by convexity of the soft tissues of the roof of the nasopharynx and its presence in youth. It is often, but not necessarily, associated with enlargement of the palatine tonsils. In general, soft-tissue fullness in the roof of the nasopharynx alone is probably normal in childhood. A soft-tissue mass in this region before 1 month of age, however, should be considered abnormal (Capitanio and Kirkpatrick, 1970). In children, lymphoid-tissue structures should be detectable after 1 month of age; in fact, they were always detectable in the series of Capitanio and Kirkpatrick (1970). These and other authors (Margulis et al., 1957) described decreased lymphoid tissues in immune-deficiency states in childhood.

In adults, until proved otherwise, a soft-tissue fullness in the roof of the nasopharynx should be considered abnormal, even when bone is not destroyed. On occasion adenoid hyperplasia appears in the adult (Jönsson, 1941; Ho, 1967b).

Sarcoidosis. Sarcoidosis of the nasopharynx is said to occur in 50% of patients with generalized disease (Larsson, 1951). Usually the mass is in the region of the pharyngeal tonsil, although the lateral wall alone may be involved. The abnormality appears as a mass, which varies from a slight irregularity in the roof to a large swelling that simulates malignant neoplasm.

Tuberculosis. Tuberculosis of the nasopharynx is most common in the posterosuperior portion of the nasopharynx; but it may be present in the posterior margin of the eustachian orifice and floor (Szanto and Hollender, 1944). When the disease causes excavation, an irregular mass is produced; but diffuse swelling may result from inflammatory infiltration (Jönsson, 1941). With bone involvement the appearance can be identical to that of malignant tumor (Mayer, 1928). Biopsy may be necessary to establish the diagnosis.

Thornwaldt's cyst. This infected cystic remnant of the fetal notochord is a small well-defined broad-based mass without adjacent infiltration (James et al., 1968). Its location is posterosuperior in the midline. The peak age of occurrence is 15 to 30 years. No predilection for either sex has been noted. The usual appearance is that of a sessile polyp 1 to 2 cm in diameter. No adjacent soft-tissue infiltration or bone involvement is seen (James et al., 1968).

Other rare benign lesions of the nasopharynx are neoplasms of the connective tissues (Stout, 1941), odontoma (McClure, 1946), and transsphenoid encephaloceles (Ingraham and Matson, 1943). (See Chapter 27.)

DIFFERENTIAL DIAGNOSIS

A large number of diseases may affect the nasopharynx. Difficulty often arises in distinguishing masses that arise outside the nasopharynx, which may resemble primary intranasopharyngeal tumors.

When bone destruction is extensive and a large soft-tissue mass is present, it may be impossible to state whether the tumor is primary in the nasopharynx or primary in a related structure. Malignant neoplasms of the nasal fossa, sphenoid, or maxillary sinuses may produce such an appearance (Miller et al., 1969).

Lethal midline granuloma is a process in which a soft-tissue mass may be in the nose, nasopharynx, and paranasal sinuses, associated with bone destruction. This entity should be considered in the differential diagnosis of extensive malignant nasopharyngeal tumor.

Occasionally a pituitary adenoma attains large size; and after breaking through the sphenoid sinus, it appears as a nasopharyngeal mass (Jönsson, 1934; Lenz, 1942) Craniopharyngioma may act similarly (Hill, 1940; Scanlon et al., 1958).

Choanal polyps may be mistaken for nasopharyngeal tumor on a lateral roentgenogram. Often careful examination reveals that the upper border is outlined by air, indicating the nasal rather than the nasopharyngeal origin of the polyp (Miller et al., 1969). Similar confusion may arise in hypertrophy of the inferior turbinate (Hill, 1940).

Masses of the palatine tonsil (Fig. 13-14) may be confused with tumors of the nasopharyngeal floor. Since these structures are in proximity, such confusion is not surprising.

Other tumors in the vicinity of the nasopharynx are chondrosarcoma, osteogenic sarcoma, and neurilemmoma, affecting the nasopharynx mainly by displacement.

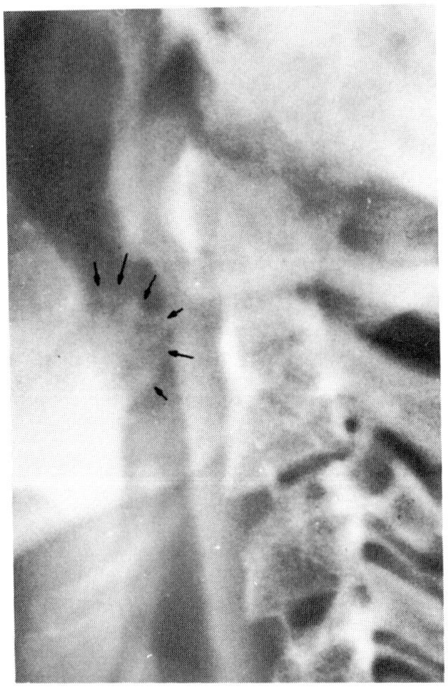

Fig. 13-14. Fibrosarcoma of palatine tonsil. Ill-defined mass arises from tonsil (arrows) and extends into inferior portion of nasopharynx.

REFERENCES

Ackerman, L. V., and del Regato, J. A.: Cancer, diagnosis, treatment and prognosis, St. Louis, 1962, The C. V. Mosby Co.

Baclesse, F., and Dulac, G.: The radiodiagnosis of malignant tumors of the rhinopharynx, J. Radiol. Electr. **29**:24-36, 1948.

Bailar, J. C., III: Nasopharyngeal cancer in white populations —a world survey. In Muir, C. S., and Shanmugaratnam, K., editors: Cancer of nasopharynx; symposium, International Union Against Cancer, Flushing, N. Y., 1967, Medical Examination Publishing Co., vol. 1.

Baylin, G. J., Reeves, R. J., and Kerman, H. D.: A roentgen and clinical study of nasopharyngeal malignancy (lymphoepithelioma and transitional cell carcinoma), Southern Med. J. **42**:467-476, 1949.

Belanger, W. G., and Dyke, C. G.: Roentgen diagnosis of malignant nasopharyngeal tumors, Amer. J. Roentgen. **50**: 9-18, 1943.

Bloch, S., and Quantrill, J. R.: The radiology of nasopharyngeal tumors including positive contrast nasopharyngography, S. Afr. Med. J. **42**:1030-1036, 1968.

Capitanio, M. A., and Kirkpatrick, J. A.: Nasopharyngeal lymphoid tissue, Radiology **96**:389-391, 1970.

Dahlin, D. C., and MacCarty, C. S.: Chordoma: study of 59 cases, Cancer **5**:1170-1178, 1952.

Deaver, J. B.: Surgical anatomy of the head and neck, Philadelphia, 1904, P. Blakiston's Son & Co.

Dobben, G. D.: Leiomyosarcoma of the nasopharynx, Arch. Otolaryng. **68**:211-213, 1958.

Epstein, B. S.: Laminagraphy in the diagnosis of nasopharyngeal tumors, Radiology **56**:355-362, 1951.

Fitzpatrick, P. J.: The nasopharyngeal angiofibroma, Clin. Radiol. **18**:62-68, 1967.

Fletcher, G. H., and Million, R. R.: Malignant tumors of the nasopharynx, Amer. J. Roentgen. **93**:44-55, 1965.

Godtfredsen, E.: Ophthalmologic and neurologic symptoms at malignant nasopharyngeal tumours; clinical study comprising 454 cases, with special reference to histopathology and possibility of earlier recognition, Acta Psychiat. Neurol., supp. 34, pp. 1-323, 1944.

Greenfield, M. M.: Malignant plasmocytoma of nasopharynx, Radiology **50**:661-665, 1948.

Groth, K. E.: The roentgen picture of the epipharynx of children under normal conditions and by adenoid vegetations, Acta Radiol. **14**:463-469, 1933.

Grunebaum, M., and Moskowitz, G.: The retropharyngeal soft tissues in young infants with hypothyroidism, Amer. J. Roentgen. **108**:543-545, 1970.

Hill, F. T.: Diagnostic pitfalls of the nasopharynx, J.A.M.A. **115**:662-665, 1940.

Ho, H. C.: Nasopharyngeal carcinoma in Hong Kong. In Muir, C. S., and Shanmugaratnam, K., editors: Cancer of nasopharynx; symposium, International Union Against Cancer, Flushing, N. Y., 1967a, Medical Examination Publishing Co., vol. 1.

Ho, H. C.: Radiological diagnosis of nasopharyngeal carcinoma with special reference to its spread through the base of the skull. In Muir, C. S., and Shanmugaratnam, K., editors: Cancer of nasopharynx; symposium, International Union Against Cancer, Flushing, N. Y., 1967b, Medical Examination Publishing Co., vol. 1.

Holman, C. B., and Miller, W. E.: Juvenile nasopharyngeal fibroma, Amer. J. Roentgen. **94**:292-298, 1965.

Ingraham, F. D., and Matson, D. D.: Spina bifida and cranium bifidum: unusual nasopharyngeal encephalocele, New Eng. J. Med. **228**:815-820, 1943.

James, A. E., Macmillan, A. S., Macmillan, A. S., Jr., and Momose, K. J.: Thornwaldt's cyst, Brit. J. Radiol. **41**:902-904, 1968.

Jóhannesson, S.: Roentgenologic investigation of the nasopharyngeal tonsil in children of different ages, Acta Radiol. [Diagn.] **7**:299-304, 1968.

Jönsson, G.: Roentgenological findings in malignant tumors of the nasopharynx, Acta Radiol. **15**:1-7, 1934.

Jönsson, G.: The roentgenographic diagnosis of pathologic conditions in the nasopharynx, Acta Radiol. **22**:651-663, 1941.

Khoo, F. Y., Chia, K. B., and Nalpon, J.: A new technique of contrast examination of the nasopharynx with cinefluorography and roentgenography, Amer. J. Roentgen. **99**:238-248, 1967.

Larsson, G.: Nasopharyngeal lesions in sarcoidosis, Acta Radiol. **36**:361-373, 1951.

Lederman, M.: Cancer of the nasopharynx; its natural history and treatment, Springfield, Ill., 1961, Charles C Thomas, Publisher.

Lederman, M.: Cancer of the nasopharynx, Proc. Roy. Soc. Med. **57**:740-742, 1964.

Lenz, M.: Roentgen therapy of primary cancer of the nasopharynx, Amer. J. Roentgen. **48**:816-832, 1942.

MacComb, W. S., and Fletcher, G. H.: Cancer of the head and neck, Baltimore, 1967, The Williams & Wilkins Co.

Mani, R. L., and Smith, M. F. W.: Rhabdomyosarcoma simulating nasopharyngeal angiofibroma, Oncology **22**:74-80, 1968.

Margulis, A. R., Feinberg, S. B., Lester, R. G., and Good, R. A.: Roentgen manifestations of congenital agammaglobulinemia, Radiology **69**:354-359, 1957.

Martin, H. E.: Cancer of the head and neck in children. In Dargen, H. W., editor: Cancer in childhood and a discussion of certain benign tumors, St. Louis, 1940, The C. V. Mosby Co. Cited by Prior, J. T., and Stoner, L. R.: Cancer **10**: 957-963, 1957.

Martin, H. E., and Blady, J. V.: Cancer of nasopharynx, Arch. Otolaryng. **32**:692-727, 1940.

Massoud, G. E., and Awwad, H. K.: Naso-pharyngeal fibroma: its malignant potentialities and radiation therapy, Clin. Radiol. **11**:156-161, 1960.

Mayer, E. G.: Roentgenographic examination of the base of the cranium in the presence of basal tumors, Radiology **10**: 319-341, 1928.

McClure, G.: Odontoma of the nasopharynx, Arch. Otolaryng. **44**:51-60, 1946.

Melot, G. J., Potvliege, R., Brihaye, J., and Martin, Ph.: Les extensions intracrâniennes des tumeurs de l'ethmoide, de l'orbite et du cavum, Acta Radiol. **50**:137-150, 1958.

Miller, D.: Nasopharyngeal cancer, Laryngoscope **61**:187-214, 1951.

Miller, W. E., Holman, C. B., Dockerty, M. B., and Devine, K. D.: Roentgenologic manifestations of malignant tumors of the nasopharynx, Amer. J. Roentgen. **106**:813-823, 1969.

Miyaji, T.: Carcinoma of the nasopharynx and related organs in Japan based on mortality, morbidity and autopsy studies. In Muir, C. S., and Shanmugaratnam, K., editors: Cancer of nasopharynx; symposium, International Union Against Cancer, Flushing, N. Y., 1967, Medical Examination Publishing Co., vol. 1.

Muir, C. S., and Shanmugaratnam, K.: The incidence of nasopharyngeal cancer in Singapore. In Muir, C. S., and Shanmugaratnam, K., editors: Cancer of nasopharynx; symposium, International Union Against Cancer, Flushing, N. Y., 1967, Medical Examination Publishing Co., vol. 1.

Oon, C. L.: Some sagittal measurements in the neck in normal adults, Brit. J. Radiol. **37**:674-677, 1964.

Pantangco, E. E., Basa, G. F., and Canlas, M.: A survey of nasopharyngeal cancers among Filipinos: review of 203 cases. In Muir, C. S., and Shanmugaratnam, K., editors: Cancer of nasopharynx; symposium, International Union Against Cancer, Flushing, N. Y., 1967, Medical Examination Publishing Co., vol. 1.

Potter, G.: The pterygopalatine fossa and canal, Amer. J. Roentgen. **107**:520-525, 1969.

Potter, G.: Sclerosis of the base of the skull as a manifestation of nasopharyngeal carcinoma, Radiology **94**:35-38, 1970.

Potter, G. D., and Seaman, W. B.: Tomography of extracerebral tumors of the head, Ann. Otol. **75**:235-246, 1966.

Prior, J. T., and Stoner, L. R.: Sarcoma botryoides of the nasopharynx, Cancer **10**:957-963, 1957.

Quisenberry, W. B., and Reimann-Jasinski, D.: Ethnic differences in nasopharyngeal cancer in Hawaii. In Muir, C. S., and Shanmugaratnam, K., editors: Cancer of nasopharynx; symposium, International Union Against Cancer, Flushing, N. Y., 1967, Medical Examination Publishing Co., vol. 1.

Rosen, L., Hanafee, W., and Nahum, A.: Nasopharyngeal angiofibroma: an angiographic evaluation, Radiology **86**: 103-107, 1966.

Scanlon, P. W., Devine, K. D., and Woolner, L. B.: Malignant lesions of the nasopharynx, Ann. Otol. Rhinol. Laryng. **67**: 1005-1021, 1958.

Schmidt, M. C.: Cancer of nasopharynx, Radiology **78**:751-759, 1962.

Stout, A. P.: Symposium on nasopharyngeal tumors. The pathological diagnosis of nasopharyngeal tumors, Laryngoscope **51**: 446-450, 1941.

Szanto, P. B., and Hollender, A. R.: Tuberculosis of the nasopharynx, Ann. Otol. Rhinol. Laryng. **53**:508-521, 1944.

Tan, B. C., and Oon, C. L.: Bone metastases in carcinoma of the nasopharynx, Clin. Radiol. **18**:69-73, 1967.

Teoh, T. B.: Epidermoid carcinoma of the nasopharynx among Chinese. In Muir, C. S., and Shanmugaratnam, K., editors: Cancer of nasopharynx; symposium, International Union Against Cancer, Flushing, N. Y., 1967, Medical Examination Publishing Co., vol. 1.

Weitz, H. L.: Roentgenography of adenoids, Radiology **47**: 66-70, 1946.

Whalen, J. P., and Berne, A. S.: The roentgen anatomy of the lateral walls of the orbit (orbital line) and the maxillary antrum (antral line) in the submentovertical view, Amer. J. Roentgen. **91**:1009-1011, 1964.

Wilson, G. H., and Hanafee, W. N.: Angiographic findings in 16 patients with juvenile nasopharyngeal angiofibroma, Radiology **92**:279-284, 1969.

Windeyer, B. W.: Chordoma, Proc. Roy. Soc. Med. **52**:1088-1100, 1959.

Wood, E. H., and Himadi, G. M.: Chordomas: roentgenologic study of 16 cases previously unreported, Radiology **54**:706-716, 1950.

Yeh, S.: Histology of nasopharyngeal cancer. In Muir, C. S., and Shanmugaratnam, K., editors: Cancer of nasopharynx; symposium, International Union Against Cancer, Flushing, N. Y., 1967, Medical Examination Publishing Co., vol. 1.

CHAPTER 14

Craniovertebral junction

Donald L. McRae

NORMAL JUNCTION

Anatomy

The craniovertebral junction is an area with indefinite boundaries. It extends from the bone around the foramen magnum down to and including the second cervical vertebra.

Foramen magnum

The bone around the foramen magnum forms the upper border of the craniovertebral junction. The foramen magnum is a round or slightly oval hole in the base of the posterior fossa. Its margins are formed by the four parts of the occipital bone: the basilar part, the two condylar parts, and the squamous part. The synchondroses between the four parts of the occipital bone must be known, and standard texts and atlases of anatomy show them well. In newborn children the synchondroses between the squamous part of the occipital bone and the two condylar parts come together near the center of the posterior margin of the foramen magnum. At this point there is usually an unossified area 6 or 8 mm wide. Occasionally an accessory ossification center appears in this small gap. The foramen magnum is oval in infants. In neonates it measures about 20 mm from front to back and about 15 mm from side to side. Usually in adults it is round and about 35 mm in diameter. On roentgenograms it appears larger because of magnification and distortion. The occipital condyles sometimes encroach slightly on the anteromesial aspects of the foramen magnum. Occasionally they are low and flat, which causes the atlas to be close to the occiput. This condition may be called a high atlas and must not be misdiagnosed as basilar invagination.

The foramen magnum is best demonstrated on lateral and anteroposterior roentgenograms of the skull (AP + 30°, using orbitomeatal base line). On well-penetrated lateral views the anterior and posterior edges of the foramen are the points at which the inner cortex of the skull turns around to become the outer cortex. In some instances, particularly abnormal cases, a midsagittal tomogram may be necessary to show these points. On anteroposterior occipital views the posterior half of the foramen is seen and the posterior arch of the atlas is projected through it. With more angulation of the tube, or in patients who can lower the chin to touch the chest, the entire foramen magnum may be demonstrated on anteroposterior occipital views. Tomograms of the base of the skull in the submentovertex view show the foramen magnum.

Atlas and axis

The anatomy of the atlas and axis is well described in standard anatomic texts, but some features are worthy of emphasis. A point of relative weakness exists in the posterior arch of the atlas at the grooves for the vertebral arteries. In some apparently normal persons the posterior arch of the atlas seems unusually close to the anterior arch. This condition is more common in females than in males (Hinck et al., 1962). Other points deserving of emphasis concern the second cervical vertebra. At birth the synchondroses between the ossification centers of the body of the second cervical vertebra and the odontoid process form parts of the superior articulating facets. The superior facets of the vertebra lie anterior to the pedicles of the vertebra, but the inferior facets lie behind the pedicles. The pars interarticularis is relatively narrow and weak. Usually its inferior facets are the smallest of all cervical facets, but its laminae and spinous processes are large. The blood supply of the odontoid process is mainly from the body of the axis. For this reason fractures through the odontoid often result in nonunion between the odontoid and the body of the axis.

Atlanto-occipital and atlantoaxial joints

It may be difficult to demonstrate the atlanto-occipital and atlantoaxial joints on open-mouth views of the atlas in patients with a high atlas. In such patients these joints are sometimes shown well on heavily exposed anteroposterior or posteroanterior views of the skull. For such views the central ray is parallel to the anthropologic base line.

Most patients flex and extend the head at the atlanto-occipital joint. A few asymptomatic patients do not move at this joint. In some this lack of motion is the result of bony union of the skull and atlas (occipitalization of the atlas). In others it is not. Patients who cannot flex and extend the head at the atlanto-occipital joint nod their heads by flexion and extension at the levels between the first cervical and first thoracic vertebrae.

The main function of the atlantoaxial joint is rotation around the odontoid process. Therefore the opposing facets of the first and second cervical vertebrae glide on each other for considerable distances. The capsular ligaments, the ligamenta flava, and the interspinous ligament at this level are long or elastic, or both. Most textbooks state that no flexion or extension exists at the atlantoaxial joint. This is incorrect; for these motions are present in about 12% of patients (Jones, 1960). Motion is best appreciated by comparing the distances between the laminae of the first and second cervical vertebrae on roentgenograms obtained on flexion and extension. Marked flexion or extension, or both, of the first cervical vertebra on the second can take place during certain movements of the head in normal patients (Hohl and Baker, 1964).

Measurements

Certain measurements about the craniovertebral junction are of medical importance (McGregor, 1948; Fischgold et al., 1952) (Figs. 14-1 and 14-2). Chamberlain's line joins the posterior end of the hard palate to the posterior lip of the foramen magnum. McGregor's line joins the posterior end of the hard palate to the lowermost point of the occipital squama. The digastric line joins the right and left digastric notches, and the bimastoid line joins the tips of the right and left mastoid processes. In about 50% of normal persons, the tip of the odontoid is at or below Chamberlain's and McGregor's lines. If more than half the odontoid process is above one of these lines, basilar invagination is probably present. In normal patients the digastric line is 11 mm (± 4 mm) above the middle of the atlanto-occipital joints. Basilar invagination is almost certainly present when the atlanto-occipital joint is at or above the digastric line. In addition to basilar invagination, some other conditions may cause the odontoid process to be high in relation to the lines of Chamberlain, McGregor, and Fischgold. These include occipitalization of the atlas, platybasia, a high atlas, a short clivus, or combinations of these.

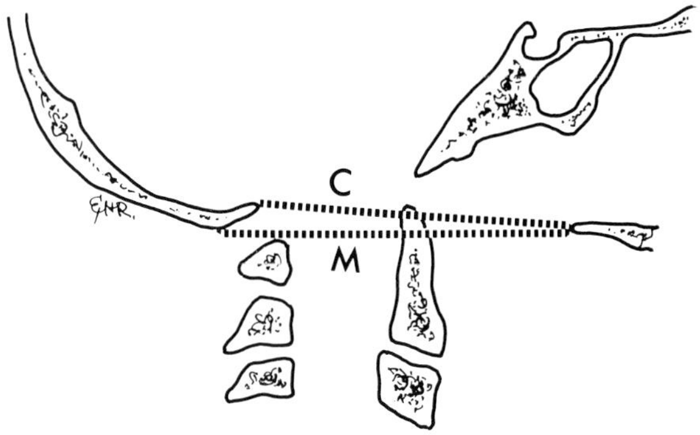

Fig. 14-1. Diagrammatic lateral view of posterior fossa, atlas, and axis in normal person. *C,* Chamberlain's line, from posterior end of hard palate to posterior lip of foramen magnum; *M,* McGregor's line, from posterior end of hard palate to lowermost point of occipital squama.

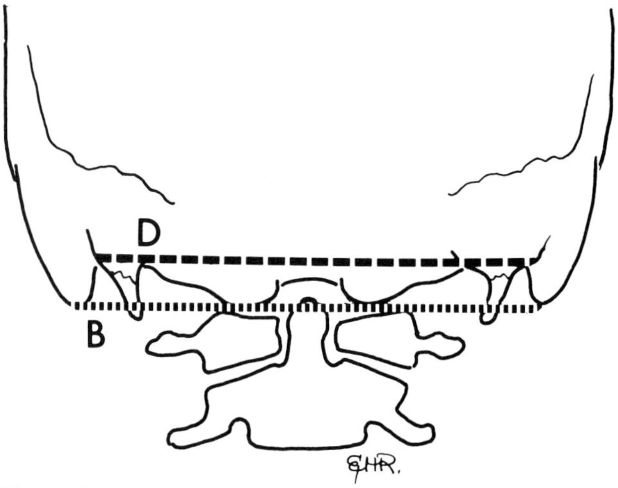

Fig. 14-2. Diagrammatic frontal view of posterior fossa, atlas, and axis. *D,* Digastric line, which is between right and left digastric notches of temporal bones; *B,* bimastoid line, between tips of right and left mastoid processes.

The basal angle is the angle between the plane of the clivus and the plane of the midline portion of the base of the anterior fossa. It is used by anthropologists in the classification of skulls. The basal angle is measured by them with an instrument called an inclinometer, which is placed inside the skull after the skullcap has been removed. Roentgenologists measure the basal angle by different methods that produce slightly different measurements. One method is to draw lines from the tuberculum sellae to the anterior lip of the foramen magnum and to the nasofrontal suture on a lateral skull roentgenogram. The angle between the two lines is then measured. Sometimes a center point is chosen in the center of the

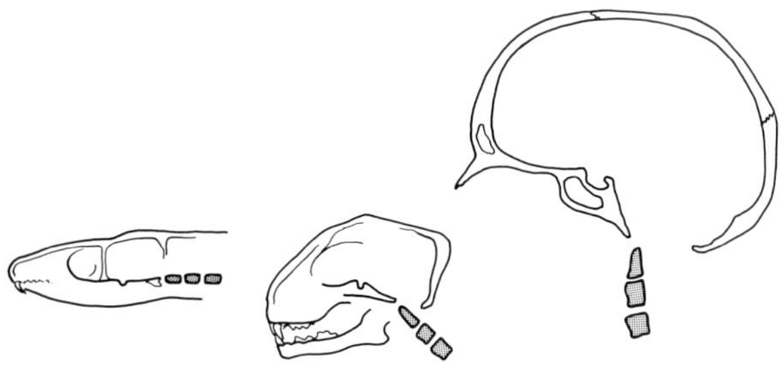

Fig. 14-3. Diagrammatic sagittal sections of skulls and upper cervical spines of reptile, lower mammal (cat), and man to illustrate relationship of planes of anterior fossa floor, clivus, and spine.

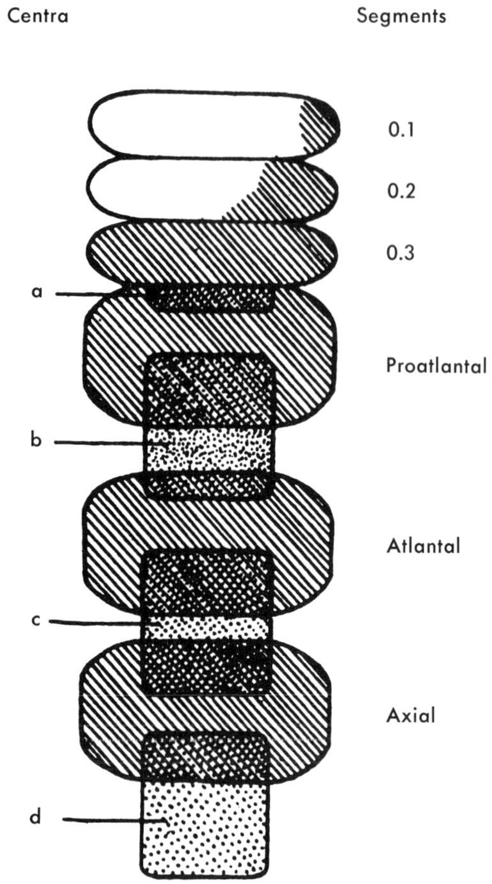

Fig. 14-4. Diagram of the three occipital and upper three cervical somites. Their relative contributions to the adult occipital bone are represented by shaded areas in the three occipital somites (*0.1, 0.2, 0.3*). Composition of centra (anlagen of vertebral bodies) of adult cervical vertebra is shown on left. Centrum of first cervical vertebra (odontoid process) is indicated by *b;* that of second cervical vertebra by *c;* that of third cervical vertebra by *d*. Area marked *a* sometimes ossifies and forms center for tip of odontoid. (Redrawn from Keith, 1949.)

sella turcica or at the tip of the dorsum sellae, both locations resulting in slightly smaller basal angles.

Anthropologists have used the angles between the spine and the skull and between the clivus and the floor of the anterior fossa as a means of placing man and the animals on a hierarchy from high to low (Fig. 14-3). Man, of course, is highest, having the smallest angle between the clivus and the anterior fossa, usually 120° to 140°. The brachycephalic races, which have the smallest basal angles, were at one time thought to be superior to the dolichocephalic races. The primates all have basal angles greater than 150°, and most mammals below the primates have basal angles close to 180°. In man the foramen magnum is approximately horizontal and is situated at the bottom of the skull so that the spinal canal is at an angle to the clivus. The apes have oblique foramina magna so that the spinal canal is more in line with the clivus. The lowest vertebrates, for example the reptiles, have the foramen magnum at the back of the skull at right angles to the clivus. The spinal canal then is in line with the clivus, which in turn is in line with the floor of the anterior fossa (Fig. 14-3).

Embryology

In the human embryo the postotic mesenchyme undergoes some degree of segmentation, with the appearance of somites. The somites in the neck and body differentiate into three portions: (1) a lateral and superficial epithelial plaque, the dermatome, which forms the dermis and adjacent subcutaneous tissues, (2) a lateral but deeper mass, the myotome, which forms the muscles, and (3) a medial and ventral mass, the sclerotome, which forms the vertebrae and intervertebral disks.

The occipital somites do not develop like spinal somites. By the end of the third week of fetal life, four occipital somites have formed but the first has already disappeared. In the remaining three somites the axial mesenchyme forms fairly typical sclerotomes, but these soon fuse into one condensed mass unlike spinal sclerotomes.

At the level of the third occipital myotome, however, the axial mesenchyme usually divides into a pale-staining cephalic (anterior) and a dense-staining caudal (posterior) portion, somewhat like a spinal sclerotome. This sclerotome is called the third occipital or third hypoglossal sclerotome. The caudal dense portion develops extensions that resemble neural and chordal processes, but no costal processes. The pale cephalic part is in relation to the last hypoglossal nerve root. Normally the posterior dense part is not associated with the pale anterior half of the first spinal sclerotome, the proatlantal sclerotome (Fig. 14-4). This dense portion remains continuous with the other tissue of its somite and with the rest of the basal plate of the anlage of the skull. Therefore the atlanto-occipital joint is truly intersegmental unlike an intervertebral joint.

In the 14 mm human embryo (gestational age about 40 days), the cartilage of the centrum of the atlas is connected with its cartilaginous arches by incompletely differentiated cartilage. Soon this poorly differentiated cartilage becomes transformed into dense blastemal tissue in which the joints above and below the lateral masses of the atlas develop. The anlage for the body of the first cervical vertebra then separates from its arches. The anlage of the body of this vertebra, however, remains in close relation to the anlage of the body of the second cervical vertebra because a normal intervertebral disk does not form between them.

During chondrification of the upper cervical vertebrae, there is condensation of tissue on the ventral surface of each of the sclerotomes. These condensed transverse bands connect the ventral ends of the blastemal neural processes; they are called hypochordal arches. They are all transitory except the first one, which is termed the hypochordal bow of the atlas. This hypochordal bow chondrifies at the time the arch of the first cervical vertebra separates from its body. The bow then joins the cartilaginous neural arch of the first cervical vertebra to form the cartilaginous atlas.

The odontoid process of the axis, therefore, comes from the anlage of the body of the first cervical vertebra. The anlagen of the bodies of the first and second cervical vertebrae unite. This union is accomplished through transformation of the anlage of the intervening intervertebral disk into hyaline cartilage, without the appearance of a nucleus pulposus.

The first spinal somite is called the proatlantal or suboccipital somite, since the nerve of this somite supplies the suboccipital muscles. The cephalic half of this sclerotome does not unite with the occipital scleromere (half of a sclerotome) in man. It probably is the anlage of the tip of the odontoid process, since there is an inconstant secondary ossification center for the tip of the odontoid. In some reptiles the anterior half of the proatlantal sclerotome unites with the occipital cartilage and later forms a bony formation called the proatlas. The word *proatlas* is incorrect if applied to human beings, in describing anomalies at the craniovertebral junction, since the development is different from that of the reptile.

The main part of the odontoid process is formed from the first spinal sclerotome (proatlantal sclerotome) together with the anterior half of the second spinal sclerotome (the atlantal sclerotome) (Fig. 14-3).

A typical spinal sclerotome in an embryo of about 5 mm proliferates in its caudal half so that this region stains more densely. The rostral less dense part and the caudal dense part become separated by a fissure. The denser caudal part of each sclerotome joins the less dense rostral half of the next caudad sclerotome. These combinations are the primordia of the primitive vertebrae. The primordia have processes that grow mesad to surround the notochord and establish the vertebral body (the chordal processes) and processes that grow dorsad flanking the neural tube (the neural processes).

The spinal nerves are situated beside the pale cephalic halves of the sclerotomes. The dense caudal half of one spinal sclerotome joins the pale cephalic half of the subjacent sclerotome. Because of the union, the spinal nerve then lies in relation to both parts of the bony vertebra. The axis is formed from the anterior pale halves of the first and second spinal sclerotomes and the posterior dense half of the first spinal sclerotome. Consequently two spinal nerves are associated with the axis, one nerve above its arch and one nerve below.

The third occipital sclerotome has a caudal scleromere with fairly well-developed neural and chordal processes. Incomplete incorporation of this scleromere in the basiocciput is considered the cause of manifestation of an occipital vertebra or vertebralization of the occiput. The bony parts involved are below the hypoglossal foramen. A complete or nearly complete ossicle here, however, is rare.

ABNORMALITIES OF JUNCTION

Abnormalities at the craniovertebral junction may involve only the bones and joints or only the meninges and nervous system, or both systems together. Some congenital anomalies of bones and joints in this region may not be associated with congenital anomalies of the meninges and central nervous system yet may gradually lead to pressure on them, either directly or indirectly, and cause secondary lesions of the central nervous system. In such instances exact diagnosis is important to plan rational therapy.

The age varies at which symptoms result from congenital abnormalities at the craniovertebral junction, depending to some extent on the type of lesion. In patients with the Chiari malformation, symptoms usually develop at birth or in early life and usually present little difficulty in diagnosis. The congenital lesions of bone and joint usually do not produce symptoms until adult life. These lesions may be misdiagnosed as multiple sclerosis, primary syringomyelia, or even disk disease. In congenital bone and joint lesions the symptoms may be pronounced in the lower extremities. When they are minimal or absent in the upper extremities, early examination of the cervical region in the search for etiologic factors may be neglected. Even when the cervical region is under suspicion, anomalies of the craniovertebral junction may be missed, unless this area is carefully inspected on the roentgenograms and additional views in flexion and extension are obtained.

Asymptomatic craniovertebral anomalies

The term asymptomatic craniovertebral anomaly means a congenital lesion or variation, which by itself is not associated with symptoms (McRae, 1960). The most common of these are areas in which bone did not develop, most frequently the atlas. The term spina bifida occulta is used most often to describe such areas; but rachischisis is a more accurate term, at least for the anterior and posterior defects.

Defects in atlas (McRae, 1960)

Isolated posterior rachischisis or spina bifida occulta of the atlas is present in some 2% of asymptomatic persons. The percentage is higher when other congenital anomalies are in the vicinity. When the anomaly occurs alone, it is of no significance. Such a potentially weak atlas, however, might be fractured by trauma that would not fracture a normal atlas. The abnormality may be recognized on lateral roentgenograms of the skull or spine. On these the thin white line that represents the posterior wall of the spinal canal at the level of the first cervical vertebra is absent. If necessary, this absence can be confirmed by anteroposterior occipital views of the skull. In such views the posterior arch of the atlas is projected through the foramen magnum. An open-mouth anteroposterior view of the first cervical vertebra also serves this purpose.

Isolated posterior rachischisis of the second cervical vertebra is rare.

Isolated anterior rachischisis of the first cervical vertebra is unusual. I have seen only one case, and the finding was incidental on skull roentgenograms obtained because the patient had complained of headache. It has the same significance as posterior rachischisis. The basal view of the skull (submentovertex projection) shows it best.

Isolated defects in the posterior arch of the first cervical vertebra away from the midline are rare, and I have seen only two cases. In both instances bone was absent from each side of the posterior arch where it was attached to the lateral mass. The center of the posterior arch was present and well developed, however. Both cases were discovered accidentally during roentgenography for head and neck injury.

Ponticuli

The normal atlas contains grooves for the vertebral arteries on the lateral and posterior surfaces of its lateral masses. The lateral part of the groove may be arched over by a spicule of bone. This bone extends from the lateral edge of the superior facet to the transverse process at the posterolateral edge of the foramen transversarium. It is called the ponticulus lateralis. A similar spicule may arch over the posterior groove and be attached to the bony edges of the groove; it is the ponticulus posticus.

Asymmetric atlanto-occipital joints (McRae, 1960)

In frontal views the atlanto-occipital joints usually appear symmetric. Occasionally one joint may be situated at a higher level than the other, but this seldom if ever produces symptoms. The higher atlanto-occipital joint usually appears to be somewhat more horizontal on the frontal roentgenograms. In basilar invagination, asymmetry of the atlanto-occipital joints is fairly common.

Asymmetric atlantoaxial joints (McRae, 1960)

In a frontal projection the slope of one atlantoaxial joint is usually the same as the slope of the other. Considerable difference in the slopes of these joints may be present without any radiologic evidence of arthritis of the joints and without symptoms.

Third occipital condyle (McRae, 1960)

A facetlike structure is occasionally seen on the anterior lip of the foramen magnum. The structure is directly above the anterior arch of the atlas, but it is separated from the arch by several millimeters. In a few instances it appears to articulate with the anterior arch of the atlas, but whether it is a true or a false joint is not clear. Usually in these latter cases the atlas is high. It is close to the base of the skull because of a short clivus or because of sessile occipital condyles, or both (Fig. 14-5). This condition should not be misdiagnosed as occipitalization of the atlas. Some authors consider it as a type of occipital vertebra (Lombardi, 1961), but others disagree (Frazer, 1940).

In some cases of basilar invagination, the anterior arch of the atlas and the anterior lip of the foramen magnum appear to be in contact. This condition should not be called a third occipital condyle.

Manifestation of an occipital vertebra

Unusual bony formations around the foramen magnum have been referred to as manifestation of an occipital vertebra. Several criteria have been advanced for differentiation between occipitalization of the atlas and manifestation of occipital vertebrae when only the dried skull is available for examination (Gladstone and Erichsen-Powell, 1915) (Table 14-1). The various criteria are not valid in all cases, however. Even the presence of the cervical spine may not help. Before the diagnosis of manifestation of an occipital vertebra is made, it is generally agreed that one must show that there is no foramen for the vertebral artery or greater occipital nerve between the abnormal ossicle and the occiput. Criteria based on the position of the hypoglossal and suboccipital nerves and the vertebral artery are probably the most reliable; but even these have been questioned (Gladstone and Erichsen-Powell, 1915; Frazer, 1940). Careful reading of the criteria of Gladstone and Erichsen-Powell (1915) suggests that only prominent edges or flanges on various sides of the foramen magnum are described. Such lesions seldom if ever produce neurologic symptoms or signs.

Logically one criterion of a normal atlas is that the atlas should not be fused to the skull *at any point*. Then,

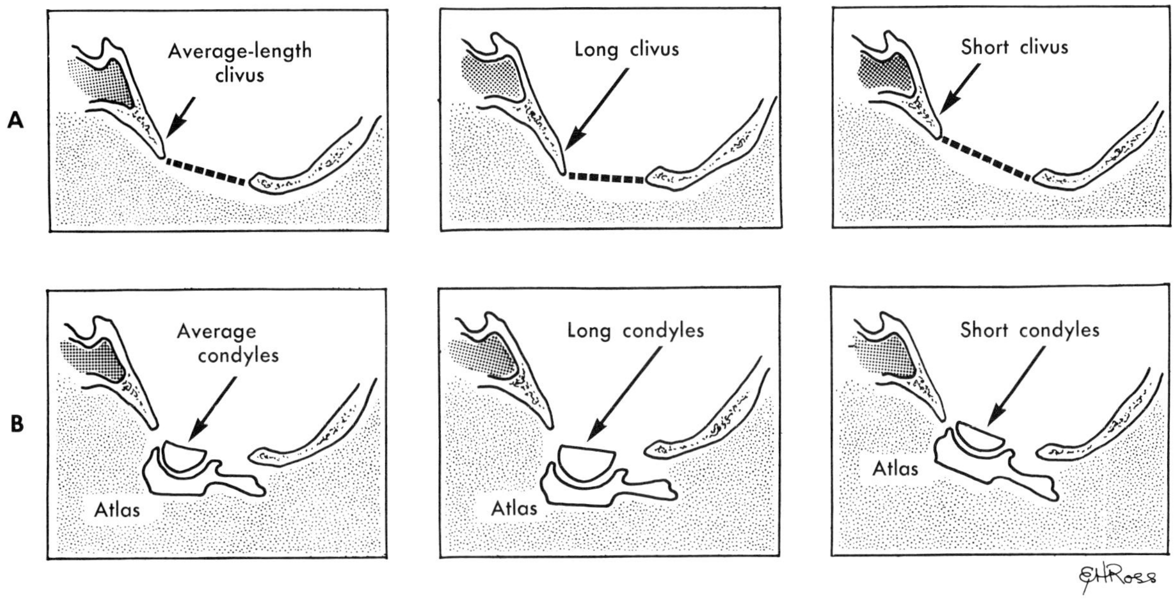

Fig. 14-5. A, Diagrammatic lateral views of clivus and foramen magnum to show variations in slope and height of foramen magnum when clivus is of different lengths. Short clivus is always present in achondroplastic dwarfs. In normal patients, short clivus indicates reduced growth or early fusion of spheno-occipital synchondrosis. Dotted line represents plane of foramen magnum as seen on lateral films. **B,** Diagrammatic lateral view of clivus, foramen magnum, and atlas with clivus of average length. Occipital condyles vary in size and shape, causing considerable variation in distance between clivus and atlas. Variation in angle between foramen magnum and atlas also results.

Table 14-1. Criteria to differentiate manifestation of occipital vertebra and occipitalization of atlas*

Manifestation of occipital vertebra	*Occipitalization of the atlas*
Condyles oval in outline, convex, converge anteriorly; surfaces directed downward and laterally; slight constriction separates anterior from posterior part of condyle; little or no encroachment of condyles on foramen magnum	Inferior articular facets nearly circular in outline, slightly concave, directed downward and mesially; lateral masses encroach considerably on the small foramen magnum; inferior articular facets may be rounded off, resembling condyles of occiput; this roundness is due to flexion and extension of head as these movements are transferred from atlanto-occipital joint to atlantoaxial joint
Anterior arch usually has no facet for the dens; occasionally a third occipital condyle may be developed; anterior arch is usually completely fused with the occipital bone	Anterior arch usually has a facet for the dens; there is usually an anterior tubercle for attachment of the longus capitis muscle; anterior arch is frequently separated by a gap from anterior edge of foramen magnum
Posterior arch not so wide as arch of atlas and less distinctly marked off from occipital bone; there is usually no gap between it and the occipital bone; also no canal for vertebral artery and suboccipital nerve between the posterior arch and the occipital bone; groove is sometimes present on the undersurface of the bone immediately behind the condyles, presumably for the vertebral artery	Posterior arch wider, forming an arc whose center would be near the pharyngeal tubercle; posterior arch is separated from occipital bone by a canal for the vertebral artery and suboccipital nerve; or there is a gap between posterior arch and occipital bone with a groove on the former (as in normal bone)
Transverse process as a rule contains no foramen for the vertebral artery and is less separated from occipital bone	Transverse process frequently free and pierced by canal for vertebral artery; costal element may be rudimentary; transverse process may be united or articulated with the occipital bone by a paraoccipital (paramastoid) process

*Modified from Gladstone, R. J., and Erichsen-Powell, W.: Manifestations of occipital vertebrae and fusion of the atlas with the occipital bone, J. Anat. Physiol. 49:190-209, 1915.

and only then, can an unusual bony formation around the foramen magnum be deleted from the group of occipitalized atlases and placed in the group of occipital vertebrae.

The third occipital condyle is considered by some authors as one type of manifestation of an occipital vertebra. Small unattached ossicles in the same position as the third occipital condyle are occasionally seen and have been called basilar processes. Bony additions, such as paracondyloid and paramastoid processes, may be lateral to the foramen magnum. These, however, are probably not manifestations of an occipital vertebra but are sometimes found in occipitalization of the atlas (McRae and Barnum, 1953). In such patients the transverse process of the occipitalized atlas on the same side is usually small or absent, suggesting that the paracondyloid or paramastoid process represents the transverse process of the atlas. Therefore the transverse process should not be considered part of an occipital vertebra.

In occipitalization of the atlas, the hypochordal arch of the atlas with its attached neural arches becomes continuous with the occipital cartilage. In spite of this, the centrum of the atlas fuses with the centrum of the axis and they separate themselves from the hypochordal bow but remain attached to the arch of the axis. In from one third to one half of patients with occipitalization of the atlas, the second and third cervical vertebrae fuse both in the bodies and in the arches.

Symptom-producing craniovertebral abnormalities

Developmental abnormalities of the brain or meninges, or of both, in the region of the craniovertebral junction usually cause hydrocephalus in early life. When congenital anomalies of the brain or meninges at the craniovertebral junction do not produce symptoms until adolescence or adult life, the clinical signs vary. In some of these patients, symptoms of low-grade increase in intracranial pressure are present. In other patients there is evidence of slowly progressive cerebellar or brainstem syndromes, often with long-tract signs in the lower extremities. In still another group, spinal cord signs may predominate but these usually are associated with a bony anomaly (McRae, 1960). Usually in the patients with predominantly intracranial symptoms and signs, roentgenograms of the skull are followed by air studies from above or below, or both. Patients with signs of spinal cord abnormality are usually investigated by roentgenography of the cervical spine and myelography. At myelography the oil must be carried to or through the foramen magnum. The patient should be examined in the supine as well as the prone position to visualize the cerebellar tonsils.

Congenital anomalies of the bones and joints of the craniovertebral junction unassociated with brain or meningeal anomalies most often produce no neurologic symptoms and signs until adult life. At that time spinal cord signs and symptoms may appear (McRae, 1960). These result from pressure on the upper cervical cord or lower medulla oblongata or from the presence of syringomyelia. The average age of onset of symptoms in such patients is 28 years. The commonest provisional diagnosis in the early stages of the disease is multiple sclerosis. Syringomyelia is the next most common diagnosis, but not all these patients have actual syringomyelia. Myelography with oil or air, or both, is usually carried out. Treatment is by decompression of the foramen magnum and upper cervical spinal canal. If atlantoaxial dislocation is present, the first and second cervical vertebrae usually need to be fused by insertion of bone grafts into the atlantoaxial joints.

Table 14-2 shows the chief complaints of sixty-eight consecutive patients with symptom-producing bony anomalies at the craniovertebral junction. The average duration and the average age at onset of each chief

Table 14-2. Chief complaints of sixty-eight patients with symptom-producing bony anomalies at craniovertebral junction

Chief complaint	*Frequency (percent)*	*Average duration* (years)*	*Average age at onset (years)*
Weakness of one or both legs	32	7 (1-20 yr)	31 (12-47 yr)
Occipital or suboccipital pain	26	3 (1 mo-9 yr)	28 (7-51 yr)
Neck pain or paresthesias	13	5 (6 mo-17 yr)	30 (16-40 yr)
Numbness/Tingling of fingers	12	2 (1-4 yr)	43 (21-57 yr)
Ataxic gait	9	18 (1-49 yr)	33 (5-50 yr)

*Figures in parentheses represent shortest and longest duration and youngest and oldest age at onset.

Table 14-3. Diagnosis in sixty-eight patients by referring physician

Diagnosis	*Percent*
Multiple sclerosis	31
Syringomyelia or syringobulbia	18
Tumor of brainstem or posterior fossa	16
Lesion of foramen magnum or Arnold-Chiari malformation	13
Cervical fracture or dislocation or cervical disk protrusion	9
Degenerative disease of cord	6
Cerebellar degeneration	4
Hysteria	3
Chronic lead poisoning	1

complaint are also shown. Uncommon chief complaints were dizzy spells, ringing in the ears, blurring of vision, diplopia, and weakness of one arm.

Exacerbations and remissions were frequent, suggesting different diagnoses at different stages to different physicians. The referring diagnoses in the sixty-eight patients are shown in Table 14-3.

Atlantoaxial dislocation

Atlantoaxial dislocation may be acute or chronic. The acute cases usually result from a single severe flexion of the head on the neck, which ruptures the transverse ligament of the atlas. The skull and atlas move forward in relation to the second cervical vertebra, pinching the upper spinal cord between the odontoid process of the axis and the posterior arch of the atlas. Sometimes tuberculous adenitis, osteomyelitis, and rheumatoid arthritis in the upper neck may lead to weakening of the transverse ligament of the atlas. In such instances relatively minor flexion or torsion of the head on the neck may result in a similar injury.

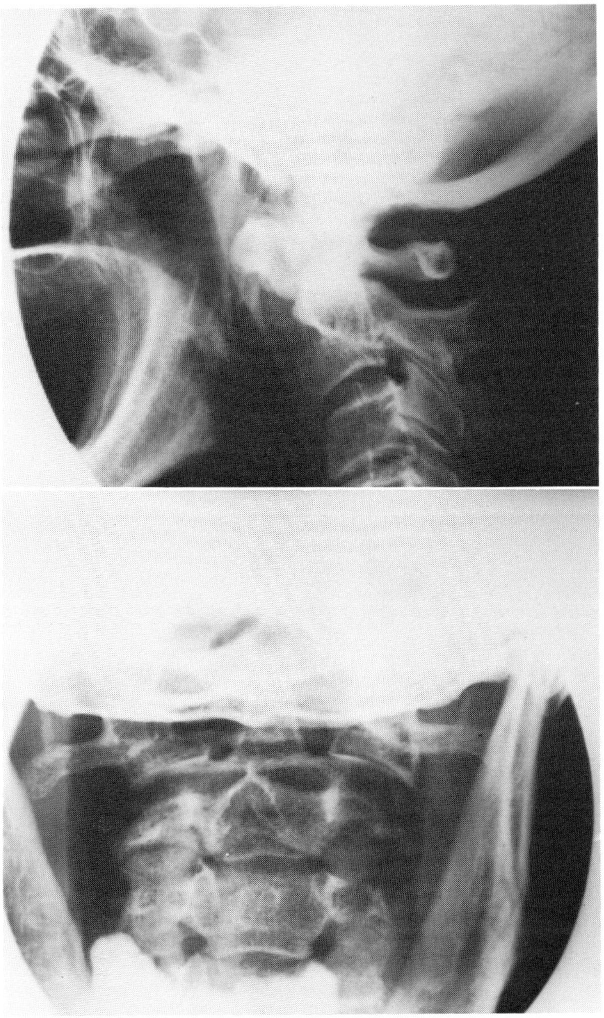

Fig. 14-6. Chronic atlantoaxial dislocation. Atlas is displaced anteriorly in relation to axis. Physician age 58 years with history of "spinal multiple sclerosis" for approximately 10 years. Fusion of first and second cervical vertebrae resulted in considerable improvement in neurologic deficit, and patient was able to return to practice.

In chronic atlantoaxial dislocation there is no history of head or neck injury or of inflammatory disease in the upper neck. Many of these cases are associated with other congenital anomalies of the bones and joints at the craniovertebral junction. The compression of the upper spinal cord or lower medulla oblongata between the posterior arch of the atlas and the odontoid process of the axis is the major cause of symptoms. Another small group of cases are those in which the lesion occurs alone. The etiology of these may be a congenital defect of the transverse ligament of the atlas. Other ligaments, of course, hold the atlas to the axis, such as the capsular ligaments of the atlantoaxial joints, the ligamentum nuchae, and the ligamenta flava. These ligaments are usually lax and do not hold the odontoid process against the anterior arch of the atlas. In chronic atlantoaxial dislocation these ligaments are abnormally lax. In fact, they may sometimes fold inward into the spinal canal and add to the pressure on the upper spinal cord.

Lateral roentgenograms of the cervical spine in flexion and extension are necessary to diagnose or exclude chronic atlantoaxial dislocation. The atlas usually glides directly forward on the axis (Fig. 14-6), but occasionally its movement is obliquely forward. The odontoid process is then allowed to slip around the side of the upper cervical cord, sparing it. Movement of the atlas on the axis may be side-to-side but is less marked than the displacement in the sagittal plane. More than half the patients with pure chronic atlantoaxial dislocation have symptoms and signs of pressure on the upper cervical cord.

Separate odontoid process

Most instances of separate odontoid process are the result of acute injury. In fact, injury is so often the cause that other etiologic factors may not be considered. There is, however, a congenital form of separate odontoid process, which is attached to the anterior lip of the foramen magnum (McRae, 1960). In some patients without history of head or neck injury, the separate odontoid processes are not fused to the skull. These may also be congenital although injury in early life, with nonunion of a fracture, cannot be excluded (Fig. 14-7). Therefore the term separate odontoid process is preferable to ununited fracture of the odontoid process when there is no history of injury.

A separate odontoid process is nearly always associated with atlantoaxial dislocation, which leads to neurologic

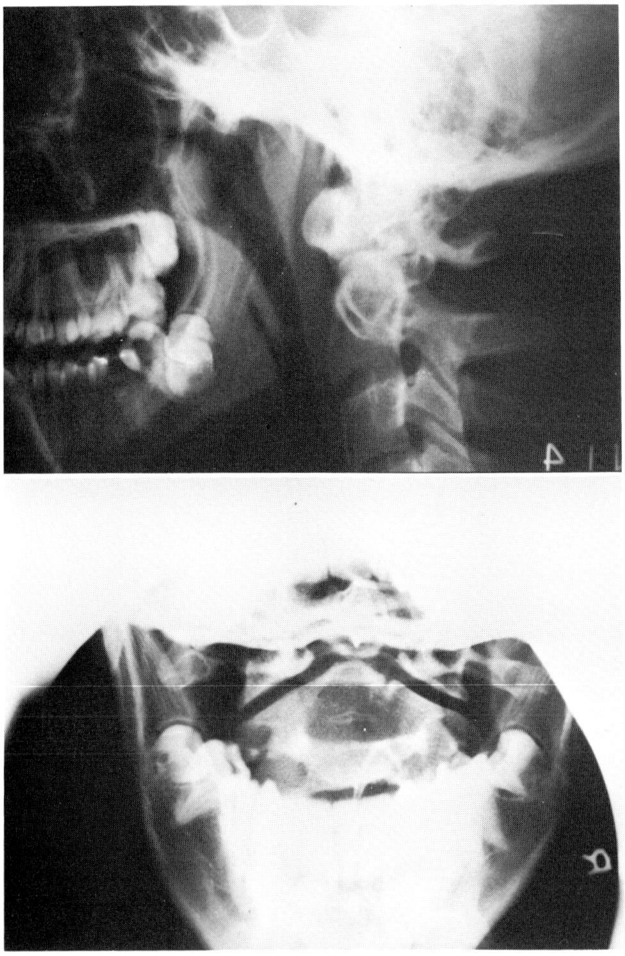

Fig. 14-7. Separate odontoid process. An 18-year-old man had had epileptic seizures since childhood but no spinal cord symptoms or signs. Separate odontoid process was first noted on skull roentgenograms and considered asymptomatic. There was no history of head or neck trauma.

symptoms and signs (Fig. 14-8). Roentgenography in flexion and extension shows that the atlas most often dislocates anteriorly on the axis. In one patient, however, the atlas dislocated posteriorly (McRae, 1960). The odontoid process usually remains close to the anterior arch of the atlas. Therefore the spinal cord is pinched between the upper posterior corner of the second cervical body and the posterior arch of the first cervical vertebra.

Absent odontoid process

Absence of the odontoid processes has been proved by tomograms or autopsy. The etiology is obscure but possibly represents congenital absence of the odontoid process. Other cases may be the result of atrophy of the odontoid process following nonunion of an odontoid fracture. Some may be examples of a separate odontoid process that is small or decalcified and is difficult to visualize.

Atlantoaxial dislocation is frequent in this condition and produces pressure on the upper cervical cord with long-tract signs similar to those produced by other bony lesions in this region.

Basilar invagination

The terms basilar invagination and basilar impression mean invagination of the margins of the foramen magnum upward into the skull. Slight upturning of the posterior edge of the foramen magnum is considered a normal variant. Platybasia, which defines a different condition, will be discussed later. The roentgenographic measurement of basilar invagination is difficult. Various lines and angles have been described that supposedly diagnose or exclude basilar invagination, but none is entirely satisfactory because normal variations are seen

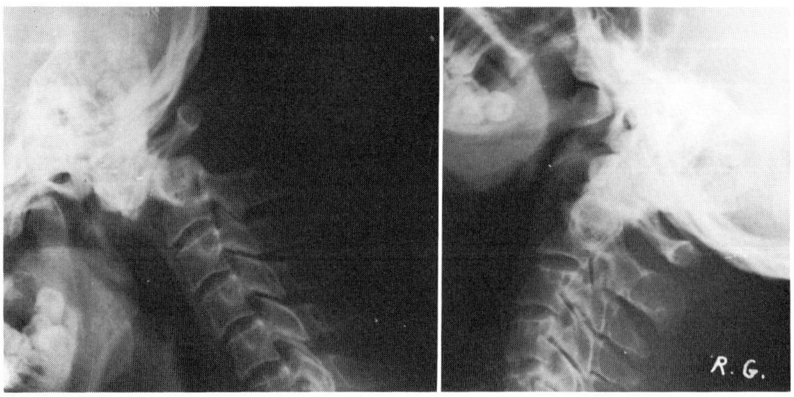

Fig. 14-8. Separate odontoid process with atlantoaxial dislocation. Man 41 years old had noted progressive weakness and sensory loss of at least 2 years' duration in legs. He denied any injury of head or neck. Tomograms (not shown) demonstrated separate odontoid process, completely surrounded by cortex and not attached to foramen magnum. Flexion films show marked atlantoaxial dislocation.

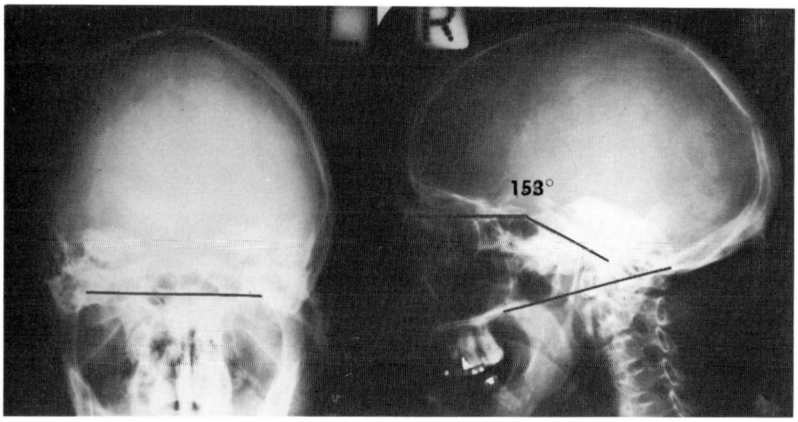

Fig. 14-9. Basilar invagination. A 30-year-old man was hospitalized because of hyperthyroidism. Asymptomatic basilar invagination was discovered on lateral views of neck. Digastric line, Chamberlain's line, and basal angle are shown in black.

A

B

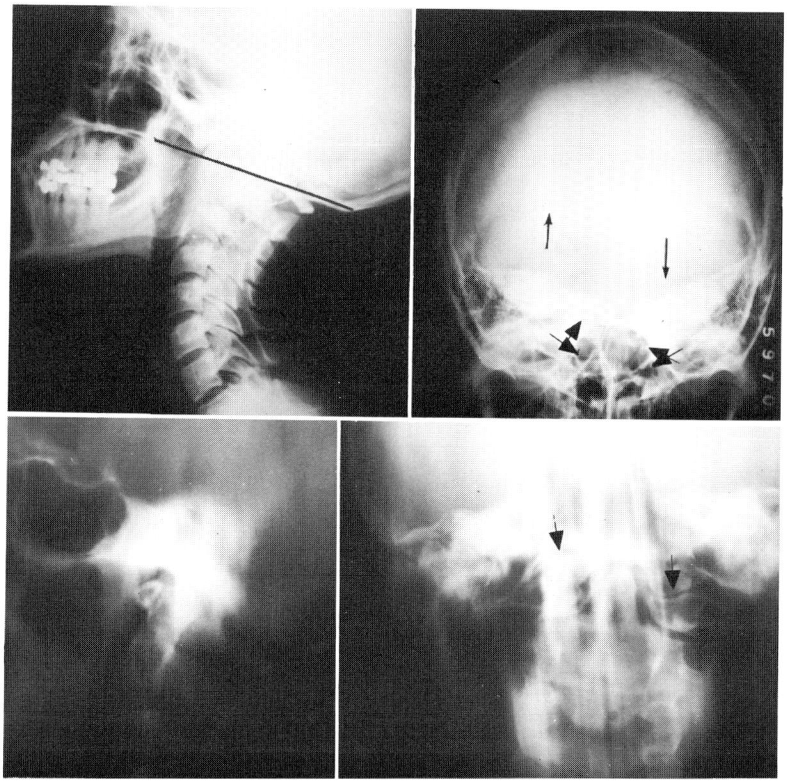

Fig. 14-10. Basilar invagination. Woman of 45 years had had dizzy spells for 12 years. Slowly progressive weakness of left leg had been noted for 7 years, and of left arm and hand for 1½ years. Recently she had noticed numbness of right leg. **A,** Lateral and frontal roentgenograms of skull do not show whether anterior arch is attached to the skull, but on frontal views atlanto-occipital and atlantoaxial joints can be seen (short black arrows). Degree of invagination of base of skull is greater on right (upward-pointing arrow) than on left (downward-pointing arrow). **B,** Tomograms show that anterior arch and lateral masses of first cervical vertebra are not fused to skull. Arrows point to atlanto-occipital joints.

in the length of the clivus, the size of the occipital condyles, and the plane of the foramen magnum (Fig. 14-5). Anteroposterior and lateral tomograms of the foramen magnum offer the best means of showing actual upward displacement of the margins of the foramen. This displacement is the absolute criterion for the diagnosis of basilar invagination. Because of their practical usefulness, Chamberlain's line (1939), McGregor's line (1948), and the digastric line are still of value; but they must be used judiciously (Fig. 14-9).

In pronounced basilar invagination the atlas may be surrounded by the occipital bone and occipitalization may be difficult to diagnose or exclude. Roentgenograms obtained in flexion often show no movement of the atlanto-occipital joint because the atlas is surrounded by the occipital bone. Laminagrams are essential in such cases (Fig. 14-10). A Towne view of the skull may allow the joints between the occipital condyles and the atlas to be seen. Another useful clue that favors basilar invagination is that the odontoid process is usually not within the foramen magnum as it is in occipitalization. In basilar invagination the tip of the odontoid process is usually directly below the anterior lip of the foramen magnum.

The cerebellar tonsils are frequently situated below the foramen magnum in basilar invagination. This low position of the cerebellar tonsils probably should not be called a Chiari malformation because the cervical nerve roots usually pass downward from the spinal cord to reach the intervertebral foramina in the normal fashion. In true Chiari malformations the brainstem and spinal cord are low and the cervical nerve roots pass upward to reach their intervertebral foramina.

When basilar invagination is present with Paget's disease, probably a secondary type of basilar invagination is indicated, which results from softening of the bones that bear the occipital condyles. The etiology is obscure when no other evidence of bone disease accompanies basilar invagination. In some instances the invagination may be a congenital abnormality; in others it may be secondary to infantile bone disease, such as rickets.

Platybasia

Platybasia is a condition in which the basal angle is greater than 142° or 144°. Platybasia by itself is an asymptomatic condition; but since it is often found in patients with basilar invagination, it is included in the present discussion. Some authors (Chamberlain, 1939) have used the terms platybasia and basilar invagination synonymously.

Occipitalization of atlas

Occipitalization of the atlas, or its assimilation to the base of the skull, implies bony union between the skull and the atlas (Figs. 14-11 and 14-12). Lack of movement between skull and atlas on roentgenographic examination is not the only criterion. Sometimes the skull does not move on the atlas when marked basilar invagination, or soft-tissue ankylosis of the skull and atlas, is present (McRae and Barnum, 1953). In occipitalization of the atlas, the most common finding is fusion between the anterior arch of the atlas and the anterior lip of the foramen magnum. Usually the anterior atlanto-occipital interval is not completely filled in with bone in the midline. In other cases small spicules of bone

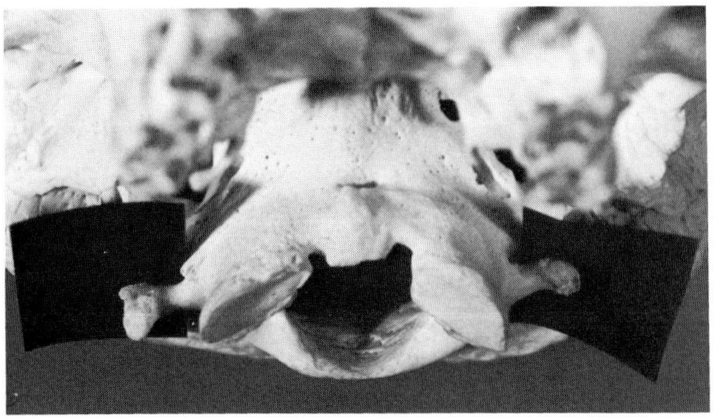

Fig. 14-11. Occipitalized atlas whose posterior arch forms curved flange around back and sides of foramen magnum. No trace of atlanto-occipital joints is visible. Transverse processes of first cervical vertebra are small, neither one having a foramen transversarium. Black paper can be slipped between them and base of skull. A small hole is seen in the anterior atlanto-occipital interval.

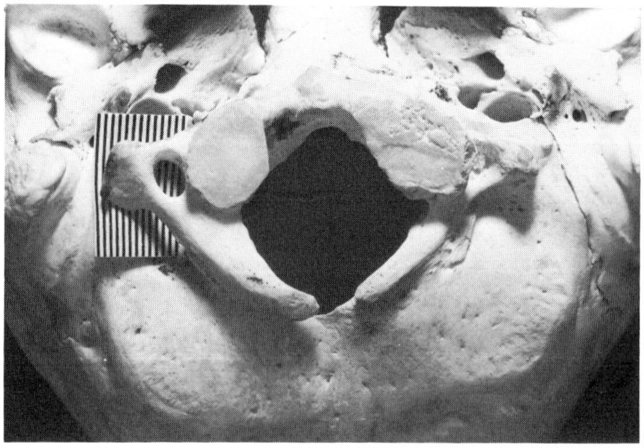

Fig. 14-12. Another occipitalized atlas with cleft posterior arch. Each side of posterior arch is fused to foramen magnum. Right transverse process is complete and not fused to skull. Left transverse process is incomplete; its tip is fused to occipital bone behind jugular foramen, where it forms a paracondyloid process. Paper could not be passed between left transverse process and base of skull.

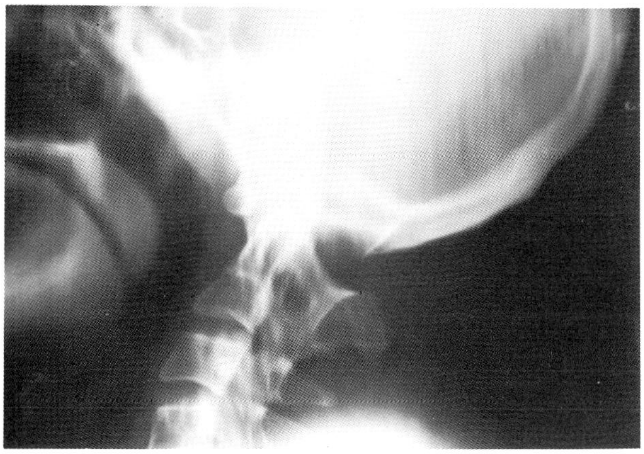

Fig. 14-13. Occipitalization of atlas. Man 44 years old had noticed weakness and ataxia of legs, and to a lesser degree of arms, for at least 1 year. Bony continuity is seen between basiocciput and anterior arch of atlas. The odontoid process lies within the effective foramen magnum and is several millimeters behind anterior arch of first cervical vertebra. Anterior arch of this vertebra does not have a facet on its posterior surface. No basilar invagination is present even though odontoid lies entirely above Chamberlain's line. Assimilated arch of first cervical vertebra forms flange on posterior edge of foramen magnum. Second and third cervical vertebrae are fused. At operation, cerebellar tonsils were below the flange on the posterior lip of the foramen magnum.

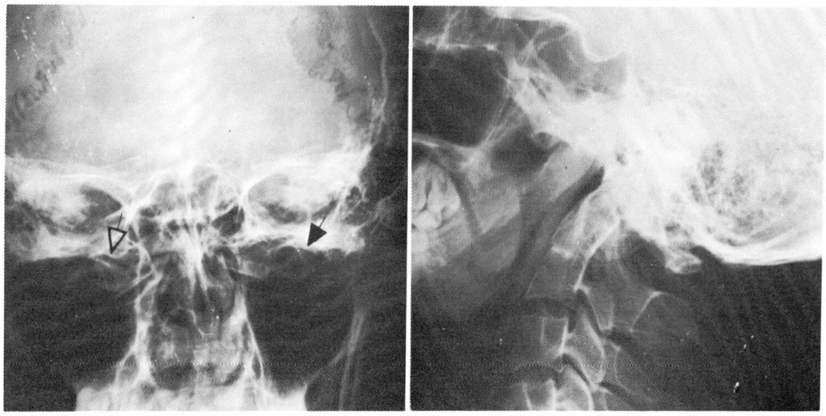

Fig. 14-14. Unilateral assimilation of atlas. Asymptomatic 24-year-old man had right atlanto-occipital joint visible (open arrow) and right transverse process of first cervical vertebra not fused to skull. No atlanto-occipital joint is seen on left. The left transverse process of first cervical vertebra is attached to base of skull (solid arrow). Neither side of posterior arch of this vertebra is attached to skull. Second and third cervical vertebrae are fused. (From McRae, D. L., and Barnum, A. S.: Amer. J. Roentgen. **70**:23-45, 1953.)

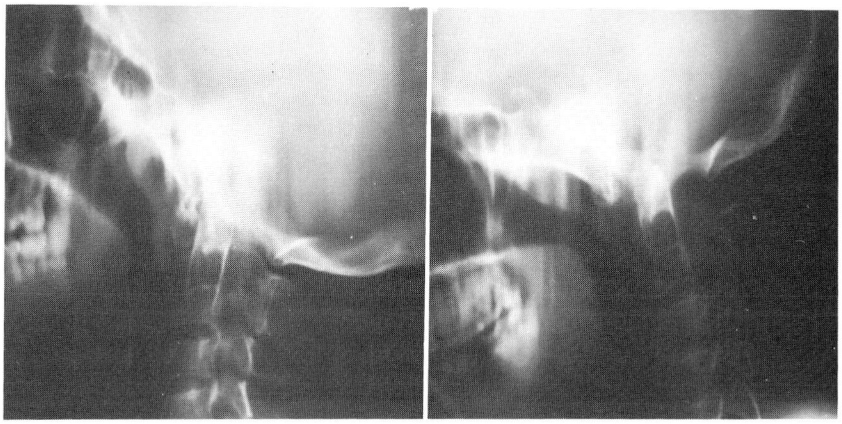

Fig. 14-15. Occipitalization of atlas with atlantoaxial dislocation. A man of 22 years had noted weakness and sensory loss of the arms for at least 1 year. The midsagittal tomograms in flexion and extension show that the assimilated atlas flexes and extends on the axis with atlantoaxial dislocation during flexion. (From McRae, D. L.: Amer. J. Roentgen. **84**:3-25, 1960.)

cross the anterior atlanto-occipital interval from top to bottom. On lateral roentgenograms and tomograms the cortex of the anterior arch of the atlas is seen to be continuous with the cortex of the basiocciput (Fig. 14-13). In still other cases the medullary cavity of the anterior arch of the atlas appears to be continuous with the medullary cavity of the basiocciput. The assimilated anterior arch of the first cervical vertebra may be close to the anterior lip of the foramen magnum. Rarely it may be as much as 6 mm below the lip, but the gap is at least partly filled in with bone. Seldom is a facet for the odontoid process obvious on the posterior surface of the fused anterior arch. Since the second cervical vertebra is closer to the skull than normal, the odontoid process is above Chamberlain's line. The atlantoaxial joints then are usually at or slightly above the digastric line. True invagination of the foramen magnum, however, is often not present.

Joint spaces between the occipital condyles and the lateral masses of the atlas are seldom demonstrated. Occasionally a unilateral joint space is seen (Fig. 14-14). Rarely one lateral half of the atlas is fused to the skull while the other half is either free or fused to the second cervical vertebra.

The transverse processes of an assimilated atlas may or may not be fused to the skull. Sometimes no transverse process is seen; instead a paracondyloid or paramastoid process is attached to the skull.

The posterior arch of the assimilated atlas is often fused to the margins of the foramen magnum, forming bony flanges on the lateral and posterior edges of the foramen. The assimilated posterior arch is often incomplete posteriorly, whether or not it is fused to the posterior edge of the foramen. These bony protuberances on the foramen magnum may not reduce its size, but there is often a thick band of dura at the level of the assimilated posterior arch. The band presses against the posterior surface of the medulla oblongata, preventing the medulla from moving away from the odontoid process.

When the atlas is occipitalized, the head no longer flexes and extends at the atlanto-occipital joint. Instead these movements must take place at the atlantoaxial joints. If the transverse ligament of the atlas has developed poorly or become stretched, atlantoaxial dislocation will occur during flexion (Fig. 14-15). Frequently in these instances neurologic symptoms and signs develop. Of course, the transverse ligament of the atlas may hold the odontoid process against the assimiliated anterior arch. In that case no atlantoaxial dislocation occurs and seldom if ever are there symptoms.

Occipitalization of the atlas is present in about 0.75% of the general population. In only one quarter to one third of this number does it cause neurologic symptoms and signs.

Chiari malformations

In 1891 and 1895 Chiari described groups of patients in whom parts of the medulla oblongata and cerebellum were below the foramen magnum. In his type I cases the cerebellar tonsils were narrow and elongated. They were closely applied to the posterior surface of the cervical portion of the medulla oblongata and upper spinal cord. The tonsils usually extended down to the posterior arch of the first cervical vertebra or occasionally slightly farther. The patients were usually older children and adults and were often asymptomatic. Rarely did they have meningoceles and myelomeningoceles. In his type II cases the deformity of the medulla oblongata and cerebellum was more pronounced. The cerebellar tonsils were often lower, and part or all of the fourth ventricle was below the foramen magnum. On the dorsal surface of the downwardly displaced medulla oblongata was a curious hump. The cervical nerve roots passed upward to reach their intervertebral foramina rather than downward as is normal (Greenfield, 1958). The type II patients all had hydrocephalus and meningoceles or myelomeningoceles, and all were infants. In 1894 Arnold reported a case similar to the type II cases of Chiari, and his name is often added to Chiari's without much justification.

The aqueduct of Sylvius in type II cases of Chiari malformation is long and narrow and forms one type of aqueduct stenosis. The foramina of Magendie and Luschka open into the spinal canal and are usually surrounded by adhesions. Hydrocephalus results from one or a combination of the following abnormalities: (1) the aqueduct may be long and narrow; (2) the foramen magnum may be obstructed by the cerebellum; (3) the foramina in the roof of the fourth ventricle may be obstructed by adhesions.

In writing about these lesions, most authors use words, such as *displacement* of the cerebellum and medulla oblongata. The word displacement connotes activity. It implies that these parts of the brain were once in a normal position and then moved into an abnormal position. There may be no such change in position. Several theories for the cause of these deformities have been advanced. The traction theory suggests that the cerebellum and medulla were once within the skull but that tethering of the spinal cord, followed by growth in length of the spine, caused them to be drawn down through the foramen magnum. Barry and his co-workers (1957) measured the fetal spinal cord, hindbrain, and midbrain. They suggested that overgrowth of the hindbrain and midbrain may have pushed the cerebellum and medulla downward. A third possibility is that a short clivus and a shallow posterior fossa caused the hindbrain to develop in an abnormally low position and it was therefore never displaced.

Type I Chiari lesions that consist mainly of low cerebellar tonsils are difficult to distinguish from tonsillar herniations that are the result of expanding intracranial lesions. On oil or air myelograms little or no cisterna magna is visible, either in the skull or in the cervical spine (Liliequist, 1960). A soft-tissue mass is seen behind the upper spinal cord. It is usually smooth and round and extends down to the posterior arch of the first cervical vertebra. Occasionally it is tongue shaped and extends to a slightly lower level (Fig. 14-16). The upper part of the spinal cord is usually anterior to the mass and is often in contact with the odontoid process. In these cases the fourth ventricle usually does not fill from below with either air or oil. Either no bony deformity is seen or a *high atlas* is present.

In the type II Chiari lesions the tonsils are usually longer, less smooth, and closely applied to the posterior surface of the upper cervical cord (Fig. 14-17). The tips of the tonsils are usually at or below the posterior arch of the second cervical vertebra. In these instances the fourth ventricle is in low position, and part of it is below the foramen magnum. The fourth ventricle usually does not fill with air or oil from below, and ventriculography may be necessary to see it. Because of the long narrow

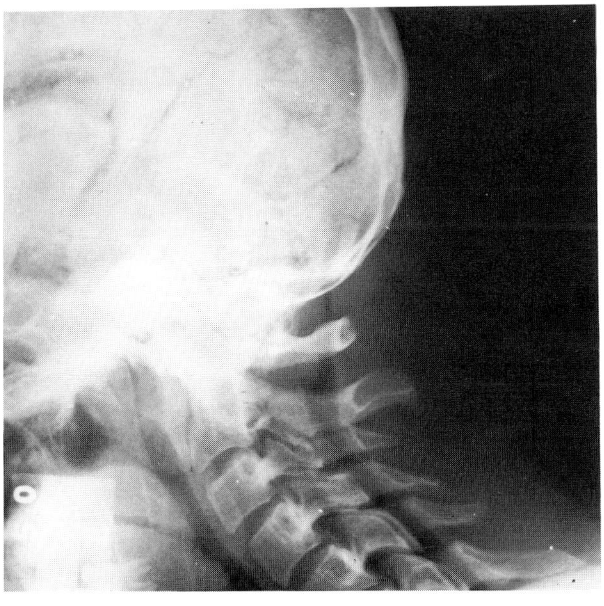

Fig. 14-16. Chiari malformation (type I). This 17-year-old man had sudden extreme occipital headaches on flexion of head and neck. Neurologic examination was negative. Air myelogram shows tips of cerebellar tonsils slightly below lower edge of arch of first cervical vertebra. This low position was confirmed at operation. Ventricular system failed to fill with air from below but did fill during air ventriculography. Ventricular system was not enlarged.

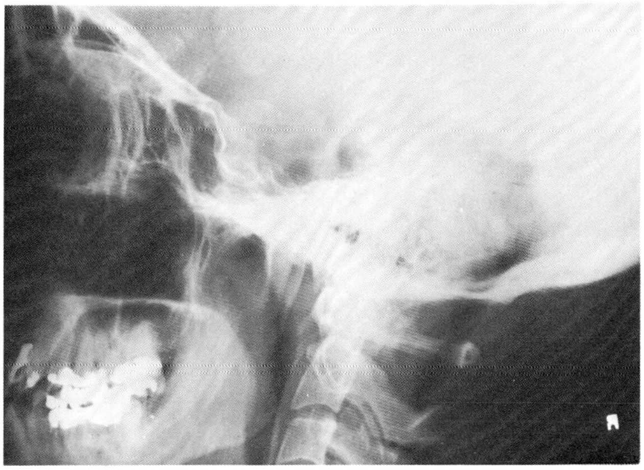

Fig. 14-17. Chiari malformation (type II). A 24-year-old man had had lumbar meningocele removed in infancy. His head was enlarged, but he was of average intelligence. He complained of headaches but had no spinal cord symptoms or signs. Air myelogram shows shallow posterior fossa containing an apparently small cerebellum. Wavy mass behind upper cervical cord extends down at least to posterior arch of second cervical vertebra. Faint round bubble of gas that overlaps posterior arch of first cervical vertebra may be in foramen of Magendie. It may also be in part of fourth ventricle, but no other ventricular gas was seen. This bubble did not move with changes in position of the patient. Note the large foramen magnum and the large spinal canal at the first and second cervical vertebrae. These findings are common in Arnold-Chiari malformation in older children and adults.

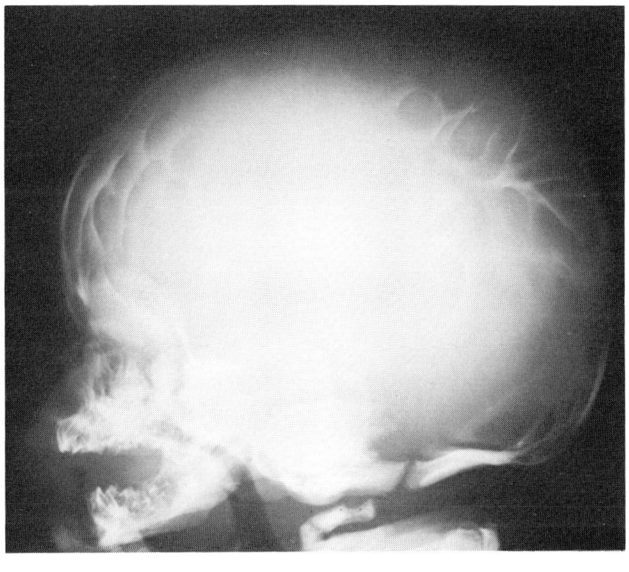

Fig. 14-18. Skull of 3-week-old child with lumbar myelomeningocele, craniolacunia, and a Chiari-type II malformation. Occipital bone behind foramen magnum is convex upward instead of downward as is normal. This is a frequent finding in newborn children with Chiari malformations.

aqueduct of Sylvius, however, its demonstration by ventricular injections of contrast material may not be possible.

In these patients the skull, the foramen magnum, and the upper cervical spinal canal are enlarged and the posterior fossa is shallow (Figs. 14-17 and 14-18).

In many newborn infants with a Chiari malformation, the normal curve of the occipital squama is reversed just behind the foramen magnum; that is, the suboccipital region is upturned (Fig. 14-18). The posterior fossa in these infants appears normal in width and normal or greater than normal in the anteroposterior diameter, but reduced in height. The high position of the foramen magnum may have caused the cerebellar tonsils and lower medulla to develop in the spinal canal rather than in the cranium.

REFERENCES

Arnold, J.: Myelocyste, Transposition von Gewebskeimen und Sympodie, Beitr. Path. Anat. **16**:1-28, 1894.

Barry, A., Patten, B. M., and Stewart, B. H.: Possible factors in the development of the Arnold-Chiari malformation, J. Neurosurg. **14**:285-301, 1957.

Chamberlain, W. E.: Basilar impression (platybasia), Yale J. Biol. Med. **11**:487-496, 1939.

Chiari, H.: Ueber Veränderungen des Kleinhirns in Folge von Hydrocephalie des Grosshirns, Deutsch. Med. Wschr. **17**: 1172-1175, 1891.

Chiari, H.: Ueber die Veränderungen des Kleinhirns, des Pons und der Medulla oblongata in Folge von congenitaler Hydrocephalie des Grosshirns, Denkschr. Akad. Wissensch. Math. Naturw. Kl. **63**:71-116, 1895.

Fischgold, H., David, M., and Brégeat, P. R.: La tomographie de la base du crâne en neuro-chirurgie et neuro-ophtalmologie, Paris, 1952, Masson & Cie.

Frazer, J. E.: The anatomy of the human skeleton, ed. 4, London, 1940, J. & A. Churchill, Ltd.

Gladstone, R. J., and Erichsen-Powell, W.: Manifestations of occipital vertebrae and fusion of the atlas with the occipital bone, J. Anat. Physiol. **49**:190-209, 1915.

Greenfield, J. G.: Neuropathology, Baltimore, 1958, The Williams & Wilkins Co.

Hinck, V. C., Hopkins, C. E., and Savara, B. S.: Sagittal diameter of the cervical spinal canal in children, Radiology **79**: 97-108, 1962.

Hohl, M., and Baker, H. R.: The atlanto-axial joint; a roentgenographic and anatomical study of normal and abnormal motion, J. Bone Joint Surg. [Amer.] **46**:1739-1752, 1964.

Jones, M. D.: Cineradiographic studies of the normal cervical spine, Calif. Med. **93**:293-296, 1960.

Keith, A.: Human embryology and morphology, ed. 6, London, 1949, Edward Arnold & Co.

Liliequist, B.: Encephalography in the Arnold-Chiari malformation, Acta Radiol. **53**:17-32, 1960.

Lombardi, G.: The occipital vertebra, Amer. J. Roentgen. **86**: 260-269, 1961.

McGregor, M.: The significance of certain measurements of the skull in the diagnosis of basilar impression, Brit. J. Radiol. **21**:171-181, 1948.

McRae, D. L.: Bony abnormalities in the region of the foramen magnum: correlation of the anatomic and neurologic findings, Acta Radiol. **40**:335-354, 1953.

McRae, D. L.: The significance of abnormalities of the cervical spine, Amer. J. Roentgen. **84**:3-25, 1960.

McRae, D. L., and Barnum, A. S.: Occipitalization of the atlas, Amer. J. Roentgen. **70**:23-46, 1953.

Russell, D. S.: Observations on the pathology of hydrocephalus, Medical Research Council. Special Report Series no. 265, London, 1949, H. M. Stationery Office.

Spillane, J. D., Pallis, C., and Jones, A. M.: Developmental abnormalities in the region of the foramen magnum, Brain **80**:11-48, 1957.

CHAPTER 15

Foramen magnum

C. G. Coin and Dennis R. Malkasian

The foramen magnum is an oval-shaped orifice in the occipital bone with a long anteroposterior diameter. It is bound anteriorly, laterally, and posteriorly by the basi-occiput, occipital condyles, and supraocciput respectively.

EMBRYOLOGY

At birth the occipital bone is in three ossified portions, the supraoccipital, exoccipital, and basioccipital. The basioccipital and exoccipital bones are separated by two

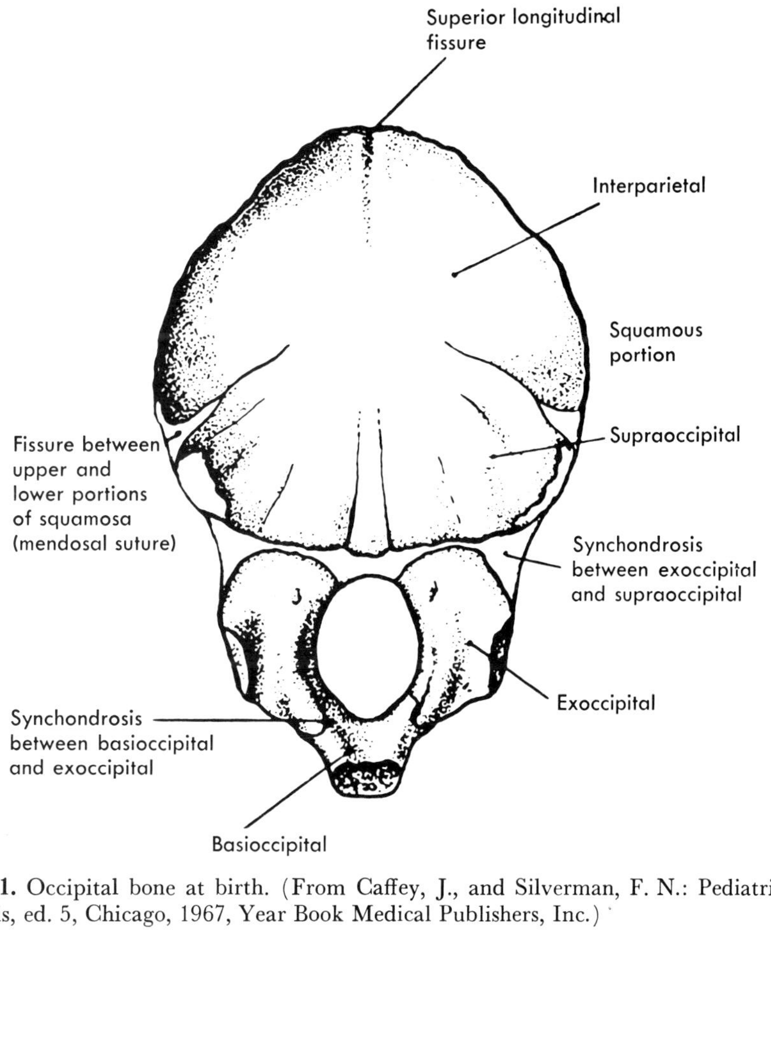

Fig. 15-1. Occipital bone at birth. (From Caffey, J., and Silverman, F. N.: Pediatric x-ray diagnosis, ed. 5, Chicago, 1967, Year Book Medical Publishers, Inc.)

anterior synchondroses, and the exoccipital and supraoccipital bones are separated by two posterior synchondroses (Figs. 15-1 and 15-2). These synchrondroses are still present at 12 months of age. They then become narrow, and after about 18 months of age their peripheral portions disappear rather rapidly. The anterior synchondrosis usually fuses between 36 and 48 months of age. The posterior synchondrosis disappears by the age of 7 years (Kruyff, 1965).

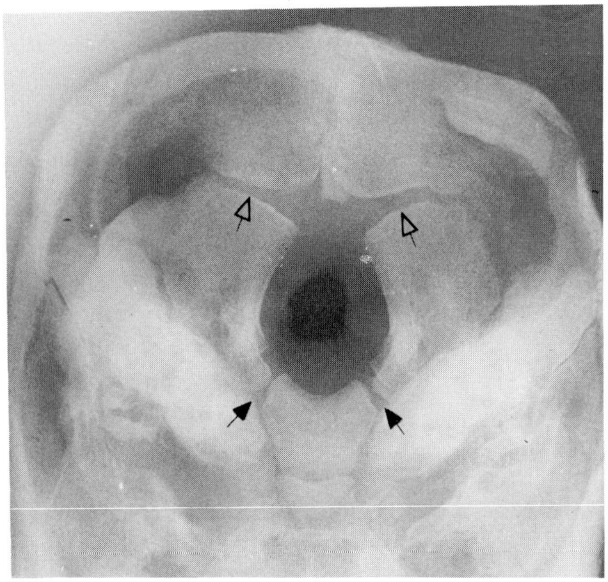

Fig. 15-2. Roentgenogram of posterior fossa specimen of infant. Innominate synchondroses (open arrows) between exoccipital and supraoccipital bones are wide. Note the anterior synchondroses between the basioccipital and exoccipital bones (solid arrows). Foramen magnum is partly occupied by diaphragm of dura. Actual opening for spinal canal (central dark area) is smaller than boundaries of ossified rim of foramen magnum. (From Kruyff, E.: Radiology **85:**501-507, 1965.)

GROSS ANATOMY

The anterior margin of the foramen magnum is formed by the basal part of the occipital bone. The anterior portion of the foramen magnum has a trapezoidal shape whereas the posterior portion is usually rounded. The medial aspect of the occipital condyle contributes to the anterior half of the lateral border of the foramen magnum (Fig. 15-3, *A*). Posterior to the occipital condyle is the condyloid fossa (Fig. 15-3, *A*). This fossa accommodates the lip of the lateral mass of

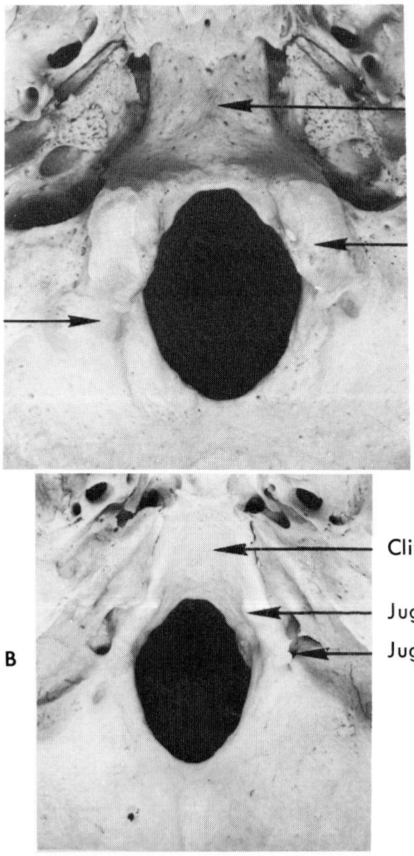

Fig. 15-3. Foramen magnum. **A,** Exocranial aspect. **B,** Endocranial aspect.

the atlas when the head is extended. Posteriorly the foramen magnum is formed by the supraoccipital segment of the occipital bone (Fig. 15-3).

The average width of the foramen magnum, measured in forty-two dried adult skulls at the level of the posterior aspect of the occipital condyle, was 2.9 cm, with a range of 2.5 to 3.4 cm. The average length of the foramen magnum was 3.4 cm, with a range of 3.2 to 3.6 cm.

The foramen magnum transmits the medulla oblongata and its meninges, the spinal portion of the spinal accessory nerve, the vertebral arteries, the anterior and posterior spinal arteries, and the veins that communicate with the internal vertebral venous plexus. The most cranial attachment of the dentate ligament (Gray, 1967) occurs at the level of the foramen magnum between the vertebral artery and the hypoglossal nerve. Slight bony roughenings on the anterior lip of the foramen magnum and the medial aspect of the occipital condyles mark the attachments of the apical, dental, and alar ligaments respectively (Figs. 15-3, *A*, and 15-4). The upper band of the cruciate ligament attaches to the anterior margin of the foramen magnum. The posterior longitudinal ligament continues through the foramen magnum as the tectorial membrane (Fig. 15-5).

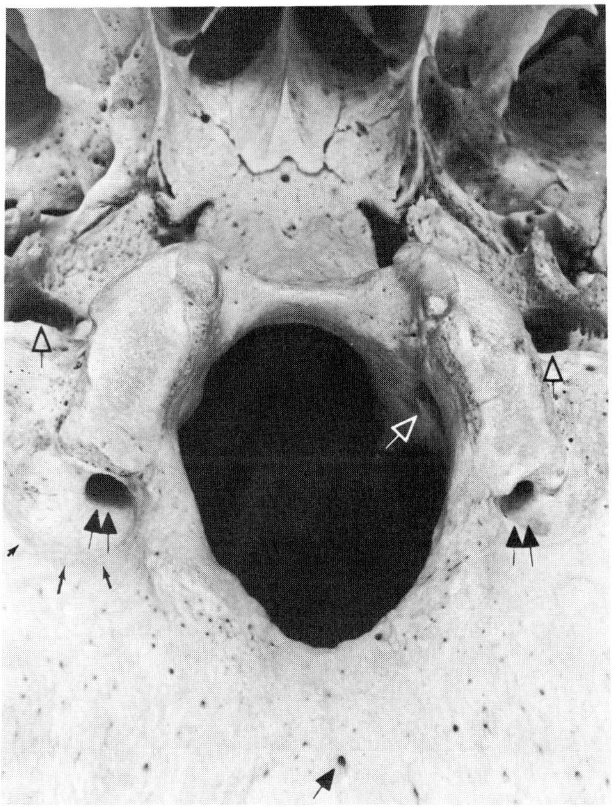

Fig. 15-4. Foramen magnum as seen from below and behind. Hypoglossal (anterior condyloid) canal is indicated by white arrow. Note the bony spicule partly traversing the hypoglossal canal. This spicule separates hypoglossal nerve from meningeal branch of ascending pharyngeal artery. Note also the condyloid fossa (small arrows), the posterior condyloid canal (double solid arrows), present on both sides in this specimen, the jugular foramen (open black arrows), and the canal for an emissary vein (solid arrow).

The base of each occipital condyle is tunneled by the hypoglossal (anterior condyloid) canal, passing forward and lateralward from the anterior lateral margin of the foramen magnum to exit medial to the exocranial opening of the jugular foramen (Fig. 15-4). The hypoglossal canal transmits the hypoglossal nerve, a meningeal branch of the ascending pharyngeal artery, and an emissary vein. On occasion the anterior condyloid canal may be divided by a bony spicule separating this meningeal artery from the hypoglossal nerve (Fig. 15-4).

The condyloid fossa is an impression on the exocranial surface immediately posterior to the occipital condyle (Fig. 15-4). A posterior condyloid canal is frequently present in the anterior margin of this fossa. It may normally be absent, or it may be found either unilaterally or bilaterally. The canals, when present, may differ in diameter. Haas (1957) stated that these canals, even when present, may not be radiographically visualized. This canal may be considered as an enlarged emissary foramen that transmits an anastomotic vein between

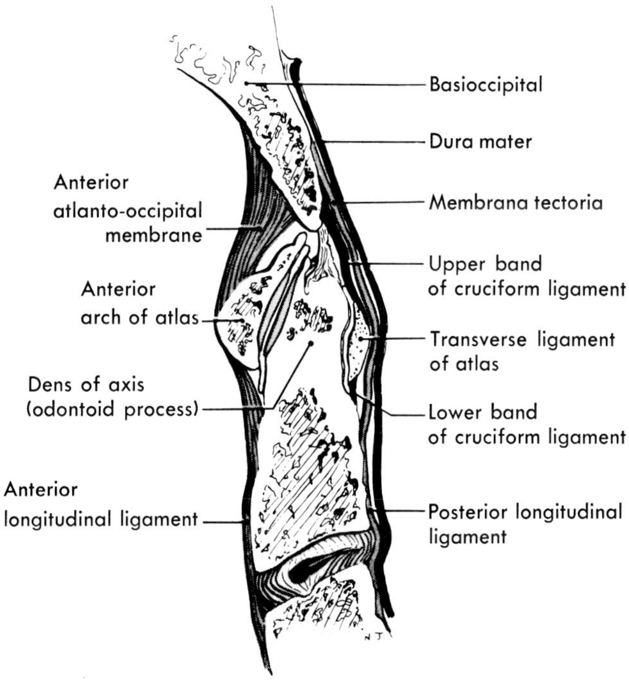

Fig. 15-5. Ligaments of atlantoaxial and atlanto-occipital joints on median section. (From Grant, J. C. B.: An atlas of anatomy, ed. 5, Baltimore, 1962, The Williams & Wilkins Co.)

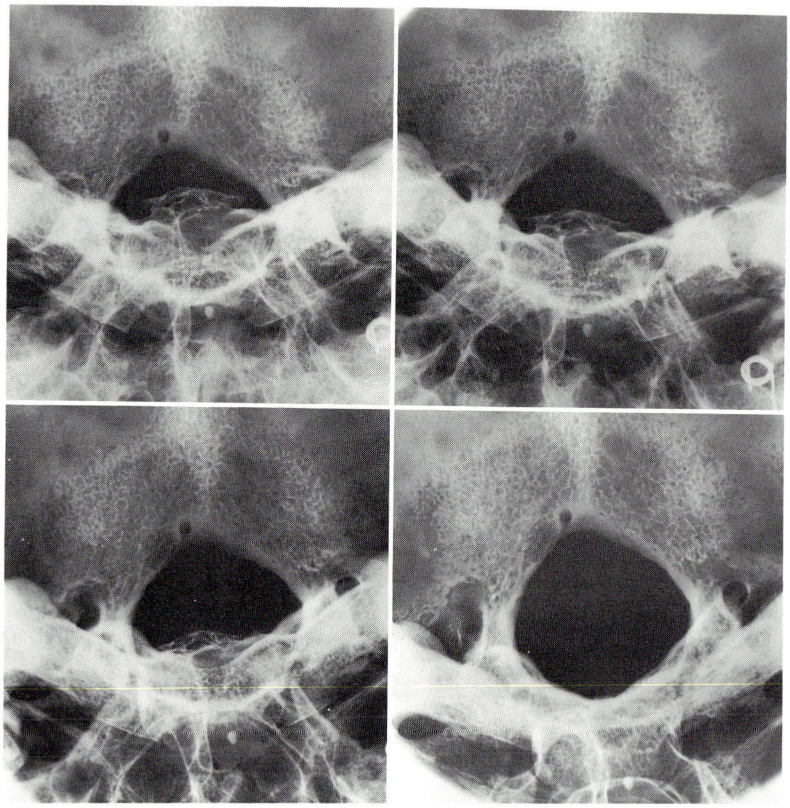

Fig. 15-6. Roentgenograms of foramen magnum in a dry skull with increasing angulation. With lesser degrees of angulation, dorsum sellae and posterior clinoid processes are projected through foramen magnum. In these cases, **A** and **B,** anterior rim of foramen magnum is obscured. With central beam directed parallel to clivus, **D,** anterior rim of foramen magnum is visualized.

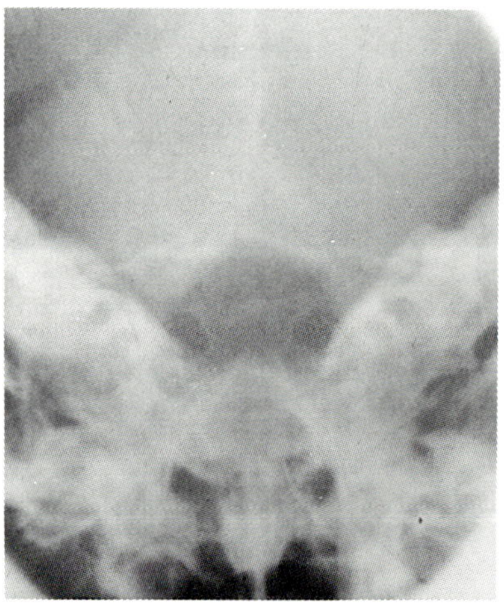

Fig. 15-7. Chamberlain-Towne projection of foramen magnum shows dorsum sellae and posterior clinoid processes projected through foramen magnum. Posterior rim of foramen magnum is well shown. Anterior rim is obscured.

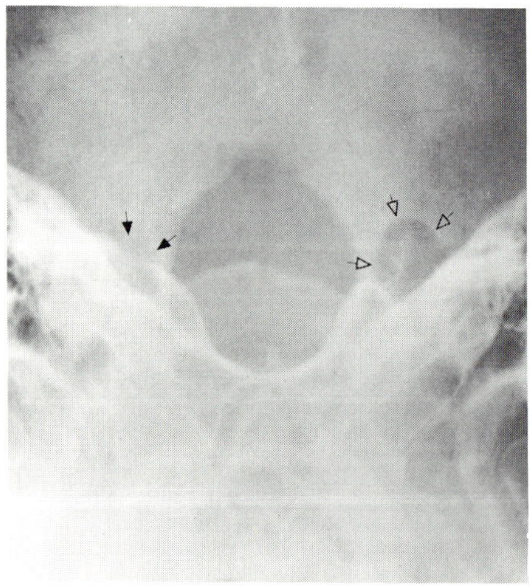

Fig. 15-8. Foramen magnum in steep Chamberlain-Towne projection. Posterior arch of first cervical vertebra is now projected across foramen magnum. Note the slight irregularity and notching of the dorsal margin of the foramen magnum. The (posterior) condyloid canal, associated with a medially coursing sigmoid sinus, is prominent (open arrows). Radiolucency on right (solid arrows) probably is a sigmoid fossa (Gathier and Bruyn, 1969).

the sigmoid sinus and the suboccipital venous plexus. The presence of this venous anastomosis may have clinical significance. Compression of the jugular veins in the Queckenstedt test in these patients may give erroneous results due to the diversion of blood through this and other emissary channels.

Occipital emissary veins traversing the supraoccipital segment of the occipital bone are frequently found in proximity to the posterior margin of the foramen magnum (Fig. 15-4). These venous channels communicate between the dural sinus and the suboccipital venous plexus and scalp veins. They represent potential routes for the spread of infection to the dural venous sinuses and are considered to be an anatomic basis for venous sinus thrombosis.

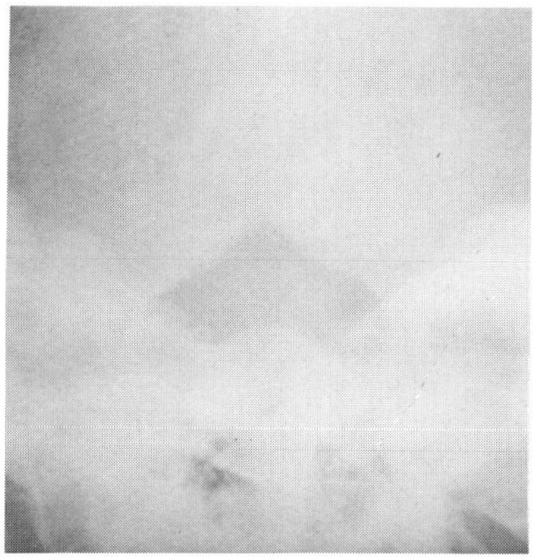

Fig. 15-9. Foramen magnum, Chamberlain-Towne projection. Posterior rim of foramen magnum has slightly pointed or notched appearance.

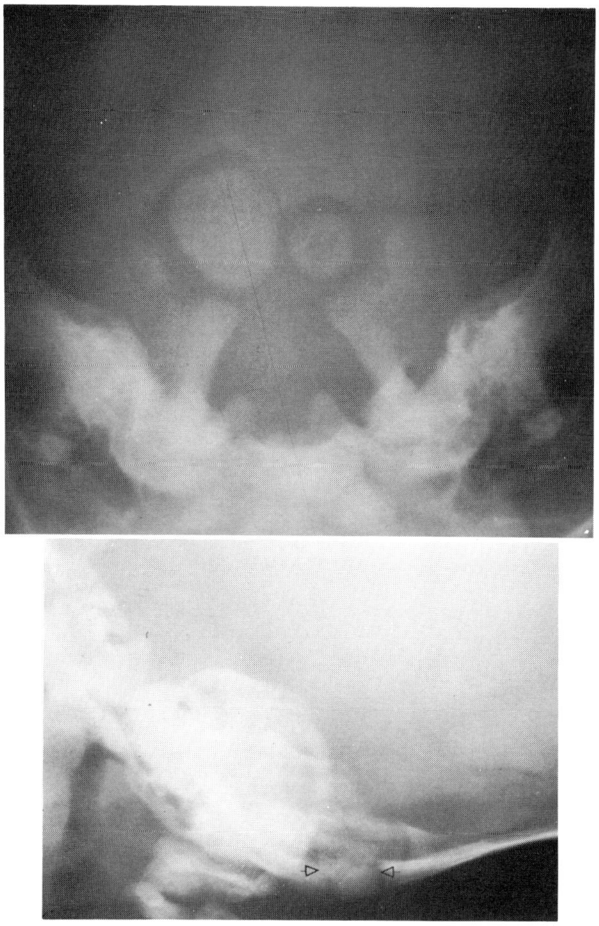

Fig. 15-10. Prominent accessory ossicles (arrows) are noted along posterior rim of foramen magnum.

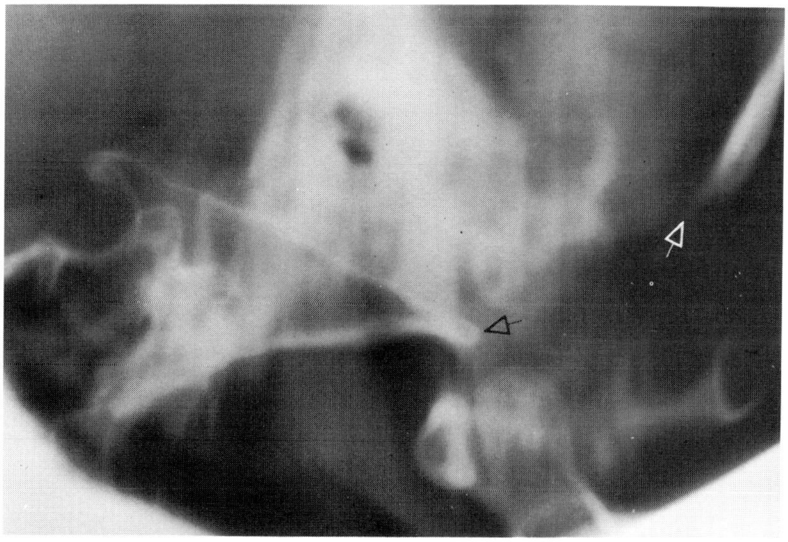

Fig. 15-11. Lateral midline tomogram of foramen magnum shows well the anterior limits of foramen (arrows) in the midsagittal plane.

ROENTGENOGRAPHIC ANATOMY

The foramen magnum is well shown in the Chamberlain-Towne projection (Fig. 15-6). With lesser degrees of angulation, the anterior portion of the foramen magnum is obscured by the overlying posterior clinoid processes and the dorsum sellae (Figs. 15-6, *A* and *B,* and 15-7). As the angulation is increased, the dorsum sellae is projected clear of the anterior rim of the foramen magnum, which then is visualized (Fig. 15-6, *C* and *D*). In this view the posterior arch of the atlas is projected across the foramen magnum, and the jugular tubercles may project over the lateral rim of the foramen (Fig. 15-8).

The condyloid fossa is not normally visible in half-axial projections. Radiolucent defects commonly attributed to the condyloid fossa are due to either the (posterior) condyloid canals or a prominent sigmoid groove (Gathier and Bruyn, 1969). The (posterior) condyloid canal, when present, may be seen as a small round radiolucency or as a crescent-shaped radiolucency at the medial margin of the foramen magnum projecting above the petrous pyramid (Fig. 15-8). The appearance of the canal in this

A B C

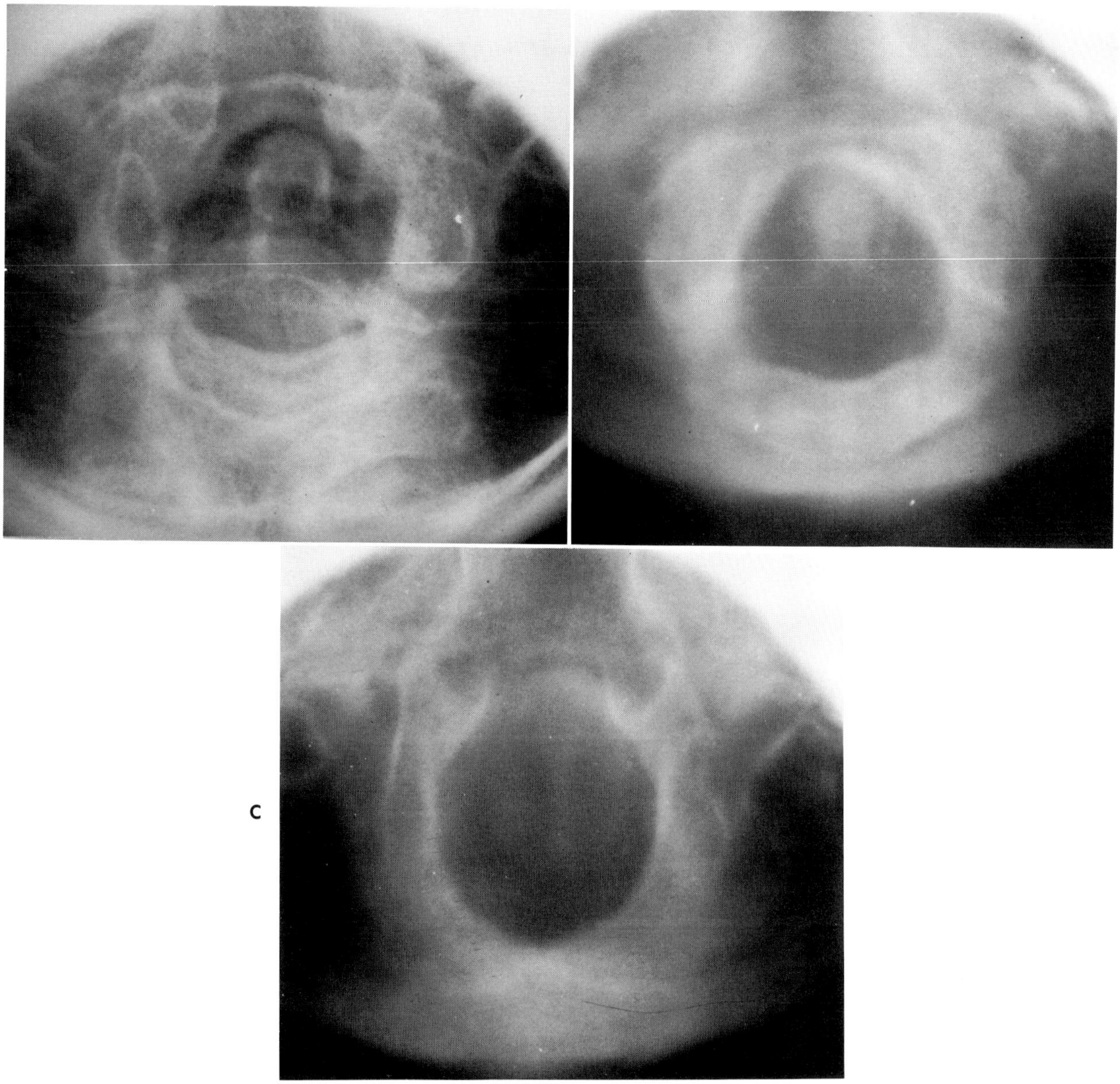

Fig. 15-12. Submentovertical projection of foramen magnum. **A,** Routine axial projection shows the foramen obscured by overlying upper cervical spine. **B,** Basal tomogram through level of first cervical vertebra shows cross-sectional view of this structure. **C,** Basal tomogram through foramen magnum demonstrates this structure in basal projection.

latter case is the consequence of a medially coursing sigmoid sinus.

The *sigmoid fossa* of Gathier and Bruyn (1969) is seen as a sharply defined round radiolucency slightly more lateral and ventral in position, projecting partially under the upper margin of the petrous pyramid (Fig. 15-8). This fossa is the result of a well-defined deepening of the sigmoid groove and is seen less frequently than the condyloid canals.

The appearance of the posterior rim of the foramen magnum varies from a smoothly round to a slightly elongated semicircle. Occasionally the posterior rim of the foramen magnum has a midline notch (incisura marginalis posterior) of varying depth (Kollmann, 1905) (Figs. 15-8 and 15-9). Other minor variations include accessory ossicles (Schultz, 1917) (Fig. 15-10) and Kerkring's processes (Caffey and Silverman, 1967).

In the lateral projection the anterior and posterior margins of the foramen magnum can be visualized, particularly when tomography is employed (Fig. 15-11). The anterior rim of the foramen magnum is easily recognized as the inferior tip of the clivus. The posterior rim of the foramen may be indistinct, but its location can often be estimated by its position relative to the posterior arch of the first cervical vertebra.

In the axial projection the foramen magnum is obscured and is often confused with the margins of the upper cervical canal (Fig. 15-12). This projection is therefore of limited value unless tomography is utilized.

The anterior rim of the foramen magnum is best visualized by frontal tomography (Fig. 15-13). In this projection the anterior rim of the foramen magnum has a smooth inferior concavity and is outlined by cortical bone. Occasionally a delta-shaped or keyhole defect is noted in the anterior rim of the foramen magnum (Fischer, 1963; Di Chiro and Anderson, 1965) (Fig. 15-14).

The anterior condyloid (hypoglossal) canal is best

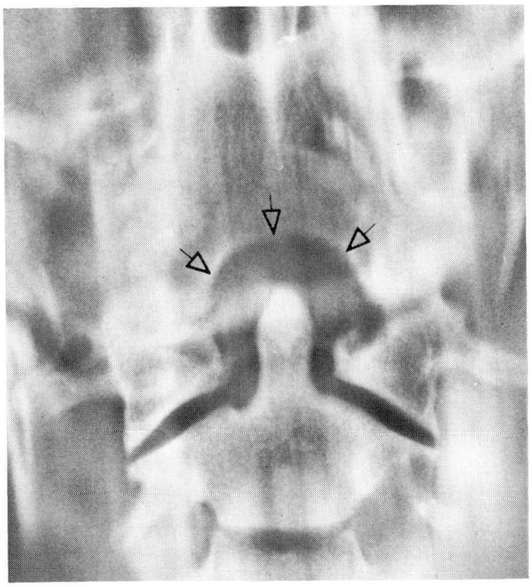

Fig. 15-13. Frontal tomogram of foramen magnum. In this projection, anterior rim of foramen magnum (arrows) has smooth inferior concavity. (From Di Chiro, G., and Anderson, W. B.: Clin. Radiol. **16:**211-223, 1965.)

A

B

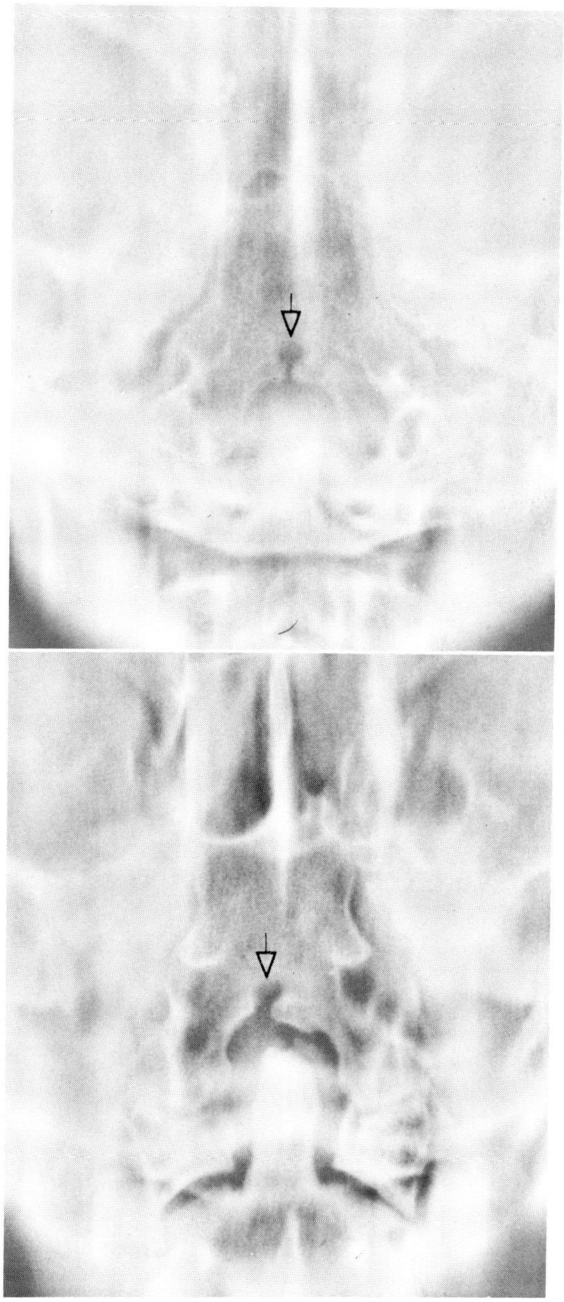

Fig. 15-14. Keyhole foramen magnum. Frontal tomograms of foramen magnum demonstrate distinct notch in anterior rim of foramen that is almost in midline in **A** and to right of midline in **B** (arrows). (From Di Chiro, G., and Anderson, W. B.: Clin. Radiol. **16:**211-223, 1965.)

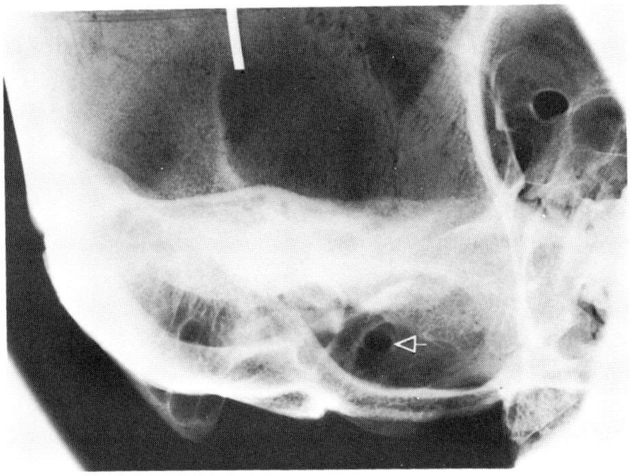

Fig. 15-15. Anterior condyloid (hypoglossal) canal (arrow) is shown in Stenvers projection. Positioning under fluoroscopic control is helpful in demonstrating this canal.

shown in the Stenvers projection (Kirdani, 1967; Gathier and Bruyn, 1969) (Fig. 15-15). Tomography in the frontal projection is helpful for a more detailed study of this region (Di Chiro and Anderson, 1965; Valvassori and Kirdani, 1967).

CLINICAL FEATURES OF FORAMEN MAGNUM LESIONS

Tumors occurring in the region of the foramen magnum present difficult diagnostic problems (Piehl et al., 1950; Craig et al., 1956; Dodge et al., 1956).

Bogordinsky (1936) reviewed the various syndromes resulting from tumors arising primarily in the foramen magnum. His principal conclusions were summarized by Cushing and Eisenhardt (1938), who stated that extramedullary tumors in this region give rise to a definite syndrome. The onset is characterized by suboccipital discomforts, protective rigidity of the cervical and occipital musculature, and sometimes pains and paresthesias in the shoulder girdle and upper extremities. At its maximum stage the clinical symptoms are as follows: (1) paralyses of the extremities, (2) rigidity and paresis of the cervical muscles, abnormal posture of the head, and paresis of the eleventh cranial nerves, (3) pains and paresthesias in the extremities and trunk, (4) pains in the occiput and the neck, (5) hemianesthesia or para-anesthesia reaching up to the upper cervical dermatomes, occasionally involving the skin field of the trigeminus, (6) sphincteric disturbances, (7) respiratory disturbances, and (8) Horner's symptom complex.

The course of the malady is slowly progressive, lasting for months and even years, though remission of isolated symptoms may occasionally be observed.

Abbott (1950) emphasized the fact that these lesions frequently simulate degenerative disease of the central nervous system. The extirpation of the tumor by surgical intervention has proved to be an efficient method of treatment in 50% of cases that were operated on.

Love and co-workers (1954) reviewed seventy-four patients with tumor of the foramen magnum encountered at the Mayo Clinic. These cases included seventy-three neoplasms and one aneurysm of the vertebral artery. The average duration of symptoms was 28 months. The age of the patients varied from 2 to 70 years. The most frequent age incidence, however, was between 31 and 50 years. Pain was a common initial complaint. It was usually suboccipital, but in a few patients it occurred in the lumbar region and lower extremities. Characteristically the pain was increased by attempted movements of the neck. Weakness of the extremity was another initial complaint. This was more common in an upper than in a lower extremity. Other primary symptoms were nausea and vomiting, peripheral paresthesias, double vision, recurrent attacks of dizziness, unsteady gait, hoarseness, and difficulty in swallowing and phonation. Several patients reported profound weakness and fatigue. Paresthesias were present in forty-five of the patients, and progressive motor weakness in forty-nine.

Blom and Ekbom (1962) reported two cases of meningioma of the foramen magnum in which the neurologic findings were pseudoathetosis (loss of sense of position) in the upper extremities and signs of a pyramidal tract lesion in the legs. They stated that these findings are an early indication of an expansive lesion in the upper cervical or foramen magnum region.

Cohen and Macrae (1962) reported four cases of tumor in the region of the foramen magnum and reviewed the literature. They emphasized the high incidence of normal myelograms frequently leading to the erroneous diagnosis of multiple sclerosis. This error can be avoided by proper myelographic examination of the foramen magnum.

ABNORMAL FORAMEN MAGNUM

Small size

Achondroplasia

The foramen magnum, which is completely formed from cartilage, is characteristically small in achondroplasia. Significant hydrocephalus, when it occurs in these patients, may be due to obstruction of the cerebrospinal fluid pathways at the level of the foramen magnum and may be associated with neurologic findings related to cord compression at this level (Caffey, 1945; Szalay, 1963; Dorst, 1964; Cohen et al., 1967) (Fig. 15-16).

Occipital dysplasia

A small or asymmetric foramen magnum is one of the early signs of craniovertebral deformity. Such a deformity may result from assimilation or fusion of a part of the first cervical vertebra to the foramen magnum (Fig. 15-17). Similar asymmetry may also be due to premature synostosis of one or more of the occipital synchondroses (Figs. 15-18 and 15-19). Kruyff (1965) described eight patients in whom the synchondrosis differed significantly from the normal. In each of his patients, either one or both synchondroses between the exoccipital and supraoccipital bones were prematurely closed. Occasionally

A

B

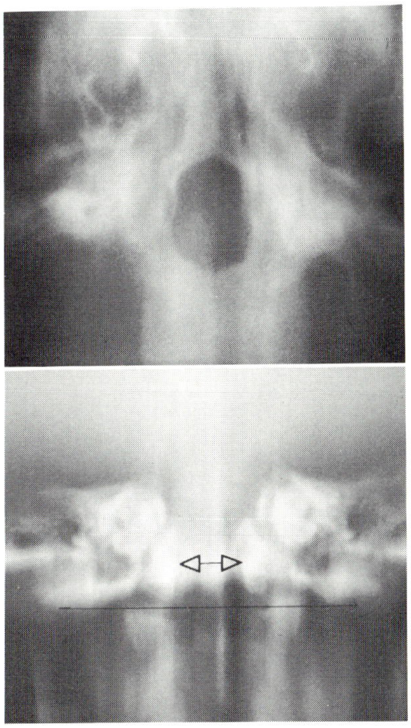

Fig. 15-16. Achondroplasia. Foramen magnum is small, as shown in both basal, **A,** and frontal, **B,** tomograms. (Courtesy Fred Sondheimer, M.D., San Francisco, Calif.)

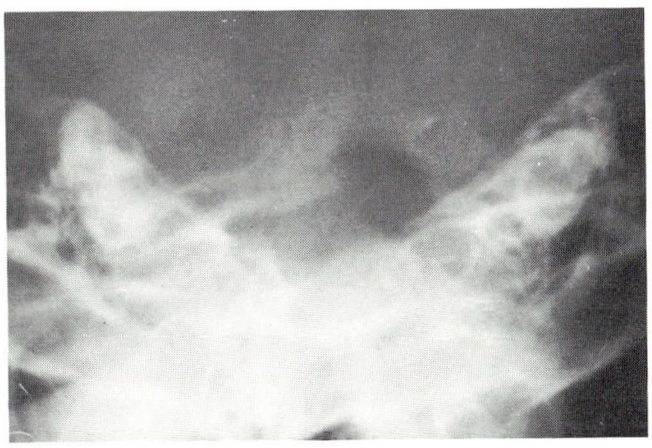

Fig. 15-17. Occipital dysplasia. Towne projection (+50°) of foramen magnum in 4-year-old boy shows posterior arch of first cervical vertebra on right incorporated into rim of foramen magnum, causing coarctation. (From Kruyff, E.: Radiology **85:**501-507, 1965.)

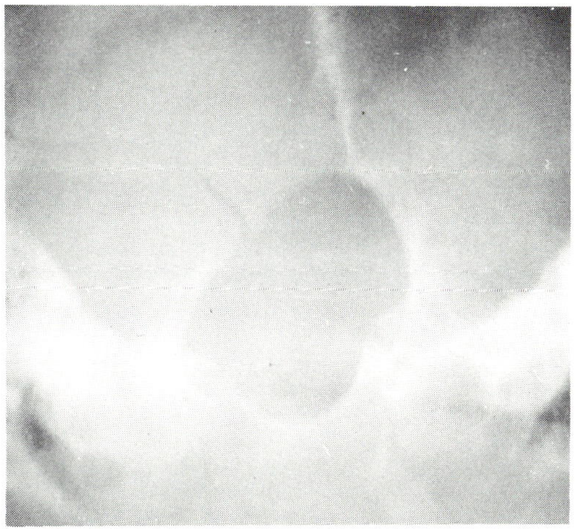

Fig. 15-18. Occipital dysplasia. Towne projection of foramen magnum in 1-year-old child with premature obliteration of posterior synchondrosis shows foramen magnum deformed. Note the asymmetry of the jugular tubercles (Courtesy E. Kruyff, M.D., Willowdale, Ontario, Canada.)

A

B

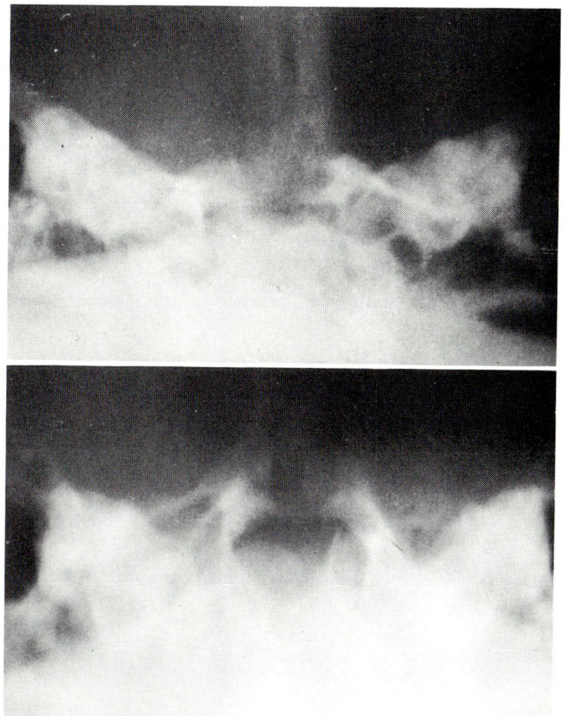

Fig. 15-19. Occipital dysplasia in 17-month-old girl. **A,** Towne projection (+40°) shows foramen magnum largely obscured. **B,** Towne projection (+50°) with strong flexion of head shows foramen magnum better. It is small with dense sclerotic margins. (From Kruyff, E.: Radiology **85:**501-507, 1965.)

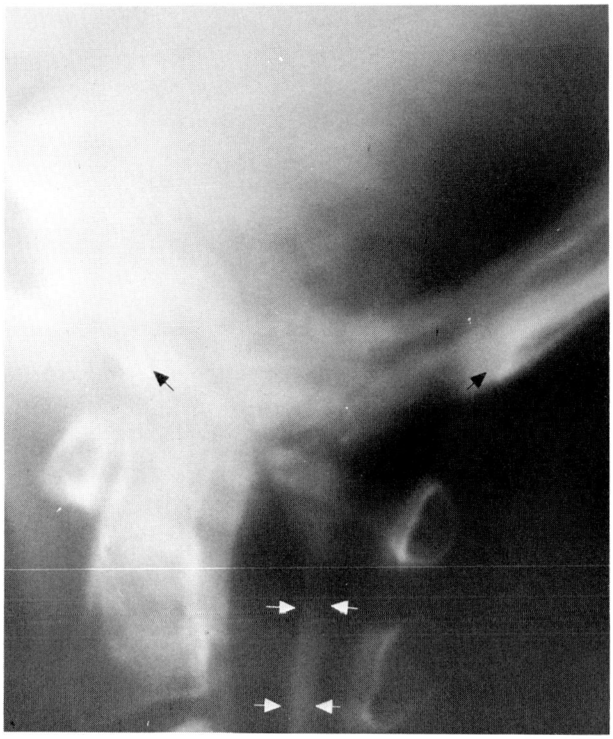

Fig. 15-20. Syringomyelia. Air myelogram, lateral midline tomogram, shows foramen magnum (black arrows) enlarged. Film taken with head slightly elevated shows narrow collapsed cord shadow (white arrows).

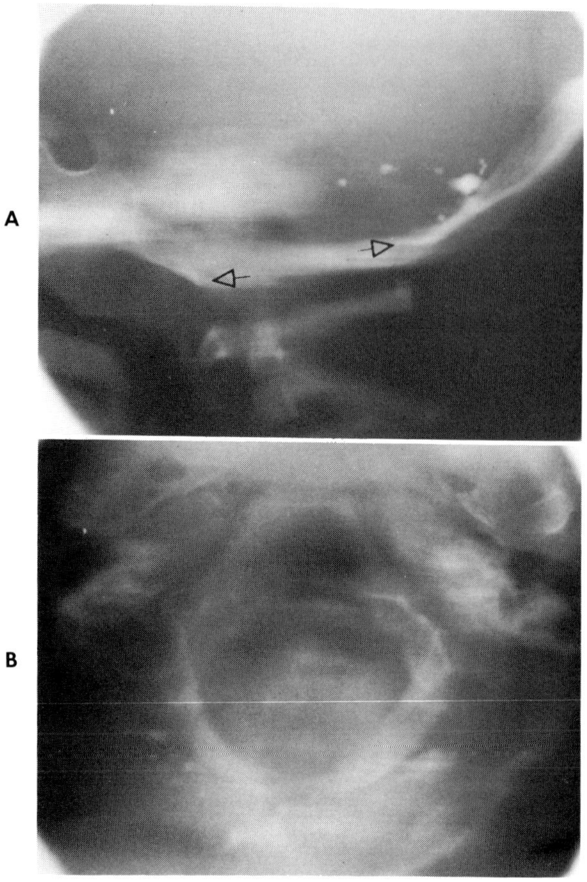

Fig. 15-21. Neurofibromatosis. **A,** Lateral midline tomogram shows foramen magnum (arrows) enlarged by neurofibroma extending through it. Upper cervical canal is also widened. **B,** Axial tomogram through level of first cervical vertebra shows expansion of cervical canal at this level.

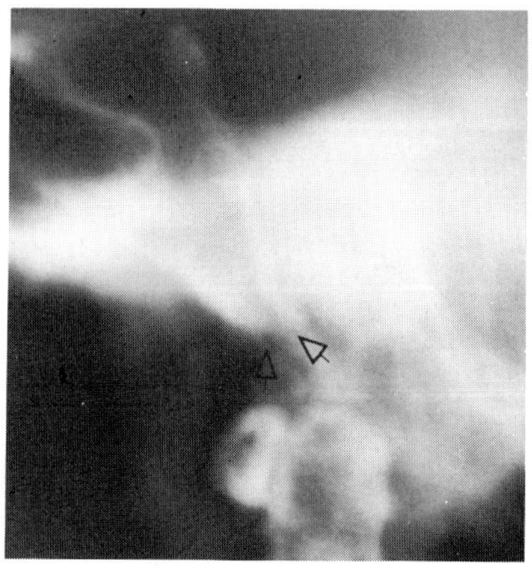

Fig. 15-22. Metastatic hypernephroma. Anterior rim of foramen magnum (inferior segment of clivus) has been destroyed (arrows).

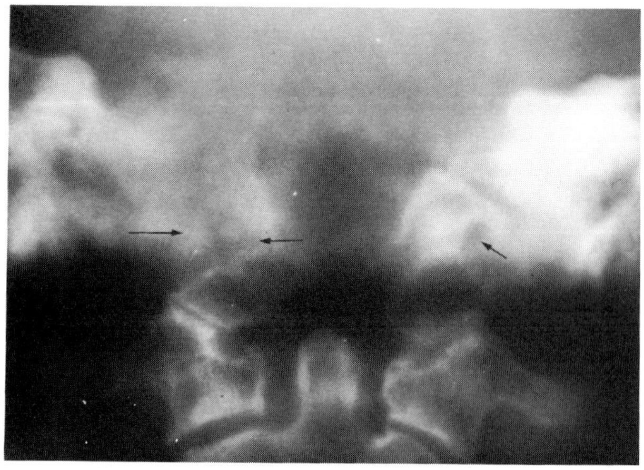

Fig. 15-23. Meningioma. Frontal tomogram shows destruction of right petrous bone, right occipital condyle, and right hypoglossal canal (horizontal arrows). Left hypoglossal canal (upward-pointing arrow) is normal. (From Valvassori, G. E., and Kirdani, M. A.: Amer. J. Roentgen. **99:**705-711, 1967.)

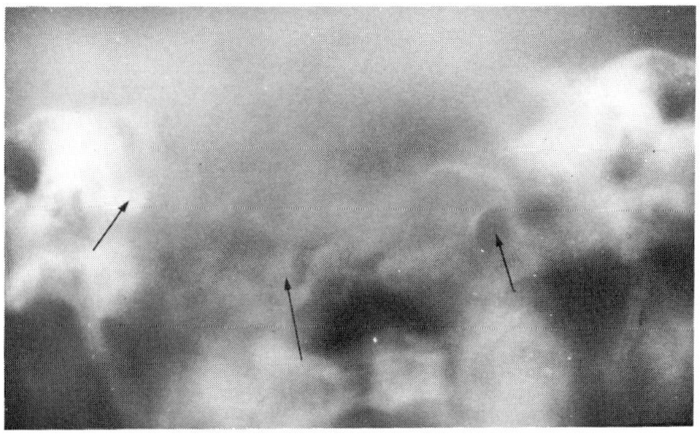

Fig. 15-24. Primary cholesteatoma. Frontal tomogram shows amputation of right petrous apex and destruction of right occipital condyle, including hypoglossal canal (arrows). Left side is normal. (From Valvassori, G. E., and Kirdani, M. A.: Amer. J. Roentgen. **99:**705-711, 1967.)

obliteration of one of the anterior synchondroses between the exoccipital and basioccipital bones had taken place. Premature obliteration of the anterior synchondrosis may interfere with the normal lateral and posterior migration of the occipital condyle. Asymmetry of these condyles causes the child to hold his head obliquely. The jugular tubercle on the affected side is usually flatter and asymmetric with respect to the contralateral side. The skulls observed by Kruyff were usually asymmetric without evidence of cerebral atrophy. Congenital heart disease was present in three of these patients. Hydrocephalus was present in one patient in whom adhesions were found at the level of the foramen magnum. None of the patients exhibited achondroplasia.

Other anomalies of the craniovertebral junction are discussed in Chapter 14.

Other causes

Endemic fluorosis (Figs. 34-2 and 34-3) and Paget's disease (Figs. 38-1 and 38-3) may cause sclerosis and narrowing of the foramen magnum.

Enlargement

Enlargement of the foramen magnum is usually a manifestation of chronic increased intracranial pressure (Di Chiro and Anderson, 1965). Enlargement may also be secondary to direct effects of an expanding process within the foramen magnum. Such enlargement is often seen in syringomyelia (Fig. 15-20) and in intramedullary and extramedullary tumors that straddle the foramen (Williams, 1969) (Fig. 15-21).

Erosion or sclerosis

Localized destruction of the foramen magnum usually indicates the presence of a neoplastic process; most commonly chordoma and metastatic malignancy (Fig. 15-

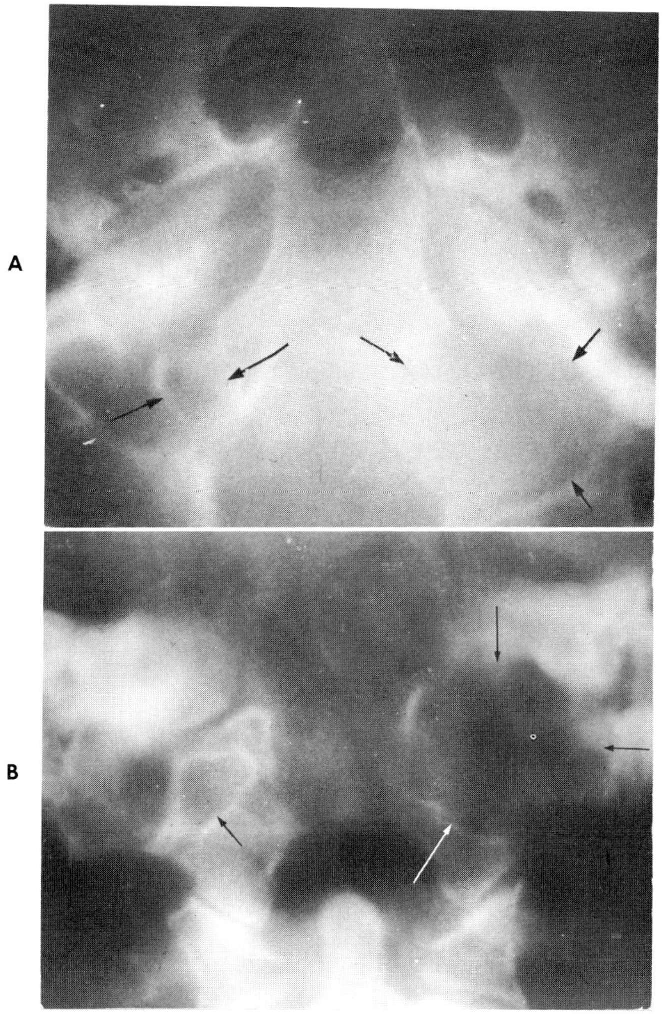

Fig. 15-25. Neurofibroma. **A,** Axial tomogram of skull shows enlargement of left and suggestive enlargement of right hypoglossal canals (arrows). **B,** Frontal tomogram shows marked expansion of left hypoglossal canal (arrows). Right canal appears moderately enlarged (arrow). (From Valvassori, G. E., and Kirdani, M. A.: Amer. J. Roentgen. **99:**705-711, 1967.)

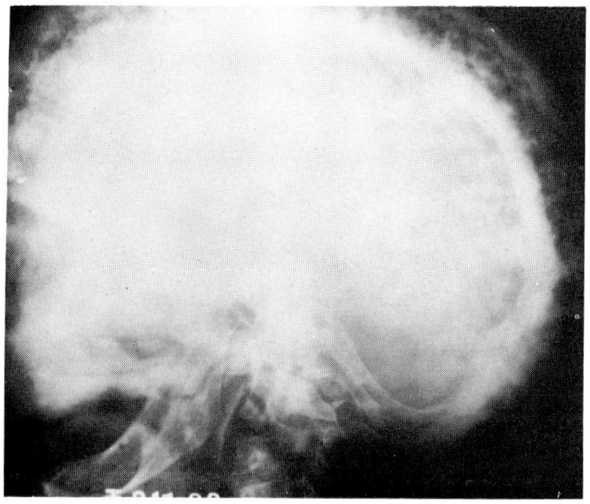

Fig. 15-26. Extensive Paget's disease of skull with basilar invagination. Foramen magnum is displaced superiorly by the marked basilar invagination.

22). The region of the anterior condyloid (hypoglossal) canal may be destroyed by a variety of lesions (Figs. 15-23 and 15-24). The canal may be expanded by a neurofibroma involving the hypoglossal nerve (Fig. 15-25).

Bony sclerosis about the foramen magnum has been observed in endemic fluorosis (Figs. 34-2 and 34-3), Paget's disease (Fig. 15-26), and osteopetrosis.

REFERENCES

Abbott, K.: Foramen magnum and high cervical cord lesions simulating degenerative disease of the nervous system, Ohio Med. J. **46**:645-651, 1950.

Blom, S., and Ekbom, K.: Early clinical signs of meningiomas of the foramen magnum, J. Neurosurg. **19**:661-664, 1962.

Bogorodinsky, D. K.: Syndrome of craniospinal tumor, Tashkent, 1936, Government Publication, U. S. S. R.

Caffey, J.: Achondroplasia. In Kelley, V. C., editor: Brennemann's practice of pediatrics, vol. 4, chap. 28, Hagerstown, Md., 1945, W. F. Prior Co., Inc.

Caffey, J., and Silverman, F. N.: Pediatric x-ray diagnosis, ed. 5, Chicago, 1967, Year Book Medical Publishers, Inc.

Cohen, L., and Macrae, D.: Tumors in the region of the foramen magnum, J. Neurosurg. **19**:462-469, 1962.

Cohen, M. E., Rosenthal, A. D., and Matson, D. D.: Neurological abnormalities in achondroplastic children, J. Pediat. **71**:367-376, 1967.

Craig, W. M., Brown, J. R., and Osborn, J. E.: Tumor of the foramen magnum, Neurology **6**:73-76, 1956.

Cushing, H., and Eisenhardt, L.: Meningiomas. Their classification, regional behaviour, life history, and surgical end results, Springfield, Ill., 1938, Charles C Thomas Publisher.

Di Chiro, G., and Anderson, W. B.: Clivus, Clin. Radiol. **16**:211-223, 1965.

Dodge, H., Love, J., and Gottlieb, C. M.: Benign tumors at the foramen magnum: surgical considerations, J. Neurosurg. **13**:603-617, 1956.

Dorst, J. P.: Functional craniology: an aid in interpreting roentgenograms of the skull, Radiol. Clin. N. Amer. **2**:347-367, 1964.

Fischer, E.: Neue Befunde am Vorderrand des Foramen occipitale magnum, Fortschr. Roentgenstr. **99**:805-808, 1963.

Gathier, J. C., and Bruyn, G. W.: The so-called condyloid foramen in the half axial view, Amer. J. Roentgen. **107**:515-519, 1969.

Gray, H.: Anatomy of the human body, C. M. Goss, editor, Philadelphia, 1967, Lea & Febiger.

Haas, L. L.: The posterior condylar fossa, foramen and canal, and the jugular foramen, Radiology **69**:546-552, 1957.

Kirdani, M. A.: The normal hypoglossal canal, Amer. J. Roentgen. **99**:700-704, 1967.

Kollmann, J.: Varianten am Os occipitale, besonders in der Umgebung des Foramen occipitale magnum, Anat. Anz. supp. 27, pp. 231-236, 1905.

Kruyff, E.: Occipital dysplasia in infancy, Radiology **85**:501-506, 1965.

Love, J. G., Thelen, E. P., and Dodge, H. W., Jr.: Tumors of the foramen magnum, London, 1954, International College of Surgeons.

Piehl, M. F., Reese, H. H., and Steelman, H. F.: The diagnostic problem of tumors at the foramen magnum, Dis. Nerv. Syst. **11**:67-76, 1950.

Schultz, A. H.: Ein paariger Knochen am Unterrand der Squama occipitalis, Anat. Rec. **12**:357-362, 1917.

Szalay, G. C.: Pseudohydrocephalus in dwarfs: the Russell dwarf, J. Pediat. **63**:622-633, 1963.

Valvassori, G. E., and Kirdani, M. A.: The abnormal hypoglossal canal, Amer. J. Roentgen. **99**:705-711, 1967.

Williams, B.: The distending force in the production of "communicating syringomyelia," Lancet **2**:189-193, 1969.

CHAPTER 16

Basal foramina and canals

Fred K. Sondheimer

FORAMEN ROTUNDUM (CANALIS ROTUNDUS, TROU GRAND ROND)

The foramen rotundum is neither a foramen nor always round. The designation of this structure has been alternating between foramen rotundum and canalis rotundus for at least 100 years. In Henle's classic anatomic text (1871) the structure was termed canalis rotundus (although in a footnote he amplified this to "foramen rotundum maxillary superior"). In 1895 the International Anatomical Nomenclature Committee designated the structure foramen rotundum. In 1935 the same committee changed the designation to canalis rotundus; and then in 1955 the same group reselected "foramen rotundum" (Leutert, 1963). The foramen rotundum is easily demonstrated as a short canal by basal tomography, and in this chapter the terms foramen and canal will both be used.

Gross anatomy

The foramen or canal is situated in the root of the greater wing of the sphenoid from 1 to 5 mm inferior to the superior orbital fissure and on the lateral aspect of the inferior margin of the fissure (Fig. 16-1). Its medial wall is commonly formed by the lateral wall of the sphenoid sinus (Figs. 16-2 and 16-3), although it may be separated from the sinus by a few millimeters. When there is a large lateral extension of the sphenoid sinus, the sinus wall also constitutes the inferior margin of the foramen (Fig. 16-4, *A*) or almost completely surrounds it (Fig. 16-4, *B*). The canal extends obliquely forward and slightly downward and connects the middle cranial and pterygopalatine fossae. It is directed laterally from posterior to anterior, at a variable angle, following the direction of the maxillary nerve (Fig. 16-3).

Measurements. Measurements of the canal obtained in twenty skulls disclosed an average lateral angulation of 8°, with a range of 3° to 20°. A medial angulation of 9° was noted in one of the foramina. In 25% of the

A

B

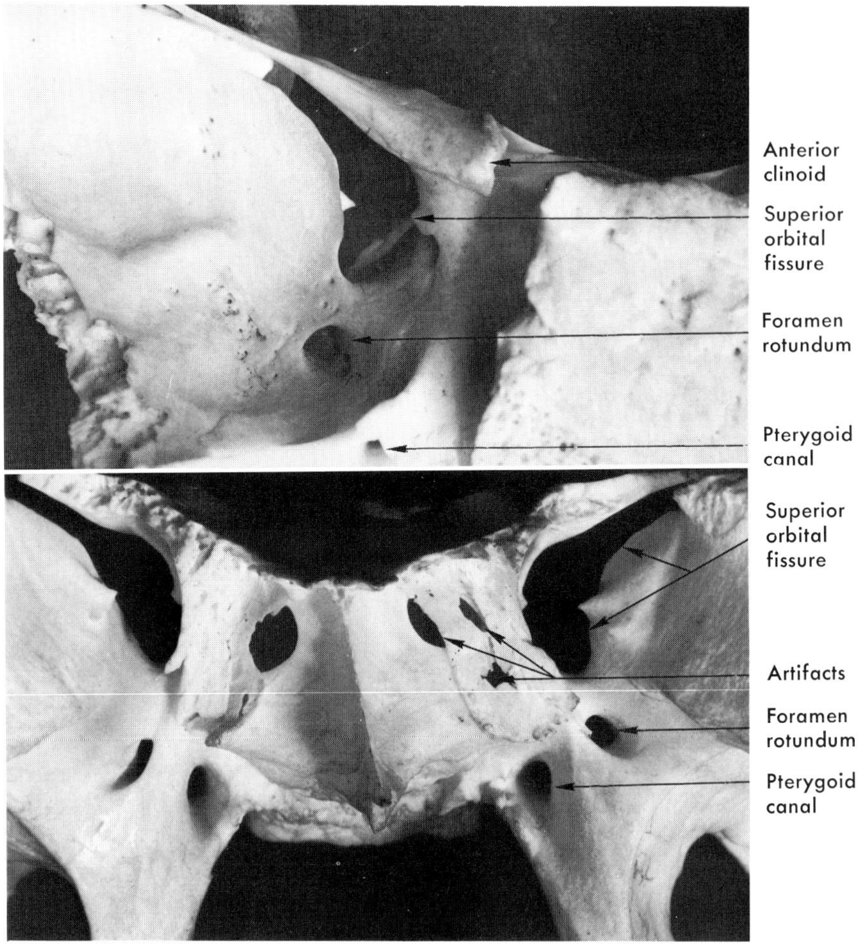

Fig. 16-1. Photographs of isolated sphenoid bone show, **A,** endocranial and, **B,** exocranial aspects of foramen rotundum and pterygoid canal. The foramen rotundum is situated at the inferolateral aspect of superior orbital fissure.

canals, the angle was less than 5° and in 25% it was more than 10°. The average length of the canal was 3.4 mm, with a range of 2 to 5 mm. The medial wall was slightly longer than the lateral. From the endocranial aspect the foramen is either round or oval; and when it is oval, the long axis is horizontal and corresponds to the curve of the greater wing of the sphenoid (Fig. 16-2, *A*). The average height noted was 2.9 mm, with a range of 2 to 4 mm, and the average width was 3.2 mm, with a range of 1.5 to 4 mm. The left side was the widest in fourteen of the fifteen specimens in which a difference was noted ($p = < 0.003$). The measurements of specimens obtained by Lindblom (1936) were 3×3 to 3.5×4 mm; and these correspond to ours.

Structures transmitted. The second division of the trigeminal nerve or *maxillary nerve* continues from its position in relation to the lateral wall of the cavernous sinus through the foramen into the pterygopalatine fossa. It is entirely sensory and supplies the skin in the middle third of the face, lower eyelid, and upper lip as well as the mucous membrane of the nasopharynx, maxillary sinus, upper gums, and teeth (Gray, 1959).

A few small *emissary veins* that connect the cavernous sinus to the pterygoid plexus sometimes pass through the canal (Gray, 1959); but according to Knott (1882) this is exceptional. Lindblom (1936) found veins in the foramen rotundum in only three specimens, and these had lumina that were "barely visible."

In Quain's case of congenital absence of the internal carotid artery cited by Fisher (1914), large branches of the internal maxillary artery entered the skull through the foramina rotundum and ovale, united in front of the trigeminal ganglion, and supplied the hemisphere.

Radiology

The *usually recommended projections* for the foramen rotundum are the Caldwell (Fig. 16-5) and Waters (Fig. 16-6, *A*) (Shapiro and Janzen, 1960) or

A

B

C

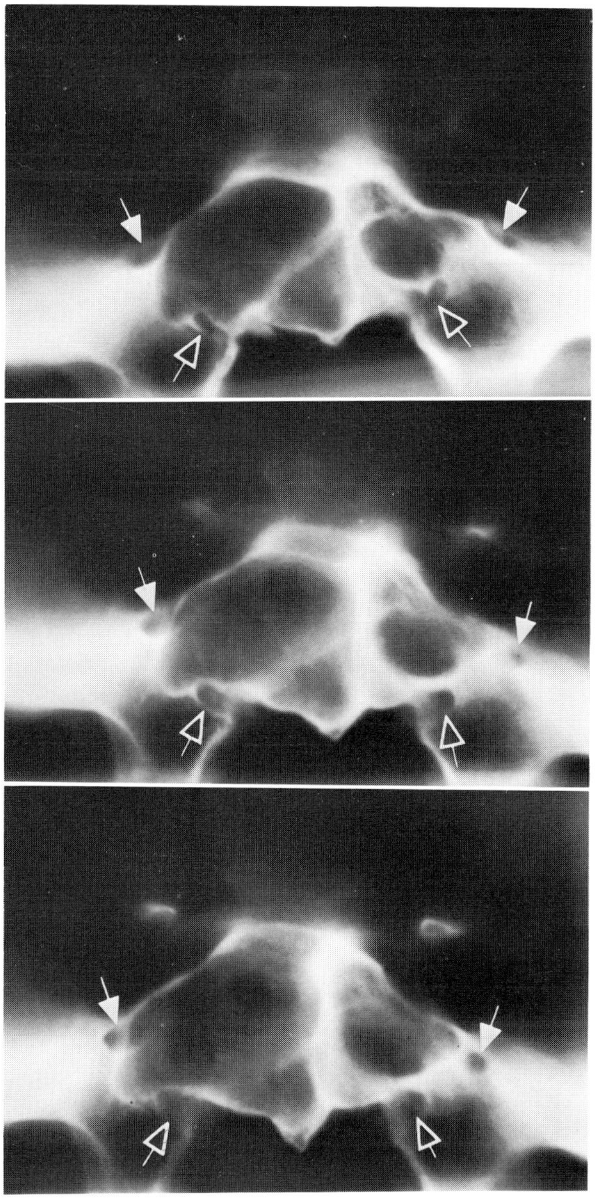

Fig. 16-2. Frontal tomograms of isolated sphenoid bone at 1 mm intervals demonstrate foramen rotundum (solid arrows) and pterygoid canal (open arrows). **A,** Most posterior plane, which corresponds to endocranial aspect. **C,** Most anterior plane, which corresponds to exocranial aspect. Note that the endocranial end (**A**) of the foramen rotundum may be oval and that the long axis of the foramen coincides with that of the greater wing of the sphenoid, which is directed upward at an angle of about 45°. In **B** and **C,** the foramen gradually assumes a rounder configuration. Sphenoid sinus frequently forms medial wall of foramen rotundum and superior wall of pterygoid canal, which is well demonstrated in these tomograms. Pterygoid canals are not seen in cross section because of their medial angulation. Posterior end of canal (**A**) is narrower than anterior end (**C**).

A

B

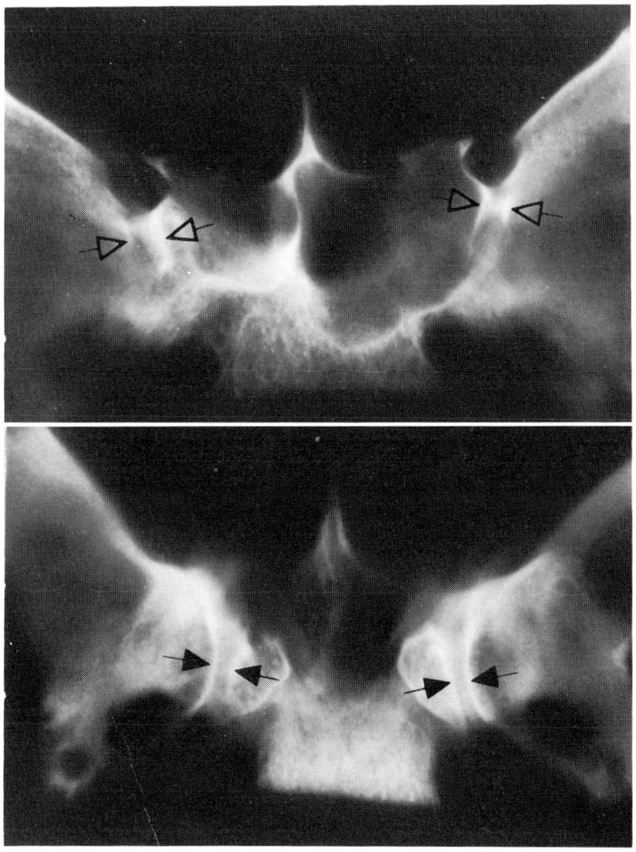

Fig. 16-3. A, Horizontal tomogram of isolated sphenoid bone shows that sphenoid sinus forms longer medial wall of foramen rotundum (arrows). Lateral angulation of foramen or short canal is also apparent. **B,** Horizontal tomogram through pterygoid canal (arrows) shows that canal is usually longer than foramen rotundum and is angled medially.

the modified Waters (Taveras and Wood, 1964). The modification suggested by the latter two authors was to decrease the angle of the orbitomeatal line from 37° to 25° (Fig. 16-6, *B*). This change may frequently be accomplished by placing the patient's nose and chin on the table, without angulation of the tube (Taveras and Wood, 1964). With this view the foramen is projected into the upper third of the maxillary antrum, relatively free of overlying shadows. This projection is the same as that described by Schaaf (1957), although he employed fluroscopy to attain the desired position of the head.

These standard projections will demonstrate the foramen rotundum if the angle of the foramen with the midsagittal plane is small or if the foramen is parallel to that plane (Figs. 16-5 and 16-6). Demonstration of the canal in these instances with posteroanterior projections is possible probably because of beam divergence.

A *new projection* has been devised for the demonstration of the foramen in those instances when the

A

B

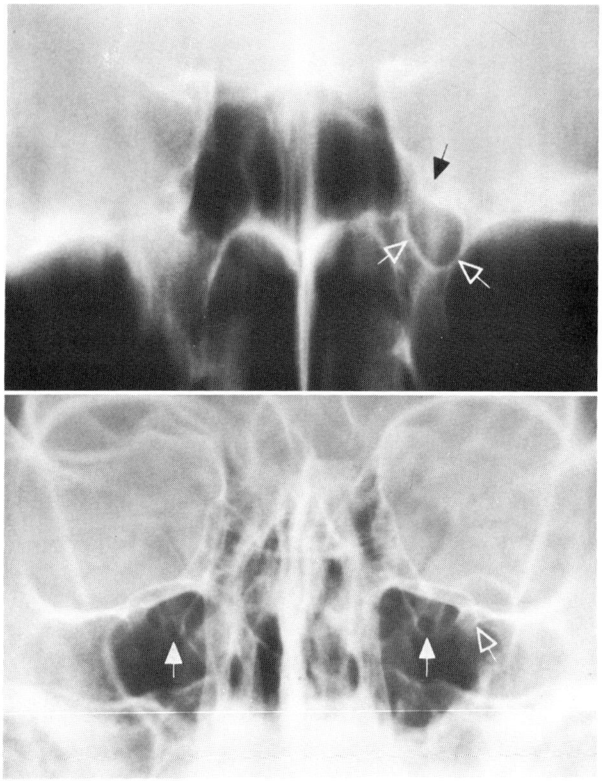

Fig. 16-4. A, Frontal tomogram at level of foramen rotundum reveals that a large extension of sphenoid sinus (open arrows) forms inferior margin of the foramen rotundum (solid arrow). **B,** Foramen rotundum (solid arrows) is almost entirely surrounded by lateral extensions of sphenoid sinus. Inferior orbital canal (open arrow) is identified for comparison.

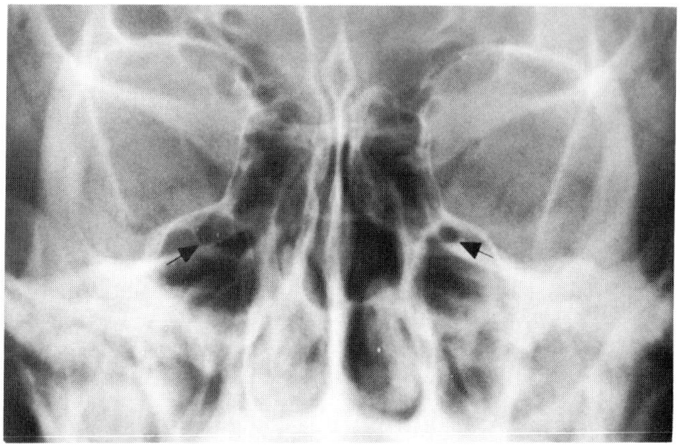

Fig. 16-5. When lateral angulation of foramen (arrows) is small, foramen is well seen in standard Caldwell projection.

A

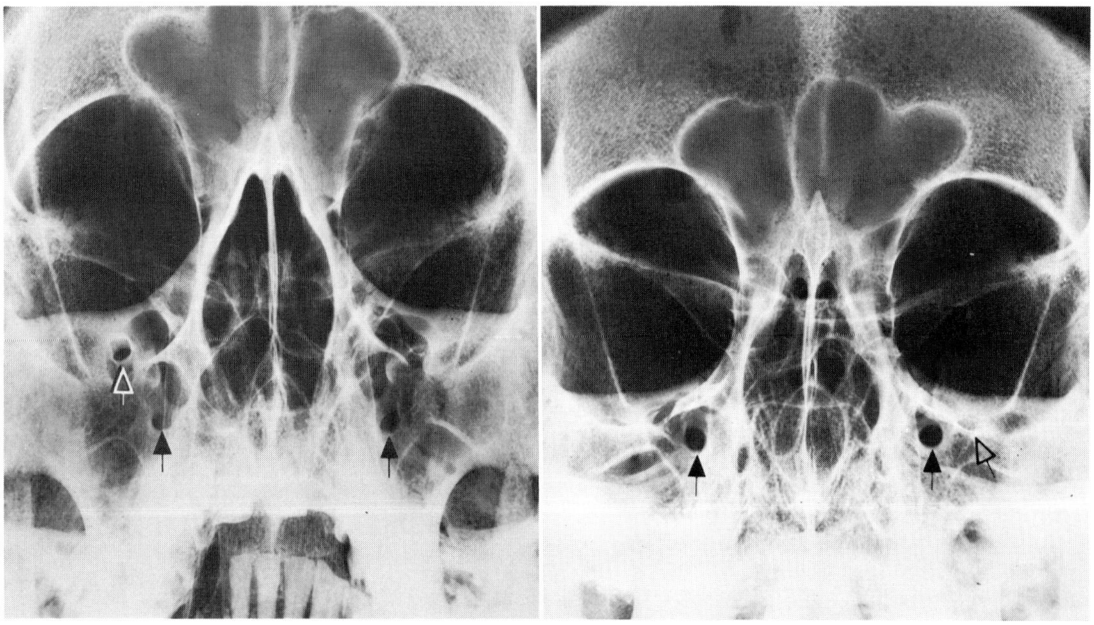

B

Fig. 16-6. A, Standard and, **B,** modified Waters projections of dry skull. **A,** In usual Waters view, the foramen rotundum (solid arrows) is seen below superior orbital fissure in the inferomedial aspect of the maxillary antrum. It should not be confused with inferior orbital foramen (open arrow). **B,** When tube is angled 25°, the foramen rotundum (solid arrows) is more easily visualized in upper third of maxillary antrum and can be distinguished from inferior orbital foramen (open arrow).

standard Caldwell view is not successful (Figs. 16-7 and 16-8). With the patient in the posteroanterior position and the tube angled about 20° for the Caldwell projection, the head is rotated approximately 10° to the contralateral side. The beam exits through the inferior margin of the orbit. This position will provide an axial projection of the canal into the inferomedial aspect of the orbit, just medial to the petrous tip (Figs. 16-7, *B,* and 16-8). Occasionally large lateral extensions of the sphenoid sinuses provide shadows that are easily confused with the foramen rotundum (Fig. 16-8).

An incidental finding has been that the cortical margins of the superior orbital fissure are better demonstrated with this slightly oblique projection than with the standard Caldwell view (Fig. 16-8). Therefore this "foramen rotundum view" is advised when questions of erosion or widening of the superior orbital fissure arise. Although angulation of the head for examination of the superior orbital fissure has been suggested previously (Kornblum and Kennedy, 1942; Gayral and Paintandre, 1952), the projection is infrequently used (Shapiro and Robinson, 1967b). Gayral and Paintandre (1952) were aware that the foramen rotundum could be seen in the inferior orbit with the projection they devised. The patient was prone with the head rotated 15° to the contralateral side and the anthropologic base line perpendicular to the film.

If the modified Caldwell view fails to demonstrate the foramen, anteroposterior tomography permits excellent definition of the cortical margins of this structure (Fig. 16-9). Tomography in the submentovertical position demonstrates the length of the canal (Fig. 16-3, *A*) in a plane about 1 cm superior to the one in which the other middle fossa foramina are contained. On frontal and basal tomograms the foramen rotundum may be distinguished from the pterygoid or Vidian canal (p. 323) by the more medial position and the smaller diameter, greater length, and medial angulation of the canal (Figs. 16-2 and 16-3).

Roentgenographic measurements of the foramen pub-

A

B

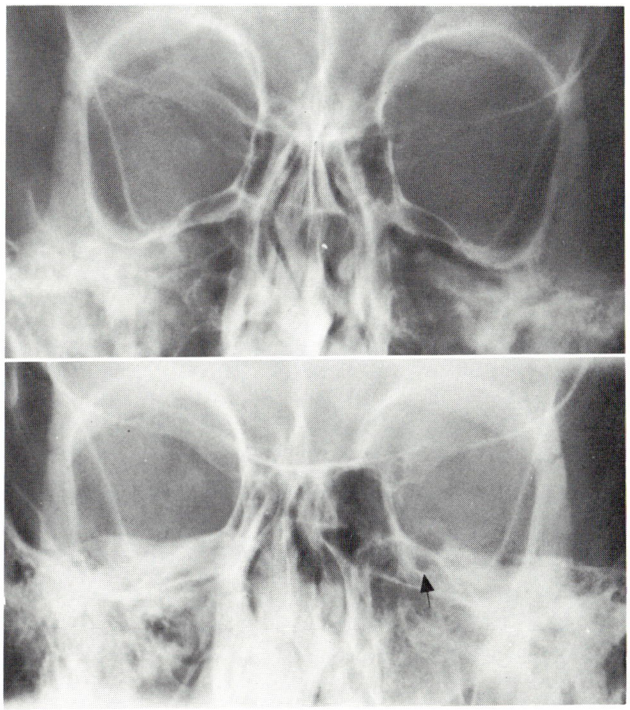

Fig. 16-7. Modified Caldwell or foramen rotundum view. **A,** Foramen rotundum is not visible in standard Caldwell projection. **B,** When head is rotated approximately 10° to contralateral side, axial view of foramen rotundum (arrow) is obtained.

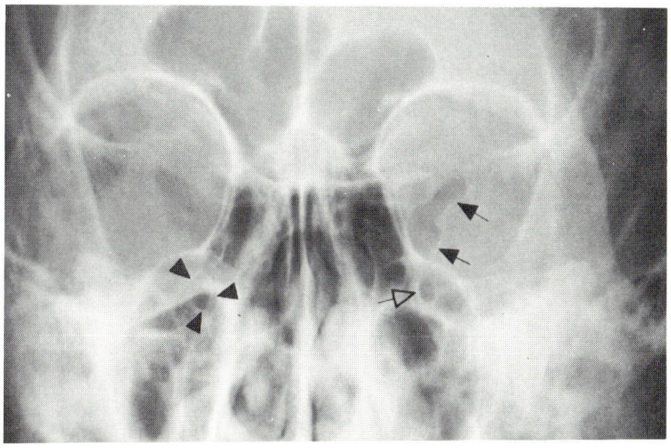

Fig. 16-8. Foramen rotundum view clearly demonstrates the foramen (open arrow), which could not be visualized in standard Caldwell projection. Cortical margin of greater wing of sphenoid (solid arrows) is also better seen than in standard Caldwell view. Lateral extensions of sphenoid sinus (arrowheads) are sometimes difficult to distinguish from the foramen rotundum.

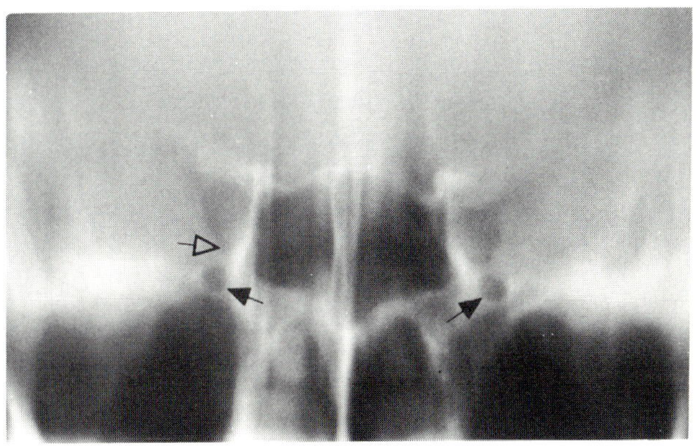

Fig. 16-9. Frontal tomogram shows relation of superior orbital fissure (open arrow) to foramen rotundum (solid arrows).

lished by Lindblom (1936) were 3 × 3 to 4 × 5 mm; and those found by Schaaf (1957) for its largest diameter averaged 3.8 mm, with a range of 2.7 to 4.8 mm.

A
B
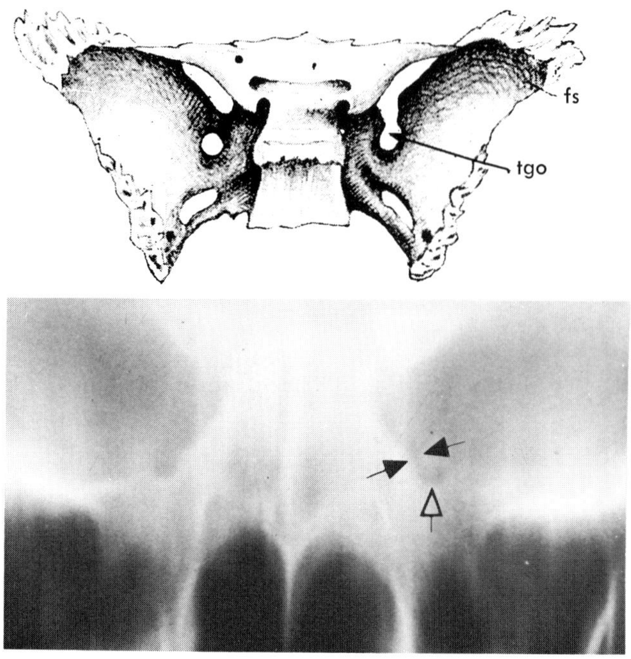

Fig. 16-10. A, Drawing from LeDouble (1903) demonstrates no separation between superior orbital fissure (*fs*) and foramen rotundum (*tgo*)—a foramen lacerum anterius—on the right. **B,** Foramen lacerum anterius, 9-year-old child. No separation exists (solid arrows) between superior orbital fissure and foramen rotundum (open arrow). (**A** from Shapiro, R., and Robinson, F.: Amer. J. Roentgen **101**:779-794, 1967.)

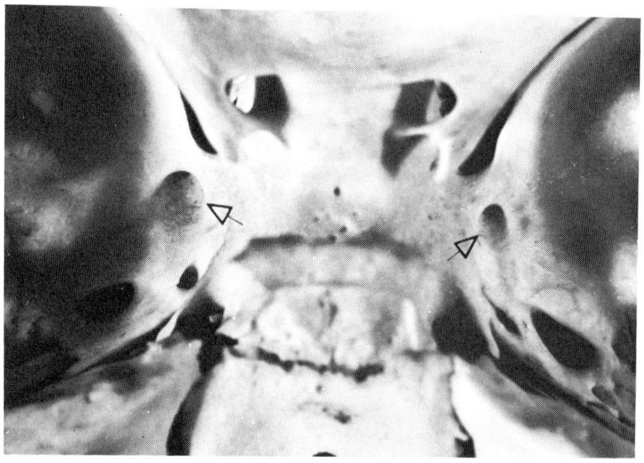

Fig. 16-11. Gross asymmetry of foramina rotunda (arrows) in skull of child. (From Shapiro, R., and Robinson, F.: Amer. J. Roentgen. **101**:779-794, 1967.)

Embryology and congenital anomalies

The *foramen lacerum anterius* is the hiatus between the orbitosphenoid (precursor of the lesser wing of the sphenoid) and the alisphenoid (precursor of the greater wing of the sphenoid). This opening has its counterpart in other mammals and is the superior orbital or sphenoid fissure in man (de Beer, 1937; Shapiro and Robinson, 1967a).

The foramen rotundum is formed when a bony spur extends from the chondral root of the greater wing to the body of the sphenoid and separates the foramen from the remainder of the sphenoid fissure. The foramen is thus entirely cartilaginous in origin (de Beer, 1937).

The foramen lacerum anterius persists in some mammals—carnivores, rodents, and ruminants. This condition may also occur in man, although it is quite uncommon (Fig. 16-10). In the normal human embryo the foramen rotundum is completely separated from the superior orbital fissure by the twelfth to sixteenth week (Shapiro and Robinson, 1967b).

Gross congenital asymmetry of the foramina is relatively infrequent (Fig. 16-11). The examination of twenty skulls disclosed inequality in the dimensions of the foramina on the two sides of more than 1 mm in only two specimens. One was 1.5 and the other 2.0 mm larger than its homologue on the opposite side. Taveras and Wood (1964) described a patient in whom symptoms compatible with a unilateral maxillary nerve tumor were associated with enlargement of the foramen rotundum on that side. Surgical exploration revealed no tumor, and the asymmetry of the two foramina was considered to be a congenital anomaly.

A small (1 to 3 mm) opening in the inferomedial wall of the foramen rotundum (Fig. 16-12, *A*) was discovered in five of fifty skulls (10%); in one specimen it was bilateral. A needle placed in this "foramen within a foramen" ended in the pterygoid process (Fig. 16-12, *B* and *C*). To our knowledge this small foramen has not been previously described and its function is not known. It may provide passage for an emissary vein from the cavernous sinus into the diploic space of the pterygoid, since anatomic studies have demonstrated that the sphenoid emissary foramen (p. 321) may end in bone.

Orbital dysplasia in *neurofibromatosis* unassociated with an actual neurofibroma was first detailed by Le Wald (1933). Since then it has been thoroughly reviewed by many authors (Peyton and Simmons, 1946; Goetsch, 1955; Meinardus, 1958; Burrows, 1963; Davidson, 1966; Tänzer, 1966). None of these, however, has noted the occasional absence of the foramen rotundum in association with the defects in the sphenoid wings, although the absence is apparent in some of their illustrations. The foramen is absent when the

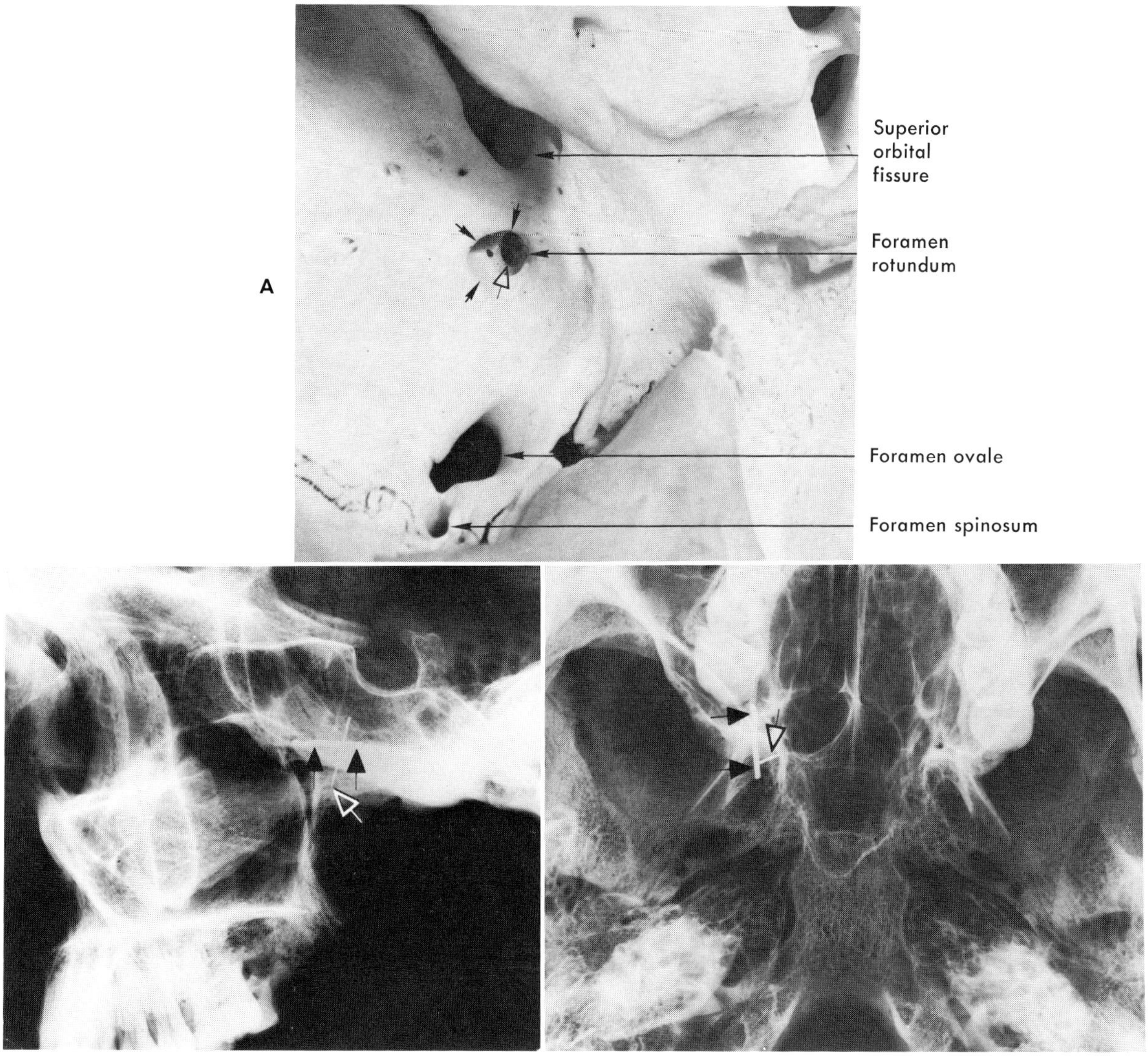

Fig. 16-12. Small foramen or canal extending downward from foramen rotundum. **A,** Photograph of dry skull demonstrates several foramina (open arrow) in medial wall of foramen rotundum. Roentgenograms of this specimen in lateral, **B,** and submentovertical, **C,** projections after large pin (solid arrows) had been placed in foramen rotundum and small pin (open arrow) had been inserted into foramen in medial wall of foramen rotundum. Small pin is seen to end in the root of the pterygoid process.

anteroinferior aspect of the greater wing is missing (Fig. 16-13, *A*) or in the rare instances of complete aplasia of the greater wing (Peyton and Simmons, 1946; Tänzer, 1966). A foramen may be seen, however, despite considerable enlargement of the superior orbital fissure, with this abnormality (Fig. 16-13, *B*).

Pathology

Enlargement. Pathologic enlargement of the foramen rotundum is rare and may be difficult to distinguish from congenital asymmetry in the absence of cortical erosion.

A *neurofibroma of the maxillary nerve* in a case of generalized neurofibromatosis reported by Tänzer (1966) resulted in massive enlargement of the foramen rotundum with a sclerotic margin. In reviewing the skull changes in neurofibromatosis, Meinardus (1958) noted enlargement of the foramen rotundum in some cases but did not cite the cause.

Raised intracranial pressure may enlarge foramina that do not contain extensions of the subarachnoid space (p. 311). Effacement of the margins of the foramen rotundum was associated with advanced skull changes

A

B

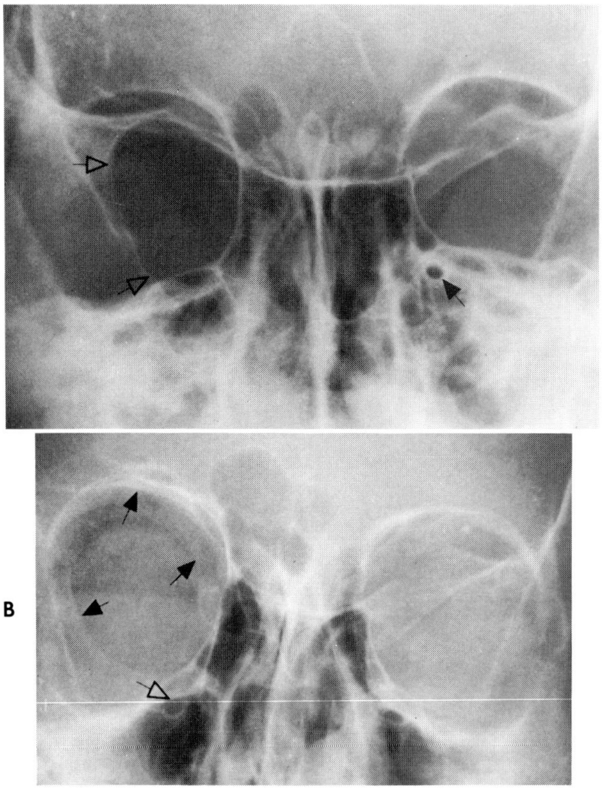

Fig. 16-13. Foramen rotundum in neurofibromatosis. **A,** Large defect in greater wing of sphenoid (open arrows) with absent foramen rotundum on the right. Foramen is normal on the left (solid arrow). **B,** Typical defect in greater and lesser sphenoid wings (solid arrows) but with intact foramen rotundum (open arrow).

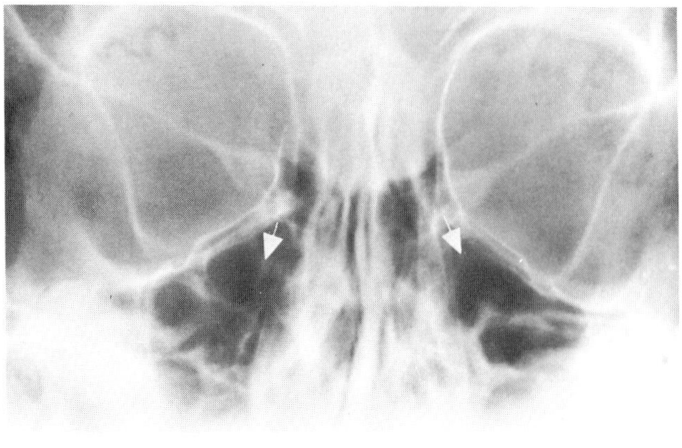

Fig. 16-14. Foramen rotundum is not visible bilaterally (arrows) in a case of long-standing raised intracranial pressure. Pronounced generalized skull changes included thinning of cortical margins of anterior clinoids and lesser wings.

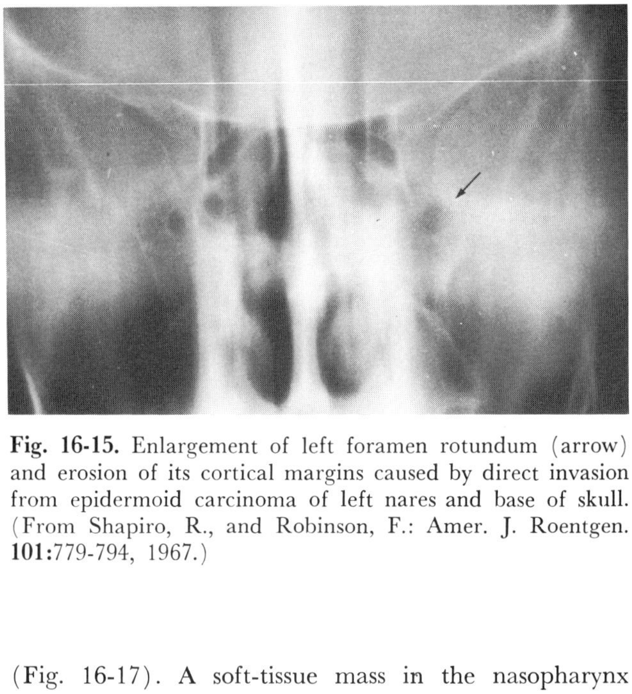

Fig. 16-15. Enlargement of left foramen rotundum (arrow) and erosion of its cortical margins caused by direct invasion from epidermoid carcinoma of left nares and base of skull. (From Shapiro, R., and Robinson, F.: Amer. J. Roentgen. **101**:779-794, 1967.)

of raised intracranial pressure in a young girl. In this patient the foramen of Monro was obstructed by a septal glioma (Fig. 16-14).

Enlargement is also possible by extension of *meningiomas* of the middle fossa, which may cause erosion of bone by infiltration, or by direct extension of *nasopharyngeal tumors* through the foramen (Shapiro and Robinson, 1967a) (Fig. 16-15). Holman and Miller (1965) noted enlargement of the foramen rotundum with demineralization of its rim in two of eighteen juvenile *nasopharyngeal fibromas*. In these fibromas associated enlargement of the superior orbital fissure, as well as anterior bowing of the posterior wall of the maxillary antrum, is diagnostic (Holman and Miller, 1965).

Destruction. The most common cause of destruction of the foramen rotundum is *metastatic tumor*. The destruction may be the result of a hematogenous metastasis (Fig. 16-16) or the direct extension of a *nasopharyngeal tumor* (Figs. 16-15 and 16-17). Nasopharyngeal tumors not only produce erosive changes (Miller et al., 1969) but can also result in sclerosis of the base (Fig. 16-17). A soft-tissue mass in the nasopharynx should suggest the diagnosis of these tumors.

The effect of *intracavernous aneurysms* of the internal carotid artery or carotid cavernous fistulae on the superior orbital fissure has been well reviewed recently (Shapiro and Robinson, 1967b). It is also described in Chapter 22. Briefly the inferior aspect of the superior orbital fissure is widened; and the inferolateral wall of the optic canal and the anterior clinoid process are both eroded. These findings associated with a calcific rim are diagnostic of an aneurysm in the anterior aspect of the cavernous sinus. When these aneurysms become large, they may also erode the foramen rotundum (Fig. 16-18), a fact not

A

B

C

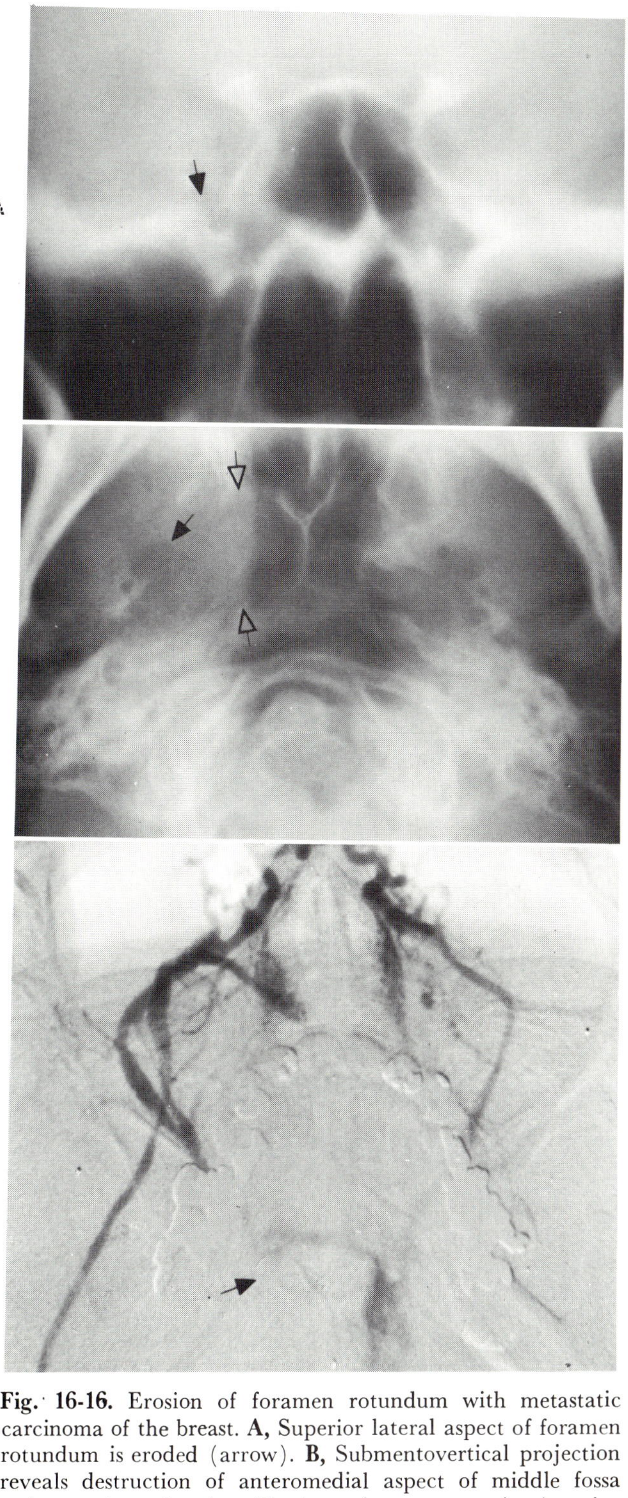

Fig. 16-16. Erosion of foramen rotundum with metastatic carcinoma of the breast. **A,** Superior lateral aspect of foramen rotundum is eroded (arrow). **B,** Submentovertical projection reveals destruction of anteromedial aspect of middle fossa and margins of sphenoid sinus (open arrows). Anterior margin of foramen ovale (solid arrow) is eroded, whereas medial margin is intact. **C,** Orbital venogram demonstrates occlusion of right cavernous sinus (arrow).

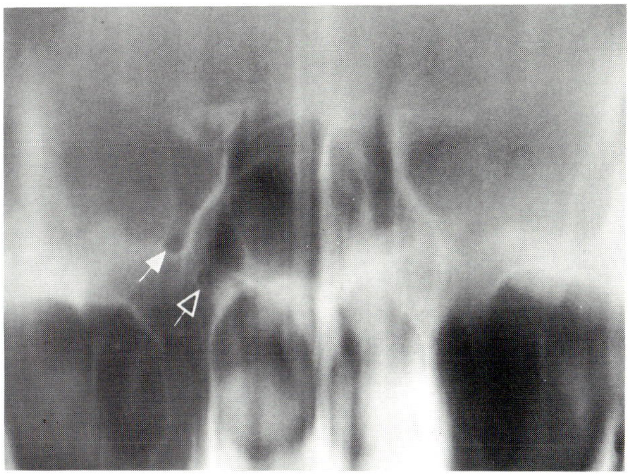

Fig. 16-17. Foramen rotundum (solid arrow) and pterygoid canal (open arrow) are normal on the right. On the left, they have been destroyed by undifferentiated nasopharyngeal carcinoma, which has caused sclerotic reaction in this case.

indicated by previous authors (Sosman and Vogt, 1926; McKinney et al., 1936; Jefferson, 1938; Rischbieth and Bull, 1958; Lombardi et al., 1963). An illustration of such a case, however, has been published (Fischgold et al., 1952).

Since one wall of the foramen rotundum is frequently formed by the sphenoid sinus (Figs. 16-2 and 16-3), erosion of the foramen by sphenoid sinus mucoceles might be expected. Associated erosion of the floor of the sella turcica, clouding of the sinuses, and widening of the superior orbital fissure are helpful in the diagnosis (Lombardi et al., 1963; Nugent et al., 1970).

Although pituitary and orbital tumors, chondromas, reticuloendotheliosis, and space-occupying lesions of the middle fossa produce widening of the superior orbital fissure, erosion of the adjacent foramen rotundum has not been reported. Destruction of the foramen has, however, been depicted in a chondroma of the sphenoid (Fischgold et al., 1952) and in a trigeminal neurinoma (Holman et al., 1961) (Fig. 16-19).

Narrowing and sclerosis. Sclerosis and narrowing of the foramen rotundum in osteopetrosis and fibrous dysplasia have been described by Shapiro and Robinson (1967a) in their comprehensive article on the middle fossa foramina. Sclerosis without narrowing may take place in fibrous dysplasia (Fig. 16-20) and sphenoid sinus mucoceles (Fig. 16-21). Paget's disease, sphenoid wing meningiomas, and thalassemia major have produced narrowing of the superior orbital fissure (Shapiro and Robinson, 1967b), but I have not seen such narrowing in the adjacent foramen rotundum.

Trauma. Fractures that involve the anterior and middle fossae may pass through the foramen rotundum (Schaaf, 1957).

A

B

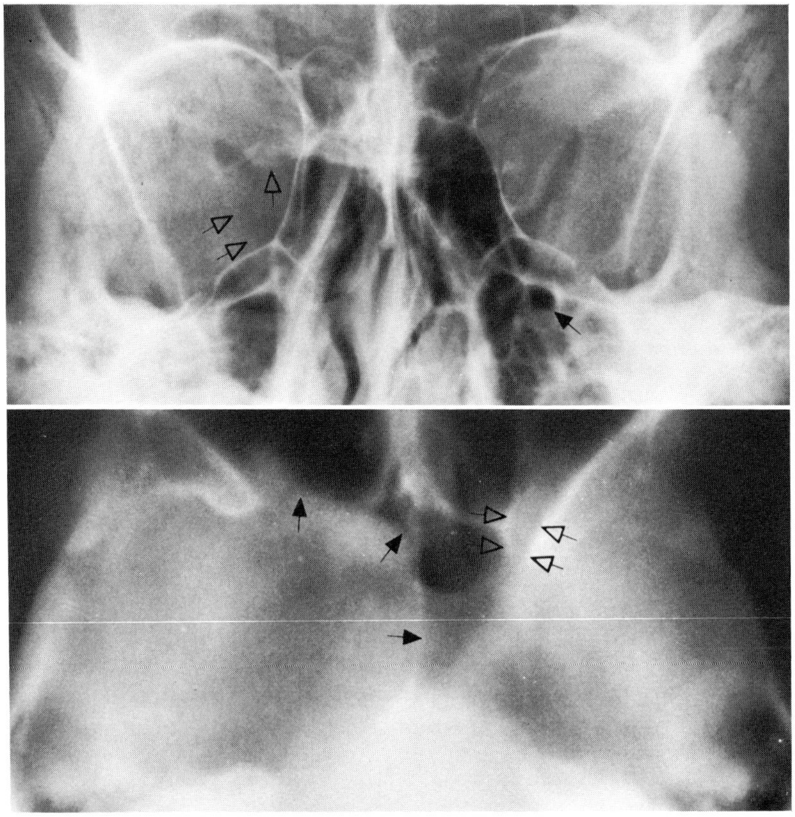

Fig. 16-18. Large intracavernous aneurysm of right internal carotid artery. **A,** Foramen rotundum is normal on the left (solid arrow) but destroyed on the right. Note the undercutting of the right anterior clinoid (single open arrow) and the widening of the superior orbital fissure (double open arrows). **B,** Submentovertical tomogram reveals normal left foramen rotundum (open arrows). Foramen rotundum on the right is destroyed by aneurysm that has almost completely replaced right sphenoid sinus (solid arrows).

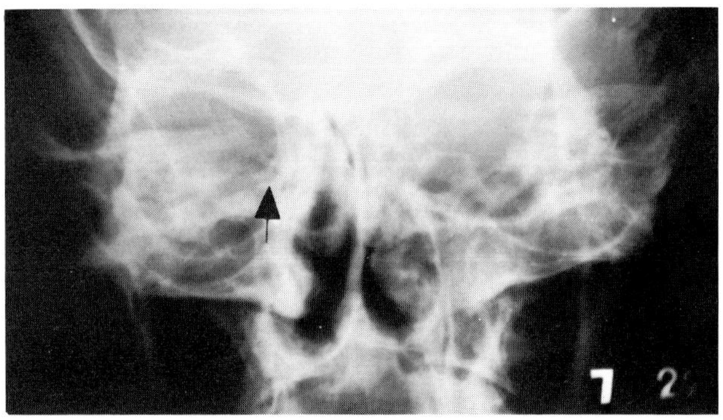

Fig. 16-19. Trigeminal neurinoma with amputation of petrous apex, and erosion of left greater and lesser sphenoid wings. Left foramen rotundum is also destroyed; that on the right (arrow) is normal. (From Holman, C. B., Olive, I., and Svien, H. J.: Amer. J. Roentgen. **86:**148-153, 1961.)

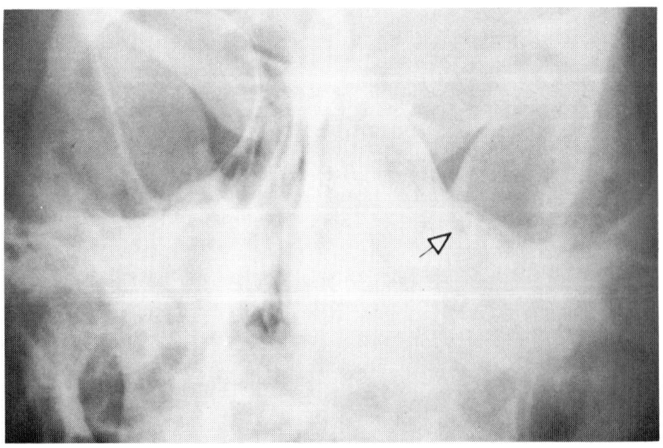

Fig. 16-20. Extensive fibrous dysplasia of facial bones with sclerosis of left foramen rotundum (arrow) and superior orbital fissure. (Courtesy Arthur T. Gronner, M.D., Lafayette, Calif.)

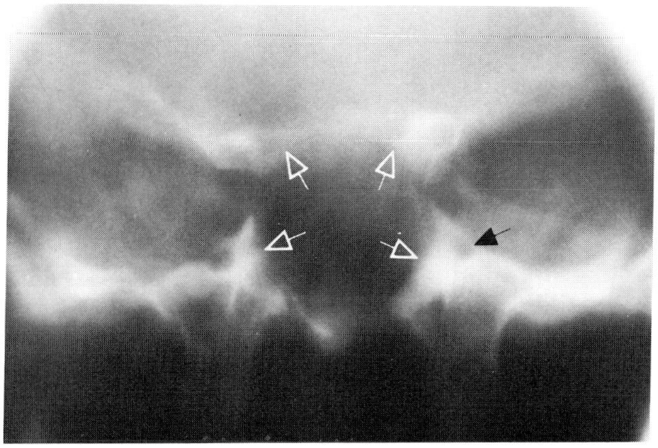

Fig. 16-21. Tomogram, frontal projection, shows mucocele of sphenoid sinus (open arrows) with sclerosis of wall of sphenoid sinus and left foramen rotundum (solid arrow).

FORAMEN OVALE

Gross anatomy

The foramen ovale is situated in the medial aspect of the greater wing of the sphenoid and connects the posteromedial aspect of the middle fossa with the infratemporal fossa. From the exocranial aspect the foramen is found at the base of the lateral pterygoid plate, anteromedial to the sphenoid spine (spina angularis) and foramen spinosum (Fig. 16-22). From the endocranial aspect it is about 1 to 1.5 cm posterolateral to the posterior border of the foramen rotundum (Fig. 16-23). The axis of the foramen ovale corresponds to that of the trigeminal nerve. It extends downward anteriorly and laterally from the petrous apex to this foramen and then follows the course of the third division of the trigeminal nerve. If this line were continued, the exit point on the cheek would be between the maxillary tuberosity (immediately behind the last molar) and the ascending ramus of the mandible. The distance from the cheek to the foramen ovale is about 6 cm (Härtel, 1921).

The size and shape of the foramen ovale vary considerably. Lindblom (1936) found that the variability in size is not related to age or to the thickness or character of the surrounding bone. He noted an inverse relationship between the size of the foramina spinosum and ovale. This relationship has also been mentioned by other authors (Greig, 1929; Shapiro and Janzen, 1960), but it was not confirmed by our measurements of roentgenograms. Variations in the size of the accessory meningeal artery would not be expected to influence materially the diameter of the foramen ovale since the artery occupies only a fraction of the area of the foramen.

Measurements. Lindblom's (1936) measurements of the foramen in skulls averaged 4 × 7 mm, with a minimum of 3 × 6 and a maximum of 4 × 10 mm. These compared well with roentgenographic measurements, when magnification of 13% was considered. The measurements of the foramen by Radoïévitch and his collaborators (1956) in 300 specimens averaged 3 to 4 × 4 to 8 mm, with a range of 1 to 6 × 5 to 10 mm.

Structures transmitted. The largest structure traversing the foramen ovale is the *mandibular nerve,* the third division of the trigeminal. It is both sensory and motor, representing the entire motor root of the trigeminal. The motor fibers supply the muscles of mastication and several other smaller muscles. The sensory fibers supply the skin of the temporal region and lower part of the face and lips, the lower teeth and gums, the mandible and temporomandibular joints, and a portion of the dura. On leaving the skull through the foramen ovale, the motor root of the nerve lies medial to the sensory root, and the two are separated by a fibrous band known as the pterygospinous ligament. The roots unite just outside the skull and are here in proximity to the otic ganglion (Gray, 1959).

The cross-sectional dimension of the mandibular nerve is quite constant (14 mm^2). Therefore the major factors in the determination of variability of size and shape of the foramen ovale are the presence and number of *veins* that pass through it (Wood-Jones, 1931; Lindblom, 1936; Henderson, 1966). These venous communications connect the cavernous sinus with the pterygoid plexus and impart the characteristic oval shape to the foramen. Henderson (1965, 1966) showed that these structures, formerly considered to be veins (Wood-Jones, 1931; Lindblom, 1936), are actually dural sinuses. Histologically they consist of a wall of dura with an endothelial lining. By injections of colored alcohol into the foramen ovale, Henderson was always able to demonstrate an 8 to 12 mm long *ovale emissary sinus,* whose lumen varied from 2 to 5 mm. In the foramen the sinus was always situated on the anteromedial aspect of the mandibular nerve (Fig. 16-24), and occasionally it caused a groove on the medial edge of the foramen (Henderson, 1965). The sinus left the skull through the foramen of Vesalius (p. 321) in only one of the 100 specimens studied by Henderson (1966). He expressed the belief that, because of its constant position, the sinus is of clinical importance in regard to injections of the gasserian ganglion. When alcohol was injected into the sinus, a strictly peripheral nerve distribution of sensory loss in the first two divisions was produced. No instances of related thrombosis of the cavernous sinus were noted (Henderson, 1965).

When present, the *accessory meningeal branch* of the internal maxillary artery enters the skull through the posterolateral portion of the foramen ovale. This artery

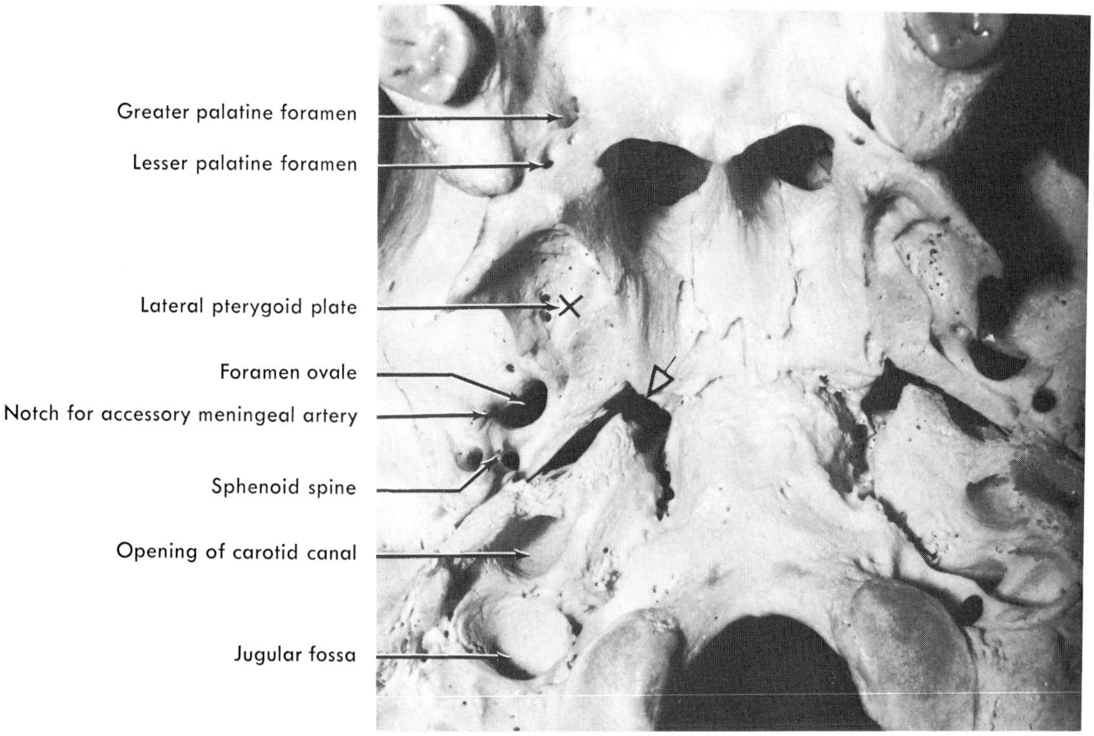

Fig. 16-22. Photograph of inferior aspect of skull demonstrates relation of foramen ovale to base of lateral pterygoid plate and sphenoid spine. In this specimen the bar that separates foramen ovale from foramen lacerum (arrow) is quite thick. Small notch for accessory meningeal artery is present on posterolateral aspect of foramen ovale. Sphenoid spine is situated between "duplicate" foramina spinosa.

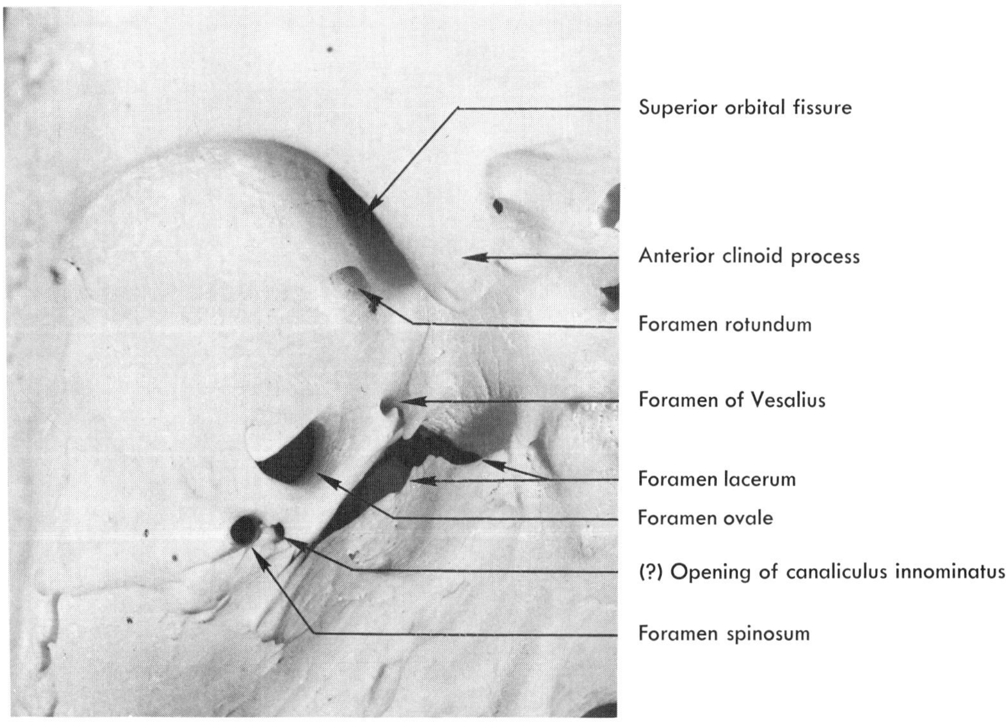

Fig. 16-23. Photograph of floor of middle fossa of skull shows relation of foramen ovale to foramina of middle fossa. Foramen of Vesalius is present, and its separation from the foramen ovale is somewhat greater than usual.

A

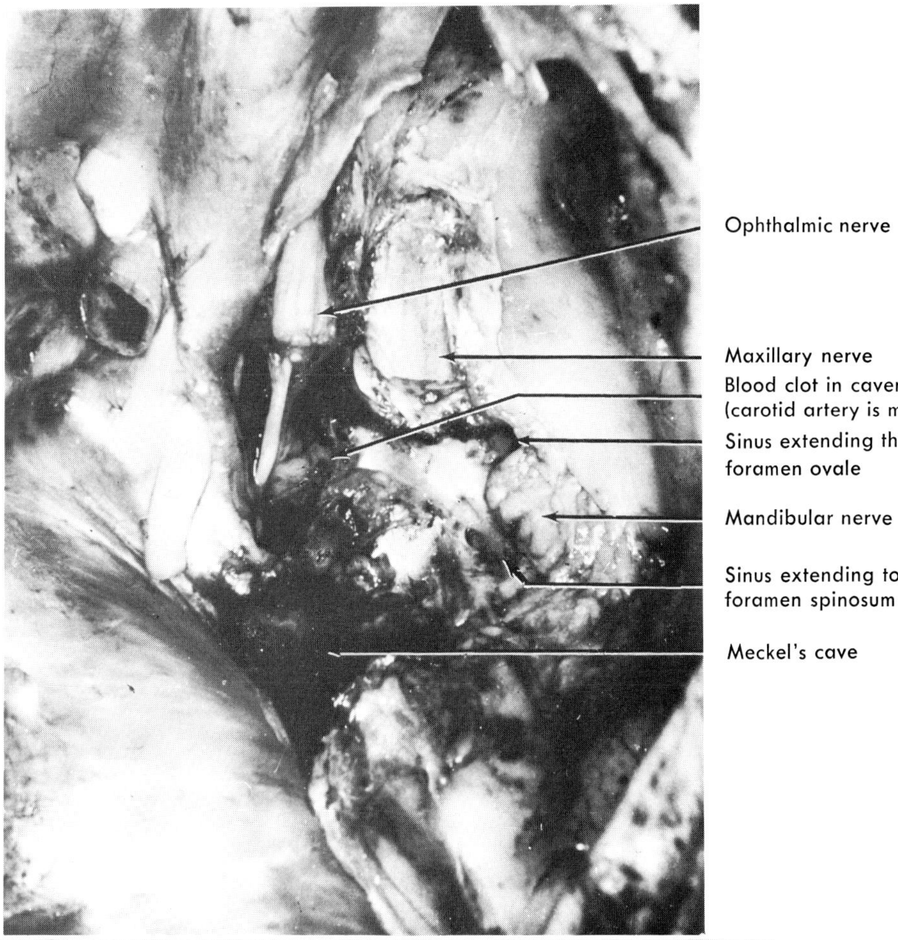

B

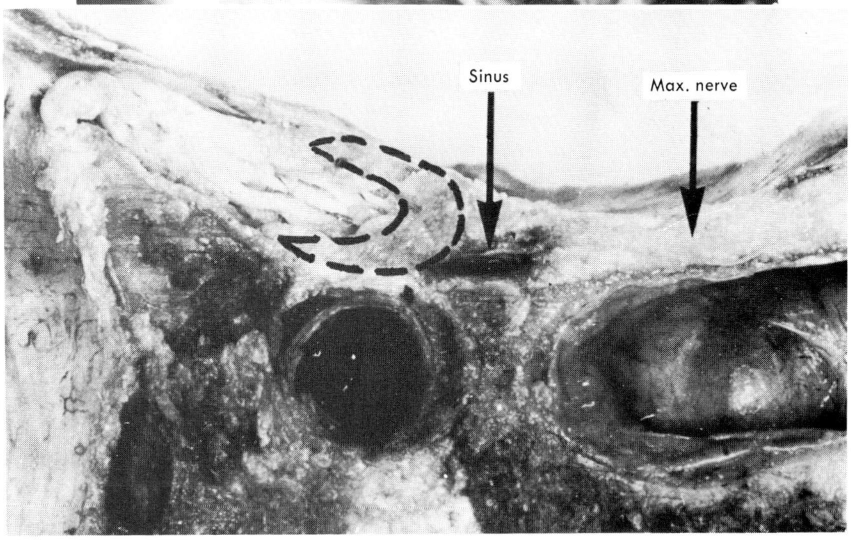

Fig. 16-24. A, Right middle fossa after injection of alcohol into Meckel's cave and removal of gasserian ganglion. Floor of wide unstained sinus, lying transversely under maxillary nerve, contains thin blood clot along its anterior wall, between foramen ovale and cavernous sinus. Branch of this sinus continues below cut end of mandibular nerve toward foramen spinosum. **B,** Vertical section through petrous bone shows emissary venous sinus under junction of maxillary nerve and ganglion (outlined). (From Henderson, W. R.: J. Anat. **100:**905-908, 1966.)

A

B

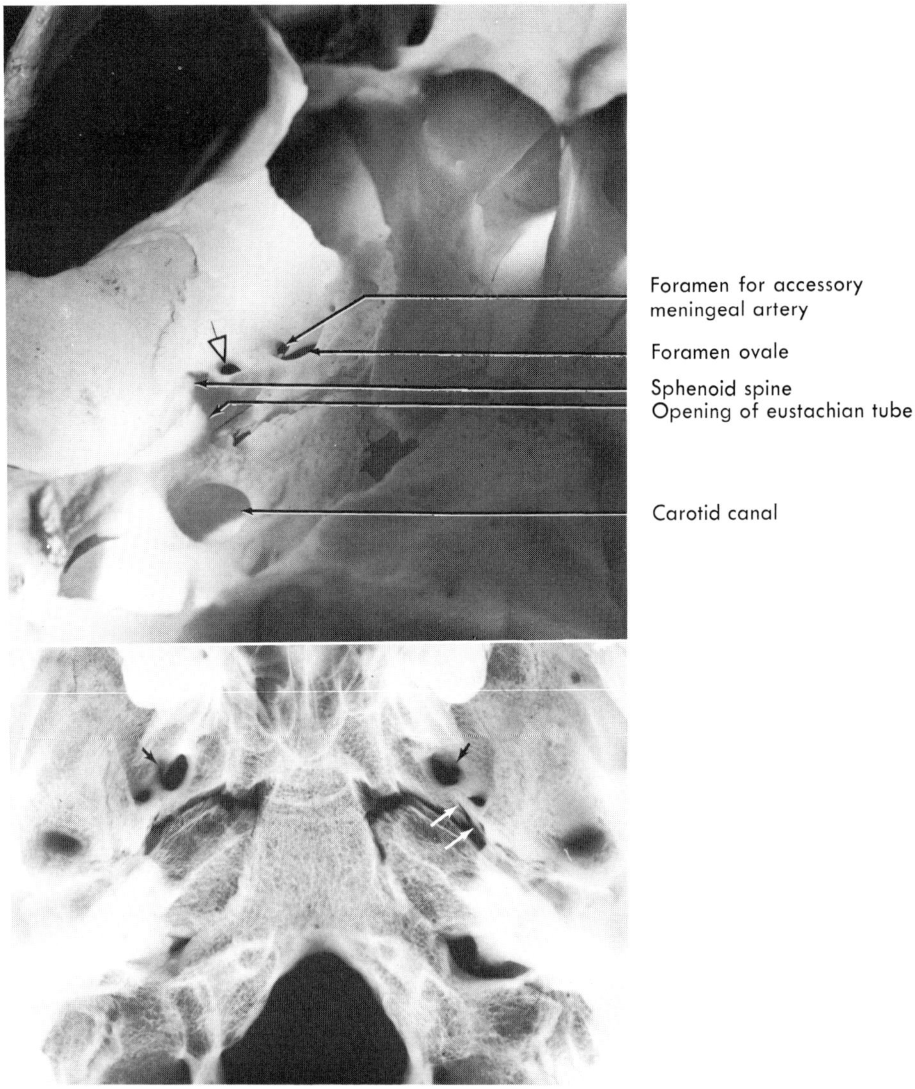

Fig. 16-25. A, Photograph of inferior aspect of base of skull shows separate foramen for accessory meningeal artery in posterolateral aspect of foramen ovale. Relation of osseous portion of eustachian tube and carotid canal may also be appreciated. Foramen spinosum is indicated by open arrow. **B,** Roentgenogram of this specimen demonstrates separate foramina for accessory meningeal artery (black arrows) on both sides. Canaliculus innominatus (white arrows) is present on the left.

supplies the gasserian ganglion and a portion of the dura. Occasionally there may be a separate foramen or slit for the artery on the lateral aspect of the foramen ovale (Fig. 16-25). Lindblom (1936) did not find that arterial grooves lead from this foramen. A groove extending anterolaterally from the posterolateral aspect of the foramen ovale, however, was found in association with a small foramen spinosum (Fig. 16-26).

Middle meningeal veins also occasionally pass through the foramen (Knott, 1882; Lindblom, 1936; Henderson, 1966) and, if so, occupy a posterior position in it.

The *lesser superficial petrosal nerve* leaves the skull through the posterior aspect of the foramen ovale when the canaliculus innominatus (p. 322) is not present.

Radiology

The foramen ovale is commonly examined in the submentovertical projection (Fig. 16-27, *A*), as originally described by Schüller (1905) and popularized by Hirtz (1922). Because the foramen is slanted downward and anteriorly, however, an axial view is obtained with a 10° to 13° caudad angulation of the central ray (Fig. 16-27, *B* and *C*). On a review of basal roentgenograms,

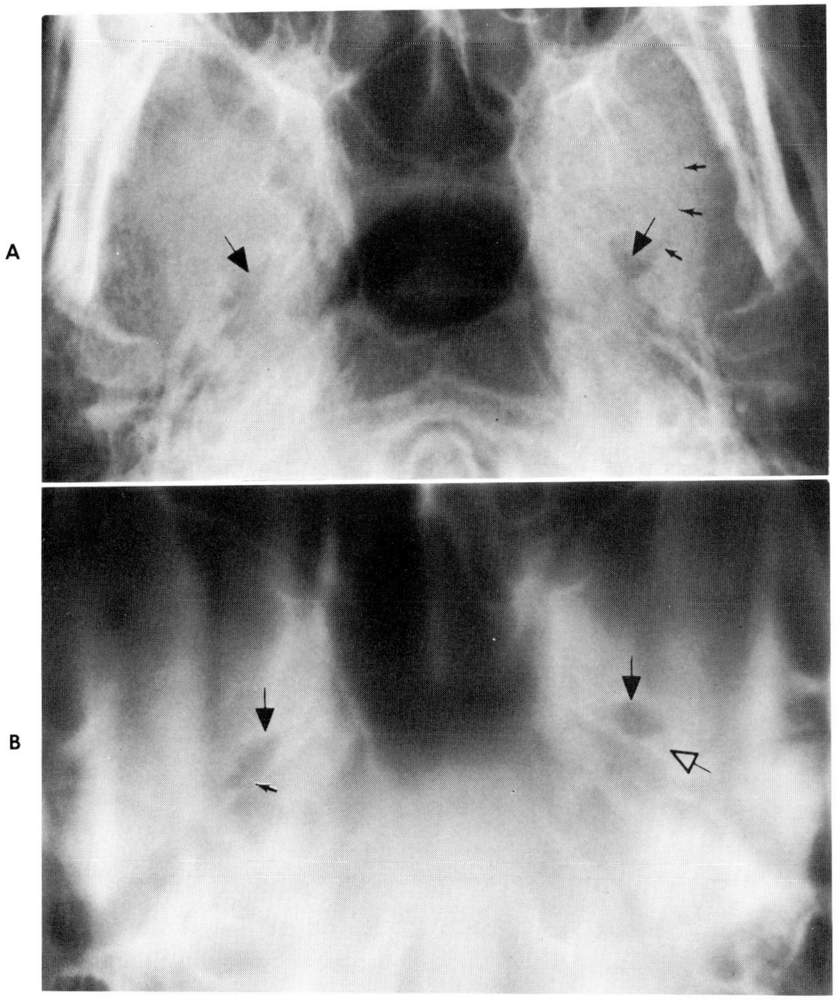

Fig. 16-26. A, Basal view of skull does not permit adequate visualization of either foramen ovale (large arrows). On left, foramen spinosum appears to be absent. A groove leads to posterior edge of foramen ovale (small arrows). Accessory meningeal artery apparently provided a large portion of the dural arterial supply. **B,** Basal tomogram clearly demonstrates foramen ovale bilaterally (solid arrows) and a tiny left foramen spinosum (open arrow). Separation of foramina spinosum and ovale on right by thin bony ridge is evident only with tomography. Canaliculus innominatus (small solid arrow) is present on right.

the cortical margins of the foramina ovale and spinosum were more clearly apparent on those views in which the angle was 75° to 80°; that is, the inferior edge of the mandible projected just anterior to the foramina (Figs. 16-27, *C,* and 16-28).

Basal tomography permits still better definition. Tomograms obtained in the plane passing through the external auditory meatus and 0.5 cm superior and inferior to it nearly always demonstrate the formina ovale and spinosum (Fig. 16-26, *B*). The foramen ovale can also be seen on frontal (Fig. 16-29) and lateral tomograms (Fig. 16-30), on which its margins appear surprisingly thick. In 20% of the 600 foramina examined by Radoïévitch and his co-workers (1956), the height of the foramen ovale was at least 0.5 cm and the term small canal was therefore applied to these foramina.

Measurements of the foramen ovale from submentovertical views by Lindblom (1936) averaged 5 × 8.5 mm and varied from a minimum of 3 × 5.5 to a maximum of 7 × 11 mm. Orley's (1949) measurements of the foramen from roentgenograms ranged from 5 to 11 mm for the length and from 2 to 7.5 mm for the width.

The foramen ovale was measured on fifty unselected submentovertical projections obtained with a focal spot–film distance of 40 inches. The canthomeatal line was not always parallel to the film, which can influence the diameter by as much as 30% (Fig. 16-27). The longest and widest diameters were recorded. The range

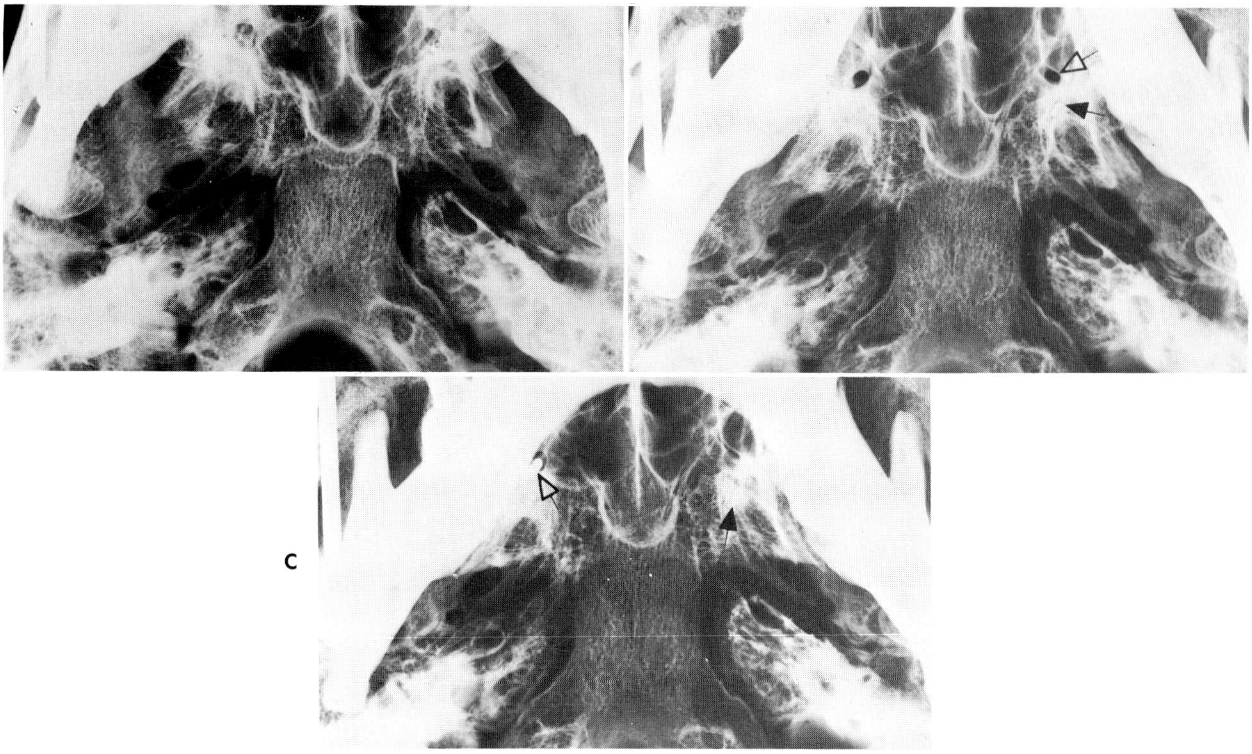

Fig. 16-27. Submentovertical roentgenograms of dry skull demonstrate effect of different tube angles on size and visibility of middle fossa foramina. As caudad angle increases, foramen ovale becomes larger and its margins are more distinct. When tube is perpendicular to canthomeatal line, **A,** foramen ovale is 3 mm wide and its cortical margins are indistinct. With 10° caudad angulation of tube, **B,** foramina are slightly larger and cortical margins are seen more clearly. In **C,** caudad angle is approximately 13°. Width of foramen ovale is now 4 mm. In **B** and **C,** there are pins in lesser (solid arrow) and greater (open arrow) palatine foramina.

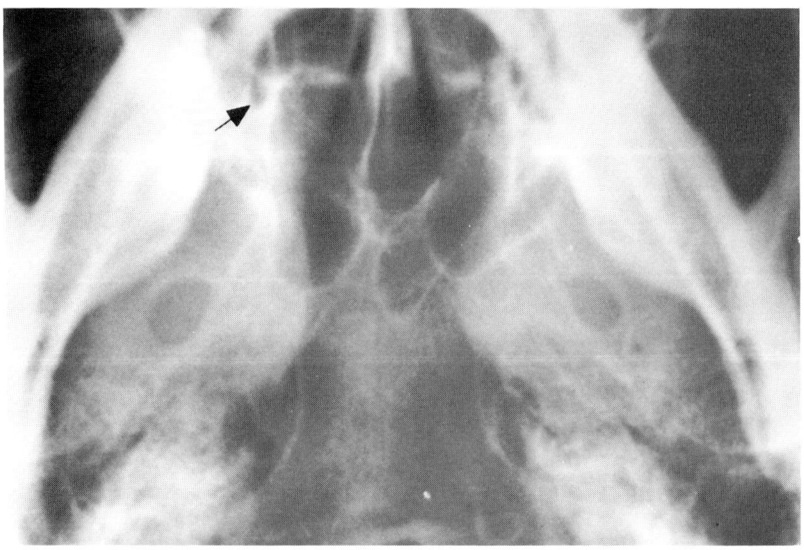

Fig. 16-28. Basal view of skull obtained with caudad angulation of central ray. Cortical margins of foramen ovale are well visualized. Foramen spinosum is small bilaterally. Greater palatine foramen (arrow) is also seen.

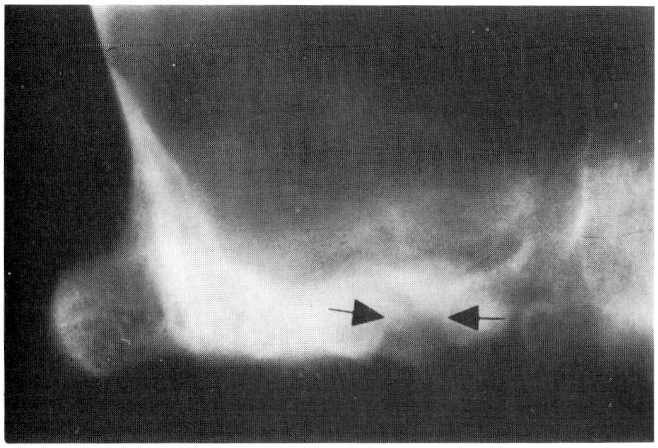

Fig. 16-29. Frontal tomogram of dry skull demonstrates tomographic appearance of foramen ovale (arrows) and thickness of middle fossa around it.

was somewhat greater than that noted by Lindblom and Orley, but the average of 5 × 9.5 mm compares closely with the measurements by Lindblom. The width varied from 3 to 10 mm, and the length from 6 to 14 mm. The smallest foramen was 3 × 7, and the largest 8 × 14 mm. The foramina did not differ by more than 4 mm in any dimension; and this discrepancy was observed only four times. The foramina were otherwise symmetric, with a difference of less than 2 mm in 80%.

Härtel (1921) devised a true axial view that conformed to the downward and anterolateral course of the trigeminal nerve and orientation of the foramen. With the patient prone, the head extended, and the affected cheek next to the film, the central ray entered 4 cm above the lambda, 2 cm from the midline toward the opposite side. It exited through the open mouth in the region of the upper second molar, projecting the foramen ovale between the zygoma, the coronoid process, and the maxillary antrum (Härtel, 1921). Brücke (1934) modified this view by examination of the patient with the mouth closed in the sitting or supine positions (Fig. 16-31). This view was more in keeping with the purpose of the projection (i.e., in preparation for percutaneous gasserian ganglion blocks). Perl and Ecker (1963) have further modified the projection for these injections. The patient lies on his back with the canthomeatal line at an angle of 65° to the vertical and the head rotated 15° to the healthy side. With the submentovertical projection the exact depth of penetration of the needle into the foramen ovale may be appreciated. For selective injection of the mandibular or maxillary branches, the angles of the midsagittal and orbitomeatal lines are altered (Ecker and Perl, 1969). These authors reported a 95% success rate in the treatment of tic douloureux with their method of alcohol injections under roentgenographic control.

A

B

C

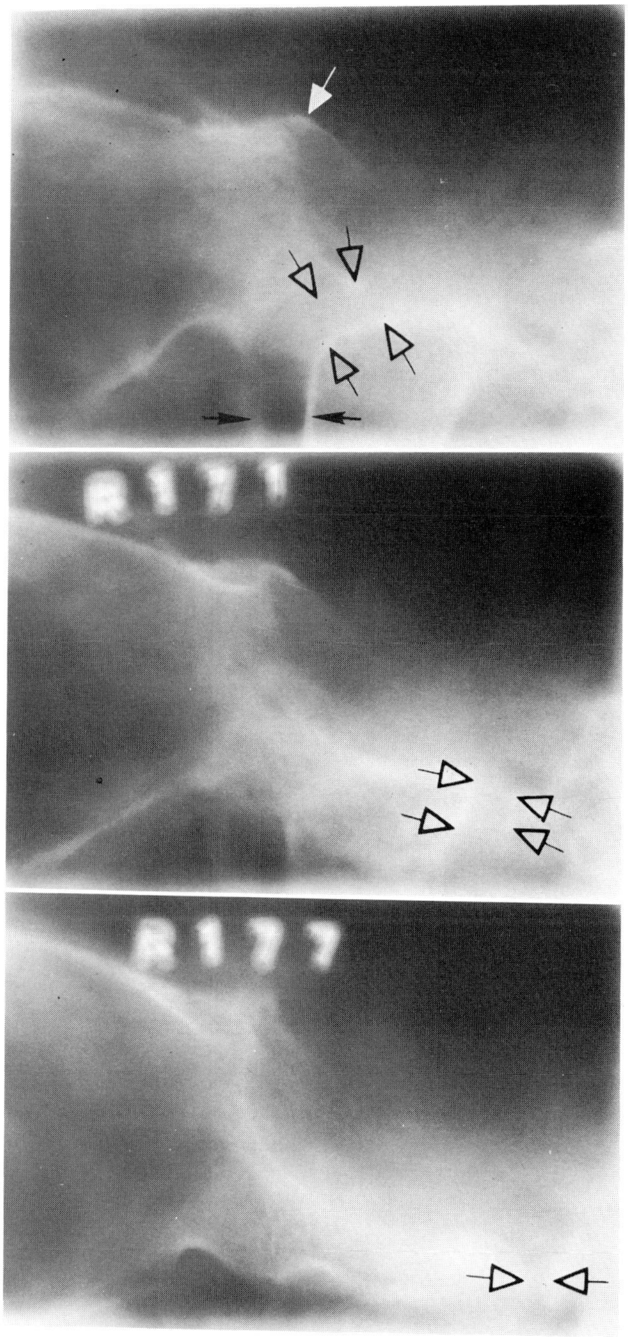

Fig. 16-30. Lateral tomograms of dry skull. **A,** Foramen rotundum (open arrows) extends forward horizontally into pterygopalatine fossa (black arrows) at level of anterior clinoid (white arrow). **B,** Foramen ovale (open arrows) is a few millimeters lateral. **C,** Six millimeters more laterally, foramen spinosum (open arrows) is visualized.

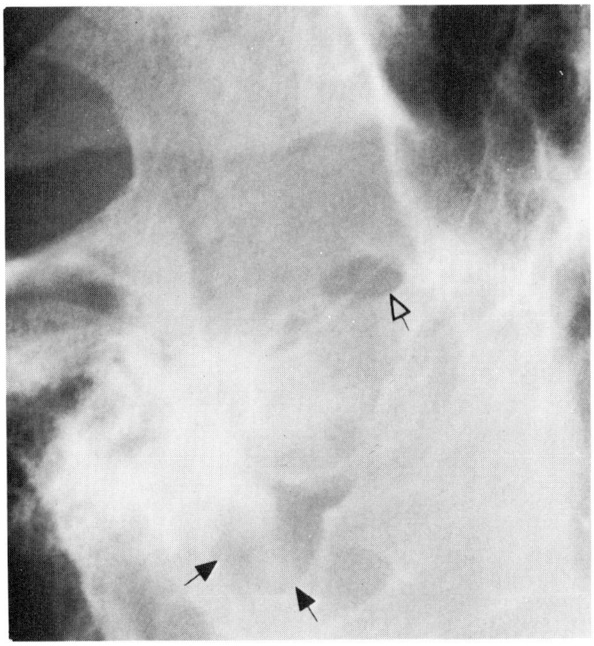

Fig. 16-31. Transmaxillary view of foramen ovale (open arrow) projects the foramen between maxillary antrum and mandible and below zygoma. Thin pterygospinous bar crosses foramen ovale. Axial projection of jugular foramen (solid arrows) is also obtained in this view.

A courageous Yugoslavian (Jelašić, 1955) has performed basal cisternography by percutaneous injection of positive contrast medium into the interpeduncular or pontine cisterns through the foramen ovale.

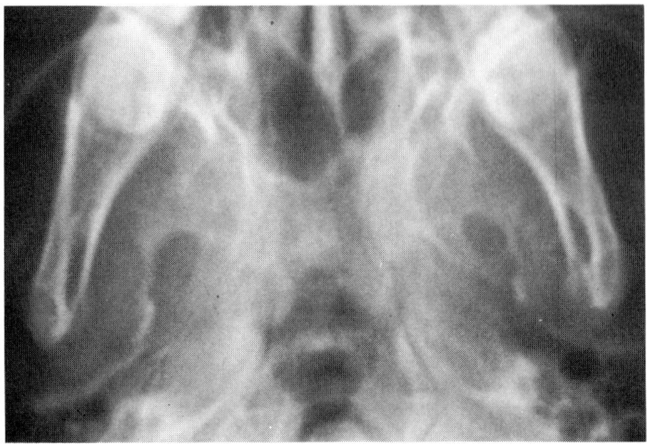

Fig. 16-32. Primitive foramen lacerum medius. Foramina spinosum and ovale are not discernible as separate structures on the right but are confluent with foramen lacerum. Sharp cortical margins on anterior and lateral aspects of foramina distinguish these anomalies from erosion by tumor.

A

B

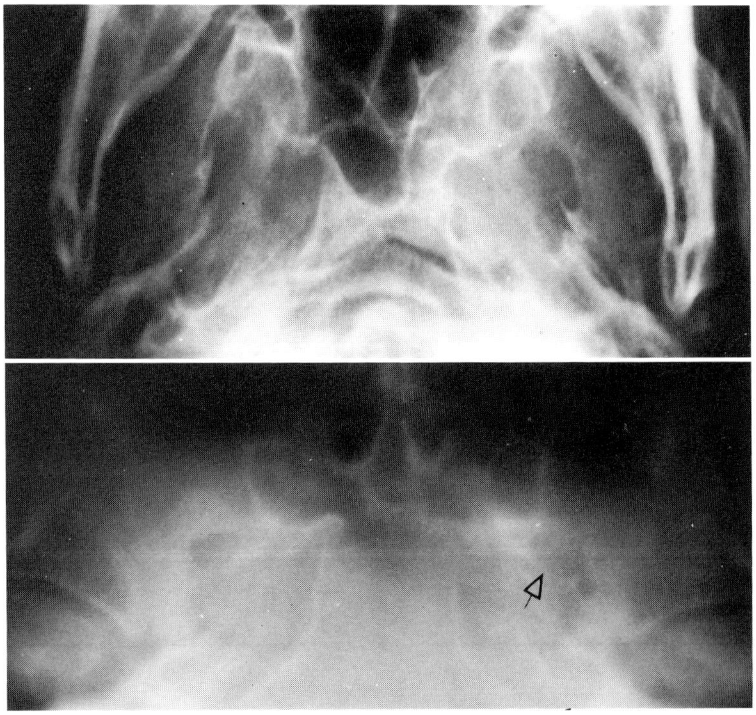

Fig. 16-33. Erosion of base of skull, especially left foramen ovale, was suspected on routine submentovertical view, **A,** of patient in whom diagnosis of nasopharyngeal carcinoma was considered. With basal tomography, **B,** however, thin rim of bone (arrow) could be demonstrated on medial aspect of foramen ovale.

Embryology and congenital anomalies

The phylogenetic development of the foramen ovale has been elegantly traced by Wood-Jones (1931), de Beer (1937), and more recently Shapiro and Robinson (1967a).

The alicochlear commissure, or primitive foramen lacerum medius, is situated between the post- or basisphenoid (precursor of the sella turcica and body of the sphenoid) and the periotic capsule. In man this commissure or fissure persists as the foramen lacerum. It is further divided into two portions by the lingulae sphenoidales (precursors of the cartilagenous segment of the greater wings). The more medial aspect becomes the carotid canal, and the more lateral the petrosphenoid fissure (on top of which the greater superficial petrosal nerve may be found).

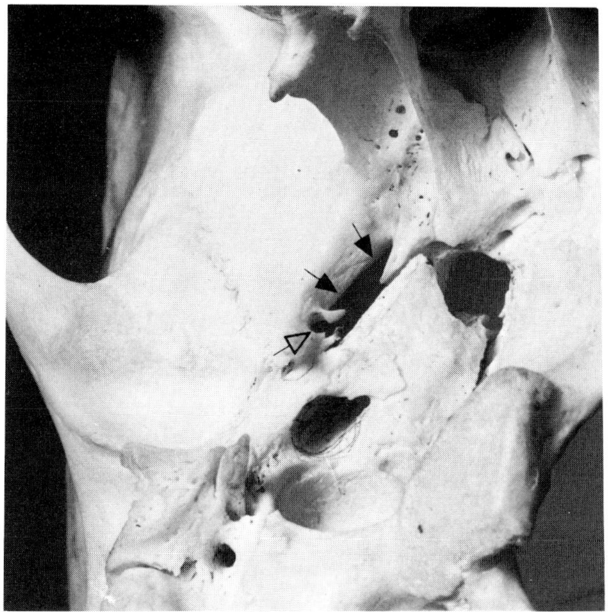

Fig. 16-34. Photograph of inferior aspect of base of skull demonstrates incomplete foramen ovale (solid arrows) and foramen spinosum (open arrow). This is pithecoid form of foramen lacerum medius. (Compare with Fig. 16-22.)

Primitively the foramen ovale is merged with the foramen lacerum medius, and under these circumstances the mandibular nerve is situated between the carotid and the stapedial arteries. (See discussion of congenital anomalies of the foramen spinosum, p. 316, and Fig. 16-54.) As the mandibular nerve sinks into the greater wing, at first a groove, later a notch, and finally a foramen develop. Various stages in this development persist in man and also account for many of the described anomalies (Wood-Jones, 1931):

1. The foramen ovale may be completely confluent with the foramen lacerum and foramen spinosum, thereby forming a primitive foramen lacerum medius (Fig. 16-32). We encountered this confluence in 4% of fifty basal roentgenograms. To be certain of such a finding without tomography is a difficult task because a thin rim of bone, which can represent the only separation, may not be visible on the routine roentgenograms (Fig. 16-33). The bony bar that separates the foramen ovale from the foramen lacerum is usually about 6 mm, but occasionally it may be much wider.

2. The foramen ovale may be present as a notch or as an incomplete foramen in the greater wing of the sphenoid. This condition persists in monkeys and apes

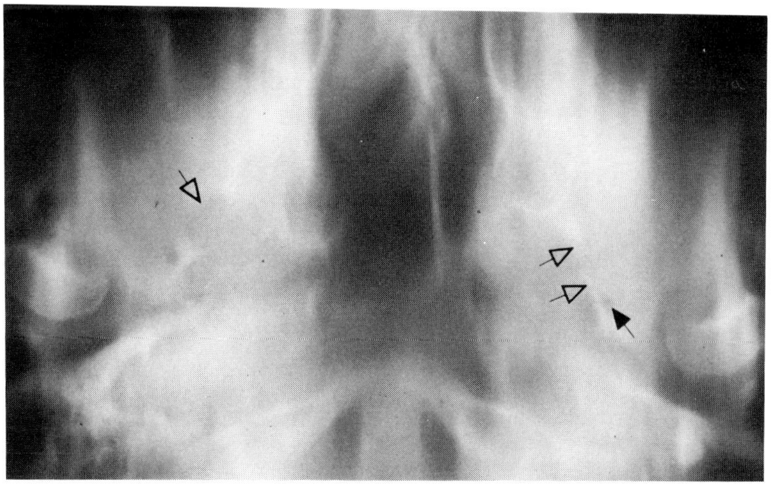

Fig. 16-35. Submentovertical tomogram demonstrates foramen lacerum medius. Right foramen ovale (single open arrow) is confluent with foramen lacerum. On the left, pterygospinous bar (double open arrows) attaches to medial aspect of foramen spinosum (solid arrow).

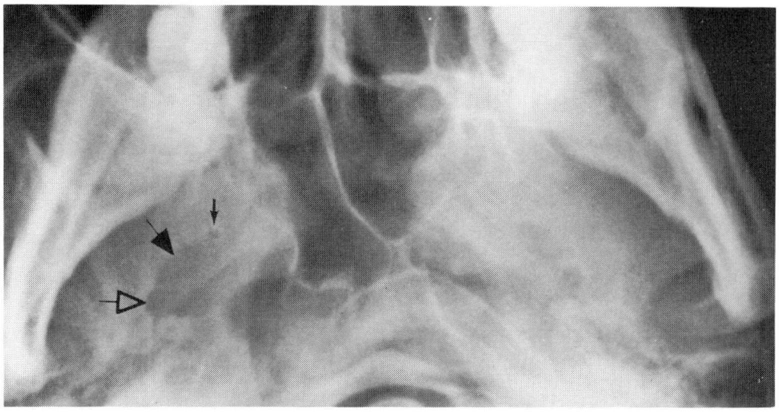

Fig. 16-36. Foramen ovale (large solid arrow) and foramen spinosum (open arrow) are confluent. Foramen ovale is also joined with foramen of Vesalius (small solid arrow) anteromedially.

and is therefore termed pithecoid (Figs. 16-34 and 16-35); it was present on 16% of the *roentgenograms* reviewed. The reported incidence of this anomaly is about 1% (Radoïévitch et al., 1956); however, we have seen the anomaly in only one of the fifty *skulls* personally examined. Such a difference would indicate that the much higher radiographic incidence represents a roentgenographic artifact that tomography and tube angulation might avoid (p. 301). The differentiation between this anomaly and erosion of the foramen by tumor may be possible only if the erosion is anterior or if the tumor has resulted in contiguous destruction (Fig. 16-16).

3. The point of entry of the nerve into the foramen may be identifiable as a suture that passes through the posterior border of the foramen.

4. The foramen ovale may communicate with the foramen spinosum by a small channel or be entirely confluent with the latter (Fig. 16-36). There was a 2% incidence of this anomaly in the material of Radoïévitch and his collaborators (1956).

5. The foramen ovale may be confluent with the foramen of Vesalius (p. 321) anteromedially (Fig. 16-36).

6. The venous portion of the foramen ovale may be separated from the remainder of the foramen by a bony spicule (Fig. 16-37). In these cases the foramen ovale has been called *duplicate,* although the anteromedial portion is actually the foramen of Vesalius. This type of separation was noted in about 0.5% of various anatomic studies (Radoïévitch et al., 1956).

7. The size and shape of the foramen may vary greatly on one or both sides. The larger more oval foramen is related to the presence of a large anterior emissary venous sinus (Lindblom, 1936; Henderson, 1966). When the sphenoid emissary foramen is well

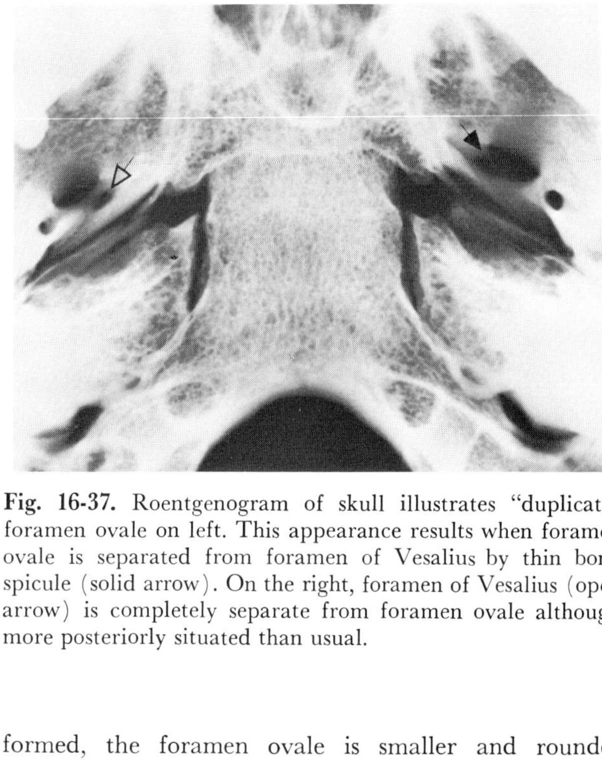

Fig. 16-37. Roentgenogram of skull illustrates "duplicate" foramen ovale on left. This appearance results when foramen ovale is separated from foramen of Vesalius by thin bony spicule (solid arrow). On the right, foramen of Vesalius (open arrow) is completely separate from foramen ovale although more posteriorly situated than usual.

formed, the foramen ovale is smaller and rounder (Wood-Jones, 1931; Shapiro and Robinson, 1967a). A small foramen ovale is sometimes associated with large lateral extensions of the sphenoid sinus, which "push back" the anterior wall of the foramen (Radoïévitch et al., 1956).

8. The thin (1 mm) bony wall of a lateral extension of the sphenoid sinus formed the anterior margin of the foramen ovale in 8% of the series of Radoïévitch and his co-workers (1956). These authors postulated that the concomitant proximity of the sphenoid sinus to the mandibular nerve might explain certain cases of isolated mandibular neuritis.

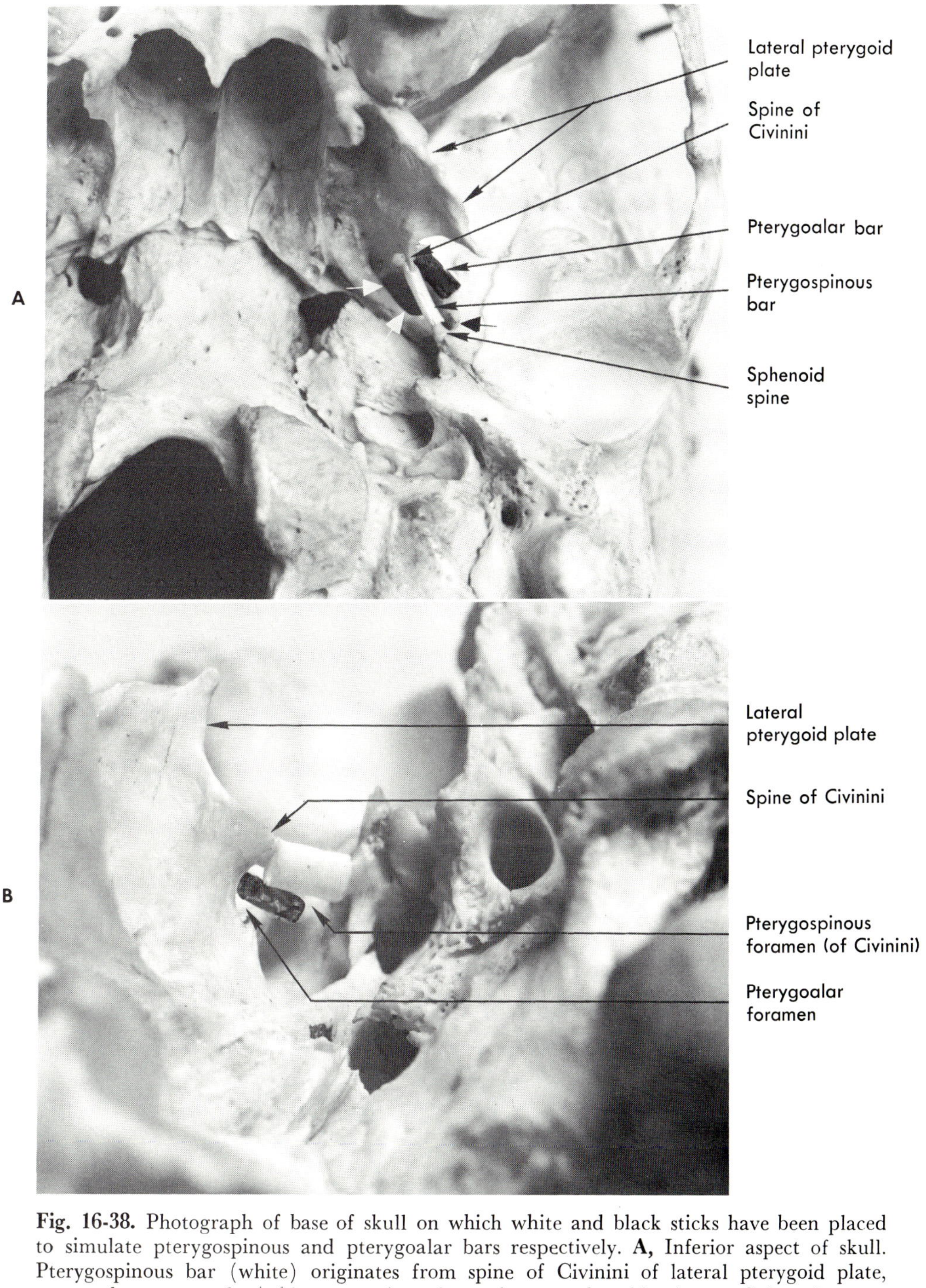

Fig. 16-38. Photograph of base of skull on which white and black sticks have been placed to simulate pterygospinous and pterygoalar bars respectively. **A,** Inferior aspect of skull. Pterygospinous bar (white) originates from spine of Civinini of lateral pterygoid plate, crosses foramen ovale (white arrows), and attaches to sphenoid spine medial to foramen spinosum (black arrow). Pterygoalar bar (black) also originates in region of spine of Civinini anteriorly but is attached to greater wing of sphenoid lateral to foramen spinosum. **B,** Lateral view of inferior surface of skull to indicate foramina formed by these bars.

A

B

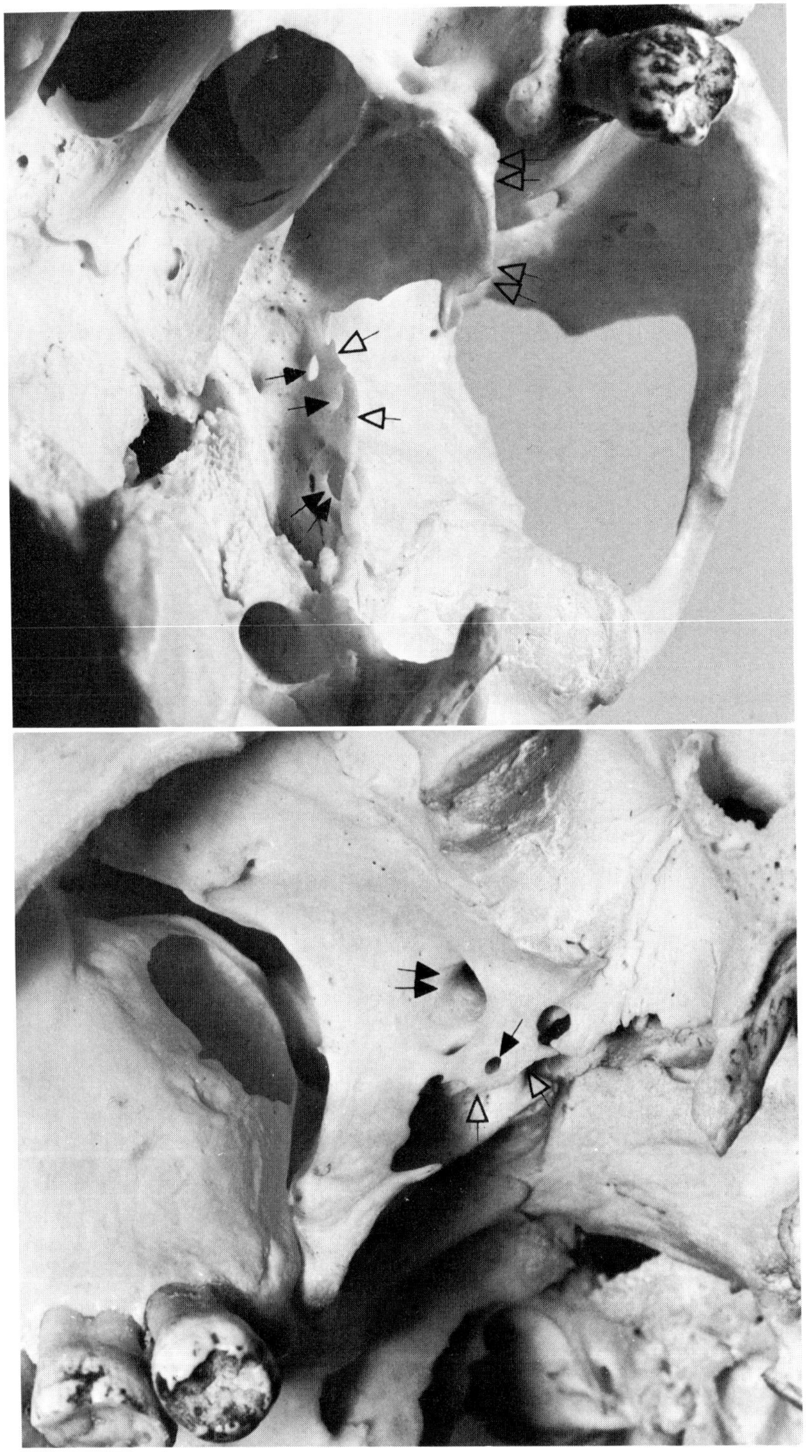

Fig. 16-39. Photographs (**A** and **B**) and roentgenograms (**C** and **D**) of large pterygospinous bar (open arrows). In **A,** origin from the lateral pterygoid plate (double open arrows) and course of the bar medial to foramen spinosum (double solid arrows) are apparent. Single solid arrows indicate pterygospinous foramina. In oblique view, **B,** foramen ovale is indicated by double solid arrows. **C,** Submentovertical roentgenogram demonstrates that pterygospinous bar (arrows) partially obscures foramen ovale. **D,** Pterygospinous bar (open arrows) and pterygospinous foramen (solid arrow) in lateral projection.

C

D

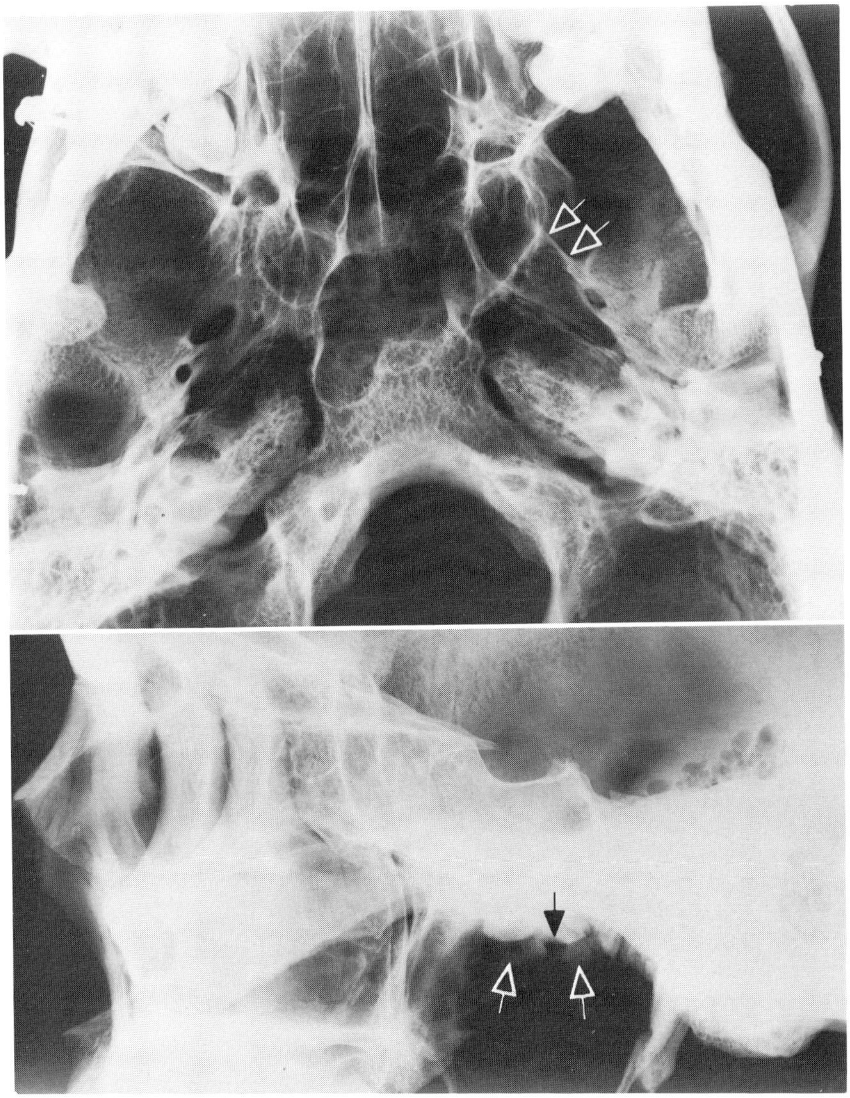

Fig. 16-39, cont'd. For legend see opposite page.

9. Rarely the foramen ovale is located posterolaterally near the sphenosquamosal suture, as in the gorilla (Shapiro and Robinson, 1967a).

Pterygospinous and pterygoalar bars. The fascia that separates the internal and external pterygoid muscles is thickened at its cranial attachments, and the resultant fibrous bands are known as the pterygospinous and pterygoalar ligaments. These may calcify or ossify, in which case they are known as the pterygospinous and pterygoalar bars and become roentgenographically visible. These bars are projected over, or lateral to, the foramen ovale in the submentovertical projection and may interfere with percutaneous injection of the mandibular nerve.

The *pterygospinous bar* is attached anteriorly to a small spur on the root of the posterior margin of the lateral pterygoid plate known as the spine of Civinini. Posteriorly the bar is attached to the angular spine of the sphenoid (Fig. 16-38). It thus passes *medial* to the foramen spinosum and crosses the foramen ovale at an angle of 20° to 40° to the sagittal plane (Priman and Etter, 1959). The small opening created between the undersurface of the skull and the pterygospinous bar is known as the *pterygospinous foramen* (of Civinini, or foramen of Civinini), which transmits the nerve and vessels of the internal pterygoid muscle (Chouké, 1946; Priman and Etter, 1959). The size of this foramen varies from 2 to 12 mm (Tebo, 1968). When ossification of the bar extends to the undersurface of the skull, there may be multiple foramina within it (Fig. 16-39). The pterygospinous ligament was completely ossified in 3% and partially ossified in 8% of the dry

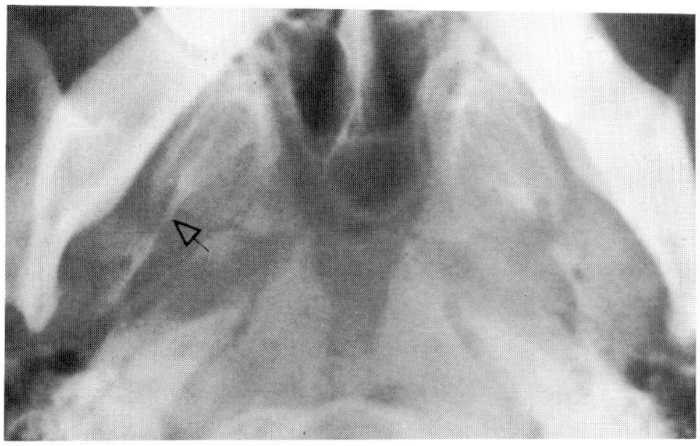

Fig. 16-40. Submentovertical roentgenogram demonstrates pterygospinous bar (arrow).

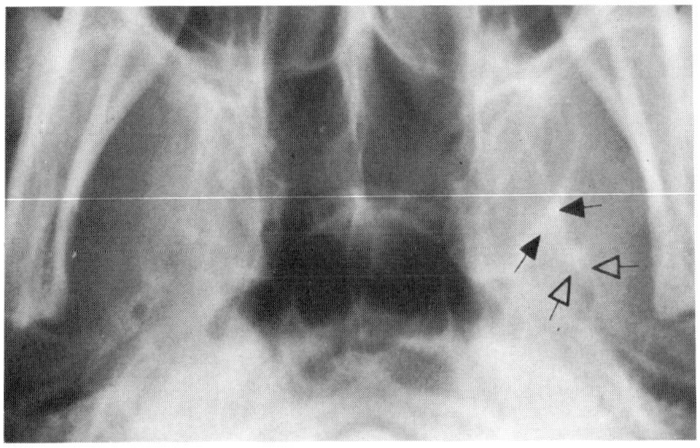

Fig. 16-41. Pterygoalar bar is attached anteriorly to lateral pterygoid plate (solid arrows) and posteriorly to greater sphenoid wing (open arrows) lateral to foramen spinosum.

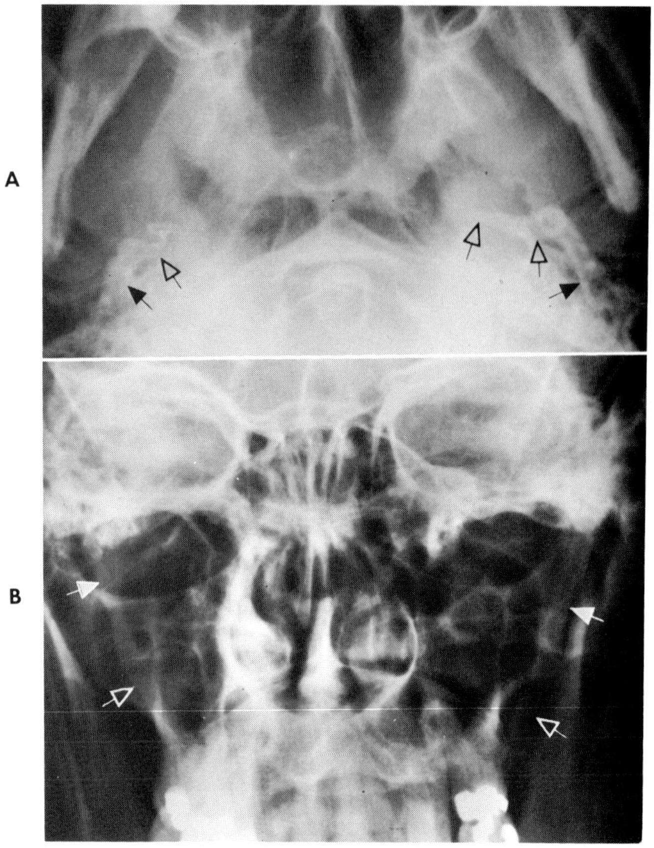

Fig. 16-42. Submentovertical (**A**) and frontal (**B**) roentgenograms demonstrate ossification of stylohyoid ligaments. More posterior attachments of these structures to the styloid process (solid arrows) and their more medial attachments anteriorly (open arrows) differentiate the ligaments from the pterygoalar and pterygospinous bars.

skulls examined by Priman and Etter (1959). In a recently collected series of 10,000 skulls, the incidence of complete ossification was 4.3% (Tebo, 1968). When present, the pterygospinous bar is visible in the basal view as a 1 to 2 mm wide linear density that extends across the foramen ovale from the lateral pterygoid plate to the medial edge of the foramen spinosum (Figs. 16-35 and 16-40). The bar may also be visible on Panorex (Tebo, 1968) and transmaxillary views (Fig. 16-31).

The *pterygoalar bar* extends from the root of the lateral pterygoid plate to the posterior attachment of the bar on the greater wing of the sphenoid at the anterolateral margin of the foramen spinosum (Fig. 16-38). In a recent comprehensive review the pterygoalar bar was referred to as the innominate bar (Lepp and Sandner, 1968). The relation of the posterior attachments of these two bars to the foramen spinosum serves to distinguish between the bars: The pterygospinous bar is always *medial,* and the pterygoalar bar always *lateral,* to the foramen. The space enclosed by the pterygoalar bar was originally given the ungainly name of *porus crotaphitico-buccinatorius,* by Hyrtl, but has more recently been called the pterygoalar foramen (Chouké, 1946; Priman and Etter, 1959). This foramen transmits the major motor branches of the mandibular nerve to the muscles of mastication. Complete ossification of the pterygoalar bar was noted in 7% of a large series of skulls (Chouké and Hodes, 1951). However, incomplete ossification was noted in 14% of the material studied by Priman and Etter (1959). This bar may be as wide as 4 mm and is visible as an increased density over the lateral margin of the foramen ovale (Chouké and Hodes, 1951; Shapiro and Robinson, 1967a) in the basilar projection (Fig. 16-41).

Only the pterygoalar bar is clinically important because of its more lateral position. It may prevent or cause more difficulty in the horizontal or lateral approaches for mandibular nerve injections (Chouké and Hodes, 1951; Priman and Etter, 1959); and it may interfere with the transmalar ascending approaches for these injections (Lepp and Sandner, 1968). Further, a pterygoalar bar may also prevent penetration of the foramen ovale for injection of the gasserian ganglion (Priman and Etter, 1959).

The appearance of an ossified stylohyoid ligament (Fig. 16-42) should not cause confusion with that of either the pterygospinous or the pterygoalar bar because of the more medial and posterior attachments of the ligament.

Pathology

Enlargement

Generalized increased intracranial pressure. Intracranial hypertension may cause enlargement of the foramina of the middle fossa, with effacement of their cortical outlines (Fig. 16-43). du Boulay (1965) reported this phenomenon and found that other signs of increased intracranial pressure also are invariably present. In the light of Henderson's work (1965, 1966), the foraminal enlargement may be caused partly by enlargement of the ovale emissary sinus. Wheeler and Honda (1965) reported bilateral symmetric enlargement of the foramen ovale secondary to intracranial hypertension in a patient with an ependymoma of the fourth ventricle. The foramina were previously roentgenographically normal.

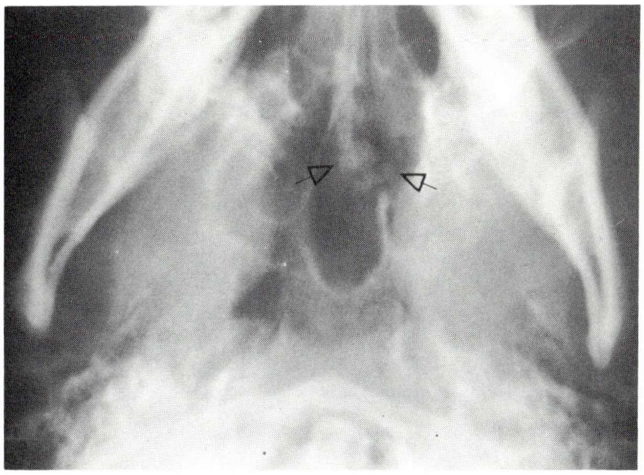

Fig. 16-43. Basal foramina are effaced in a patient with advanced skull changes of raised intracranial pressure secondary to calcified septal glioma (arrows). (See Fig. 16-14.)

Neurinoma of mandibular nerve. These neurinomas are rare—certainly less common than tumors of the trigeminal ganglion itself, of which about ninety-five cases have been reported (Glasauer and Tandon, 1969). Mandibular neurinomas are always associated with neurofibromatosis and result in uniform smooth enlargement of the foramen ovale (Fig. 16-44). The anterior aspect of the greater wing may be absent in neurofibromatosis, but Shapiro and Robinson (1967a) stated that the foramen ovale does not enlarge in the absence of a neural tumor. Meinardus (1958), however, reported a case of bilateral enlargement of the foramen ovale in a patient with neurofibromatosis but without symptoms of mandibular nerve dysfunction. He postulated that the foraminal enlargement was the result of dysplasia of the sphenoid bone.

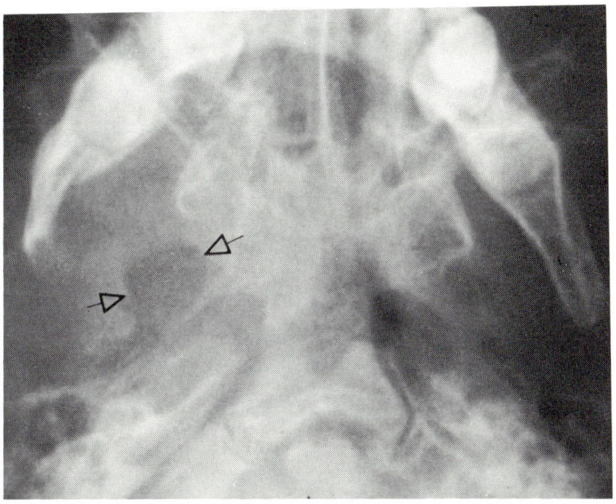

Fig. 16-44. Marked enlargement of foramen ovale (arrows) in a patient with generalized neurofibromatosis and neurofibroma of mandibular nerve. Note the smooth outline of the foramen. (Courtesy Charles A. Gooding, M.D., San Francisco, Calif.)

Erosion of floor of middle fossa. Such erosions may begin as an isolated enlargement of the foramen ovale, as illustrated by du Boulay (1965) in a carcinoma metastatic to the cavernous sinus and Meckel's cave and by Schmidt and Driesen (1957) in a metastatic cylindroma.

Chordoma. A chordoma that grew through the foramen ovale and caused enlargement of the foramen was reported in a 38-year-old woman with a long history of cranial neuropathies (Lafon et al., 1953).

Large vein. A large vein was found in the foramen ovale of a patient with mandibular neuritis of 7 years' duration. Smooth enlargement of the foramen ovale on the basal skull roentgenogram had prompted surgical exploration (Schmidt and Driesen, 1957).

Destruction. A large variety of diseases may cause erosion or destruction of the floor of the middle fossa and foramina ovale and spinosum.

Vascular lesions

ANEURYSM. Aneurysms of the cavernous portion of the internal carotid artery not infrequently cause large areas of bone destruction in the contiguous middle fossa. The bony margins are usually sharply defined, and calcification in the perimeter often helps to identify the lesion (Fig. 16-45).

A

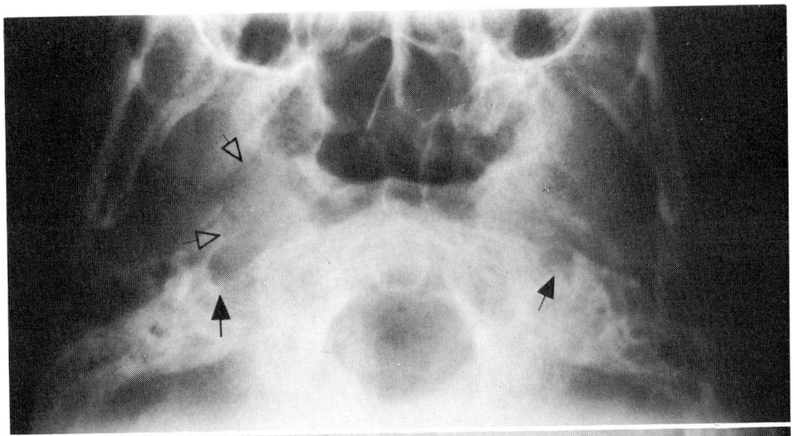

B

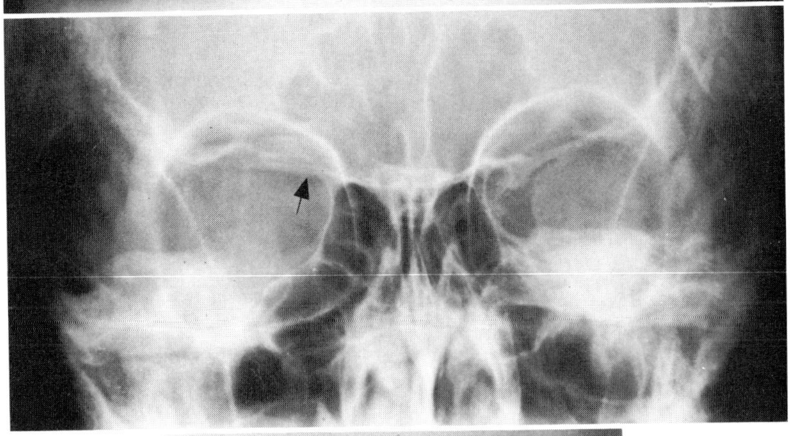

C

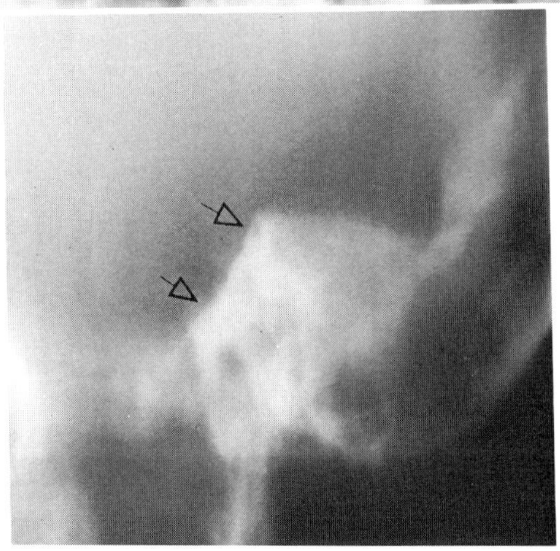

Fig. 16-45. Erosion of floor of middle fossa and petrous apex by large intracavernous aneurysm of internal carotid artery. **A,** Submentovertical projection reveals characteristically sharp margins (open arrows) of erosion. Enlarged right and normal left carotid canals are indicated by solid arrows. **B,** Undercutting of right anterior clinoid is evident (arrow). Superior orbital fissure is enlarged. **C,** Tomogram of petrous bone in Stenvers position reveals that anterior half of petrous bone has been eroded by aneurysm (arrows).

CAROTID CAVERNOUS FISTULA. Vascular erosion may also occur with carotid cavernous fistulae (Shapiro and Robinson, 1967a).

Tumors

CARCINOMA. The most common tumor to erode the floor of the middle fossa is extension from a nasopharyngeal or paranasal sinus carcinoma. These tumors cause bone destruction with ill-defined margins. They may cause extensive defects (Fig. 16-46), but they can also be manifested by mixed lytic and sclerotic changes (Fig. 16-17).

MENINGIOMA. Meningiomas in this region usually are

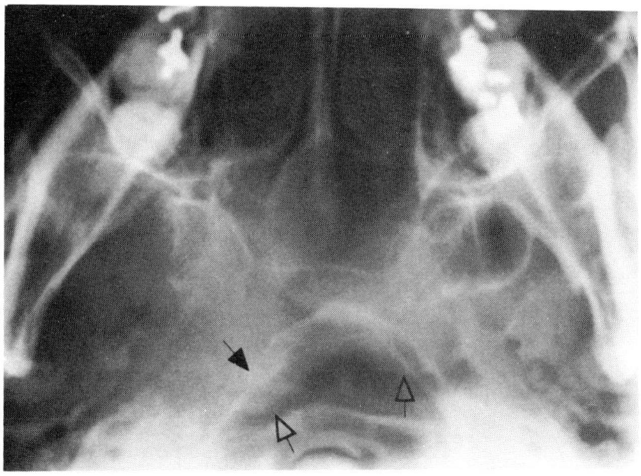

Fig. 16-46. Nasopharyngeal carcinoma with erosion of foramina of middle fossa, petrous apex, and sphenoid sinus. There is large soft-tissue mass in nasopharynx (open arrows). Anterior aspect of hyoid bone (solid arrow) is also eroded. The hyoid bone is well visualized because clivus was completely destroyed.

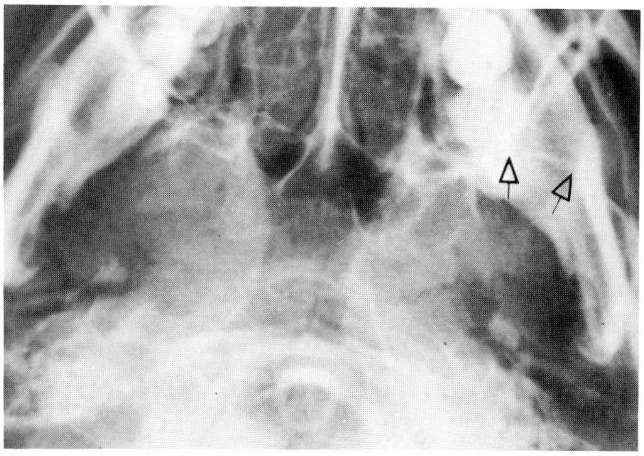

Fig. 16-48. Effacement of foramina of middle fossa in a patient with long-standing right temporal lobe glioma. Anterior margin of left middle fossa is clearly seen (arrows) but that on the right is no longer visible. (From du Boulay, G. H.: Principles of x-ray diagnosis of the skull, London, 1965, Butterworth & Co., Ltd.)

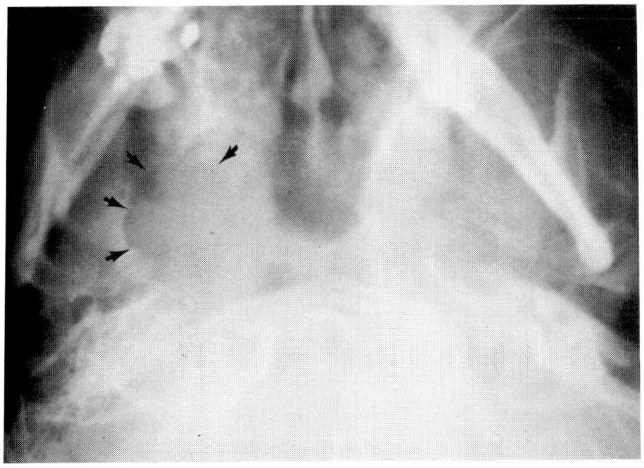

Fig. 16-47. Sharply marginated erosion of middle fossa (arrows), with destruction of basal foramina in a patient with trigeminal neurinoma. (From Holman, C. B., Olive, I., and Svien, H. J.: Amer. J. Roentgen. **86**:148-153, 1961.)

manifested by hyperostosis, but occasionally they may be purely lytic. In this event, distinction from other tumors is frequently not possible.

NEURINOMA OF GASSERIAN GANGLION. These lesions produce a variety of bone changes, depending on their size and primary route of extension into either the middle or the posterior fossa.

Erosion of the region of the foramen ovale (Taveras and Wood, 1964) (Fig. 16-47) or actual widening of the foramen (Glasauer and Tandon, 1969) is the most common finding on roentgenograms of the skull. Holman and his co-workers (1961), however, found that the most characteristic roentgen finding produced by these tumors is erosion of the petrous tip medial to the internal auditory meatus. The structures of the middle fossa were eroded in more than 50% of their cases. These tumors may attain considerable size in the absence of the characteristic symptoms of facial numbness without pain, because they develop in the nerve sheath and only secondarily cause pressure on the nerve fibers (Holman et al., 1961).

EPIDERMOID OR CHOLESTEATOMA. These lesions may cause erosion of the middle fossa and basal foramina. The erosion is usually well-defined and occasionally may be scalloped. A ring of calcification sometimes surrounds the larger tumors (Bloom and Keohane, 1965; du Boulay, 1965; Shapiro and Robinson, 1967a).

GLIOMA. Very long-standing temporal lobe gliomas rarely produce thinning of the middle fossa to the extent that the basal foramina are no longer clearly delineated (du Boulay, 1965) (Fig. 16-48).

Miscellaneous lesions

RETICULOENDOTHELIOSIS. These lesions, especially histiocytosis X, may cause scalloped defects in the floor of the middle fossa (Fig. 16-49). In the healing phase the lesions may exhibit a sclerotic reaction (Shapiro and Robinson, 1967a).

FRACTURE. Fractures of the middle fossa are infrequently seen on basal roentgenograms. As in the vault, however, a bony defect with smooth margins may develop in association with a leptomeningeal cyst (Shapiro and Robinson, 1967a).

A

B

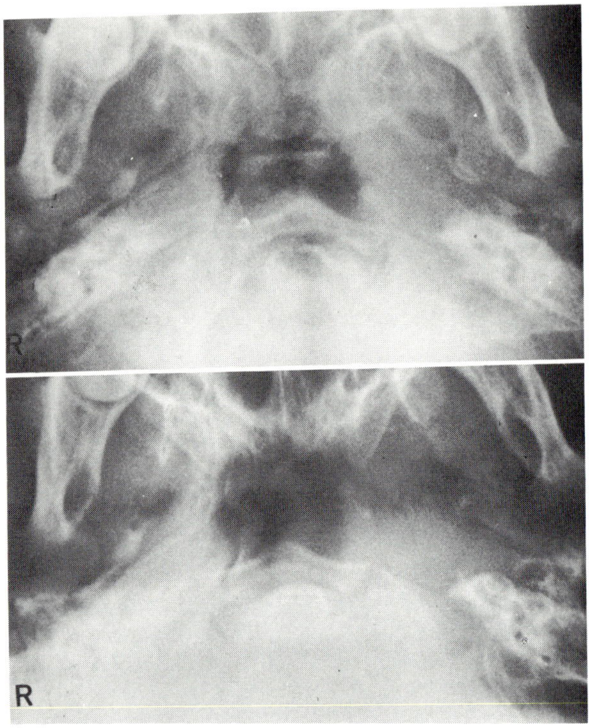

Fig. 16-49. Histiocytosis X with destruction of floor of left middle fossa. **A,** Foramina ovale and spinosum are still intact. **B,** Reexamination 1 year later shows progressive bone destruction with loss of margins of foramina of middle fossa on left side. (From Shapiro, R., and Robinson, F.: Amer. J. Roentgen. **101**:779-794, 1967.)

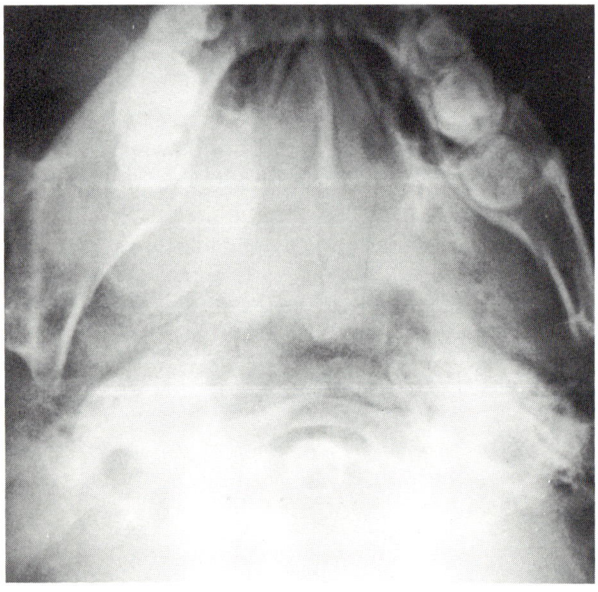

Fig. 16-50. Fibrous dysplasia involving right sphenoid and temporal bones. Middle fossa foramina are no longer visible. (Courtesy Arthur T. Gronner, M.D., Lafayette, Calif.)

Narrowing and sclerosis

Osteopetrosis. When the density of the bones of the base and vault is markedly increased, the foramina are difficult to see; and when visible, they may be narrowed. A diagnosis with roentgenograms of the skull alone may be possible; however, a skeletal survey may be required (du Boulay, 1965; Shapiro and Robinson, 1967a).

Fibrous dysplasia. Involvement of the base of the skull is usually accompanied by changes in the vault and facial bones. When the base is affected, isolated involvement of the greater wing of the sphenoid is rare (Leeds and Seaman, 1962). The bone changes may be purely sclerotic or a mixture of sclerosis and increased lucency. Enlargement or narrowing of the middle fossa foramina is therefore theoretically possible, or the foramina may be obscured (Fig. 16-50).

Paget's disease. Involvement of the floor of the middle fossa is by the sclerotic form of the disease and is usually accompanied by changes in the vault. The foramina are difficult to visualize, or they may be constricted (du Boulay, 1965; Shapiro and Robinson, 1967a).

FORAMEN SPINOSUM (TROU PETIT ROND)

Gross anatomy

The foramen spinosum is a small opening in the posteromedial aspect of the greater wing of the sphenoid that connects the infratemporal fossa with the middle cranial fossa. From the endocranial aspect (Fig. 16-23) the foramen is situated just posterolateral to the foramen ovale and a few millimeters lateral to the petrosphenoid fissure. On the undersurface of the skull, the eustachian (pharyngotympanic) tube is medial to the foramen spinosum; and the spine of the sphenoid (spina angularis) forms the posterolateral border of the foramen (Fig. 16-25, *A*). The foramen is sometimes incorporated into this spine, thereby forming a canal that may be as long as 1 cm.

Measurements. The foramen or short canal is usually 2 to 4 mm long (Lindblom, 1936) and oval or round in cross section. Its long diameter is almost always in line with the axis of the foramen ovale, but it may be at a right angle to this axis. Lindblom's (1936) measurements of the short axis of the foramen in skeletal specimens averaged 2 mm, with a minimum of 1.5 and a maximum of 3 mm. The difference between the long and short diameters averaged 0.5 mm.

Structures transmitted. The *middle meningeal artery,* a branch of the internal maxillary artery, enters the skull through the foramen spinosum and supplies most of the supratentorial dura mater. After it enters the skull, it also gives off branches to the trigeminal ganglion as well as the superficial petrosal, superior tym-

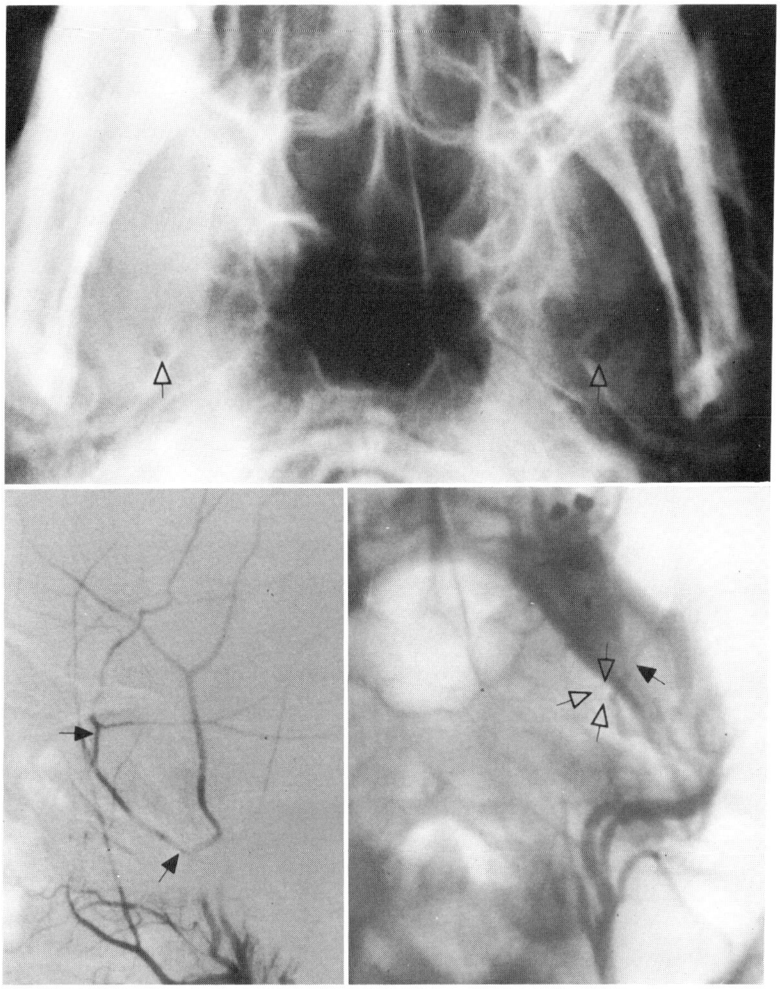

Fig. 16-51. A, Enlarged left foramen spinosum (arrows) was found in a woman with symptoms of left hemisphere lesion. Left foramen spinosum measured 4.5 × 5 mm and was 2 mm larger than right. Discrepancy was larger than had been previously reported (see text). Selected external carotid angiography in lateral, **B,** and submentovertical, **C,** projections revealed normal middle meningeal artery (solid arrows). In this case, artery traversed lateral aspect of foramen spinosum (open arrows).

panic, orbital, and temporal branches (Gray, 1959). The middle meningeal artery usually fills the foramen from side to side, across the short diameter of the foramen (Lindblom, 1936), but the artery may be situated in the posterior angle of the foramen (Fig. 16-51, *C*).

The remainder of the foramen is usually occupied by the *middle meningeal vein or veins,* which drain the dura and empty into the pterygoid plexus. The veins are commonly in front of, but may be behind, the artery (Lindblom, 1936). These veins are sometimes connected to the cavernous sinus by an extension of the ovale emissary sinus described by Henderson (1966); and therefore cavernous blood may drain through the foramen spinosum. (See discussion of the structures transmitted through the foramen ovale, p. 297 and Fig. 16-24, *A*).

The *recurrent or meningeal branch of the mandibular nerve* (nervus spinosus) enters the skull through the foramen with the middle meningeal artery and supplies the dura. It also sends a branch to the mucous membrane of the mastoid air cells (Gray, 1959).

Radiology

The foramen spinosum is usually clearly demonstrated in the full axial projection (Fig. 16-27, *A*). The foramen or canal is sometimes not directed vertically but rather is slanted upward and posteriorly at an angle of 30°. Therefore a comparable caudad tube angle may be necessary to demonstrate it adequately

(Lindblom, 1936) (Fig. 16-27, *B* and *C*). Hyperextension of the head may also cause spurious absence of the foramen for the same reason (Shapiro and Robinson, 1967a). Basal tomography through the plane of the external auditory canal or 0.5 cm superior and inferior to that level demonstrates the foramen when the plain roentgenograms are not conclusive.

Lindblom (1936) found the width of the foramen to average 2 mm (1 mm minimum; 3.5 mm maximum) on basal roentgenograms. He also noted in his evaluation of roentgenograms that the dimensions of the foramina on the two sides differed by 1.5 mm in only 1% and by 1 mm in only 2%.

Our measurements of the foramina on fifty basal projections (100 foramina) obtained with a focal spot–film distance of 40 inches were as follows: average = 2.3 × 3.0 mm; smallest = 1 × 1 mm; largest and longest = 3 × 5 mm; widest = 3.5 × 2.5 mm. A difference of more than 1 mm between the foramina on the two sides was found in 12% of the roentgenograms (1.5 mm in 8%; 2 mm in 4%). The difference was 1 mm in 20%, and the remainder differed by 0.5 mm or were equal in size.

An inverse relationship between the size of the foramen ovale and the size of the foramen spinosum has been noted (Greig, 1929; Lindblom, 1936; Shapiro and Janzen, 1960). This relation was not confirmed in our material. Considerable asymmetry may exist in the normal (Fig. 16-51). However, a patient with a foramen spinosum larger than 5 mm in diameter or a foramen that differs from its homologue on the opposite side by more than 2 mm should be evaluated for other roentgen signs of pathology associated with an enlarged middle meningeal artery.

Embryology and congenital anomalies

Anomalies of the foramen spinosum may be related to atavistic defects in osteogenesis, as described with the foramen ovale (p. 305), or they may be caused by variations in the development of the middle meningeal artery.

Defects in osteogenesis (Wood-Jones, 1931)

1. The foramen lacerum medius may be complete, in which case a separate foramen spinosum is not discernible (Fig. 16-32).
2. Separation from the foramen ovale may be incomplete, with a narrow channel connecting the two foramina (Fig. 16-52); or the foramina spinosum and ovale may be entirely confluent (Fig. 16-36).
3. The foramen spinosum may be incomplete above or below.
4. The medial aspect of the foramen spinosum may be defective, in which case there will be communication with the petrosphenoid fissure (Fig. 16-53). This anomaly was present in 4% of the fifty basal roentgenograms reviewed by us.

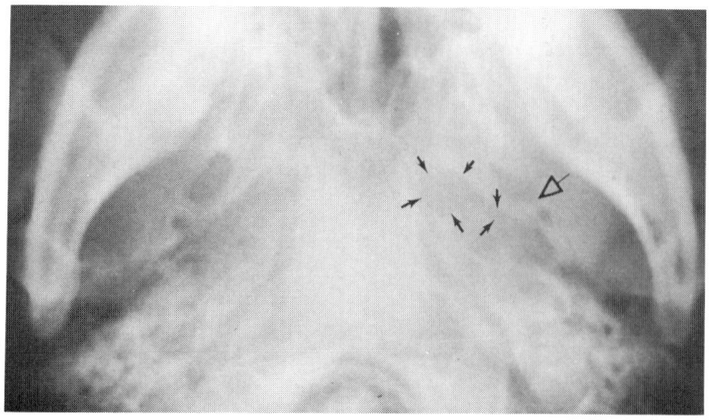

Fig. 16-52. Narrow channel (open arrow) connects left foramina ovale and spinosum. Foramen lacerum (small arrows) is well seen.

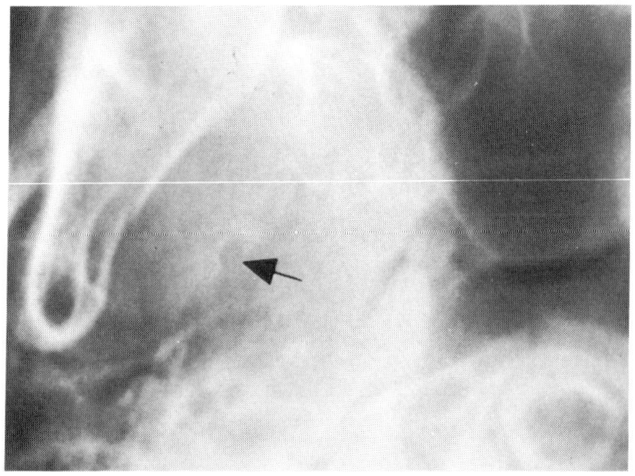

Fig. 16-53. Foramen spinosum is open medially (arrow) and communicates with petrosphenoid fissure.

5. The relation of the foramen spinosum to the sphenoid spine is variable. The foramen may perforate the apex of the spine (Fig. 16-38, *A*). The spine may also form the posterior, lateral, or rarely the medial wall of the *canalis spinosus* (a term suggested by Wood-Jones); or it may be some distance medial to the spine.
6. The foramen spinosum may communicate with the canaliculus innominatus (p. 322).

Variations in development of middle meningeal artery

1. Especially in dry skulls (Figs. 16-22 and 16-54), but also on clinical roentgenograms, the foramen may be duplicated. Lindblom (1936) suggested that anterior and posterior foramina were related to early bifurcation of the meningeal artery and that a second more medial foramen existed for the superficial petrosal nerve. This observation was not confirmed by our examination of the arterial grooves in fifty skulls. Duplica-

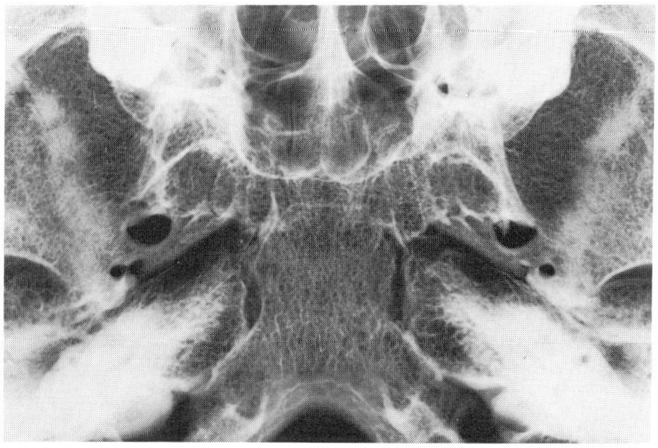

Fig. 16-54. Roentgenogram of specimen illustrated in Fig. 16-22. Foramen spinosum is duplicated on the right.

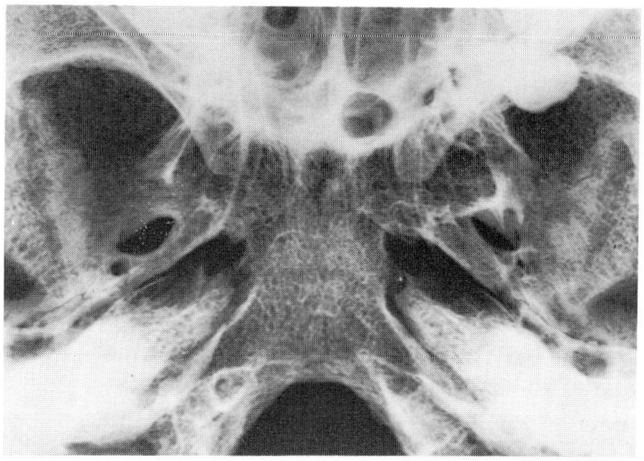

Fig. 16-55. Basal roentgenogram of skull illustrates tiny left foramen spinosum.

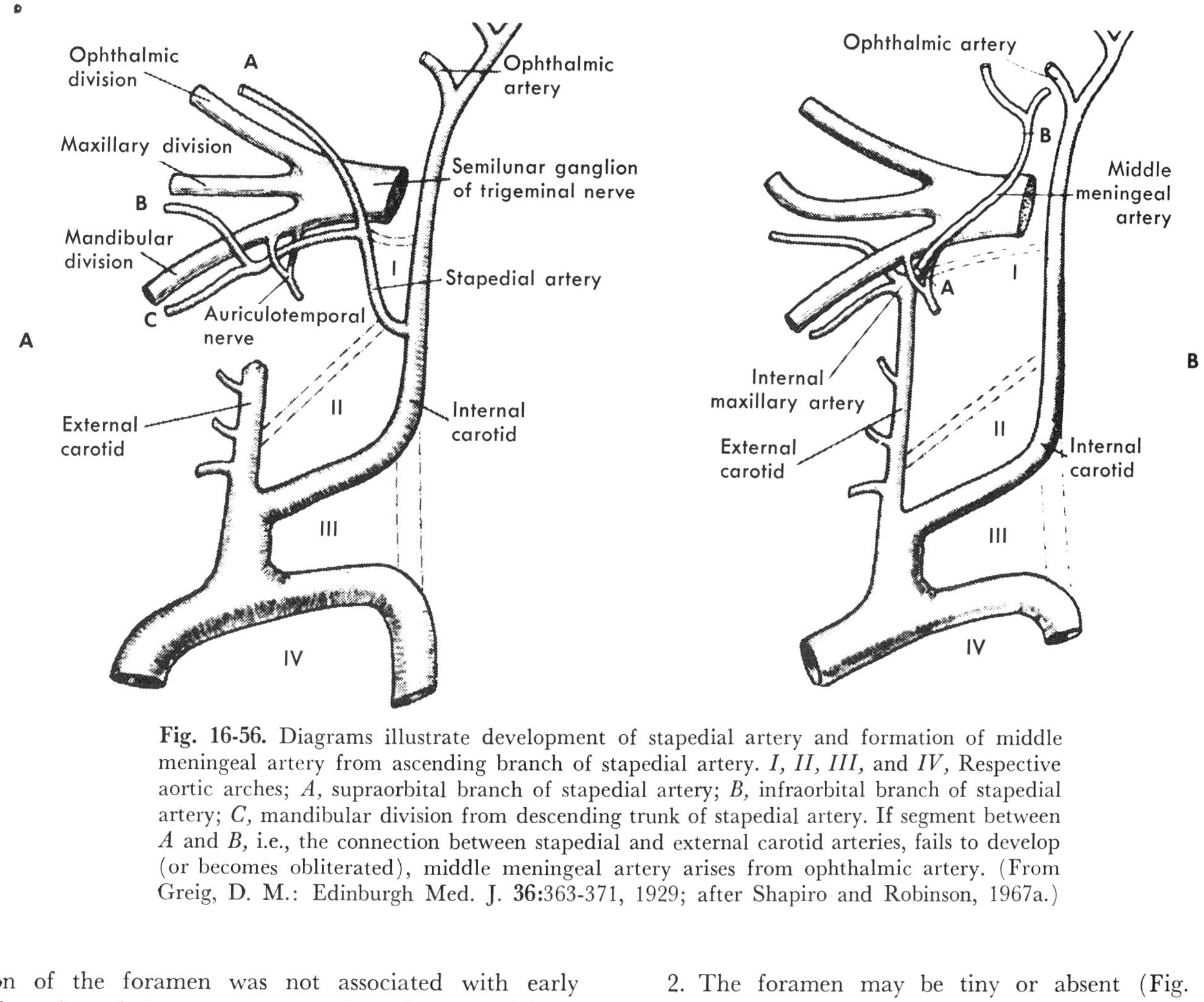

Fig. 16-56. Diagrams illustrate development of stapedial artery and formation of middle meningeal artery from ascending branch of stapedial artery. *I, II, III,* and *IV,* Respective aortic arches; *A,* supraorbital branch of stapedial artery; *B,* infraorbital branch of stapedial artery; *C,* mandibular division from descending trunk of stapedial artery. If segment between *A* and *B,* i.e., the connection between stapedial and external carotid arteries, fails to develop (or becomes obliterated), middle meningeal artery arises from ophthalmic artery. (From Greig, D. M.: Edinburgh Med. J. **36**:363-371, 1929; after Shapiro and Robinson, 1967a.)

tion of the foramen was not associated with early bifurcation of the artery, even when the second foramen was much larger (Figs. 16-22 and 16-54) than necessary to accommodate the lesser superficial petrosal nerve, which is usually minute. (See discussion of the canaliculus innominatus, p. 322.)

2. The foramen may be tiny or absent (Fig. 16-55). It was absent in 0.4% of Lindblom's (1936) roentgenographic series. Curnow (1873) originally described the association of a minute foramen spinosum with ophthalmic origin of the middle meningeal artery. Fisher (1914) and Greig (1929), who also described

A

B

C

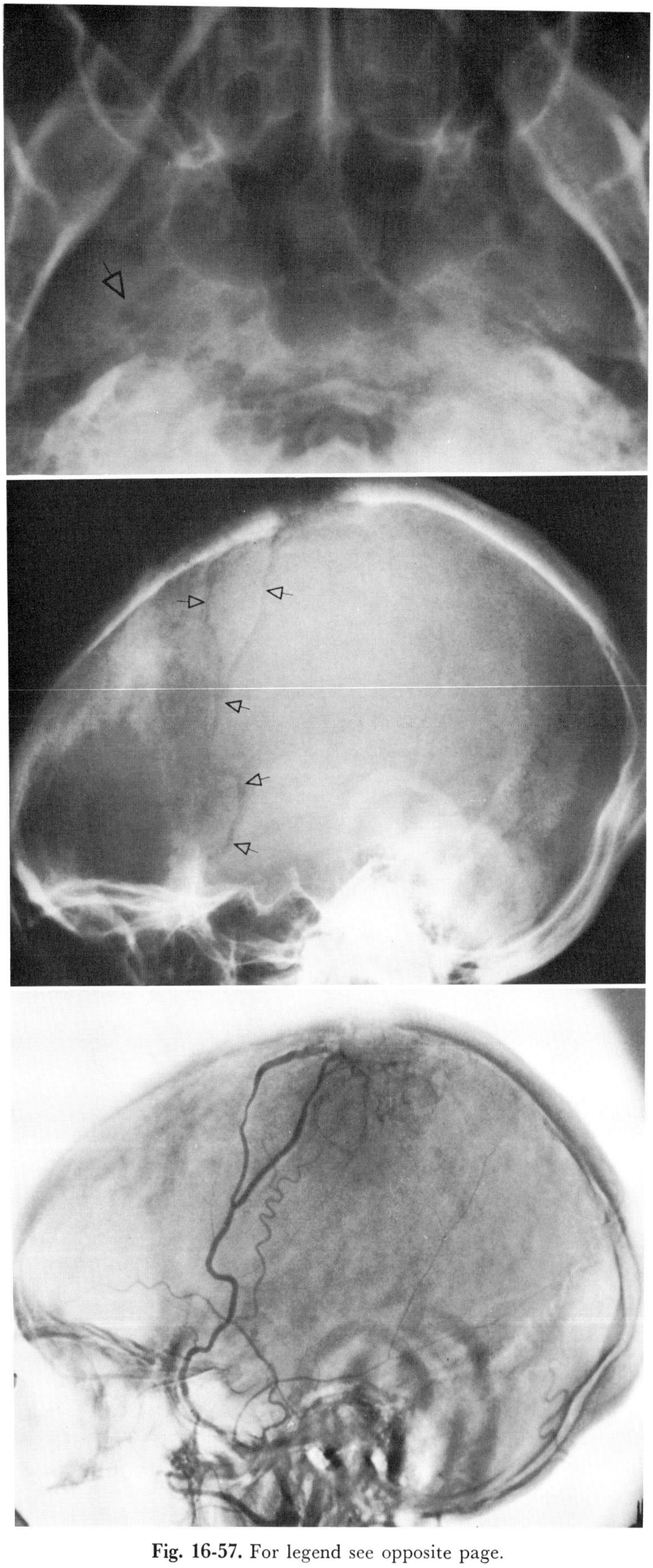

Fig. 16-57. For legend see opposite page.

Fig. 16-57. Right parasagittal meningioma in 61-year-old woman. **A,** Submentovertical roentgenogram reveals enlarged right foramen spinosum (arrow). It was about 2 mm larger than the left. **B,** Lateral projection reveals enlarged middle meningeal vascular channels (arrows) leading to lytic lesion in vertex of skull. **C,** Selective external carotid angiogram demonstrates that hypertrophied anterior branch of middle meningeal artery fills these grooves and supplies the meningioma.

A

B

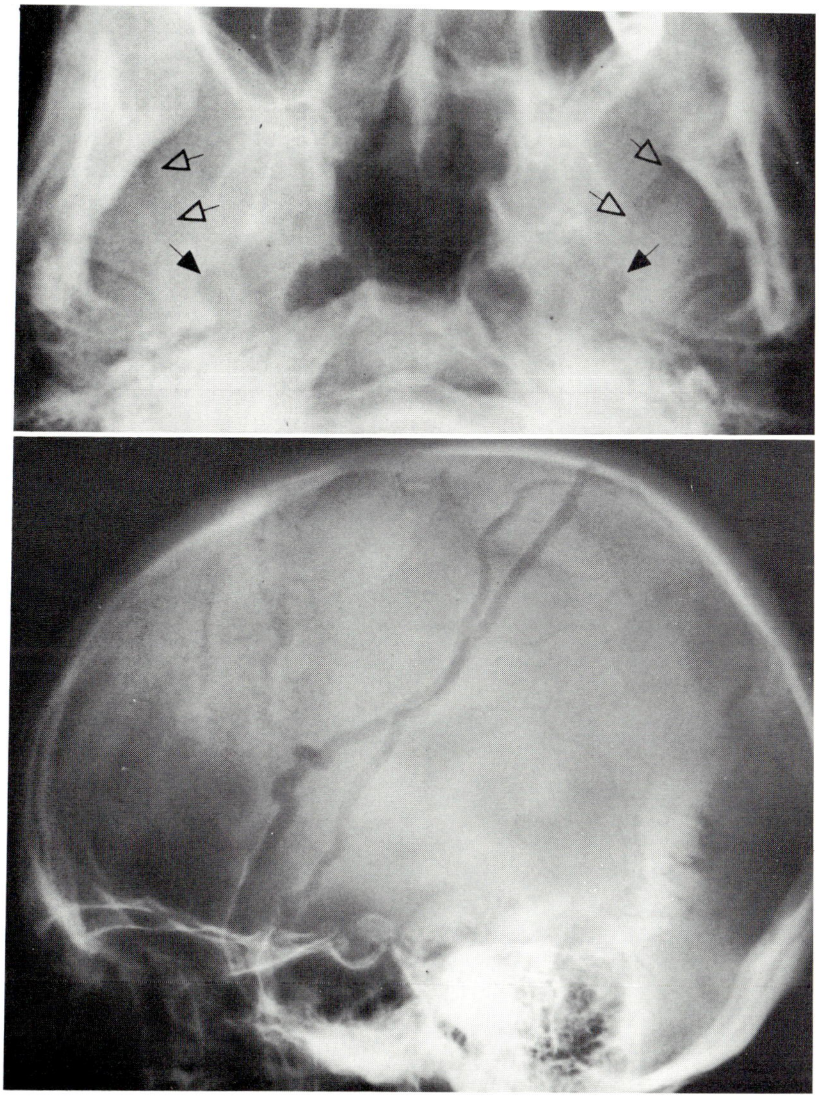

Fig. 16-58. Primarily dural arteriovenous malformation in region of superior longitudinal sinus supplied by middle meningeal arteries. **A,** Submentovertical view demonstrates huge foramina spinosa (solid arrows), which measured 4.5 × 6 mm and 4 × 4.5 mm. Large vascular grooves (open arrows) are evident in both submentovertical and lateral, **B,** projections. These grooves were almost entirely filled by markedly enlarged middle meningeal arteries.

such cases, and Wood-Jones (1931) related this association to the development of the stapedial artery. Embryologically the stapedial artery is derived from the dorsal portion of the second aortic arch and at this stage (6.5 mm embryo) is connected to the internal carotid artery via the hyoid artery between the first and second arches. The stapedial artery later develops supraorbital and infraorbital branches that accompany the respective divisions of the trigeminal nerve (Fig. 16-56, *A*). Later these branches lose their connection to the internal carotid artery and fuse with the external carotid artery, forming the internal maxillary branches of the latter (Fig. 16-56, *B*). The middle meningeal artery thus develops from the supraorbital or ascending branch of the stapedial artery. When the connection of the stapedial artery to the external carotid artery fails to develop (or becomes obliterated), the middle meningeal artery arises from the ophthalmic artery. In this event, the foramen spinosum is tiny or absent and the meningeal artery enters the cranial cavity through the superior orbital fissure (Fisher, 1914; Greig, 1929; Wood-Jones, 1931; Lie, 1968).

3. The accessory meningeal artery occasionally provides a large portion of the supply to the dura. In this event, the foramen spinosum is small and the groove for the meningeal vessels extends from the posterior aspect of the foramen ovale (Fig. 16-26).

Pathology

Widening of the foramen spinosum with anterior and middle third parasagittal as well as frontal and parietal convexity meningiomas has been appreciated for some time (Sosman and Putnam, 1925). Lindblom (1936) also noted widening of the foramen with occasional meningiomas of the sphenoid wings and anterior fossa. Most observers, however (Traub, 1961; Taveras and Wood, 1964; Rumbaugh and Potts, 1966), have concluded that because of frequent normal asymmetry enlargement of the foramen spinosum must be accompanied by a widened middle meningeal groove on the same side to have pathologic significance (Fig. 16-57). This widening may be appreciated only in the basal projection with pterion meningiomas (Lindblom, 1936). Even though a convexity tumor is quite large, hypertrophy of the meningeal artery may not be commensurate because of the supply from the internal carotid artery.

Dural or combined dural and cerebral arteriovenous malformations may be associated with enlargement of the foramen spinosum (Lindblom, 1936; Holmgren, 1946; Rumbaugh and Potts, 1966). In a case with bilateral foraminal enlargement (Fig. 16-58), as well as in previously reported instances of dural vascular malformations, significant widening of the meningeal grooves of the calvarium was a concomitant finding. Conversely, however, an enlarged foramen spinosum may focus attention on a certain vascular channel and thereby indicate that the channel is arterial rather than venous (Lindblom, 1936). Differentiation between meningiomas and arteriovenous malformations is not possible on the basis of the appearance of the bony vascular channels.

Although hypertrophy of the middle meningeal artery in Paget's disease may be accompanied by enlargement of the foramen spinosum, usually this fact is not appreciated because extensive sclerotic changes in the vault obscure the foramen on basal roentgenograms.

Other pathologic alterations of the foramen spinosum are related to changes in the floor of the middle fossa. (See previous discussion of the pathology of the foramen ovale.)

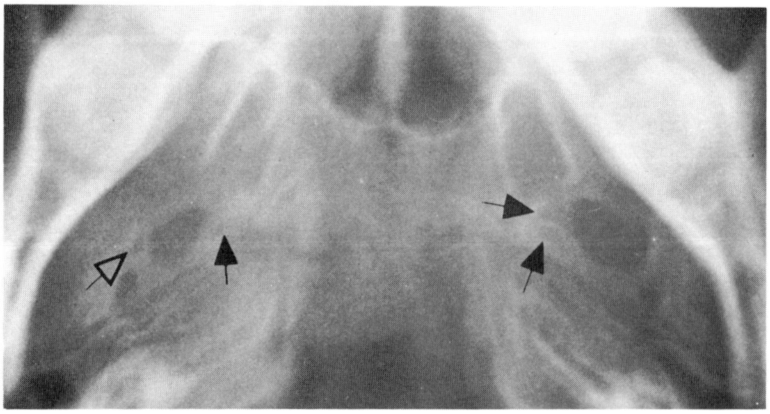

Fig. 16-59. Submentovertical roentgenogram shows two foramina of Vesalius (solid arrows) on the left and one on the right. Notion that a small foramen ovale is associated with a large foramen of Vesalius obviously is not valid in this patient. Separate foramen for accessory meningeal artery (open arrow) is evident on the right.

FORAMEN OF VESALIUS (SPHENOID EMISSARY FORAMEN, FORAMEN VESALII, CANALICULUS SPHENOIDALIS)

Gross anatomy

The foramen of Vesalius is a small inconstant opening in the medial aspect of the greater wing of the sphenoid anteromedial to the foramen ovale (Fig. 16-23). It connects the medial aspect of the middle fossa with the region of the scaphoid fossa, in which the tensor veli palatini originates.

Measurements. Lindblom (1936) found that the foramen sometimes ends in the diploic space, and he noted that it was never larger than 1 mm in diameter. It was larger than 1 mm in 5% of the specimens examined by Boyd (1930), however, and as large as 2 mm in four instances. The foramen was bilateral in 15% of these specimens and unilateral in about 22%.

Structures transmitted. As its name implies, the sphenoid emissary foramen transmits a *vein* that connects the cavernous sinus and the pterygoid plexus. Henderson (1966) showed that occasionally this may be a venous sinus rather than a vein. It leaves the skull through the anterior aspect of the foramen ovale when the foramen of Vesalius is absent.

The meningeal branch of the ascending pharyngeal artery entered the skull through this foramen in a case of congenital absence of the internal carotid artery (Fisher, 1914).

Radiology

Schüller (1938) recognized the presence of the foramen of Vesalius, which he termed the canaliculus sphenoidalis, on the standard axial view. He indicated that frequently two foramina appear on one side (Fig. 16-59). The foramen is visible only in the submentovertical projection (Fig. 16-36), on which it is seen as a 1 to 2 mm well-circumscribed lucency a few millimeters anteromedial to the foramen ovale. When unilateral, the ipsilateral foramen ovale is smaller than the foramen ovale on the opposite side (Wood-Jones, 1931; Shapiro and Robinson, 1967a). The foramen of Vesalius was visualized in 15% of fifty basal views.

Embryology and congenital anomalies

According to Wood-Jones (1931) the foramen of Vesalius exists in no other primate and its presence therefore is a distinctive feature of man. It may be variously situated in relation to the foramen ovale. Only a bony spicule may separate it from the foramen ovale (Fig. 16-37), and in these cases the foramen ovale has been called "duplicate." At the other extreme the separation may be as much as 1 cm (Fig. 16-23).

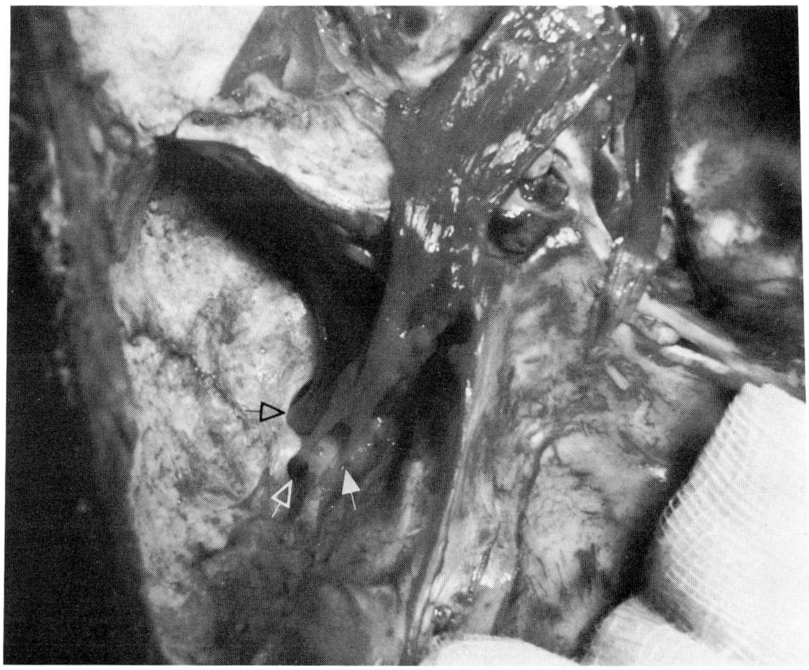

Fig. 16-60. Photograph of floor of middle fossa at necropsy. Dura has been stripped from the middle fossa but not from vessels that are reflected forward. Lesser superficial petrosal nerve (solid white arrow) enters canaliculus innominatus between foramen spinosum (open white arrow) and foramen ovale (open black arrow).

CANALICULUS INNOMINATUS (CANAL OF ARNOLD)

Gross anatomy

The canaliculus innominatus is a small canal occasionally found a few millimeters posterior to the foramen ovale and medial to the foramen spinosum (Fig. 16-60).

Structures transmitted. When present, this canal transmits the lesser superficial petrosal nerve, which is a continuation of the tympanic branch of the glossopharyngeal nerve but also contains a few filaments from the facial nerve. In addition, the canal carries preganglionic parasympathetic fibers to the parotid gland via the otic ganglion. When the canal is absent, the lesser superficial petrosal nerve leaves the skull through the foramen ovale (Gray, 1959).

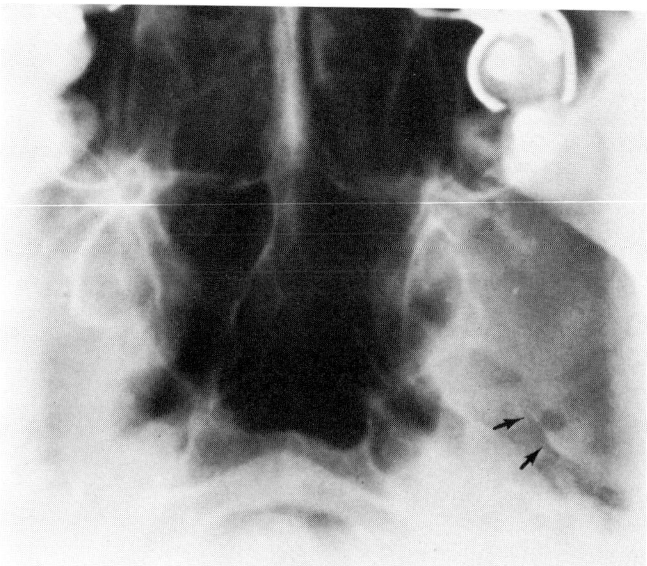

Fig. 16-61. Small canaliculus innominatus (arrows) is seen medial to the foramen spinosum.

Radiology

In the submentovertical projection the small canaliculus innominatus is sometimes seen as a slitlike opening extending toward the foramen ovale between the petrosphenoid synchondrosis and the foramen spinosum (Figs. 16-25, *B*, and 16-61). The canaliculus was seen in about 20% of the fifty submentovertical projections reviewed. A notch can appear in the usual location of the canaliculus (Fig. 16-62). This defect is probably related to the lateral *hook* (Gray, 1959) of the cartilaginous eustachian tube and perhaps also to the lesser superficial petrosal nerve.

FORAMEN LACERUM

Gross anatomy

In the fresh skull the foramen lacerum is actually not a foramen but rather an aperture, whose inferior aspect is filled with fibrocartilage. It is located at the base of the medial pterygoid plate and is bounded anteriorly and laterally by the greater wing of the sphenoid. Posteriorly its boundary is the apex of the petrous portion of the temporal bone, and medially the body of the sphenoid and basiocciput (Figs. 16-22 and 16-23). The posterior end of the pterygoid canal opens in front of the foramen, and the rostral opening of the carotid canal ends on its posterior aspect (Gray, 1959).

The size of the foramen lacerum is quite variable and depends on the extent of the development of the chondral root of the greater sphenoid wing and foramina ovale and spinosum (Figs. 16-32 to 16-35).

Structures transmitted. Until fairly recently anato-

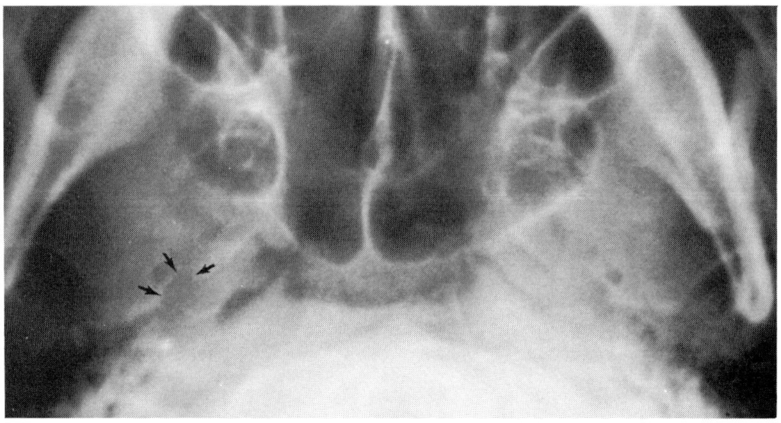

Fig. 16-62. Submentovertical view demonstrates notch (arrows) in usual location of canaliculus innominatus. This defect may be related to the eustachian tube (see text).

mists held the belief that the internal carotid artery entered the skull through the foramen lacerum (Jefferson, 1938). In fact, in the illustrations in Schüller's book on the roentgenology of the skull base published in 1905, the structure is labeled "foramen caroticum." There is now universal agreement that after it leaves the carotid canal the artery merely rests on the endocranial aspect of the cartilage that fills the foramen lacerum.

The structures actually piercing this cartilage, and therefore going through the foramen, are the *meningeal branch of the ascending pharyngeal artery* and *the nerve of the pterygoid canal,* and sometimes a vein that connects the cavernous sinus and pterygoid plexus.

The nerve is described in the discussion of the pterygoid canal (p. 324).

Radiology

The foramen lacerum is seen occasionally in the submentovertical projection as an irregularly shaped lucency between the lateral border of the greater wing of the sphenoid and the petrous apex (Fig. 16-52). The margins of the foramen are frequently difficult to identify because of the cancellous nature of the surrounding bone and the overlying nasopharyngeal air shadows (Fig. 16-28).

PTERYGOID CANAL (VIDIAN CANAL)

Gross anatomy

The pterygoid canal is situated in the body of the sphenoid and connects the foramen lacerum with the pterygopalatine fossa. Its posterior opening is situated below the foramen rotundum in the fused mass of the greater wing and body of the sphenoid and pterygoid plates, that is, the inferior aspect of the front wall of the foramen lacerum (Fig. 16-63) (Frazer, 1965). As the canal extends horizontally forward and medially, it is either straight or curvilinear (Fig. 16-64). The canal frequently has a relation to the floor of the sphenoid sinus (Radoïévitch and Jovanovitch, 1955). The canal widens as it extends forward, and the anterior opening into the pterygopalatine fossa flares like a trumpet (Fig. 16-1, *B*).

In a study of 700 canals, Radoïévitch and Jovanovitch (1955) found that the length averages 14.5 mm with a range of 6 to 20 mm. They found that the width

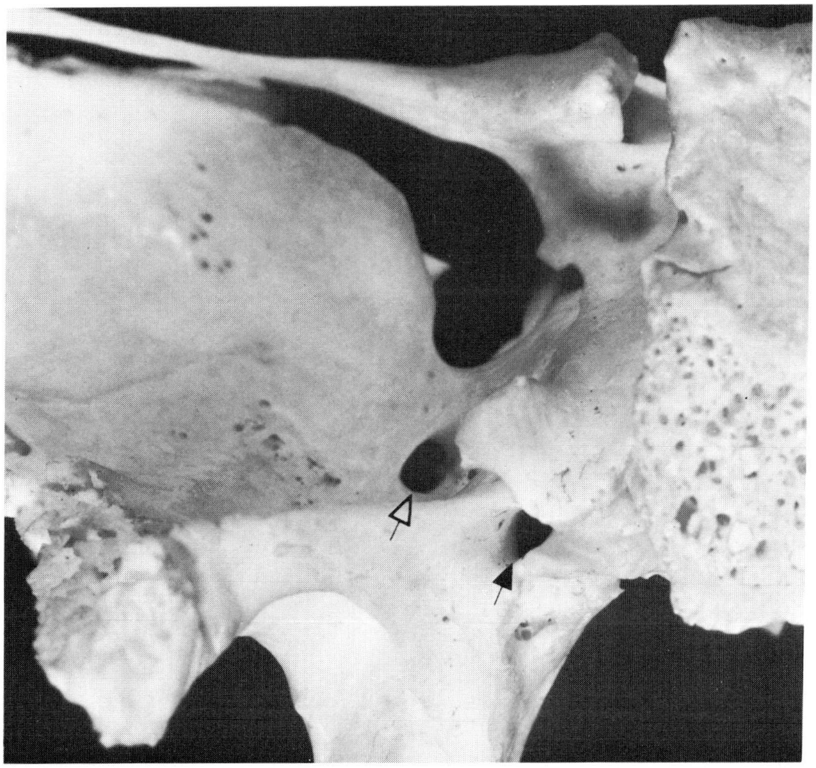

Fig. 16-63. Photograph of endocranial aspect of isolated sphenoid bone. Pterygoid canal (solid arrow) is situated below and medial to foramen rotundum (open arrow) at anterior margin of foramen lacerum. Note that the foramen rotundum is directed laterally and the pterygoid canal medially.

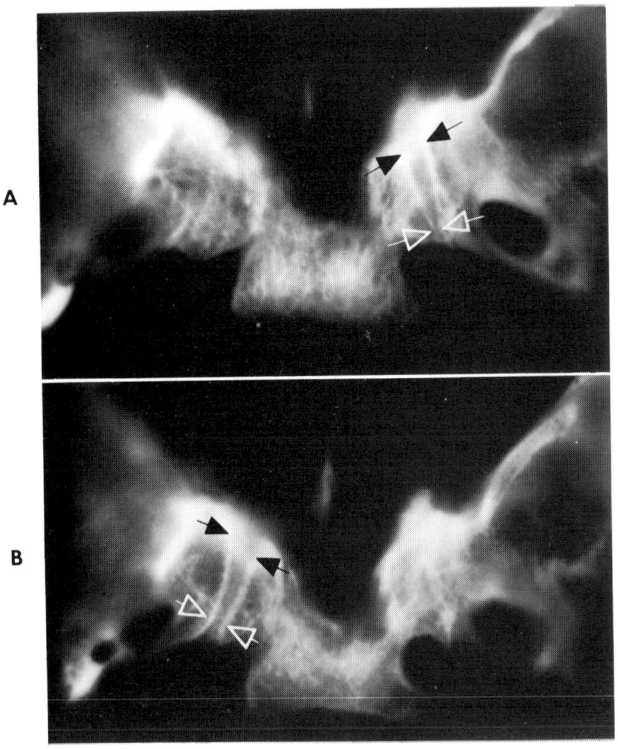

Fig. 16-64. Submentovertical tomograms of two sphenoid bones. In first specimen, **A,** pterygoid canal follows a curvilinear course. In second specimen, **B,** the course is straight. Note that the anterior end of the canal (solid arrows) is wider than the posterior end (open arrows) and that the canal is in the same plane as the foramina ovale and spinosum.

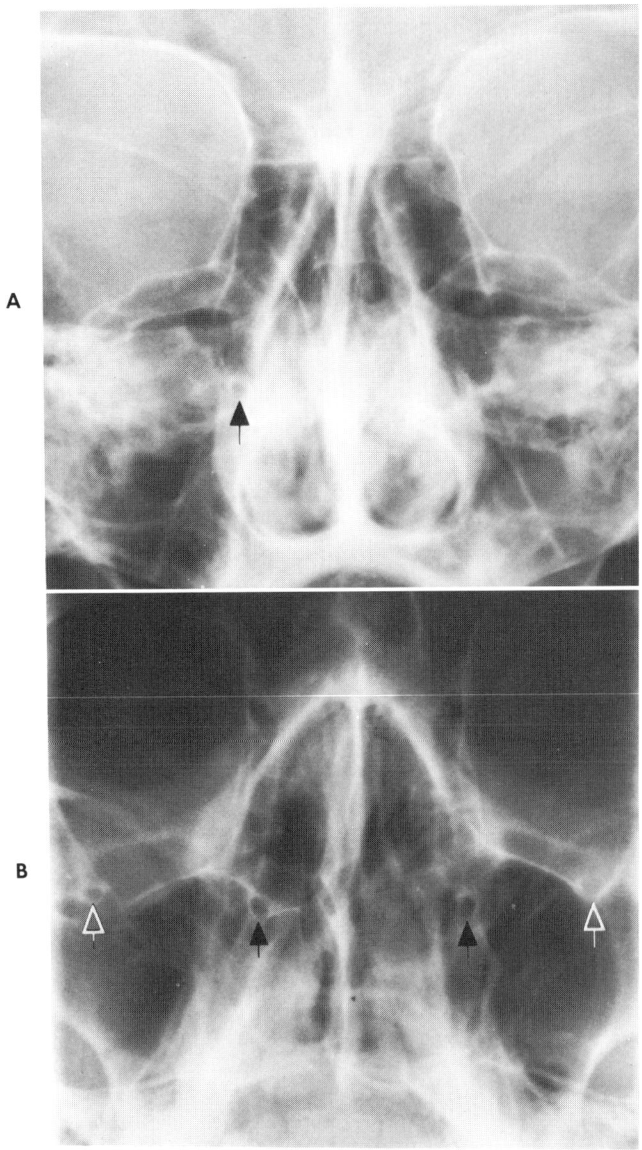

Fig. 16-65. Pterygoid canal (solid arrows) is sometimes visible on standard Caldwell, **A,** and Waters, **B,** views. **A,** Small osteoma is seen in left ethmoid sinus. **B,** More laterally placed inferior orbital foramina (open arrows) may also be seen.

of the canal was most frequently 1.5 mm, ranging from 0.5 to 2.5 mm. The size of the canal in children and adults was not significantly different.

Structures transmitted. The *nerve of the pterygoid canal* (vidian nerve) is an autonomic nerve formed by the union of the greater superficial petrosal and deep petrosal nerves and is joined in the canal by a small ascending branch from the otic ganglion. The greater superficial petrosal nerve contains both sensory and parasympathetic fibers and arises from the geniculate ganglion of the facial nerve. The deep petrosal nerve is a sympathetic nerve and is a branch of the internal carotid plexus. After it exits from the canal, the vidian nerve enters the sphenopalatine ganglion. Fibers from this ganglion are distributed to the lacrimal gland and to the mucous membranes of the nose, pharynx, and palate (Gray, 1959).

The *artery of the pterygoid canal* (vidian artery) arises from the third portion of the internal maxillary artery and is distributed to the upper pharynx and eustachian tube. An inconstant branch from the petrous portion of the internal carotid artery sometimes anastomoses with this vessel and is also called the artery of the pterygoid canal (Gray, 1959).

Radiology

The pterygoid canal can be visualized on routine Caldwell (Fig. 16-65, *A*) and Waters (Fig. 16-65, *B*) projections, on which it appears as a 1 to 2 mm round lucency with sclerotic margins. It is more clearly seen with frontal tomography (Fig. 16-2). Its relation to the foramen rotundum and its curvilinear course may both be appreciated on submentovertical tomograms (Figs.

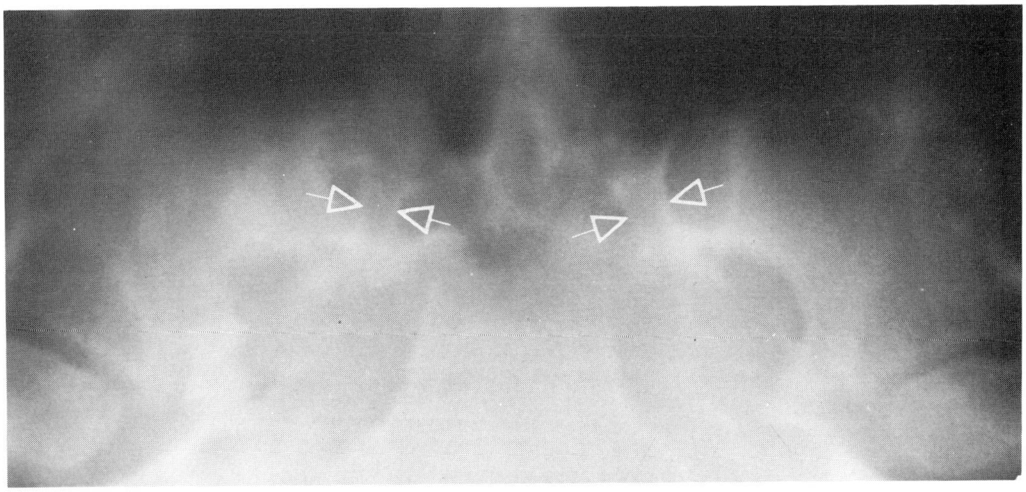

Fig. 16-66. Submentovertical tomogram demonstrates that pterygoid canals (arrows) may be correctly identified by their medial angulation although they are unusually short. Optic and rotund canals (foramina) are projected in same region but are both directed laterally.

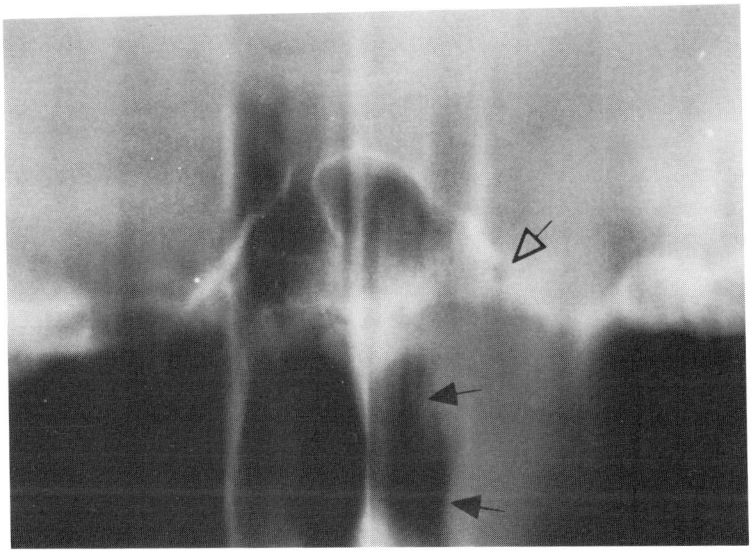

Fig. 16-67. Carcinoma of nasopharynx displaces nasopharyngeal air column medially (solid arrows) and has caused sclerotic reaction around left pterygoid canal (open arrow) and sphenoid sinus.

16-64, *A*, and 16-66), on which the medial angulation is also evident.

Embryology and congenital anomalies

In the embryonic skull the two pterygoid processes are separate. These fuse to enclose the neurovascular bundle of pterygoid vessels and thus form the pterygoid canal (Frazer, 1965).

In 95% of skulls, the pterygoid canal has a forward and medial angulation (Radoïévitch and Jovanovitch, 1955). The angulation of the canal is not generally appreciated (Gray, 1959). In the remaining 5% the canal is straight. The medial angulation varied from 15° to 25° in a few of our specimens.

In 33% of the skulls studied by Radoïévitch and Jovanovitch (1955), the roof of the pterygoid canal was formed by the floor of the sphenoid sinus (Fig. 16-2). This proximity occurred most frequently in association with large lateral extensions of the sinus. The canal may cause an elevation on the floor of the sinus. With pneumatization of the medial pterygoid plate, the pterygoid canal is almost completely surrounded by the sphenoid sinus, a finding in 3% of the material of Radoïévitch and Jovanovitch (1955). In 7% of skulls,

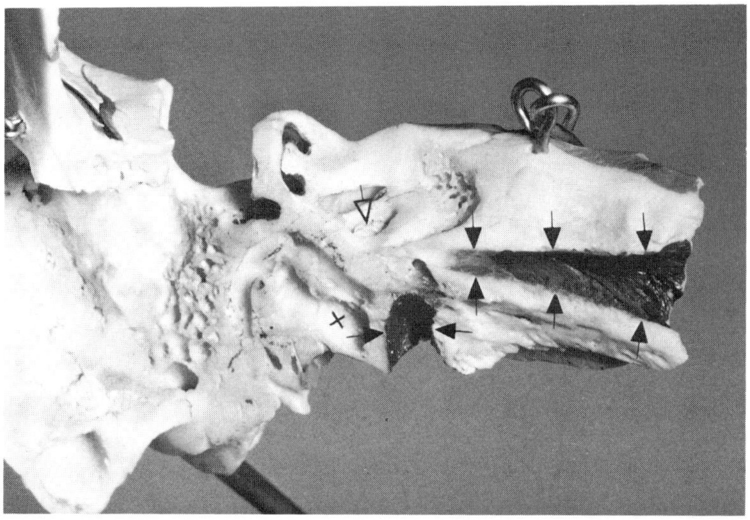

Fig. 16-68. Photograph of dissected petrous bone that has been opened along axis of facial and carotid canals and tympanum. Relation of carotid canal (solid arrows) to cochlea (open arrow) and tympanum (X) is shown.

A

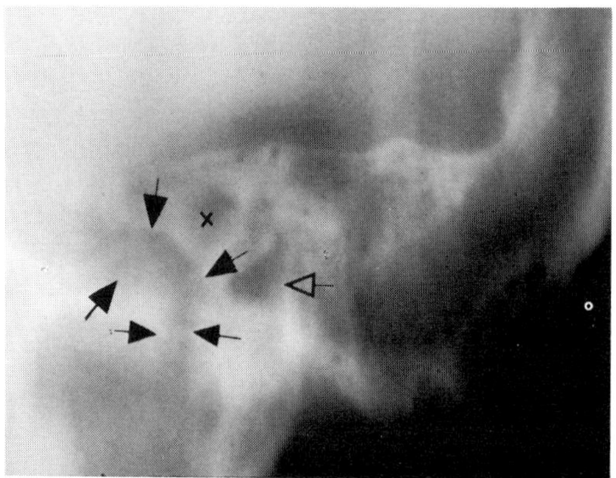

B

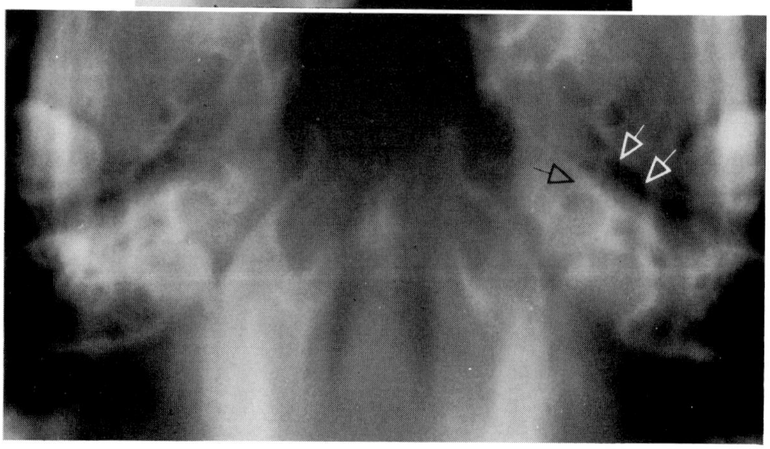

Fig. 16-69. Tomograms of petrous bone demonstrate relation of carotid canal to adjacent structures. **A,** In tomogram obtained in Stenvers projection, carotid canal (solid arrows) is closely related to cochlea (X), near bend of canal, and to jugular fossa (open arrow). **B,** In submentovertical view, lateral wall of carotid canal (open black arrow) forms medial wall of osseous portion of eustachian tube (open white arrows).

these workers also found a close relation between the posterior ethmoid cells and the pterygoid canal. The superior wall of the canal was deficient in 6% of their specimens, but the vessels within the canal were still surrounded by periosteum. These authors therefore postulated that sphenoid or ethmoid sinus disease may occasionally cause "vidian neuralgia" (Vail, 1932).

Pathology

The pterygoid canal is sometimes eroded by nasopharyngeal tumors, which may also result in sclerotic reaction (Fig. 16-67). Internal carotid artery aneurysms sometimes erode its walls.

CAROTID CANAL

Gross anatomy

The carotid canal is situated in the inferior aspect of the petrous portion of the temporal bone and leads from the neck to the middle fossa (Fig. 16-68). Its exocranial opening is situated just anteromedial to the jugular foramen (Figs. 16-22 and 16-25, *A*). The canal first ascends vertically a few millimeters in front of and medial to the tympanic cavity and cochlea (Fig. 16-69, *A*). It then bends 90° and continues medially, anteriorly, and slightly downward, medial to the osseous portion of the eustachian tube (Figs. 16-25, *A,* and 16-69, *B*). The horizontal portion of the canal is wider anteriorly although, of course, the carotid artery does not change caliber within it (Figs. 16-68 and 16-70). Ossification of the roof of this segment of the canal varies considerably in extent and may be incomplete. The endocranial opening and termination of the canal are at the petrous apex, adjacent to the posterior border of the foramen lacerum (Fig. 16-71). At this point the carotid artery enters the cranial cavity (middle fossa) between the lingula and the petrosal process of the body of the sphenoid.

Measurements. In skulls the average width of the

A

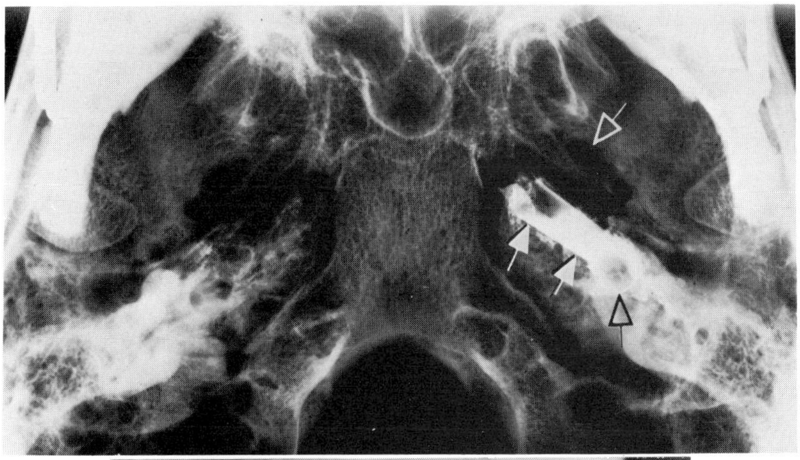

B

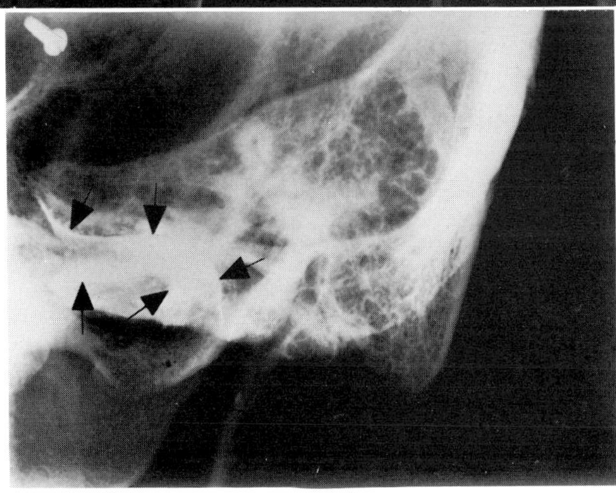

Fig. 16-70. Roentgenograms of skull in which left carotid canal has been filled with barium in submentovertical, **A,** and Stenvers, **B,** projections. **A,** Axial view of vertical segment of canal (open black arrow) is obtained in basal projection. Horizontal portion (solid arrows) widens anteriorly and ends at coronal level of foramen ovale (open white arrow). **B,** Both the vertical and the horizontal segments of canal (solid arrows) are seen in Stenvers projection.

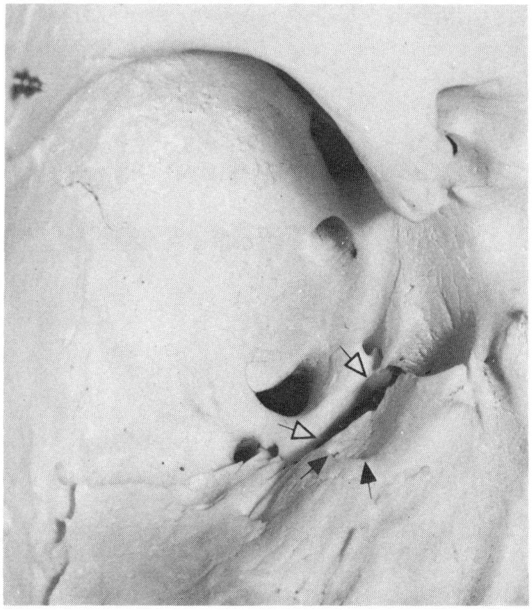

Fig. 16-71. Photograph of middle fossa of skull demonstrates endocranial opening (solid arrows) of carotid canal at posterior aspect of foramen lacerum (open arrows).

carotid canal at the bend is 5.5 mm (range 5 to 6.5 mm). This measurement correlates with measurements of the carotid artery on angiograms after correction for magnification (4 to 5 mm) and addition of 0.5 mm for the thickness of the wall of the artery. The length of the canal is 3 to 4 cm (Lindblom, 1936).

Structures transmitted. The *internal carotid artery* passes from the neck to the middle fossa through the carotid canal. During its course in the canal, the carotid artery gives rise to one or two caroticotympanic branches, which enter the tympanic cavity, as well as the artery of the pterygoid canal, or vidian artery. An extension of the dura mater surrounds the carotid artery in the canal.

Several small veins, which begin as extensions from the cavernous sinus, surround the carotid artery in the canal and drain from the cavernous sinus into the internal jugular vein (Knott, 1882; Gray, 1959). At the bend the veins are situated on the inner aspect of the artery (Lindblom, 1936).

The *internal carotid nerve,* a continuation of the superior cervical ganglion of the sympathetic trunk, divides into two branches in the canal. These branches lie on the medial and lateral aspects of the artery. The medial branch becomes the cavernous plexus, which is distributed with the cerebral arteries and the third, fourth, and fifth cranial nerves. The lateral branch forms the internal carotid plexus, which sends branches to the artery and to the abducent and trigeminal nerves and gives rise to the deep petrosal nerve. The latter joins the greater superficial petrosal nerve to form the vidian nerve (Gray, 1959).

Radiology

The full axial view (Figs. 16-45 and 16-70, *A*) is the only standard projection that demonstrates the carotid canal. The full length of the canal is visible in the Stenvers projection (Fig. 16-70, *B*). In both of these views, the canal is more clearly visible on tomograms (Fig. 16-69). A more detailed presentation of the tomographic anatomy of the canal is available in Chapter 19, where its appearance in the mastoid views is also discussed. In the standard basal projection the vertical portion of the canal is not always visible and sometimes appears as a foramen (Fig. 16-72). Occasionally a 30° caudad angulation of the central ray in the axial view may show the canal to better advantage (Lindblom, 1936). The more medial or horizontal portion of the canal may not be visible in the basal projection because it is surrounded by a spongy bone. Decker (1960) suggested a 10° to 15° rotation of the head to the same side in order to enhance the image of this segment of the canal.

Rumbaugh and Potts (1966) devised an axial view of this portion of the canal. In the lateral projection the head is rotated 30° to the contralateral side (Fig. 16-73). Because of the variable course of the canal, fluoroscopy may sometimes be necessary to obtain this projection.

Lindblom (1936) noted that the narrowest point in the canal is the transverse diameter of the bend. In adults he found the values for the width of the carotid canal at this point to be: axial projection, average 6.5 mm (range 5.5 to 7.0 mm); frontal projection, average 7.5 mm (range 6.5 to 9.0 mm). In children less than 10 years of age, the values were about 1 mm less. On fifty basal projections the vertical portion of the canal was seen well enough for measurement unilaterally in 28% and bilaterally in 40%. Most of the canals were 6 mm wide. This dimension also represented the average, with a range of 5 to 8 mm. When the canal is measured, note should be made of the fact that the osseous segment of the eustachian tube may occasionally be as wide as the proximal horizontal carotid canal and therefore be confused with it (Fig. 16-69, *B*).

Embryology and congenital anomalies

The development of the carotid canal in the alicochlear commissure has been described. (See discussion of embryology and the foramen ovale, p. 305, and also Chapter 7.)

Complete absence of the carotid canal is associated with agenesis of the internal carotid artery (Evans,

A

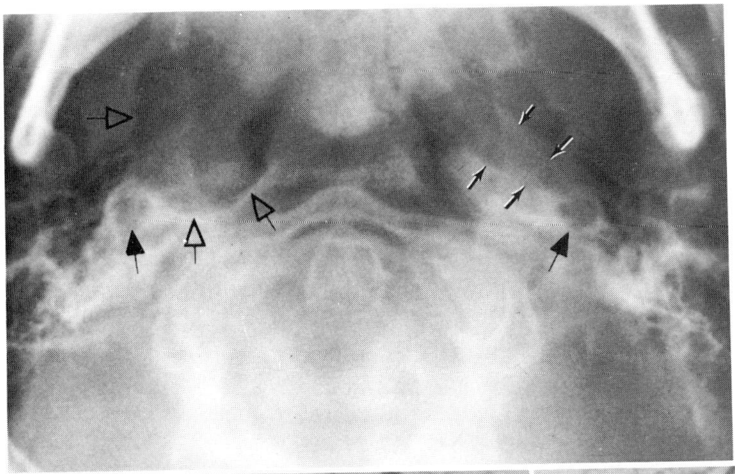

Fig. 16-72. Middle and posterior fossa meningioma in 16-year-old boy. **A,** Submentovertical roentgenogram reveals lytic defect (open arrows) involving medial aspect of floor of middle fossa and petrous apex. Vertical portion of carotid canal (solid arrows) is not affected and appears as a foramen bilaterally. Horizontal segment of canal is normal on the left (small arrows) but destroyed on the right. Selective internal carotid angiograms in frontal, **B,** and lateral, **C,** projections reveal downward displacement of horizontal segment of petrous portion of internal carotid artery (open arrows). Extradural portion of internal carotid is displaced medially and stretched.

B

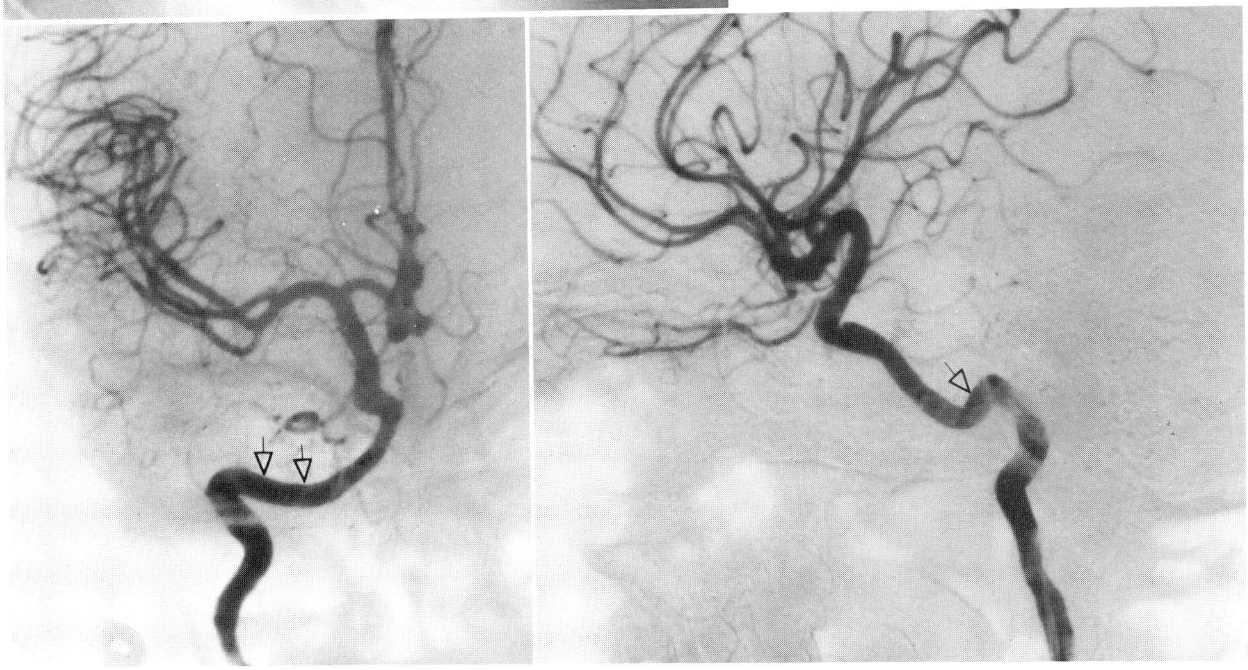

C

A

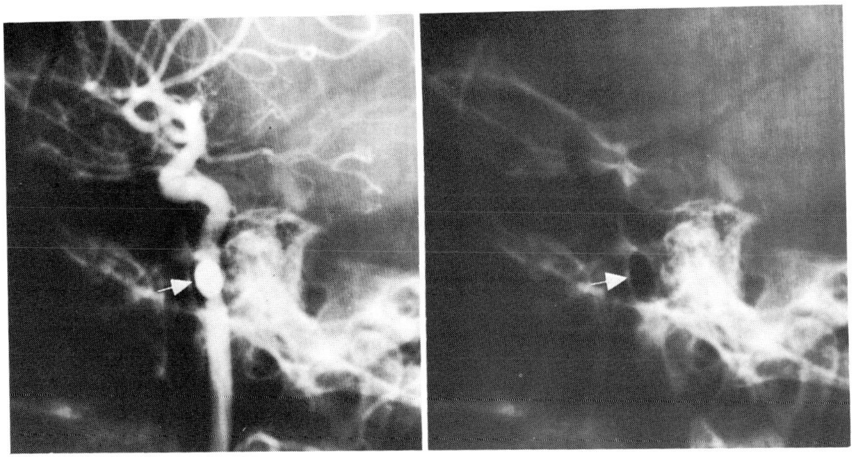

B

Fig. 16-73. Axial study of medial portion of carotid canal in rotated lateral view. **A,** Arteriogram provides axial projection of internal carotid artery as it passes forward in petrous bone (arrow). **B,** Plain roentgenogram in position of angiography demonstrates axial view of carotid canal (arrow). Head is rotated 30° away from injected side. (From Rumbaugh, C. L., and Potts, D. G.: Amer. J. Roentgen. **98:** 525-534, 1966.)

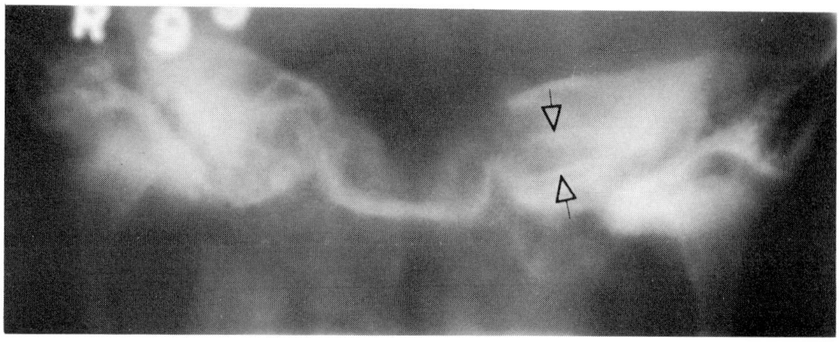

Fig. 16-74. Frontal tomogram through petrous bone demonstrates normal left carotid canal (arrows). Structure is not visible on the right. Complete congenital absence of right internal carotid artery was demonstrated angiographically. (Courtesy David O. Davis, M.D., Salt Lake City, Utah.)

1956) (Fig. 16-74). Only four examples of bilateral absence of the internal carotid arteries and canals, which were proved by dissection of the petrous bones, have been reported by Lie (1968). In the case reported by Fisher (1914), the basilar artery was enlarged and supplied the anterior and middle cerebral arteries through the posterior communicating arteries bilaterally. The ophthalmic arteries arose from the posterior communicating and middle cerebral arteries. Several cases of unilateral absence of the internal carotid artery and carotid canal are also cited by Lie (1968). In one of these, dysplasia rather than absence of the canal was described.

A clinically important, but previously unrecognized, anomaly of the carotid artery and canal has recently been described by Scanlan (in press). The internal carotid artery may pass through the middle ear in the petrous portion of its course (Fig. 16-75, *A*). The artery is tapered in the upper cervical region; it enters the cranium posterior to the external auditory meatus and ascends between the facial canal and the jugular bulb (Fig. 16-75, *B*). It then enters the middle ear and bends sharply forward to reach the carotid canal. The vertical portion of the carotid canal is absent in these patients. The horizontal segment has a crescent shape and a sclerotic rim on lateral tomograms.

A

B

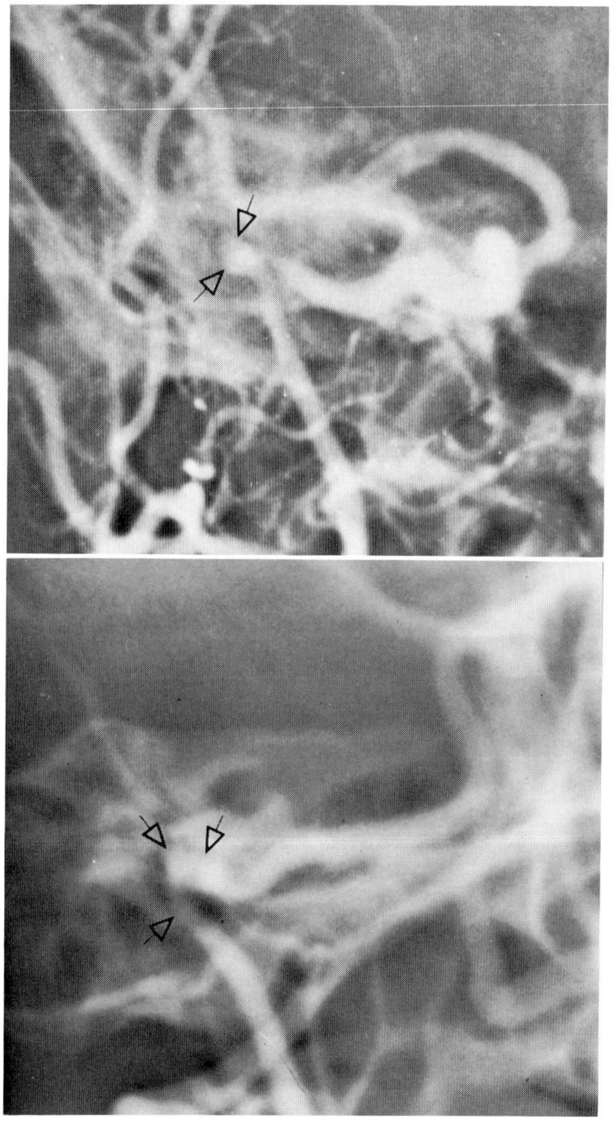

Fig. 16-75. Anomalous course of internal carotid artery through middle ear. **A,** Frontal projection of right common carotid angiogram demonstrates that internal carotid artery enters skull lateral to its usual position. The artery first ascends higher than horizontal portion and at this point is within tympanic cavity (arrows). It narrows within temporal bone and then widens intracranially. **B,** Stenvers projection from brachial angiogram of another patient shows internal carotid artery again narrowing in temporal bone and making hairpin turn in middle ear (arrows). (Courtesy Robert Scanlan, M.D., Los Angeles, Calif.)

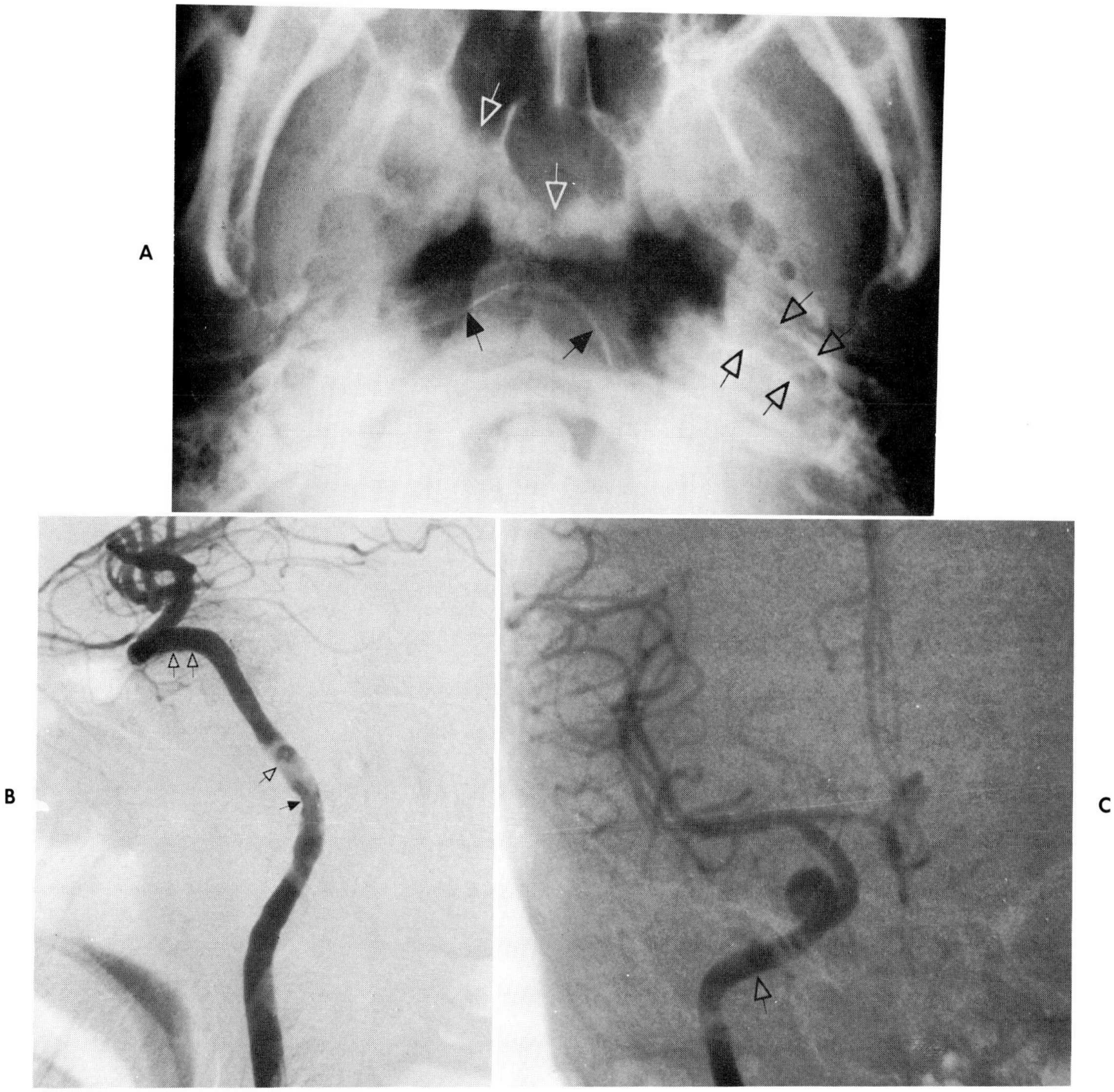

Fig. 16-76. Nasopharyngeal carcinoma with extensive destruction of base of skull. **A,** Submentovertical view shows erosion of posterior aspect of sphenoid sinus (open white arrows). Horizontal portion of left carotid canal (open black arrows) is normal but destroyed on the right. Hyoid bone (solid arrows) is well seen because of erosion of base. Selective internal carotid angiogram in magnified lateral, **B,** and frontal, **C,** projections reveals marked upward displacement of horizontal segment (single open arrow) of petrous portion of internal carotid artery. In lateral projection, irregularity of carotid artery in region of bend (solid arrow) is apparent. Cavernous portion of internal carotid artery (double open arrows) is also elevated.

Pathology

Enlargement. In *arteriovenous malformations* predominantly supplied by the carotid artery, enlargement of the carotid canal can be seen on basal roentgenograms (Rumbaugh and Potts, 1966). This enlargement may be most evident in the vertical portion of the canal, since it has been shown that the width of the canal corresponds quite closely to the width of the carotid artery at this point. Enlargement of the carotid canal may also take place with *aneurysms* of the cavernous portion of the internal carotid artery (Fig. 16-45).

Lindblom (1936) described bilateral enlargement of the carotid canals in a case of *trigeminal neurinoma.* The tumor extended under the lesser wing of the sphenoid and apparently compressed the more rostral internal carotid arteries. Enlargement of the petrosal segments of the arteries was confirmed angiographically.

Table 16-1. Intrapetrous internal carotid artery aneurysms

Authors	*Age*	*Sex*	*Clinical presentation*	*Roentgen findings*	*Pathology*	*Comment*
Pierini and Agra (1954)	52	M	Epistaxis, hearing loss, tinnitus, right facial atrophy and hypesthesia; history of syphilis	Angiogram—aneurysm at bend	—	Possible luetic origin; preganglionic section right fifth and ninth nerves 7 years prior to current symptoms
Barrett and Lawrence (1960)	26	M	Profuse left aural hemorrhage 6 weeks after mastoidectomy for chronic ear infection	Angiogram—saccular aneurysm extending from proximal carotid canal to operative defect	—	Chronic infection may have exposed artery to operative trauma
Pecker et al., (1960)	20	M	Extraocular palsies following fall on occiput	Destruction floor middle fossa and petrous apex; angiogram—huge intrapetrous aneurysm	—	Traumatic aneurysm
Guirguis and Tadros (1961)	19	M	Left temporal headaches, dysphagia, diplopia, tinnitus, deafness, paralysis left sixth through ninth and twelfth nerves	Erosion left petrous apex	4 cm saccular aneurysm; endothelium eroded, media replaced by fibrous tissue	Apparently congenital aneurysm
Hiranandani et al. (1962)	40	M	Intermittent hemorrhage right ear; 6-year history otitis media	Sclerosis right temporal bone; angiogram—"normal"	4 × 3 × 3 cm aneurysm eroding carotid canal; histology: arteriosclerotic changes	Questionable influence of infection; authors thought etiology was arteriosclerotic
Harrison et al. (1963)	34	M	Left-sided headache and facial numbness; complete fifth nerve palsy	Erosion of petrous apex and adjacent middle fossa; angiogram—lobulated saccular aneurysm extending to petrous tip	—	Aneurysm smaller after clamping of common carotid artery
Allen (1967)	43	F	Progressive hearing loss; surgery for suspected otosclerosis	Erosion floor middle fossa; postoperative angiogram—aneurysm petrous and cavernous portions, primitive trigeminal artery	—	Apparently congenital aneurysm
Busby et al. (1968)	29	M	Profuse epistaxis, right deafness, and sixth nerve palsy 2 years after fall	Temporal and basal skull fracture; angiogram—"lesion in petrous canal"	3 × 4 aneurysm in middle of canal	History chronic otitis
Conley and Hildyard (1969)	7	F	Tinnitus, vascular mass in left middle ear; tympanotomy revealed dehiscence in region of jugular bulb	Angiogram—connection between middle ear mass and internal carotid artery	Biopsy of mass: vessel wall	Possible anomalous course internal carotid artery through tympanum
Stallings and McCabe (1969)	9	F	Copious bleeding following myringotomy for purulent otorrhea with cholesteatoma	Angiogram (postoperative)—2 × 3 cm aneurysm arising at lateral portion of bend	—	Although reported as congenital, infection may have been etiologic

Destruction. As the anterior aspect of the petrous bone forms a border of both the middle and the posterior fossae, lesions that arise in either region may cause erosion of the carotid canal. These include meningiomas (Fig. 16-72, *A*), tumors of the gasserian ganglion and clivus, and tumors originating in the region of the jugular foramen.

The petrous portion of the internal carotid artery may be displaced downward when the canal is eroded by *intracranial tumors* (Fig. 16-72, *B* and *C*). Conversely, when the canal is destroyed by *extracranial neoplasms,* upward displacement of the petrous segment of the carotid artery may occur (Fig. 16-76).

Only ten *aneurysms* of the petrous portion of the internal carotid artery have been reported. The patients reported by Rousseau and Spillman (1951) are also described as examples of this entity, but the documentation is not adequate. The ten cases are tabulated (Table 16-1) since they have not been previously collected. The most common predisposing circumstances to the development of an intrapetrous aneurysm are trauma and chronic otitis media. Only a thin bony plate separates the vertical portion of the carotid canal and tympanum (Fig. 16-68). Chronic middle ear infection may therefore lead to erosion of this bone with consequent exposure, or actual erosion, of the carotid artery. Harrison and his co-workers (1963) indicated that the clinical and roentgen findings of these aneurysms depend on the direction of expansion of the aneurysms into the middle ear, posterior fossa, cavernous sinus, or Meckel's cave. Hearing loss, paralysis of different combinations of the third through the twelfth cranial nerves, and aural hemorrhage are the most frequent clinical manifestations. Epistaxis may occur due to erosion of the adjacent eustachian tube. Erosion of the petrous apex and adjacent middle fossa is the most common roentgenographic abnormality.

Fractures. Fractures of the canal may result in the formation of aneurysms; but they may also lead to thrombosis of the internal carotid artery within the canal (Thomson, 1963). Fractures can also be associated with trauma to the cochlea and internal auditory canal (Fig. 39-36, *C* and *D*).

General. The canal is subject to all the metabolic, infectious, and neoplastic processes seen elsewhere in the petrous portion of the temporal bone (Chapter 19).

JUGULAR FORAMEN (FORAMEN LACERUM POSTERIUS, TROU DÉCHIRÉ POSTÉRIEUR)

Gross anatomy

The jugular foramen is a bird-shaped opening in the base of the skull between the lateral edge of the occipital bone and the inferomedial aspect of the petrous pyramid. It is actually a short canal that is oriented anteriorly, laterally, and inferiorly, and it connects the posterior fossa with the upper cervical region. From the endocranial aspect (Fig. 16-77, *A*) it is related to the cerebellum above, the hypoglossal canal medially, the petro-occipital fissure and inferior petrosal sinus anteriorly, and the internal auditory meatus superiorly and laterally. The lateral portion of the exocranial aspect of the foramen is formed by the jugular fossa, which is directly below the thin bony floor of the middle ear (Fig. 16-77, *B*). The stylomastoid foramen and styloid process are lateral to the foramen; the occipital condyle is medial; and the exocranial opening of the carotid canal is anterior. The foramen is separated from the carotid canal by a thin bony ridge in which is situated the opening of the inferior tympanic canaliculus for the tympanic branch of the ninth nerve (Gray, 1959).

The foramen is anatomically divided into an anterior *pars nervosa* and a posterior *pars vascularis* by a fibrous or bony septum. This septum connects the jugular spine of the petrous pyramid with the jugular process of the occipital bone (Di Chiro et al., 1964) (Fig. 16-78). Some authors (Lindblom, 1936; Gray, 1959) have subdivided the foramen into three compartments: the anterior (medial), for the inferior petrosal sinus; the intermediate, synonymous with the pars nervosa; and the posterior (lateral), synonymous with the pars vascularis. The anterior and intermediate portions are frequently not clearly demarcated from each other.

The size and shape of the jugular foramen vary considerably. In their excellent study of this structure, Di Chiro and his co-workers (1964) reviewed the previously recorded measurements. Since the endocranial and exocranial dimensions differ, only the results of those authors (Aubaniac, 1951; Di Chiro et al., 1964) who have measured both diameters are tabulated (Table 16-2). Frequent asymmetry between the foramina was noted, with the right side equal to or larger than the left in 70% to 90% of the cases. Di Chiro and his co-workers (1964) attributed the differences in size of the foramina primarily to the dimensions of the pars vascularis, which in turn was determined by the size of the transverse sinus. They established this relationship by comparing the size of the transverse sinus on angiograms with the size of the jugular foramen on submentovertical roentgenograms. The foramen on the side with the larger transverse sinus was either larger than or the same size as the contralateral foramen; it was never smaller. By obtaining the sum of the width of the pars nervosa (*a* in Fig. 16-79), the pars vascularis (*b*), and the length of the entire foramen (*c*), Di Chiro and his collaborators (1964) established an index for the overall size of the foramen. They found that the range of differences between the two sides was 1 to 8 mm and that the asymmetry was less than

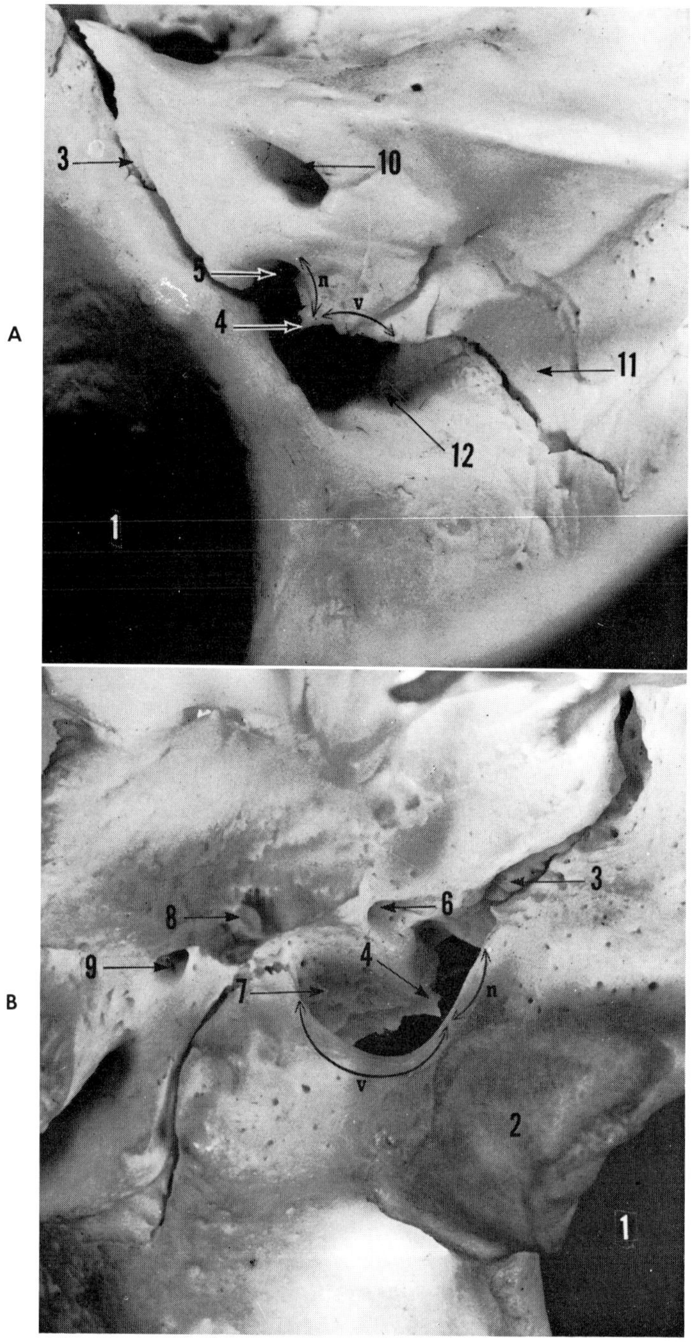

Fig. 16-77. Photographs of base of skull demonstrate endocranial, **A**, and exocranial, **B**, openings of normal jugular foramen. Several structures are identified: *1*, Foramen magnum; *2*, occipital condyle; *3*, petro-occipital fissure; *4*, jugular spine of petrous bone; *5*, pyramidal notch of petrous bone; *6*, pyramidal fossette; *7*, jugular fossa; *8*, styloid process; *9*, stylomastoid foramen; *10*, internal auditory meatus; *11*, groove for lateral sinus; *12*, jugular fossette of occipital bone; *v*, pars vascularis; *n*, pars nervosa. (From Di Chiro, G., Fisher, R. L., and Nelson, K. B.: J. Neurosurg. **21**:447-460, 1964.)

Table 16-2. Size of jugular foramen

	Number	Right				Left			
	of	Length (mm)		Width (mm)		Length (mm)		Width (mm)	
Author	*cases*	*Average*	*Range*	*Average*	*Range*	*Average*	*Range*	*Average*	*Range*
Aubaniac (1951)									
Exocranial	100	16.8	10 to 26	10.2	5 to 15	16.1	11 to 21	9.0	4 to 14
Endocranial	100	15.0	9 to 20	6.7	3 to 16	14.4	10 to 20	6.0	3 to 14
Di Chiro et al. (1964)									
Exocranial	129	16.6	8 to 25	10.7	5 to 15	16.2	6 to 21	9.0	4 to 16
Endocranial	71	14.5	7 to 20	8.2	5 to 14	14.1	6 to 19	7.7	4 to 13

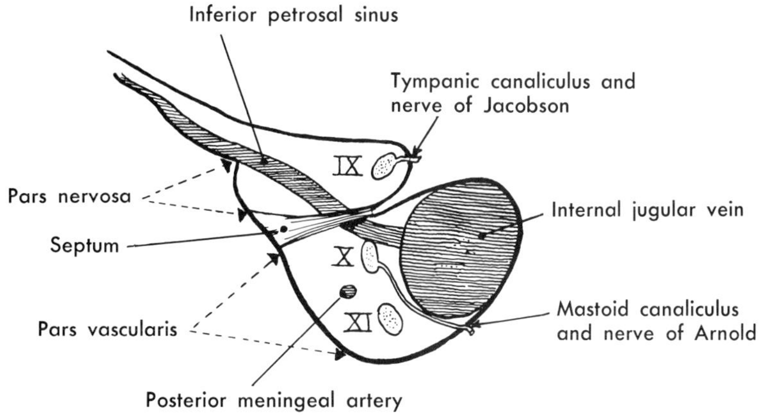

Fig. 16-78. Structures within and passing through jugular foramen. Note that the tenth and eleventh nerves pass through the pars vascularis. (From Di Chiro, G., Fisher, R. L., and Nelson, K. B.: J. Neurosurg. **21**:447-460, 1964.)

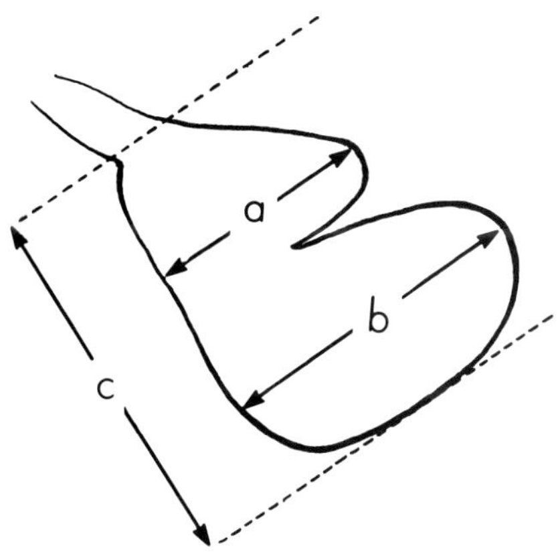

Fig. 16-79. Method of measuring size of jugular foramen. *a,* Width of pars nervosa; *b,* width of pars vascularis; *c,* total length of jugular foramen. (From Di Chiro, G., Fisher, R. L., and Nelson, K. B.: J. Neurosurg. **21**:447-460, 1964.)

12 mm in 95%. A difference of more than 20 mm is considered pathologic.

Structures transmitted

PARS NERVOSA. The *inferior petrosal sinus* leaves the skull through the anterior portion of the jugular foramen. It passes through the pars nervosa between the ninth and tenth nerves (Hayek, 1929) and joins the internal jugular vein within or slightly below the jugular foramen (Knott, 1882).

The *glossopharyngeal (ninth) nerve* is a mixed nerve with both general and special afferent and efferent fibers. It leaves the skull through the pars nervosa and gives off the tympanic nerve (of Jacobson) within the jugular foramen. The tympanic nerve supplies fibers to the parotid gland and mucous membrane of the middle ear and continues as the lesser superficial petrosal nerve. (See discussion of the canaliculus innominatus, p. 322.) The other branches of the ninth nerve are sensory to the pharynx, tonsil, and posterior tongue. Visceral branches supply the carotid body and parotid and mucous glands in the pharynx and posterior portion of the tongue (Gray, 1959).

PARS VASCULARIS. The *internal jugular vein* originates in the lateral portion of the jugular foramen in the form of an expansion called the jugular bulb. The bulb, which occupies the jugular fossa, is a continuation of the transverse sinus and is joined by the inferior petrosal sinus.

The *vagus (tenth) nerve* leaves the skull through the

posterior portion of the jugular foramen in a dural sheath with the accessory nerve but separate from the glossopharyngeal nerve (Fig. 16-78). It is a mixed nerve with both general and visceral afferent and efferent fibers. Its branches are widely distributed to the viscera of the neck, thorax, and abdomen. Within the jugular foramen the vagus gives rise to the *nerve of Arnold,* its auricular branch. The latter then passes posterior to the internal jugular vein to enter the mastoid canaliculus. From here it continues through the petrous bone and communicates with the facial nerve. It is a somatic afferent nerve to the skin behind the auricle and external auditory meatus (Gray, 1959).

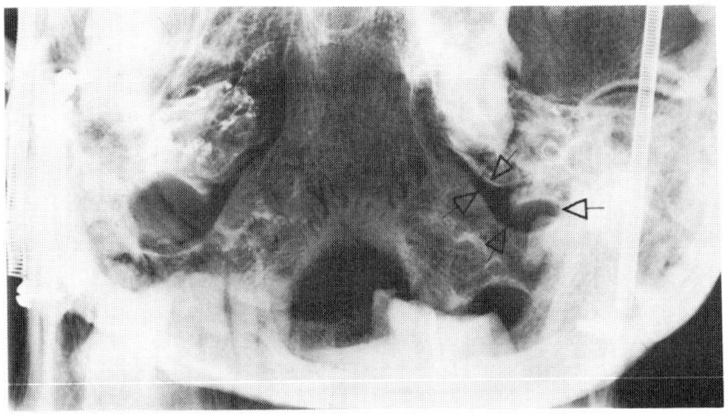

Fig. 16-80. Chaussé II view of dry skull. With skull rotated 10° to the right, axial view of left jugular foramen (arrows) is obtained through the open mouth.

The *accessory (eleventh) nerve* is a motor nerve that is divided into a cranial portion and a spinal portion. The two parts are usually united within the jugular foramen, where they are also in a common sheath with the vagus. After leaving the foramen the cranial portion separates from the spinal and joins the vagus, with which it is distributed to the muscles of the pharynx and larynx. The spinal portion enters the skull through the foramen magnum. It pierces the dura over the jugular bulb and joins the cranial portion for a short distance. It then leaves the skull through the jugular foramen and is distributed to the sternocleidomastoid and trapezius muscles (Gray, 1959).

Meningeal branches of the ascending pharyngeal and occipital arteries enter the skull through the jugular foramen and are distributed to the dura of the posterior fossa.

Radiology

The normal jugular foramen is not visible on standard roentgenograms of the skull, including the full basal or axial view.

For this reason more than twenty different special

A

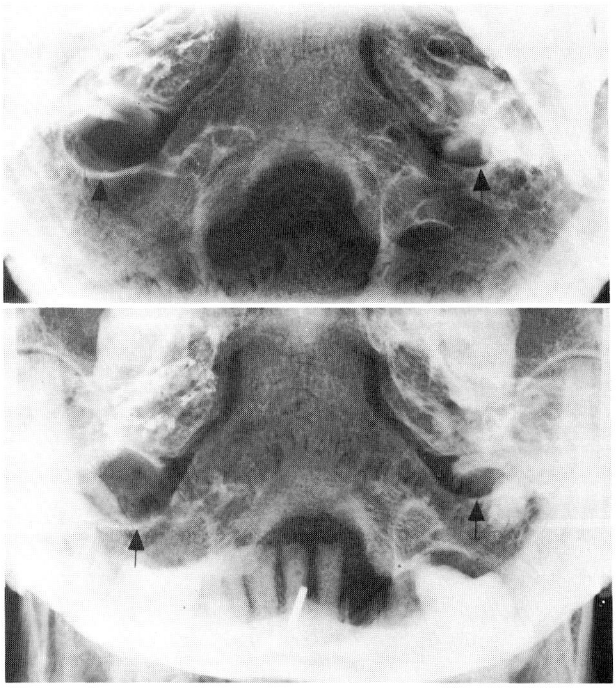

B

Fig. 16-81. Bilateral symmetric projections of jugular foramina (arrows). **A,** Canthomeatal line makes angle of 25° with perpendicular (Eraso projection). **B,** Exposed with mouth open and an angle of 37° (Kim and Capp, 1966). A more axial view is obtained with the larger angle.

projections have been devised for the examination of the jugular foramen. Di Chiro and his group (1964) classified these projections into four groups, which they tabulated: the oblique unilateral (either with or without tomography) and the symmetric bilateral (with or without tomography). The Chaussé II (Fig. 16-80) is an example of a standard oblique unilateral projection. The head of the supine patient is turned 10° toward the side to be examined and extended so that the central ray can be directed through the open mouth at a line that joins the external auditory meatuses (Chaussé, 1950). Three films are exposed with slightly different centration. Fischgold and his co-workers (1954) and Hawkins (1966) utilized unilateral oblique projections with tomography. The patient is examined in the supine position with the median sagittal plane turned 60° (Fischgold et al.) or 45° (Hawkins) away from the side being examined. Lateral tomography has recently been suggested as another useful method for examination of the foramen (Wilner, 1970).

The ideal projection would be coincident with the long axis of the canal. Since the axis may differ on the two sides, however, reproduction of projections is difficult. For this reason symmetric bilateral standard projections (Eraso, 1961; Hawkins, 1966; Kim and Capp, 1966; Strickler, 1966) are preferred (Fig. 16-81), especially in combination with tomography (Csàkàny and Donàth, 1958; Di Chiro et al., 1964). These projections are designed as axial projections of the foramen, which has a downward and forward angulation of approximately 45°. In the tomographic technique of Csàkàny and Donàth (1958), the patient is supine with the head extended so that the canthomeatal line is at a 45° angle to the film. The central ray passes through the open mouth, and the plane of the tomograms passes through the external auditory meatus and 0.5 and 1.0 cm inferior to it (Di Chiro et al., 1964). The projection of Kim and Capp (1966) utilizes the standard 37° angle for the Waters view, which is modified by keeping the patient's mouth open and directing the central ray through the external auditory meatus. The views suggested by Strickler (1966) may be more difficult to reproduce since the angle for the position of the canthomeatal line is not specified. Instead the central ray passes through the open mouth and infratragal notch.

Embryology and congenital anomalies

The space between the basiocciput and the auditory capsule—the foramen lacerum posterius—persists as the jugular foramen in man (Shapiro and Robinson, 1967a).

The septum that separates the jugular foramen into two compartments may ossify (Fig. 16-82). Ossification was complete unilaterally in 13% and bilaterally in 5% of the skulls examined by Di Chiro and his group (1964). The jugular foramen may also be completely surrounded by a bony ring, and in this case it does not communicate with the petro-occipital synchondrosis (Khoo, 1946).

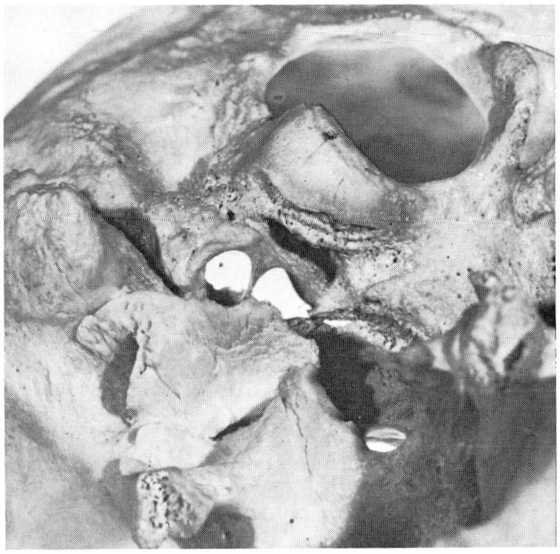

Fig. 16-82. Complete ossification of septum that normally divides jugular foramen into two compartments. (From Di Chiro, G., Fisher, R. L., and Nelson, K. B.: J. Neurosurg. **21**:447-460, 1964.)

The situation of the nerves that pass through the jugular foramen is variable. Hayek (1929) was one of the first to indicate that the orientation in man differs from that of the crocodile, in which the ninth, tenth, and eleventh nerves exit together. He indicated that only the glossopharyngeal nerve leaves the skull through the pars nervosa and that it sometimes notches or actually passes through a separate foramen in the petrous bone.

Inequality in size of the jugular foramina is apparently a late phylogenetic development not exhibited by monkeys but present in anthropoid apes (Wood-Jones, 1931). Two cases of giant jugular fossae were reported by Khoo (1946), in which this structure was approximately 2 cm wide and 2.5 cm deep.

Pathology

Vascular. The vascular portion of the jugular foramen may enlarge in association with *arteriovenous malformations* and aneurysms of the vein of Galen (Di Chiro et al., 1964; Rumbaugh and Potts, 1966). Expansion of the pars vascularis is smooth, with intact cortical margins (Fig. 16-83), and is the result of increased blood flow through the transverse sinus.

Aneurysms of the petrous portion of the internal carotid artery may erode the foramen (Guirguis and Tadros, 1961).

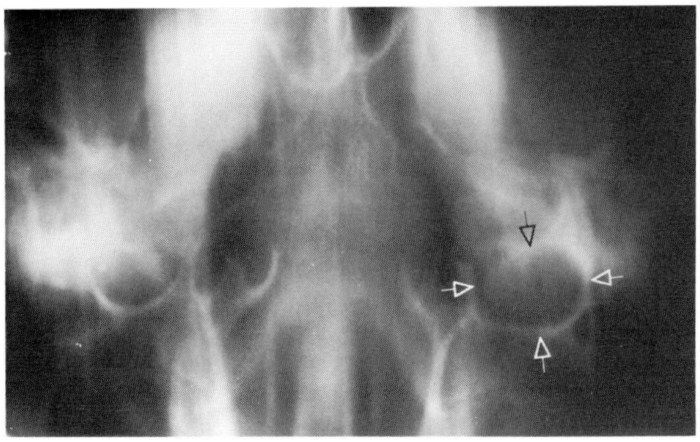

Fig. 16-83. Submentovertical tomogram illustrates marked enlargement of pars vascularis (arrows) of left jugular foramen in a patient with arteriovenous malformation. (From Rumbaugh, C. L., and Potts, D. G.: Amer. J. Roentgen. **98:** 525-534, 1966.)

Neoplasms. *Glomus jugulare tumors* (chemodectomas, nonchromaffin paragangliomas) are the most common tumors to affect the jugular foramen. They arise from small (0.1 to 1.5 mm) glomus bodies of which usually one to three are present in each ear (Guild, 1953). Histologically they are composed of many small capillaries surrounded by epithelioid cells. More than half of these glomera are located in the adventitia of the jugular bulb, but they are also found along the course of the ninth, Arnold's, and Jacobson's nerves. Approximately 25% of them are situated in the mucosa of the cochlear promontory (Guild, 1953). The tumors may thus originate within the jugular foramen (glomus jugulare) or middle ear (glomus tympanum). They may be bilateral; and in one patient simultaneous development with a carotid body tumor was reported (Palacios, 1970).

Clinically they have been found to affect women three times as frequently as they do men. In 316 pa-

A

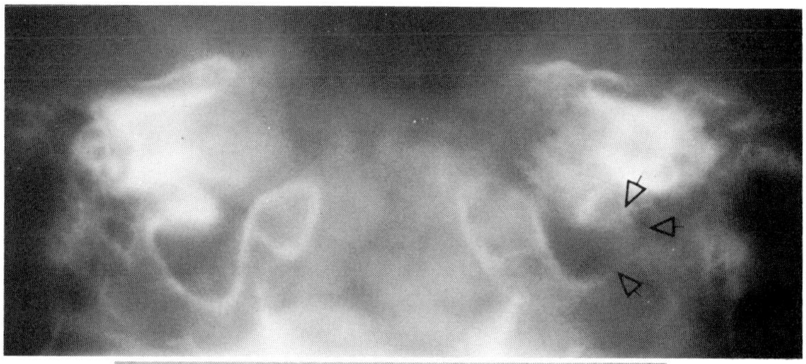

B

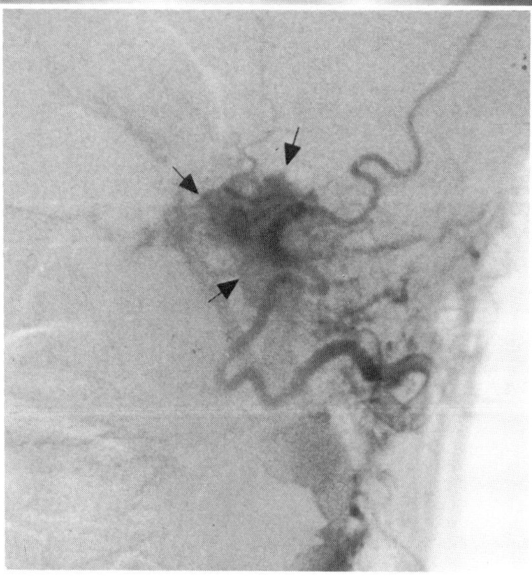

Fig. 16-84. Glomus jugulare tumor. **A,** Frontal tomograms through jugular foramina reveal erosion of cortical margin of left jugular foramen (arrows). Cortical margin of right foramen is well defined. **B,** Selective external carotid angiogram, frontal projection, reveals small uniform tumor stain in area of osseous defect.

tients (Alford and Guilford, 1962) the average age was 49 years and the range was 17 to 85 years. The tumors are characteristically slow growing, with an average symptomatic period of 6 to 7 years prior to diagnosis (Hawk and McCormack, 1959; Alford and Guilford, 1962). The presenting symptoms may be primarily otic, combined otic and neurologic, and (less commonly) primarily neurologic. The most common initial findings are hearing loss, tinnitus, otorrhea, facial paralysis, pain, aural polyps, and palsy of the ninth, tenth, and eleventh nerves (Hawk and McCormack, 1959; Alford and Guilford, 1962). Paralysis of these nerves has been termed the syndrome of the jugular fossa or Vernet's syndrome. It consists of loss of taste

A

B

C

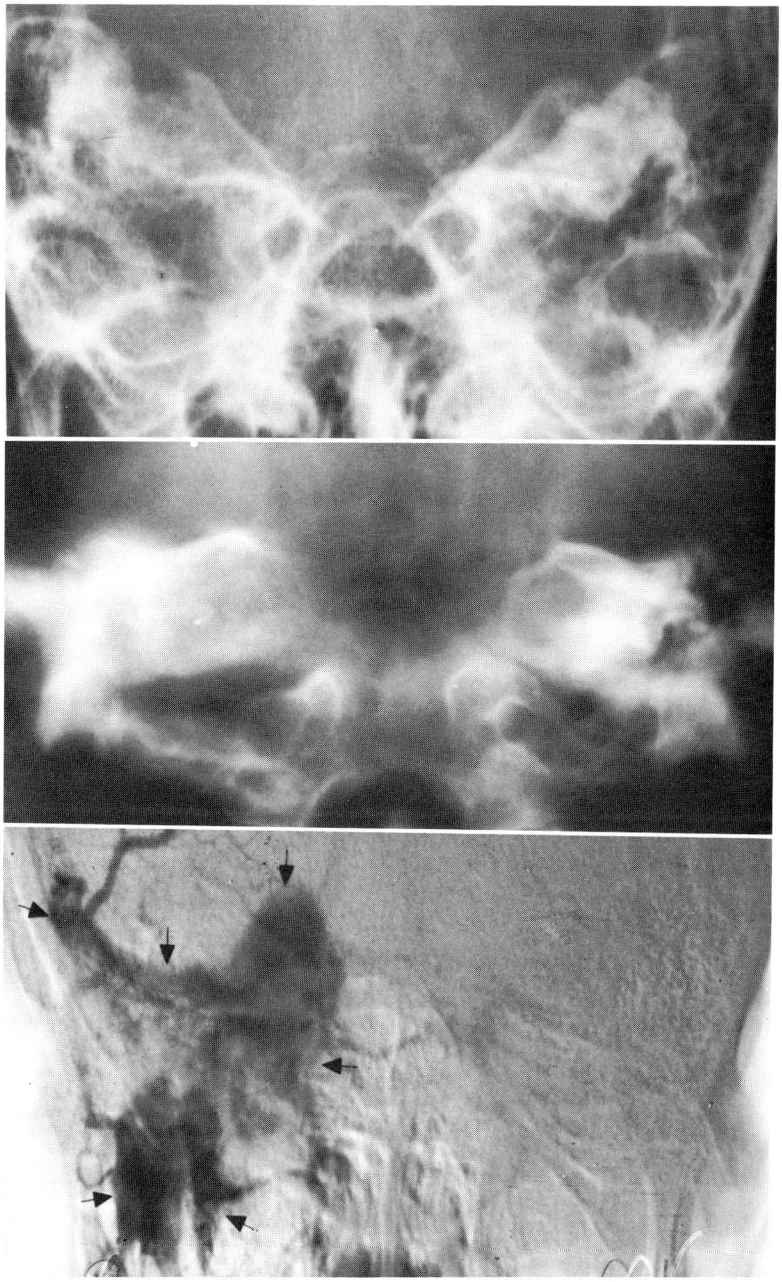

Fig. 16-85. Glomus jugulare tumor. **A,** In Towne projection, irregular destruction of inferior aspect of right petrous bone is apparent. **B,** Anteroposterior tomogram further delineates this erosion. Right jugular foramen is no longer visible. **C,** Selective external carotid angiogram reveals that tumor blush corresponds to area of bone involvement (arrows).

in the posterior third of the tongue (ninth nerve), paralysis of the vocal cord and palate (tenth nerve), and weakness of the trapezius and sternocleidomastoid muscles (eleventh nerve) (Svien et al., 1963). With medial extension of these tumors into the hypoglossal canal, twelfth nerve palsy may also appear in addition to paralysis of the ninth, tenth, and eleventh nerves. The resultant symptom complex is known as the Collet-Sicard syndrome. One of the patients described by Hawkins (1966) presented with a subarachnoid hemorrhage.

The *roentgenology* of glomus tumors has been reviewed by Rice and Holman (1963), Di Chiro and co-workers (1964), Hawkins (1966), Miller and co-workers (1969), Palacios (1970), and others. The roentgenographic features depend on the site of origin (i.e., tympanic or jugular) and the route of invasion; but they do not correlate with the severity or duration of symptoms (Rice and Holman, 1963). The accurate tomographic and angiographic localization of these tumors is important since those arising in the tympanum are much smaller and more easily resectable than those originating in the jugular foramen (Kohut and Lindsay, 1965). When glomus jugulare tumors are examined early, erosion of the margins of the jugular foramen may be the only roentgen finding (Fig. 16-84). As they continue to grow, the jugular foramen becomes enlarged by erosion (Alford and Guilford, 1962; Rice and Holman, 1963; Di Chiro et al., 1964). The erosion characteristically involves the inferior aspect of the medial portion of the petrous bone, and this is optimally demonstrated in the Towne projection (Rice and Holman, 1963) (Fig. 16-85). Erosion may extend anteriorly, into the middle fossa or temporomandibular joint, or

A

B

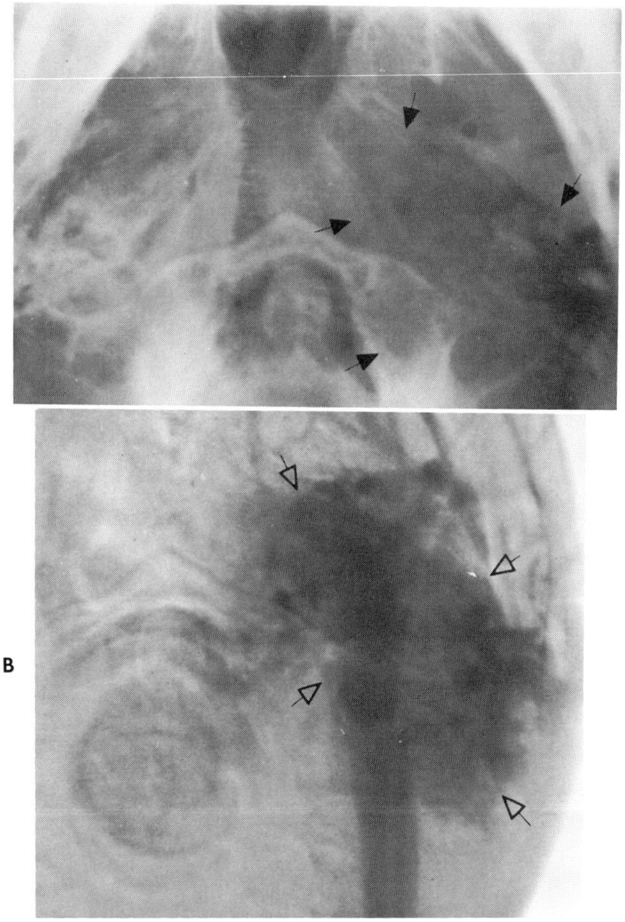

Fig. 16-86. Huge glomus jugulare tumor demonstrates correspondence of tumor blush and bony erosion. **A,** In slightly oblique submentovertical projection, extensive area of reticular bony destruction (arrows) extends from region of jugular foramen to foramen lacerum and petrosphenoid fissure. **B,** Common carotid angiogram in submentovertical view reveals large tumor stain (arrows), which appears to fill interstices of destroyed bone and corresponds to shape of area of destruction.

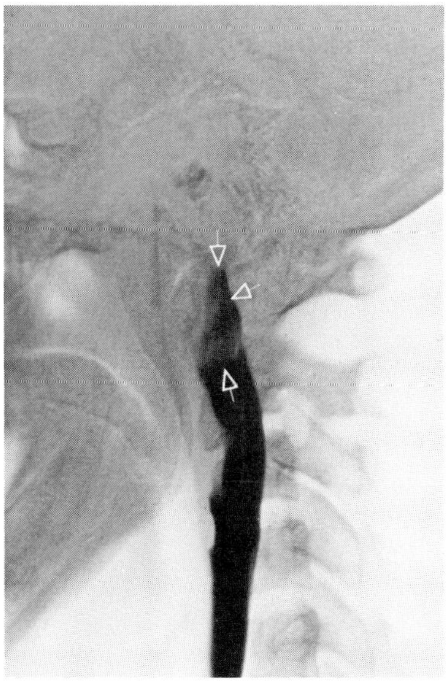

Fig. 16-87. Inferior aspect of glomus jugulare tumor (arrows) is outlined on a jugular phlebogram, lateral projection.

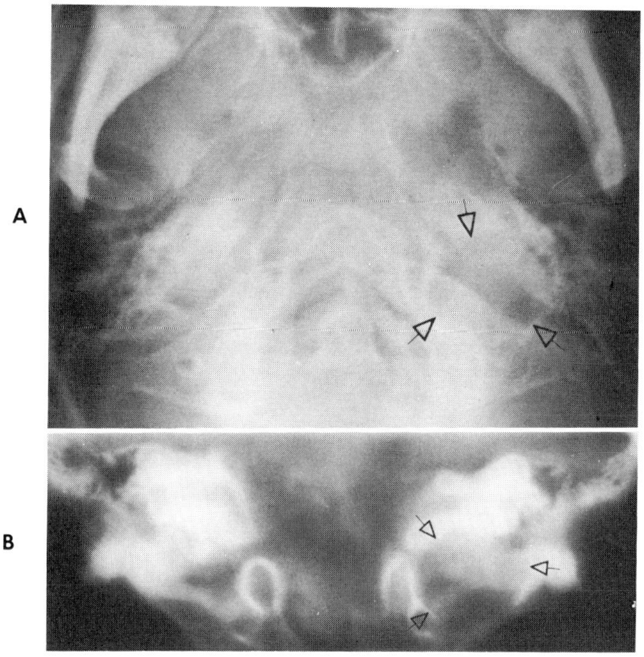

Fig. 16-88. Neurinoma of ninth, tenth, or eleventh cranial nerve in patient with jugular foramen syndrome. **A,** In submentovertical view, large defect (arrows) extends posteriorly from petrous bone. **B,** Frontal tomogram illustrates sharp smooth margins of defect (arrows), which retains a sclerotic border. (Courtesy David O. Davis, M.D., Salt Lake City, Utah.)

posteriorly, to destroy the jugular tubercle of the foramen magnum and the hypoglossal canal (Hawkins, 1966). The erosion is usually infiltrative instead of purely lytic and results in a lacework of bone (Figs. 16-85 and 16-86) rather than a sharply marginated filling defect. Angiography confirms the presence of tumor between the remaining bony trabeculae (Figs. 16-85, *C,* and 16-86, *B*). Clouding or sclerosis of the mastoid air cells has been reported in many of these patients, but the significance of this finding is in question because of the high incidence of the finding in the general population (Di Chiro et al., 1964). Clouding or sclerosis may sometimes occur after destruction of the tympanic membrane (Palacios, 1970).

The blood supply of these tumors frequently arises from the tympanic branch of the ascending pharyngeal artery. Therefore selective angiography of the external as well as of the internal carotid and vertebral arteries is necessary for complete evaluation of these tumors. A characteristic uniform blush outlines the extent of the tumor (Decker, 1960; Hawkins, 1966; Allen, 1967; Palacios, 1970). Jugular venography (Hamberger and Gejrot, 1964; Cornell, 1969) helps to outline the inferior limits of the tumor (Fig. 16-87). These authors have described instances in which fairly large downward extensions were not suspected prior to venography.

Neuromas (neurilemmomas) of the ninth, tenth, and eleventh cranial nerves represent a relatively rare cause of enlargement of the jugular foramen. Fewer than thirty cases have been reported, and reviews have been published by Columella and co-workers (1959) and by Di Chiro and co-workers (1964). These authors found that the exact nerve of origin is difficult to define at surgery and that the tumors may be associated with neurofibromatosis. Smooth uniform enlargement of the jugular foramen, with erosion of the jugular spine, is the characteristic roentgen finding (Di Chiro et al., 1964). The erosion may extend beyond the confines of the foramen (Fig. 16-88), but a smooth sclerotic margin will still be evident. Enlargement of the medial aspect of the foramen may be accompanied by widening of the petro-occipital fissure. The defects produced by these tumors rarely mimic those of glomus jugulare tumors (Fig. 16-89).

Other neoplasms that may sometimes resemble primary tumors of the jugular foramen are *chondromas* (Minagi and Newton, 1969) (Fig. 16-90) and *nasopharyngeal carcinomas* (Fig. 16-91). Other characteristics of these tumors, such as calcification and routes of invasion, are useful in the differential diagnosis.

Many other lesions may involve the jugular foramen. Some of these have been cited by Di Chiro and his group (1964) and include meningioma, chordoma, metastatic carcinoma, cholesteatoma, carcinoma of the tympanic cavity, and vagal body chemodectoma. An osteoclastoma of the jugular foramen was recently reported (Moyes et al., 1970).

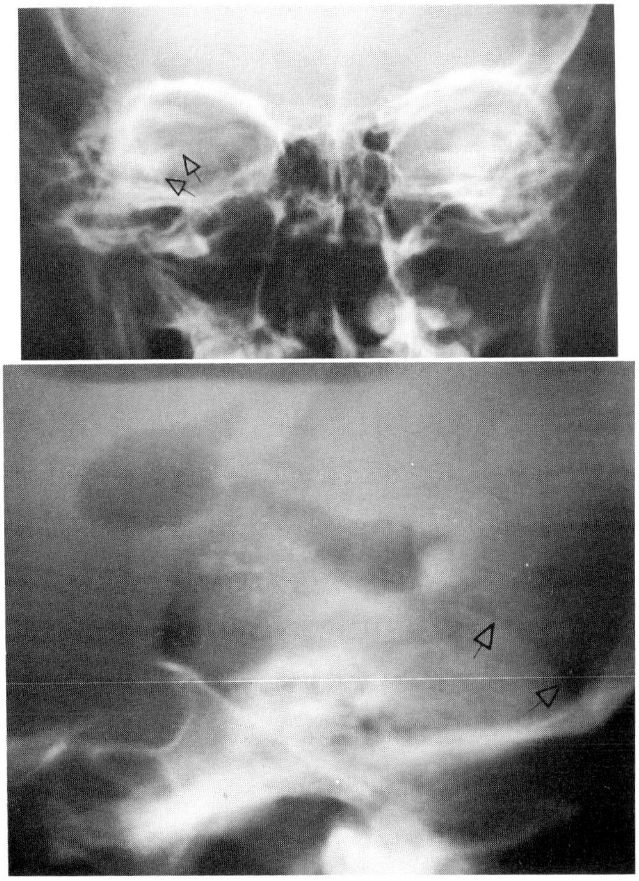

A

B

Fig. 16-89. Neurinoma of eleventh cranial nerve. **A,** Perorbital view of petrous pyramid discloses erosion of inferior aspect of right petrous bone (arrows). Appearance is similar to that of defect caused by glomus jugulare tumors. **B,** Lateral tomogram from pneumoencephalogram reveals upward displacement of air in vallecula and foramen magnum (arrows) by the tumor.

Fractures of the skull base may extend through the jugular foramen (Fig. 39-34, *B*).

GREATER PALATINE FORAMEN

Gross anatomy

The greater palatine foramen is situated in the posterior angle of the palate and connects the pterygopalatine canal with the oral cavity (Fig. 16-22).

Structures transmitted. The greater (descending) palatine artery and the greater (anterior) palatine branch of the sphenopalatine nerve pass through the canal. The nerve and artery supply the gums and mucous membranes of the hard palate and adjacent soft palate (Gray, 1959).

Radiology

The foramen is included in this chapter because it may be visualized on underangulated submentovertical projections (Fig. 16-27, *B* and *C*) in the lateral aspect of the palate anterior to the medial pterygoid plate and lesser palatine foramen. The foramen is angulated downward anteriorly about 20° (Fig. 16-92) and is therefore not visualized in the standard submentovertical projection. It appears as a round or oval lucency approximately 2 mm in diameter (Fig. 16-28).

LESSER PALATINE FORAMEN

Gross anatomy

The lesser palatine foramen, which may be multiple, is situated in the pyramidal process of the palatine bone posterior to the greater palatine foramen (Fig. 16-22).

Structures transmitted. The foramen transmits the lesser palatine nerve and twigs from the greater palatine artery. The nerve and artery are distributed to the soft palate, uvula, and tonsil (Gray, 1959).

Radiology

The foramen is included in this chapter because it is sometimes visualized on standard axial projections just anterior to the medial pterygoid plate (Figs. 16-27, *B*

A

B

C

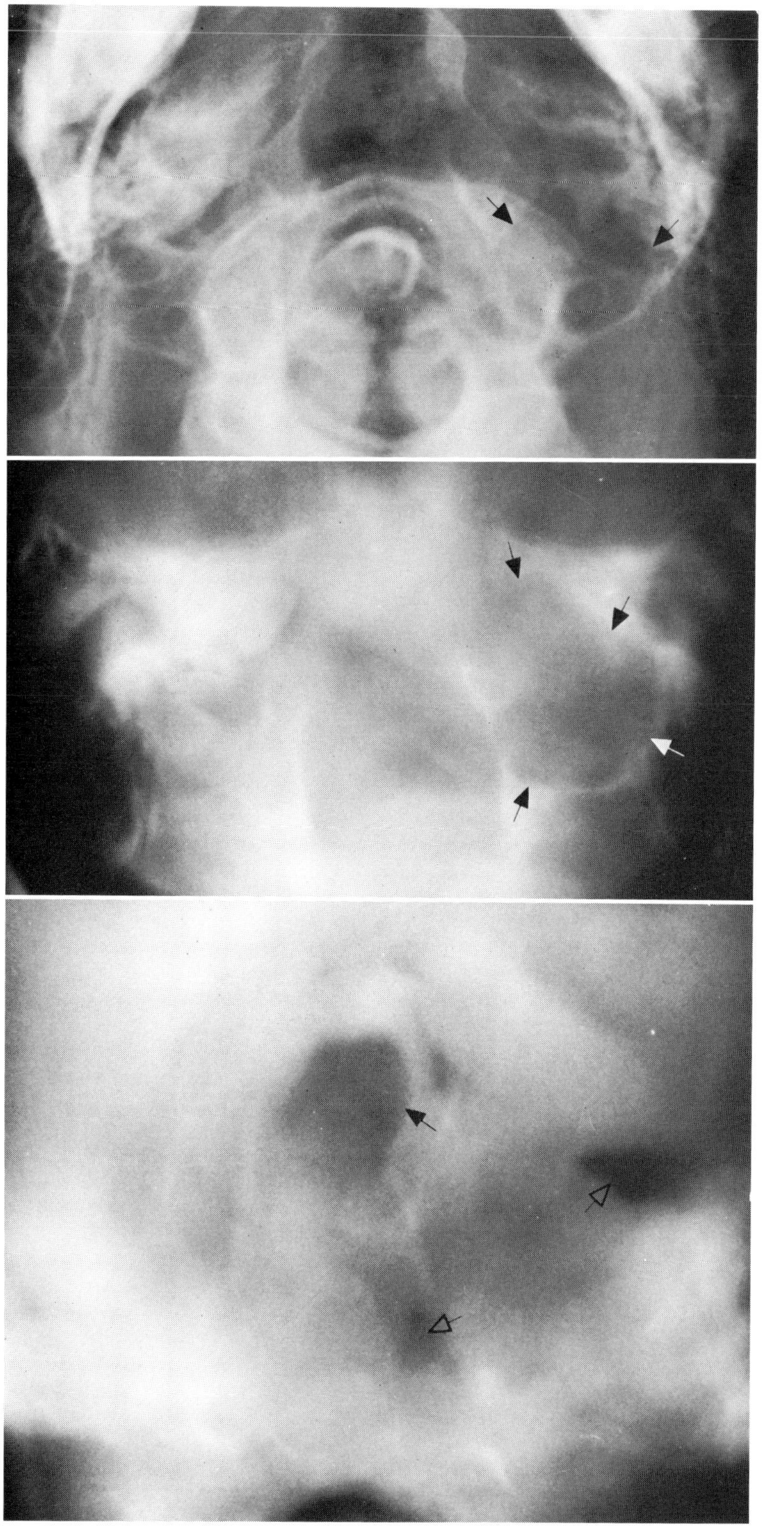

Fig. 16-90. Chondroma of region of jugular foramen. Erosion of left petrous and occipital bones centered on jugular foramen is demonstrated in both the conventional submentovertical projection, **A,** and a submentovertical tomogram, **B.** Smooth margins of defect (arrows) simulate appearance of neurinoma. **C,** Upright tomogram, frontal projection, from pneumoencephalogram shows mass projecting into cerebellopontine angle cistern (open arrows) and distorting lateral aspect of fourth ventricle (solid arrow).

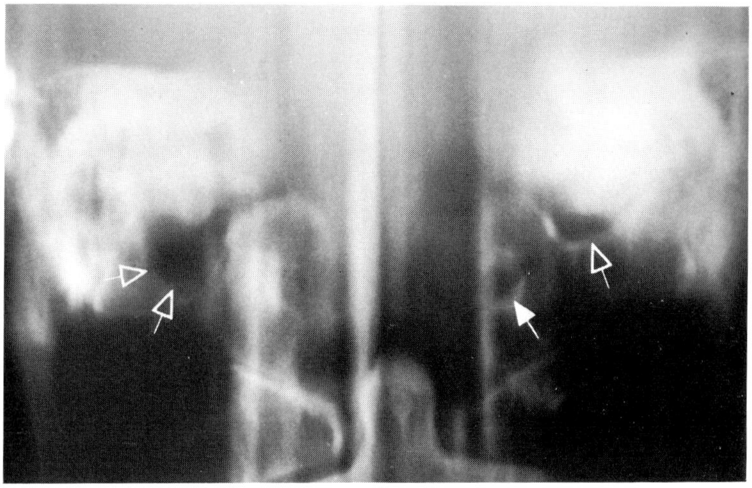

Fig. 16-91. Nasopharyngeal carcinoma simulates appearance of early glomus jugular tumor. (Compare with Fig. 16-84.) Cortical margins of inferior aspect of right jugular foramen (double open arrows) are no longer visible. On left, cortical margins are normal (single open arrow). Left hypoglossal canal is normal (solid arrow). Canal on the right has been eroded by the same tumor.

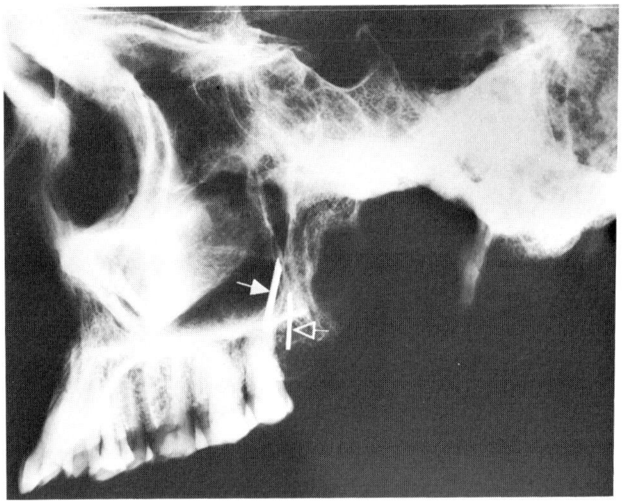

Fig. 16-92. Lateral view of skull in which large pin (solid arrow) has been placed in greater palatine foramen and small pin (open arrow) has been placed in lesser palatine foramen. Forward angulation of the greater palatine foramen is larger than that of the lesser palatine foramen.

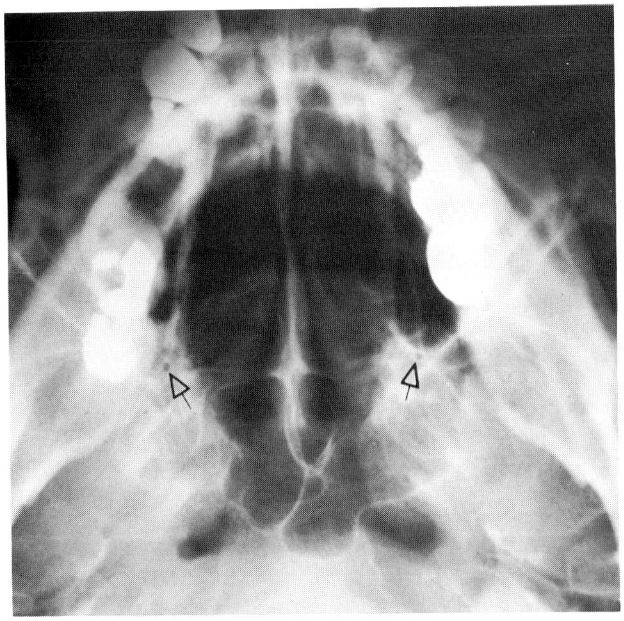

Fig. 16-93. Small lesser palatine foramina (arrows) are visible just anterior to pterygoid process in submentovertical projection.

and *C,* and 16-93). One or two foramina may be seen on each side, where they appear as lucencies about 1 mm in diameter with well-defined sclerotic margins. A greater or a lesser palatine foramen was apparent in twenty of the fifty basal projections reviewed by us. Although smaller, the lesser palatine foramen is seen more frequently than the greater because its forward angulation is smaller: 5° to 10° as opposed to 20° for the greater palatine foramen (Fig. 16-92).

REFERENCES

Alford, B. R., and Guilford, F. R.: A comprehensive study of tumors of the glomus jugulare, Laryngoscope **72**:765-787, 1962.

Allen, G. W.: Angiography in otolaryngology, Laryngoscope **77**:1909-1961, 1967.

Aubaniac, R.: Les variations du canal déchiré postérieur, Trav. Lab. Anat. Fac. Med. Alger, pp. 23-33, 1951 (cited by Di Chiro et al., 1964).

Barrett, J. H., and Lawrence, V. L.: Aneurysm of the internal carotid artery as a complication of mastoidectomy, Arch. Otolaryng. **72**:366-368, 1960.

Bloom, D. L., and Keohane, M. F.: Epidermoid tumors of the skull and brain, Radiology **85**:485-493, 1965.

Boyd, G. I.: Emissary foramina of cranium in man and anthropoids, J. Anat. **65**:108-121, 1930.

Brücke, H.: Ueber die Röntgendarstellung des Foramen ovale, Roentgenpraxis **6**:603-606, 1934.

Burrows, E. H.: Bone changes in orbital neurofibromatosis, Brit. J. Radiol. **36**:549-561, 1963.

Busby, D. R., Slemmons, D. H., and Miller, T. F.: Fatal epistaxis via carotid aneurysm and eustachian tube, Arch. Otolaryng. **87**:295-298, 1968.

Chaussé, C.: Trois incidences pour l'examen du rocher, Acta Radiol. **34**:274-287, 1950.

Chouké, K. S.: On the incidence of the foramen of Civinini and the porus crotaphitico-buccinatorius in American Whites and Negroes. I. Observations on 1544 skulls, Amer. J. Phys. Anthrop. **4**:203-226, 1946.

Chouké, K. S., and Hodes, P. J.: Pterygo-alar bar and its recognition by roentgen methods in trigeminal neuralgia, Amer. J. Roentgen. **65**:180-182, 1951.

Columella, F., Delzanno, G. B., and Nicola, G. C.: Les neurinomes des quatre derniers nerfs craniens, Neurochirurgie **5**:280-295, 1959.

Conley, J., and Hildyard, V.: Aneurysm of the internal carotid artery presenting in the middle ear, Arch. Otolaryng. **90**: 35-38, 1969.

Cornell, S. H.: Jugular venography, Amer. J. Roentgen. **106**: 303-307, 1969.

Csàkàny, G., and Donàth, T.: Vergleichende röntgenanatomische Untersuchung der beiderseitigen Foramina jugularia, Fortschr. Roentgenstr. **88**:439-446, 1958.

Curnow, J.: Two instances of irregular ophthalmic and middle meningeal arteries, J. Anat. Physiol. **8**:155-156, 1873.

Davidson, K. C.: Cranial and intracranial lesions in neurofibromatosis, Amer. J. Roentgen. **98**:550-556, 1966.

de Beer, G. R.: The development of the vertebrate skull, Oxford, 1937, Clarendon Press.

Decker, K.: Klinische Neuroradiologie, Stuttgart, 1960, Georg Thieme Verlag.

Di Chiro, G., Fisher, R. L., and Nelson, K. B.: The jugular foramen, J. Neurosurg. **21**:447-460, 1964.

du Boulay, G. H.: Principles of x-ray diagnosis of the skull, London, 1965, Butterworth & Co., Ltd.

Ecker, A., and Perl, T.: Selective gasserian injection for tic douloureux; technical advances and results, Acta Radiol. **9**: 38-48, 1969.

Eraso, S. T.: Roentgen and clinical diagnosis of glomus jugulare tumors; four cases and a new radiographic technic, Radiology **77**:252-256, 1961.

Evans, T. H.: Carotid canal anomaly; other instances of absent internal carotid artery, Med. Times **84**:1069-1072, 1956.

Fischgold, H., David, M., and Brégeat, P.: La tomographie de la base du crâne en neurochirurgie et neuro-ophthalmologie, Paris, 1952, Masson & Cie.

Fischgold, H., Metzger, J., and Korach, G.: Tomographie de la region pétro-sphéno-occipitale; incidence des quatre dernières paires crâniennes, Acta Radiol. **42**:56-64, 1954.

Fisher, A. G.: Case of complete absence of both internal carotid arteries with a preliminary note on development of stapedial artery, J. Anat. Physiol. **48**:37-46, 1914.

Frazer, J. E.: Anatomy of the human skeleton, ed. 6, A. S. Breathnach, editor, London, 1965, J. & A. Churchill, Ltd.

Gayral, L., and Paintandre: Appareil nouveau pour effectuer des radiographies symétriques des fentes sphénoidales en incidence oblique, J. Radiol. Electr. **33**:192-197, 1952.

Glasauer, F. E., and Tandon, P. N.: Trigeminal neurinoma in adolescents, J. Neurol. Neurosurg. Psychiat. **32**:562-568, 1969.

Goetsch, E.: Schädelveränderungen bei Neurofibromatose Recklinghausen, Fortschr. Roentgenstr. **83**:225-229, 1955.

Gray, H.: Anatomy of the human body, ed. 27, C. M. Goss, editor, Philadelphia, 1959, Lea & Febiger.

Greig, D. M.: Congenital anomalies of the foramen spinosum, Edinburgh Med. J. **36**:363-371, 1929.

Guild, S. R.: The glomus jugulare, a nonchromaffin paraganglion in man, Ann. Otol. **62**:1045-1071, 1953.

Guirguis, S., and Tadros, F. W.: An internal carotid aneurysm in the petrous temporal bone, J. Neurol. Neurosurg. Psychiat. **24**:84-85, 1961.

Hamberger, C. A., and Gejrot, T.: A contribution to the diagnosis of glomus jugulare tumors, Laryngoscope **74**:1029-1036, 1964.

Harrison, T. H., Odom, G. L., and Kunkle, E. C.: Internal carotid aneurysm arising in carotid canal; report of a case with extension to the gasserian ganglion, Arch. Neurol. **8**: 328-331, 1963.

Härtel, F.: Röntgenographische darstellung des Foramen ovale des Schädels, Fortschr. Roentgenstr. **27**:493-495, 1921.

Hawk, W. A., and McCormack, L. J.: Nonchromaffin paraganglioma of the glomus jugulare; review of the literature and report of six cases, Cleveland Clin. Quart. **26**:62-80, 1959.

Hawkins, T. D.: Radiological investigation of glomus jugulare tumors, Acta Radiol. **5**:201-210, 1966.

Hayek, H.: Ueber Teilung des Foramen jugulare, Anat. Anz. **68**:65-70, 1929.

Henderson, W. R.: The anatomy of the gasserian ganglion and the distribution of pain in relation to injections and operations for trigeminal neuralgia, Ann. Roy. Coll. Surg. Eng. **37**:346-373, 1965.

Henderson, W. R.: A note on the relationship of the human maxillary nerve to the cavernous sinus and to an emissary sinus passing through the foramen ovale, J. Anat. **100**:905-908, 1966.

Henle, J.: Handbuch der systematischen Anatomie des Menschen, Brunswick, Germany, 1871, F. Viewig & Son, vol. 1.

Hiranandani, L. H., Chandra, O., Malpani, N. K., and Ahuja, K. K.: An internal carotid aneurysm in the petrous temporal bone, J. Laryng. **76**:703-706, 1962.

Hirtz, E. J.: La radiographie de la base du crâne, J. Radiol. Electr. **6**:253-263, 1922.

Holman, C. B., and Miller, W. E.: Juvenile nasopharyngeal fibroma; roentgenologic characteristics, Amer. J. Roentgen. **94**:292-298, 1965.

Holman, C. B., Olive I., and Svien, H. J.: Roentgenologic features of neurofibroma involving the gasserian ganglion, Amer. J. Roentgen. **86**:148-153, 1961.

Holmgren, B. S.: Radiographic changes produced by intracranial arterio-venous aneurysms, Acta Psychiat. Neurol., supp. 46, pp. 145-155, 1946.

Jefferson, G.: On the saccular aneurysms of the internal carotid artery in the cavernous sinus, Brit. J. Surg. **26**:267-302, 1938.

Jelašić, F.: Ueber die röntgenologische Darstellung der basalen Zisternen mittels direkter Applikation des Kontrastöls durch das Foramen ovale, Nervenarzt **26**:139-145, 1955.

Khoo, F. Y.: Giant jugular fossa with brief notes on the anatomical variations of the jugular fossa, Amer. J. Roentgen. **55**:333-336, 1946.

Kim, S. K., and Capp, M. P.: Jugular foramen and early roentgen diagnosis of glomus jugulare tumor, Amer. J. Roentgen. **97**:597-600, 1966.

Knott, J. F.: On the cerebral sinuses and their variations, J. Anat. **16**:27-42, 1882.

Kohut, R. I., and Lindsay, J. R.: Glomus jugulare tumors—new techniques for determining operability, Laryngoscope **75**:750-762, 1965.

Kornblum, K., and Kennedy, G. R.: The sphenoidal fissure; an anatomical, roentgenological, and clinical study, Amer. J. Roentgen. **47**:845-858, 1942.

Lafon, R., Gros, C., Labange, R., Cadilhac, J., Minvielle, J., Paleirac, R., and Vlahovitch, B.: Tumeur du foramen ovale, confrontations anatomo-radiologiques, J. Radiol. Electr. **34**: 258-260, 1953.

Le Double, A. F.: Traité des variations des os du crâne de l'homme et de leur signification au point de vue de l'anthropologie zoologique, Paris, 1903, Vigot Frères.

Leeds, H., and Seaman, W. B.: Fibrous dysplasia of the skull and its differential diagnosis; a clinical and roentgenographic study of 46 cases, Radiology **78**:570-582, 1962.

Lepp, F. H., and Sandner, O.: Anatomic-radiographic study of ossified pterygospinous and "innominate" ligaments, Oral Surg. **26**:244-260, 1968.

Leutert, G.: Die anatomischen Nomenklaturen von Basel, Jena, Paris in dreifacher Gegenüberstellung, Stuttgart, 1963, Georg Thieme Verlag.

Le Wald, L. T.: Congenital absence of the superior orbital wall associated with pulsating exophthalmos, Amer. J. Roentgen. **30**:756-764, 1933.

Lie, T. A.: Congenital anomalies of the carotid arteries, Amsterdam, 1968, Excerpta Medica Foundation.

Lindblom, K.: A roentgenographic study of the vascular channels of the skull, Acta Radiol., supp. 30, 1936.

Lombardi, G., Passerini, A., and Migliavacca, F.: Intracavernous aneurysms of the internal carotid artery, Amer. J. Roentgen. **89**:361-371, 1963.

McKinney, J. M., Acree, A., and Soltz, S. E.: The syndrome of the unruptured aneurysm of the intracranial portion of the internal carotid artery, Bull. Neurol. Inst. N. Y. **5**:247-277, 1936.

Meinardus, K.: Ueber Schädelveränderungen bei Neurofibromatosis Recklinghausen, Radiol. Clin. **27**:357-364, 1958.

Miller, W. E., Holman, C. B., Dockerty, M. B., and Devine, K. D.: Roentgenologic manifestations of malignant tumors of the nasopharynx, Amer. J. Roentgen. **106**:813-823, 1969.

Minagi, H., and Newton, T. H.: Cartilaginous tumors of the base of the skull, Amer. J. Roentgen. **105**:308-313, 1969.

Moyes, P. D., Bratty, P. J. A., and Dolman, C. L.: Osteoclastoma of the jugular foramen: case report, J. Neurosurg. **32**:255-257, 1970.

Nugent, G. R., Sprinkle, P., and Bloor, B. M.: Sphenoid sinus mucoceles, J. Neurosurg. **32**:443-451, 1970.

Orley, A.: Neuroradiology, Springfield, Ill., 1949, Charles C Thomas, Publisher.

Palacios, E.: Chemodectomas of the head and neck, Amer. J. Roentgen. **110**:129-140, 1970.

Pecker, J., Hoel, J., Javalet, A., and Fournier, H.: Paralysie du moteur oculaire externe par aneurysme intra-petreux traumatique de la carotide interne, Presse Med. **68**:1023-1024, 1960.

Perl, T., and Ecker, A.: Radiologically controlled injections through the foramen ovale for relief of tic douloureux and of Parkinsonism, Acta Radiol. [Diagn.] **1**:901-912, 1963.

Peyton, W. T., and Simmons, D. R.: Neurofibromatosis with defect in wall of orbit; report of 5 cases, Arch. Neurol. Psychiat. **55**:248-265, 1946.

Pierini, E. A. A., and Agra, A.: Epistaxis como signo de hemorrhagia de la carotide interne en su porcion timpanica; probable aneurisma intrapetroso, Prensa Med. Argent. **41**: 945-948, 1954.

Priman, J., and Etter, L. E.: Pterygospinous and pterygoalar bars, Med. Radiogr. Photogr. **35**:2-6, 1959.

Radoïévitch, S., and Jovanovitch, S.: La morphologie du canal Vidien et ses rapports avec les sinus paranasaux chez l'homme adulte et l'enfant, Rev. Laryng. **76**:481-492, 1955.

Radoïévitch, S., Jovanovitch, S., and Lotritch, N.: La morphologie du trou ovale et les rapports du nerf maxilaire inférieur avec le sinus sphénoidal, Rev. Laryng. **77**:11-19, 1956.

Rice, R. P., and Holman, C. B.: Roentgenographic manifestations of tumors of the glomus jugulare (chemodectoma), Amer. J. Roentgen. **89**:1201-1208, 1963.

Rischbieth, R. H. C., and Bull, J. W. D.: The significance of enlargement of the superior orbital (sphenoidal) fissure, Brit. J. Radiol. **31**:125-135, 1958.

Rousseau, F., and Spillman, J.: Deux cas d'epistaxis incoercible avec cécité homolatérale par lésion de la carotide interne intracrânienne après chute sur la tête, Ann. Otolaryng. **68**:461-465, 1951.

Rumbaugh, C. L., and Potts, D. G.: Skull changes associated with intracranial arterio-venous malformations, Amer. J. Roentgen. **98**:525-534, 1966.

Scanlan, R.: Anomalous course of the internal carotid artery through the middle ear, Radiology. (In press.)

Schaaf, J.: Die röntgenologische Darstellung des Foramen rotundum (canalis rotundus), Fortschr. Roentgenstr. **86**: 102-104, 1957.

Schmidt, H., and Driesen, W.: Einseitige Erweiterung eines Foramen ovale des Schädels, Fortschr. Roentgenstr. **86**:508-511, 1957.

Schüller, A.: Die Schädelbasis im Röntgenbilde, Hamburg, 1905, L. Graefe u. Sillem.

Schüller, A.: Die röntgenographische Darstellung einiger Nervenkanale des Schädelbasis, Fortschr. Roentgenstr. **57**: 640-641, 1938.

Shapiro, R., and Janzen, A. H.: The normal skull; a roentgen study, New York, 1960, Paul B. Hoeber, Inc.

Shapiro, R., and Robinson, F.: The foramina of the middle fossa: a phylogenetic, anatomic, and pathologic study, Amer. J. Roentgen. **101**:779-794, 1967a.

Shapiro, R., and Robinson, F.: Alterations of the sphenoidal fissure produced by local and systemic processes, Amer. J. Roentgen. **101**:814-827, 1967b.

Sosman, M. C., and Putnam, T. J.: Roentgenologic aspects of brain tumors—meningiomas, Amer. J. Roentgen. **13**:1-12, 1925.

Sosman, M. C., and Vogt, E. C.: Aneurysms of the internal carotid artery and the circle of Willis from a roentgenological viewpoint, Amer. J. Roentgen. **15**:122-134, 1926.

Stallings, J. O., and McCabe, B. F.: Congenital middle ear aneurysm of the internal carotid, Arch. Otolaryng. **90**:39-43, 1969.

Strickler, J. M.: New and simple techniques for demonstration of the jugular foramen, Amer. J. Roentgen. **97**:601-606, 1966.

Svien, H. J., Baker, H. L., and Rivers, M. H.: Jugular foramen syndrome and allied syndromes, Neurology **13**:797-809, 1963.

Tänzer, A.: Die Veränderungen am Schädel bei der Neurofibromatosis Recklinghausen; Versuch einer Einteilung, Fortschr. Roentgenstr. **105**:50-62, 1966.

Taveras, J. M., and Wood, E. H.: Diagnostic neuroradiology, Baltimore, 1964, The Williams & Wilkins Co.

Tebo, H. G.: The pterygospinous bar in panoramic roentgenography, Oral Surg. **26**:654-657, 1968.

Thomson, J. L. G.: Traumatic thrombosis of the internal carotid artery in the carotid canal, Brit. J. Radiol. **36**:840-842, 1963.

Traub, S. P.: Roentgenology of intracranial meningiomas, Springfield, Ill., 1961, Charles C Thomas, Publisher.

Vail, H. H.: Vidian neuralgia, Ann. Otol. **41**:837-856, 1932.

Wheeler, P. S., and Honda, M.: Enlargement of the foramina ovale by increased intracranial pressure, Neurology **15**:785-786, 1965.

Wilner, H. I.: (editorial) The neuroradiologist and the ear, Amer. J. Roentgen. **110**:190-191, 1970.

Wood-Jones, F.: The non-metrical morphological characters of the skull as criteria for racial diagnosis. Part I. General discussion of the morphological characters employed in racial diagnosis, J. Anat. **65**:179-195, 1931.

CHAPTER 17

Clivus

C. G. Coin and Dennis R. Malkasian

GROSS ANATOMY

The term clivus was used by von Sömmerring (1791), Blumenbachii (1807), and Virchow (1857) to describe that part of the inner skull base between the foramen magnum and the dorsum sellae. The boundaries of the clivus are not well defined. Common radiologic usage indicates that the definition should include the entire thickness of the basioccipital bone and the body of the sphenoid bone. The lateral margins of the clivus are formed by the petro-occipital fissure superiorly and by the synchondrosis between the basioccipital and exoccipital bones inferiorly (Fig. 17-1). The posterior boundary slopes downward and inferiorly from the base of the dorsum sellae to the anterior margin of the foramen magnum. The anterior margin of the clivus is not well defined, since it blends with the sphenoid sinus. The inferior boundary represents the nasopharyngeal surface of the lower portion of the sphenoid and the basiocciput. The inferior or exocranial surface is roughened by the attachments of the fibrous raphe of the pharynx and the muscles of the nasopharynx. In contrast, the posterior or endocranial surface of the clivus is usually smooth.

The surfaces of the clivus are composed of cortical bone. The central portion is composed of cancellous bone that may be pneumatized to a variable degree by the sphenoid sinus (Fig. 17-2).

The endocranial surface of the clivus is usually slightly concave, occasionally flat, and rarely convex. The depth of the clivus is defined as the maximum distance of the cortex of the clivus above or below a line that connects the dorsum sellae and the anterior margin of the foramen magnum (Fig. 17-3). Kruyff and Munn (1963) studied the depth of the clivus in 500 normal children whose ages ranged from birth to 15 years. In 488 (97.6%) the clivus was slightly concave or flat. A concavity with a depth of 2 mm was seen in eight patients (1.6%). In four patients (0.8%) a concavity measuring 3 mm in depth was noted. No clivus had a posterior convexity. Di Chiro and Anderson (1965) examined ninety-four dry skulls and roentgenograms of the skull in seventy-two normal adults and thirty-seven normal children. In 77% the clivus was slightly concave; in 19% it was flat; and in 14% it was convex posteriorly. In none was the concavity greater than 3 mm.

The basal angle, which is formed by the intersection of the plane of the clivus and the plane of the anterior fossa, measures an average of 137°, with a range of from 123° to 152° (McRae, 1953; Poppel et al., 1953).

The length of the clivus from the base of the dorsum sellae to the anterior margin of the foramen magnum was measured in forty-two adult skulls. The average length was 3.4 cm, with a range of from 3.1 to 4 cm.

The jugular tubercles are small bony protuberances that project superiorly and posteriorly from the lateral inferior margin of the clivus. Di Chiro and Anderson (1965) found these tubercles to be inconstant, with one or both sides too flat or poorly defined for satisfactory appraisal in twenty of ninety-four specimens. The interjugular distance, defined as the distance between the two jugular tubercles, is an index of the width of the inferior portion of the clivus (Fig. 17-4). The average interjugular distance is 2 cm in the dry skull, with a range of from 1.5 to 3.0 cm (Di Chiro and Anderson, 1965).

The inferior petrosal sinuses extend along the lateral margin of the clivus and drain into each jugular bulb lateral to the jugular tubercles. The basilar venous plexus lies on the endocranial surface of the clivus and is covered by dura. The belly of the pons and the ven-

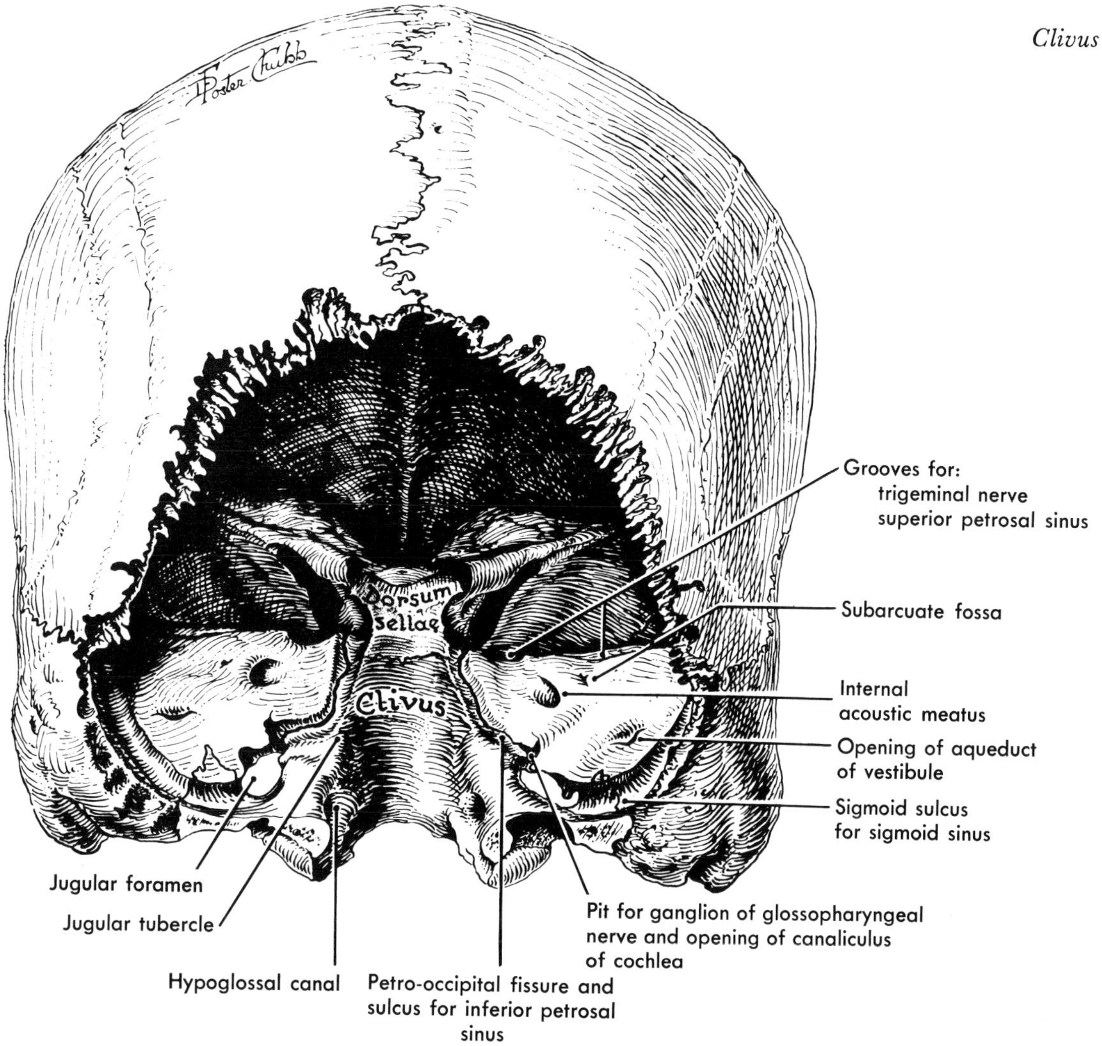

Fig. 17-1. Posterior cranial fossa from behind. Squamous part of occipital bone has been removed. (From Grant, J. C. B.: An atlas of anatomy, ed. 5, Baltimore, 1962, The Williams & Wilkins Co.)

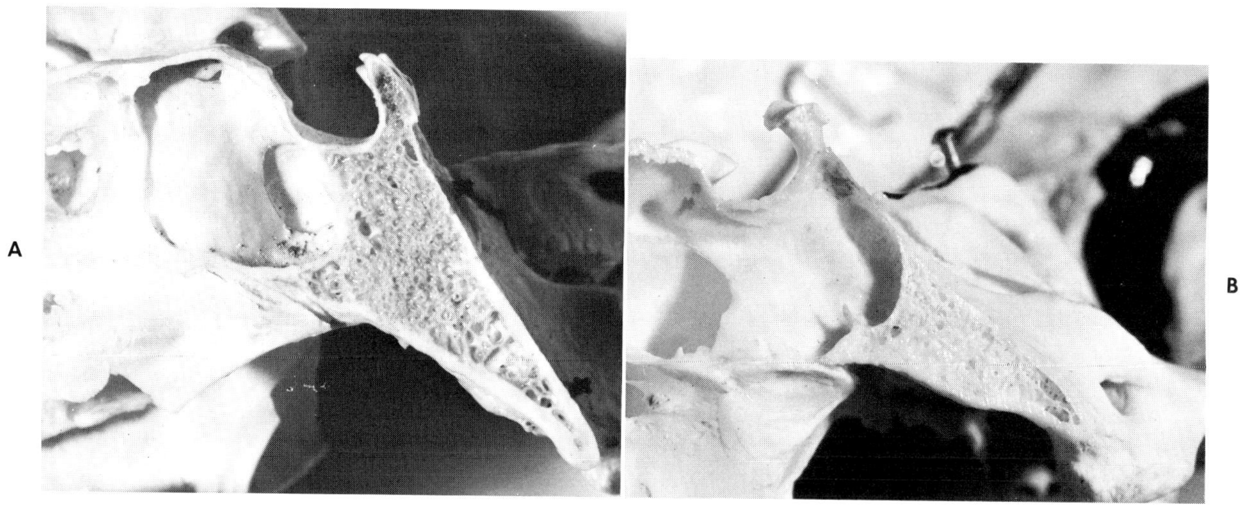

Fig. 17-2. Midline sagittal section of clivus and sphenoid. In **A,** margins of clivus are composed of cortical bone, and central segment of cancellous bone. In **B,** clivus is partly pneumatized by sphenoid sinus. Note the very thin cortical bone along the upper posterior boundary of the clivus.

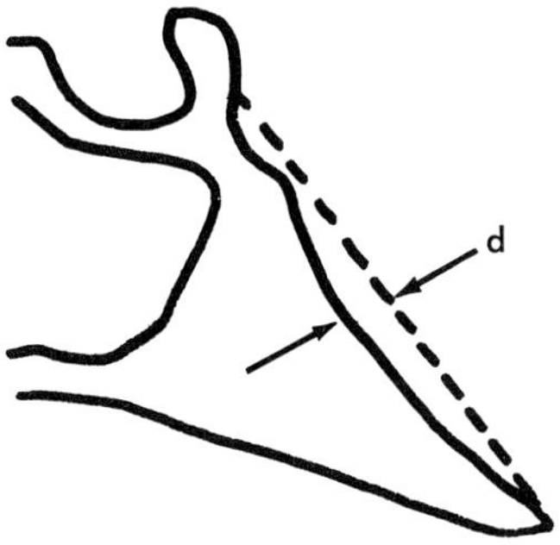

Fig. 17-3. Measurement of depth of clivus (*d*).

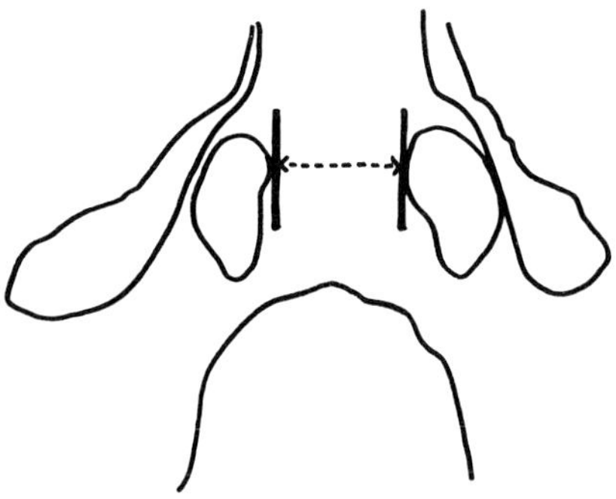

Fig. 17-4. Measurement of interjugular distance.

tral surface of the medulla oblongata lie in close relation to the clivus and may contribute to impressions on its surface. The pons and medulla are separated from the clivus by the pontine and medullary cisterns.

EMBRYOLOGY

The clivus develops by enchondral bone formation. By the third week of gestation, the notochord in the cephalic region of the fetus has begun to develop (Arey, 1965). As ontogenesis progresses, condensations of mesenchyme presage chondrocranium formation. During the sixth week chondrogenesis of the mesenchymal model appears (Hamilton et al., 1952). Chondrification centers begin in the presumptive basiocciput and spread superiorly to unite with cartilaginous centers in the region of the future basisphenoid (Gray, 1967). Subsequently a parachordal cartilaginous plate migrates medially around the notochord and about the roots of the hypoglossal nerve (Gray, 1967). By the eighth week chondrification has reached the height of development. The basal portion of the sphenoid bone contains one or two ossification centers by the sixth week of fetal life (Gray, 1967).

At birth the clivus consists of partially ossified components of the basiocciput and sphenoid body, separated by the spheno-occipital synchondrosis (Caffey, 1963). In the lateral view of the skull or in the sagittal tomogram, these components are well seen. The ossi-

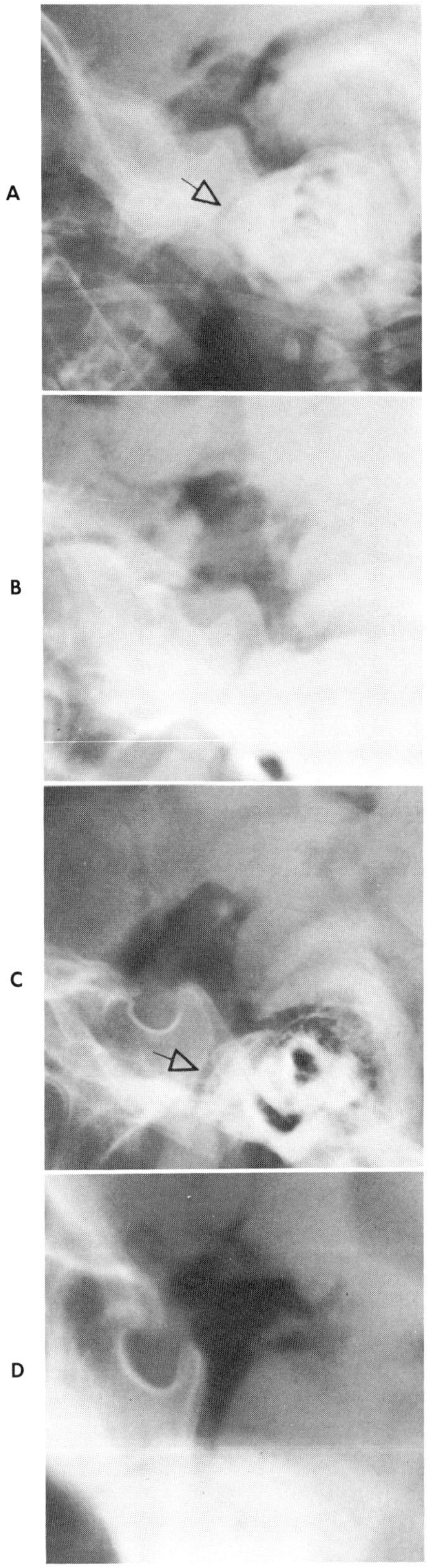

Fig. 17-5. Pneumoencephalogram in lateral brow up position. Mantle of cartilage, outlined by air in the pontine and interpeduncular cistern, lies adjacent to posterior aspect of ossified clivus. Thickness of cartilage decreases with age. **A,** Three months. **B,** Nine months. **C,** Three years. **D,** Five years. Arrow indicates spheno-occipital synchondrosis.

fied portion of the clivus is separated from the pontine and medullary cisterns by a mantle of cartilage (Fig. 17-5). The spheno-occipital synchondrosis fuses at about 14 years in females and 16 years in males. The time of fusion may vary; however, the synchondrosis does not persist beyond 21 years of age (Grant, 1962).

ROENTGEN ANATOMY

Roentgenograms of the skull in the standard projections rarely provide adequate views of the clivus. Petrous pyramids and mastoid air cells partially obscure the clivus on lateral views. This may be partly overcome by overpenetrated and high-kilovolt film. The dorsal surface of the clivus is seen in tangent on the Chamberlain-Towne projection; however, it is usually partly obscured by the dorsum sellae (Fig. 17-6).

The clivus is best depicted by sagittal tomography in the lateral projection and by frontal tomography in which the plane of the cut is parallel to the slope of the clivus (Fig. 17-7).

On a midsagittal tomogram the clivus is depicted as a triangle whose base passes through the dorsum sellae and whose apex is at the anterior margin of the foramen magnum. The dorsal and ventral surfaces are outlined by a white line of cortical bone. The base of this triangle (from base of dorsum sellae to endocranial surface of clivus) measures from 1.5 to 2.5 cm, and the sides of the triangle (endo- and exocranial surfaces of clivus) measure from 2.5 to 5.0 cm. The shape of

A

B

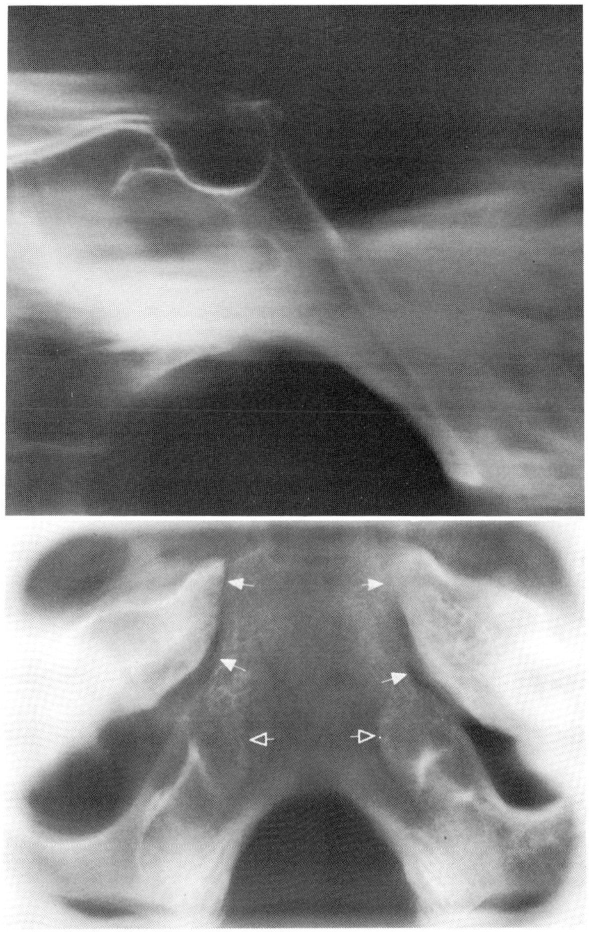

Fig. 17-7. A, Midsagittal tomogram of clivus shows triangular shape of clivus and its cortical margins well. Sphenoid sinus does not extend to posterior margin of clivus, which is therefore composed primarily of cancellous bone. **B,** Frontal tomogram of clivus shows medial aspect of jugular tubercles (open arrows) and petro-occipital fissure (solid arrows) well.

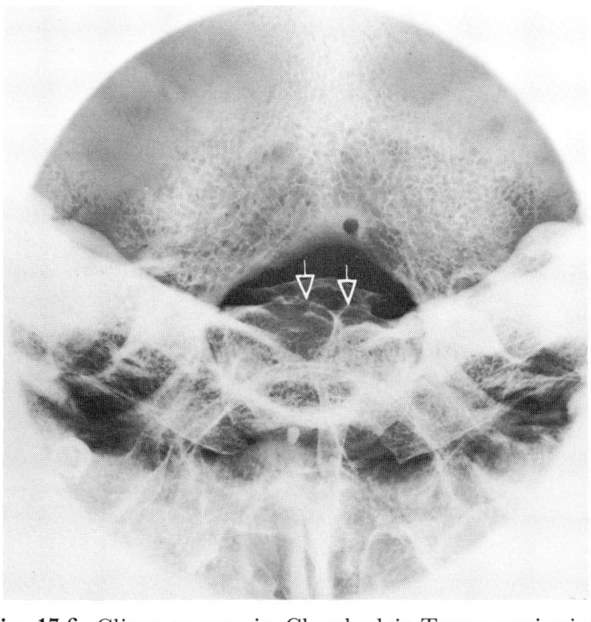

Fig. 17-6. Clivus as seen in Chamberlain-Towne projection. Posterior surface of clivus (arrows) is projected anterior to dorsum sellae.

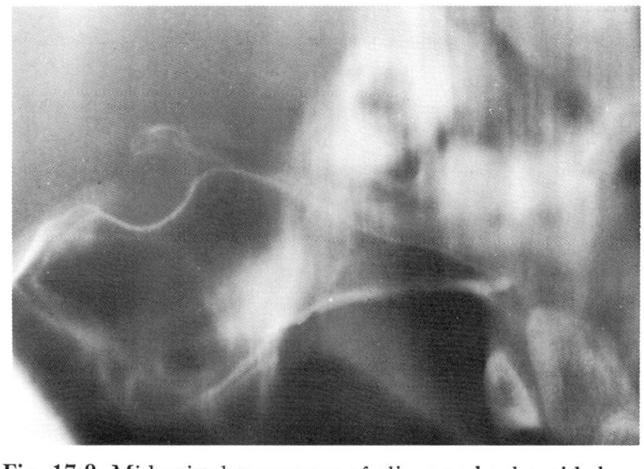

Fig. 17-8. Midsagittal tomogram of clivus and sphenoid shows clivus in this patient extensively pneumatized by sphenoid sinus.

the posterior surface of the clivus varies. The clivus usually is slightly concave posteriorly, which in most instances does not exceed 3 mm. The clivus is flat in about 25% of the cases, whereas in 10% it has a slight posterior convexity (Di Chiro and Anderson, 1965).

The interjugular distance, as measured on frontal tomograms, is 2.5 cm (2.2 to 3.2 cm) in adults and 2.3 cm (1.8 to 3.3 cm) in children (Di Chiro and Anderson, 1965).

Compact cortical bone, recognized as a sharp well-demarcated white line on sagittal tomography, forms the anterior and posterior boundaries of the clivus. The central portion of the clivus inferiorly is usually composed of cancellous bone. The sphenoid sinus does not penetrate into the body of the sphenoid until about the fourth year of life. From the fourth to the twelfth year, pneumatization may extend into the clivus for a variable distance (Vidic, 1968). The clivus may become completely pneumatized (Fig. 17-8). When pneumatization is present, the bony margins of the clivus may be thin (Figs. 17-2, *B,* and 17-8).

PATHOLOGY

Changes in size or shape

In 1939, Rossier reported increased concavity of the clivus of greater than 3 mm as suggestive of a space-occupying lesion of long duration in the posterior fossa. Stern (1964) reported a concavity greater than 2 mm in 50% of patients with lesions at the tentorial notch or in the posterior fossa. Di Chiro and Anderson (1965) found a posterior concavity of the clivus of 4 mm in posterior fossa tumors, obstructive hydrocephalus, pinealomas, and supratentorial tumors. They emphasized that an increased posterior concavity does not necessarily indicate a mass in the posterior fossa but merely represents long-standing increased intracranial pressure (Figs. 17-9 and 17-10).

A convex clivus is a common finding associated with platybasia and basilar impression. A hump at the spheno-occipital synchondrosis was associated with a short basioccipital portion in four patients who had assimilation of the atlas, slight basilar invagination, or platybasia (McRae, 1953).

The clivus is significantly shortened in achondroplasia because of little or no longitudinal bone growth at the spheno-occipital synchondrosis.

The jugular tubercles may be spread apart, with a resultant increase in the interjugular distance, in patients with chronic increased intracranial pressure. This increased distance has relatively little significance because of the inconstancy of these two eminences and the difficulty in recognizing them (Kryuff and Munn, 1963; Di Chiro and Anderson, 1965).

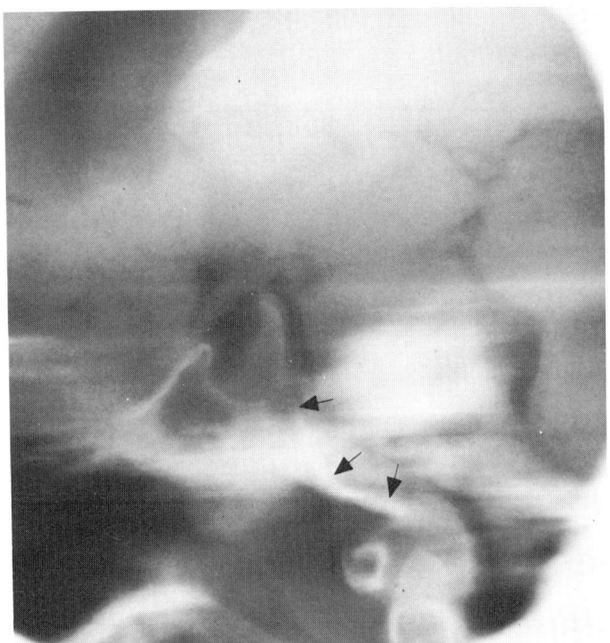

Fig. 17-9. Crouzon's disease. Pneumoencephalogram, brow up lateral midline tomogram, shows that clivus (arrows) has deep posterior concavity. This change may be related to chronic increased intracranial pressure.

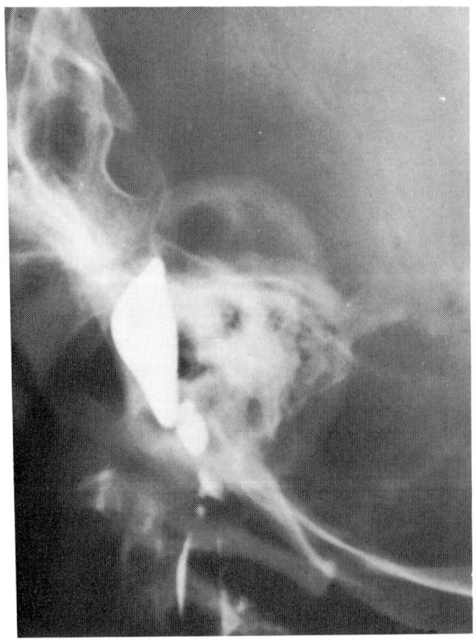

Fig. 17-10. Neurofibromatosis in 7-year-old boy. Large neurofibroma straddled foramen magnum and caused chronic increased intracranial pressure. Clivus shows marked posterior concavity, which at the time of cervical myelography is filled with Pantopaque. (Same case as Fig. 15-21.)

Specific lesions involving the clivus

Clivus chordoma (Boldrey and McNally, 1941; Congdon, 1952; Stevenson et al., 1966; Guiot, 1968)

Chordoma is the most common tumor of the clivus. This tumor, believed to originate from a notochordal remnant, is invasive and destructive and capable of distant metastasis. The position of the notochordal remnant varies within the clivus (Fig. 17-11). Higinbotham and co-workers (1967) reported on forty-six chordomas from all sites studied at Memorial Hospital from 1930 to 1965. The origin of 35% of these tumors was in the region of the clivus. Chordoma may develop in any age group; it was reported as early as the seventh month of fetal life by Henning (1900) and as late as 82 years of age by Plaut and Blatt (1967). Headache and cranial nerve palsies are the most frequent presenting symptoms. The growth rate of the tumor varies. The average survival is about 3 years and may be as long as 18 years.

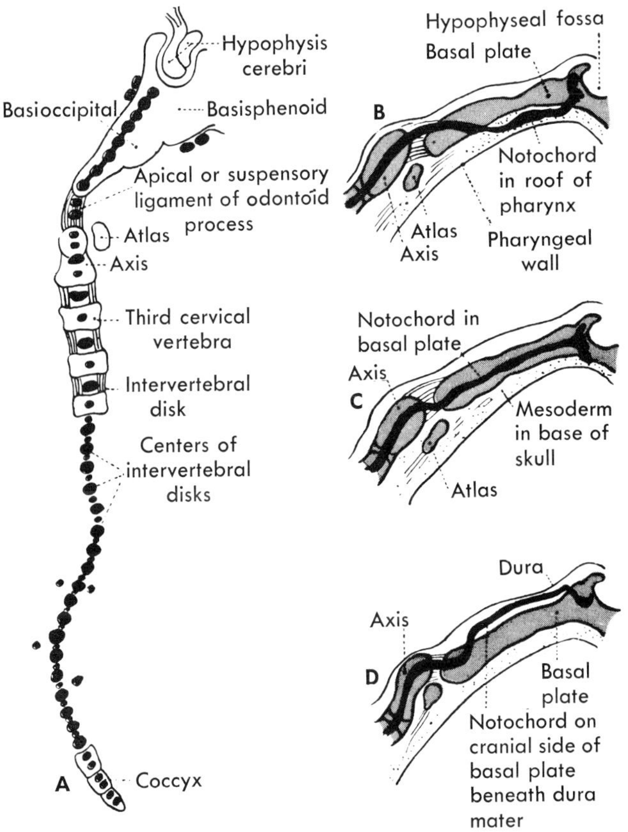

Fig. 17-11. A, Sites where remnants of notochord may persist in adult and give rise to chordomas, indicated in black. **B** to **D,** Sagittal sections of head end of the embryonic notochord (in black). Positions that notochord may occupy in relation to basal or parachordal plate of cartilage are illustrated. Relation in **B** would appear to be commonest, and in **D** the least common. (From Pendergrass, E. P., Schaeffer, J. P., and Hodes, P. J.: Head and neck in roentgen diagnosis, ed. 2, Springfield, Ill., 1956, Charles C Thomas, Publisher, vol. 2.)

Wood and Himadi (1950), Lindgren and Di Chiro (1951), Schisano and Tovi (1962), and Zingesser and Schechter (1964) all have described dense nodular calcification associated with bone erosion in a high percentage of patients with clivus chordoma. Di Chiro and Anderson (1965) studied nine cases of clivus chordoma in which retrosellar calcification was found in seven and bone erosion in eight. They stated that dense retrosellar calcification with bone destruction of the clivus, dorsum sellae, and petrous bones is practically pathognomonic of clivus chordoma (Figs. 17-12 and 17-13).

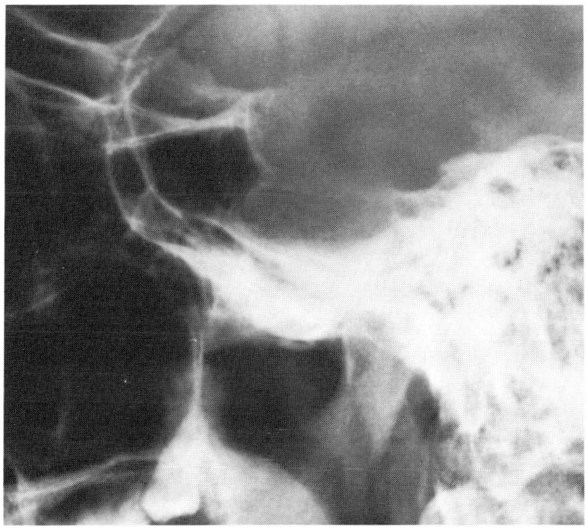

Fig. 17-12. Chordoma. Clivus, dorsum sellae, and posterior floor of sella have been destroyed. Soft-tissue mass projects into sphenoid sinus.

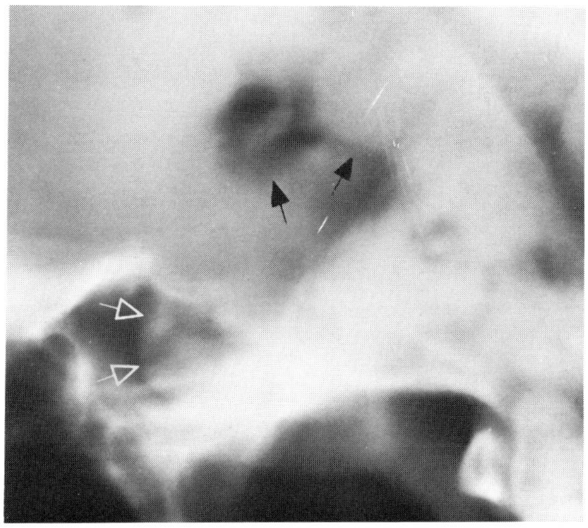

Fig. 17-13. Chordoma. Pneumoencephalogram, lateral projection, shows that superior portion of clivus, dorsum sellae, and posterior segment of floor of sella have been destroyed. Soft-tissue mass projects into sphenoid sinus (open arrows). Prepontine and interpeduncular cisterns are displaced posteriorly (solid arrows).

A

B

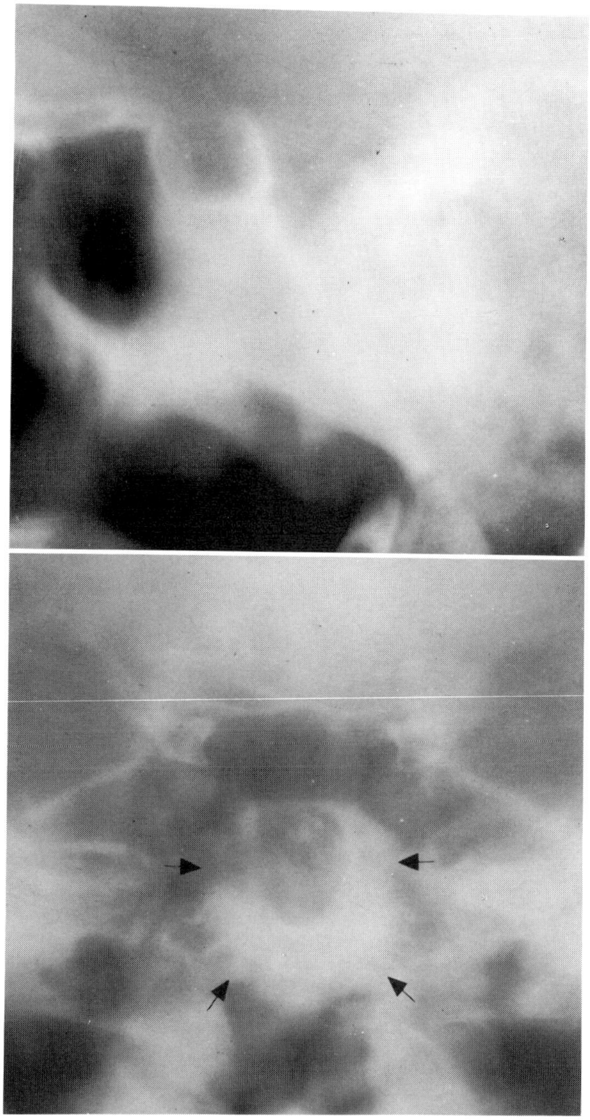

Fig. 17-14. Clivus meningioma. **A,** Lateral midsagittal tomogram. **B,** Frontal tomogram. Extensive sclerosis of clivus is noted (arrows). Central radiolucency is the sphenoid sinus.

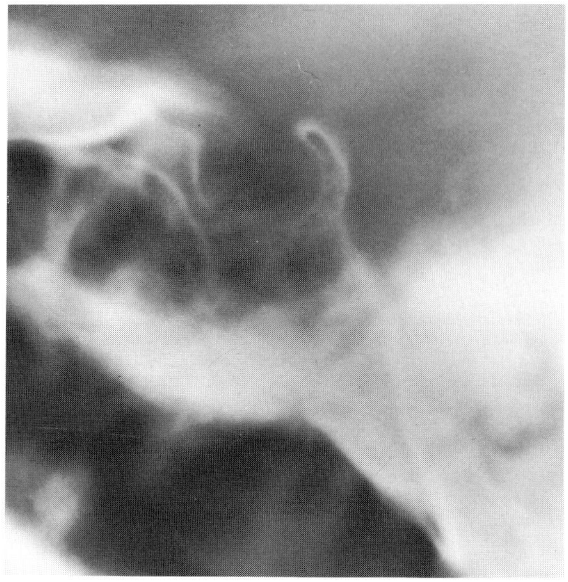

Fig. 17-15. Clivus meningioma. Irregular sclerosis and destructive changes involve the clivus. Floor of sella has been destroyed.

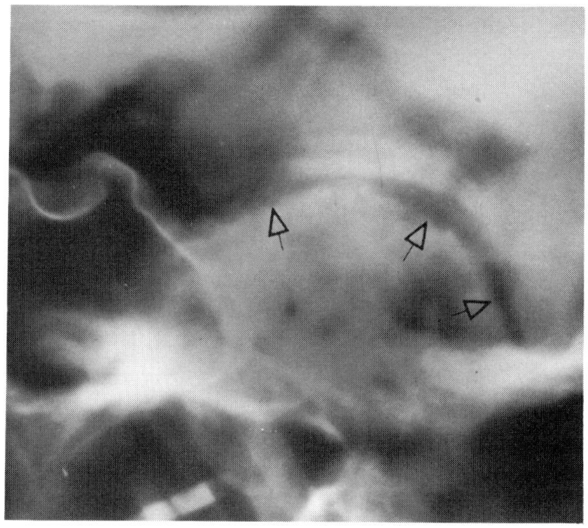

Fig. 17-16. Clivus meningioma. Pneumoencephalogram, lateral midline tomogram, shows that clivus is apparently intact. Meningioma has caused marked posterior displacement of lower portion of pontine and medullary cisterns (arrows).

Clivus meningioma

Meningioma of the clivus comprised 11.2% of meningiomas of the posterior fossa in the series of Olivecrona (1927). Castellano and Ruggiero (1953) reported on eight cases of clivus meningioma. When detected, these tumors were relatively large and had formed deep indentations into the belly of the pons. The clinical findings were remarkably varied and minimal despite the large sizes of the neoplasm. They were usually related to cranial nerve involvement.

On plain roentgenograms hyperostosis appears as the most characteristic finding in meningioma of the clivus. The hyperostosis may consist of a generalized increased bony density (Fig. 17-14) or may be irregularly sclerotic (Fig. 17-15). The yield of positive findings on plain roentgenographic studies is often relatively low and would be increased by tomography. Even tomography, however, may show no bone changes with large clivus meningiomas (Fig. 17-16). Bone erosion and sellar changes are rare, and some authors have stated that clivus meningioma does not effect such changes (Di Chiro and Anderson, 1965).

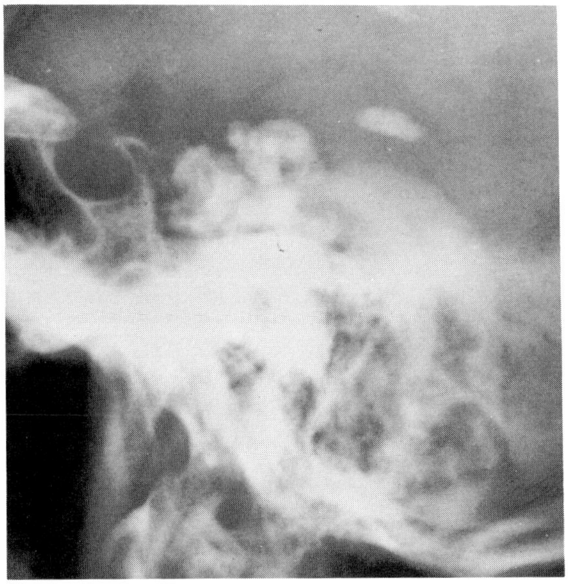

Fig. 17-17. Clivus chondroma. Large lobulated calcified mass lying adjacent to an intact clivus is well shown.

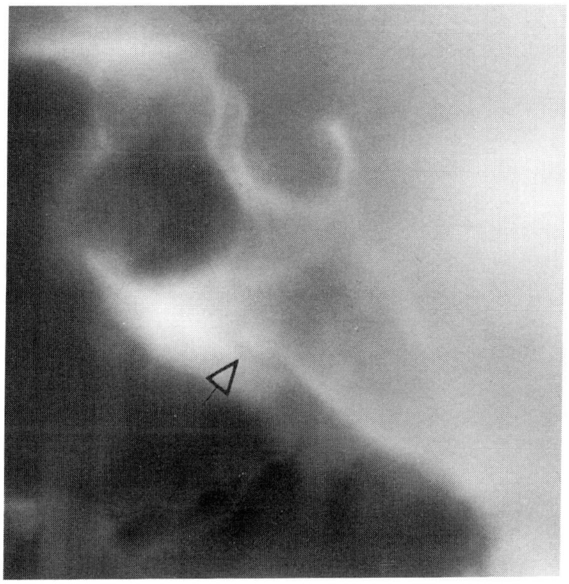

Fig. 17-18. Metastatic carcinoma of breast. Lateral midsagittal tomogram shows irregular destruction of cancellous portion of clivus. Localized destructive process also involves cortical margin inferiorly (arrow).

A

B

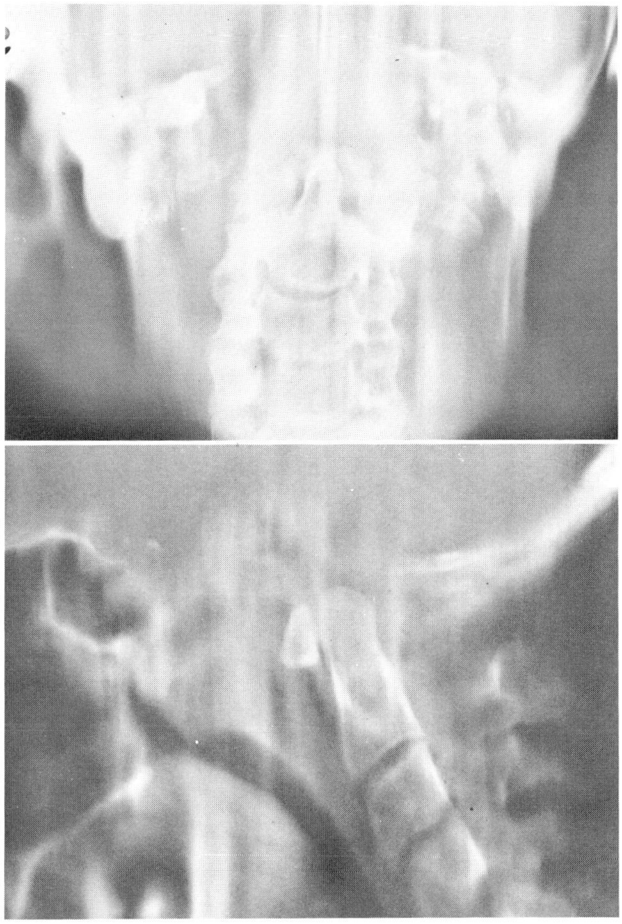

Fig. 17-19. Plasmocytoma. **A,** Frontal tomogram. **B,** Sagittal tomogram. Clivus and dorsum sellae are completely destroyed. (From Di Chiro, G., and Anderson, W. B.: Clin. Radiol. **16:**211-223, 1965.)

Cartilaginous tumors (List, 1943; King and Butcher, 1944; Klinger, 1951; Gabrielson and Kingman, 1964)

Cartilaginous tumors of the base of the skull are rare. Acquaviva and his co-workers (1965) found ninety-nine cases of intracranial chondromas reported in the literature and added two additional cases. In sixty-six of these patients, the tumor involved the base of the skull; in the remainder the tumor was situated at various other intracranial sites. The tumors at the skull base were more common in females. Cartilaginous tumors of the skull base are noted most commonly between the second and fifth decades.

In their review Acquaviva and his collaborators (1968) noted that of the fifty-three cartilaginous tumors of the skull base studied with plain roentgenograms, thirty were calcified. The calcification was massive in thirteen, whereas it was more granular in seventeen. Tumor calcification was apparent in two of three patients reported by Minagi and Newton (1969). These authors reported a clivus chondroma associated with coarse conglomerates of dense retroclival calcification (Fig. 17-17). Acquaviva and his associates (1968) noted bone destruction in twenty-four of the fifty-three patients with chondromas of the skull base. The combination of dense retrosellar calcification and bone destruction has been considered as practically pathognomonic of clivus chordoma. Plaut and Blatt (1967),

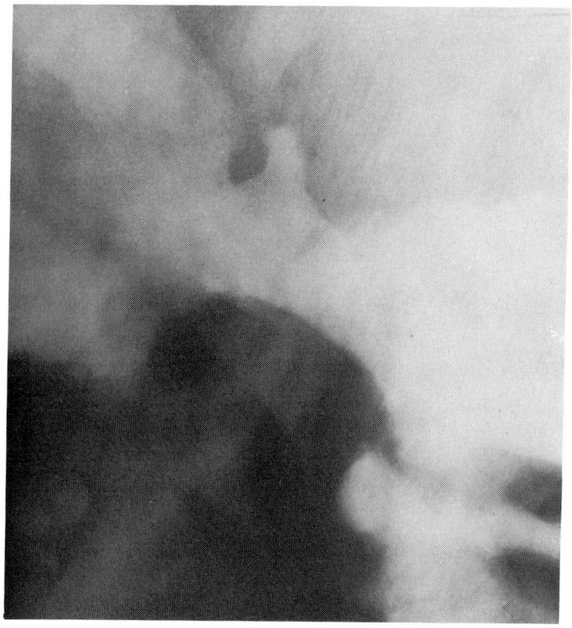

Fig. 17-20. Osteopetrosis. Extensive sclerosis of clivus and adjacent bones is evident.

however, concluded that the differential diagnosis of chondroma and chordoma of the clivus is often difficult and may be impossible.

Other lesions involving the clivus (Echols, 1945)

The clivus may be involved by a variety of osteolytic lesions: infections, reticuloendotheliosis, metastatic neoplasm (Fig. 17-18), direct extension from adjacent neoplasm, plasmocytomas, giant cell tumors (Fig. 17-19), and others. Bone sclerosis that involves the clivus may also be seen with Paget's disease and osteopetrosis (Fig. 17-20).

REFERENCES

Acquaviva, R., Tamic, P. M., Thevenot, C., Fournie, R., Grau, P., Bru, P., LeBascle, J., and Esplan, J. F. R.: Los condromas intracraneales. Revisión de la literatura a propósito de dos casos, Rev. Esp. Otoneurooftal. **24**:15-34, 1965.

Arey, L. B.: Developmental anatomy: a textbook and laboratory manual of embryology, Philadelphia, 1965, W. B. Saunders Co.

Blumenbachii, J. F.: Geschichte und Beschreibung der Knochen des menschlichen Korpers, Gottingen, 1807, Dieterich.

Boldrey, E. B., and McNally, W. J.: Chordoma of the basi-occiput and basisphenoid: report of 4 cases, Arch. Otolaryng. **33**:391-400, 1941.

Caffey, J.: Pediatric x-ray diagnosis, ed. 4, Chicago, 1963, Year Book Medical Publishers, Inc.

Castellano, F., and Ruggiero, G.: Meningiomas of the posterior fossa, Acta Radiol., supp. 104, pp. 136-153, 1953.

Congdon, C. C.: Benign and malignant chordomas: a clinical anatomical study of twenty cases, Amer. J. Path. **28**:793-821, 1952.

Di Chiro, G., and Anderson, W. B.: Clivus, Clin. Radiol. **16**: 211-223, 1965.

Echols, D. H.: Giant cell tumor of the sphenoid bone: case report, J. Neurosurg. **2**:16-20, 1945.

Gabrielsen, T. O., and Kingman, A. F., Jr.: Osteocartilaginous tumors of base of skull: report of unique case and review of literature, Amer. J. Roentgen. **91**:1016-1023, 1964.

Grant, J. C. B.: An atlas of anatomy, ed. 5, Baltimore, 1962, The Williams & Wilkins Co.

Gray, H.: Anatomy of the human body, C. M. Goss, editor, Philadelphia, 1967, Lea & Febiger.

Guiot, G.: The rhinoseptal route for the removal of clivus chordomas, Johns Hopkins Med. J. **122**:329-335, 1968.

Hamilton, W. J., Boyd, J. D., and Mossman, H. W.: Human embryology, Cambridge, 1952, W. Heffer & Sons, Ltd.

Henning, L.: Ueber congenitale echte Sacraltumoren, Beitr. Path. Anat. **23**:593-619, 1900.

Higinbotham, N. L., Phillips, R. F., Farr, H. W., and Hustu, H. O.: Chordoma: thirty-five year study at Memorial Hospital, Cancer **20**:1841-1850, 1967.

King, I. S., and Butcher, J.: Osteochondroma of base of skull, Arch. Path. **37**:282-285, 1944.

Klinger, M.: Cartilage tumors of the base of the skull with intracranial extension, Acta Neurochir. **1**:337-380, 1951.

Kruyff, E., and Munn, J. D.: Posterior fossa tumors in infants and children, Amer. J. Roentgen. **89**:951-965, 1963.

Lindgren, E., and Di Chiro, G.: Radiographic findings in 14 cases of Sturge-Weber syndrome, Acta Radiol. **35**:387-399, 1951.

List, C. F.: Osteochondromas arising from the base of the skull, Surg. Gynec. Obstet. **76**:480-492, 1943.

Minagi, H., and Newton, T. H.: Cartilaginous tumors of the base of the skull, Amer. J. Roentgen. **105**:2:308-313, 1969.

McRae, D. L.: Bony abnormalities in the region of the foramen magnum: correlation of the anatomic and neurologic findings, Acta Radiol. **40**:335-354, 1953.

Olivecrona, A. H.: Die chirurgische Behandlung der Gehirntumoren. Eine klinische Studie, Berlin, 1927, Julius Springer.

Plaut, H. F., and Blatt, E. S.: Chordoma of clivus: report of four cases, Amer. J. Roentgen. **100**:639-649, 1967.

Pendergrass, E. P., Schaeffer, J. P., and Hodes, P. J.: Head and neck in roentgen diagnosis, ed. 2, Springfield, Ill., Charles C Thomas, Publisher, vol. 2.

Poppel, M. H., Jacobson, H. G., Duff, B. K., and Gottlieb, C.: Basilar impression and platybasia in Paget's disease, Radiology **61**:639-644, 1953.

Rossier, J.: Un symptôme radiologique des tumeurs de la fosse postérieure, Rev. Neurol. **71**:289-297, 1939.

Schisano, G., and Tovi, D.: Clivus chordomas, Neurochirurgia **5**:99-120, 1962.

von Sömmerring, S. T.: Vom Baue des menschlichen Korpers, Frankfurt, 1791-1796, Varrentrapp & Wenner, vol. 1 to 5.

Stern, W. E.: Personal communication, 1964.

Stevenson, G. C., Stoney, R. J., Perkins, R. K., and Adams, J. E.: A transcervical transclival approach to the ventral surface of the brainstem for removal of clivus chordoma, J. Neurosurg. **24**:544-551, 1966.

Vidic, B.: The postnatal development of sphenoid sinus and its spread into dorsum sellae and posterior clinoid processes, Amer. J. Roentgen. **104**:177-183, 1968.

Virchow, R. L. K.: Untersuchungen über die Entwickelung des Schädelgrundes im gesunden und krankhaften Zustande und über den Einfluss derselben auf Schädelform, Gesichtsbildung und Gehirnbau, Berlin, 1857, Reimar.

Wood, E. H., Jr., and Himadi, G. M.: Chordomas: roentgenologic study of 16 cases previously unreported, Radiology **54**: 706-716, 1950.

Zingesser, L. H., and Schechter, M. M.: The radiology of masses lying within and adjacent to the tentorial hiatus, Brit. J. Radiol. **37**:486-510, 1964.

CHAPTER 18

Sella turcica

Henry W. Pribram and George H. du Boulay

The history of mankind is an immense sea of errors in which a few obscure truths may here and there be found.
C. B. di Beccaria

At a meeting of the Society for Psychiatry and Nervous Diseases in Berlin on November 13, 1899, Oppenheim described the abnormal deepening and expansion of the sella in a patient with a pituitary tumour. Since then many papers on the anatomy and pathology of the sella have been published (Camp, 1924; Schaeffer, 1924; Kornblum, 1932; Mahmoud, 1958; and many others).

NORMAL SELLA

Henry W. Pribram

The sella turcica is the central depression within the sphenoid bone. Anteriorly its bony landmarks include the planum sphenoidale, the limbus sphenoidale, the chiasmatic sulcus, and the tuberculum sellae (Fig. 18-1). Anterolateral landmarks include the optic canal, the anterior clinoid processes, and the optic strut, which forms the floor of the optic canal (Fig. 18-2). The floor of the sella is the roof of the sphenoid sinus. Posteriorly the sella is bounded by the dorsum sellae and the posterior clinoid processes; its lateral margins are the carotid sulci; and its superior boundary is the diaphragma sellae.

Development of sella

The body of the sphenoid bone is developed in cartilage and consists of two main parts until the seventh or eighth month of fetal life. One part, the presphenoid, is in front of the tuberculum sellae; and one part, the postsphenoid, is behind. The presphenoid leads to formation of the anterior part of the sella turcica and the lesser wings of the sphenoid, whereas the postsphenoid forms the remainder of the sella turcica, the dorsum sellae, and the greater wings of the sphenoid. Cartilage formation begins posteriorly and extends forward around the pituitary to form the cartilaginous presphenoid. At birth the sella consists only of a small depression. The ossification center for the sella appears shortly after birth, and ossification takes place in the basisphenoid and presphenoid (Fig. 18-3). Although the tuberculum sellae is present at birth, the planum sphenoidale is not yet formed. The dorsum sellae is absent and develops from a separate ossification center. During the first year of life, ossification of the middle portion of the presphenoid center leads to an increase in height and the formation of the planum. The planum continues to enlarge but remains separate from the presphenoid. Posterior growth of the planum leads to overlapping of the presphenoid by the limbus and determines the shape and length of the chiasmatic sulcus. A narrow planum results in a wide chiasmatic sulcus, and vice versa. The normal notch between the limbus and the presphenoid (Fig. 18-4) should not be mistaken for the intersphenoid synchondrosis, which is located below the tuberculum sellae (Kier, 1968) (Fig. 18-5). The limbic notch has been mistakenly referred to as the J sella (Kier, 1969) (Fig. 18-4). The intersphenoid synchondrosis is formed by fusion of the presphenoid and the postsphenoid, and it is seen occasionally as a thin canal

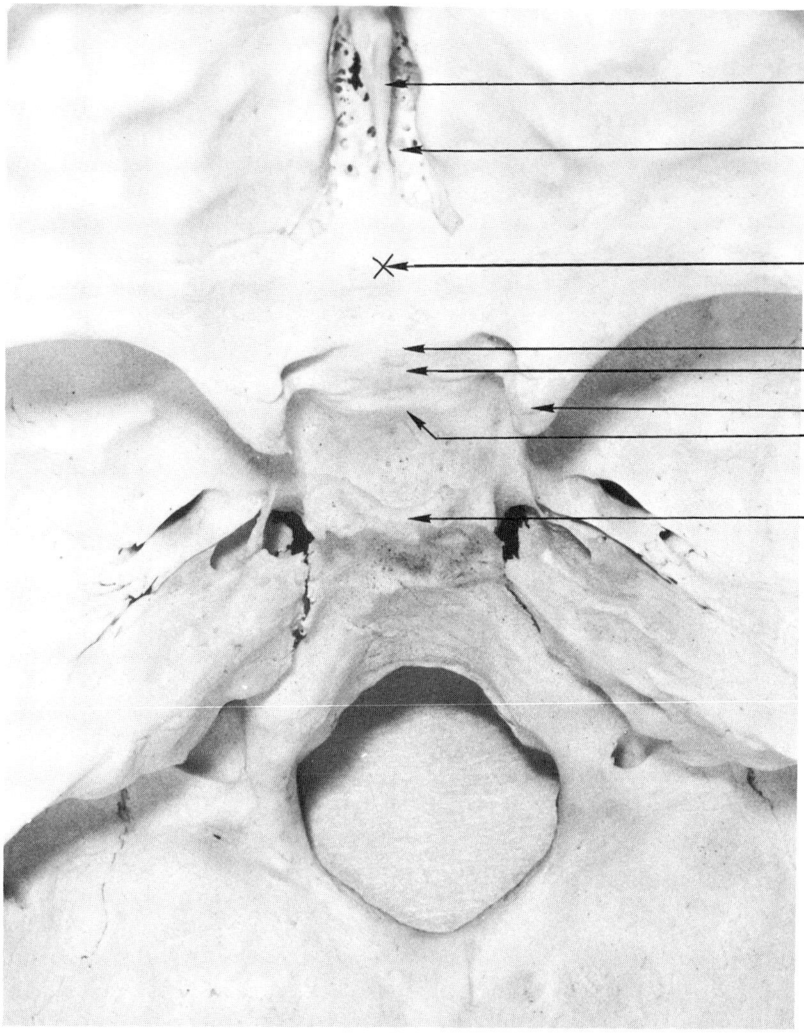

Fig. 18-1. View of skull base seen from above to show relation of sella turcica to anterior, middle, and posterior fossae.

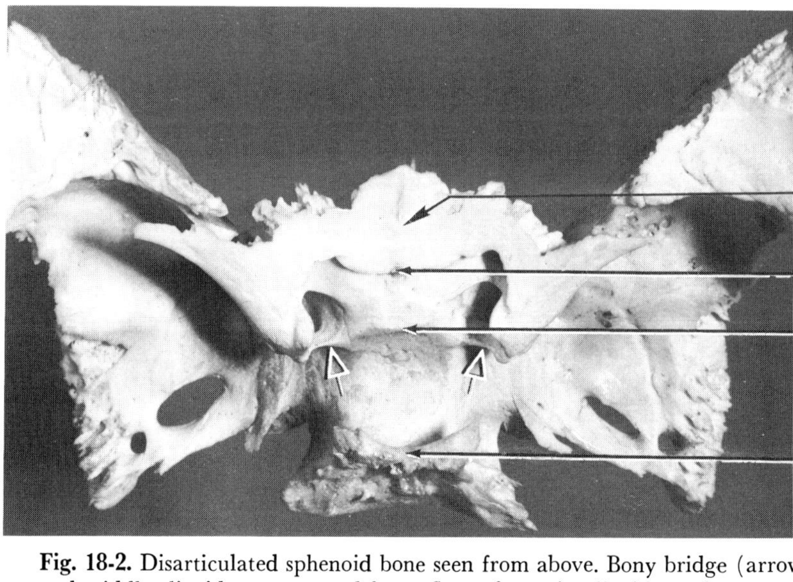

Fig. 18-2. Disarticulated sphenoid bone seen from above. Bony bridge (arrows) joins anterior and middle clinoid processes and forms floor of caroticoclinoid canal.

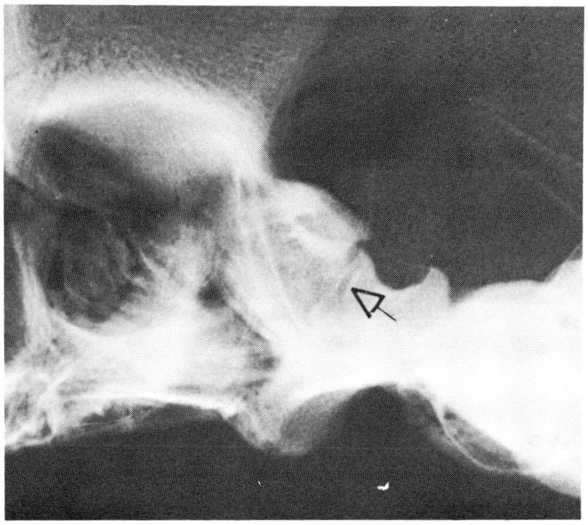

Fig. 18-3. Lateral roentgenogram of fetal skull shows that sella is small because dorsum is still partly cartilaginous. Planum sphenoidale is slightly concave. The concave chiasmatic sulcus is overshadowed by somewhat bulbous anterior clinoid processes. Intersphenoid synchondrosis is prominent (arrow).

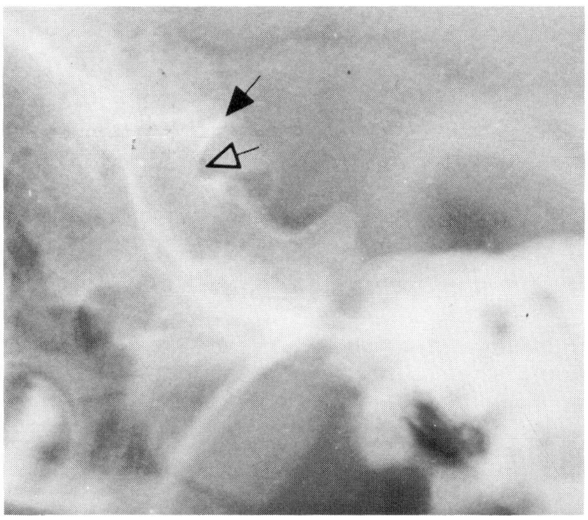

Fig. 18-4. Normal sella in an infant. Limbus (solid arrow) and chiasmatic sulcus (open arrow) are prominent. Sella is shallow. Dorsum sellae is not completely ossified.

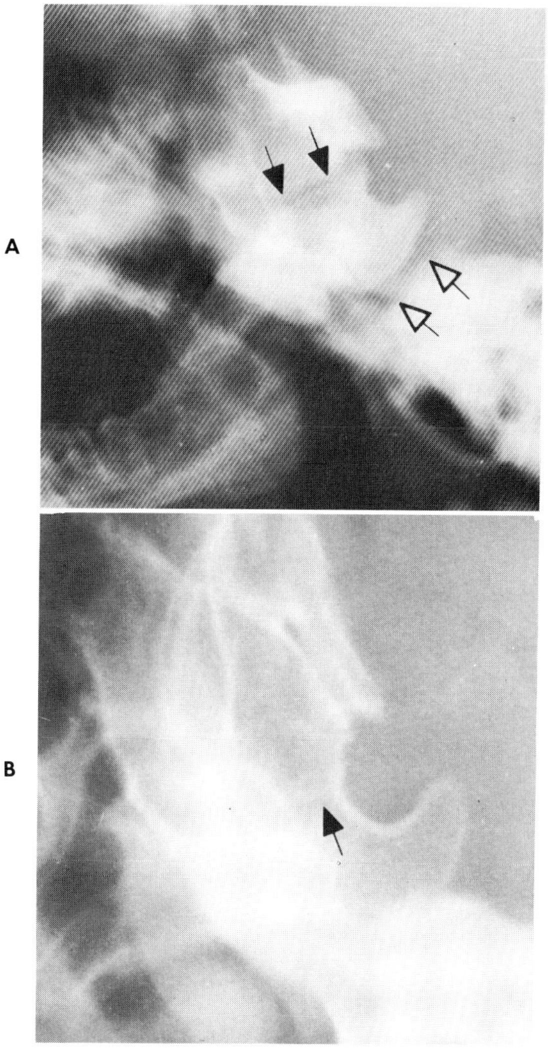

Fig. 18-5. A, Well-marked intersphenoid synchondrosis (solid arrows) in newborn infant. Spheno-occipital synchondrosis (open arrows) is prominent. **B,** At 9 months of age, intersphenoid synchondrosis is closing and is much less prominent (arrow).

extending forward and downward from the margin of the tuberculum sellae (Fig. 18-5, *B*). It should not be confused with the craniopharyngeal canal, which is not visible after birth (Lowman et al., 1966; Kier, 1968). The craniopharyngeal canal arises from the lowest portion of the sella. Kaufman (1969) claims to have identified it in cases of cerebrospinal fluid rhinorrhea. Posteriorly the dorsum sellae and adjacent sphenoid unite with the occipital bone to form the clivus. The spheno-occipital synchondrosis (Fig. 18-5) disappears between the fourteenth and twentieth years, but fusion may be delayed until the twenty-fifth year or fail to occur at all.

Normal anatomy (gross and roentgenologic)

Planum sphenoidale

The planum sphenoidale (Figs. 18-1 and 18-2) is a thin well-defined plate of bone that extends from the cribriform plate to the limbus sphenoidale. The central portion, which extends forward and articulates with the cribriform plate, has been termed the ethmoid plate. Its lateral extensions form the roofs of the optic canals (Fig. 18-2) and blend with the anterior clinoid processes. The planum sphenoidale has a smooth upper surface that may be slightly concave.

In the frontal projection the planum is identified

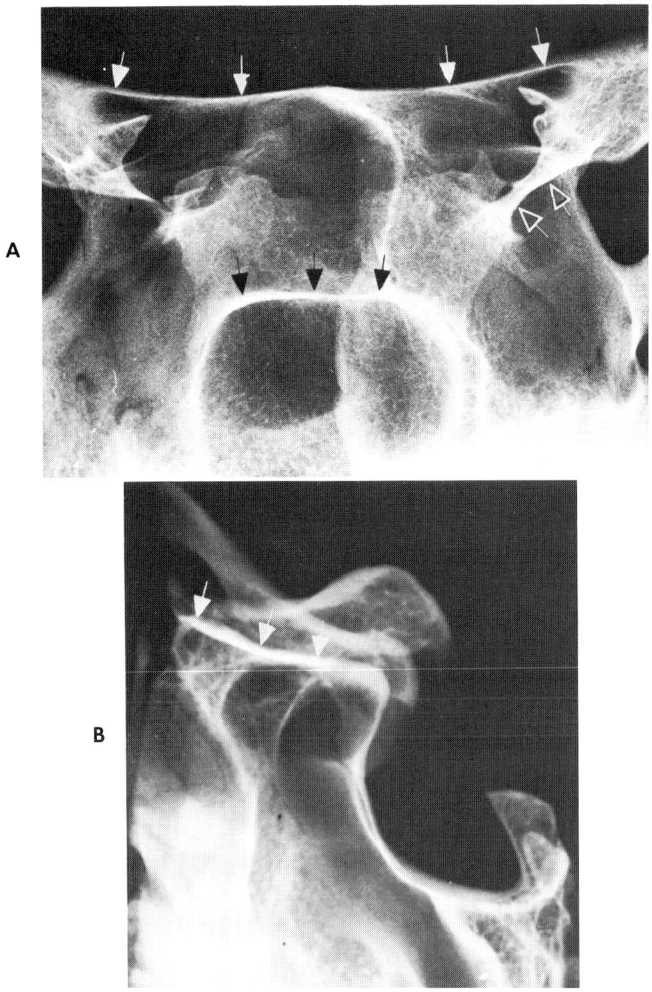

Fig. 18-6. Roentgenogram of sphenoid bone. **A,** Frontal projection. **B,** Lateral projection. Planum sphenoidale (solid white arrows) joins two lesser wings of sphenoid. (Floor of sella is indicated by solid black arrows; interclinoid ligament by open arrows.)

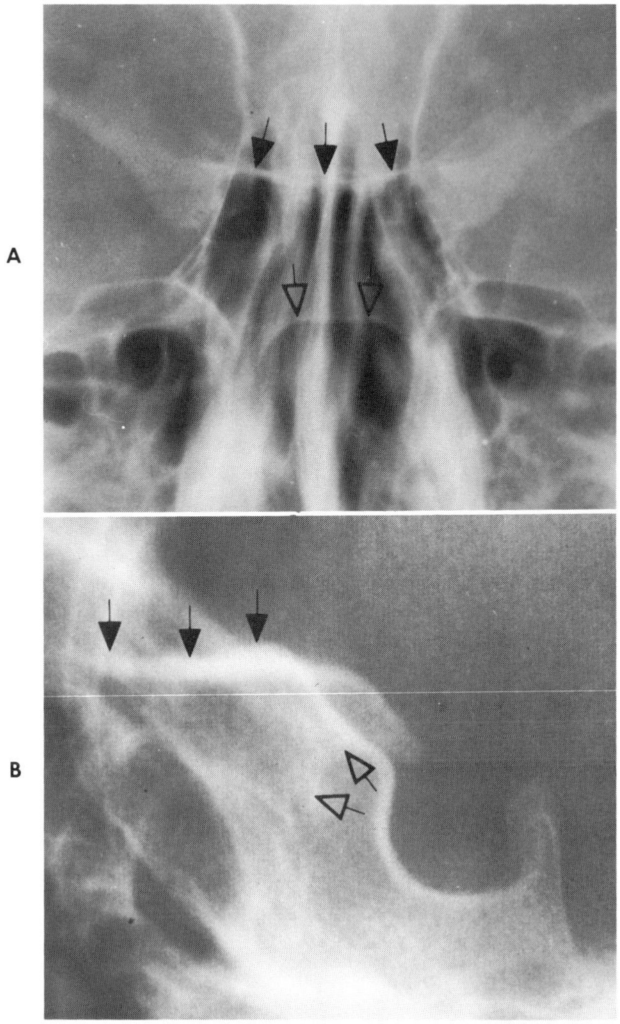

Fig. 18-7. Planum sphenoidale (solid arrows) shown as well-defined plate of cortical bone in both frontal, **A,** and lateral, **B,** projections. Optic strut (open arrows), superimposed on chiasmatic sulcus, is faintly shown in lateral projection. Floor of sella (open arrows) in frontal projection is limited laterally by carotid sulcus.

as the jugum that joins the two lesser wings of the sphenoid (Figs. 18-6, *A*, and 18-7, *A*). The width of the planum is determined by the degree of separation between the two orbits. The crista galli is seen as a linear vertical density above the planum. In the lateral projection the planum is identified below the orbital roofs as a well-defined density extending to the limbus sphenoidale (Figs. 18-6, *B*, and 18-7, *B*). Tomography in the lateral and frontal projections defines it more clearly.

Limbus sphenoidale

The limbus sphenoidale marks the posterior boundary of the planum sphenoidale (Fig. 18-8). The appearance of the limbus varies with the shape of the chiasmatic sulcus. When the chiasmatic sulcus is concave, the limbus sphenoidale is prominent (Fig. 18-9). On the other hand, when the chiasmatic sulcus is convex, the limbus is barely discernible (Fig. 18-6, *B*). The limbus can be identified only in the lateral projection, and it is found at the intersection of the orbital roofs and the planum sphenoidale. It is overlapped by the anterior clinoid processes.

Chiasmatic sulcus

The chiasmatic sulcus is a depression of variable depth, spanning the distance between the cranial openings of the optic canals (Fig. 18-2). Anteriorly it is bounded by the limbus sphenoidale, and posteriorly by the tuberculum sellae. The chiasmatic sulcus is

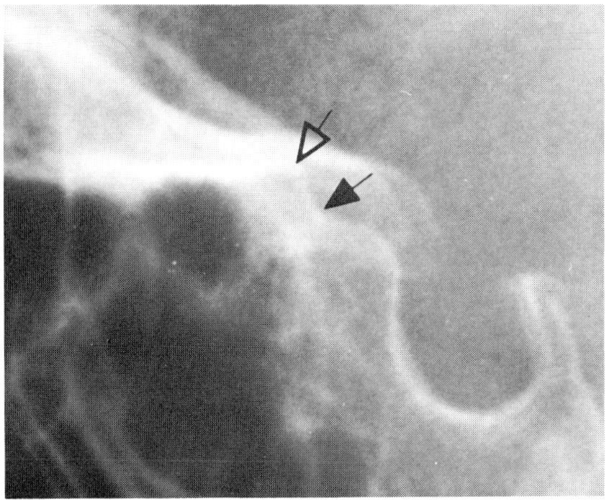

Fig. 18-8. Chiasmatic sulcus (solid arrow) is convex, and there is a marked step at the point of fusion between limbus (open arrow) and presphenoid.

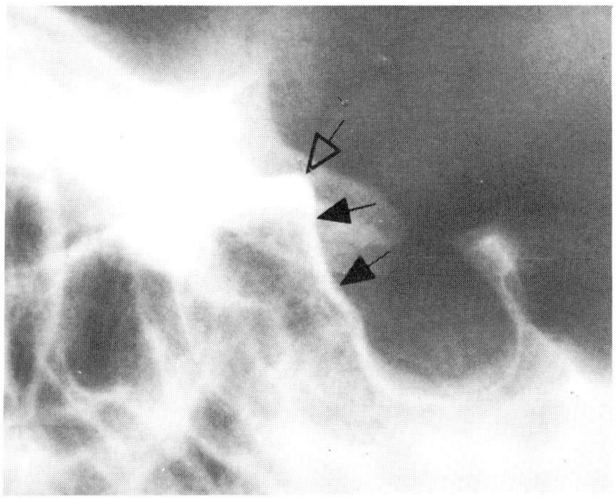

Fig. 18-9. Slightly concave chiasmatic sulcus (solid arrows) with much longer vertical component than usual. Prominent limbus sphenoidale is indicated by open arrow.

usually horizontal, but it may at times be almost vertical (Fig. 18-9). Its shape is affected by the degree of pneumatization of the sphenoid. When pneumatization is extensive, the shape of the chiasmatic sulcus tends to be convex (Fig. 18-10, *A*). With lesser degrees of pneumatization, the chiasmatic sulcus may be flat (Fig. 18-10, *B*) or concave (Fig. 18-9). A poorly pneumatized sphenoid has been termed an infantile sphenoid (Holman, 1959). The width of the chiasmatic sulcus is determined by the width of the planum sphenoidale in an inverse relationship. Thus a wide planum leads to a narrow chiasmatic sulcus. The optic strut and the roof of the optic canal may be seen on the lateral roentgenogram of the skull and may simulate enlargement of the chiasmatic sulcus (Kier, 1968) (Figs. 18-4 and 18-11). This appearance is particularly common in infants and children.

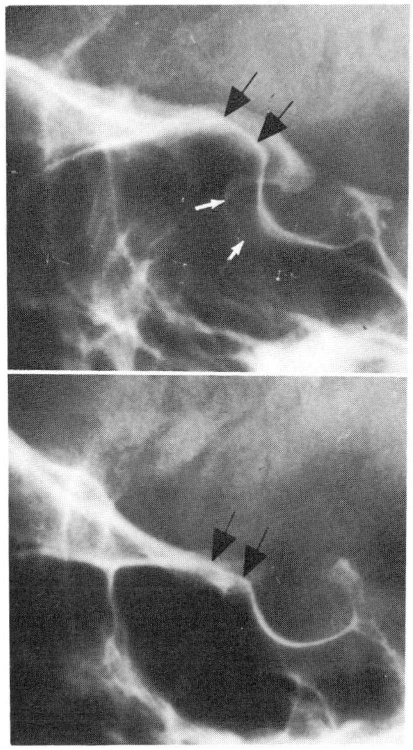

Fig. 18-10. Variation in normal appearance of chiasmatic sulcus (black arrows). **A,** Convex. **B,** Flat. Carotid sulcus is indicated by white arrows.

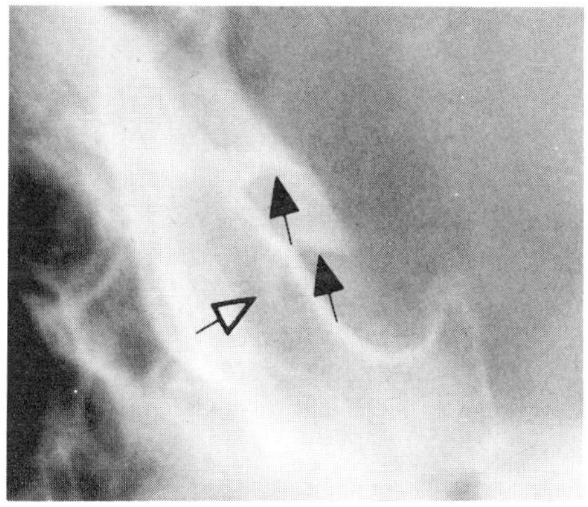

Fig. 18-11. Normal sella in 3-year-old child. Lateral roentgenogram shows that dorsum sellae is partially ossified. Chiasmatic sulcus is flat. Roofs of two optic canals (solid arrows) and optic struts (open arrows) can be seen in slightly rotated projection.

Despite the name, the optic chiasm seldom lies within the chiasmatic sulcus. It is situated either above the diaphragma sellae or at a variable distance from the diaphragma. In relation to the hypophysis, the chiasm

A B C D

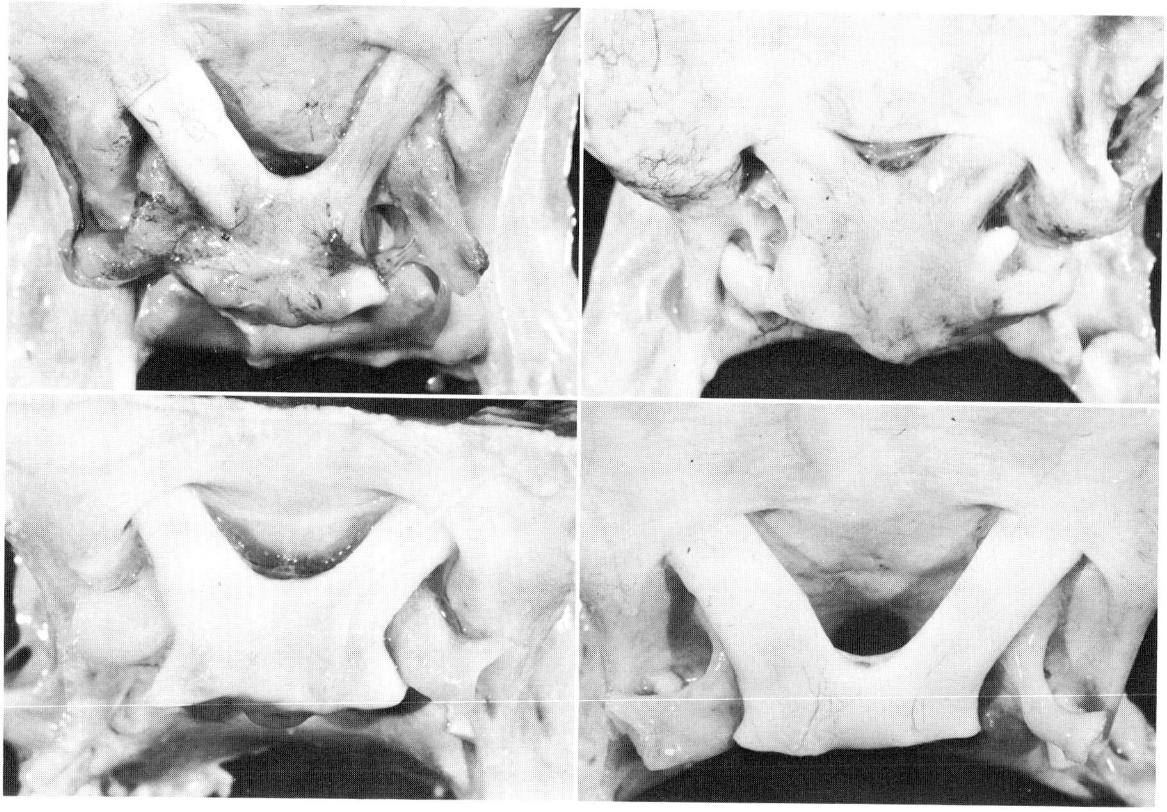

Fig. 18-12. Relation of optic chiasm to sella. **A,** Normal (79%). Optic chiasm is located almost completely over diaphragma sellae, only a small portion projecting over dorsum sellae. **B,** Pre-fixed (5%). Optic chiasm is partly located in chiasmatic sulcus. **C,** Overlying diaphragma sellae (12%). **D,** Post-fixed (4%). Optic chiasm is located on dorsum sellae.

may be prefixed or postfixed (Schaeffer, 1924). The prefixed chiasm (5%) overlies the tuberculum sellae (Fig. 18-12, *B*), whereas the postfixed chiasm (4%) overlies the dorsum sellae (Fig. 18-12, *D*). In the remainder the optic chiasm is wholly (79%) or almost wholly (12%) related to the diaphragma sellae (Fig. 18-12, *A* and *C*). Findings from autopsy studies by Schaeffer were confirmed in the living by Bull (1956) and by Mahmoud (1958). Bull (1956) found that the insertion of the optic chiasm into the third ventricle, which he termed the chiasmatic point, was situated 10 to 23 mm from the chiasmatic sulcus. Bergland and his associates (1968) found that the position of the chiasm is related to the length of the tuberculum. The length varied from 3 to 12 mm, with an average of 7 mm. (By "tuberculum" they meant the distance of the tuberculum sellae from a line drawn between the optic nerves at the point where the nerves enter the optic canal.) A short tuberculum was associated with the postfixed chiasm, and vice versa. The chiasmatic sulcus can be identified only in the lateral projection as the intervening groove between the limbus sphenoidale and the tuberculum. It is frequently overshadowed

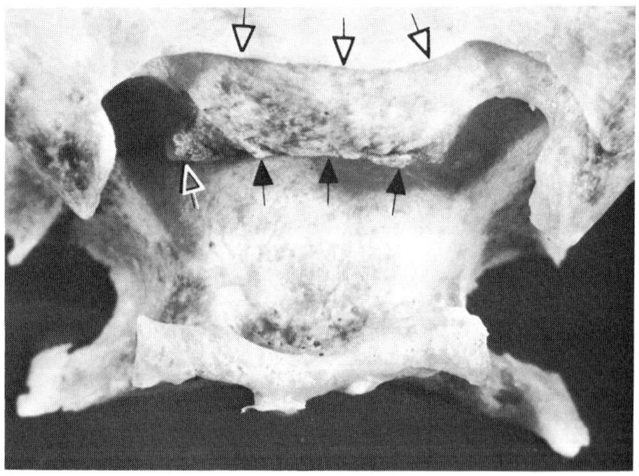

Fig. 18-13. Disarticulated sphenoid bone seen from above. Well-demarcated limbus (open black arrows) and tuberculum sellae (solid arrows) are shown. Well-formed middle clinoid process (open white arrow) is seen on the left. Dorsum sellae is hollowed in its central portion, which is often extremely thin. It is curved and its lateral borders, particularly on the left, extend farther forward than its central portion. Note the well-formed carotid sulcus on the left.

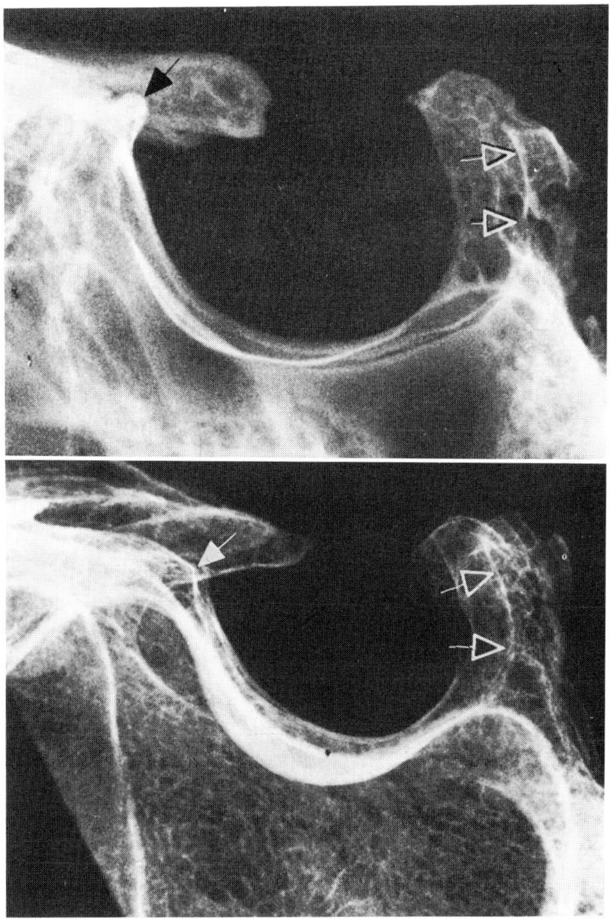

Fig. 18-14. Lateral roentgenograms of sella. Tuberculum sellae (solid arrow) is better defined in **A,** where chiasmatic sulcus is concave. In **B,** tuberculum sellae (solid arrow) is less well defined and chiasmatic sulcus is convex. Lamina dura lining central portion of dorsum sellae (open arrows) is projected behind lateral strut of dorsum.

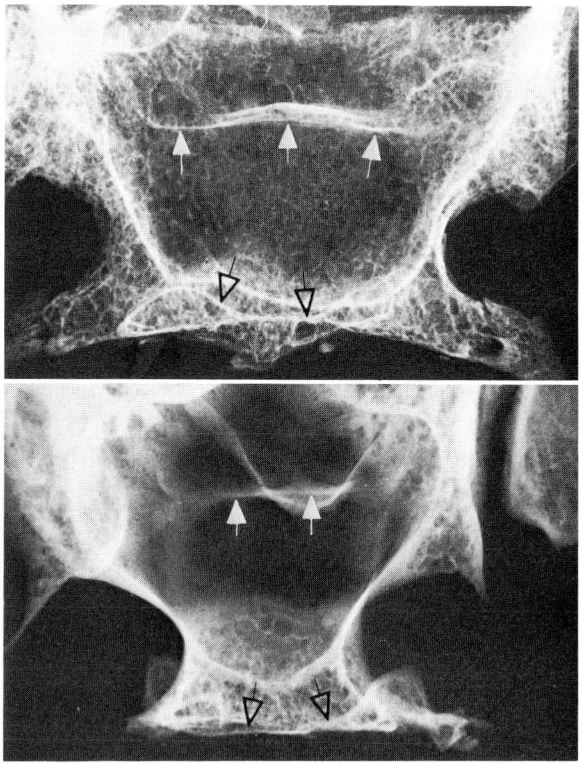

Fig. 18-15. Basal roentgenograms show well-defined tuberculum sellae (solid arrows) and dorsum sellae (open arrows). Thick cortical margin of sphenoid sinus extends anteriorly to dorsum sellae.

by the anterior clinoid processes and forms part of the roof of the sphenoid sinus.

Tuberculum sellae

The tuberculum sellae is a transverse ridge that forms the posterior margin of the chiasmatic sulcus as well as the anterior margin of the pituitary fossa (Fig. 18-13). It spans the distance between the anterior limits of the carotid sulci. This distance is variable and determines the length of the tuberculum sellae. The prominence of the tuberculum sellae is related to the shape of the chiasmatic sulcus (Fig. 18-14). The tuberculum sellae can be identified in the lateral and basal projections (Figs. 18-14 and 18-15). In the lateral projection it is partly obscured by the anterior clinoid processes (Fig. 18-14).

Anterior clinoid processes

The anterior clinoid processes are the posterior medial extensions of the lesser wings of the sphenoid (Fig. 18-1). They form the anterior and lateral borders of the carotid sulcus. Their appearance, shape, and thickness vary considerably (Figs. 18-5, 18-6, *B,* and 18-14). They are frequently asymmetric, and occasionally one may be vestigial or absent. Pneumatization of the sphenoid sinus may extend into the anterior clinoid processes. The tips of the anterior clinoid processes are situated slightly lateral to the posterior clinoid processes (Figs. 18-1, 18-2, and 18-13). The optic strut is a bony ridge that arises from the anteroinferior margin of the anterior clinoid process (Fig. 18-16). It forms the floor of the optic canal and separates the floor from the superior orbital fissure and the internal carotid artery (Fig. 18-2). The anterior clinoid processes may be identified in the frontal and lateral projections. In the frontal projection they are situated lateral to the dorsum sellae and above the roof of the sphenoid sinus. In the true lateral projection the two anterior clinoid processes are superimposed on each other; but if the film is rotated, one may be seen above the other. Under these circumstances

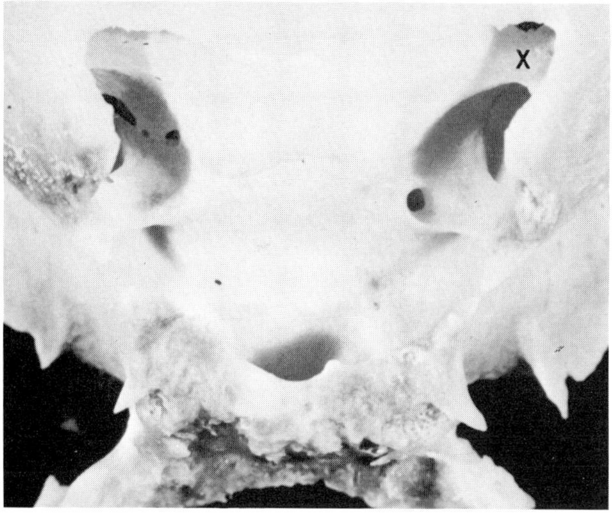

Fig. 18-16. Sella seen from above. Optic strut (X) forms lateral and inferior margin of optic canal.

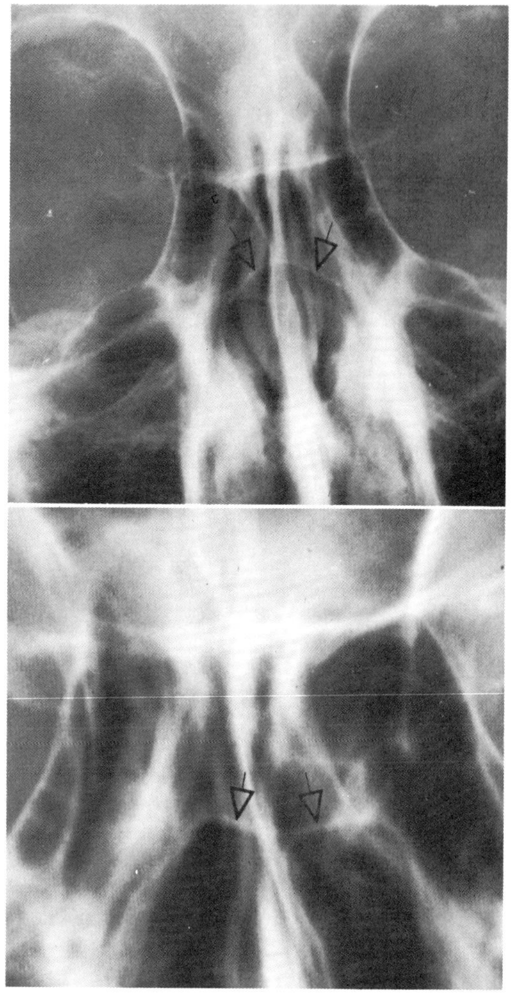

Fig. 18-17. Floor of sella, frontal projection. **A,** Convex. **B,** Concave.

part of the optic strut and the optic canal roof may be brought into view, simulating enlargement of the chiasmatic sulcus. Identification of the optic strut rests on continuation of the strut with the anterior clinoid process. Since the strut is normally superimposed on the chiasmatic sulcus, it may be seen as a curved linear density (Fig. 18-7, *B*), which has been mistaken for the intersphenoid synchondrosis. The latter is found caudal to the tuberculum sellae (Fig. 18-5, *A*).

Middle clinoid processes

The middle clinoid processes are inconstant elevations on the anterior wall of the pituitary fossa, medial to the carotid artery (Fig. 18-13). At this level the internal carotid arteries pierce the dura mater and become intradural. Ossification of the intraclinoid bridge between the anterior and middle clinoid processes leads to the formation of the caroticoclinoid canal (Fig. 18-2). This canal is believed to be a developmental anomaly (Kier, 1968). Middle clinoid processes can be identified only in the lateral view as a slight spur on the anterior margin of the pituitary fossa just below the tuberculum sellae.

Floor of sella turcica

For purposes of description, the floor of the sella turcica will include portions of the anterior and the posterior walls of the pituitary fossa. The floor of the sella turcica is therefore considered to extend from the tuberculum to the dorsum sellae. In the sagittal plane the floor usually has a rounded appearance (Fig. 18-10, *B*), but its horizontal portion may be relatively straight (Fig. 18-10, *A*). In the coronal section the horizontal portion of the floor usually has a slightly convex (Fig. 18-17, *A*) or flat appearance (Figs. 18-6, *A*, and 18-7, *A*). Occasionally it has a slight downward concavity (Fig. 18-17, *B*). The sellar floor may be asymmetric, sloping downward more on one side than on the other. The horizontal portion of the carotid sulcus forms the lateral margin of the floor. The boundary between the floor and the carotid sulcus is normally rounded (Figs. 18-6, *A*, 18-7, *A*, and 18-17). In the lateral projection the floor of the pituitary fossa is well defined; the cortical bone that lines it has been termed lamina dura. The lamina dura continues posteriorly on to the dorsum sellae. The sphenoid sinus extends for a variable distance beneath the sellar floor. The cortical lining of the sphenoid sinus is much thicker and better defined than that of the cancellous bone (Fig. 18-14, *B*). Consequently the lamina dura is thickest over the sinus and thinnest on the inner aspect of the dorsum sellae.

A

B

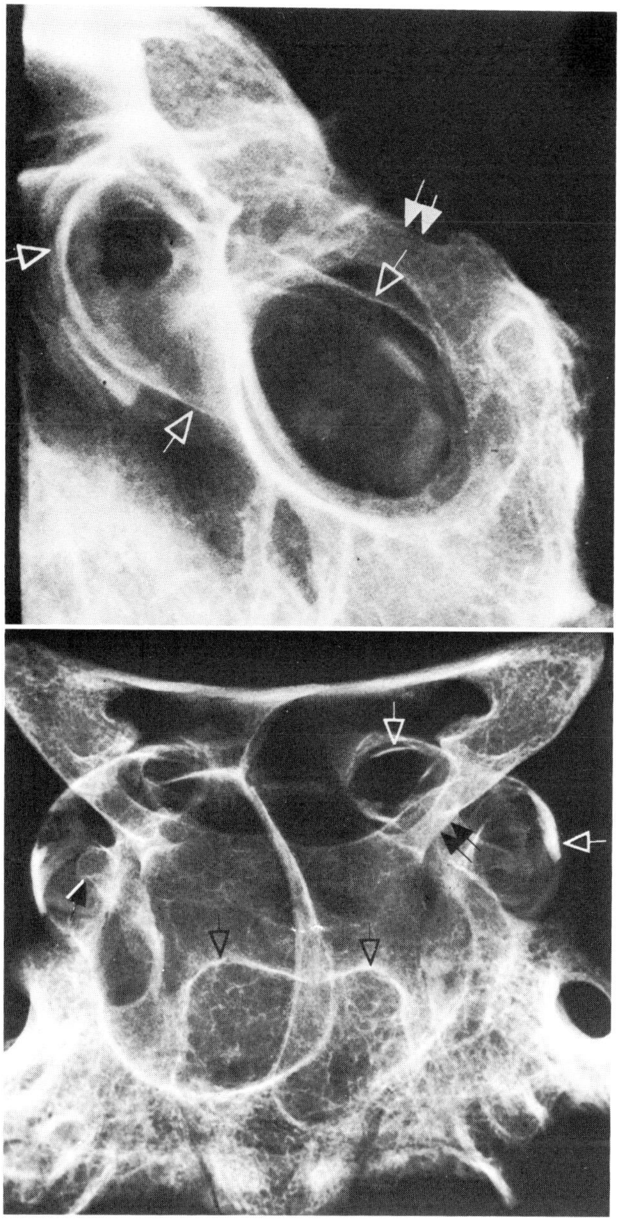

Fig. 18-18. Roentgenograms of sella with calcification in cavernous portion of internal carotid artery (open white arrows). Interclinoid ligament is ossified (double solid arrows). Floor of sella is concave and slightly asymmetric (open black arrows). **A,** Lateral projection. **B,** Frontal projection.

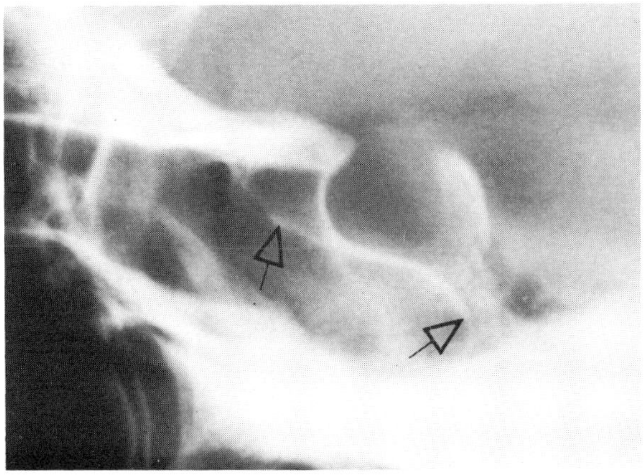

Fig. 18-19. Prominent carotid sulcus (arrows).

A

B

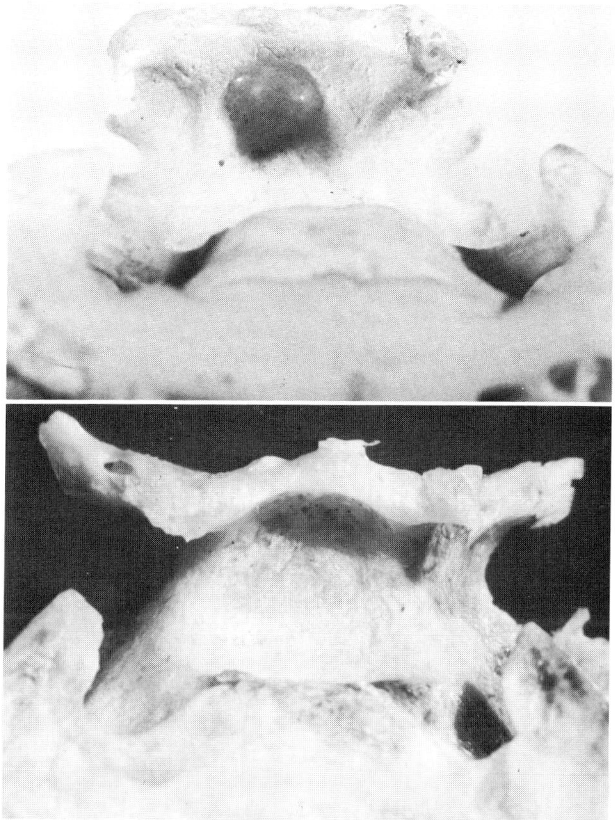

Fig. 18-20. Closeup view of dorsum sellae seen from front, **A,** and above, **B.** Note the lateral and horizontal struts surrounding the central depression within the dorsum sellae.

The appearance of the cortical lining of the pneumatized and unpneumatized portions of the floor of the sella is strikingly different. In the normal sella the lamina dura is preserved and neither age nor osteoporosis will affect it (Nordmark, 1949; Lindgren and Di Chiro, 1951; Fry and du Boulay, 1965). The only possible exceptions are arterial hypertension (Jefferson, 1955; Fry and du Boulay, 1965) or alcoholism (Albert and LeMay, 1968). A sloping or asymmetric floor may give the appearance of a double or even a triple floor on the lateral projection.

Carotid sulcus

The carotid sulcus is a shallow groove along the superolateral aspect of the sphenoid sinus that is formed by the cavernous portion of the internal carotid artery (Figs. 18-2 and 18-18). The depth of the carotid sulcus varies. The sulcus is usually shallow but may have a prominent inferior border. In the lateral projection the carotid sulcus is identified as an S-shaped groove projected below the level of the floor of the sella (Engels, 1958) (Fig. 18-19). In the frontal projection it appears as a shallow indentation on either side of the floor of the sella. When calcified, the cavernous portion of the internal carotid artery can be identified within the carotid sulcus on both frontal and lateral projections (Fig. 18-18).

Dorsum sellae

The dorsum sellae (Figs. 18-1 and 18-2) is the vertical posterior boundary of the sella and is formed by two lateral struts topped by a horizontal strut (Fig. 18-20). It varies greatly in shape and thickness. Mahmoud (1958) found that the thickness of the dorsum ranges from 2 to 7 mm but that only the lateral portions are thick. The central portion is a well-defined hollow between the sturdier lateral pillars and forms a bed for the posterior portion of the pituitary gland (Fig. 18-20). The central portion is often extremely thin (Scheuermann, 1932; Fry and du Boulay, 1965). It may even be absent so that a foramen is found within the dorsum sellae (Laschi, 1931). The lateral aspect of the dorsum sellae may be grooved by the sixth nerve or by a persistent trigeminal artery (Fig. 18-82). The anterior wall of the dorsum sellae is smooth, whereas the posterior aspect is rough. The roughness of the posterior aspect of the dorsum is due to the dural venous plexus in this location. The posterior clinoid processes are the lateral and superior extensions of the dorsum sellae. The tips of the posterior clinoid processes are usually rounded, and they project forward and slightly laterally (Fig. 18-21). Occasionally the tips are pointed and may extend forward to join with the anterior clinoid processes (bridged sella) (Fig. 18-21, *C*).

In the lateral projection the dorsum sellae is seen as a vertical plate of bone with well-defined anterior and posterior cortical margins (Fig. 18-14). The lamina dura overlying the central portion of the dorsum sellae is often projected behind that of the lateral pillars of the dorsum (Figs. 18-14 and 18-22). In this respect the appearance of the dorsum sellae is rather like that of an armchair (Fig. 18-23). Pneumatization of the sphenoid sinus may extend into the dorsum sellae and the posterior clinoid processes. An exostosis may arise from the posterior aspect of the dorsum (Fig. 18-24). In the frontal view the dorsum sellae is best identified in the Towne projection (Fig. 18-21). In this projection the appearance varies greatly. The dorsum sellae may be seen as a quadrilateral plate of bone, or it may

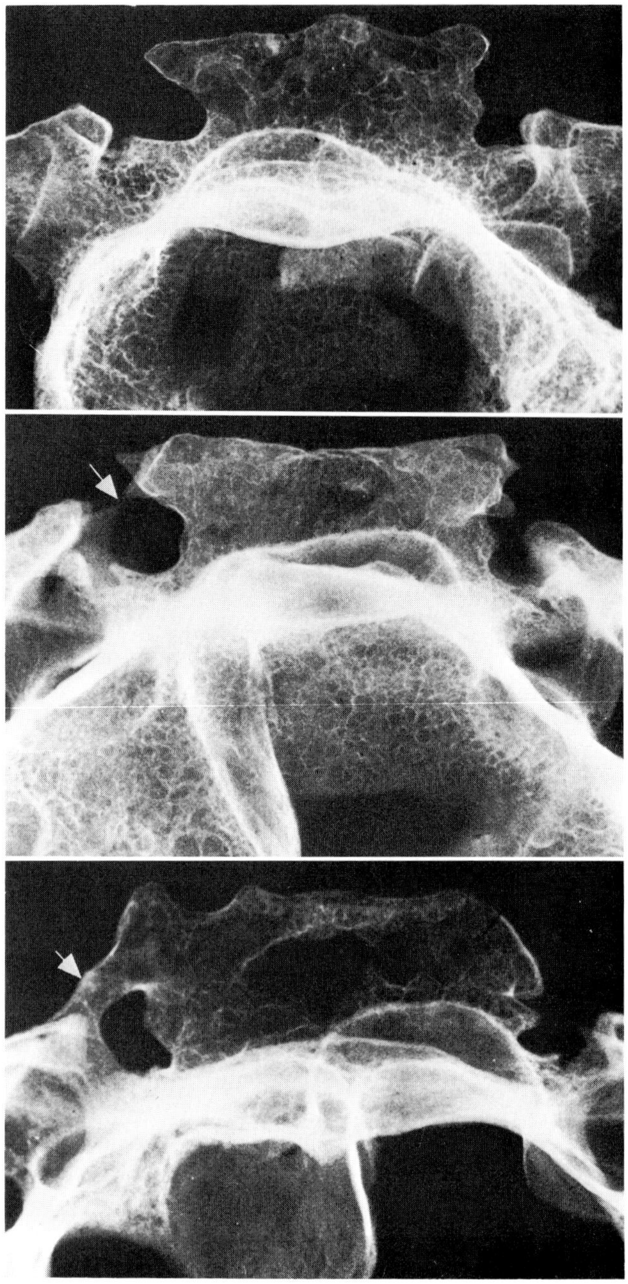

Fig. 18-21. Roentgenograms of dorsum sellae in frontal projection. Interclinoid ligament (arrow) is partly ossified in **B** and completely ossified in **C.** Central portion of dorsum is thin in **C.**

have a narrow waist. The posterior clinoid processes, too, may be bulbous or pointed. The dorsum sellae can usually be identified in the base view and, when so seen, is often curved with a concavity anteriorly (Fig. 18-23).

Dural attachment of sella

The diaphragma sellae is the dural fold formed by the anterior extension of the tentorium (Fig. 18-25).

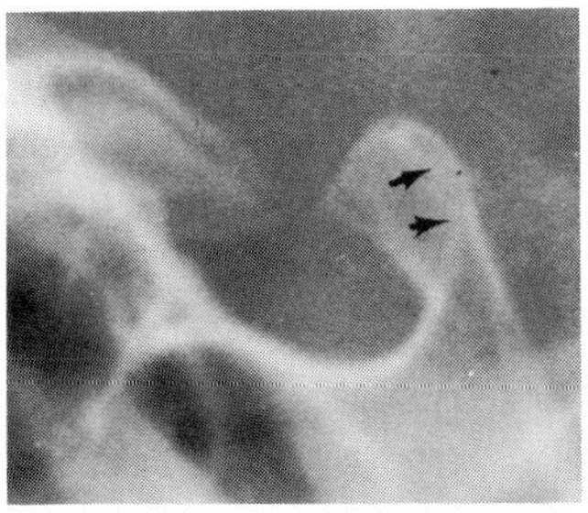

Fig. 18-22. Normal sella. Lateral roentgenogram reveals central portion of dorsum (arrows) lying posterior to lateral portion. Central portion of dorsum is thin.

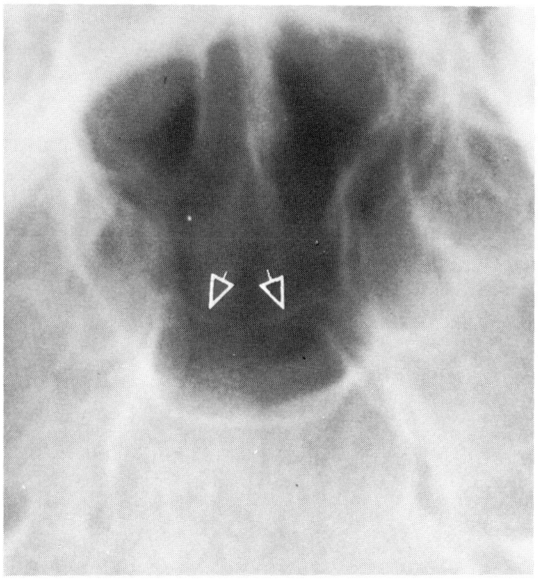

Fig. 18-23. Normal sella. Basal projection shows normal curvature of dorsum sellae (arrows).

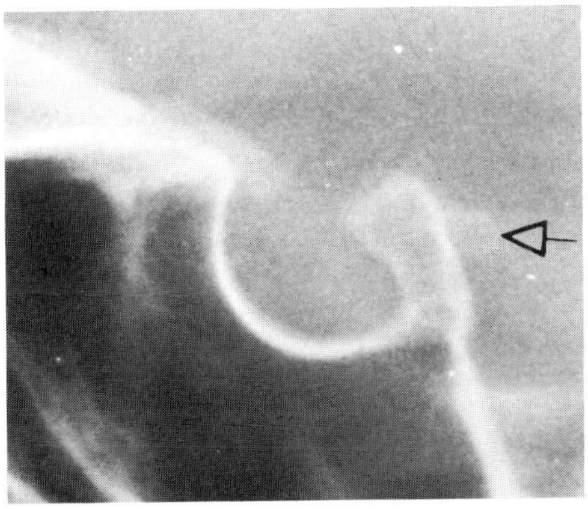

Fig. 18-24. Normal sella. Lateral roentgenogram shows that sphenoid is well pneumatized. Exostosis arises from posterior aspect of dorsum sellae (arrow).

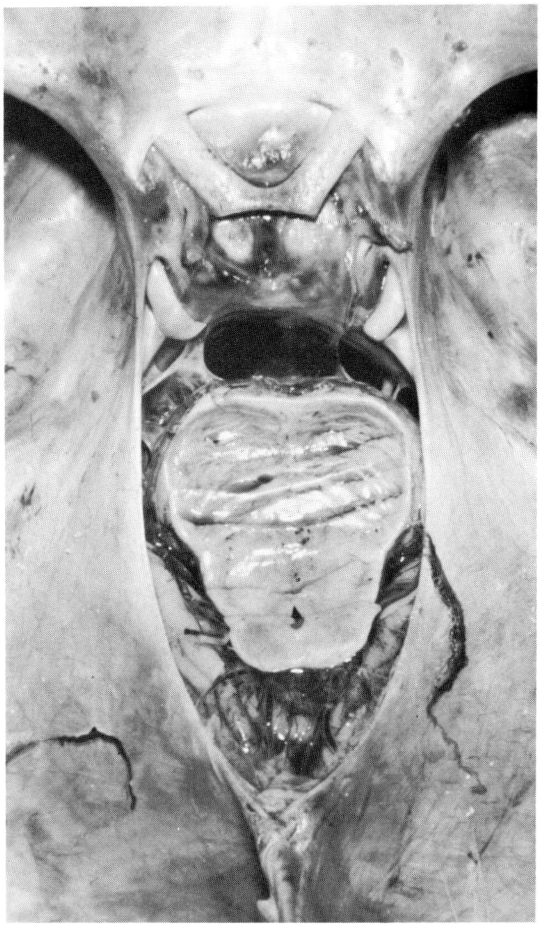

Fig. 18-25. Tentorial incisura seen from above. Tentorium is attached anteriorly to the anterior clinoid processes and tuberculum sellae.

It is attached anteriorly to the tuberculum, posteriorly to the dorsum, and laterally to the interclinoid ligament, which joins the anterior and posterior clinoid processes. The diaphragma sellae has a central opening that transmits the pituitary stalk. The thickness of the diaphragma, as well as the size of the opening, varies. The diaphragma sellae was studied in detail by Busch (1951), who examined 788 sellae turcicae. He described three main types: (1) the diaphragma forms a complete covering with only a small opening for the pituitary stalk (41.9%) (Figs. 18-26, *A* and *B,* and 18-27); (2) the diaphragma is incomplete, with an opening for the stalk less than 3 mm (37.6%); and (3) the diaphragma is represented by only a rim of tissue less than 2 mm in width (20.5%) (Fig. 18-26, *C* and *D*). In a similar study the opening for the pituitary stalk was noted to be greater than 5 mm in 39% of the cases (Bergland et al., 1968). In sagittal section the diaphragma sellae usually slopes slightly downward into the sella (Fig.

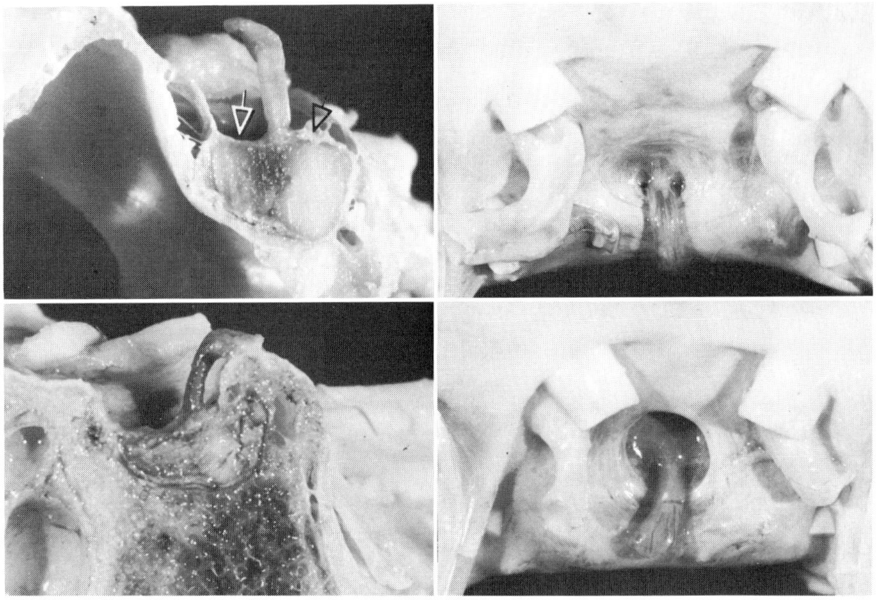

Fig. 18-26. Normal variations in size of opening of diaphragma sellae. **A** and **B,** Well-developed diaphragma with small opening for hypophyseal stalk. **C** and **D,** Large central opening in diaphragma.

18-26). The interclinoid ligament may calcify or ossify (Fig. 18-28).

Ligamentous attachments may also bridge the anterior and middle clinoid processes (Fig. 18-2). Ossification of this ligament leads to the formation of the caroticoclinoid canal. The petroclinoid ligament extends from the posterior clinoid processes inferolaterally to the petrous apex (Fig. 18-29). The calcified petroclinoid ligament may be seen posterior to the sella extending laterally to the petrous ridges (Fig. 18-30).

Measurement of sella

Careful examination of the changes within the sella is far more rewarding than measuring the sella. There are times, however, when measuring the sella may be valuable in the analysis of sellar abnormalities. It has been shown that about 80% of the sella is occupied by the pituitary gland and that the gland may increase in size during pregnancy (Di Chiro and Nelson, 1962; McLachlan et al., 1968). It has also been suggested that the sella increases in size with age (Israel, 1970).

Length

Camp (1924) suggested that a distance exceeding 16 mm between the tuberculum sellae and the dorsum sellae (with a 40-inch anode-to-film distance) probably indicates an enlarged sella. Taveras and Wood (1964) measured the greatest anteroposterior diameter and

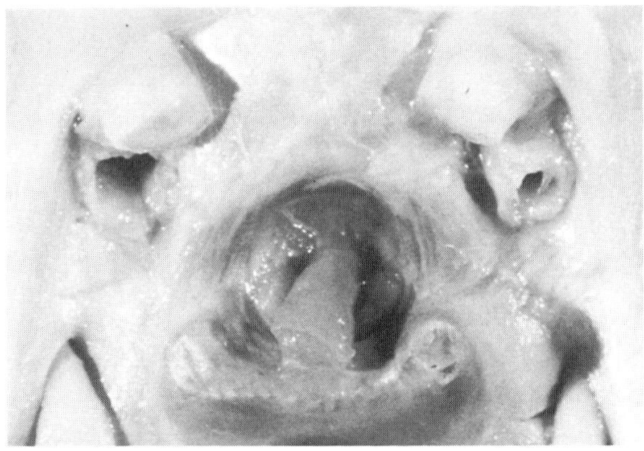

Fig. 18-27. Sella seen from above. Diaphragma sellae is complete but very thin.

regarded 17 mm as the upper limits of normal. They too used a 40-inch anode-to-film distance and positioned the head 2 inches from the Potter-Bucky tray.

Depth

To measure the depth, a line is drawn from the tuberculum sellae to the top of the dorsum sellae. The lowest point in the pituitary fossa is then joined to this line. If the distance along the second line measures 14 mm or more, the sella is considered to be abnormally deep (anode-film distance 40 inches).

A

B

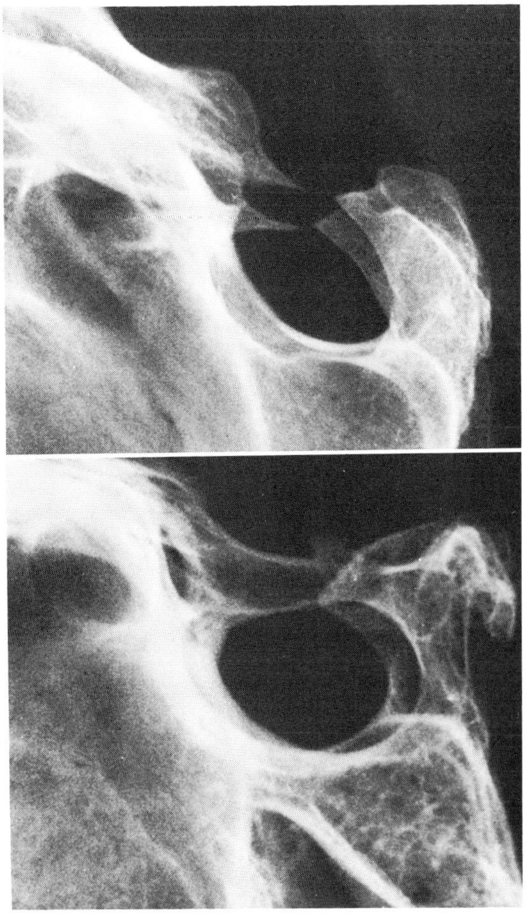

Fig. 18-28. Lateral roentgenogram of sphenoid bone. **A,** Interclinoid ligament is almost entirely ossified and posterior clinoid processes are pointed. **B,** Completely ossified interclinoid ligaments.

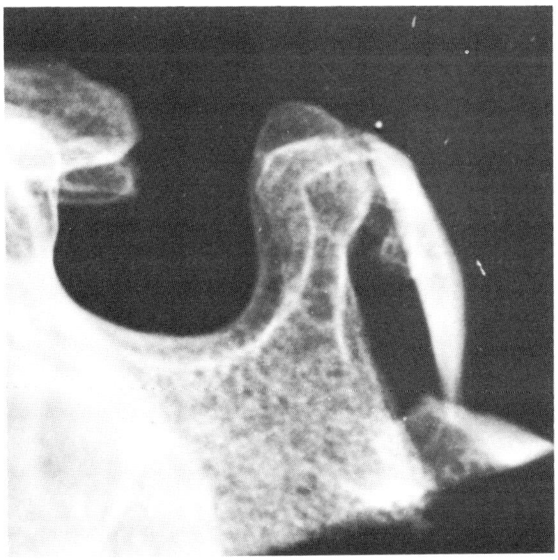

Fig. 18-29. Lateral roentgenogram of sphenoid bone. Densely calcified petroclinoid ligament extends from posterior clinoid process to petrous apex.

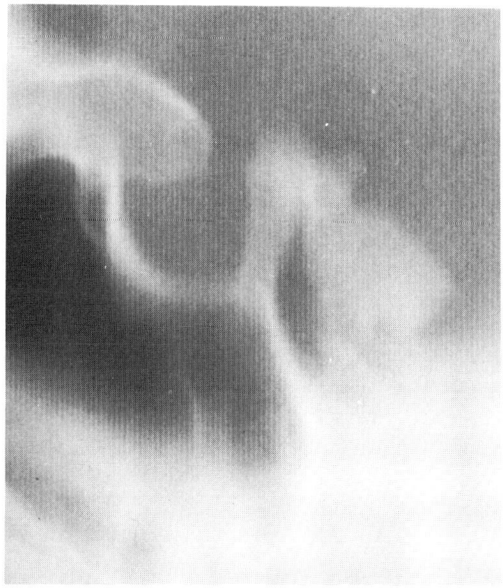

Fig. 18-30. Lateral roentgenogram of sella. Petroclinoid ligament is calcified.

Area

The area of the sella may be measured on lateral projections of the skull by means of a compensating planimeter or by multiplying the length by the depth. The upper limit of normal is said to be 130 mm^2 at 28-inch anode-to-film distance (Hare et al., 1941; Mahmoud, 1958).

Width

The width of the sella affects the volume of the sella. The width is measured in frontal views or in frontal tomograms. The normal sella varies in width from 10 to 15 mm, with a maximum of 19 mm at a 36-inch anode-to-film distance (Di Chiro, 1960). When the floor cannot be identified, an idea of the sellar width may be obtained from the width of the dorsum sellae.

Volume

Di Chiro and Nelson (1962) suggested that the volume of the pituitary fossa be calculated as follows:

$$\text{Volume } (mm^3) = \text{One half } (\text{length} \times \text{depth} \times \text{width}) \ (mm)$$

With this calculation they obtained a mean value of 594 mm^3 at 30-inch anode-to-film distance, with a range of 233 to 1,092 mm^3, in 173 adults. Again considerable overlap was noted between the normal and the abnormal. Oon (1963) estimated the normal volume as between 700 and 2,000 mm^3 at 28-inch anode-to-film distance. He measured the area in 250 adults and multiplied this measurement by the width to calculate the volume.

Tables showing the increase in size of the sella in childhood have been published by Silverman (1957). He also published observations of the mean area, as measured with a compensating planimeter, in relation to the length and depth of the pituitary fossa.

Radiography

Routine roentgenography

Routine roentgenograms of the skull obtained in the following projections demonstrate the sella turcica.

Lateral view. The lateral view allows examination of the planum, the chiasmatic sulcus, the anterior clinoid processes, the tuberculum, the pituitary fossa and sellar floor, the dorsum sellae, and the posterior clinoid processes. The sphenoid sinus, the carotid sulcus, and the clivus are included in the assessment of the sella. The cortical bone lining the sella (lamina dura) should be examined with great care. It is helpful to contrast the appearance of the cortical bone in three different areas: the planum, the portion overlying the sphenoid sinus, and the portion lining the dorsum sellae and floor of the sella at its junction with the dorsum. As was pointed out in the foregoing discussion of normal anatomy, the dorsum sellae is a quadrilateral plate of bone with very strong sturdy lateral pillars joined by an equally strong pillar at the top. In between is the central concavity of the dorsum sellae, which is often extremely thin. The cortical bone lining this concavity should therefore be sought posterior to the cortical lining of the lateral pillars. This is where the early changes of increased intracranial pressure or intrasellar tumor are found. It is also where the early changes are missed because the cortical lining of the lateral pillars is mistakenly examined and found to be normal. Additional difficulty is caused by the fact that the lateral pillars may obscure the cortical lining of its central portion.

Towne view. The Towne view allows examination of the dorsum sellae, which should be projected through the foramen magnum.

Frontal projection. The frontal projection (PA 0) allows specific examination of the anterior clinoid processes and the dorsum sellae. The cribriform plate and floor of the sella are also identified. Particular attention should be paid to the junction of the floor and the lateral walls of the sphenoid sinus. The junction is normally rounded whether the floor is concave, flat, or convex. One of the early signs of enlargement of the sella is a sharpening and deepening at this junction.

Posteroanterior projection. The posteroanterior film with the tube angle 25° (PA 25) toward the patient's feet projects the petrous pyramids through the maxillary antra. This position allows examination of the planum sphenoidale, the floor of the sella, and the sphenoid sinus as well as the superior orbital fissure. On occasion, it might allow assessment of the optic canals. This projection is specifically useful for examination of the sphenoid sinus and the floor of the sella.

Basal view. The sella may be identified in the basal view (AP –90). However, identification is often difficult and is perhaps easier when the sella is abnormal. Careful correlation between the lateral and basal views allows identification of the length of the sella, the dorsum sellae, the tuberculum, and the lateral walls of the floor of the sella.

Coned and magnification views. Coned and magnification views of the sella may be helpful. Generally speaking, if the lateral skull film is of good quality and cones are used as well as fine grids, high-definition screens, and meticulous positioning, a coned view of the sella is not necessary. Magnification views may, on occasion, clarify points of interest noted on the routine skull film.

Tomography

Tomography may be invaluable in the assessment of the sella, and one should not hesitate to use it. However, I feel that easy access to tomography has resulted in neglect of the plain films, even by experienced neuroradiologists. It is surprising how much may be learned from plain films and how much is missed by not studying the films carefully. If tomography is required, anteroposterior and lateral tomograms should be obtained. The procedure is particularly useful to demonstrate the width of the sella, which must be assessed accurately before transsphenoidal surgery. Lateral tomography better delineates the length of the sella and the size of the intracranial portion of the optic canal.

Special studies

The subject of special studies is covered in detail in volumes 2 and 3. Bilateral carotid angiography is indicated to exclude an aneurysm. Angiography may also give valuable information about the size and extent of a mass in the region of the sella turcica. Suprasellar extension may be recognized by upward displacement of the anterior cerebral arteries (60% to 80% of the cases) and by lateral or posterior displacement of the supracavernous internal carotid artery. Lateral displacement of the cavernous portion, however, is best assessed in the basal view, which indicates the size of the intrasellar mass. In the venous phase upward displacement of the internal cerebral vein and venous angle may be shown. Gross lateral extension of a pituitary tumor results in upward displacement of the middle cerebral artery and basal vein. The cavernous branches of the internal carotid artery and a tumor blush may be demonstrated.

Encephalography with tomography will define a mass that has arisen in the suprasellar region or a mass that has extended from inside the sella turcica to the suprasellar region. It will also show whether the sella is empty. Subarachnoid air lateral to the tumor may lead to the impression that no suprasellar mass is present unless the anterior end of the third ventricle is shown (Pribram and Swann, 1960).

Ventriculography is unnecessary in the assessment of sellar or suprasellar masses unless the encephalogram is unsuccessful or the foramen of Monro is obstructed. Ventriculography does not allow differentiation between extrinsic, intrinsic, and intraventricular masses.

Venography of the cavernous sinus allows more precise delineation of the lateral extent of an intrasellar tumor than is possible with carotid angiography. This procedure is valuable before transsphenoidal surgery, particularly since a tumor may enlarge asymmetrically.

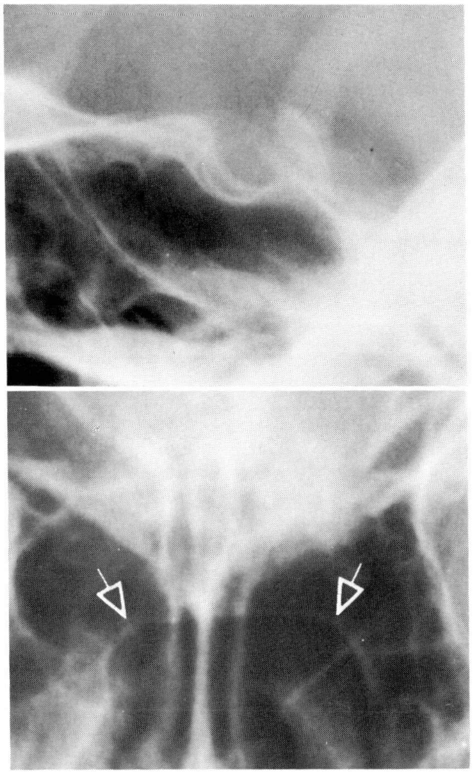

A

B

Fig. 18-31. Normal sella. **A,** In lateral projection, sella appears small. **B,** Posteroanterior view, however, shows broad floor of sella (arrows). Sella is therefore normal in volume.

ABNORMAL SELLA

Henry W. Pribram

Abnormal size

Small sella

It is very unusual for the sella to be abnormally small. The sella that appears small in the lateral projection may nevertheless be normal because of its greater than average width (Fisher and Di Chiro, 1964) (Fig. 18-31). A well-pneumatized sella is most apt to show this finding. A small sella may be found in primary hypopituitarism (Riach, 1966; Hubble, 1967) (Fig. 18-32) and growth hormone deficiency (Fisher and Di Chiro, 1964) (Fig. 18-33) if the onset of the disease is before the age of 6 years. This finding of an abnormally small sella may therefore be of therapeutic importance. Fisher and Di Chiro (1964) found the sella to be small in 56.8% of forty-four patients with hypopituitarism. In three patients in whom the onset was after the age of 7 years, the sella was normal. Fisher and Di Chiro (1964) also found a small sella in 13.5% of patients with genetic dwarfism. Unusual familial hypopituitary dwarfism in two mentally retarded sisters was reported by Ferrier and Stone (1969). In each the sella was small. The sisters differed from the usual pituitary dwarf, in whom the sella is normal. Other members of the family were normal physically and their sellae were normal. The sella was also reported to be small in a 13½-year-old boy with Cushing's syndrome due to an adrenocortical adenoma (Steinbach et al., 1963). The boy had a bone age of 10 years and a sella that measured 9.5 × 6.3 mm, with a mean area of 49 mm². Two and one half years after surgery his bone age and height became normal. The sella at that time measured 81.9 mm². These workers concluded that the initial small size of the sella had been due to inhibition of the anterior pituitary by the adrenal adenoma. A small sella was also reported in Sheehan's syndrome (Meador and Worrell, 1966; Harlin and Givens, 1968). These authors, however, considered only the lateral profile of the sella and failed to consider its width. I have seen calcification in a small sella in

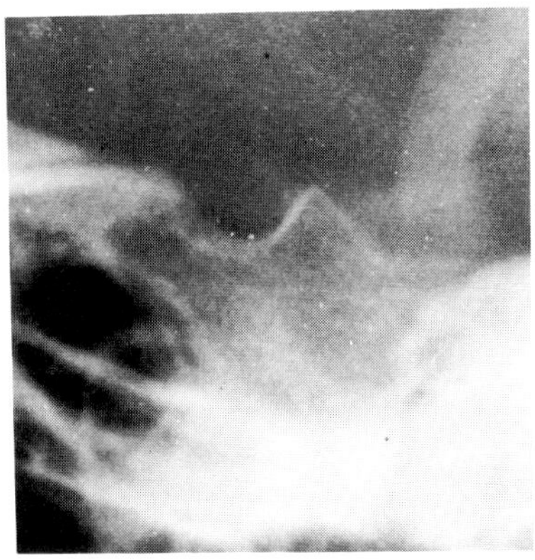

Fig. 18-32. Hypopituitarism. Lateral roentgenogram shows vestigial sella.

a patient with Sheehan's syndrome. A small sella in lateral profile may also be found in dystrophia myotonica but is not diagnostic of this condition (Caughey, 1952; Isherwood and Mawdsley, 1963).

The sella may be vestigial (Fig. 18-33). This interesting entity has been termed dysplasia of the sella (Lundberg and Gemzell, 1966). In the three cases that Lundberg and Gemzell described, evidence of pituitary insufficiency was noted. The sella measured 16 mm² in one patient, 30 mm² in another, and 39 mm² in the third. These measurements correspond to the normal sella at birth, at 6 months, and at 1 year respectively (Silverman, 1957). In all three patients the volume was less than 240 mm³, which is the lowest normal value described by Di Chiro and Nelson (1962).

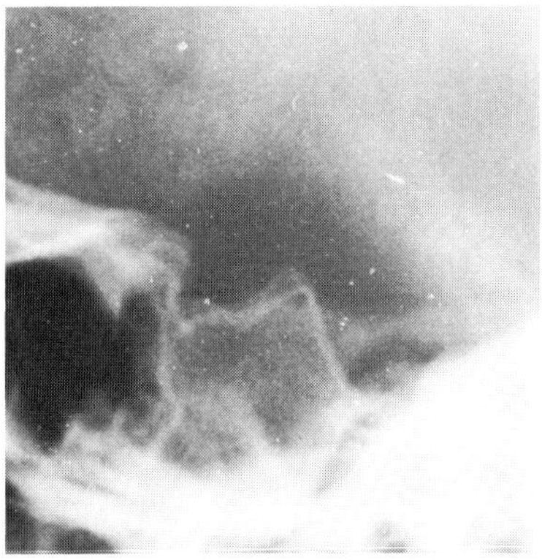

Fig. 18-33. Growth hormone deficiency. Sella is small and irregular in a 10-year-old boy with growth hormone deficiency.

Large sella without local bone destruction

Intrasellar masses may cause enlargement of the sella with preservation of cortical bone (Figs. 18-34 and 18-35). In these instances there is uniform enlargement with a deepening of the floor, and thinning, as well as posterior displacement of the dorsum. These changes are first seen in the posteroinferior aspect of the sella. The dorsum sellae becomes curved due to direct pressure of the tumor on its thin central portion. As the tumor enlarges, the thicker lateral struts of the dorsum become thinned and displaced caudally. The dorsum, although thinned and displaced, usually can be identified on roentgenograms of the skull (Fig. 18-36). Ordinarily the posterior clinoid processes are preserved even when displaced posteriorly. This displacement results in an increase in the distance between the tuber-

A B C D

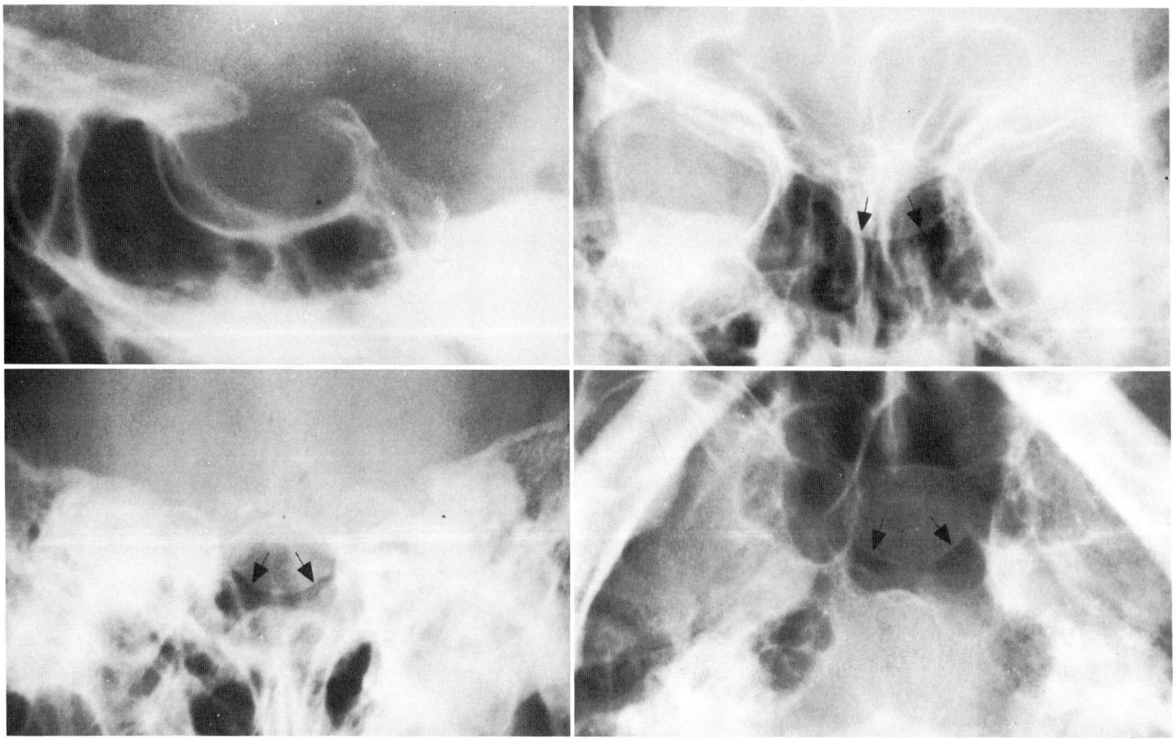

Fig. 18-34. Chromophobe adenoma with large sella. **A,** Lateral projection. **B,** Frontal projection. **C,** Towne projection. **D,** Basal projection. Floor (arrows) is deepened into sphenoid sinus by intrasellar tumor.

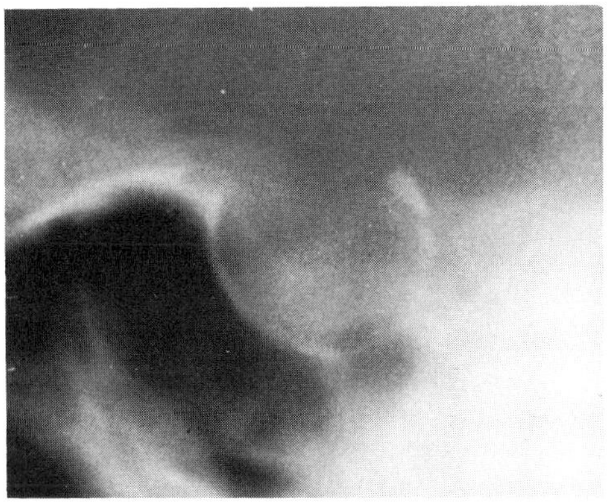

Fig. 18-35. Pituitary adenoma. Sella is uniformly enlarged.

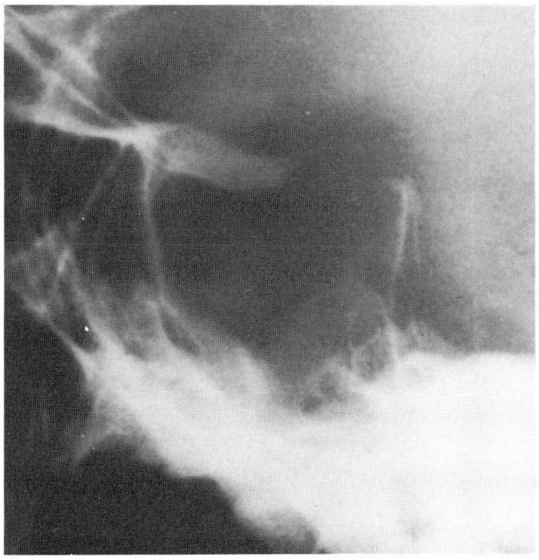

Fig. 18-36. Chromophobe adenoma. Lateral view of skull shows destruction of posteroinferior aspect of dorsum sellae and floor of sella. Upper segment of dorsum sellae is straightened. Note the forward expansion of the anterior and vertical component of the sella.

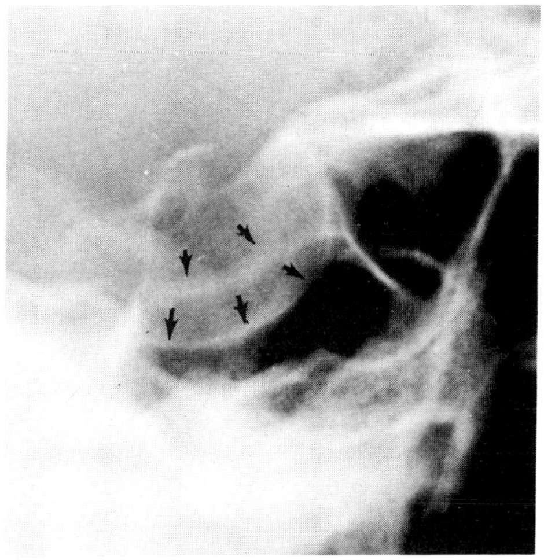

Fig. 18-37. Chromophobe adenoma. Lateral roentgenogram of sella shows asymmetric expansion. Floor (arrows) on one side is deepened more than on the other. Dorsum sellae is straightened.

culum sellae and the posterior clinoid processes. Enlargement is at times quite asymmetric so that one side of the sella may remain relatively normal (Figs. 18-37 and 18-38). In the frontal projection deepening of the sellar floor is recognized by an increase in the concavity of the sella and a sharpening at the junction between the floor and the carotid sulcus (Fig. 18-39). Deepening of the floor may be asymmetric (Fig. 18-38). The cortical bone lining the floor is destroyed with increasing intrasellar pressure. The anterior clinoid processes are often elevated and may be eroded on the undersurface. These changes too are often asymmetric (Fig. 18-40).

Uniform enlargement of the sella is most commonly seen in pituitary tumors and in the empty sella syndrome; less commonly in craniopharyngioma and intrasellar aneurysm.

Pituitary tumors

Chromophobe adenoma. This is the most common pituitary tumor to cause enlargement of the sella. In a study of fifty chromophobe adenomas, the youngest patient was 15 years and the oldest 58 years of age (Pribram and Swann, 1960). Most patients were between the ages of 30 and 60. Thirty-two were male and eighteen female. Visual failure and hypopituitarism are usually the presenting symptoms of a patient with chromophobe adenoma. Bitemporal hemianopsia is the most common finding, but unilateral loss of vision may occur (Walsh and Hoyt, 1969). The loss of vision in the majority of patients develops slowly, but there are cases in which loss of vision is extremely rapid (Walsh and Hoyt, 1969). Visual field defects are the result of upward extension of the tumor and pressure on the blood supply to the optic nerves and chiasm (Schneider et al., 1970). The location of the chiasm is therefore of considerable importance in the clinical presentation of pituitary tumors. A prefixed chiasm with short optic nerves allows extension of the pituitary tumor between the optic tracts so that visual field defects may not be found even though a large suprasellar mass is present. On the other hand, if the chiasm is postfixed with long optic nerves, visual field defects appear early. Signs of pituitary insufficiency are another common feature of this tumor. They consist of changes in the growth and distribution of hair, a dry skin, obesity, and hypogonadism. Fröhlich's syndrome and Levi-Lorain dwarfism may be encountered (Pribram and Swann, 1960).

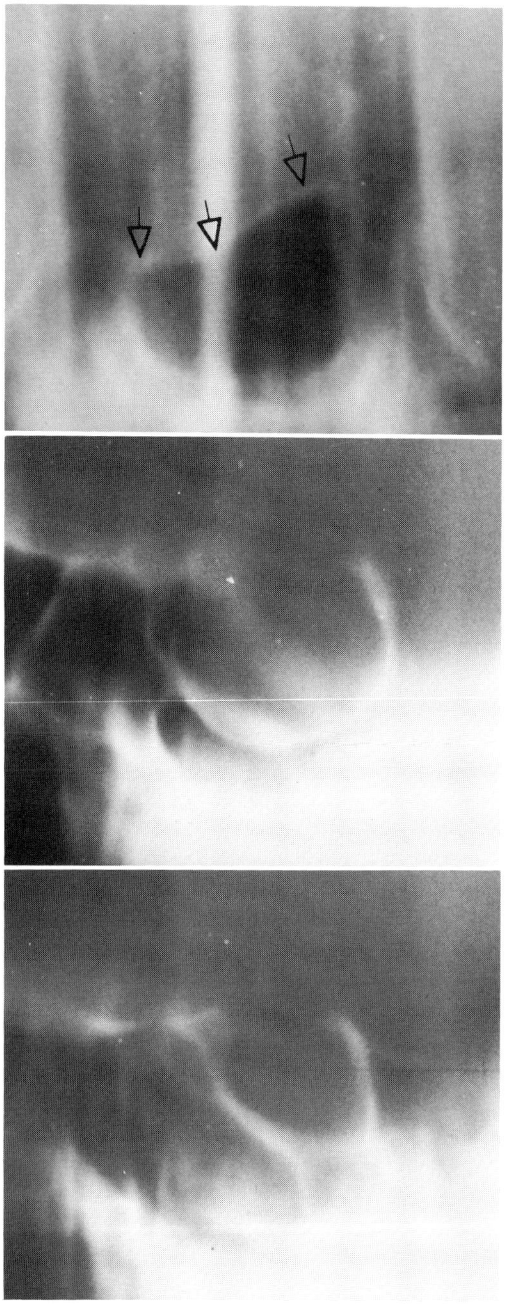

A

B

C

Fig. 18-38. Chromophobe adenoma. **A,** Frontal tomogram shows marked depression of floor on right (arrows). **B** and **C,** Lateral tomograms show cut made to right of midline. Note the marked expansion of the sella in **B.** Note also that the cut made to the left of the midline in **C** shows a more normal appearance.

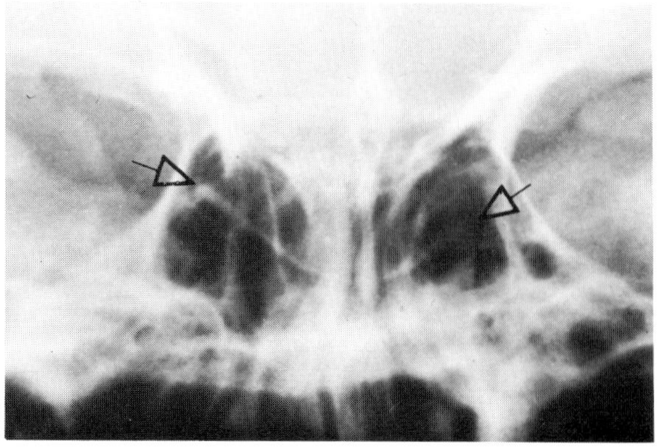

Fig. 18-39. Chromophobe adenoma. Posteroanterior view of skull shows deepening and expansion of floor of sella. Arrows indicate junction between floor and carotid sulcus.

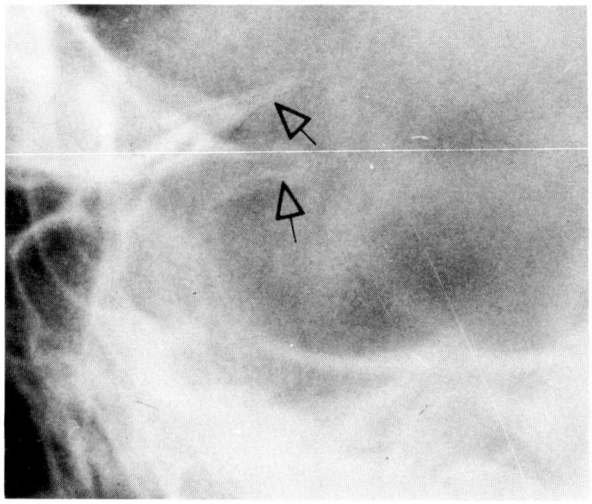

Fig. 18-40. Chromophobe adenoma. Lateral view of sella shows extreme expansion. Note the elevation of one of the anterior clinoid processes (arrows).

Clinical signs of pituitary insufficiency were present in 42% of chromophobe adenomas described by Pribram and Swann (1960), which is in agreement with the findings of other authors (Bakay, 1950; Mogensen, 1957). Changes of hypopituitarism may also occur with intrasellar aneurysm (Dussault et al., 1969) or the empty sella syndrome (Caplan and Dobben, 1969). Radiographic changes of hypopituitarism include calcification of the auricular cartilage (Pribram et al., 1971).

The sella is almost always abnormal in the presence of a chromophobe adenoma (Fig. 18-41). During the early stages of tumor growth, the sella enlarges but cortical bone is preserved. Thus the sella becomes more globular and its floor is somewhat depressed. Frequently this depression is more marked on one side than on the other, a finding best appreciated in the frontal projection (Figs. 18-38 and 18-39). The dorsum sellae becomes curved because of the direct pressure of the tumor on the thin midline portion of the dorsum sellae. Destruction of the posteroinferior aspect of the dorsum sellae, with loss of cortical bone, then follows. This re-

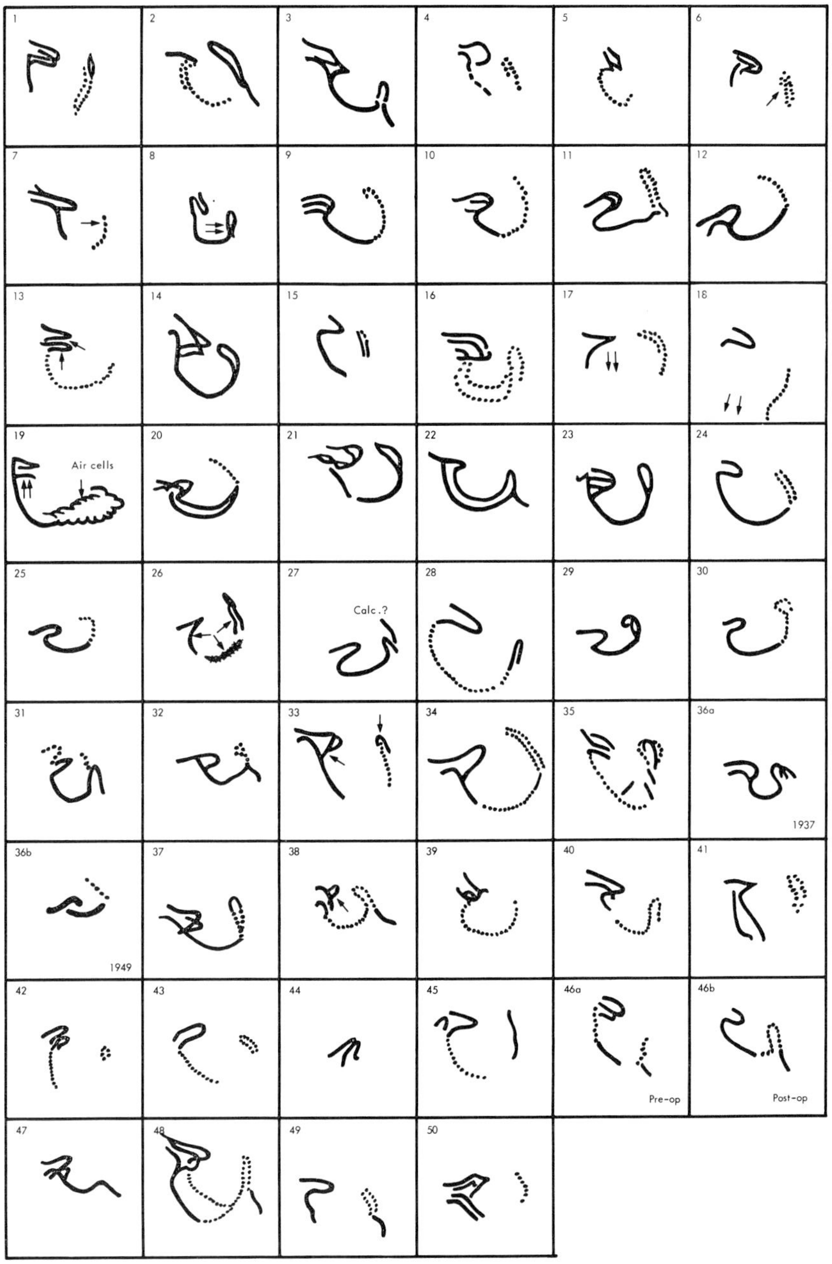

Fig. 18-41. Chromophobe adenomas. Chart of tracings of changes in sella in fifty cases. Destruction is indicated by dotted line or by absence of solid line. Expansion is indicated by change in contour of the sella.

gion is the most vulnerable area since it is frequently poorly pneumatized and the lining cortical bone is thin. Cancellous bone has been shown to be physiologically less resistant than compact or cortical bone (Jefferson, 1940). Once the protection of the cortical bone is lost, destruction of cancellous bone progresses more rapidly and the tumor expands downward and backward. Expansion of the floor into the sphenoid sinus (Figs. 18-34 and 18-39) is common and has been reported in 50% of patients with pituitary tumors (Frazier, 1930; Mahmoud, 1958). Such extension was also present in twenty-five of fifty of our patients (Pribram and Swann, 1960). As the tumor escapes through the diaphragma sellae, the posterior clinoid processes are displaced backward and the anterior clinoid processes may be elevated. The diaphragma sellae is believed to be resistant to pressure. Therefore possibly suprasellar extension may be determined in part by the size of the opening for the pituitary stalk. Pituitary tumors frequently appear to grow like mushrooms, with a thin stalk where the

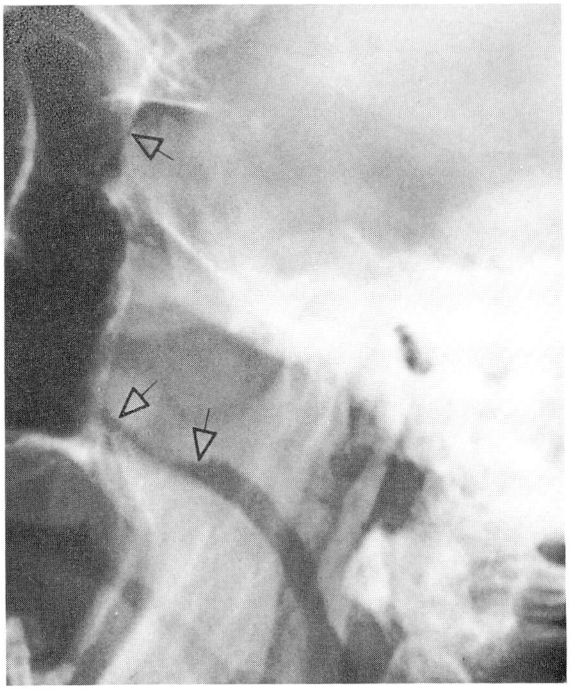

Fig. 18-42. Chromophobe adenoma. Lateral roentgenogram shows destruction of sella and large nasopharyngeal mass (arrows).

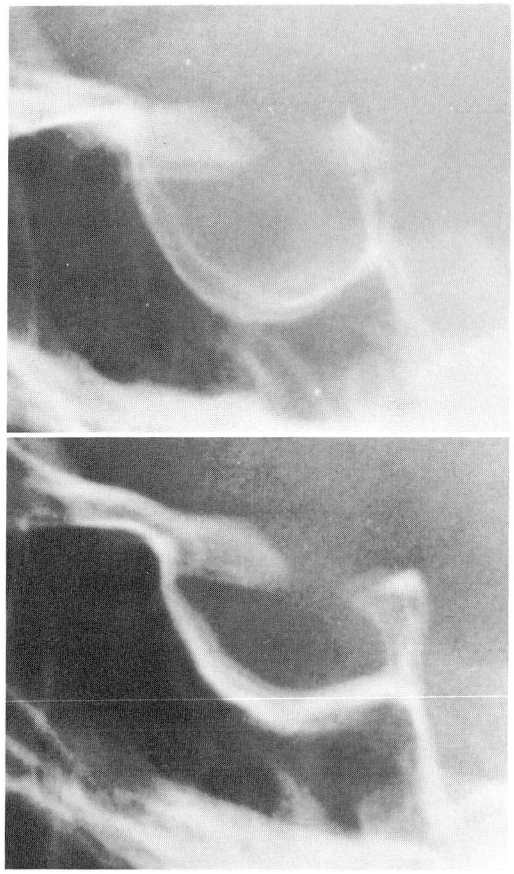

Fig. 18-43. Chromophobe adenoma. **A,** Sella is asymmetrically expanded. Cortical lining is preserved and dorsum sellae is straightened. **B,** After radiotherapy, sella is smaller and now has unusually thick cortical lining. Dorsum sellae is reconstituted.

tumor pierces the diaphragma sellae and then becomes free to expand above the diaphragma. Because air may be seen on either side of the tumor at encephalography, this mushroomlike appearance may be an illusion. Large tumors may enlarge the superior orbital fissure and erode the optic canal. The tumor may extend into the middle and posterior fossae. Parasellar extension is best appreciated when the sphenoid is well pneumatized. In these cases a soft-tissue mass will be seen. Large tumors may extend into the nasopharynx (Fig. 18-42). A tight diaphragma sellae or calcification of the diaphragma might encourage this downward extension. A faint remnant of the posterior clinoid processes frequently remains even when the sella has been entirely destroyed. Once all the landmarks of the sella have been obliterated, it is impossible to determine whether an intrasellar or suprasellar tumor or an enlarged third ventricle has been the cause. Calcification is rare (du Boulay and Trickey, 1962) but is more likely in cystic tumors (Lindgren and Di Chiro, 1951). The incidence of calcification was reported as 6% by Deery (1929) in a survey of 285 cases. Pituitary calculi are said to be characteristic of the eosinophilic adenomas. A ballooned sella is a common finding, but chromophobe adenomas frequently enlarge asymmetrically and produce a double floor. This asymmetric enlargement may be confirmed in the frontal projection or by tomography (Figs. 18-38 and 18-39). After radiotherapy the outline of the sella may be restored (Fig. 18-43). The bone is usually more dense than normal and the sella does not regain its normal shape.

Eosinophilic adenomas. These tumors of the pituitary usually present with symptoms of gigantism, if they occur in childhood, or acromegaly, if they occur after the epiphyses have fused. The earliest changes are a slight increase in the thickening of the soft tissues. At this time the growth hormone levels are raised but the features of acromegaly are still reversible. Measurement of the heel pad was proposed as a simple way to show the soft-tissue thickening (Steinbach and Russell, 1964). Steinbach and Russell (1964) found that the heel pad beneath the calcaneum measured 13 to 21 mm, and they considered measurements above 23 mm to indicate acromegaly.

The changes in the sella are usually more subtle than in chromophobe adenoma (Fig. 18-44). Enlargement of the sella is usually less although nonsecretory, mixed,

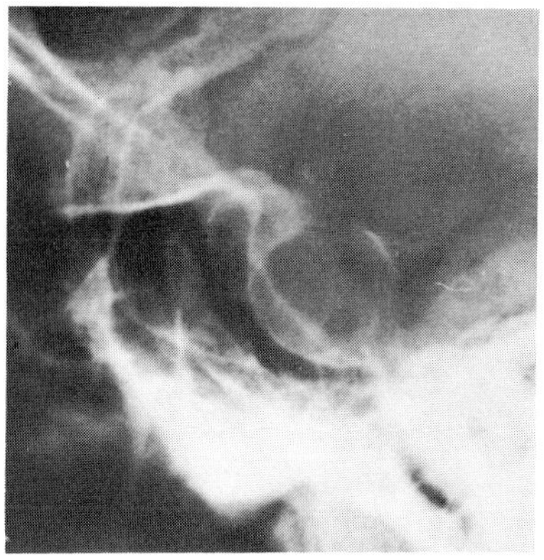

Fig. 18-44. Eosinophilic adenoma. Sella shows asymmetric expansion of floor and anterior wall. Dorsum sellae is slightly straightened.

or cystic eosinophilic tumors may attain considerable size. The sella is ballooned but may be asymmetric. Eosinophilic tumors are more prone to undercut the anterior clinoid processes. Changes of acromegaly are frequently found in the skull and consist of enlargement of the frontal sinuses and the maxillary antra as well as thickening of the frontal and parietal bones. The jaws become prominent, and the space between the teeth increases. Changes of acromegaly have also been reported in association with an intrasellar aneurysm (Fathie, 1965).

Basophilic adenoma. These adenomas only rarely cause enlargement of the sella. Cushing's syndrome may be caused by benign and malignant adrenal tumors, or by hyperplasia, of the adrenal cortex. Pituitary adenomas also may cause the disease, and in these cases the tumors may be basophilic, chromophobe, or mixed. When the sella is abnormal, the changes are the same as those found in chromophobe adenoma.

Nelson's syndrome. In 1958, Nelson and collaborators described an ACTH-secreting chromophobe adenoma in a patient who at the age of 24 years had undergone bilateral adrenalectomy for Cushing's syndrome. This same patient has been the subject of several other papers (Nelson et al., 1958, 1960; Minagi and Steinbach, 1968). The patient is still in good health although with somewhat dark pigmentation. Since the original report (Nelson et al., 1958), it has become clear that in many patients ACTH-secreting tumors may first become manifest after bilateral adrenalectomy for Cushing's syndrome. The tumors develop from 1 to 10 years after surgery and are commonly chromophobe adenomas, although basophilic and mixed adenomas as well as carcinomas have been reported. Most of the patients were female, reflecting the greater incidence of Cushing's syndrome in that sex. The roentgenographic changes are those of an intrasellar tumor whose

A

B

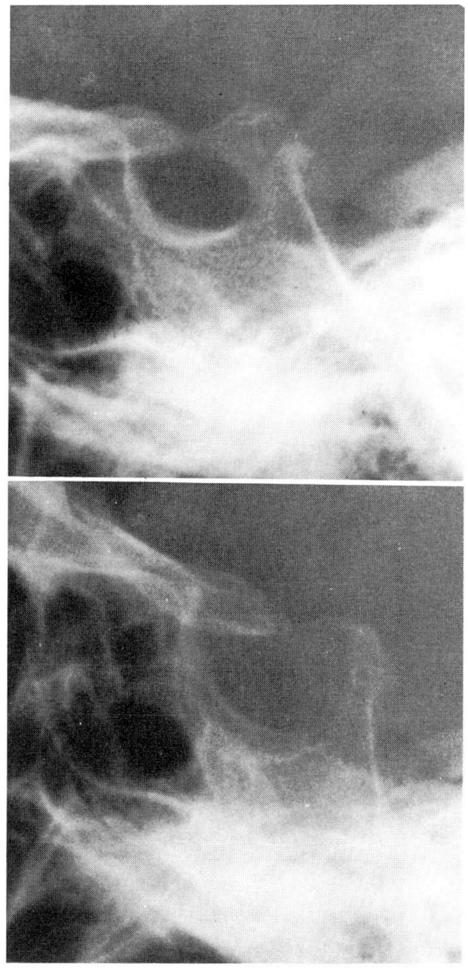

Fig. 18-45. Nelson's syndrome. **A,** Sella is normal at time of bilateral adrenalectomy. **B,** Two years later. Sella shows classic changes of intrasellar tumor with enlargement, deepening of floor, loss of normal lamina dura, and erosion of inner aspect of dorsum.

growth is often rapid, and extension into the sphenoid sinus is common. The importance of noting the condition has emphasized the need for clinical and radiologic follow-up examinations of these patients (Fig. 18-45). In many patients (Salassa et al., 1959) evidence of an ACTH-secreting tumor is present when the patient is first seen. In others the tumor lies dormant until after adrenalectomy, when it begins to grow aggressively. Increased pigmentation is the first sign of such growth.

Polyadenomatosis. This syndrome is hereditary, caused by a dominant mutated gene (Wermer, 1954, 1963). It is characterized by tumors of several endocrine glands and peptic ulceration. Tumors of the anterior pituitary gland, the parathyroid, the thyroid, the pancreas, and the adrenal cortex are found. The pituitary tumor may be chromophobe, eosinophilic,

A

B

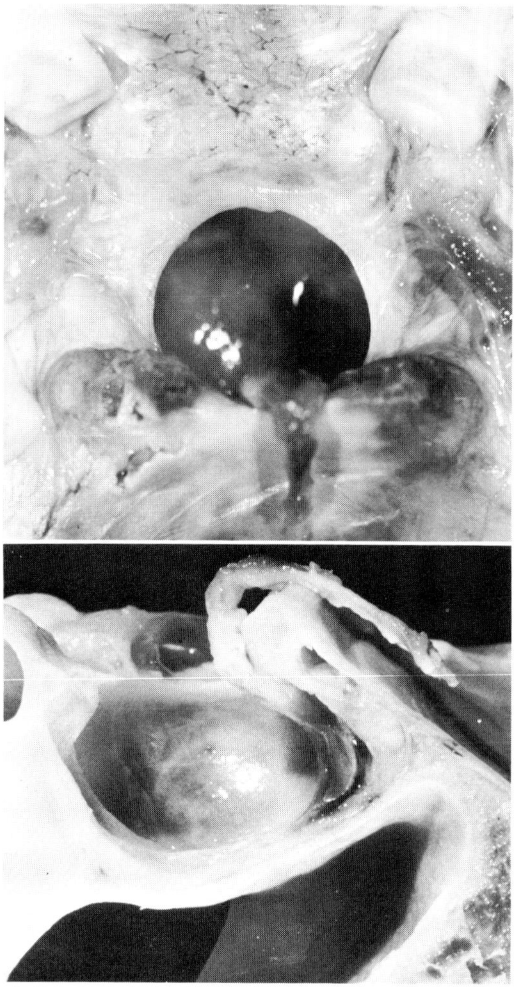

Fig. 18-46. Empty sella. **A,** Seen from above. Note the large defect in the diaphragma. Arachnoid can be seen glistening within the sella. Infundibulum is posterior in position. **B,** Midsagittal section shows pituitary compressed against posterior wall of sella. Note the posterior position of the infundibular stalk.

A

B

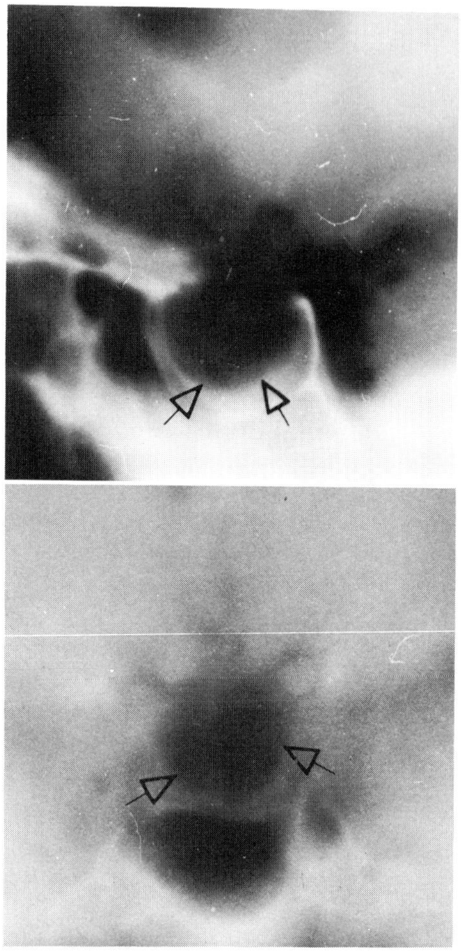

Fig. 18-47. **A,** Pneumoencephalogram, lateral brow up tomogram, shows that sella is ballooned. Air from suprasellar cisterns extends into pituitary fossa (arrows). **B,** Pneumoencephalogram, frontal tomogram, shows air within sella (arrows).

basophilic, or mixed adenomas. The changes in the sella are those of an intrasellar tumor.

Carcinoma of pituitary. This is a rare condition (Bakay, 1950; Newton et al., 1962). Diagnosis may be suggested clinically by either an extremely rapid enlargement of the sella or the development of the cavernous sinus syndrome. However, these findings are not diagnostic, since rapid growth may occur with benign adenoma. The sellar changes are often indistinguishable from those caused by benign adenoma.

Empty sella. The term empty sella was coined by Busch (1951) to describe a deficient diaphragma sellae, a slightly enlarged sella, and no visible pituitary gland (Fig. 18-46). He described three types of diaphragma sellae: (1) the type that forms a complete covering with only a small opening for the pituitary stalk (41.9%), (2) the type that is incompletely closed but in which the opening for the stalk is less than 3 mm, and (3) the type that forms only a peripheral rim. Schaeffer (1924) had made similar observations, and more recently Bergland and his co-workers (1968) found that in 39% of cases the opening in the diaphragma sellae was greater than 5 mm. Obviously such cases predispose to ballooning of the subarachnoid space into the sella (Fig. 18-47). Bergland and associates (1968) found that the subarachnoid space extended into the sella in 20% of patients. Spontaneous cerebrospinal fluid fistula may follow; and persistence of the craniopharyngeal canal has been so incriminated by Kaufman (1969) (Fig. 18-48). Stereotactic transsphenoidal surgery of

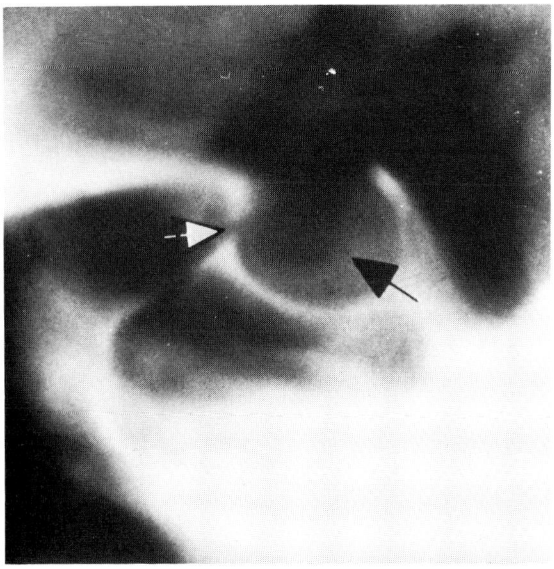

Fig. 18-48. Empty sella and cerebrospinal fluid rhinorrhea. Encephalogram (lateral brow up position) shows air extending into sella (black arrow). Defect in region of tuberculum sellae (white arrow) was the site of the cerebrospinal fluid leak.

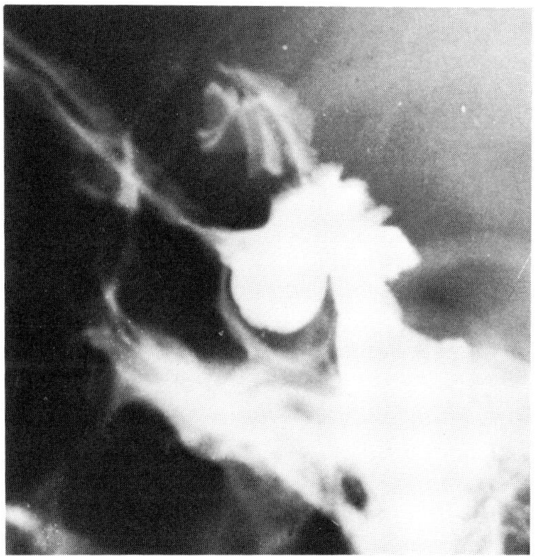

Fig. 18-49. Empty sella. Subarachnoid space within sella was intentionally filled at time of Pantopaque myelography.

the pituitary may also lead to cerebrospinal fluid rhinorrhea when the subarachnoid space extends into the sella (Brisman et al., 1969).

In recent years the empty sella syndrome has received much attention, which has led to numerous publications (Ring and Waddington, 1966; Calkins et al., 1968; Gabriele, 1968; Kaufman, 1968; Lee and Adams, 1968; Zatz et al., 1969). The diagnosis should be considered in any patient with an enlarged sella who has no endocrine symptoms or visual abnormality. However, symptoms or signs of endocrine insufficiency have been reported in some cases of the empty sella syndrome (Caplan and Dobben, 1969). Visual field symptoms have also been reported in some cases (Mortara and Norrell, 1970). For the most part, the finding of an enlarged sella is coincidental when the skull is examined for some other reason, for example, for head injury or headache. The enlargement of the sella in the empty sella syndrome differs in no way from enlargement caused by any other intrasellar mass, and the diagnosis is possible only on pneumoencephalography or Pantopaque encephalography (Fig. 18-49). Therefore, whenever an air study is performed, a deliberate attempt should be made to demonstrate the intrasellar subarachnoid space (Fig. 18-47).

General agreement has been reached that one of the major factors in the etiology of the empty sella is a deficiency in the diaphragma sellae. In addition, Kaufman (1968) has suggested that increased intracranial pressure may be a factor. In many instances the cerebrospinal fluid pressure was not measured, and therefore this point has not been clarified. Nevertheless, cerebrospinal fluid pressure was normal in many patients. In addition to a deficiency in the diaphragma, the position of the optic chiasm may be relevant. A postfixed chiasm may be a factor in that the contents of the sella are not protected by the optic chiasm. In this respect a review of the tracings of the encephalograms in the article by Zatz and his co-workers (1969) suggests that these were patients with postfixed chiasms.

Craniopharyngioma. Craniopharyngiomas arise from the epithelial rests of the craniopharyngeal duct. The tumor may be solid or cystic, or both. The ages in fifty unselected cases (Pribram and Swann, 1960) ranged from 6½ to 67 years; eight patients were more than 50, twenty-eight were less than 20, and twenty-five were younger than 16; almost half were more than 20. The range of ages was similar in a series of sixty patients reported by Barnett (1959). He included one 2-year-old patient and eight over the age of 50 years. In contrast, with chromophobe adenoma the greatest incidence is in the age group 30 to 60 years and is rare below the age of 15.

Endocrine changes often accompany these tumors and were present in thirty of the fifty cases of Pribram and Swann (1960). Evidence of hypopituitarism was present in twenty-eight, endocrine overactivity in one, and a mixture of both in another. Endocrine changes are somewhat more florid than those found in chromophobe adenomas. Changes in the hair and skin are the most common, followed by hypogonadism. Polyuria and polydipsia are frequent in patients with craniopharyngioma, whereas in chromophobe adenoma these two

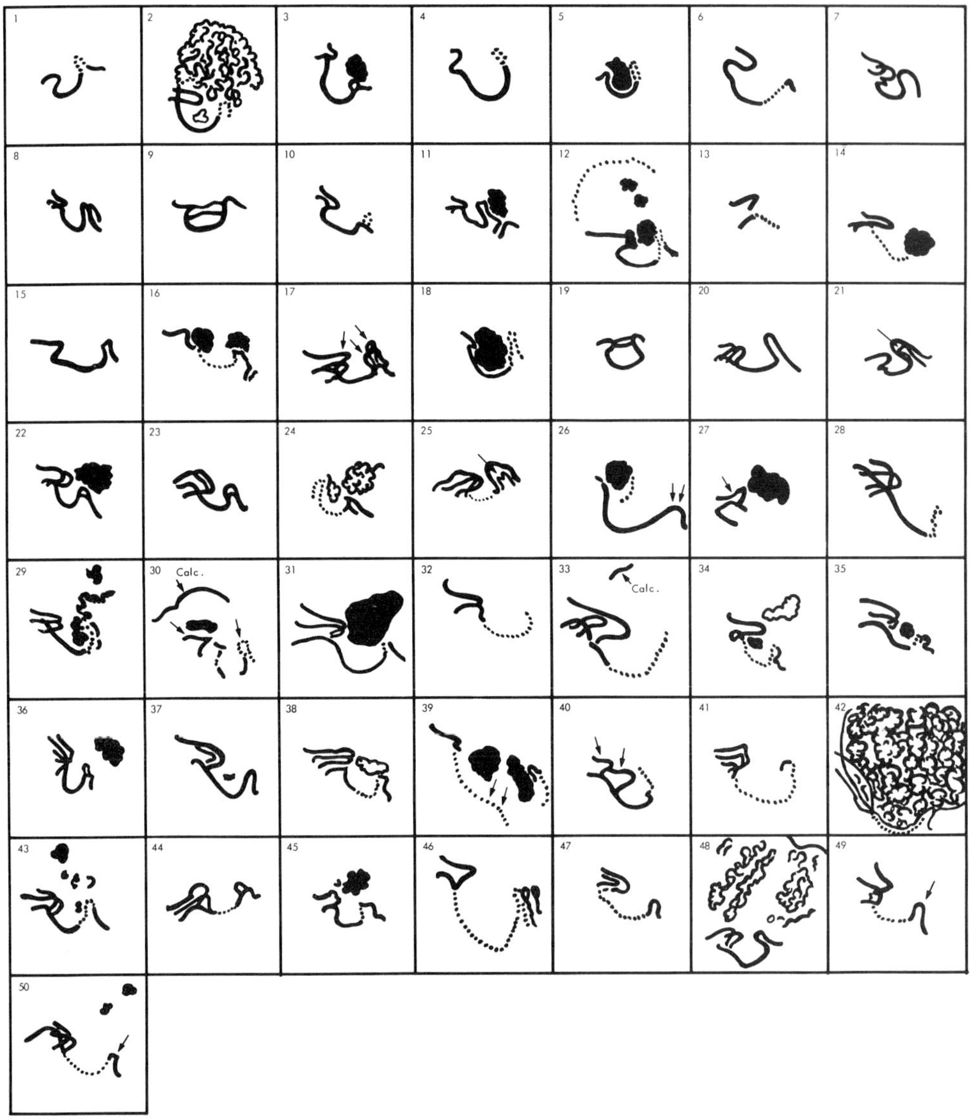

Fig. 18-50. Craniopharyngiomas. Chart of tracings of sella and suprasellar region in fifty cases of craniopharyngioma. Calcification is indicated by solid black areas or lines. Destruction of sella is indicated by dotted line, and erosion without destruction either by arrows or by deformity of the sella.

disturbances are uncommon. Retarded bone age, or Levi-Lorain dwarfism, may be an associated finding of craniopharyngioma. Occasionally it is the first finding that leads to a roentgenogram of the skull. Loss of vision may also be an early symptom.

Calcification is extremely common (Fig. 18-50). In a series of fifty patients (Pribram and Swann, 1960), calcification was seen in twenty-eight (56%). It was present in seventeen (68%) of the twenty-five patients under the age of 16 years, and in eleven (44%) of those over 16. These findings agree closely with those of Lindgren and Di Chiro (1951), who found calcification in thirty out of fifty-four patients (55%). In a review of the literature, they found that calcification was described in 139 of 238 craniopharyngiomas (58%). Previous authors had reported calcification in a much higher percentage of patients, ranging from 71% to 80% (McKenzie and Sosman, 1924; Deery, 1929; Cushing, 1932). Calcification is rare in patients younger than 2 years and occurs in approximately 20% in this age group. Calcification may be curvilinear, nodular, or flocculent (Fig. 18-50). It may be intrasellar, suprasellar, or remote from the sella (Fig. 18-50). The tumor is frequently larger than the area of calcification would indicate and may be so large as to obstruct the foramen of Monro. The tumor may

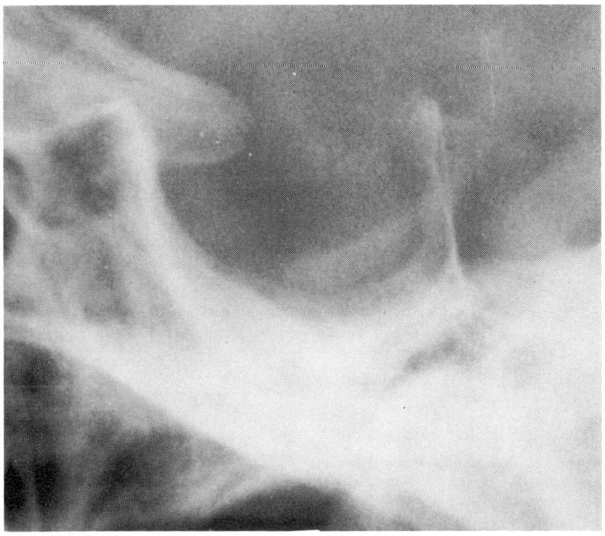

Fig. 18-51. Craniopharyngioma. Lateral roentgenogram of sella shows expansion and destruction of posteroinferior aspect. Dorsum sellae is straightened.

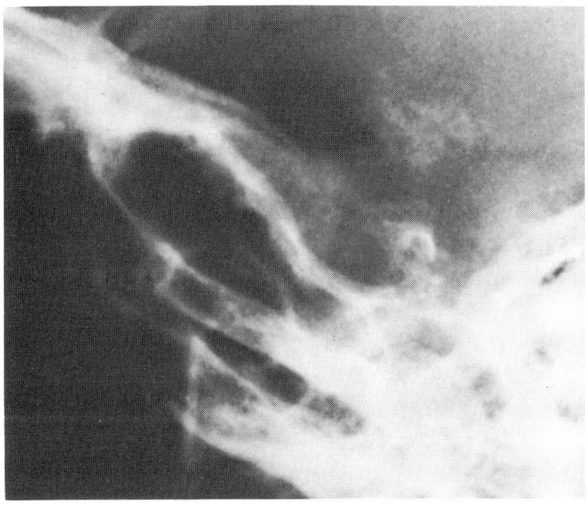

Fig. 18-52. Craniopharyngioma. Lateral roentgenogram of sella shows irregular suprasellar calcification. Posterior clinoid processes and upper portion of dorsum sellae are destroyed. Floor of sella is thickened and sclerotic.

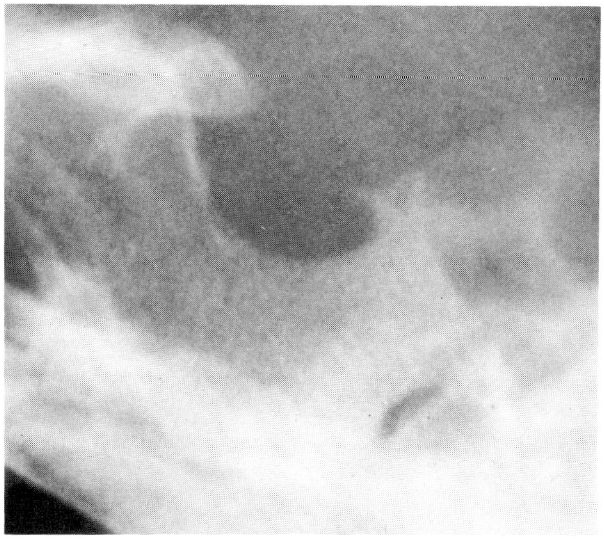

Fig. 18-53. Craniopharyngioma. Posterior clinoid processes are destroyed, and dorsum sellae is scalloped. Lamina dura has been destroyed. Optic strut is seen anteriorly through convex chiasmatic sulcus.

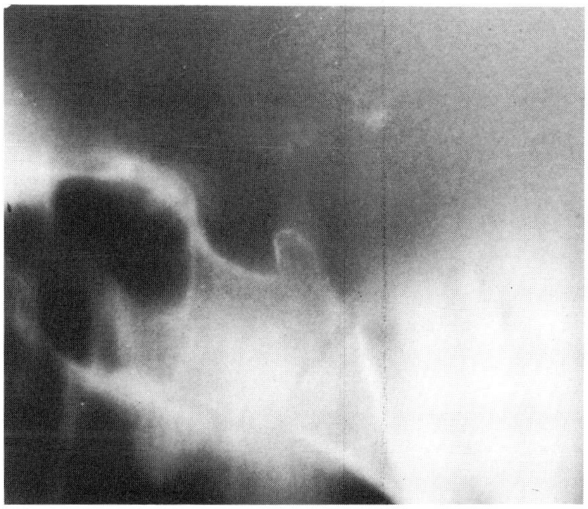

Fig. 18-54. Craniopharyngioma. Lateral midsagittal tomogram of sella shows faint suprasellar calcifications. Posterior clinoid processes and upper part of dorsum sellae are destroyed.

even be located in the interpeduncular fossa (cases *3, 11, 22* and *36* in Fig. 18-50). Curvilinear calcification in a craniopharyngioma is more commonly associated with a tumor that is entirely cystic. Calcification may also be seen in an optic chiasm glioma or a hypothalamic glioma, in which the calcification is usually stippled. With a chordoma, which is usually more destructive, the calcification is more dense. Enlargement of the sella may be present in craniopharyngioma but is less marked and less common than in pituitary tumors. Sellar enlargement was reported in 74% (Barnett, 1959) and was present in 62% of our patients (Pribram and Swann, 1960). The floor of the sella was involved less frequently than in the chromophobe adenomas. The *open* sella is a favorite descriptive term that has been applied to the separation of the anterior clinoid processes from the dorsum sellae and the posterior clinoid processes (Fig. 18-51). Extension into the sphenoid sinus is less common in craniopharyngioma; it is more characteristic of pituitary tumors. Destruction of the dorsum sellae begins from above and gradually whittles away the posterior clinoid processes and the dorsum (Figs. 18-52 to 18-54). Similar changes may take place in the anterior clinoid processes. The changes result from direct pressure of the tumor and, in general, cause flattening of the sella rather than the ballooning found in an intrasellar tumor. Increase in density of the sella was reported by Barnett (1959) in about 11% of cases (Fig. 18-52). Such increased density was noted neither by us (Pribram and Swann, 1960) nor by others (du Boulay, 1970).

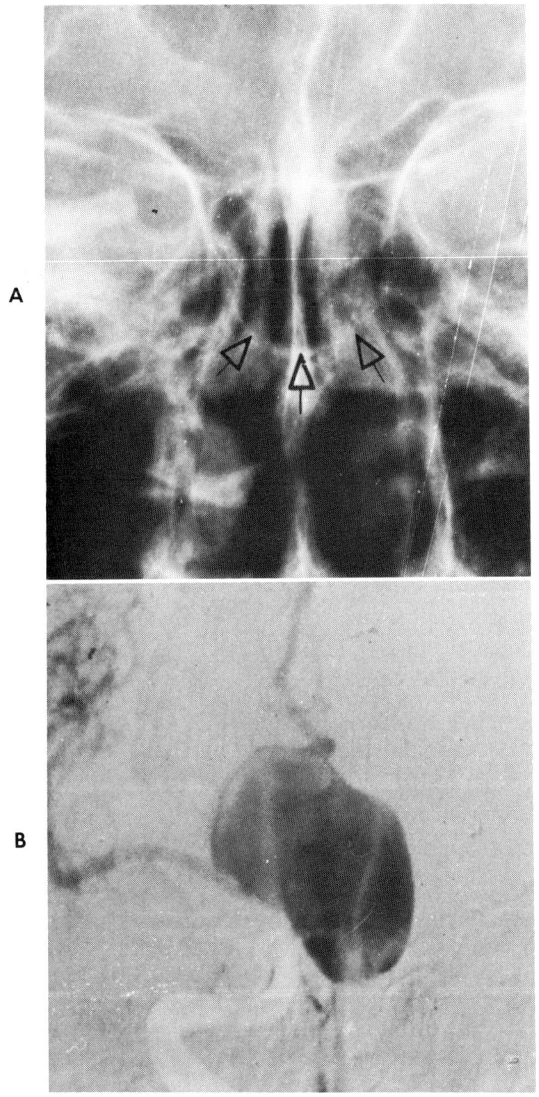

Fig. 18-55. Internal carotid artery aneurysm. **A**, Anteroposterior roentgenogram of skull shows deepening of floor of sella (arrows). This appearance simulates chromophobe adenoma. **B**, Internal carotid arteriogram, frontal projection, shows that changes in sella are caused by large internal carotid artery aneurysm that extends into sella.

The suprasellar mass may be demonstrated by angiography or by encephalography. Curvilinear calcification requires investigation by bilateral carotid angiography to exclude an aneurysm. Vertebral angiography may be required when the mass extends to the interpeduncular and pontine cisterns, for its results govern the choice of surgical approach. If the carotid angiogram appears normal, encephalography is performed since a normal angiogram does not exclude a suprasellar mass.

Intrasellar aneurysm. An aneurysm of the cavernous internal carotid artery may cause sellar enlargement that resembles enlargement of a pituitary adenoma (Lodge et al., 1927; Zollinger and Cutler, 1933) (Fig. 18-55). The first case of intrasellar aneurysm was recorded by Mitchell in 1888. Heuer and Dandy (1916) reported an aneurysm of the internal carotid artery that destroyed the sella. Careful examination of the sella often reveals erosion of the lateral aspect of the floor and dorsum, whereas a normal sella is faintly seen on the side distant from the aneurysm. The carotid sulcus may be distorted, and a soft-tissue mass may be seen in the lateral and basal views (Fig. 18-56). These changes are best appreciated when the sphenoid sinus is well pneumatized. Undercutting of the anterior clinoid processes (Sosman and Vogt, 1926), enlargement of the superior orbital fissure (Rischbieth and Bull, 1958), and calcification may also take place. An alleged classic sellar enlargement produced by a chromophobe adenoma was illustrated in the textbook of Holmes and Robbins (1955). The lesion proved to be an intrasellar aneurysm at surgery and at necropsy (White and Ballantine, 1961). White and Ballantine (1961) described

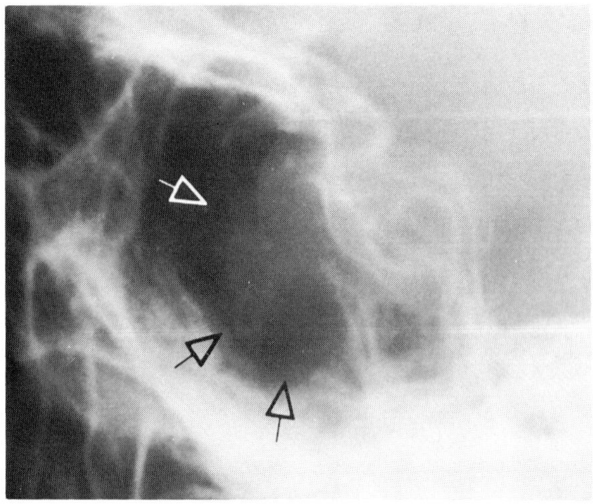

Fig. 18-56. Aneurysm of cavernous portion of internal carotid artery. Lateral projection of sella shows soft-tissue mass overlying sphenoid sinus anteriorly and distorting carotid sulcus (arrows).

three of their own patients with intrasellar aneurysm and found nineteen in the literature. Surgeons reported to them an additional thirteen cases. Twenty-nine of the thirty-five cases had been diagnosed as pituitary tumor, and an aneurysm was found at surgery or necropsy. Distortion of the carotid sulcus may also be caused by a tortuous internal carotid artery as in patients with arteriovenous malformations (Fig. 18-57). Arteriosclerotic elongation of the internal carotid artery and its proximal intra-arterial branches may cause visual defects simulating a suprasellar tumor (Hilton and Hoyt, 1966).

Hypothyroidism. The sella may enlarge in cretinism (Fig. 18-58) due to failure of the feedback mechanism (Nièpce, 1851; Middlemass, 1959). After treatment the

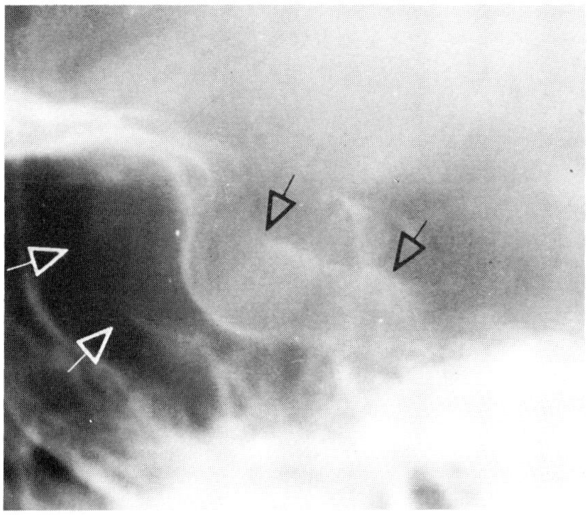

Fig. 18-57. Arteriovenous malformation. Carotid groove is enlarged by dilated internal carotid artery (arrows).

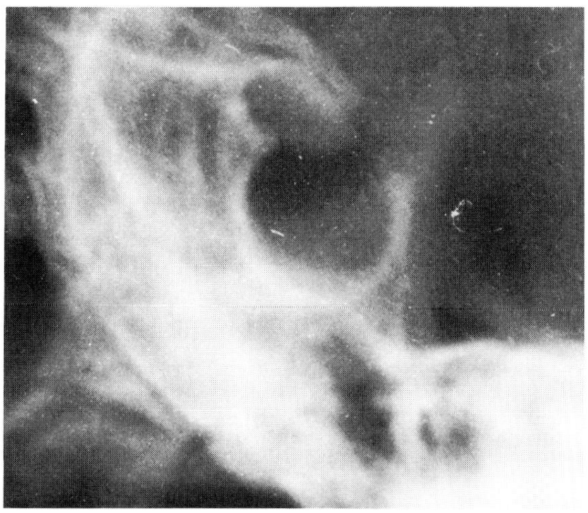

Fig. 18-58. Hypothyroidism. Lateral roentgenogram shows slightly enlarged sella.

sella may revert to normal (Taveras and Wood, 1964). In a case of cretinism reported by Hadden and Alexander (1968), autopsy revealed a normal pituitary gland and an intrasellar aneurysm.

Hypogonadism. Sellar enlargement may occur with untreated hypogonadism (Bower, 1968).

Neurofibromatosis. Asymmetric sellar enlargement (Fig. 18-62) may be associated with a defect in the posterior wall of the orbit. These changes are related to the skeletal dysplasia of neurofibromatosis.

Oxycephaly. Grundy and his co-workers (1970) reported three patients with oxycephaly and visual failure. Roentgenograms of the skull showed a large and deepened sella in lateral profile. No mention of the sella in the frontal projection was made, however. Our experience is that the sella in such cases is narrow and therefore normal in volume.

Local destruction or erosion

Erosion of undersurface of anterior clinoid process and chiasmatic sulcus

Glioma of optic chiasm. Piloid astrocytomas of the optic nerve and chiasm are most frequent in childhood and in patients with neurofibromatosis. Nevertheless gliomas of the optic chiasm do occur in adults (Fig. 18-59, *C*) and in patients without neurofibromatosis. The triad of optic nerve pallor, loss of visual acuity, and visual field defects should suggest this diagnosis (Evans et al., 1963). Optic chiasm gliomas may be associated with precocious sexual development, whereas craniopharyngiomas are often associated with retarded skeletal development. The optic chiasm glioma is a slow-growing tumor essentially suprasellar. It may be associated with enlargement of the optic canal. Optic canal enlargement was present in eighteen of twenty-seven optic chiasm gliomas reported by Evans and his co-workers (1963), and in seven it was bilateral. Enlargement of the intracranial portion of the optic canal is best appreciated on the lateral film with or without tomography (Fig. 18-59). The slow growth of the tumor results in the formation of a compartment anterolateral to the sella. This local excavation is formed by enlargement of the optic canal at the lateral aspect of the chiasmatic sulcus underneath the anterior clinoid process. The anterior clinoid process is excavated on its inferior and medial aspect (Fig. 18-59). In addition, the optic chiasm glioma may excavate the chiasmatic sulcus. The slow growth of the tumor contributes to the preservation of the cortical bone. In the series of Evans and his group (1963), these changes were seen in seventeen of thirty, and in four it was the only finding. These authors also reported similar findings in six patients with orbital neurofibromatosis. In other respects the changes caused by optic chiasm glioma are

A

B

C

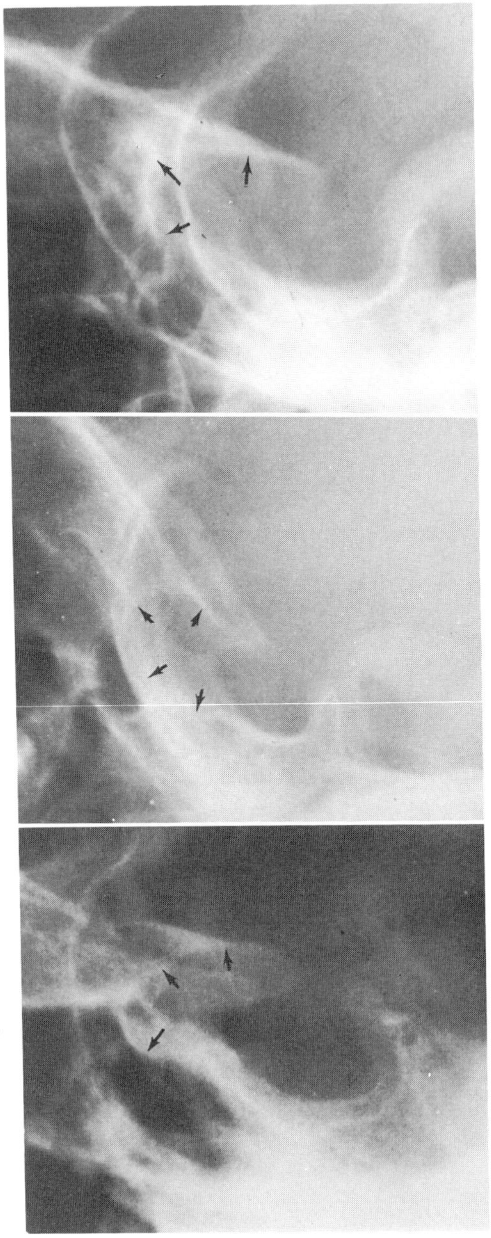

Fig. 18-59. Optic chiasm gliomas. Excavation and deepening of chiasmatic sulcus and undercutting of anterior clinoid processes are noted in these three cases.

those of a suprasellar mass, with erosion of the posterior clinoid processes and the dorsum sellae from above. The sella may be enlarged, but this occurs only after destruction of the dorsum sellae. Calcification resembling that of a craniopharyngioma may be found occasionally. It was reported in one patient by Heuer and Dandy in 1916 and in another by Cushing in 1929. Lindgren and Di Chiro (1951) reported calcification in three of nine optic chiasm gliomas. Calcification is usually nodular and may be indistinguishable from that seen in a craniopharyngioma or a hypothalamic glioma.

Optic nerve glioma and J sella. The clinical presentation of an optic nerve glioma is the same as just discussed with regard to optic chiasm glioma. Air studies are invaluable in determining whether the tumor is confined to the optic nerve or involves the optic chiasm. A characteristic deformity is caused by enlargement of the cranial end of the optic canal (Fig. 18-59) and may be defined as follows: The cranial end of the optic canal is deepened beneath the anterior clinoid process, and the undersurface of the anterior clinoid process is eroded and scalloped (Fig. 18-59); the cortical floor remains intact and is often thicker than normal because of the slow growth of the tumor; the process may extend to involve the chiasmatic sulcus. In this case the pituitary fossa extends farther forward than normal to form a rounded compartment (Fig. 18-59). The well-defined cortex and the rounded anterior end are essential components of the deformed sella. These changes must not be confused with a normally developed chiasmatic sulcus (Kier, 1968, 1969) (Fig. 18-4). Improper positioning may result in the projection of the optic strut or the optic canal roof above the chiasmatic sulcus, leading to a mistaken impression of an excavated chiasmatic sulcus (Fig. 18-11).

The term J sella has been attributed erroneously to Martin and Cushing (1923); they did not coin the term but merely described the characteristic erosion seen in optic nerve glioma. The long and heated controversy concerning the J sella (Davidoff and Epstein, 1950; Burrows, 1964; Kier, 1968) has led to the suggestion that the term be abandoned (Kier, 1969). According to du Boulay and Trickey (1970) the confusion arose because in aqueduct stenosis the sulcus chiasmaticus may remain large and be assimilated in the true sella. In addition, the sulcus is more vertical than normal as a result of the deformity of the whole skull. The dorsum is short and the anterior clinoid processes are large. Thus in profile the sella really does look like a "J." Common usage has led to the application of the term to other conditions where the deformity resembles a J lying on its side. In the past the normally developing limbus has often been called a J sella, leading to considerable additional confusion (Kier, 1968).

Optic nerve sheath tumor. Neurofibroma and meningioma of the optic nerve may produce enlargement of the optic canal and erosion of the anterior clinoid process in the same way as an optic nerve glioma. Meningiomas, in addition, often cause sclerosis of the optic canal and the anterior clinoid process.

Pituitary adenoma. Pituitary adenomas may elevate and erode one and sometimes both anterior clinoid processes. They may also erode the optic canal and enlarge the superior orbital fissure.

Aneurysm. An internal carotid artery aneurysm, when large, frequently erodes the undersurface of the anterior clinoid process and excavates the chiasmatic sulcus in the same way as an optic nerve glioma (Wren, 1969). Distortion of the carotid sulcus and a soft-tissue mass with, or without, calcification may be noted.

Dilated third ventricle. A dilated third ventricle acts as a mass. Particularly, increased intracranial pressure of long standing, such as is found in aqueduct stenosis, will cause excavation of the chiasmatic sulcus and undercutting of the anterior clinoid processes. These changes are usually associated with enlargement of the sella and destruction of the dorsum sellae and the posterior clinoid processes. These changes are found only in obstructive, and not in communicating, hydrocephalus.

Craniopharyngioma. A craniopharyngioma, particularly when it is intrasellar, may cause erosion of the anterior clinoid processes. Craniopharyngioma is sometimes closely related to the chiasmatic sulcus and, under these circumstances, may cause excavation of the chiasmatic sulcus.

Frontal lobe tumor. A frontal lobe tumor (Fig. 18-60), particularly when it is slow growing, may excavate the chiasmatic sulcus and the planum sphenoidale.

Gargoylism. Many of the changes described in gargoylism have been based on fiction rather than fact. However, abnormalities of the presphenoid are found under certain circumstances in gargoyles. Elongation and excavation of the chiasmatic sulcus may occur in patients with increasing head size (Kier, 1968) (Fig. 18-61). Neuhauser and co-workers (1968) described the association of arachnoid cysts in gargoyles and demonstrated changes in the chiasmatic sulcus due to pressure erosion from the cysts (see p. 387).

Neurofibromatosis. Many bony abnormalities are found in neurofibromatosis. These include absence of the greater wing of the sphenoid and an enlarged and deformed sella turcica (Fig. 18-62). Additional changes in the chiasmatic sulcus probably occur only in association with an optic nerve glioma, neurofibroma, or optic sheath meningioma (Evans et al., 1963).

Carotid cavernous fistula. A soft-tissue mass usually overlies the sphenoid sinus. This soft-tissue density may

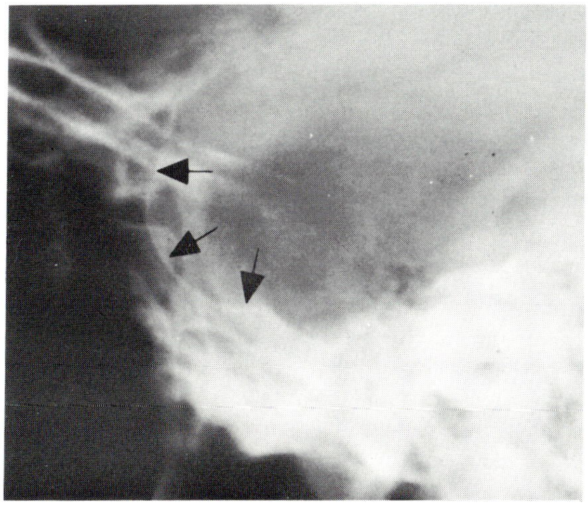

Fig. 18-60. Ependymoma of frontal lobe. Planum and chiasmatic sulcus show marked excavation (arrows). Anterior clinoid processes are pointed. Posterior clinoid processes and dorsum sellae have been destroyed. Such a sella has been erroneously termed "J" sella. It merely represents changes due to a long-standing suprasellar mass.

A

B

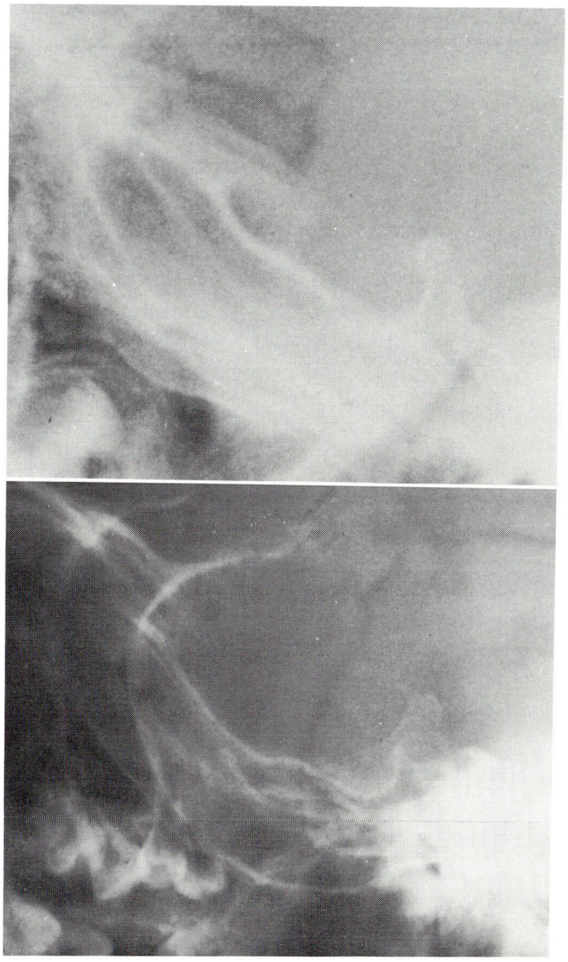

Fig. 18-61. Hurler-Hunter syndrome (gargoyle). **A,** Chiasmatic sulcus is concave. This change results in apparent elongation of sella. **B,** Dorsum sellae is hollowed out. Anterior clinoid processes are sharpened.

A

B

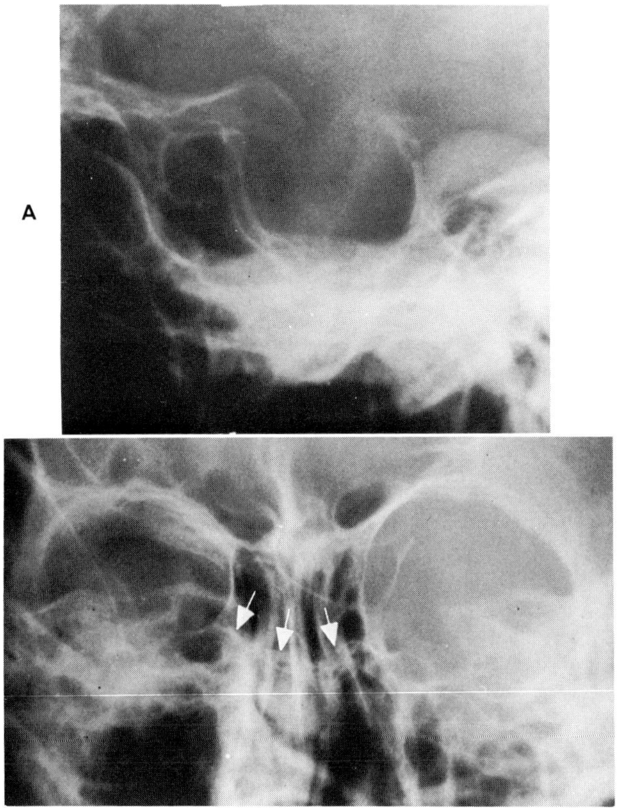

Fig. 18-62. Neurofibromatosis. **A,** Lateral roentgenogram shows that sella is large with asymmetric deepening of floor. Dorsum sellae is thin and rounded. **B,** Frontal roentgenogram of sella shows asymmetric floor (arrows). Defect in posterior wall of left orbit and asymmetry of orbit are also shown.

be visible in the lateral and basal views. Erosion of the undersurface of the anterior clinoid processes might be expected, but we have not seen it.

Erosion of upper surface of anterior clinoid processes

Suprasellar meningioma. Meningiomas may arise from the cribriform plate, the planum (Fig. 18-63), the tuberculum, or the anterior clinoid processes. Suprasellar meningiomas may show calcification or hyperostosis (Figs. 18-64 and 18-65). The calcification is usually homogeneous or granular and is present in about 7% (Cushing and Eisenhardt, 1938; Lindgren and Di Chiro, 1951). Occasionally only a fleck of calcification is seen (Fig. 18-66). Spongy thickening of the planum sphenoidale may take place (Fig. 18-64) and differentiation from fibrous dysplasia (Fig. 18-68) may be difficult (Leeds and Seaman, 1962). The bone of fibrous dysplasia does not contain trabeculae and for its thickness is not very dense. The changes may be more widespread, or evidence of fibrous dysplasia may be found elsewhere in the skull. The

A

B

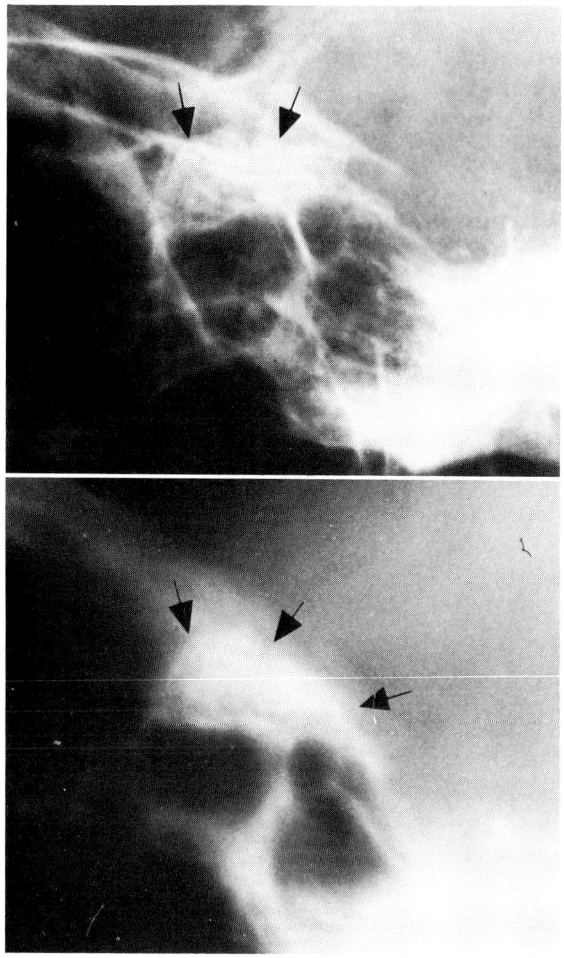

Fig. 18-63. Meningioma, planum sphenoidale. **A,** Lateral roentgenogram of skull with slight rotation. **B,** Lateral tomogram. Hyperostosis of planum (arrows) is shown more clearly on tomogram. Posterior clinoid processes and dorsum sellae have been eroded from above.

tumor mass of a meningioma is frequently larger than the area of calcification or hyperostosis. The sella is deformed from above, with a hollowing out of the anterior clinoid processes and destruction of the posterior clinoid processes and the dorsum. The anterior clinoid processes may be thickened or hyperostotic (Figs. 18-63 to 18-65), which occasionally may be in response to a distant meningioma. Enlargement of the sella may result when the tumor extends into it (Figs. 18-65, *A,* and 18-67). Extension or proximity of a meningioma to the sella may result in increased density of the sella. The most useful investigation usually is selective internal and external carotid angiography supplemented with subtraction techniques. Meningiomas of the tuberculum may show no abnormal blood supply. At encephalography the tumor can be outlined with air and commonly is seen to deform the anterior third ventricle.

A

B

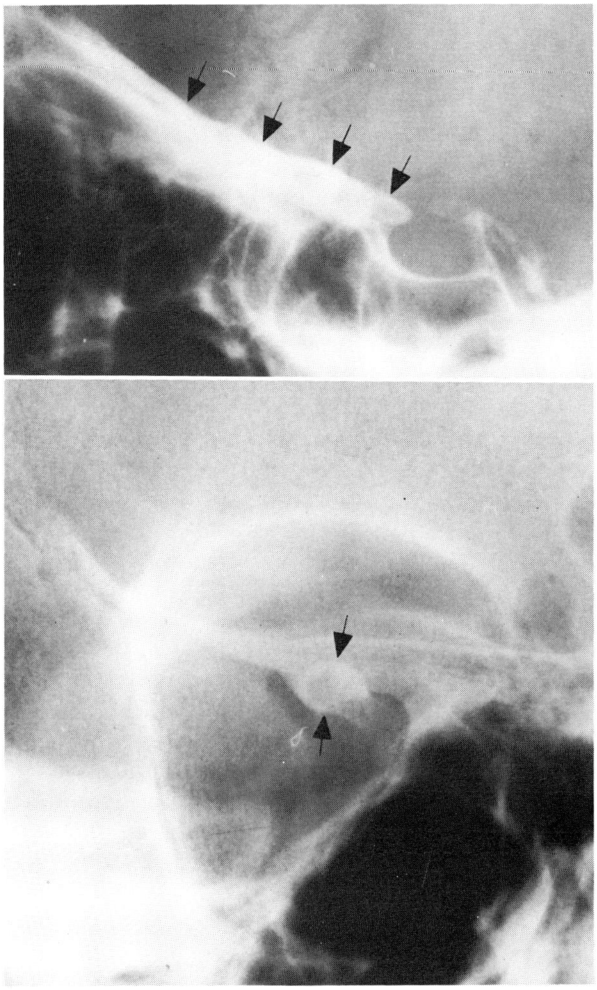

Fig. 18-64. Meningioma, planum sphenoidale. **A,** Lateral roentgenogram of skull shows thickening of planum sphenoidale (arrows). **B,** Optic foramen view. Bone sclerosis also involves anterior clinoid process (arrows).

A

B

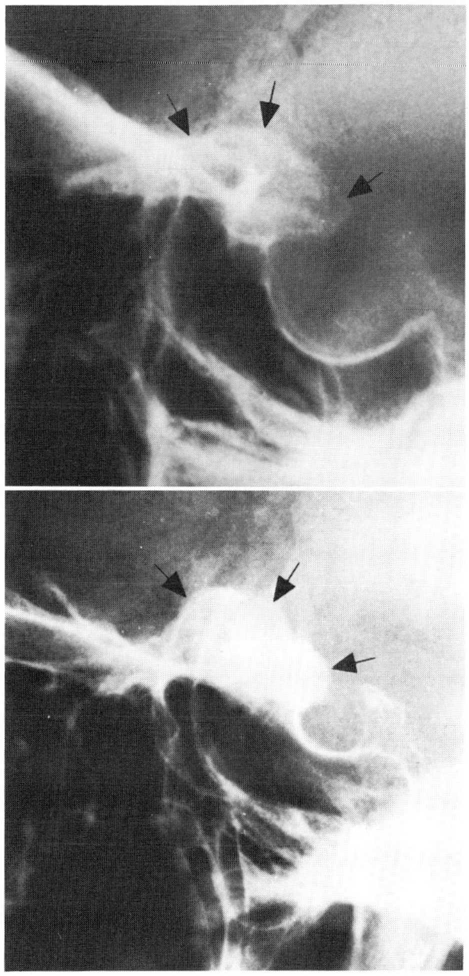

Fig. 18-65. Meningioma, planum sphenoidale. **A,** Bulbous hyperostosis of planum sphenoidale and anterior clinoid processes. Posterior clinoid processes of dorsum sellae are destroyed. **B,** Dense hyperostosis of planum sphenoidale and tuberculum sellae. Remainder of sella is normal.

Increased intracranial pressure due to dilated third ventricle. Increased intracranial pressure with a dilated third ventricle causes pressure erosion of the anterior clinoid processes and sometimes the planum sphenoidale. These changes are usually accompanied by destruction of the dorsum sellae and the posterior clinoid processes. The bone changes are dependent on the location of the third ventricle, which location, in turn, is related to the length of the optic nerves and the position of the optic chiasm. These changes are discussed in further detail in the ensuing pages.

Frontal tumor. A slow-growing frontal tumor (Fig. 18-60) may cause pressure erosion of the upper surface of the anterior clinoid processes and the planum sphenoidale.

Aneurysm. A suprasellar aneurysm may cause hollowing out of the planum sphenoidale and the anterior clinoid processes.

Suprasellar arachnoid cysts in gargoylism. Neuhauser and his co-workers (1968) reported twelve patients with the Hurler-Hunter syndrome each of whom had an arachnoid cyst with associated changes in the sella and the sphenoid bone. These authors described progressive depression of the planum sphenoidale and the chiasmatic sulcus as well as thinning, truncation, and separation of the anterior clinoid processes. The posterior clinoid processes and the dorsum were spared, but the body and lesser wings of the sphenoid were occasionally affected. In each instance ventricular dilatation and thickening of the meninges were present. Arachnoid cysts that deformed the sphenoid bone were demonstrated at necropsy.

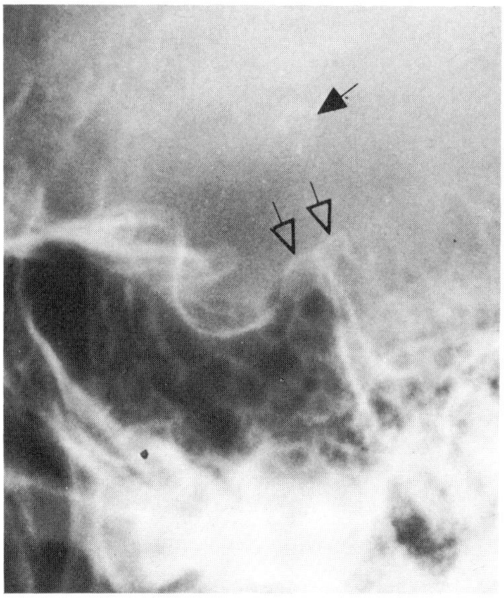

Fig. 18-66. Meningioma, dorsum sellae. Posterior clinoid processes and upper portion of dorsum sellae are destroyed (open arrows). Note the faint circular calcification above the sella (solid arrow).

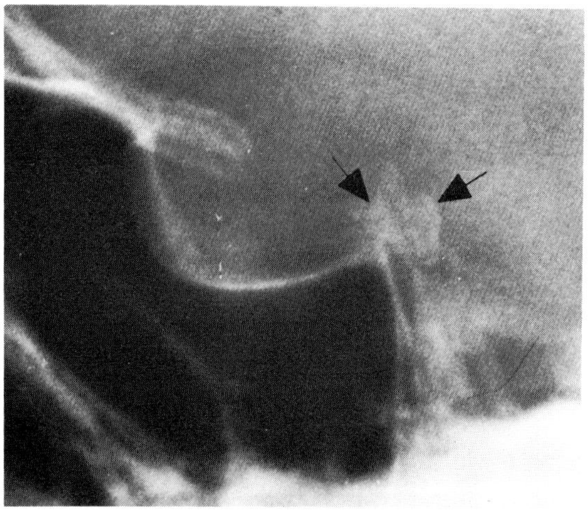

Fig. 18-67. Meningioma, dorsum sellae. There is irregular hyperostosis (arrows) of posterior clinoid processes and dorsum sellae. Sella is deepened anteriorly, and anterior clinoid processes are undermined.

A

B

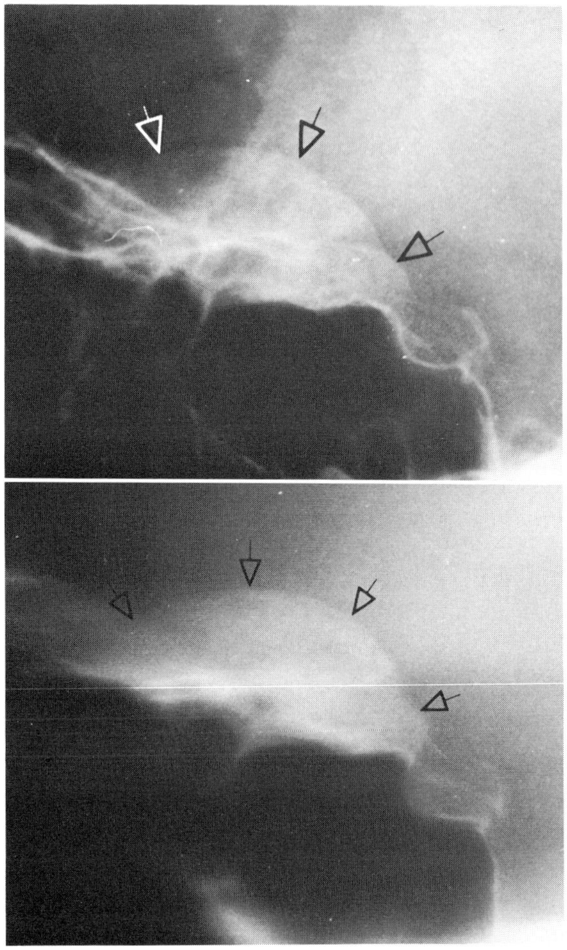

Fig. 18-68. Fibrous dysplasia. **A,** Lateral roentgenogram of sellar region. **B,** Lateral tomogram. Note the homogeneous, sharply demarcated, increased bony density involving the planum sphenoidale.

Localized erosion of floor

Nasopharyngeal tumor. Tumors of the paranasal sinuses (ethmoid, maxillary, or sphenoid) may involve the sella (Fig. 18-69). These tumors may be carcinomas, adenocarcinomas, sarcomas, lymphoepitheliomas, or plasmocytomas (Fig. 18-70). The destruction of the sella begins in the floor and may then involve the entire pituitary fossa. A lymphoepithelioma (Fig. 18-71) may give rise to irregular sclerotic changes in the sphenoid bone. Nasopharyngeal carcinomas are more destructive than benign tumors. After treatment with radiotherapy, the destroyed bone may be restored. This bone is frequently more dense than normal bone and the sella does not regain its normal shape (Fig. 18-72).

Sphenoid sinus mucocele. A mucocele may be formed by blockage of the ostium of a paranasal sinus. The contents may be mucus or pus. In the latter the term pyocele is probably more appropriate. Sphenoid sinus mucoceles are rare; they may lead to destruction of the floor of the sella and apparent enlargement of the pituitary fossa (Fig. 18-73). As a mucocele expands, it first destroys the septa within the sinus (Figs. 18-74 and 18-75) and later the walls of the sinus. The floor of the sella is pushed up and subsequently may even be destroyed (Fig. 18-74). The cause of the destructive process

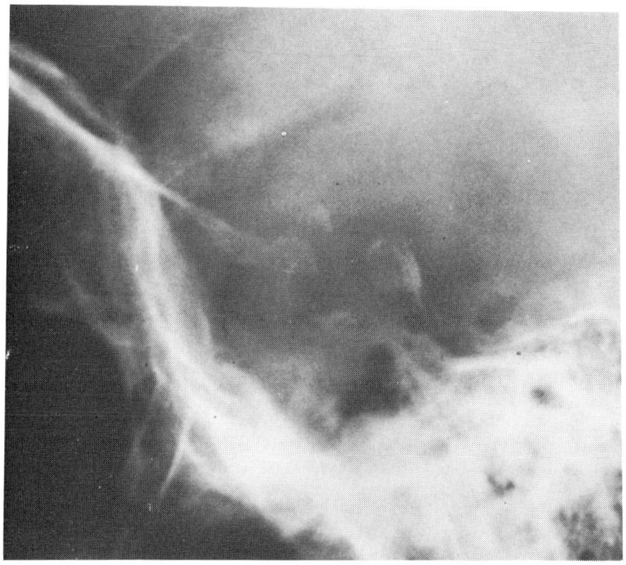

Fig. 18-69. Nasopharyngeal carcinoma. Lateral roentgenogram of sellar region shows ill-defined soft-tissue mass obscuring sphenoid sinus. There is no enlargement of sella, but sellar floor shows irregular destruction.

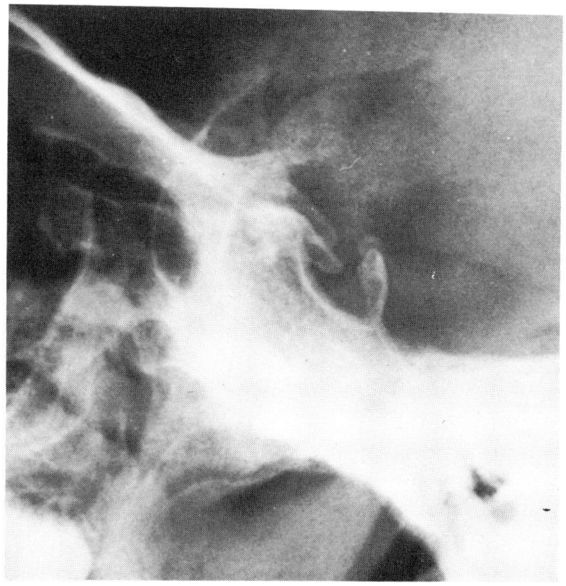

Fig. 18-71. Lymphoepithelioma of nasopharynx. Lateral film of skull shows irregular sclerosis of sphenoid sinus. Sella is normal.

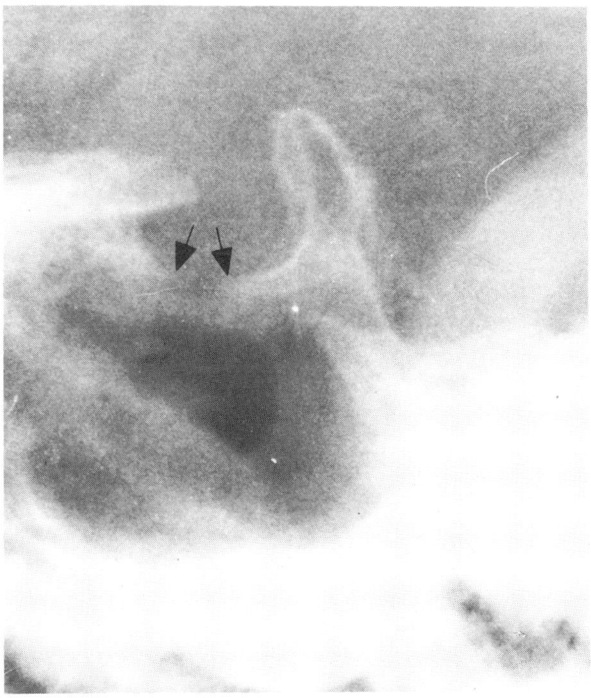

Fig. 18-70. Plasmocytoma. Sphenoid sinus is partially obscured by mass within. Note the localized destruction of the floor of the sella (arrows).

A

B

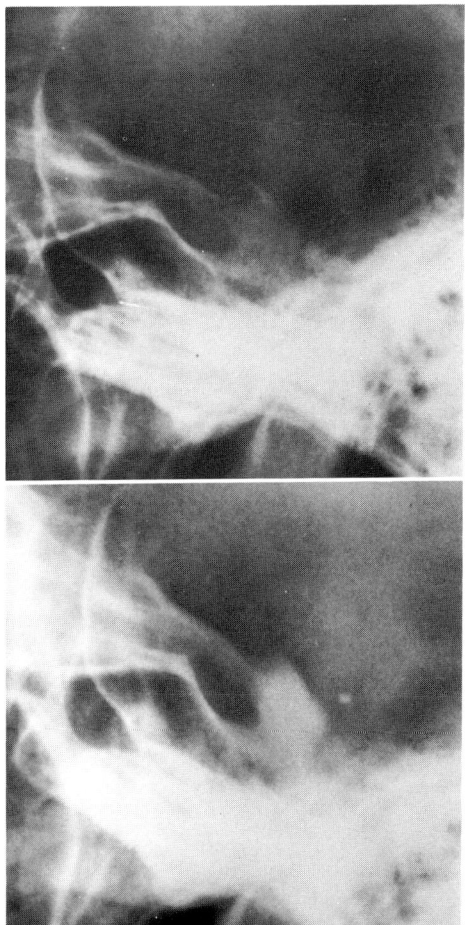

Fig. 18-72. Adenocystic carcinoma. **A,** Dorsum sellae and superior portions of clivus show irregular destruction. **B,** After irradiation an increased density in previously destroyed region is noted.

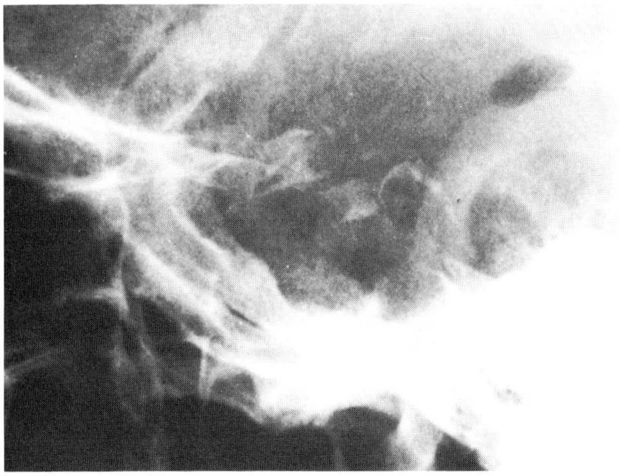

Fig. 18-73. Sphenoid sinus mucocele. Sella shows irregular destructive changes.

A

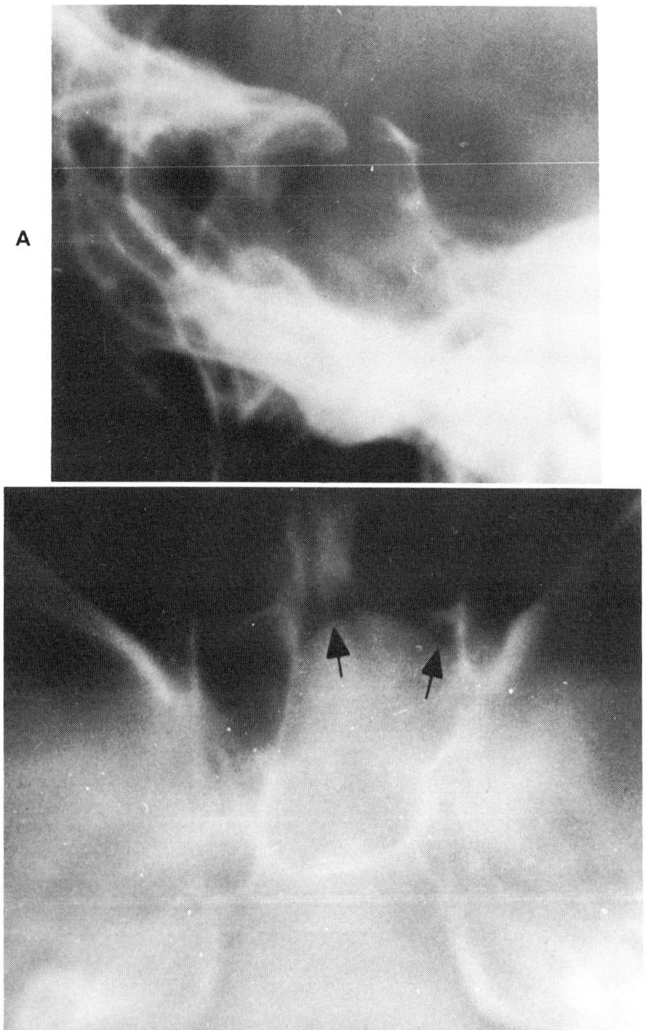

B

Fig. 18-74. Sphenoid sinus mucocele. **A,** Lateral projection shows sphenoid sinus to be partially opacified. Floor of sella has been destroyed. **B,** Basal projection shows soft-tissue mass within sphenoid sinus sharply demarcated anteriorly (arrows).

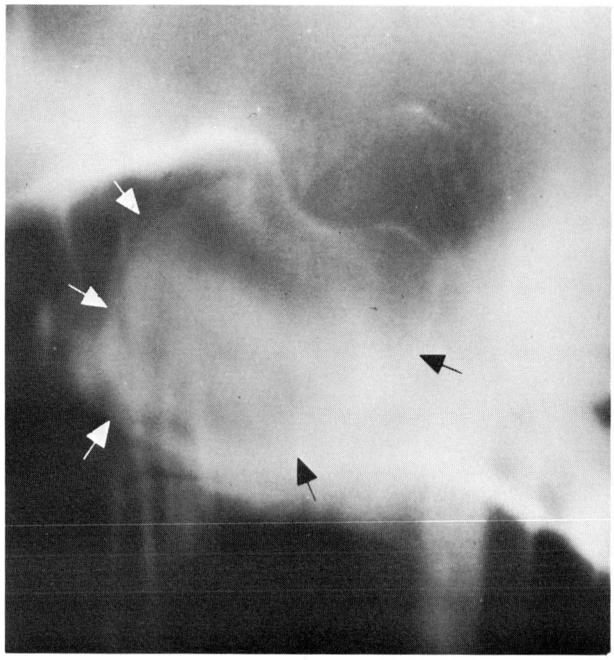

Fig. 18-75. Sphenoid sinus mucocele. Lateral midline tomogram of sellar region shows sphenoid sinus expanded by sharply demarcated soft-tissue mass within it (arrows).

may then be difficult to determine. Nugent and his coworkers (1970) in an analysis of sixty-three sphenoid sinus mucoceles found that thirty-eight involved the sella, of which twenty-nine destroyed the floor. Whether the mass arose within the sella or below it in many instances was difficult to determine. By tomography these workers were able to demonstrate the expanded but nevertheless intact roof of the sphenoid sinus in one of their patients. The presence of an intact roof of the sphenoid sinus is the most important feature in the differentiation between intrasellar and infrasellar lesions (Fig. 18-75). The tuberculum sellae, the planum, the optic canal, and the medial wall of the orbit were involved in about 10%.

Metastasis. Metastases may spread to the pituitary fossa and may simulate a pituitary tumor. This possibility should be remembered in patients with a known malignant neoplasm who develop signs of a pituitary tumor. Evidence of bone destruction rather than expansion may be found. Metastatic prostatic carcinoma may cause sclerosis of the sphenoid sinus and the anterior fossa (Fig. 18-76).

Basal encephalocele. Basal encephaloceles are rare

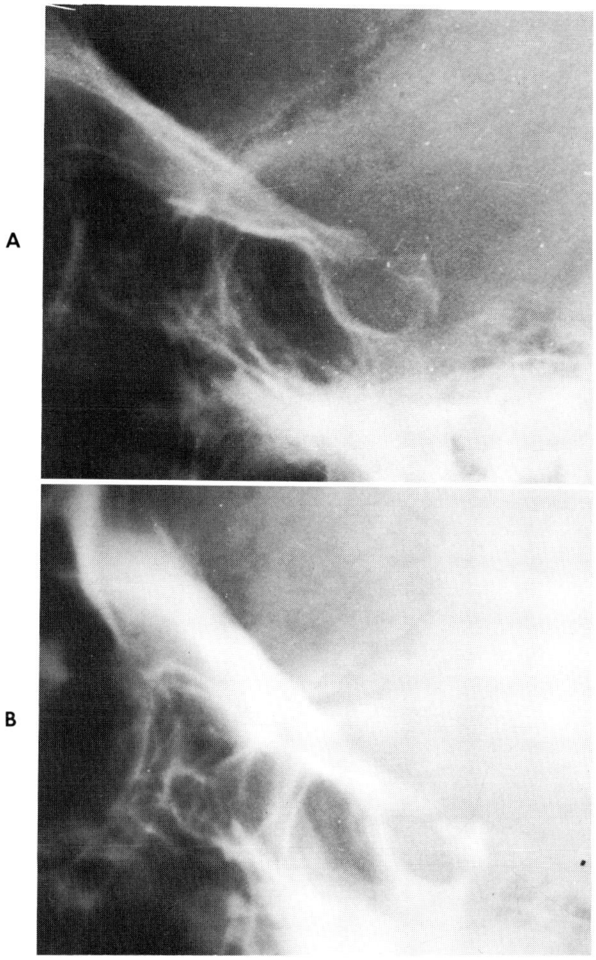

Fig. 18-76. Carcinoma of prostate. **A,** Planum sphenoidale and sella appear normal. **B,** Lateral roentgenogram of skull obtained 2 years later shows extensive sclerosis of sphenoid bone and anterior fossa due to metastasis from carcinoma of prostate.

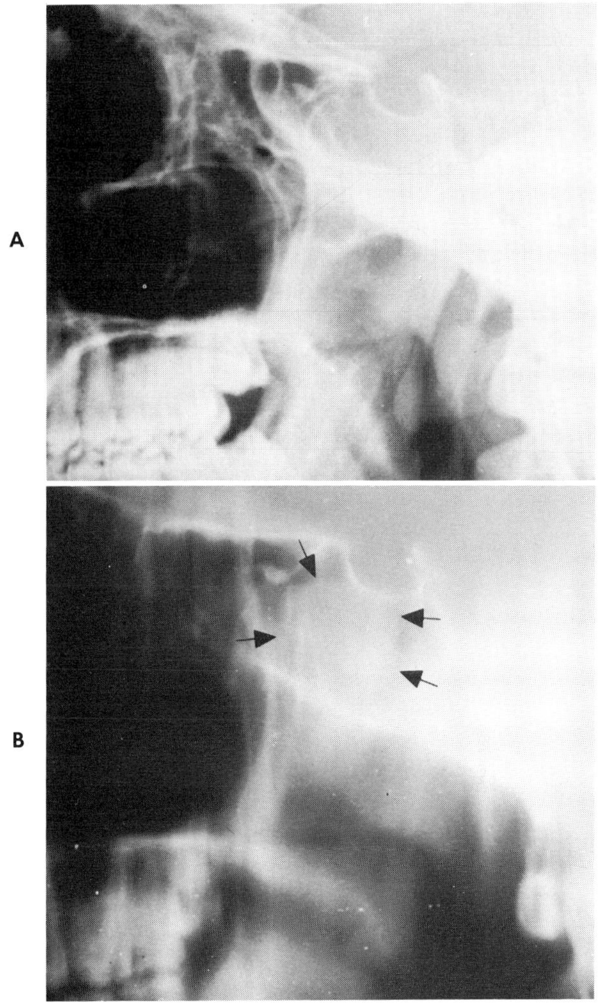

Fig. 18-77. Juvenile nasopharyngeal angiofibroma. **A,** Lateral roentgenogram of sellar region. **B,** Lateral midline tomogram shows sharply circumscribed mass within nasopharynx extending into sphenoid sinus (arrows).

lesions characterized by herniation of intracranial contents through a defect in the base of the skull. The transsphenoid encephalocele is recognized by a sharply circumscribed defect in the floor of the sella seen in the basal skull film. Such a defect was present in all five patients reported by Pollock and co-workers (1968) and was associated with a nasopharyngeal mass. Pneumoencephalography and arteriography are particularly helpful in delineating the extent of the encephalocele. (See Chapter 27.)

Giant cell tumor. Giant cell tumors have been reported in the skull and nasal sinuses and, on rare occasions, in the sphenoid bone. Geissinger and his co-workers (1970) reported a 20-year-old pregnant housewife with destruction of the floor of the sella and the dorsum. Biopsy showed the neoplasm to be a giant cell tumor. In reviewing the literature these authors found that eight of eleven patients were women. Multiple cranial nerve palsies and destruction of the sella were the usual findings.

Leiomyoma. A patient with intrasellar leiomyoma was reported by Kroe and his co-workers (1968). Tumors of mesodermal elements have been reported elsewhere in the brain and are believed to arise from embryonic rests. In the case of intrasellar leiomyoma, the tumor was thought to have arisen possibly from vascular smooth muscle. The changes due to an intrasellar leiomyoma are those of an intrasellar mass, with erosion of the floor and the dorsum sellae.

Juvenile nasopharyngeal angiofibroma. Juvenile nasopharyngeal angiofibroma is a highly vascular benign neoplasm of the nasopharynx that develops almost exclusively in the adolescent male. Although these tumors rarely metastasize, or invade adjacent structures,

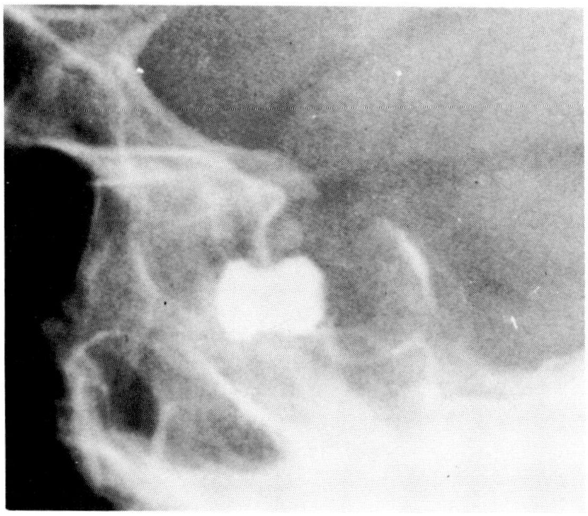

Fig. 18-78. Postoperative sella. Lateral roentgenogram of sella shows Silastic plug traversing anterior portion of floor of sella after transsphenoidal hypophysectomy.

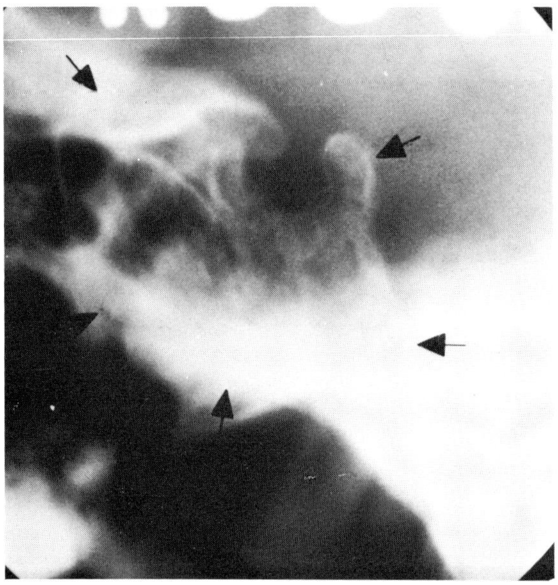

Fig. 18-79. Meningioma of clivus. Lateral film of sella shows irregular calcification and destruction of sphenoid and floor of sella. Meningioma extended into sphenoid sinus and cerebellopontine angle.

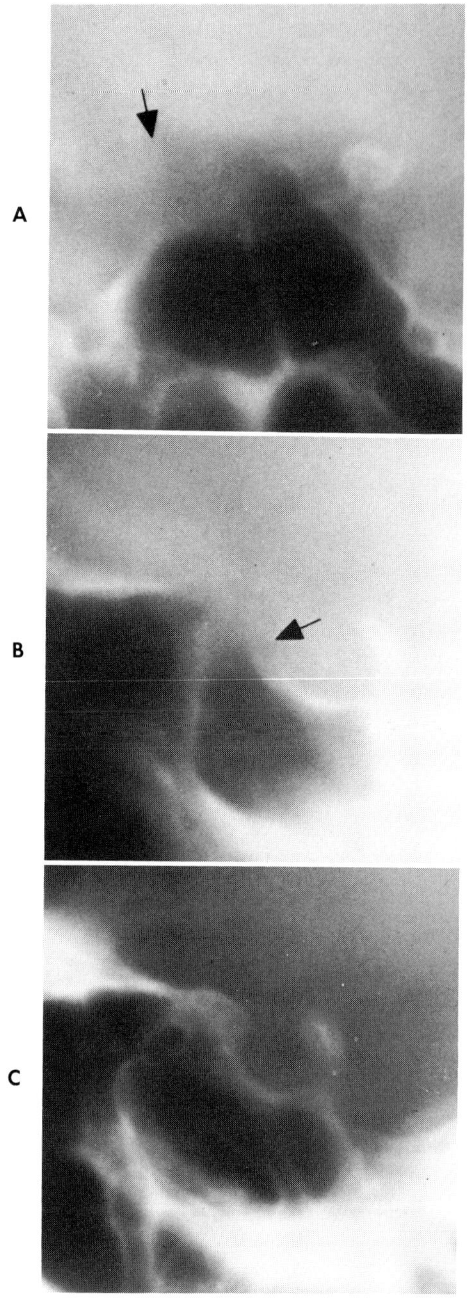

Fig. 18-80. Meningioma of cavernous sinus. **A,** Frontal tomogram shows right anterior clinoid process and lateral wall of sphenoid sinus destroyed (arrow). **B,** Lateral tomogram to right of midline shows destruction of anterior clinoid process and adjacent floor of sella and planum sphenoidale (arrow). **C,** Lateral tomogram to left of midline shows normal left half of sella. Left anterior clinoid process is intact.

they do cause pressure erosion. A soft tissue mass may be seen in the nasopharynx and sphenoid sinus (Fig. 18-77). The sphenoid bone may become eroded or sclerosed, and the superior orbital fissure enlarged. A characteristic feature reported by Holman and Miller (1965) was anterior bowing of the posterior wall of the maxillary sinus. This anterior bowing is best seen in the lateral or the basal view. Investigation of these tumors requires common carotid as well as selective internal and external carotid angiography (Wilson and Hanafee, 1969).

Postoperative sella. Transsphenoidal surgery is frequently undertaken for chromophobe and eosinophilic pituitary adenomas. Yttrium implants may be used in the treatment of acromegaly, and the implant may be retained with a screw. Alternatively, after transsphenoidal surgery, a Silastic plug (Fig. 18-78) may be used to repair the defect in the floor of the sella to prevent a possible postoperative cerebrospinal fluid fistula.

Erosion of dorsum and posterior clinoid processes

Lateral surface

Parasellar meningoma. Meningiomas of the middle fossa or of the lesser wing of the sphenoid may involve the cavernous sinus; and they may destroy the sella on its lateral aspect (Figs. 18-79 and 18-80). We have seen two meningiomas and one pituitary adenoma that involved the anterior, middle, and posterior fossae; we termed them triple fossa tumors.

Neurofibroma. Tumors of the fifth nerve (e.g., neurofibroma or sarcoma) may also appear as parasellar masses and destroy the lateral aspect of the sella. The floor of the middle fossa and the medial aspect of the petrous apex may also become eroded (Holman et al., 1961). A nasopharyngeal mass may be present.

Chordoma. These arise from remnants of the notochord and appear predominantly at either end of the vertebral column. Thus intracranially they arise in the clivus and the sella in the region of the spheno-occipital synchrondrosis. According to Wood and Himadi (1950) about 37% of the tumors involve the skull. These are tumors of low malignancy and are more common in males than females by a ratio of about 2:1. They are most frequent in the third and fourth decades of life. They grow to involve the sella and spread upward, forward, and downward. A soft-tissue mass may be found in the nasopharynx. The presence of both an intracranial and an extracranial mass should suggest the diagnosis of chordoma, nasopharyngeal carcinoma, or large pituitary tumor. In the early stages neither destruction nor calcification is seen, but later both may be present. Calcification is often extremely dense or vacuolated. Destruction of the base of the skull may be evident (Fig. 18-81).

Aneurysm of internal carotid artery. In addition to undercutting the anterior clinoid processes, an aneurysm may erode the lateral aspect of the pituitary fossa and the dorsum sellae. A soft-tissue mass with or without calcification may be seen on lateral and basal views (Fig. 18-56).

Anomalous vessels. The trigeminal artery may pass through the dorsum sellae or lateral to it (Lamb and Morris, 1961). On occasion the lateral aspect of the dorsum sellae may be eroded (Fig. 18-82).

Miscellaneous conditions. Epidermoid and subarachnoid cysts may on occasion erode the lateral aspect of the sella.

A

B

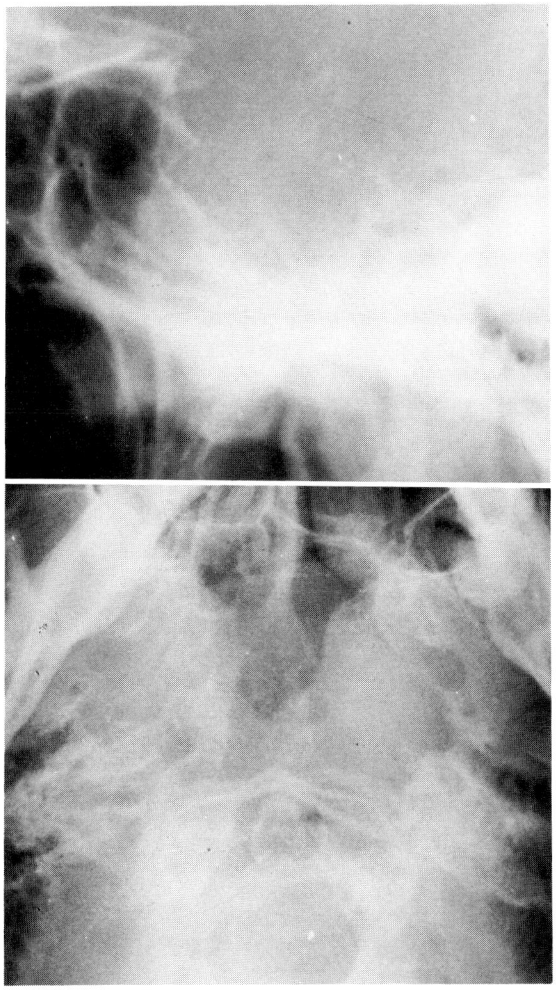

Fig. 18-81. Chordoma. **A,** Lateral roentgenogram of sella shows dorsum sellae and floor of sella and adjacent clivus to be destroyed. Note the faint retrosellar calcification. **B,** Basal view shows asymmetric destruction of base of skull on left involving petrous temporal apex.

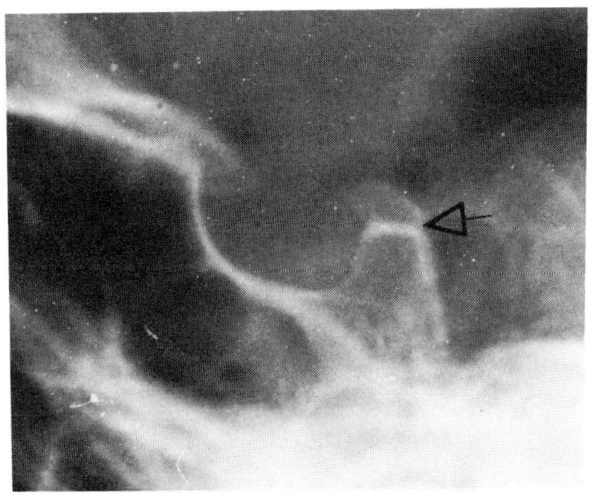

Fig. 18-82. Trigeminal artery. Note the unilateral erosion of the dorsum sellae (arrow).

Anterior surface of dorsum

Intrasellar masses. The changes associated with intrasellar masses have already been discussed.

Upper surface of dorsum and posterior clinoid processes

Suprasellar masses

CRANIOPHARYNGIOMA. These too have already been discussed.

OPTIC CHIASM GLIOMA. Gliomas of the optic chiasm, in addition to excavating the chiasmatic sulcus, may also destroy the posterior clinoid processes and the dorsum sellae and may cause enlargement of the pituitary fossa.

HYPOTHALAMIC TUMOR. These tumors may cause roentgenographic changes similar to those of craniopharyngiomas (Fig. 18-83). Bony erosion, when present, occurs from above and affects one or both posterior clinoid processes and the dorsum sellae. I have noted, when evaluating parasellar calcification, that craniopharyngiomas cause these changes more frequently than do hypothalamic gliomas. The deformity of the dorsum and the calcification may be indistinguishable from craniopharyngioma (Hamby, 1934). Even air studies may be confusing since the tumor may extend into the interpeduncular cistern (Lindgren and Di Chiro, 1951).

A

B

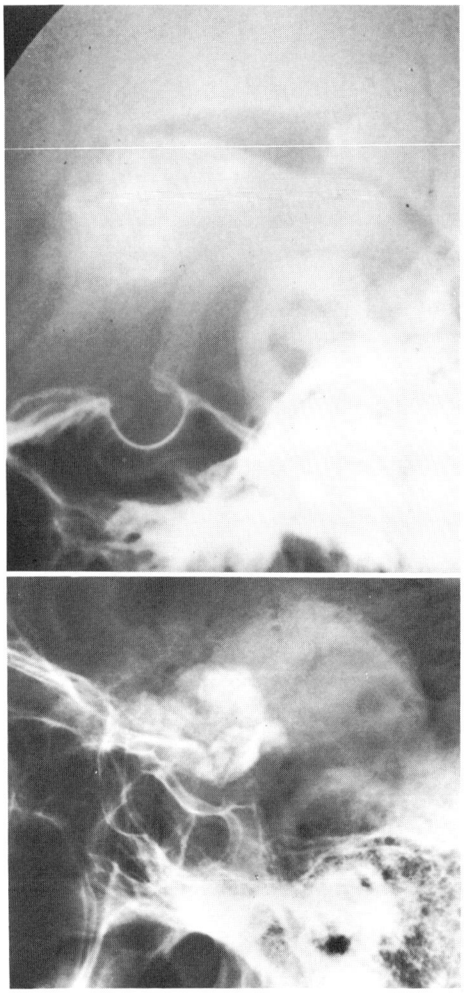

Fig. 18-83. Hypothalamic glioma. **A,** Pneumoencephalogram, lateral sitting position, shows that sella is normal. Calcified suprasellar mass projects into floor of third ventricle. **B,** Densely calcified suprasellar mass with destruction of dorsum sellae in another patient. This appearance simulated a craniopharyngioma.

MENINGIOMA. Classically, suprasellar meningiomas erode the anterior clinoid processes from above. Similar changes in the posterior clinoid processes and the dorsum sellae also occur.

SUBARACHNOID CYST. Sansregret and associates (1969) reported three patients with suprasellar subarachnoid cysts with findings of a suprasellar mass. These workers postulated two types: one that develops from the suprasellar subarachnoid cisterns and one that arises from the third ventricle, possibly on an inflammatory basis. Erosion of the dorsum and scalloping of the clivus were noted. The dorsum sellae was destroyed from above, and the anterior clinoid processes were elevated.

ANEURYSM. Suprasellar aneurysm may destroy the posterior clinoid processes and the dorsum sellae from above. It also can enlarge the pituitary fossa and thus simulate an intrasellar tumor (Fig. 18-55).

HISTIOCYTOSIS X. This condition may involve the hypothalamus. In the one biopsy-proved case that I have seen, the radiologic findings were those of a suprasellar mass. Serial roentgenograms were available for review since 1965, which was when the symptoms first developed. Roentgenograms of the sella at that time showed a well-formed and thick lamina dura. Some thinning, pointing, and erosion of the upper part of the dorsum sellae were also noted (Fig. 18-84). By February 1966 the lamina dura was much less dense than it had been at the original examination. The lamina dura in the upper part of the dorsum was less thick, and the anterior clinoid processes were demineralized. By August of the same year, further loss of lamina dura and further destruction of the dorsum sellae were observed. In March 1967 the lamina dura was fuzzy and poorly seen, and there had been further destruction of the dorsum from above. After radiation therapy the lamina dura and the dorsum sellae became reconstructed (Fig. 18-84).

ATYPICAL TERATOMA (ECTOPIC PINEALOMA). This rare tumor, which appears as a suprasellar mass, has caused considerable argument among neuropathologists. It may follow seeding from a pinealoma in the subarachnoid space or be a direct extension from tumor in the pineal

A

B

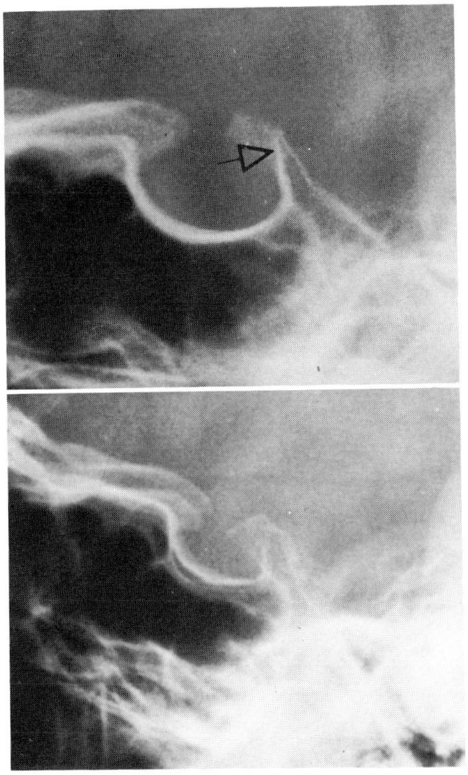

Fig. 18-84. Histiocytosis X. **A,** Upper part of dorsum sellae is slightly pointed and sharpened (arrow). Lamina dura is well defined and thick. **B,** After radiotherapy, floor of sella has been reconstituted. Sella is now smaller than before treatment.

region. In these cases a mass may be demonstrated in the suprasellar region as well as in the posterior end of the third ventricle. In some patients with such a suprasellar tumor, the pineal gland is normal. For this reason the suprasellar tumor has been classified as an atypical teratoma. A small and somewhat dense sella has been noted in four patients, but whether this is of diagnostic significance is doubtful.

LIPOMA. I have seen two suprasellar lipomas at necropsy but never one that produced symptoms.

DERMOID CYST. Dermoid cysts or epidermoids may also develop in the suprasellar region, and changes of a suprasellar mass may be shown.

FRONTAL GLIOMA. A slow-growing frontal tumor occasionally causes erosion of the planum, the anterior clinoid processes, the posterior clinoid processes, and the dorsum sellae from above.

Dilated third ventricle. A dilated third ventricle due to obstructive hydrocephalus behaves as a tumor and erodes the dorsum sellae and the posterior clinoid processes from above. It usually results in enlargement of the sella. (See ensuing discussion on the sella in increased intracranial pressure.)

Posterior surface

Posterior fossa tumor. A characteristic scalloping and erosion of the clivus as a result of benign posterior fossa tumors was described by Kruyff and Munn (1963). These changes are usually found only in children and are most commonly the result of an astrocytoma. The scalloping usually exceeds 3 mm in depth and must be distinguished from a normal curve of the dorsum sellae and the clivus.

Metastasis. Erosion and scalloping of the clivus and dorsum, indistinguishable from that just described for the more benign posterior fossa tumors, may result from metastases to the dorsum sellae. I have seen one patient with a metastasis from a colloid carcinoma of the colon who had such changes on the posterior surface of the dorsum sellae.

Arachnoid cyst. An arachnoid cyst may produce erosion of the posterior aspect of the dorsum sellae.

Basilar artery aneurysm. I have not seen erosion secondary to a basilar artery aneurysm, but erosion due to a vertebral artery aneurysm was reported at necropsy by Wells (1922).

Local bony sclerosis and change in texture

Fibrous dysplasia

Fibrous dysplasia may cause cystic, sclerotic, or mixed bony changes. The sclerotic form usually involves the skull base (Fig. 18-68), and the cystic form the vault. If the sella is involved, the changes of fibrous dysplasia are nearly always more widespread (Fig. 18-85) and found in the younger age groups.

Ossifying fibroma

Ossifying fibroma is a variant of fibrous dysplasia that may superficially resemble chordoma (Fig. 18-86). It may be enclosed by a paranasal sinus, which it may enlarge. The fibroma is better defined than a chordoma even when neighboring bone is involved in the process.

Meningioma

Changes in the planum range from a barely discernible hyperostosis to massive calcification (Figs. 18-63 to 18-65). The thickening in the planum is sometimes best appreciated on tomography. The meningioma is frequently larger than hyperostosis would indicate.

The anterior clinoid processes may show sclerosis and thickening secondary to a meningioma (Fig. 18-65), but I have seen similar as yet unexplained changes with a convexity meningioma.

The tuberculum sellae or the posterior clinoid processes (Fig. 18-67) may also become sclerotic when invaded by meningioma.

Irregular sclerosis with or without destructive changes

A

B

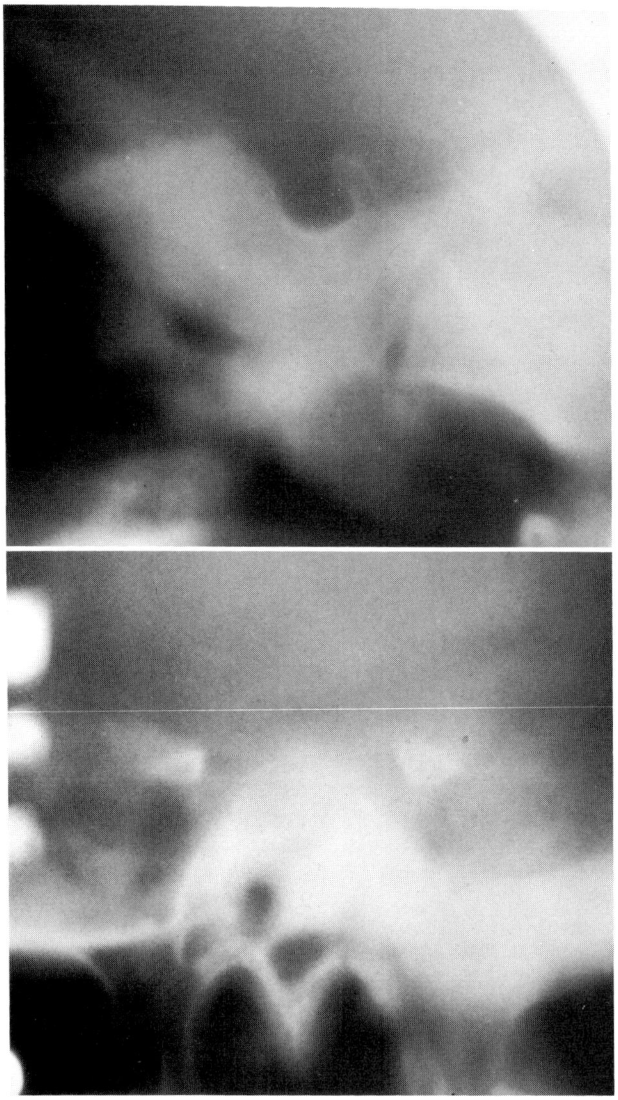

Fig. 18-85. Fibrous dysplasia. A, Lateral projection. B, Frontal tomogram. Sphenoid bone, dorsum sellae, and anterior clinoid processes are densely sclerotic.

may be found in a parasellar meningioma invading the cavernous sinus. These meningiomas may be very large and may extend from the anterior fossa to the posterior fossa.

Metastatic tumor

Metastatic tumors to the skull are sometimes osteoblastic and, when they involve the sella, may cause an increase in density (Fig. 18-76).

Suprasellar tumor

I have seen generalized increase in density of the sella in cases of atypical teratoma but am not convinced that this sclerosis is any more real than that described as secondary to craniopharyngioma.

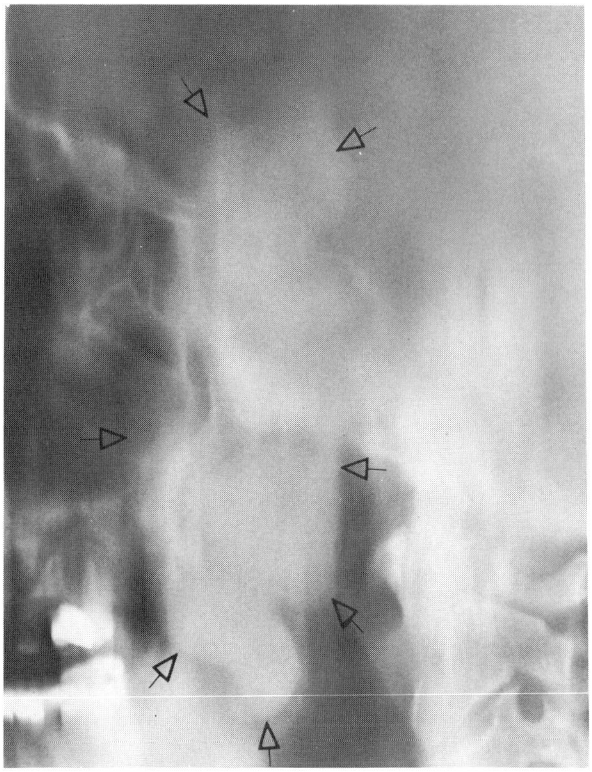

Fig. 18-86. Ossifying fibroma. Lateral tomogram of parasellar region shows well-defined suprasellar, intrasellar, and nasopharyngeal mass (arrows). Sella is slightly enlarged.

Osteochondroma, osteoma, chondroma

Osteochondroma, osteoma, and chondroma develop in the base of the skull, the clivus, the cerebellopontine angle, and the planum (Fig. 18-87). In a review of 113 cartilaginous tumors of the skull, fifty-seven were reported as sphenoid in origin (Berkmen and Blatt, 1968). Bone destruction and calcification occur in over half the tumors. Calcification has not been reported in tumors arising in the cerebellopontine angle (Minagi and Newton, 1969), but I have seen one case. The appearance of chondroma is that of a honeycomb with lucent areas formed by noncalcified cartilage (Fig 18-88).

Soft-tissue masses

Soft-tissue masses may be seen within the sphenoid sinus. Such masses may be secondary to an intrasellar tumor extending into the sphenoid sinus (Figs. 18-34 and 18-39). Soft-tissue masses within the sphenoid sinus are also found in nasopharyngeal angiofibroma or tumors of the nasopharynx. Aneurysms of the cavernous portion of the internal carotid artery also produce soft-tissue masses in the parasellar region (Chynn, 1966). In these instances distortion of the carotid sulcus, enlargement of the superior orbital fissure, and calcifi-

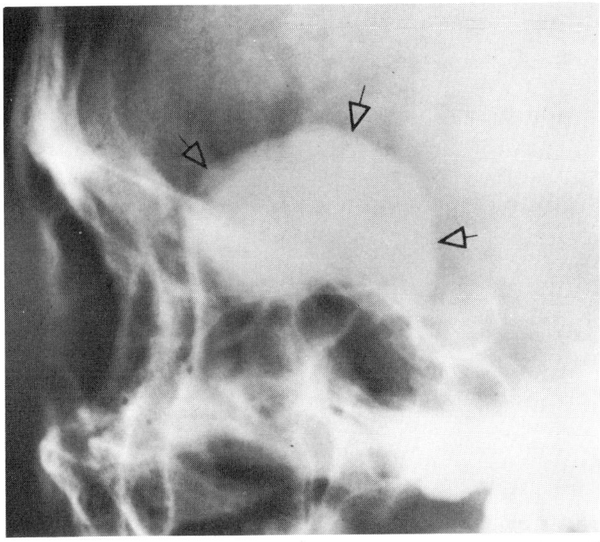

Fig. 18-87. Osteoma of planum. Sharply delineated, well-defined, bony density projects superiorly from planum sphenoidale (arrows).

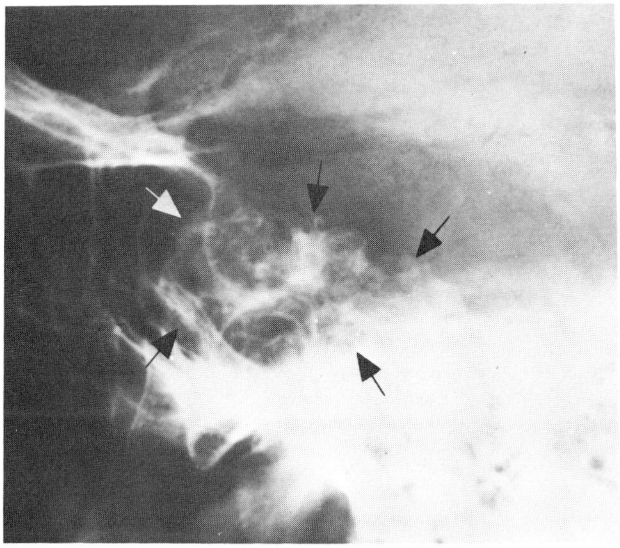

Fig. 18-88. Parasellar chondroma. Lateral roentgenogram of skull shows honeycombed irregular calcification overlying sellar region (arrows). Sella itself is normal.

cation may also be appreciated. Another cause of the parasellar or nasopharyngeal soft-tissue mass is a carotid cavernous fistula (Unger et al., 1969).

Miscellaneous conditions

Infection. Tuberculosis, coccidioidomycosis, or pyogenic abscess may affect the sella. I have seen coccidioidomycosis in one patient in whom the sella was destroyed. A case of aspergillosis of the sella was reported by Wollschlaeger and co-workers in 1970. The sella

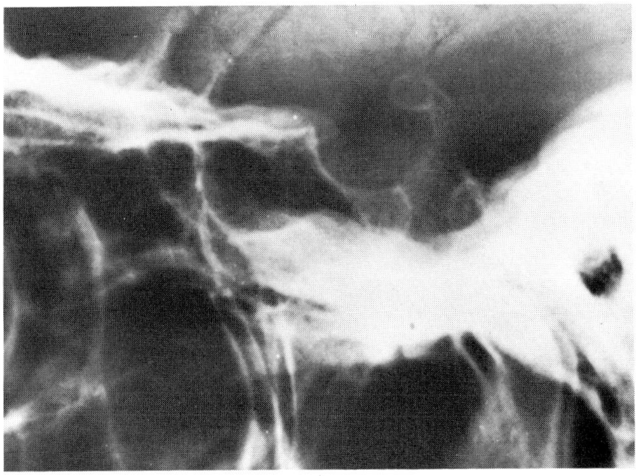

Fig. 18-89. Destruction of lamina dura in posterior part of floor of pituitary fossa. This loss of lamina dura within the cavity of the sella was called category I erosion by du Boulay and El Gammal (1966). In this case (a 52-year-old patient) it was the result of cerebral metastasis.

was of normal size but the floor was demineralized and indistinct. There was no evidence of destruction.

Trauma. Fracture of the sella is indeed rare. Fractures of the dorsum sellae and the floor of the sella were described by Engels (1961) in five patients, and a fracture of the dorsum sellae was reported by Busch (1963). Entrapment of the basilar artery by a fracture of the clivus has been reported by Loop and his collaborators (1964).

SELLA IN RAISED INTRACRANIAL PRESSURE AND HYDROCEPHALUS

George H. du Boulay

The alterations in the sella turcica that result from intracranial pressure and hydrocephalus have been well described. Most of the fundamental observations were contributed by Kornblum and Osmund (1935), Twining (1939), Schüller (1941), Nordmark (1949), Epstein (1951), Lindgren and Di Chiro (1951), and Tönnis and co-workers (1954). Mahmoud (1958) provided helpful necropsy and histologic studies. These various contributions have resulted in detailed descriptions of the following abnormalities.

Changes in sella in increased intracranial pressure

Erosion of sellar cortex. Erosion of the cortical bone that lines the pituitary fossa (Fig. 18-89) is usually seen earliest at the anterior part of the base of the dorsum. The erosion often spreads to involve most of the sellar floor but occasionally is first recognized more anteriorly. Mahmoud (1958) showed that the process is truly an erosion caused by osteoclasts and that the pits produced in the lamina dura (a convenient name for the cortex) tend to coalesce. Consequently the roentgenographic appearance depends not only on the extent and chronicity of the process but also on the optical resolution achieved in the roentgenographic image; it also depends on the positioning of the patient, which may or may not allow a good tangential view of the affected bone.

Further, the appearance may vary with the thickness of the eroded portion of the lamina dura. The cortex overlying cancellous bone is thin, and interruption is seen early. Over the sphenoid sinus the lamina dura, which forms the walls of the sella and sinus, is of double thickness, and detection of erosion is more difficult.

In the earlier stages optimal roentgenograms may reveal pinpoint interruptions of the white line of the lamina dura. However, unless high-definition intensifying screens, a grid of maximum efficiency, and perfect processing have been employed, minute alterations from the normal should be ignored.

As erosion progresses, the roentgenographic appearance becomes more obviously abnormal. The outlines of the sella (i.e., the lamina dura) are described as rubbed out or osteoporotic. Loss of the white line is usually most severe where erosion first began, near the posterior part of the sellar floor. Frequently, however, much more than that area is involved; even the whole sella may be destroyed. The erosion may reach a point at which bony separation between the sphenoid sinus and the soft-tissue contents of the pituitary fossa is no longer detectable.

The lamina dura overlying cancellous bone is perhaps more easily penetrated (Mahmoud, 1958); but comparatively few sellae are extensively encased in cancellous bone except in childhood. When cancellous bone is exposed because of loss of the lamina dura, deep pitting and confluence of pits may become visible eventually on roentgenograms of good quality.

Erosion of the sellar lamina dura is an example of a widespread process easily visible in a particular location. In chronic raised intracranial pressure the process may affect the entire lining of the cranium or any part of it. This fact should be remembered, although it is not discussed here except insofar as the immediately adjacent areas are concerned. The most important of these areas are the planum sphenoidale, the sulcus chiasmaticus, and the tuberculum sellae. The white lines that represent these structures may undergo exactly the same change as the sellar lamina dura. The chronology and significance are described in the succeeding pages.

Erosion of top of dorsum sellae. Erosion of the top of the dorsum sellae (Fig. 18-90) should be distinguished from that of the sellar lining, just described. Destruction of the top of the dorsum includes, moreover, in some instances, loss of those rough elements of bone that are the site of attachment of the petroclinoid ligaments; it is not merely a process centered on the cavity of the sella.

As a result of erosion of the posterior clinoid processes, the dorsum in the lateral view may appear as a truncated cone with a flattened top or as a thin spike. In both cases the upper margins are poorly demarcated unless all that remains is a single flake of bone.

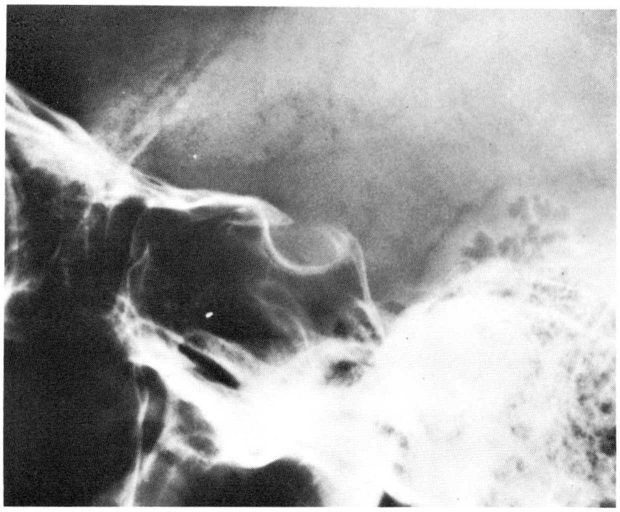

Fig. 18-90. Top of dorsum sellae has lost its clear-cut outline. Category II erosion (du Boulay and El Gammal, 1966) resulted from posterior frontal glioma that caused direct pressure.

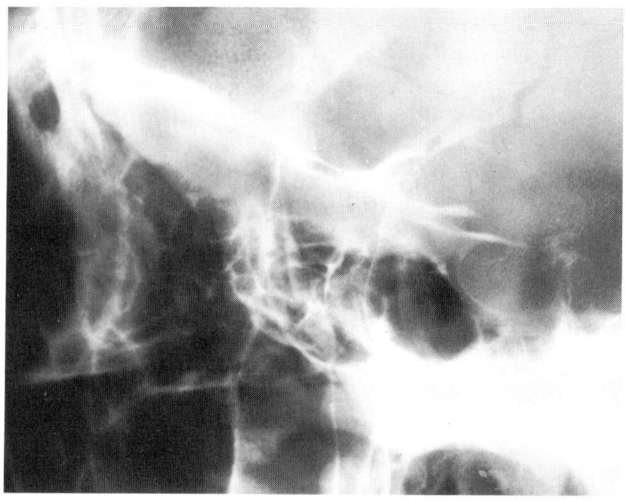

Fig. 18-91. Tentorial meningioma. This lateral oblique view shows how anterior clinoid processes may become thin as a result of raised intracranial pressure over many months.

A thin dorsum sellae eroded in this way under pressure from a dilated third ventricle may be angled anteriorly. With erosion of the sellar floor, near its base, and with sellar enlargement (discussed later), this appearance of forward angulation is even more pronounced.

Changes in anterior clinoid processes. The anterior clinoid processes are affected late and in ways different from those of the posterior (Fig. 18-91). In long-standing hydrocephalus the entire base of the skull may be thin. The anterior fossa may even grow into a more spherical cavity. The anterior clinoid processes are not spared but become thinner and sharper, and in lateral views they may be difficult to recognize. In the postero-anterior inclined projection the anterior clinoid processes and the lesser wings of the sphenoid form frail and indistinct lines.

Local perisellar tumors often produce local and characteristic erosions. Long-standing temporal or frontal lobe tumors may also cause erosion, more on one side of the sella than on the other. Consequently asymmetric thinning of the anterior clinoid processes results. In these cases roentgenograms usually also show abnormalities in the rest of the sella.

Enlargement of sella. Discussions about enlargement of the sella always result in questions regarding the normal size of a sella and sellar measurements. These measurements and their significance are discussed in the preceding sections of this chapter. When the sella enlarges as a result of raised intracranial pressure or hydrocephalus, invariably some erosion or alteration of shape occurs.

In raised intracranial pressure the sella may become enlarged in one of three ways: (1) the lamina dura may be destroyed so completely that it no longer has the strength to withstand intracranial pressure; as a result the sellar floor herniates downward into the sphenoid sinus (Fig. 18-92); (2) coalescence of erosions in cancellous bone, particularly at the base of the dorsum sellae, may cause the cavity of the sella to extend downward into the clivus; this extension may be appreciated in histologic sections but the cavity does not reach sufficient size to be recognized easily on roentgenograms; (3) enlargement may take place by less dramatic stages in long-standing conditions. Erosion is not a feature; but growth under abnormal stimuli causes a peculiar shape of the sella. The commonest of these peculiarities is seen sufficiently often to be considered characteristic of chronic obstructive (noncommunicating) hydrocephalus (Fig. 18-93). It is not a true enlargement of the sellar cavity itself. The dorsum is short, indeed sometimes extremely so. The longest axis of the sella turcica in the lateral view is more or less in line with the clivus. The reason for this appearance is that the anterior sellar wall is elongated upward into the chiasmatic sulcus, which itself is enlarged. The general line of the anterior wall and the chiasmatic sulcus forms an angle with the planum sphenoidale of 270° or more. Commonly the anterior clinoid processes, presumably because of unusual torsion on their ligaments, are blunt and massive. The upper cavity, limited anteriorly by the chiasmatic sulcus, is occupied

A

B

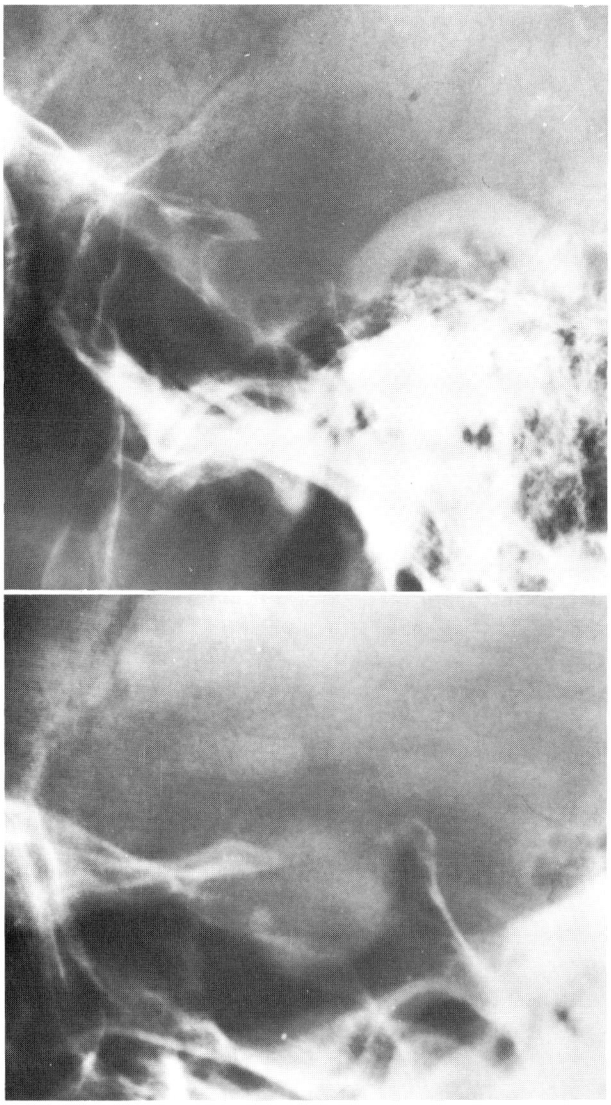

Fig. 18-92. A, Same tumor as in Fig. 18-90, 6 months later. Frontal glioma has extended considerably. Dorsum sellae is greatly damaged, and entire lamina dura of sella has been destroyed. Planum sphenoidale has also been eroded. This combination of erosions (category III) has resulted in herniation of whole region downward into sphenoid sinus (i.e., enlargement of the sella). **B,** Similar situation in another patient (with frontal oligodendroglioma). Top of dorsum sellae is only slightly affected.

A

B

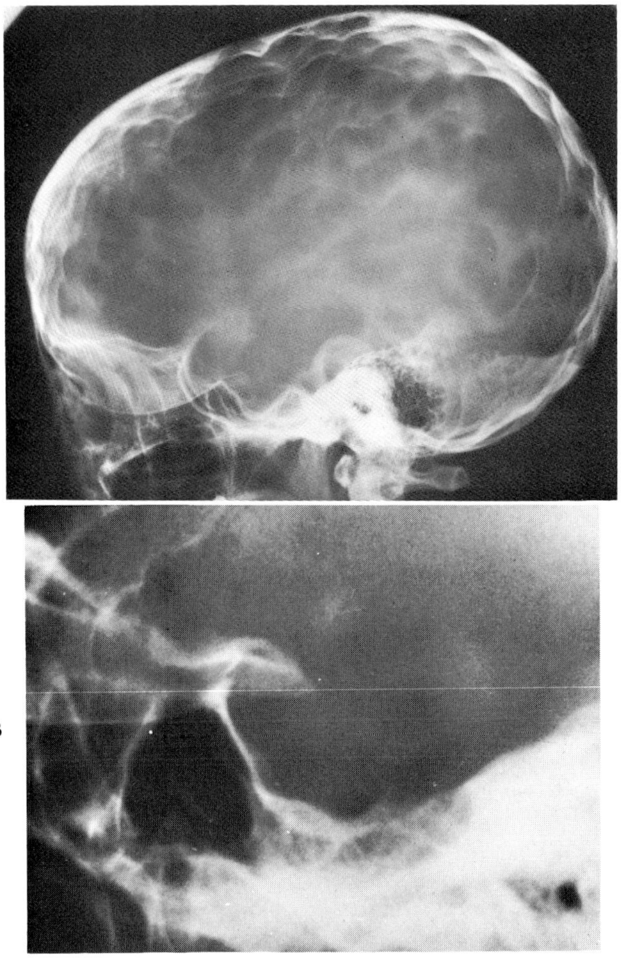

Fig. 18-93. A, Aqueduct stenosis. Extreme erosion of dorsum sellae. Sulcus chiasmaticus is large and vertical and appears to form part of pituitary fossa. Lamina dura is intact. Note the large anterior clinoid processes. The skull is expanded, the floor of the anterior fossa is depressed, convolutional markings are increased, and transverse sinuses are low. **B,** Similar sella. In this patient, it is the result of hydrocephalus caused by slow-growing quadrigeminal plate tumor. Note that the upper half of what appears to be the anterior wall of the sella is in reality the sulcus chiasmaticus.

by the dilated third ventricle. The cortex is often well formed and without erosions.

Those familiar with the literature will realize that what has just been described is sometimes called a J sella. The term J sella, however, is also commonly used to describe a different appearance, which may be associated with glioma of the optic chiasm. The term was erroneously attributed to Martin and Cushing (1923), and it has often been used synonymously with "omega" sella (a more suitable description of the sella of optic chiasmal glioma). Another inaccurate designation, "slipper" sella, describes a normal appearance in infancy and also the exaggerated appearance in an expanded skull in hydrocephalus. Because these inadequate descriptive names have caused so much confusion, the *J sella* should be dropped, as Kier (1968) also suggested. The shape of the sella described previously in this section, however, is seen in 50% of cases of aqueduct stenosis after infancy (du Boulay and Trickey, 1970).

The main confusion about the so-called J sella was introduced by those authors who thought that the double concavity of the anterior wall was its main feature.

Significance of these abnormalities

The significance of some of the described abnormalities is based on analyses by du Boulay (1957, 1965, 1969), by Fry and du Boulay (1965), by du Boulay and El Gammal (1966), and by du Boulay and Trickey (1967, 1970).

Pressure changes of some sort may be noted in about one third of patients with tumors distant from the sella. Of these, 20% do not have papilledema. In this 20% are many who, despite short clinical histories and the absence of other signs of raised intracranial pressure, have long-standing and operable tumors.

The earliest detectable abnormality is usually a loss of the lamina dura. Under ideal circumstances this loss is occasionally detected within a few weeks after the onset of raised pressure (Tönnis et al., 1954; du Boulay and El Gammal, 1966).

Erosion of lamina dura. As an isolated sign, without any other abnormality of the sella turcica, erosion of the lamina dura (Figs. 18-89 and 18-92) was found in about 12% of intracranial tumors (category I erosion, du Boulay and El Gammal, 1966). Whether the tumor was above or below the tentorium made no difference.

In about twice this number of patients with either infra- or supratentorial tumors, erosion of the lamina dura and some additional sellar abnormality were seen. Such erosion occurs in many cases of aqueduct stenosis, but virtually never in communicating hydrocephalus.

Erosion of top and back of dorsum sellae. Tumors of the posterior fossa cause erosion of the top and back of the dorsum sellae (category II erosion, du Boulay and El Gammal, 1966) (Fig. 18-90) about twice as often as do supratentorial tumors. Even so, however, only 10% of posterior fossa tumors are associated with such erosion. In patients with supratentorial tumors, category II change is usually associated with other sellar abnormalities, particularly an extensive erosion of the lamina dura. With hydrocephalus resulting from infratentorial masses, it may be seen alone, however. Still more commonly this type of erosion results from a suprasellar tumor.

Erosion of planum sphenoidale. After many months of raised intracranial pressure, erosion of the lamina dura may have extended to the planum sphenoidale (Fig. 18-92). The usually crisp white line of that structure blurs or disappears. Nearly always before this disappearance, the top of the dorsum sellae has also been damaged. The combination of erosion of the top of the dorsum sellae, of the lamina dura, and of the planum sphenoidale (category III sellar change, du Boulay and El Gammal, 1966) is nearly always caused by a slow-growing frontal or posterior frontal tumor. Often this tumor is a glioma, sometimes a meningioma.

I have also seen this combined erosion in one patient with chronic frontal subdural hematoma. Few posterior fossa masses are capable of producing such a degree of bone destruction, although it has occasionally been observed with tentorial meningiomas. With frontal tumors, however, that erode the top of the dorsum sellae, the planum sphenoidale is damaged in almost half the cases.

Differential diagnosis from pituitary tumors

Destruction of the cortical lining of the pituitary fossa may also accompany the growth of tumors, particularly pituitary tumors, within the sella. After thorough examination of the plain roentgenograms of the skull, only about 3% of all pituitary tumors cause confusion regarding diagnosis. The majority of the plain roentgenograms present fairly obvious evidence of the true nature of the tumor.

Ballooning of the pituitary fossa is the most common of the additional and specific signs in pituitary adenoma (Fig. 18-35). Sclerosis of bone betrays a meningioma or occasionally a chordoma. Rarely gliomas of the optic chiasm cause a characteristic excavation in the anterior part of the sellar region (Fig. 18-59). Craniopharyngioma is usually suprasellar and retrosellar. Although a fair number of these tumors protrude into the cavity of the pituitary fossa as well, half of all craniopharyngiomas cause a shortened and extremely flat dorsum. The cortical top of the dorsum in these cases is usually preserved. The abnormality may therefore be distinguished from that caused by frontal tumors and from those producing hydrocephalus.

Differentiation between the changes of pressure in adults and the effect of local tumor and disease is more difficult in the following circumstances: (1) when there is apparently complete destruction of the dorsum sellae; in these situations one should search for displacement of fragments, away from the cavity of the sella (intrasellar tumor), or toward it (hydrocephalus and craniopharyngioma); (2) when, occasionally, erosion of the lamina dura by pituitary adenoma is accompanied by enlargement of the sella, which nevertheless is not characteristically ballooned in shape; (3) rarely, when metastatic carcinoma has spread from the pituitary fossa or the suprasellar region; destruction, or at least an obvious change in texture, extends more deeply into the bone than is the case with raised intracranial pressure; (4) when the lesion, usually an aneurysm of the internal carotid, is truly parasellar; in these situations the lateral roentgenogram may suggest at first glance an enlargement and osteoporosis. Careful examination of all views reveals the true state. A faint but sharply outlined dorsum (of which as much as one lateral half may be missing), destruction of one lateral half of the sellar floor, and destruction usually of an anterior clinoid process are all visible.

Changes in sella in childhood

Much that has been said applies equally to the sella in children. The lamina dura is eroded in similar situations and after a similar length of time. It may be overlooked because diastasis of the sutures attracts the attention of the radiologist. Destruction of the top of the dorsum results particularly from tumors of the posterior fossa that cause hydrocephalus. Rarely destruction may be seen as a result of long-standing frontal and frontoparietal masses that push the base of the brain against the base of the skull.

In children, however, opportunities for the more chronic sellar changes are fewer. Moreover, slow-growing frontal tumors, which in adults cause many of the most severely damaged sellae, are exceptional before the age of 30. Consequently *chronic* sellar changes in children tend to be restricted to those suffering from developmental abnormalities, especially aqueduct stenosis. In infancy, changes resulting from communicating hydrocephalus are confined to a simple elongation of the sella, which may accompany a general expansion of the head.

Changes in sella with relief of raised intracranial pressure

Roentgenograms obtained after excision of cerebral tumors and after operative procedures for the relief of hydrocephalus have been studied. These indicated that osteoclastic resorption ceases rapidly and is replaced by increased new bone formation. Within a few weeks the lamina dura reappeared and some evidence of repair of the dorsum sellae and posterior clinoid processes was seen (Fig. 18-94). The fact that bone (e.g., the posterior clinoid processes) should reappear, must mean that some periosteal or osteoid tissue had not been destroyed entirely. Total destruction and displacement, however, cannot be corrected, so the reformed bone in advanced cases is abnormal in shape. The dorsum may be short, or the cavity of the sella enlarged.

From observation of patients with recurrent symptoms, the susceptibility to erosion of the reformed lamina dura appears to be much less than that of the original bone lining. A second episode of raised intracranial pressure rarely causes erosion.

These documented observations of recovery probably illustrate the physiologic processes at work in *arrested*

A

B

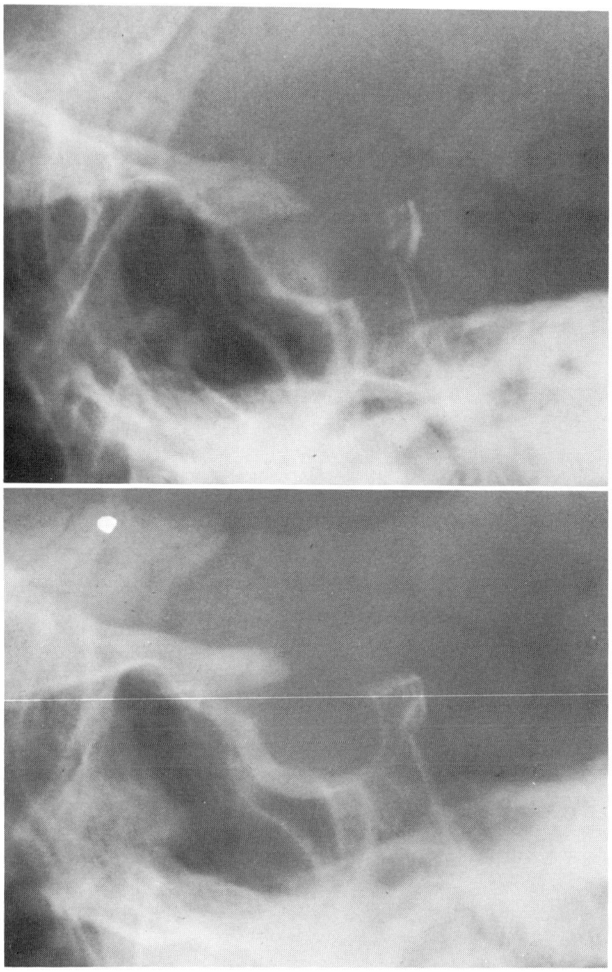

Fig. 18-94. A, Frontal glioma with category I and category II erosions. **B,** Same case 3 months later, after partial excision of the tumor. Lamina dura and cortex at top of dorsum sellae have both reappeared. Top of dorsum sellae, however, is abnormally flat.

noncommunicating hydrocephalus. They may explain why the sella, although abnormal in shape, sometimes has a strikingly thick cortex.

Just as sellar erosion is a particular example of the effect of pressure on the whole inner table of the skull, so are the corrective processes that lead to thickening. Roentgenograms of the calvarium often show similar new bone formation.

REFERENCES

Albert, M., and LeMay, M.: Demineralisation of the dorsum sellae associated with alcoholism, Brit. J. Radiol. **41:**331-332, 1968.

Bakay, L.: Results of 300 pituitary adenoma operations, J. Neurosurg. **7:**240-255, 1950.

Barnett, D. J.: Radiologic aspects of craniopharyngiomas, Radiology **72:**14-18, 1959.

Bergland, R. M., Ray, B. S., and Torack, R. M.: Anatomical variations in the pituitary gland and adjacent structures in 225 human autopsy cases, J. Neurosurg. **28:**93-99, 1968.

Berkmen, Y. M., and Blatt, E. S.: Cranial and intracranial cartilaginous tumours, Clin. Radiol. **19:**327-333, 1968.

Bower, B. F.: Pituitary enlargement secondary to untreated primary hypogonadism, Ann. Intern. Med. **69:**107-109, 1968.

Brisman, R., Hughes, J. E. O., and Mount, L. A.: Cerebrospinal fluid rhinorrhea and empty sella, J. Neurosurg. **31:**538-543, 1969.

Bull, J.: The normal variations in the position of the optic recess of the third ventricle, Acta Radiol. **46:**72-80, 1956.

Burrows, E. H.: So-called J-sella, Brit. J. Radiol. **37:**661-669, 1964.

Busch, G.: Fraktur der Sella turcica, Fortschr. Roentgenstr. **99:**420-421, 1963.

Busch, W.: Die Morphologie der Sella turcica und ihre Beziehungen zur Hypophyse, Arch. Path. Anat. **320:**437-458, 1951.

Calkins, R. A., Pribram, H. F. W., and Joynt, R. J.: Intrasellar arachnoid diverticulum. A case report, Neurology **18:**1037-1040, 1968.

Camp, J. D.: Normal and pathological anatomy of sella turcica as revealed by roentgenograms, Amer. J. Roentgen. **12:**143-156, 1924.

Caplan, R. H., and Dobben, G. D.: Endocrine studies in patients with the "empty sella syndrome," Arch. Intern. Med. **123:** 611-619, 1969.

Caughey, J. E.: Bone changes in the skull in dystrophia myotonica, J. Bone Joint Surg. **34B:**343-351, 1952.

Chynn, K. Y.: Neuroradiologic exploration in intra- and parasellar conditions, Radiol. Clin. N. Amer. **4:**93-116, 1966.

Cushing, H.: The chiasmal syndrome of primary optic atrophy and bitemporal field defects in adult patients with a normal sella turcica, Trans. XIII Concilium Ophthalmologicum Hollandia **3:**97-184, 1929.

Cushing, H.: Basophilic adenomas of pituitary body, their clinical manifestations (pituitary basophilism), Bull. Johns Hopkins Hosp. **50:**137-195, 1932.

Cushing, H., and Eisenhardt, L.: Meningiomas, Springfield, Ill., 1938, Charles C Thomas, Publisher.

Davidoff, L. M., and Epstein, B. S.: The abnormal pneumoencephalogram, Philadelphia, 1950, Lea & Febiger.

Deery, E. M.: Note on calcification in pituitary adenomas, Endocrinology **13:**455-458, 1929.

Di Chiro, G.: The width (third dimension) of the sella turcica, Amer. J. Roentgen. **84:** 26-37, 1960.

Di Chiro, G., and Nelson, K. B.: The volume of the sella turcica, Amer. J. Roentgen. **87:**989-1008, 1962.

du Boulay, G. H.: The radiological evidence of raised intracranial pressure in children, Brit. J. Radiol. **30:**375-377, 1957.

du Boulay, G. H.: Principles of x-ray diagnosis of the skull, London, 1965, Butterworth & Co., Ltd.

du Boulay, G. H.: In Shanks, S. C., and Kerley, P., editors: A text-book of x-ray diagnosis, by British authors, ed. 4, London, 1969, H. K. Lewis & Co., Ltd., vol. 1.

du Boulay, G. H.: Personal communication, 1970.

du Boulay, G. H., and El Gammal, T.: Classification, clinical value, and mechanism of sella turcica changes in raised intracranial pressure, Brit. J. Radiol. **39:**422-442, 1966.

du Boulay, G. H., and Trickey, S. E.: Case reports: calcification in chromophobe adenoma, Brit. J. Radiol. **35:**793-795, 1962.

du Boulay, G. H., and Trickey, S. E.: The choice of radiological investigation in the management of tumors around the sella, Clin. Radiol. **18**:349-365, 1967.

du Boulay, G. H., and Trickey, S. E.: The sella in aqueduct stenosis and communicating hydrocephalus, Brit. J. Radiol. **43**:319-326, 1970.

Dussault, J., Plamondon, C., and Volpe, R.: Aneurysms of the internal carotid artery simulating pituitary tumours, Canad. Med. Ass. J. **101**:785-790, 1969.

Engels, E.: The roentgen appearance of the carotid sulcus of the sphenoid bone, Acta Radiol. **49**:113-116, 1958.

Engels, E.: Basal skull fractures involving the sella turcica, Clin. Radiol. **12**:177-178, 1961.

Epstein, B. S.: Shortening of the posterior wall of the sella turcica caused by dilatation of the third ventricle or certain suprasellar tumors, Amer. J. Roentgen. **65**:49-55, 1951.

Evans, R. A., Schwartz, J. F., and Chutorian, A. M.: Radiologic diagnosis in pediatric ophthalmology, Radiol. Clin. N. Amer. **1**:459-495, 1963.

Fathie, K.: Large aneurysm of internal carotid artery simulating an eosinophilic adenoma, J. Iowa Med. Soc. **55**:246-249, 1965.

Ferrier, P. E., and Stone, E. F., Jr.: Familial pituitary dwarfism associated with an abnormal sella turcica, Pediatrics **43**:858-865, 1969.

Fisher, R. L., and Di Chiro, G. H.: The small sella turcica, Amer. J. Roentgen. **91**:996-1008, 1964.

Frazier, C. H.: Series of pituitary pictures. Commentaries on pathologic, clinical and therapeutic aspects, Arch. Neurol. Psychiat. **23**:656-695, 1930.

Fry, K. I., and du Boulay, G. H.: Some observations on the sella in old age and arterial hypertension, Brit. J. Radiol. **38**:16-22, 1965.

Gabriele, O. F.: The empty sella syndrome, Amer. J. Roentgen. **104**:168-170, 1968.

Geissinger, J. D., Siqueira, E. B., and Ross, E. R.: Giant cell tumors of the sphenoid bone, J. Neurosurg. **32**:665-670, 1970.

Grundy, L., Goree, J. A., and Jimenez, J. P.: Oxycephaly in the adult simulating pituitary tumor. Clinical and roentgenologic manifestations, Amer. J. Roentgen. **108**:762-766, 1970.

Hadden, D. R., and Alexander, F.: Adult cretinism with lingual thyroid and pituitary fossa enlargement, Proc. Roy. Soc. Med. **61**:655-656, 1968.

Hamby, W. B.: Spongioblastoma bipolare in region of hypothalamus associated with infantilism and without dwarfism, Arch. Neurol. Psychiat. **31**:1258-1265, 1934.

Hare, H. F., Silveus, E., and Smedal, M. I.: Roentgenologic diagnosis of pituitary tumors, Radiology **52**:193-198, 1941.

Harlin, R. S., and Givens, J. R.: Sheehan's syndrome associated with eclampsia and a small sella turcica, Southern Med. J. **61**:909-911, 1968.

Heuer, G. J., and Dandy, W. E.: Roentgenography in the localization of brain tumor, Bull. Johns Hopkins Hosp. **27**:311-322, 1916.

Hilton, G. F., and Hoyt, W. F.: An arteriosclerotic chiasmal syndrome, J.A.M.A. **196**:1018-1020, 1966.

Holman, C. B.: Roentgenologic manifestations of glioma of optic nerve and chiasm, Amer. J. Roentgen. **82**:462-471, 1959.

Holman, C. B., and Miller, W. E.: Juvenile nasopharyngeal fibroma—roentgenologic characteristics, Amer. J. Roentgen. **94**:292-298, 1965.

Holman, C. B., Olive, I., and Svien, H. J.: Roentgenologic features of neurofibromas involving the gasserian ganglion, Amer. J. Roentgen. **86**:148-153, 1961.

Holmes, G. W., and Robbins, L. L.: Roentgen interpretation, ed. 6, Philadelphia, 1955, Lea & Febiger.

Hubble, D.: Diagnosis of hypopituitarism in childhood, Arch. Dis. Child. **42**:228-231, 1967.

Isherwood, I., and Mawdsley, C.: Familial aspects of radiologic changes in dystrophia myotonica, Acta Radiol. **1**:110-117, 1963.

Israel, H.: Continuing growth in sella turcica with age, Amer. J. Roentgen. **108**:516-527, 1970.

Jefferson, A.: Hypertensive cerebral vascular disease and intracranial tumour; a study in diagnosis, Quart. J. Med. **24**:245-268, 1955.

Jefferson, G.: Extrasellar extensions of pituitary adenomas; president's address, Proc. Roy. Soc. Med. **33**:433-458, 1940.

Kaufman, B.: The "empty" sella turcica—manifestation of the intrasellar subarachnoid space, Radiology **90**:931-941, 1968.

Kaufman, B., Sandstrom, P. H., and Young, H. F.: Alteration in size and configuration of the sella turcica as the result of prolonged cerebrospinal fluid shunting, Radiology **97**:537-542, 1970.

Kaufman, H. H.: Nontraumatic cerebrospinal fluid rhinorrhea, Arch. Neurol. **21**:59-65, 1969.

Kier, E. L.: The infantile sella turcica. New roentgenologic and anatomic concepts based on a developmental study of the sphenoid bone, Amer. J. Roentgen. **102**:747-767, 1968.

Kier, E. L.: "J" and "omega" shape of sella turcica; anatomic clarification of radiologic misconceptions, Acta Radiol. **9**:91-94, 1969.

Kornblum, K.: Alterations in structure of sella turcica as revealed by roentgen ray, Arch. Neurol. Psychiat. **27**:305-321, 1932.

Kornblum, K., and Osmund, L. H.: Effect of intracranial tumors on the sella turcica. An analysis of 446 cases of verified intracranial tumor, Arch. Neurol. Psychiat. **34**:111-123, 1935.

Kroe, D. J., Hudgins, W. R., Simmons, J. C. H., and Blackwell, C. F.: Primary intrasellar leiomyoma, J. Neurosurg. **29**:189-191, 1968.

Kruyff, E., and Munn, J. D.: Posterior fossa tumors in infants and children, Amer. J. Roentgen. **89**:951-965, 1963.

Lamb, J., and Morris, L.: Carotid-basilar artery: report and discussion of five cases, Clin. Radiol. **12**:179-186, 1961.

Laschi, G.: Un caso di foramen dorsi sellae, Radiol. Med. **18**:707-712, 1931.

Lee, W. M., and Adams, J. E.: The empty sella syndrome, J. Neurosurg. **28**:351-356, 1968.

Leeds, N., and Seaman, W. B.: Fibrous dysplasia of the skull and its differential diagnosis, Radiology **78**:570-582, 1962.

Lindgren, E., and Di Chiro, G.: Suprasellar tumours with calcifications, Acta Radiol. **36**:173-195, 1951.

Lodge, S. D., Walker, G. F., and Stewart, M. J.: Aneurysm of the left internal carotid artery simulating pituitary tumour, Brit. Med. J. **2**:1179-1180, 1927.

Loop, J. W., White, L. E., and Shaw, C. M.: Traumatic occlusion of the basilar artery within a clivus fracture, Radiology **83**:36-40, 1964.

Lowman, R. M., Robinson, F., and McAllister, W. B.: Craniopharyngeal canal, Acta Radiol. [Diagn.] **5**:41-54, 1966.

Lundberg, P. O., and Gemzell, C.: Dysplasia of the sella turcica: clinical and laboratory investigations in three cases, Acta Endocrinol. **52**:478-488, 1966.

Mahmoud, M. S.: The sella in health and disease: value of the radiographic study of the sella turcica in morbid anatomical and topographic diagnosis of intracranial tumours, Brit. J. Radiol., supp. 8, pp. 1-100, 1958.

Martin, P., and Cushing, H.: Primary gliomas of chiasm and optic nerves in their intracranial portion, Arch. Ophthal. **52**:209-241, 1923.

McKenzie, K. G., and Sosman, M. C.: The roentgenological diagnosis of craniopharyngeal pouch tumors, Amer. J. Roentgen. **11**:171-176, 1924.

McLachlan, M. S. F., Williams, E. D., Fortt, R. W., and Doyle, F. H.: Estimation of pituitary gland dimensions from radiographs of the sella turcica, Brit. J. Radiol. **41**:323-330, 1968.

Meador, C. K., and Worrell, J. L.: The sella turcica in postpartum pituitary necrosis (Sheehan's syndrome), Ann. Intern. Med. **65**:259-264, 1966.

Middlemass, I. B. D.: Bone changes in adult cretins, Brit. J. Radiol. **32**:685-688, 1959.

Minagi, H., and Newton, T. H.: Cartilaginous tumors of the base of the skull, Amer. J. Roentgen. **105**:308-313, 1969.

Minagi, H., and Steinbach, H. L.: Roentgen aspects of pituitary tumors manifested after bilateral adrenalectomy for Cushing's syndrome, Radiology **90**:276-280, 1968.

Mitchell, S. W.: Aneurysm of an anomalous artery causing antero-posterior division of the chiasm of the optic nerves and producing bitemporal hemianopsia, Trans. Amer. Neurol. Ass., pp. 239-251, 1968.

Mogensen, E. F.: Chromophobe adenoma of the pituitary gland; a follow-up study on 60 surgical patients with special reference to endocrine disturbances, Acta Endocr. **24**:135-152, 1957.

Mortara, R., and Norrell, H.: Consequences of a deficient sellar diaphragm, J. Neurosurg. **32**:565-573, 1970.

Nelson, D. H., Meakin, J. W., Dealy, J. B., Jr., Matson, D. D., Emerson, K., Jr., and Thorn, G. W.: ACTH-producing tumor of the pituitary gland, New Eng. J. Med. **259**:161-164, 1958.

Nelson, D. H., Meakin, J. W., and Thorn, G. W.: ACTH-producing pituitary tumors following adrenalectomy for Cushing's syndrome, Ann. Intern. Med. **52**:560-569, 1960.

Neuhauser, E. B. D., Griscom, N. T., Gilles, F. H., and Crocker, A. C.: Arachnoid cysts in the Hurler-Hunter syndrome (Kystes arachnoidiens dans le syndrome de Hurler-Hunter), Ann. Radiol. **11**:453-469, 1968. (Société Europaenne de Radiologie Pediatrique, Basel, April, 1967.)

Newton, T. H., Burhenne, H. J., and Palubinskas, A. J.: Primary carcinoma of the pituitary, Amer. J. Roentgen. **87**: 110-120, 1962.

Nièpce, B.: Enlarged sella due to cretinism (hypothyroidism). Traité du goître et du crétinisme, Paris, 1851, J. B. Ballière.

Nordmark, B.: Pressure changes in the sella turcica in the presence of glioma in the cerebral hemispheres, Acta Radiol. **32**:461-467, 1949.

Nugent, G. R., Sprinkle, P., and Bloor, B. M.: Sphenoid sinus mucoceles, J. Neurosurg. **32**:443-451, 1970.

Oon, C. L.: The size of the pituitary fossa in adults, Brit. J. Radiol. **36**:294-299, 1963.

Pollock, J. A., Newton, T. H., and Hoyt, W. F.: Transsphenoidal and transethmoidal encephaloceles: a review of clinical and roentgen features in 8 cases, Radiology **90**:442-453, 1968.

Pribram, H. F. W., and Swann, G. F.: The radiological changes and clinical incidence of endocrine effects in sellar and parasellar tumours, Radiology **75**:877-884, 1960.

Riach, I. C. F.: The pituitary fossa in childhood with particular reference to hypopituitarism, Brit. J. Radiol. **39**:241-248, 1966.

Ring, B. A., and Waddington, M.: Primary arachnoid cysts of the sella turcica, Amer. J. Roentgen. **98**:611-615, 1966.

Rischbieth, R. H. C., and Bull, J. W. D.: Significance of enlargement of superior orbital (sphenoidal) fissure, Brit. J. Radiol. **31**:125-135, 1958.

Salassa, R. M., Kearns, T. P., Kernohan, J. W., Sprague, R. G., and MacCarty, C. S.: Pituitary tumors in patients with Cushing's syndrome, J. Clin. Endocr. **19**:1523-1539, 1959.

Sansregret, A., Ledoux, R., Duplantis, F., Lamoureux, C., Chapdelaine, A., and Leblanc, P.: Suprasellar subarachnoid cysts —radioclinical features, Amer. J. Roentgen. **105**:291-297, 1969.

Schaeffer, J. P.: Some points in regional anatomy of optic pathway with especial reference to tumors of hypophysis cerebri and resulting ocular changes, Anat. Rec. **28**:243-279, 1924.

Scheuermann, H.: The roentgenological picture of the normal and the pathological sella turcica, Acta Radiol. **13**:404-432, 1932.

Schneider, R. C., Kriss, F. C., and Falls, H. F.: Prechiasmal infarction associated with intrachiasmal and suprasellar tumors, J. Neurosurg. **32**:197-208, 1970.

Schüller, A.: X-ray symptoms of intracranial hypertension, Confin. Neurol. **3**:253-256, 1941.

Silverman, F. N.: Roentgen standards for size of the pituitary fossa from infancy through adolescence, Amer. J. Roentgen. **78**:451-460, 1957.

Sosman, M. C., and Vogt, E. C.: Aneurysms of the internal carotid artery and the circle of Willis, from a roentgenological viewpoint, Amer. J. Roentgen. **15**:122-134, 1926.

Steinbach, H. L., Noetzei, M., and Ozonoff, M. B.: Small pituitary fossa in Cushing's syndrome due to adrenal neoplasm, New Eng. J. Med. **269**:1286-1289, 1963.

Steinbach, H. L., and Russell, W.: Measurement of the heel pad as an aid to diagnosis of acromegaly, Radiology **82**: 418-423, 1964.

Taveras, J. M., and Wood, E. H.: Diagnostic neuroradiology, Baltimore, 1964, The Williams & Wilkins Co.

Tönnis, W., Schiefer, W., and Rausch, F. J.: Sellaveränderungen bei gesteigerten Schädelinnendruck, Deutsch. Z. Nervenheilk. **171**:351-369, 1954.

Twining, E. W.: In Shanks, S. C., Kerley, P., and Twining, E. W., editors: A text-book of x-ray diagnosis. By British authors, London, 1939, H. K. Lewis & Co., Ltd.

Unger, J. D., Unger, G. F., and Nora, D.: Carotid cavernous fistula presenting as a nasopharyngeal mass, Amer. J. Roentgen. **106**:376-380, 1969.

Walsh, F. B., and Hoyt, W. F.: Clinical neuro-ophthalmology, ed. 3, Baltimore, 1969, The Williams & Wilkins Co.

Wells, H. G.: Intracranial aneurysm of the vertebral artery, Arch. Neurol. Psychiat. **7**:311-320, 1922.

Wermer, P.: Genetic aspects of adenomatosis of endocrine glands, Amer. J. Med. **16**:363-371, 1954.

Wermer, P.: Endocrine adenomatosis and peptic ulcer in a large kindred, Amer. J. Med. **35**:205-212, 1963.

White, J., and Ballantine, H. T., Jr.: Intrasellar aneurysms simulating hypophyseal tumours, J. Neurosurg. **18**:34-50, 1961.

Wilson, G. H., and Hanafee, W. N.: Angiographic findings in 16 patients with juvenile nasopharyngeal angiofibroma, Radiology **92**:279-284, 1969.

Wislocki, G. B.: The meningeal relations of the hypophysis cerebri. II. An embryological study of the meninges and blood vessels of the human hypophysis, Amer. J. Anat. **61**: 95-130, 1937.

Wollschlaeger, G., Wollschlaeger, P. B., Lopez, V. F., and Zemel, H. J.: A rare cause of occlusion of the internal carotid artery, Neuroradiology **1**:32-38, 1970.

Wood, E. H., and Himadi, G. M.: Chordomas: a roentgenological study of 16 cases previously unreported, Radiology **54**:706-716, 1950.

Wren, M. W. G.: Significance of the so-called J-shaped sella in the diagnosis of intracranial aneurysm, Brit. J. Ophthal. **53**:307-309, 1969.

Zatz, L. M., Janon, E. A., and Newton, T. H.: The enlarged sella and the intrasellar cistern, Radiology **93**:1085-1091, 1969.

Zollinger, R., and Cutler, E. C.: Aneurysm of the internal carotid artery. Report of a case simulating tumor of the pituitary, Arch. Neurol. Psychiat. **30**:607-611, 1933.

CHAPTER 19

Temporal bone

David O. Davis and Calvin L. Rumbaugh

NORMAL FEATURES

Gross and roentgenographic anatomy

General relationships

The temporal bone consists of four components: squamous, petrous, mastoid, and tympanic. It has two major processes: the zygomatic, which articulates with the zygoma to form the malar arch, and the styloid, to which several muscles and ligaments are attached.

Squamous portion. The squamous segment is a thin sheet of bone resembling a sail. It extends superiorly to form the lateral part of the main temporal bone mass (Fig. 19-1) and is part of the calvarium; it will not be described in detail here.

Petrous portion. The petrous portion is a wedge-shaped bone that extends forward and medially. Its apex is closely apposed to the clivus and is therefore in proximity to the dorsum sellae and cavernous sinus (Figs. 19-1 and 19-2). The base of the petrous portion is fused with the internal surfaces of the squamous and mastoid portions. Anterolaterally it is related to the sphenoid bone and posteromedially to the occipital bone.

Surfaces. The petrous temporal bone has three surfaces: superior, posterior and inferior (Fig. 19-1).

The superior surface forms the posterior part of the floor of the middle cranial fossa. The inferomedial portion of the superior surface lies above the carotid canal. A minor depression on the anterior surface slightly lateral to the apex contains the trigeminal ganglion. Another slight depression related to the internal auditory canal and cochlea lies slightly lateral to the trigeminal impression and is separated from it by an irregular ridge. The arcuate eminence, a slight elevation caused by the underlying superior semicircular canal, lies on the lateral aspect of the superior surface. The tegmen tympani, the thin roof of the tympanic antrum, forms the most lateral portion of the superior surface of the petrous temporal bone. It is located between the arcuate eminence and the squamous portion of the temporal bone (Figs. 19-1, *B,* and 19-3, *B*).

The posterior surface of the petrous temporal bone is vertical and forms the anterior wall of the posterior cranial fossa (Figs. 19-1, *B,* and 19-2). The opening of the internal auditory canal (porus acusticus internus) lies midway between the medial apex and the lateral base (Fig. 19-1, *B*). The deep transverse sinus groove forms the lateral boundary of the posterior surface (Fig. 19-3, *E* and *F*). The opening for the vestibular aqueduct, which transmits the endolymphatic duct, lies approximately midway between the internal auditory meatus and the sinus groove (Figs. 19-1, *B,* and 19-2).

The inferior or basal surface, a part of the skull base, is very irregular. The inferior opening of the carotid canal is seen as a large almost circular aperture in the central portion of this surface. The carotid canal initially extends vertically upward and then turns sharply forward and medially to reach the apex of the petrous temporal bone (Fig. 19-1, *C*). The levator palati and the cartilaginous portion of the eustachian tube lie between the carotid canal opening and the apex

We would like to thank Wilson J. Sesana, M.D., and Ben Senturia, M.D., for their help and support; Gail Cissna and Norman Hente, R. T., for photographic assistance; and Mrs. Connie Staples, for typing the manuscript.

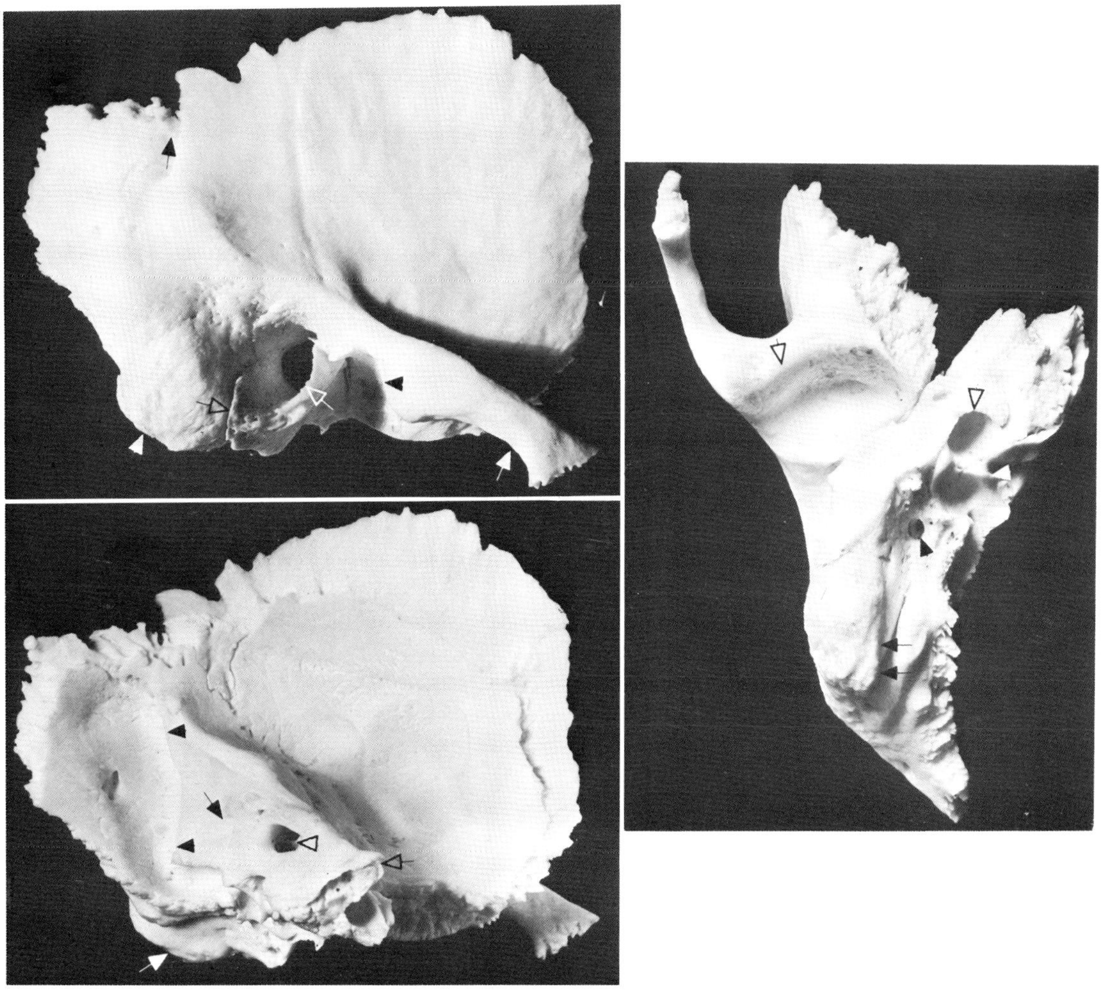

Fig. 19-1. Photographs of a disarticulated temporal bone. **A,** Lateral aspect. Mastoid, tympanic, and squamous portions of the temporal bone are shown on this projection. Petrous portion, extending medially, is hidden. Squamosa, the flat upper portion of the temporal bone, has a smooth surface crossed by a prominent vertical vascular groove. Notch (solid black arrow) for downward projection of the articular surface of the parietal bone indents the superior margin of the bone. Zygomatic process (solid white arrow) curves laterally and anteriorly. Mandibular fossa (black arrowhead) lies immediately in front of the anterior margin of the external auditory canal (open white arrow). Tympanomastoid suture is indicated by open black arrow; tip of mastoid process by white arrowhead. Styloid process is absent. **B,** Medial aspect of the squamosa is slightly roughened by vascular channels. Long free superior margin represents beveled edge of the temporal side of the squamosal suture. Zygomatic process extends anteriorly from lateral aspect of the temporal bone. Anterior margin of sigmoid sinus (black solid arrowheads) forms a small ridge along lateral aspect of the petrous bone. Note the foramen for an emissary vein in the posterior portion of the groove for the sigmoid sinus. Internal auditory canal (open arrowhead) is seen end-on. Ridge of bone, the falciform crest, is seen within the depth of this canal. Site of articulation between the petrous tip and the clivus is irregular (open black arrow). Circular opening below the petrous tip represents the medial end of the intratemporal portion of the carotid canal. Fossa for exit of the vestibular aqueduct (solid black arrow) lies anterior to the sinus groove. Inferior surface of the mastoid process is indicated by white arrow. **C,** Inferior or basal aspect. Petrous apex projects medially and forward. Entrance foramen of the carotid canal (open black arrowhead) lies on its inferior aspect. Caroticojugular spine (white arrowhead) separates the carotid canal from the jugular foramen. Stylomastoid foramen or exit of the facial canal (solid black arrowhead) lies lateral to the jugular fossa at base of the styloid. Note the rough articular surfaces, with the sphenoid bone anteriorly and the occipital bone posteriorly, along the medial aspect of the specimen. Medial aspect of the mastoid process is indicated by solid black arrows, mandibular fossa by open black arrow.

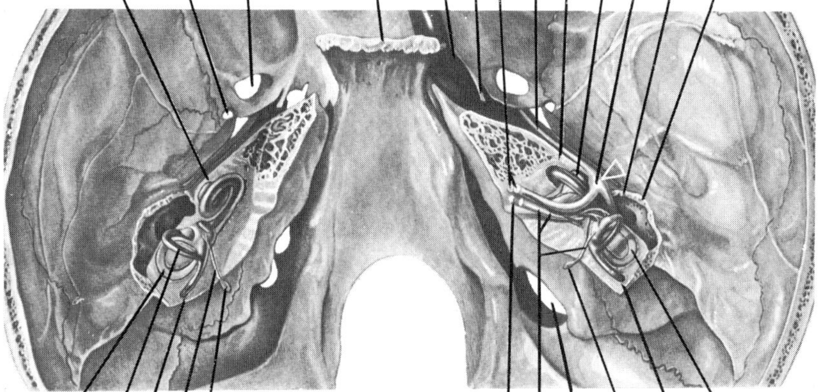

Fig. 19-2. View of base of the skull from above to show relation of the two petrous bones, with the clivus medially and the sphenoid bones anteriorly. On the left, petrous bone has been cut away to reveal the relation of the labyrinth to the bone. Endolymphatic duct is seen to extend posteriorly from the vestibule to exit on the surface of the bone. On the right, nerves in the internal auditory canal are portrayed. Bulge in the genu of the facial nerve is caused by the geniculate ganglion (arrowhead). (From Pernkopf, E.: Atlas of topographical and applied human anatomy, H. Ferner and H. Monsen, editors, Philadelphia, 1963, W. B. Saunders Co., vol. 1.)

of the petrous temporal bone. A large groove for the superior bulb of the internal jugular vein is situated immediately behind the carotid canal and inferior and medial to the middle ear (Fig. 19-1, *C*). The tympanic portion of the temporal bone is lateral to the carotid canal, and the temporomandibular joint is anterior and lateral to the canal. The lateral portion of the inferior temporal bone splits to ensheathe the upper portion of the styloid process. This process extends downward and medially. The stylomastoid foramen, which transmits the facial nerve and the stylomastoid artery, lies between the styloid and the mastoid processes (Fig. 19-1, *C*).

Borders. The petrous temporal bone also has three borders: superior, posterior, and anterior.

The superior border is the longest and is grooved by the superior petrosal sinus. The tentorium, except at its medial extremity, is attached to the superior border; at its medial extremity the tentorium is crossed by the roots of the trigeminal nerve. The posterior border extends medially to the jugular fossa. It is grooved by the inferior petrosal sinus. The anterior border adjoins the sphenoid bone.

Mastoid portion. The mastoid process of the temporal bone forms the posterior and lateral margins of the bone. The occipitofrontalis and auricularis posterior muscles are attached to the rough lateral surface of the process. The mastoid foramen, located near the posterior border of the process, transmits an emissary vein from the transverse sinus and a small dural branch of the occipital artery. The mastoid process is a large prominence extending inferiorly from the mastoid portion of the temporal bone (Figs. 19-1, *A,* and 19-3, *A* and *B*). The digastric groove lies immediately medial to the mastoid process. A shallower groove, which contains the occipital artery, lies adjacent and medial to the digastric groove. The intracranial surface of the mastoid portion is formed by the deep curved sigmoid sinus groove. In this region the sigmoid sinus is closely related to the medial mastoid air cells. The mastoid portion articulates superiorly with the parietal bone and posteriorly with the occipital bone. Superiorly and anteriorly it joins the squamous portion of the temporal bone, and medially and anteriorly it is related to the petrous portion of the temporal bone. The external auditory canal and the tympanic part of the temporal bone lie directly anterior to the mastoid portion (Figs. 19-1, *A,* and 19-3, *A* and *B*).

Tympanic portion. The tympanic portion forms the anterior wall, the floor, and a small portion of the posterior wall of the external auditory canal. Its anterior surface forms part of the articular fossa of the temporomandibular joint. Its posterior surface is curved with a concavity directed posteriorly and superiorly.

Organ of hearing (petrotympanic segment)

The organ of hearing is divided into three portions: the external ear, the middle ear, and the inner ear or labyrinth. Many of the structures concerned with hearing and balance are contained within a small part of the petrous temporal bone. As Anson (1969) has said, "Man depends, for his senses of equilibrium and hearing, upon areas of neuroanatomy whose outside dimensions are within the compass of a ten cent piece and whose space accommodates two drops of fluid." The key to successful interpretation of temporal bone radiographs is a thorough understanding of this segment of the temporal bone.

To understand the anatomy of the temporal bone properly, one must first visualize the relation of the bone to the rest of the skull. The axes of the internal and external auditory canals are almost perpendicular to the sagittal plane. A line joining the centers of the two external auditory meatuses will correspond almost exactly with the axis of the internal and external auditory canals on both sides (Fig. 19-4). The long axis of the petrous portion of the temporal bone or petrous pyramid is directed forward and medially at about a 45° angle to the axis of the canals (Fig. 19-5, *A*). If this relationship is understood, analysis of the structures of the temporal bone is facilitated.

External ear. The external ear consists of the auricle (which is relatively unimportant radiologically) and the external auditory canal. The external auditory canal is approximately 2.5 cm long and is separated from the middle ear by the tympanic membrane. The lateral portion of the canal is surrounded by cartilage, and the medial portion by bone. The inferior wall of the canal is slightly longer than the superoposterior wall. The tympanic membrane therefore has an oblique position. The anterior wall is closely related to the mandibular fossa and the parotid gland (Figs. 19-1, *A,* 19-3, *F,* and 19-5, *E*). The posterior wall separates the external canal from the mastoid air cells. The cranial cavity is closely related to the superior wall of the lateral portions of the external auditory canal. More medially the distance between the superior wall and the cranial cavity becomes greater. The floor of the canal is formed by the tympanic bone, and the roof by squamosa.

The drum spur, or scutum, a sharp projection of bone, lies at the medial termination of the external auditory canal (Figs. 19-6 to 19-9). The tympanic membrane is attached to this spur, which separates the external auditory canal from the epitympanic recess or attic.

Three sutures related to the external auditory canal should not be mistaken for fractures: the tympanomastoid suture, which lies posterior and inferior to the canal and extends obliquely upward immediately anterior to the mastoid process (Fig. 19-1, *A*); the tympanosquamosal suture, which lies superior and anterior to the canal, slightly below the root of the zygomatic process; and the petrotympanic suture, which extends through the posterior margin of the mandibular fossa.

Middle ear. The middle ear includes the tympanic cavity and the mastoid antrum. The tympanic cavity is an air-filled space that is relatively narrow from side to side (Fig. 19-10). Posteriorly it communicates with the mastoid antrum via the aditus, and anteromedially with the pharynx via the eustachian tube. Superiorly is the epitympanic recess (Figs. 19-6 and 19-7, *F*).

Ossicles. Three ossicles, the malleus, incus, and stapes, conduct airborne vibrations from the tympanic membrane to the fluid within the inner ear (Figs. 19-6 and 19-11). These ossicles are composed of enchondral bone and are formed from the first and second brachial arches.

The malleus is the most lateral and the largest ossicle (Figs. 19-4, 19-12, and 19-13). It has a head and a handle that are separated by a constriction, the neck. The handle of the malleus projects downward medially and posteriorly and is attached to the medial aspect

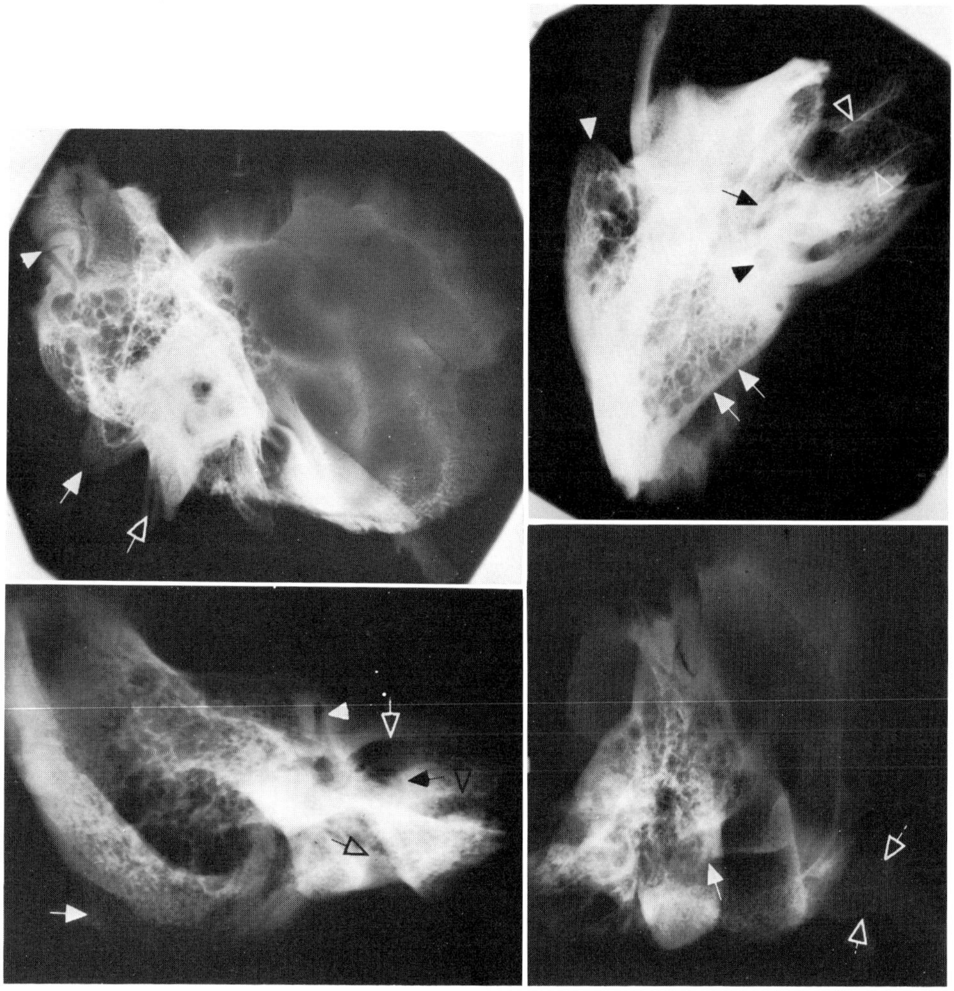

Fig. 19-3. Roentgenogram of disarticulated temporal bone. **A,** Lateral projection. Note the convolutional markings of the relatively thin squamous portion. Mastoid and portions of the petrous bone are pneumatized. Relatively little information regarding the labyrinth portion and the tympanic portion of the bone is obtained in this projection. Styloid process is indicated by open white arrow; mastoid tip by solid white arrow; emissary vein channels by solid white arrowhead. **B,** Basal projection shows the internal auditory canal extending medially between the vestibule (black arrowhead) and the anterior portion of the cochlea (black arrow). Intratympanic portion of the carotid canal (open white arrowheads) extends anteromedially. Dense bone surrounds the labyrinth contents. Pneumatization extends as far medially as petrous tip. Mastoid tip is indicated by white arrowhead; posterior wall of the petrous pyramid by white arrows. **C,** Stenvers projection. Lateral aspect is to the reader's left. Mastoid tip is indicated by solid white arrow; cochlea by solid black arrow. Roof of the internal auditory canal (open white arrow) is slightly foreshortened. Note the superior semicircular canal (solid white arrowhead) and the adjacent sclerotic bone. Note also the lateral semicircular canal. Vestibule is found inferior to the superior semicircular canal. Internal auditory canal is always projected just medial to the vestibular shadow. Carotid canal is indicated by open black arrow. **D,** Chaussé III projection. This projection is useful to identify the medial aspect of the external auditory canal, the drum spur (solid white arrow). Base of the zygomatic process is indicated by open white arrows. **E,** Mayer-Owen view. Posterior aspect of the bone is to the reader's left. Groove for the transverse and sigmoid sinus along the medial posterior aspect of the petromastoid portion of the bone is indicated by black arrowheads; cochlea by solid black arrow; drum spur by solid white arrow; external auditory canal by open white arrow; carotid canal by open black arrow. Zygomatic process and mandibular fossa for the condyle of the mandible are on the reader's right. **F,** Schüller view. External auditory canal is shown by black arrow; sinus groove by white arrow. Note the mastoid and pneumatized portions of the petrous pyramid. Squamous portion is located superiorly but is difficult to see on this projection.

E 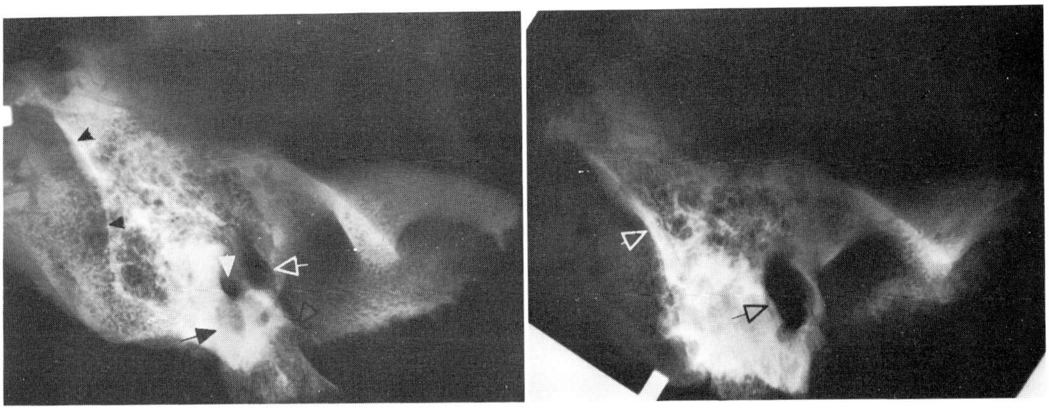 F

Fig. 19-3, cont'd. For legend see opposite page.

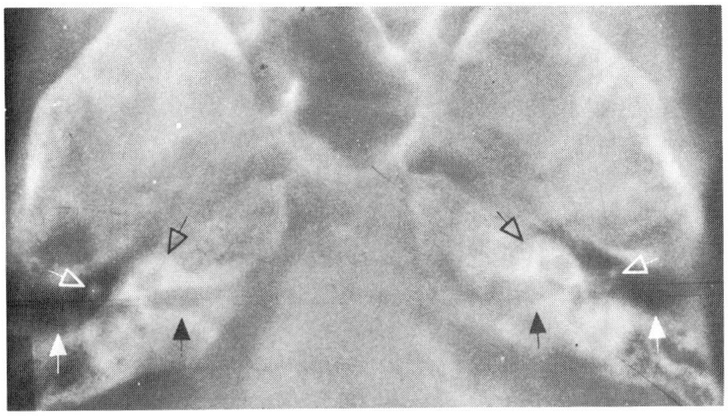

Fig. 19-4. Polytome laminagraphic section in submentovertical position shows external auditory canal (white solid arrows indicate posterior walls) and internal auditory canal (solid black arrows indicate posterior walls) forming straight line from one side to the other. Ossicles are shown by open white arrows; cochlea by open black arrows.

of the upper portion of the tympanic membrane. At this point the tympanic membrane is drawn medially toward the tympanic cavity, forming a lateral concavity. The head of the malleus lies in the epitympanic recess. It articulates posteromedially with the body of the incus at the incudomalleolar joint.

The incus lies posterior to the malleus (Figs. 19-12 and 19-13). It is divided into a body and two processes, long and short. The body is rounded and compressed from side to side. The short process projects posteriorly and is attached to a small fossa in the lower and posterior part of the epitympanic recess. The long process descends almost vertically, posteriorly and medially, to the handle of the malleus. The long process of the incus and the handle of the malleus are almost parallel. The inferior end of the long process of the incus bends medially and articulates with the head of the stapes (incudostapedial joint).

The stapes, the most medial ossicle, resembles a stirrup (Figs. 19-12 and 19-13). Medial to the head of the stapes is a narrow neck that branches into slender anterior and posterior limbs. These in turn are attached to the base. The base of the stapes is fixed to the margins of the vestibular window (fenestra vestibulae) by a ring of ligamentous fibers.

Tympanic cavity. The tympanic cavity is bounded by a roof and a floor as well as by anterior, posterior, lateral, and medial walls.

The roof of the tympanic cavity, the tegmen tympani, is a thin plate of bone that separates the tympanic cavity from the cranial cavity. The tegmen tympani also forms the roof of the mastoid antrum more posteriorly (Fig. 19-5, *D*).

The floor is a thin plate of bone that separates the tympanic cavity from the jugular fossa.

The anterior wall of the tympanic cavity is relatively short. It is perforated by two canals. The upper, and smaller, canal transmits the tensor tympani muscle. The lower canal is larger and represents the bony portion of the eustachian tube, which extends anteriorly, medially, and somewhat inferiorly to connect the middle ear with the lateral wall of the nasopharynx. The eustachian tube is partly osseous and partly cartilaginous, and its total length is about 3.5 to 4 cm. The bony part lies adjacent to the tympanic cavity and is approximately 1 cm in length. The cartilaginous portion is related to the petrosphenoid groove.

The posterior wall of the tympanic cavity has an aperture superiorly, the aditus, that leads into the mastoid antrum. A ridge formed by the canal for the facial nerve lies on the medial wall of the tympanic cavity. A bulge caused by the lateral semicircular canal lies immediately above and posterior.

The lateral wall of the tympanic cavity is formed by the tympanic membrane and the ring of bone into which it is inserted.

The medial wall of the tympanic cavity has a bulge,

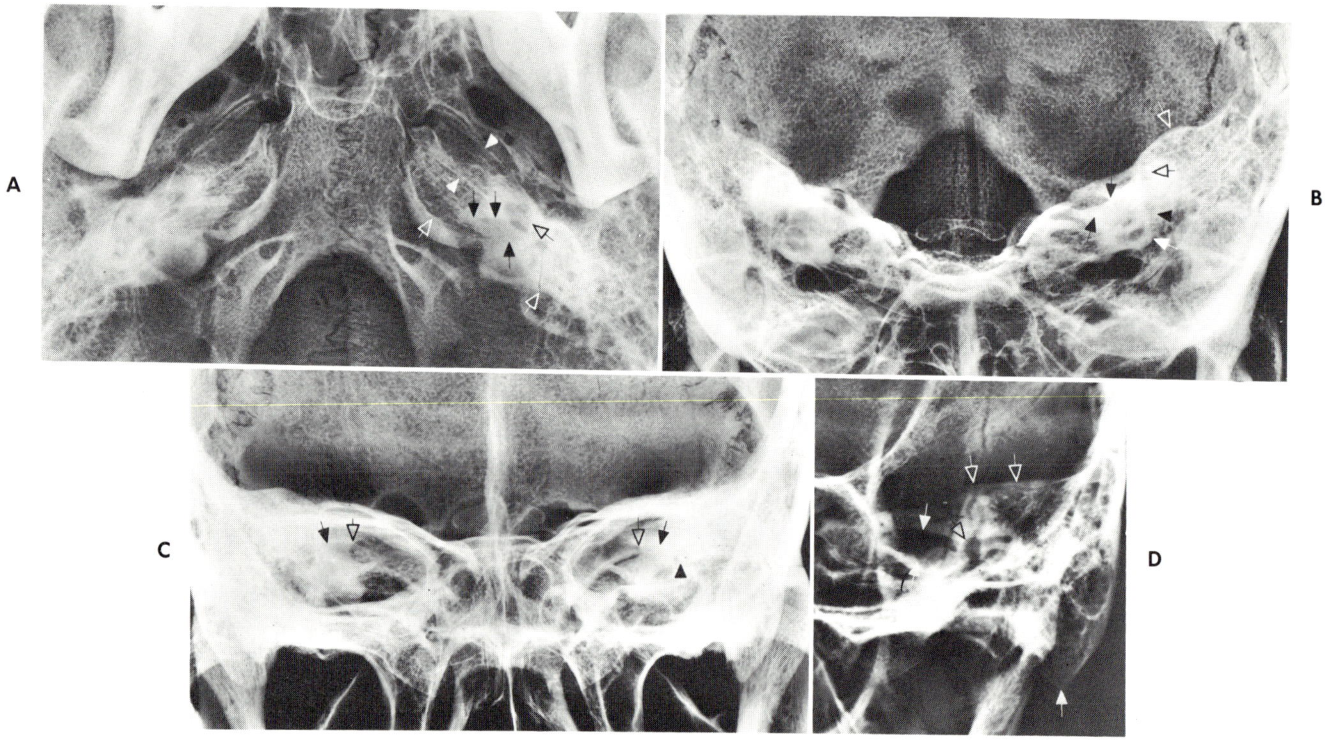

Fig. 19-5. Roentgenograms of dried skull specimens. **A,** Submentovertical view shows the relatively dense petrous pyramid projecting anteromedially. Posterior margins of the pyramid are indicated by open white arrows. Internal auditory canals (solid black arrows) have a horizontal course. Axis of the cochlea (open black arrow) is directed somewhat laterally but is almost perpendicular to axis of the petrous pyramid. Internal carotid artery canal (solid white arrowheads) extends anteromedially along the main axis of the petrous pyramid. **B,** Towne projection shows arcuate eminence (open white arrow) bulging superiorly from the petrous ridge. Internal auditory canal (solid black arrows) extends medially. Cochlea (solid white arrow) is projected slightly inferior and lateral to the medial aspect of the internal auditory canal. Superior semicircular canal (open black arrow) lies just above the lucency of the vestibule (solid black arrowhead). Note the jugular foramen below the cochlea. **C,** Straight AP view places the internal auditory canal (black arrows) approximately in the middle of the orbits. The canals can best be compared in this projection. Note the posterior wall (open arrows) of the porus acousticus. Distance from the posterior wall to the medial edge of the vestibule (black arrowhead) can easily be measured. **D,** Stenvers view shows top of petrous pyramid or petrous ridge forming a horizontal line (open white arrows). Medial arrow is at the arcuate eminence, overlying the superior semicircular canal. Lateral open arrow indicates the petrous ridge above the tegmen tympani, or roof of the tympanum. Superior and lateral semicircular canals extend from the vestibule (open black arrow). Internal auditory canal and mastoid tip are indicated by solid white arrows. **E,** Schüller view shows sinodural plate (open white arrows) marking the junction of the petrous bone and the lateral and sigmoid sinus. Auditory canal axis (solid black arrow) is seen end-on. Mandibular fossa lies immediately anterior to the auditory canal. Articular eminence (open black arrow) forms anterior boundary of the fossa. Emissary vein channel is indicated by white arrowhead.

E

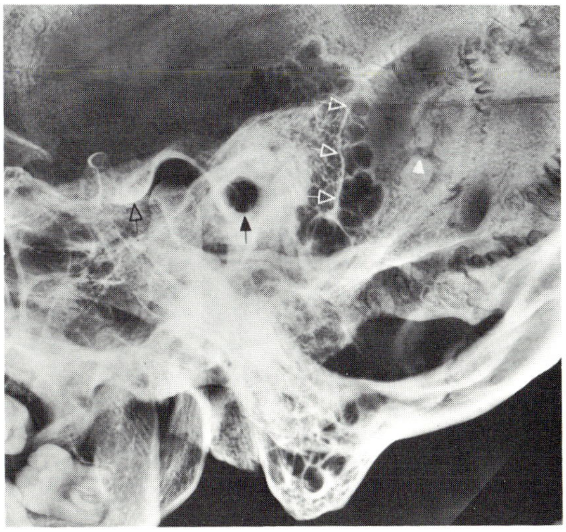

Fig. 19-5, cont'd. For legend see opposite page.

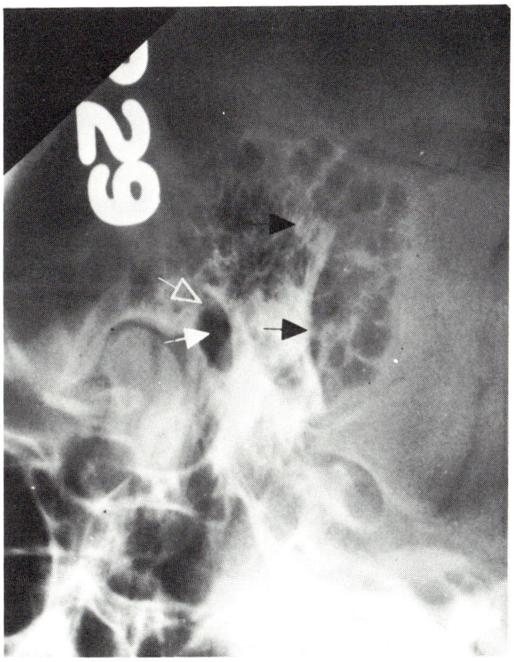

Fig. 19-6. Mayer-Owen view of normal temporal bone. This projection is designed to evaluate pneumatization of the mastoid and tympanic areas. In addition, the external auditory canal and drum spur (open arrow), which is a bony bridge separating the canal from the epitympanic recess, can be evaluated. Sinodural plate (solid black arrows) is well shown. One of the ossicular processes (solid white arrow) is faintly visualized.

the promontory, caused by the basal turn of the cochlea. The vestibular or oval window (fenestra vestibulae) lies posterior and superior to the promontory. The round window (fenestra cochleae) lies in a depression behind the promontory. The round window is closed by a membrane known as the secondary tympanic membrane. The facial nerve runs horizontally above the promontory and the oval window.

Inner ear. The inner ear consists of two parts: the bony labyrinth and the membranous labyrinth (Fig. 19-14).

The bony labyrinth consists of three parts: the vestibule, the three semicircular canals, and the cochlea. These cavities in the petrous part of the temporal bone are lined by periosteum and contain a clear fluid, perilymph. The membranous labyrinth lies within the bony labyrinth. It is surrounded by perilymph and contains fluid called endolymph. The otic capsule, which arises from fourteen separate ossification centers, surrounds this entire structure. By the fifth month of fetal life, the inner ear structures have reached the adult size. Some of the surfaces of the enchondral otic capsule convert to cancellous bone, allowing solid incorporation of the capsule into the remainder of the petrous pyramid.

The membranous labyrinth is even more complex than the bony labyrinth. Except for the endolymphatic duct, however, it is of less roentgenographic importance.

VESTIBULE. The vestibule lies behind the cochlea and in front of the semicircular canals (Fig. 19-5). It is rounded but slightly flattened from side to side, measuring about 5 mm from top to bottom and front to back and about 3 mm in width. The vestibule contains two small sacs, the utricle and the saccule, that are part of the membranous labyrinth. The utricle is in the upper and posterior part of the vestibule and is closely related to the semicircular canals, which open into it. The saccule is in the medial lower and anterior part of the vestibule and is related to the cochlea. The oval window (fenestra vestibulae) is the opening in the lateral wall of the vestibule. The aqueduct of the vestibule, which contains the ductus endolymphaticus, arises from the medial wall of the vestibule. The vestibular aqueduct extends to the posterior surface of the petrous temporal bone lateral to the internal auditory meatus. Here its opening is covered by a thin plate of bone.

SEMICIRCULAR CANALS. The three semicircular canals, superior, posterior, and lateral, lie above and behind the vestibule (Figs. 19-5, 19-7, 19-10, 19-11, 19-13, and 19-14). They vary in length from 12 to 22 mm. Each canal has a slight dilatation at one end, the ampulla. The semicircular canals open into the vestibule by five orifices, one of these being common to two canals. The superior semicircular canal lies in a vertical plane that

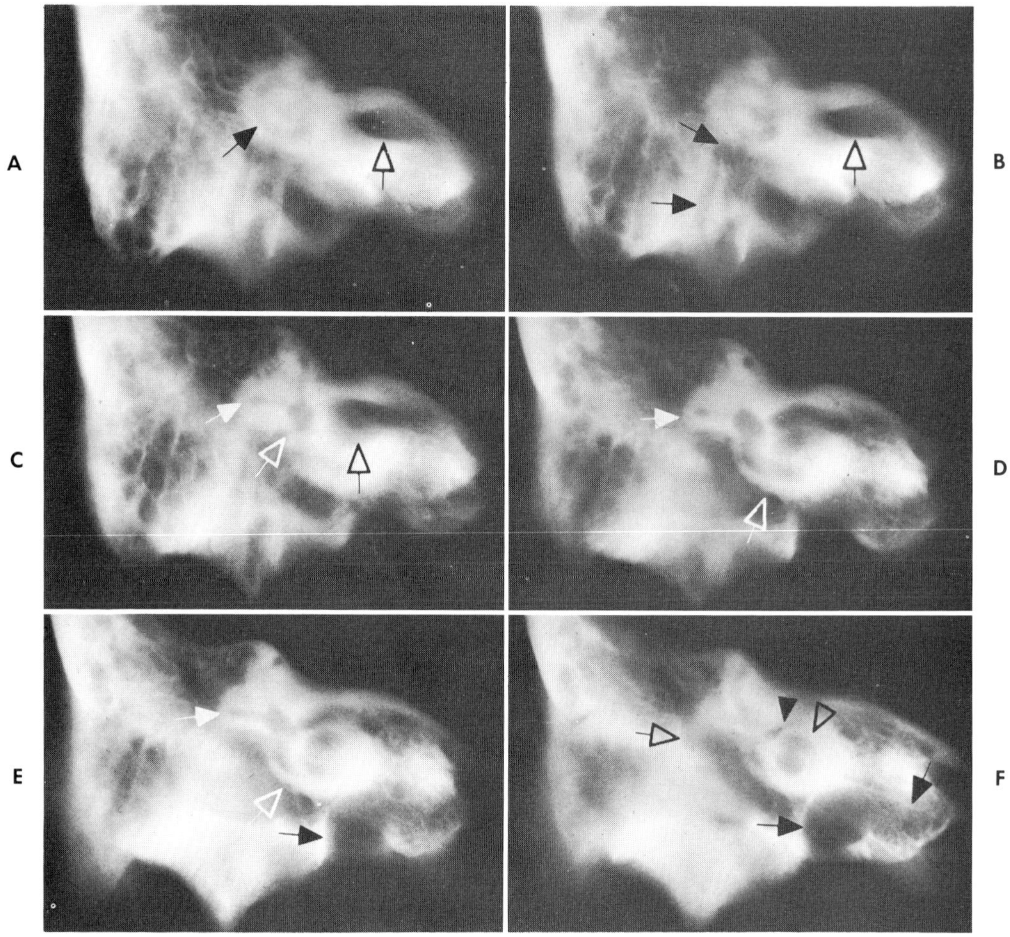

Fig. 19-7. Hypocycloidal laminagraphic sections (1 mm thickness) of dried disarticulated temporal bone in a position comparable to the standard AP projection. **A** represents the most posterior section, **G** the most anterior. **A,** Posterior semicircular canal (solid black arrow). Internal auditory canal (open black arrow) opens posteriorly on the surface of the petrous pyramid. Mastoid and lateral petrous areas are well pneumatized. **B,** Descending portion of the facial canal (solid black arrows) opens inferiorly into the stylomastoid foramen. Internal auditory canal (open black arrow) and posterior semicircular canals are still visible. **C,** Lateral bulbous portion of the internal auditory canal (open arrow) is now shown. Lateral semicircular canal (solid white arrow) is just becoming visible. Oval window in vestibule is indicated by open white arrow. **D,** Basal turn of the cochlea (open white arrow) has come into view. Lateral semicircular canal (solid white arrow) is well shown. Lucent dot in the superior surface of the petrous pyramid is part of the superior semicircular canal. **E,** Lateral margin of the internal carotid canal (black arrow) has come into view. External auditory canal is becoming visible laterally. Basal turn of the cochlea (open white arrow) and tympanum lying lateral to it are well shown. Ossicles are not present in this specimen. Lateral semicircular canal is indicated by solid white arrow. **F,** Internal carotid artery canal (solid black arrows) extends medially toward the petrous tip. Facial canal (solid black arrowhead) is seen as it turns between the cochlea (open black arrowhead) and the vestibule just after its exit from the internal auditory canal. Lateral wall of the epitympanic recess or attic is indicated by open black arrow. **G,** Drum spur or bony bridge (open black arrow) separates medial aspect of the external auditory canal from the epitympanic recess. Most of the labyrinth is now invisible. Internal carotid artery canal (solid black arrow) is still well seen.

G
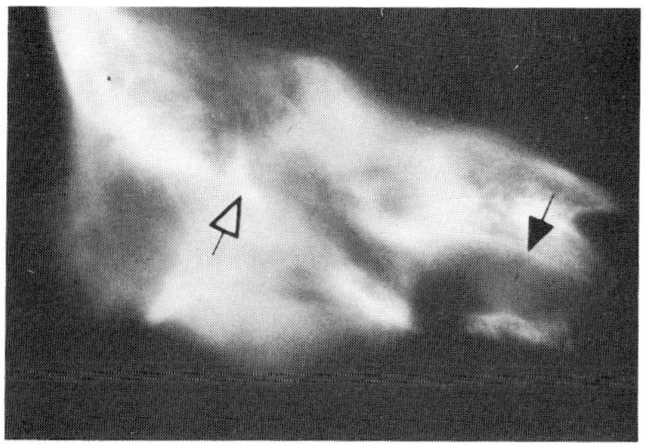

Fig. 19-7, cont'd. For legend see opposite page.

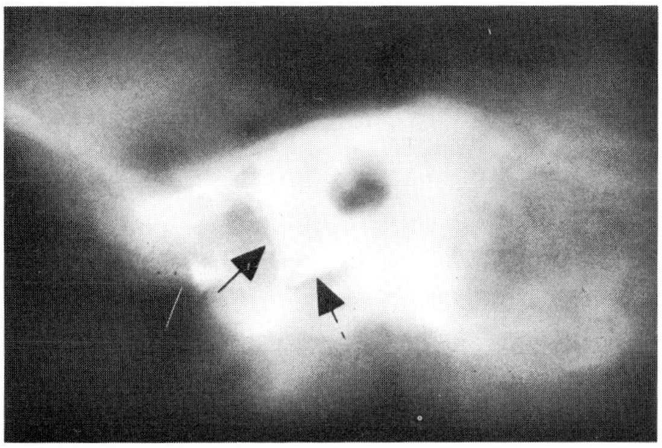

Fig. 19-8. Lateral laminagram of disarticulated temporal bone shows well the sharply defined bony spur (arrows) between the carotid canal and the jugular bulb. This bony spur is destroyed when a glomus jugulare tumor extends superiorly.

A

B

C
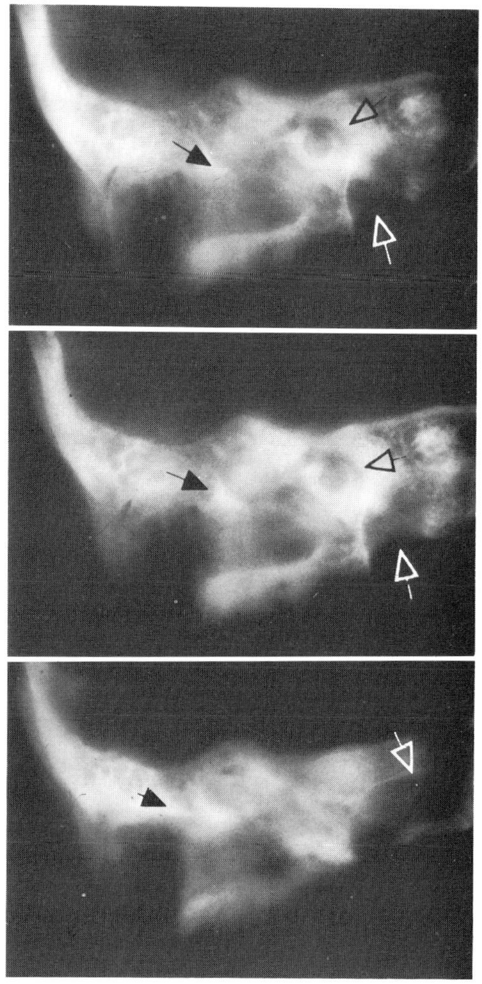

Fig. 19-9. Hypocycloidal laminagraphic sections (1 mm thickness) of dried disarticulated temporal bone placed in a rotated frontal position approaching the usual Stenvers projection. **A** is the most posterior, and **C** the most anterior, section. Drum spur is indicated by solid black arrow; cochlea by open black arrow; carotid canal by open white arrow.

is perpendicular to the long axis of the petrous temporal bone. The ampulla of the superior semicircular canal is on its anterolateral end. Its posteromedial end joins the upper limb of the posterior semicircular canal. The superior semicircular canal causes a slight bulge in the anterior surface of the petrous temporal bone, forming the arcuate eminence. The posterior semicircular canal lies in a vertical plane directed posterolaterally, almost parallel to the posterior surface of the petrous temporal bone. Its ampulla is on its inferior end. The lateral or horizontal semicircular canal curves backward and laterally in a horizontal plane. It is related to the medial wall of the epitympanic recess. Its ampulla is on its anterior end.

COCHLEA. The cochlea consists of a spiral canal that makes two and one-half turns around a cone-shaped central bony core, the modiolus (Figs. 19-7, 19-10, 19-13, and 19-14). The cochlea measures approximately 9 mm in diameter at the base and 5 mm from top to bottom. The base of the modiolus is related to the lateral portion of the internal auditory canal. The cochlea forms the anterior portion of the labyrinth, and its apex is directed anteriorly and laterally. The first turn of the cochlea bulges into the medial wall of the tympanic cavity to form the promontory. At the beginning of the basal turn of the cochlea are two main openings: (1) the round window (fenestra cochlea), which opens into the medial wall of the tympanic cavity, and (2) an elliptic opening into the vestibule. The anterior and inferior surface of the cochlea lies just behind the posterior wall of the carotid canal as the canal turns anteriorly and medially. The cochlear aqueduct is a tiny channel extending from the basal turn of the cochlea posteromedially to a deep notch immediately below the internal auditory meatus. The cochlear aqueduct is therefore more medial than the vestibular aqueduct.

Internal auditory canal. The internal auditory canal extends laterally from the central part of the posterior

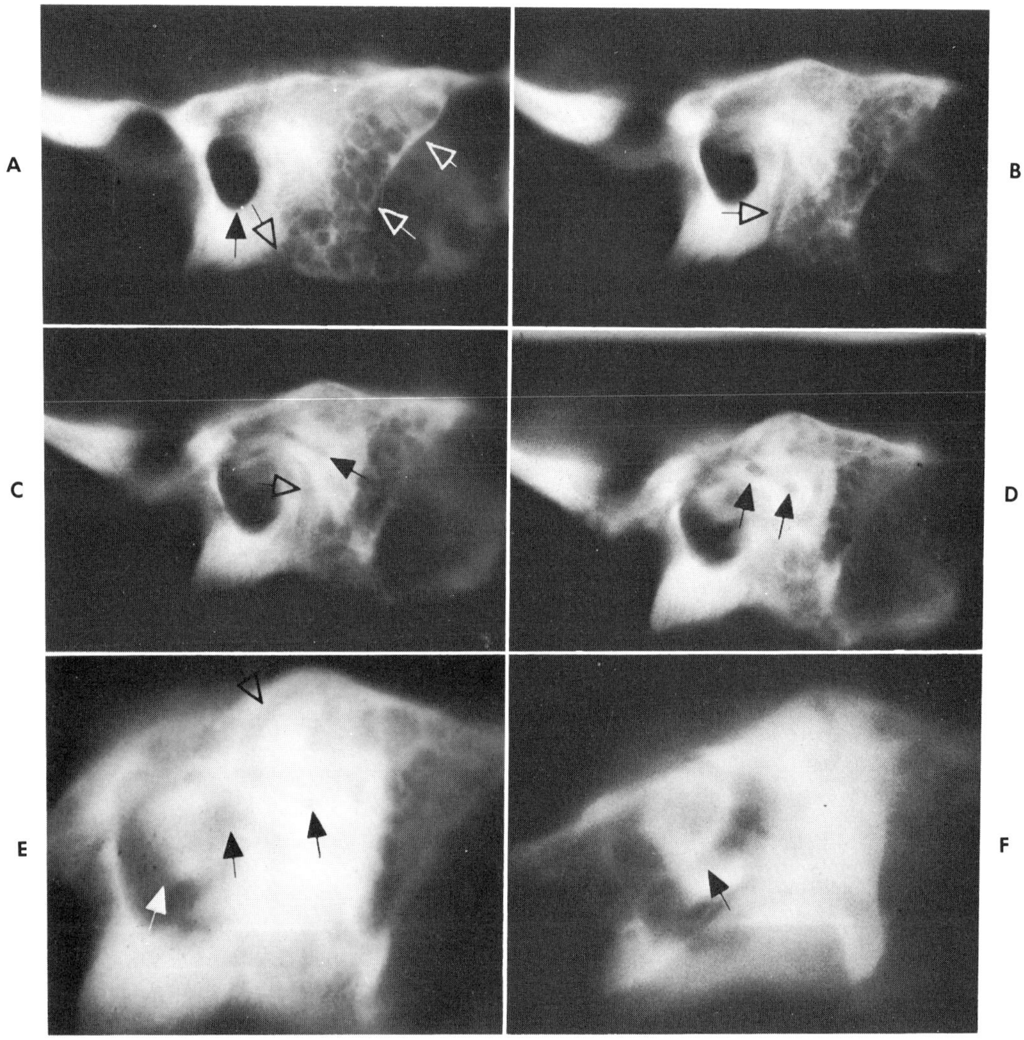

Fig. 19-10. Polytomographic sections (1 mm thickness) of dried disarticulated temporal bone, lateral projection. Interval between the cuts is 2 mm. **A** is the most lateral; **F** the most medial. **A,** Section is medial to the mastoid tip. Mandibular fossa lies immediately anterior to the external auditory canal (solid black arrow). Posterior wall of the sinus (open white arrows) and stylomastoid foramen, exit foramen of the seventh nerve (open black arrow), are well shown. **B,** Descending portion of the facial canal (open arrow) courses downward behind the external auditory canal. **C,** More superior portion of the facial canal (open arrow) is now seen. Lateral semicircular canal (solid black arrow) is also visualized. **D,** Proximal limbs of the lateral semicircular canal (arrows) curve back down toward the vestibule. Part of the cochlea lies just anterior to the anterior black arrow. Radiolucent space below the cochlea is the tympanum. **E,** More of the cochlea (white arrow) can now be seen. Lateral semicircular canal is indicated by solid black arrows; superior semicircular canal by open black arrow. **F,** Lucency behind the cochlea (arrow) represents part of the vestibule. Sharply demarcated anterior portion of the cochlea is caused by carotid canal.

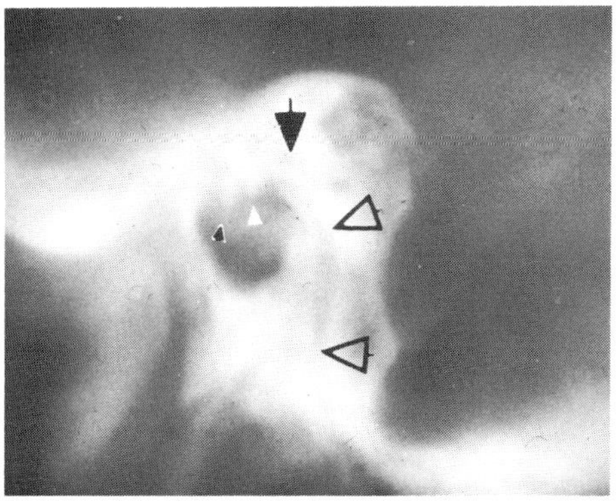

Fig. 19-11. Polytomographic section of temporal bone, lateral projection, shows normal position of the malleus or anterior ossicle (small black arrowhead) and the incus or posterior ossicle (small white arrowhead). Appearance of these two ossicles has been likened to that of a molar tooth. Facial canal passes under the lateral semicircular canal (solid black arrow). Condyle of the mandible is faintly seen anteriorly. Descending portion of facial canal is indicated by open black arrows.

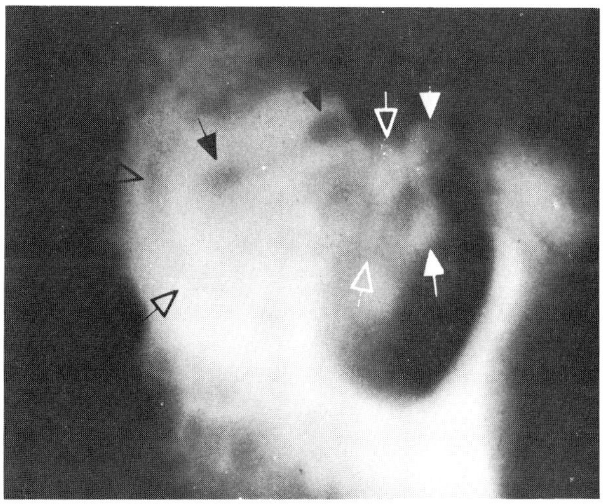

Fig. 19-12. Hypocycloidal laminagraphic section (1 mm thickness) of a freshly removed temporal bone in lateral projection. Section is at the level of the ossicular chain; anterior portion is to the reader's right. Solid white arrows indicate the malleus; superior arrow the head; inferior arrow the handle as it widens into the manubrium. Open white arrows indicate the incus; superior arrow the head; inferior arrow the long process. Short process of the incus cannot usually be identified in this projection. Two solid black arrows indicate anterior and posterior limbs of the lateral semicircular canal; open black arrows indicate posterior portion of the posterior semicircular canal. Margins of the tympanic cavity are well visualized anteriorly and posteriorly.

surface of the petrous temporal bone (Figs. 19-3, *B,* 19-5, 19-10, 19-13, and 19-14). Since the posterior surface of the petrous bone is oblique, the opening of the internal auditory canal is also oblique. The anterior margin of the opening of the canal blends with the posterior surface of the petrous temporal bone and is therefore ill defined. The posterior margin of the opening is well defined. The canal measures 5 to 7 mm from top to bottom. The central portion of the canal is slightly larger than the medial or lateral segment. A sharply defined bridge of bone and fibrous tissue, the falciform crest, divides the lateral portion of the canal or fundus into superior and inferior compartments (Fig. 19-1, *B*). Each of these in turn is divided by a vertical ridge into anterior and posterior portions. The facial nerve lies in the upper and anterior compartment, the cochlear nerve in the lower and anterior compartment. The upper and lower divisions of the vestibular nerve pass through the upper and lower posterior compartments respectively. In addition, the internal auditory canal contains several small veins and the internal auditory artery (Mazzoni and Hansen, 1970).

Facial nerve. The facial nerve consists of motor and sensory roots. The sensory root is known as the nervus intermedius. From its origin at the lower border of the pons, the facial nerve extends laterally and anteriorly to enter the internal auditory canal. At the lateral end of the canal, the facial nerve lies in the upper and anterior compartment, where it enters the facial canal. At first the facial canal courses laterally above the vestibule until it reaches the medial wall of the epitympanic recess. Here it turns backward above the promontory and the oval window and below the lateral semicircular canal. It then curves downward in the medial wall of the tympanic cavity and courses inferiorly to emerge from the stylomastoid foramen (Figs. 19-7, 19-10, 19-13, and 19-14). The chorda tympani arises from the facial nerve in the midportion of the descending course of the facial nerve. It courses anteriorly between the handle of the malleus and the long process of the incus.

Developmental anatomy

The inner ear is ectodermal in origin (Anson and Donaldson, 1967; Shambaugh, 1967). Invagination of the ectoderm leads to the formation of the otocyst, which represents the primitive labyrinth. The first ossification center appears around the cochlea during the sixteenth week of fetal life. The last (fourteenth) center appears around the semicircular canal at about the twentieth week. The inner portion of the bony otic capsule develops into the perilymph structures that surround the membranous labyrinth. Ossification is

Text continued on p. 422.

A 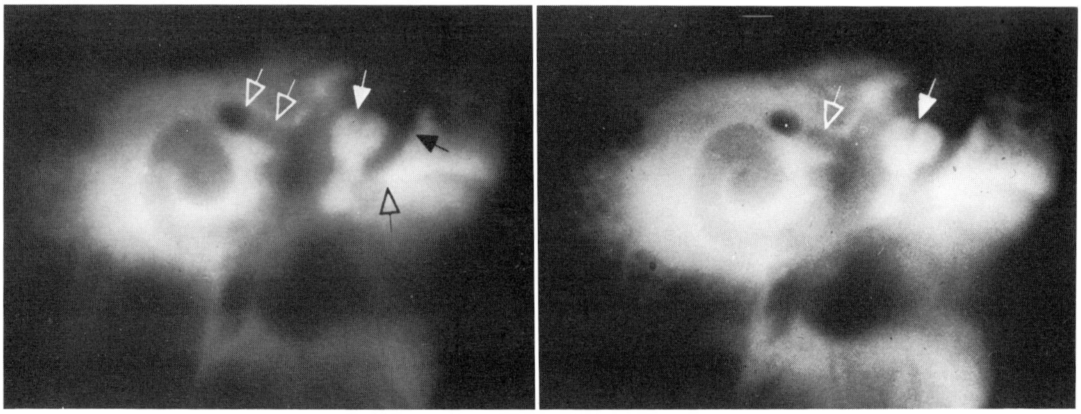 B

Fig. 19-13. Hypocycloidal laminagraphic sections (1 mm thickness) of a freshly removed left temporal bone in frontal projection. **A** is the most anterior section; **I** the most posterior. These sections illustrate labyrinthine, ossicular, and tympanic relationships. In the illustrations the patient faces the viewer, medial aspect to the reader's left and lateral aspect to the reader's right. These sections are separated by 1 mm. **A,** Spiral turns of cochlea are well seen. Anterior portion of the facial canal, the genu (open white arrows), extends laterally from internal auditory canal. Geniculate ganglion lies immediately above this portion of the canal. Head of the incus (solid white arrow) lies within the epitympanic recess, which communicates superiorly with the aditus ad antrum. Drum spur (open black arrow) marks the medial aspect of the external auditory canal at its junction with lateral wall of epitympanic recess (solid black arrow). **B,** Cochlea and its spiral laminae are well outlined. Head of the malleus lies anteromedial, and head of the incus posterolateral, to the incudomalleolar joint (solid white arrow). Facial canal is indicated by open white arrow. **C,** Promontory represents protrusion of the basal turn of the cochlea into the tympanum (open white arrow). Long process (black arrow) and head (solid white arrow) of the incus are well shown. **D,** Promontory or basal turn of the cochlea (open white arrow) is better defined in this section. Roof of the internal auditory canal (black arrows) is just coming into view. Rounded radiolucent area beneath this region is combination shadow of the base of the cochlea and the internal auditory canal. **E,** More of the internal auditory canal can now be identified, but overlying cochlear shadow is still visible. Superior semicircular canal (open black arrows) and anterior limb of the lateral semicircular canal (solid black arrow) are shown. Footplate of the stapes is indicated by small white arrowhead; arrowhead lies in the vestibular shadow. One arm or crus of the stapes can be seen medial to the incudostapedial joint (solid white arrow). Basal turn of the cochlea (open white arrow) is still visible. **F,** Entire internal auditory canal is now visualized. Its inferior margin is indicated by two solid black arrows; falciform crest by open white arrow. Two small white arrowheads are projected in the vestibule. They indicate the upper and lower margins of the footplate of the stapes and at same time show the margins of the oval or vestibular window. Facial canal (open black arrow) is seen beneath the lateral semicircular canal. **G,** Descending portion of the facial canal (open black arrow) is coming into view. Midportion of the lateral aspect of the lateral semicircular canal lies above the open black arrow. Vestibule (solid black arrow) is well shown. White arrow is projected above the posterior aspect of the tympanic cavity. **H,** Posterior limb of the superior semicircular canal extends downward from the apex (white arrow) to the vestibule. Posterior limb of the lateral semicircular canal (solid black arrow) is well shown. Descending portion of the facial canal (open black arrows) courses inferiorly toward the stylomastoid foramen. **I,** Descending portion of the facial nerve canal (open black arrows) is still well shown. Lateral aspect of jugular fossa is indicated by open white arrow; medial inferior portion of the posterior semicircular canal by solid white arrow; posterior limb of the superior semicircular canal by solid black arrow.

C D E F G H I

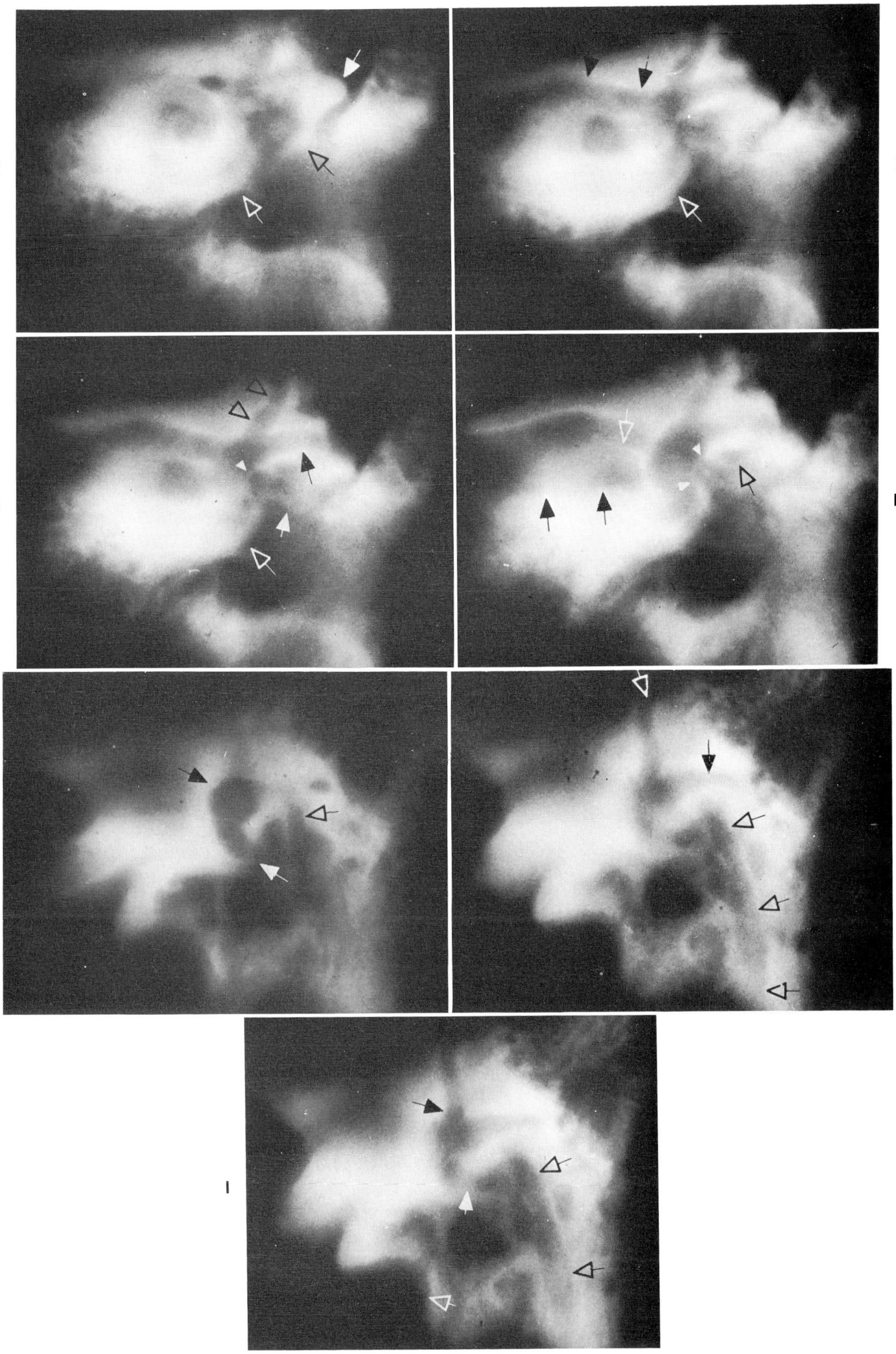

Fig. 19-13, cont'd. For legend see opposite page.

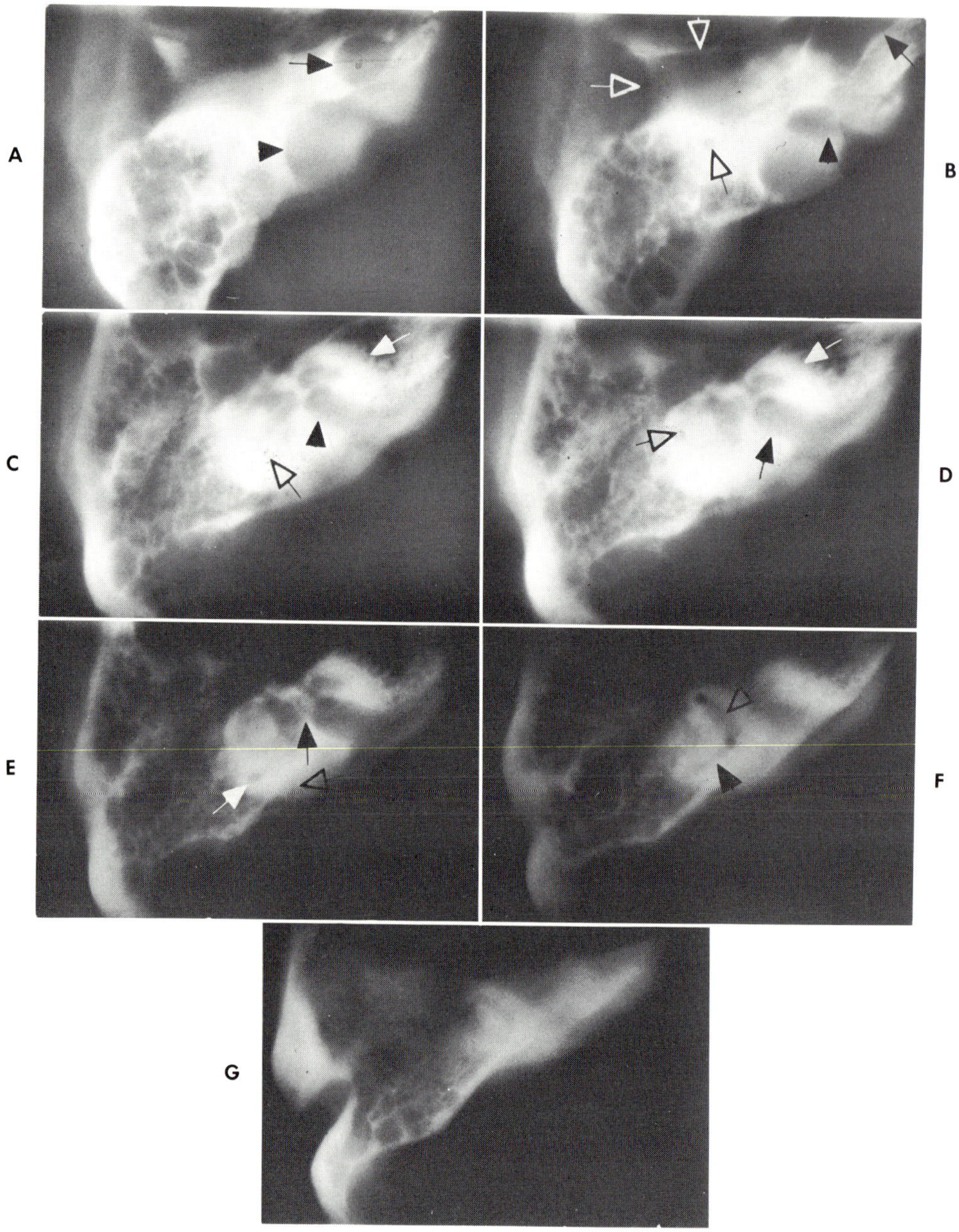

Fig. 19-14. Hypocycloidal laminagraphic section (1 mm thickness) of dried distarticulated temporal bone in the basal or axial position. **A** represents the most inferior section; **G** the most superior. Sections are cut at 4 mm intervals. **A,** External auditory canal is faintly outlined lateral to opening of the carotid canal (solid black arrow). Pneumatized mastoid tip lies lateral to anterior margin of the jugular foramen (solid black arrowhead). **B,** Descending portion of facial canal (open black arrow) is visualized as it travels behind the external auditory canal (open white arrows). Carotid canal (solid black arrow) courses anteromedially. Posterior margin of the internal auditory canal is indicated by solid black arrowhead. **C,** Cochlea is indicated by white arrow; posterior wall of the internal auditory canal by black arrowhead; posterior semicircular canal by open black arrow. **D,** Posterior wall of internal auditory canal (solid black arrow) terminates abruptly medially; anterior wall blends smoothly with the petrous pyramid medially. Horizontal semicircular canal is seen *en face* (open black arrow). Cochlea is indicated by white arrow. **E,** Cochlea and internal auditory canal are again well seen. Posterior semicircular canal is marked by white arrow; vestibule by solid black arrow; vestibular aqueduct by open black arrow. **F,** Superior (open black arrow) and posterior (solid black arrow) semicircular canals are well shown. **G,** Superior margin of the petrous pyramid with notch for articulation of parietal bone laterally and superior semicircular canal at the level of the arcuate eminence are now visualized.

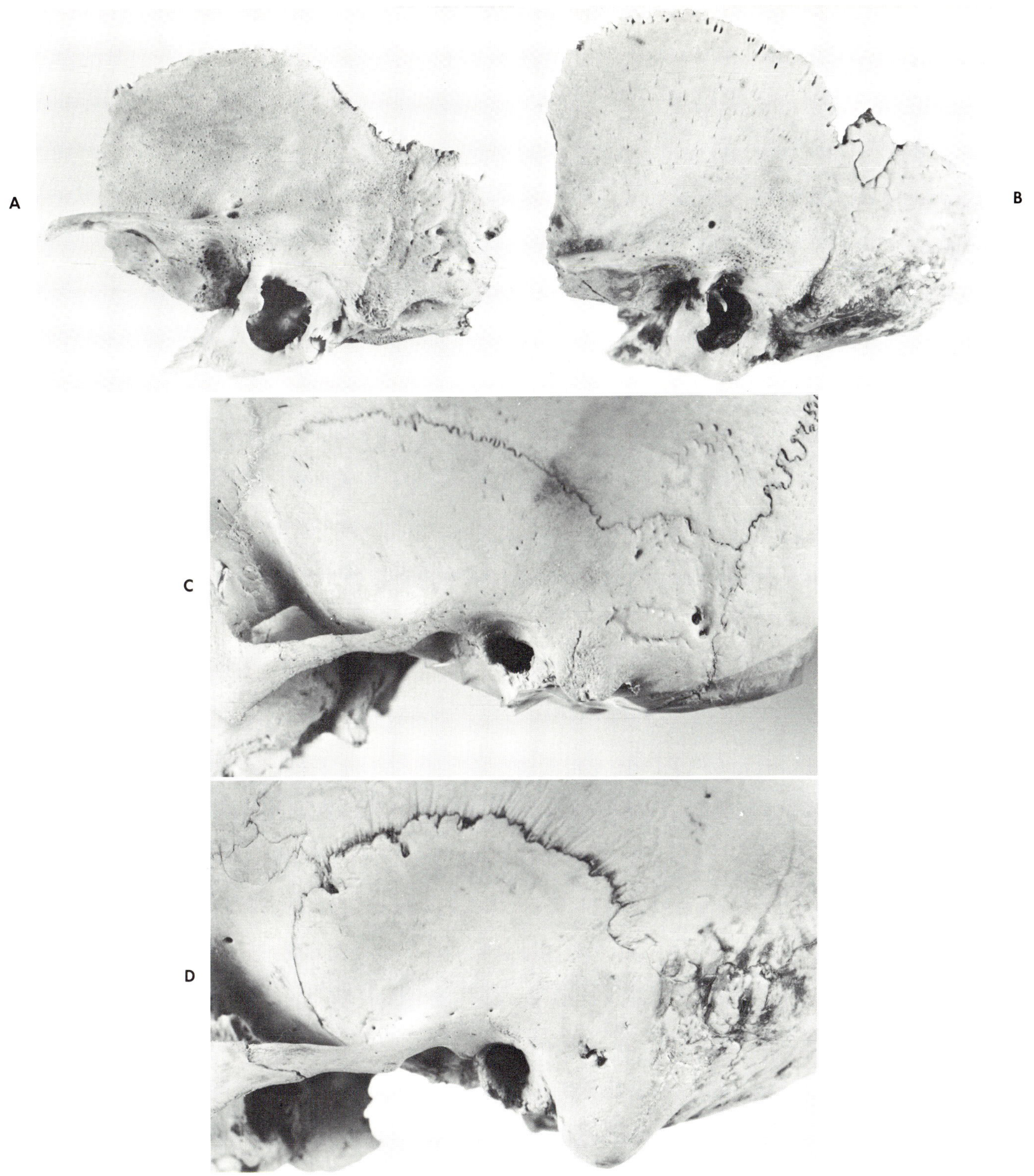

Fig. 19-15. Normal postnatal development of temporal bone. **A,** Age 6 months. Note the large cavity comprising the external auditory canal and the middle ear region. Only a rudiment of the mastoid tip is present. **B,** Age 12 months. External auditory canal cavity remains large. Some circumferential growth in the region has occurred, however. Mastoid is still undeveloped. **C,** Age 24 months. At this time, external auditory canal is more adult in configuration. Mastoid process has begun to grow downward behind the external auditory canal. **D,** Age 4 years. By this time, bone has reached essentially adult configuration. Tympanic portion is completely modified. Mastoid process may grow slightly more but is almost completely developed. (Courtesy Mildred Trotter, M.D., Washington University School of Medicine, St. Louis, Mo.)

A

B

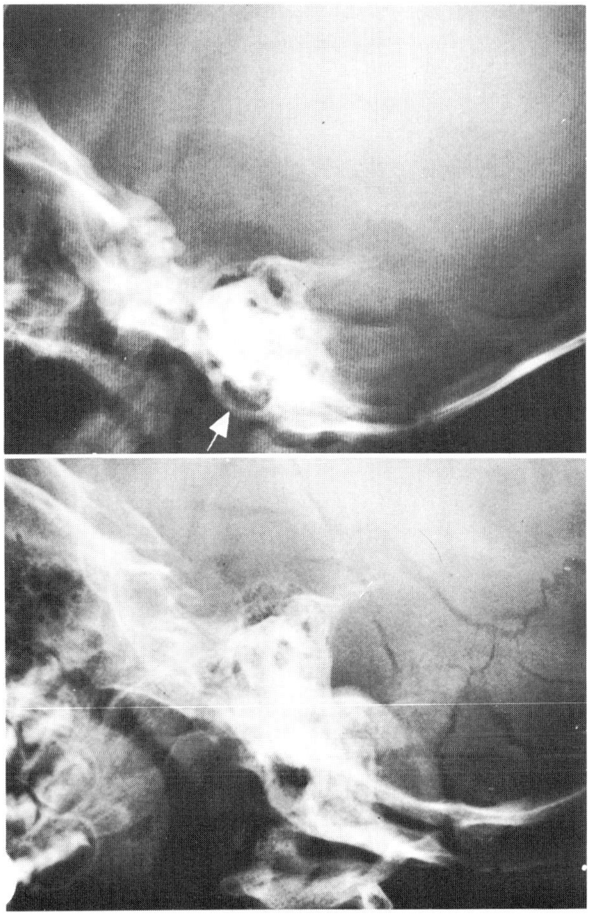

Fig. 19-16. Normal roentgenograms of postnatal temporal bone development. **A,** Age 6 months. Tympanic ring (arrow) is large, and there is no significant mastoid aeration or growth. **B,** Age 18 months. Tympanic portion of mastoid has changed toward the adult configuration. Mastoid process is not yet developed.

A

B

C

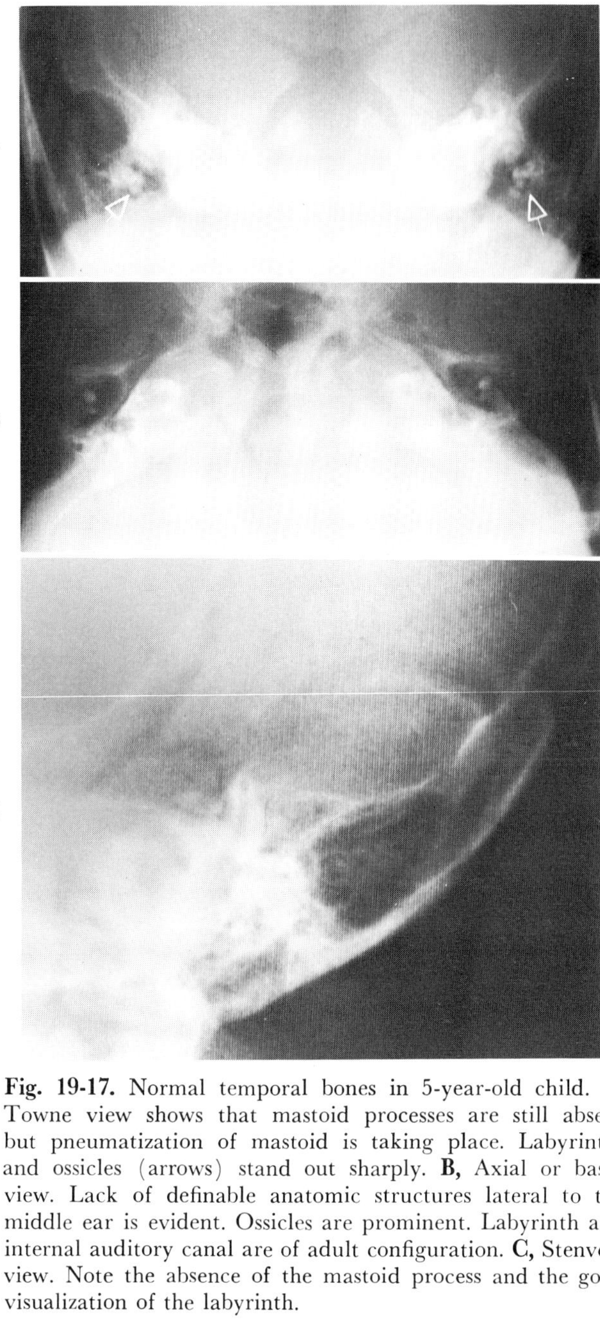

Fig. 19-17. Normal temporal bones in 5-year-old child. **A,** Towne view shows that mastoid processes are still absent but pneumatization of mastoid is taking place. Labyrinths and ossicles (arrows) stand out sharply. **B,** Axial or basal view. Lack of definable anatomic structures lateral to the middle ear is evident. Ossicles are prominent. Labyrinth and internal auditory canal are of adult configuration. **C,** Stenvers view. Note the absence of the mastoid process and the good visualization of the labyrinth.

essentially complete after 5 months of gestation, and the inner ear changes little in structure or growth into adult life. The complete development of the inner ear early in the embryonic period is a unique phenomenon.

The middle and outer ear develop from the gill or branchial structures of the embryo. At 4 weeks of gestation, the first branchial groove deepens and becomes the external auditory meatus. At the same time an evagination from the pharyngeal tissue grows outward toward the branchial cleft. Meanwhile the auricle develops from the first and second branchial arches. The first pharyngeal pouch develops into the eustachian tube and middle ear cavity. The tympanic membrane is formed of epithelial cells growing in from the first branchial groove.

The ossicles develop from the first and second branchial arches. Condensation of the first branchial arch forms the greater portion of the incus and malleus. The second branchial arch differentiates to form the stapes, the stapedial attachment to the long process of the incus, and the handle of the malleus. Each ossicle ossifies from a single center. Additional erosion and thinning in the stapes do occur, but little growth in the ossicular chain takes place after midterm. While the ossicular chain is differentiating and ossifying, the mesenchyme in the region of the middle ear loosens and is replaced by the growing epithelium of the pharyngeal pouch. Immediately after birth the loose structures of the region of the tympanic cavity expand as air enters the cavity through the eustachian tube. The cavity then becomes pneumatized in its final form.

The eustachian tube develops from the same pharyngeal pouches as the middle ear cavity; it communicates between the pharynx and the tympanic cavity. After birth, pneumatization is more rapid, extending into the mastoid area and also into the petrous bone. The mastoid processes are aerated by the projection of these pneumatized membranes into the bony structures, which replace the bone marrow. Pneumatization occasionally continues into adult years. The pneumatization of the mastoid varies considerably in different persons but tends to be symmetric from side to side.

In the newborn child the temporal bone is incompletely ossified. The osseous portion of the external auditory canal is short but develops later. The mastoid process is also absent in the neonate and does not complete its growth until the second year of life (Figs. 19-15 to 19-17).

Roentgenographic examination of temporal bone

The inadequacy of standard projections for the examination of the temporal bone is reflected in their number and diversity. Most of the views have been devised to evaluate a single part of the bone or a single type of abnormality (Compere and Valvassori, 1964). Their application, however, has often been extended to demonstrate other structures. These structures are frequently distorted by the angulation needed to displace overlying structures from the original area of interest.

The best way to evaluate the finer details of the temporal bone is by pleuridirectional tomography with a unit such as the Polytome (Brünner et al., 1961; Brünner, 1969). However, this type of study is time consuming, expensive, and technically trying, and it results in higher radiation doses than do conventional films. Its routine use therefore is difficult to justify. A compromise method is to use frontal and lateral linear tomography with a book (multilayer) cassette. In addition, one angled lateral view (Schüller) of each temporal bone is included in the examination to supply the anatomic information needed by the surgeon. These films are superior to a complete series of standard (nontomographic) films.

Many radiologists believe that standard nontomographic films of the temporal bone are required before proceeding to tomography. Such films demonstrate the gross changes; but more subtle lesions may be overlooked unless supplemental tomographic views are obtained. The following views have been suggested for the evaluation of the temporal bone (Etter and Cross, 1963; Etter, 1965).

Schüller view (or Rünstrom modification)

The Schüller projection (PA −25, +90) is an angled lateral view showing the sinodural plate, the external auditory canal, the mastoid process, the mastoid antrum, the epitympanic recess, and the drum spur (Fig. 19-5, *E*). Rünstrom (1933) recommended that the exposures be made with the mouth open to visualize the petrous apex between the anterior wall of the external auditory canal and the mandibular condyle. The ossicles are often projected into the lucent shadow of the external canal, which is seen almost end-on. Large emissary veins are often shown grooving the posterosuperior portion of the mastoid in this projection. Although useful anatomic information is obtained, the diagnostic value of these projections is minimal.

Stenvers view (Stenvers, 1917)

The Stenvers projection (PA +12, +45) gives an *en face* view of the petrous temporal bone (Fig. 19-5, *D*). It is particularly useful in the evaluation of the mastoid tip (Pendergrass et al., 1956). The internal auditory canal is foreshortened in this projection and is therefore not well demonstrated (Fig. 19-9). The hypoglossal foramen is often well shown.

Towne (half-axial) view

The Towne half-axial (AP +35) demonstrates the petrous apex, the mastoid processes, and the mastoid antrum as well as the internal auditory canal (Fig. 19-5, *B*). The density of the two mastoid processes may be compared in this projection. Increased angulation in relation to the base line demonstrates the foramen magnum and adjacent occiput.

Perorbital view

In the perorbital view of the internal auditory canals, the central ray is directed parallel to the canthomeatal line and the internal auditory canals are projected through the orbits (PA +10 or AP +10) (Fig. 19-5, *C*).

Axial view

The axial projection (AP −90) may be useful to demonstrate the internal and external auditory canals, the ossicles, and the mastoid processes (Fig. 19-5, *H*). However, finer details in the petrous temporal bone are usually difficult to evaluate in this projection. The subaxial view (AP −80) or a view with even less angulation in relation to the base line is useful to demonstrate the jugular foramina.

Mayer view

The Mayer view (AP +45, −45) or the Owen modification (AP +30, −50) is an angled oblique projection used to display the lateral wall of the epitympanic recess (drum spur) (Mayer, 1926; Owen, 1947) (Fig. 19-6). The tympanic cavity, ossicles, and mastoid antrum are also shown. The Mayer and Chaussé III views should be obtained in all patients with inflammatory or postinflammatory lesions of the middle ear.

Chaussé III

The Chaussé III view (AP +30, +15) is an excellent projection to demonstrate the drum spur and is therefore useful when cholesteatoma is suspected.

Tomography

Anteroposterior (Fig. 19-7) and lateral (Fig. 19-10) sections are usually obtained with tomography (Valvassori, 1969). Tomography is occasionally useful in the basal (Fig. 19-14), Stenvers (Fig. 19-9) or reversed Stenvers position. Each tomographic examination of the temporal bone should be closely supervised by a radiologist so that adequate correctly positioned films are obtained. A preliminary section should be obtained to check the position, coning, and exposure factors. The tomographic sections should be made no more than 2 mm apart. Sections at 1 mm intervals are needed to demonstrate finer details. Shielding of the lens of the eye is desirable to reduce the radiation dosage to the lens.

DISEASES INVOLVING TEMPORAL BONE

The temporal bone may respond to disease by showing destruction, erosion, or sclerosis. The location of a lesion involving the temporal bone often gives a clue to the nature of the lesion. (See outline.) The history and clinical findings often provide further information regarding the nature of the lesion.

Differential diagnosis of diseases affecting temporal bone (by location and type of change)

- I. Destructive (irregular marginal lucencies)
  - A. Petrous pyramid
    - 1. Inflammatory: petrositis (Gradenigo's syndrome)
    - 2. Malignant neoplasm
      - a. Nasopharyngeal carcinoma—anteromedial
      - b. Parotid tumors—anterolateral
      - c. Other metastatic neoplasia—any site
      - d. Chordoma—medial inferior
    - 3. Benign neoplasm
      - a. Glomus jugulare—inferolateral
    - 4. Other
      - a. Histiocytosis X—any site
  - B. Middle ear
    - 1. Inflammatory
    - 2. Malignant neoplasm
      - a. Squamous cell carcinoma
      - b. Sarcoma
    - 3. Glomus hypotympanicum
    - 4. Histiocytosis X
  - C. External ear and mastoid
    - 1. Inflammatory
    - 2. Malignant neoplasm
      - a. Squamous cell carcinoma
      - b. Parotid tumor
      - c. Sarcoma
- II. Erosive (lucent pressure defect, well-defined margins, with or without sclerosis)
  - A. Petrous apex
    - 1. Fifth-nerve neurinoma
    - 2. Epidermoid in cerebellopontine angle cistern
    - 3. Aneurysm (intracavernous or intrapetrous carotid)
    - 4. Meningioma (Meckel's cave)
  - B. Lateral two thirds of petrous pyramid
    - 1. Subarachnoid cyst
    - 2. Glioma
  - C. Internal auditory meatus, canal, or both
    - 1. Acoustic neuroma
    - 2. Patulous canal—normal
    - 3. Facial nerve neuroma
    - 4. Vascular
      - a. Aneurysm
      - b. Bilateral anterior inferior cerebellar artery loop
    - 5. Increased intracranial pressure
    - 6. Meningioma
  - D. Middle ear and antrum
    - 1. Cholesteatoma
    - 2. Granuloma
    - 3. Postsurgical change
  - E. Mastoid
    - 1. Cholesteatoma
    - 2. Facial nerve neuroma
    - 3. Postsurgical change
  - F. External canal
    - 1. Inclusion cyst
  - G. Jugular foramen
    - 1. Glomus jugulare
    - 2. Neuroma
    - 3. Meningioma
    - 4. Chondroma
- III. Sclerotic
  - A. Postinflammatory
  - B. Paget's disease
  - C. Otosclerosis
  - D. Fibrous dysplasia
  - E. Adult Pyle's disease (craniometaphyseal dysplasia)
  - F. Mucopolysaccharidosis
  - G. Nasopharyngeal carcinoma (usually postradiation therapy)
  - H. Osteopetrosis

Infections

The roentgenographic changes caused by infection do not depend on etiology but on duration of the disease. Otitis media and acute and subacute mastoiditis may cause no roentgenographic changes.

Acute infection

Acute infection is usually caused by organisms reaching the tympanic cavity via the eustachian tube. Quite probably organisms also reach the tympanic cavity via the external auditory meatus, the internal auditory meatus, the lymphatics, and the blood vessels. The organisms are usually streptococci, staphylococci, or pneumococci. The mucosa of the tympanic cavity may become edematous, and fluid may accumulate in the middle ear. These changes may also extend into the mastoid antrum and air cells. The eustachian tube usually becomes blocked by edema. A partial vacuum then forms in the tympanic cavity and causes retraction of the tympanic membrane.

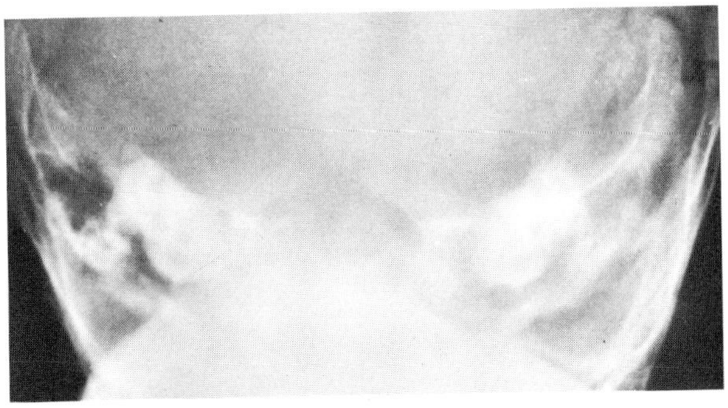

Fig. 19-18. Acute mastoiditis. A 6-month-old child with clouding of all mastoid air cells on the left. Compare with the normally developed and pneumatized right side (reader's left).

Roentgenographic examination of the ear may show no abnormality associated with otitis media. The earliest change seen in acute infection is usually an overall clouding (increased radiodensity) of the pneumatized portions of the temporal bone. This change is caused by thickening of the membranes by edema or in more advanced cases by an exudate within the air cells (MacPherson and Dunbar, 1965) (Figs. 19-18 and 19-19). If antibiotic therapy is instituted at this stage, the inflammatory changes may subside, leaving no residual roentgenographic changes. If therapy is not effective, the changes may progress to destruction of the bony cell walls, first seen roentgenographically as blurring of the septa. Focal areas of lucency indicate destruction and abscess formation. These changes are most common in the mastoid area but may be seen in other parts of the temporal bone (Figs. 19-20 and 19-21). Spread of the inflammation may lead to osteomyelitis or abscess formation in the petrous pyramid. Acute petrositis associated

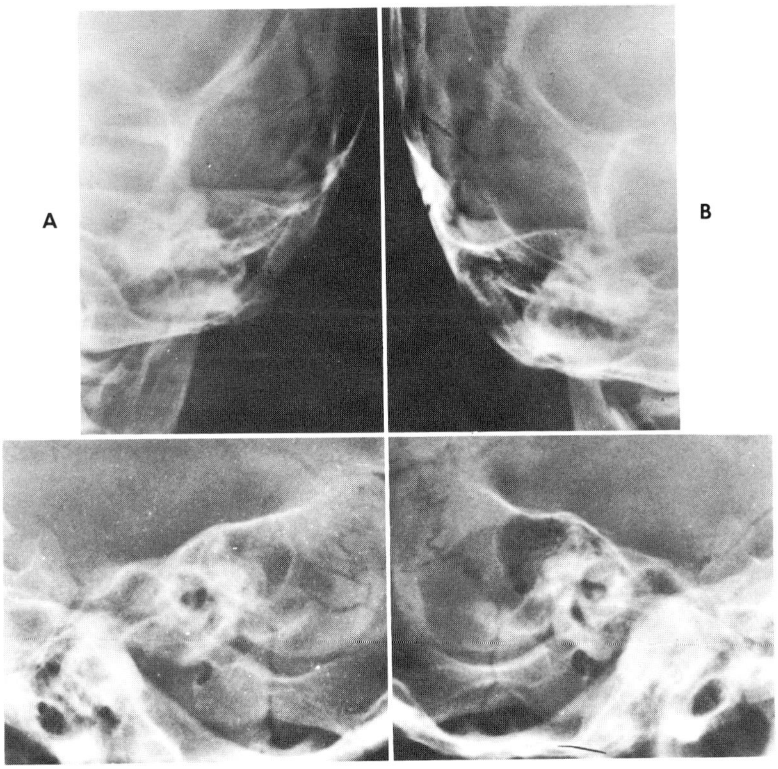

Fig. 19-19. Subacute mastoiditis. A 1-year-old child with recurrent drainage from the left ear. **A,** Stenvers view of left mastoid area shows clouding and indistinctness of the air cells secondary to edema, fluid, and possibly some decalcification of the walls of the air cells. **B,** Stenvers view of normal side, for comparison. **C,** Law projection of left side shows clouding of the petromastoid region and blurring of the septa or walls. **D,** Law view of normal side, for comparison.

A

B

C

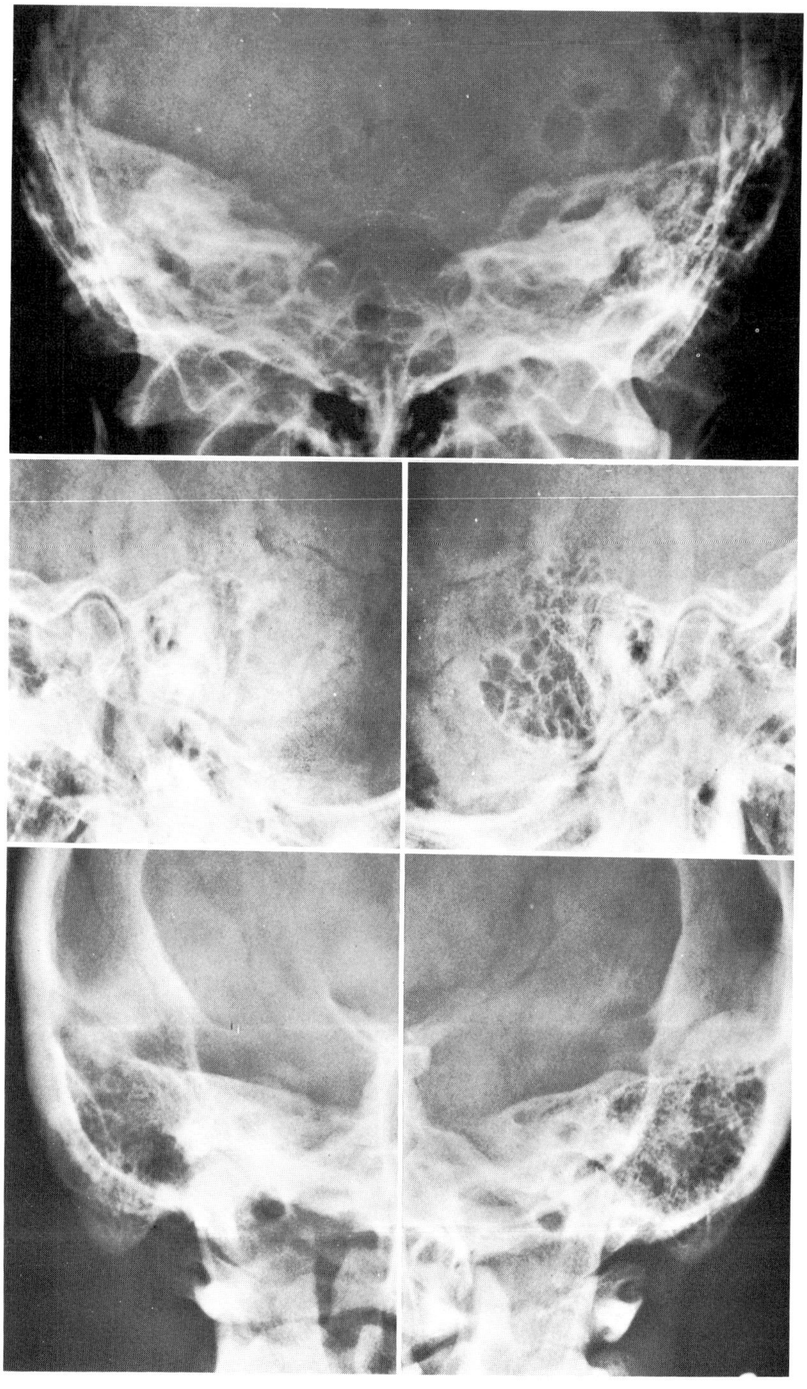

Fig. 19-20. Mastoiditis with abscess formation. **A,** Towne projection. Right side (viewer's left) shows clouding and loss of definition of the mastoid air cells. Left side is normal. **B,** Law projection. Note the destruction and clouding of the mastoid and petromastoid region on the right. Left mastoid is well aerated. **C,** Stenvers projection. Note the increased density and loss of air cell definition on the affected side (viewer's left).

A B C

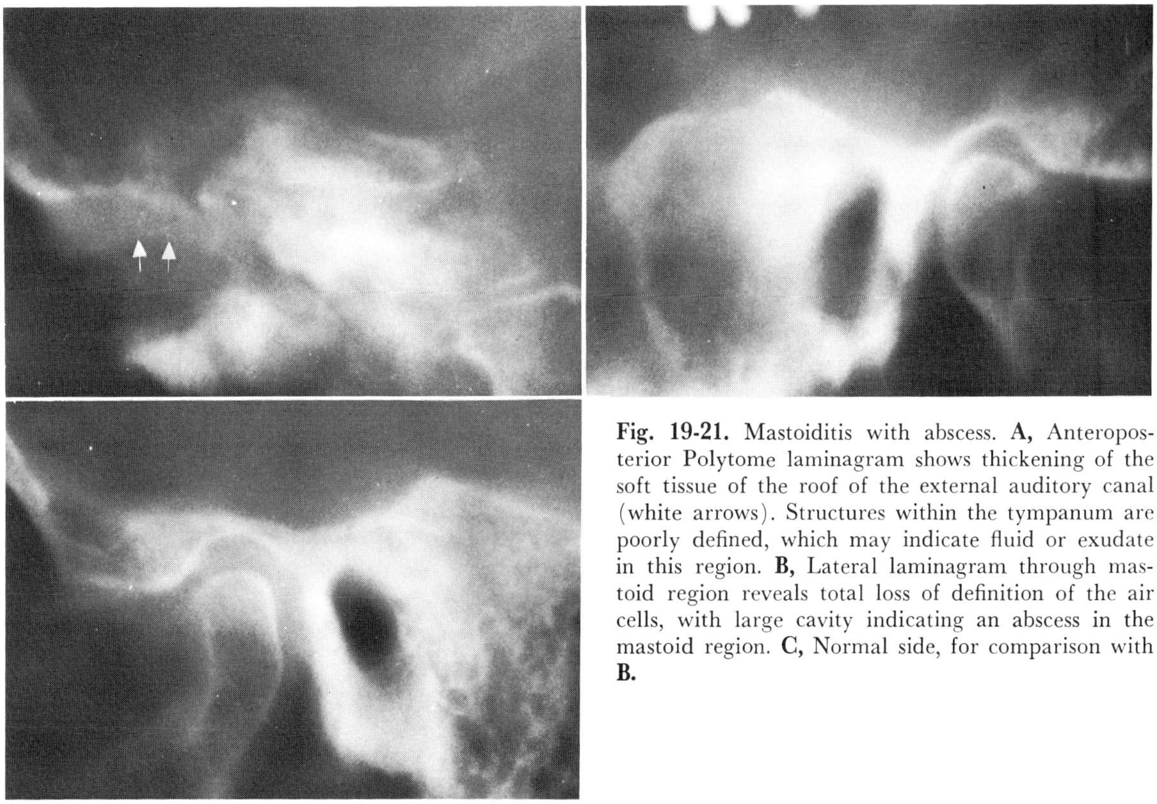

Fig. 19-21. Mastoiditis with abscess. **A,** Anteroposterior Polytome laminagram shows thickening of the soft tissue of the roof of the external auditory canal (white arrows). Structures within the tympanum are poorly defined, which may indicate fluid or exudate in this region. **B,** Lateral laminagram through mastoid region reveals total loss of definition of the air cells, with large cavity indicating an abscess in the mastoid region. **C,** Normal side, for comparison with **B.**

A B C D

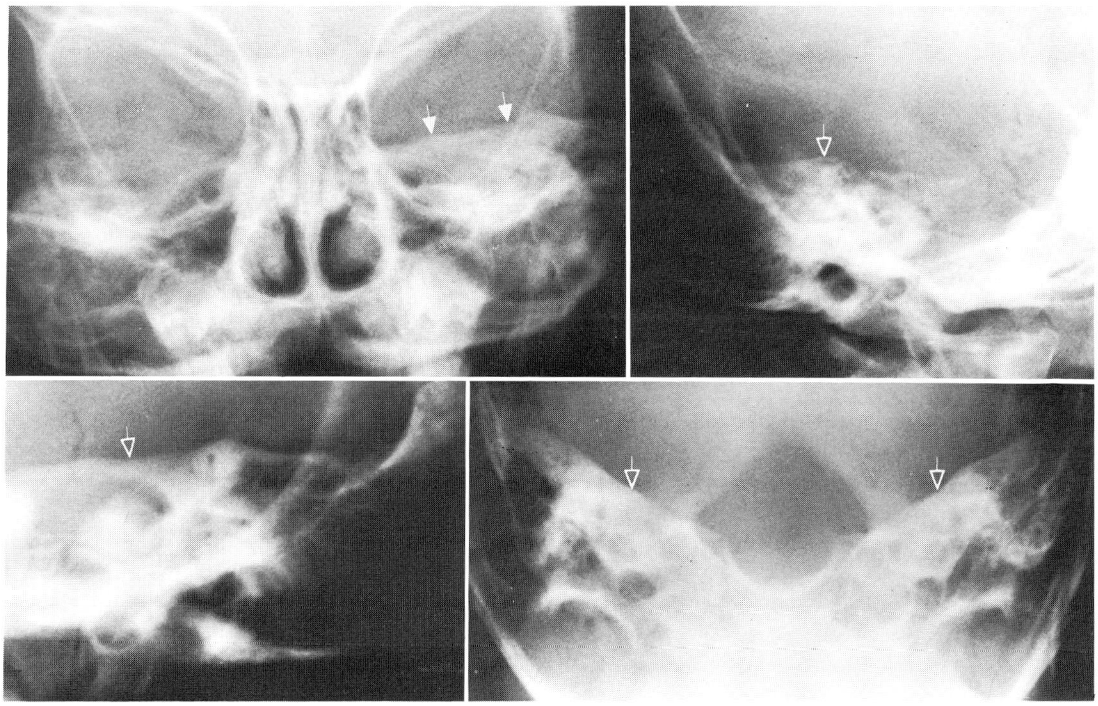

Fig. 19-22. Petrositis (Gradenigo's syndrome). **A,** Caldwell view shows the right petrous pyramid destroyed. Left petrous ridge (arrows) is normal. **B,** Stenvers view shows the petrous pyramid medial to the superior semicircular canal (arrow) destroyed. **C,** Stenvers view of normal side, for comparison. **D,** Towne view 9 months later shows reconstitution and normal calcification of the petrous pyramids. Petrous ridges are indicated by arrows. Large lucent cavity lateral to the labyrinth on the right is secondary to a mastoidectomy. Patient had been treated with antibiotic therapy and made an uneventful recovery.

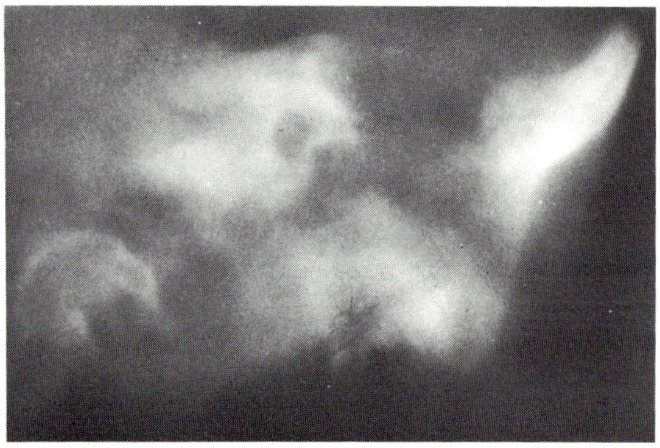

Fig. 19-23. Mastoid abscess with breakthrough into the cranial vault. AP Polytome laminagram of the left temporal bone reveals a large cavity destroying most of the petrous pyramid lateral to the labyrinth. Tympanic and external auditory canal structures are not defined. Cavity represents the large petromastoid abscess that had extended superiorly. A brain abscess was removed, and then mastoid surgery was performed.

with inflammation of the surrounding tissues leads to Gradenigo's syndrome (diplopia, periorbital pain, and otorrhea). This entity is characterized roentgenographically by irregular destruction with spotty radiolucencies scattered through the petrous pyramid (Figs. 19-22 and 19-23). Displacement of bony fragments away from their normal position may cause apparent bone enlargement.

Chronic infection

When the infection has been present for a longer period, sclerosis or increased density of the temporal bone develops. If the infection occurs in the first 2 years of life, the bone may not pneumatize, which increases the sclerotic appearance. Dense sclerosis of a completely pneumatized bone may also develop with low-grade infections (Fig. 19-24).

The history, physical examination, and clinical course give a better assessment of the activity of the infection than does the roentgenographic appearance. It is therefore better for the radiologist to give a descriptive diagnosis, such as sclerotic mastoid disease, and to indicate the amount of pneumatization rather than attempt to determine the activity of the infection or its chronicity from the roentgenographic appearance alone.

Granuloma

Subacute or chronic disease may cause a granulomatous reaction in the tympanic cavity or mastoid antrum. The granuloma first obliterates the air-containing space with soft-tissue density. This finding is best shown by tomography and by comparison of the involved with the normal side. The diagnosis may be difficult if both sides are similarly involved.

A

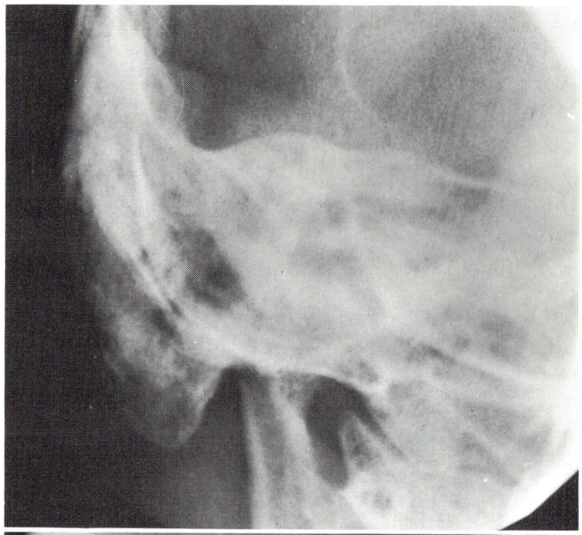

B

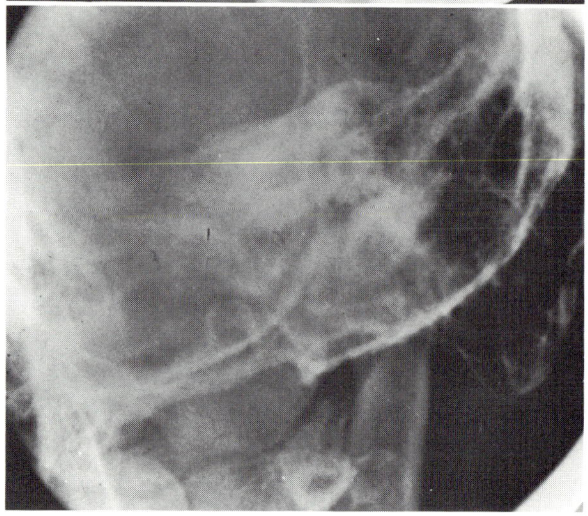

Fig. 19-24. Chronic mastoiditis in a patient with a long history of draining ear. **A,** Stenvers view shows extensive sclerosis of the entire petromastoid region, indicating osteitis secondary to the mastoiditis. Presence of some air cells indicates that the bone was initially normally pneumatized. **B,** Normal side, for comparison.

Later pressure from the expanding granuloma may erode the bony walls of the tympanic cavity or mastoid antrum, causing enlargement of these structures. The regular, smooth, and well-defined erosion indicates pressure rather than infiltrative destruction.

Postoperative changes

After a mastoidectomy the radiographic evaluation of the temporal bone may be difficult. A large amount of bone may be removed around the medial end of the external auditory canal during a radical or modified radical mastoidectomy (Figs. 19-25 and 19-26). In addition, the ossicles may be excised and the epitympanic recess and mastoid antrum may be surgically

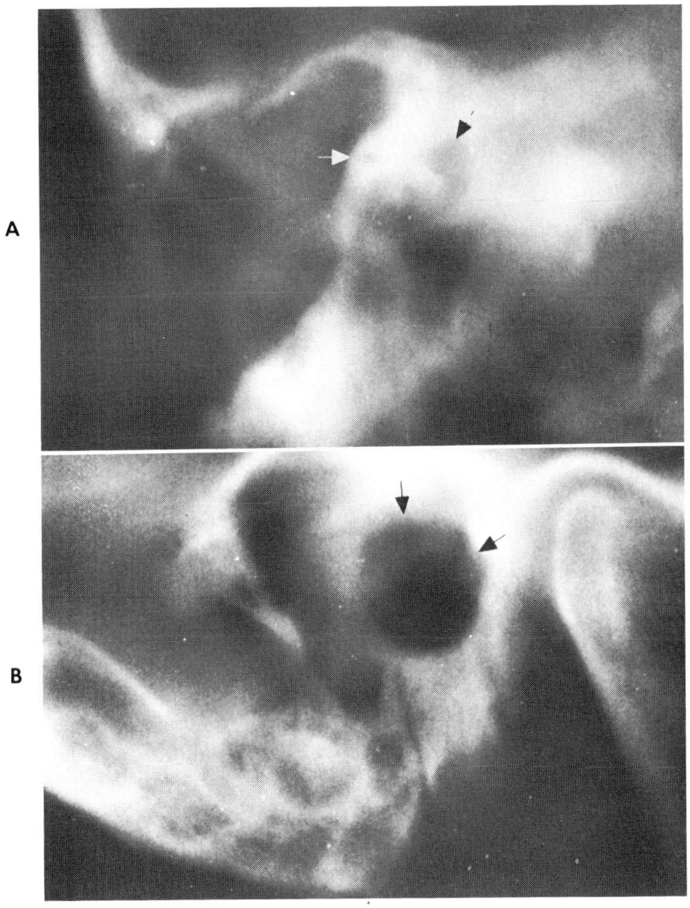

Fig. 19-25. Radical mastoidectomy. **A,** Anteroposterior laminagram of petrous bone shows the vestibule (black arrow) and lateral semicircular canal (white arrow). Large cavity lateral to these structures results from a radical mastoidectomy. Note that the ossicles are absent and that the excavation is carried up to the tegmen tympani. **B,** Lateral Polytome laminagram reveals a large mastoidectomy defect extending into the area of the tympanum (black arrows) and posteriorly to the wall of the petrous pyramid.

enlarged. In such cases evaluation of any changes when compared with previous films is important. Soft-tissue densities in the surgical cavity noted months or years after the surgery may indicate residual inflammatory tissue.

The margins of surgical defects tend to be regular, whereas those of inflammatory defects are irregular. Occasionally a surgical defect may allow downward herniation of the dura and brain through the roof of the external canal (Baron, 1969). The edges of the defect, which are beveled inward from above, suggest a downward protruding mass from the cranial cavity (Fig. 19-27).

Intracranial complications

Destructive inflammatory changes in the superior or posterior surfaces of the petrous temporal bone may lead to an abscess in either the temporal lobe or the cerebellum (Fig. 19-23). Occasionally the intracranial infection is limited to the subdural or extradural spaces. Chronic infections may also cause phlebitis of the lateral or sigmoid dural vein sinuses, which may result in sinus thrombosis. This thrombosis may extend to the opposite side.

Cholesteatoma

Cholesteatoma may be primary or secondary. Primary cholesteatomas, which are developmental in origin, are much less common (Brosnan, 1967) than secondary cholesteatomas that are the result of inflammatory ear disease. The roentgenographic changes of primary and secondary cholesteatomas are identical.

Those cholesteatomas associated with inflammatory ear disease usually follow a perforation of the tympanic membrane, most commonly in its posterior and superior portion. When the tympanic membrane is perforated, the normal reparative processes may loculate invaginated epithelial cells from the membrane to form an inclusion in the tympanic cavity. These loculated cells

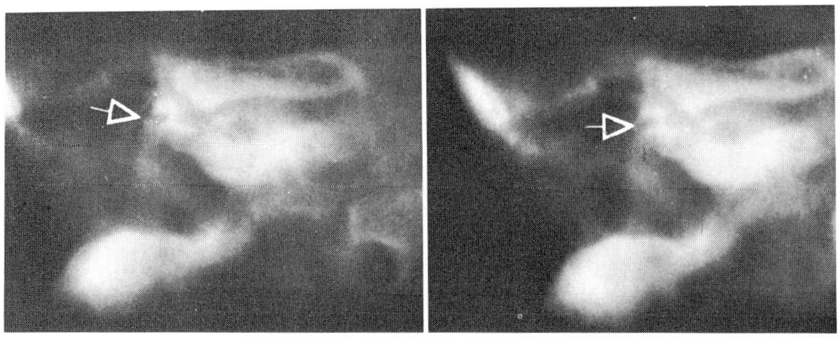

Fig. 19-26. Radical mastoidectomy with labyrinth fistula. Polytome laminagrams, frontal projection, show a cavity lateral to the labyrinth, the result of a radical mastoidectomy. Usually dense wall of the lateral semicircular canal (arrows) is absent. This indicates the presence of a fistula between the labyrinth and the mastoidectomy cavity.

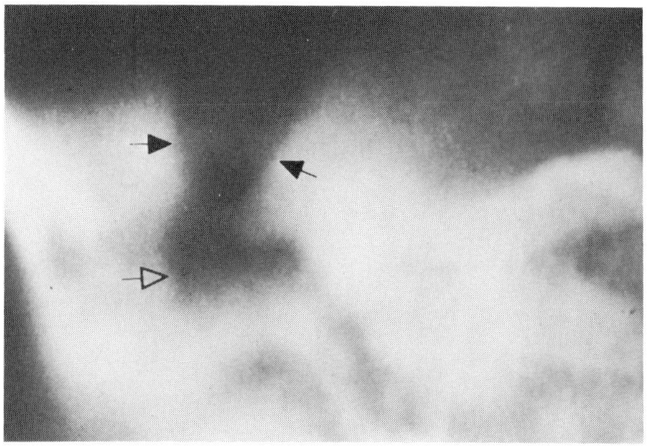

Fig. 19-27. Dural herniation through superior mastoidectomy defect. Patient had had a mastoidectomy and later developed pneumocephalus. Polytome laminagram, frontal projection, reveals a medially beveled defect (solid black arrows) in roof of the petrous bone above the external auditory canal. Air extends superiorly from the external auditory canal (open black arrow). This type of beveling suggests downward herniation of the dura. Such herniation may be a complication of mastoidectomy, which weakens the bony partition and allows eventual rupture of the dura and subarachnoid space into the ear.

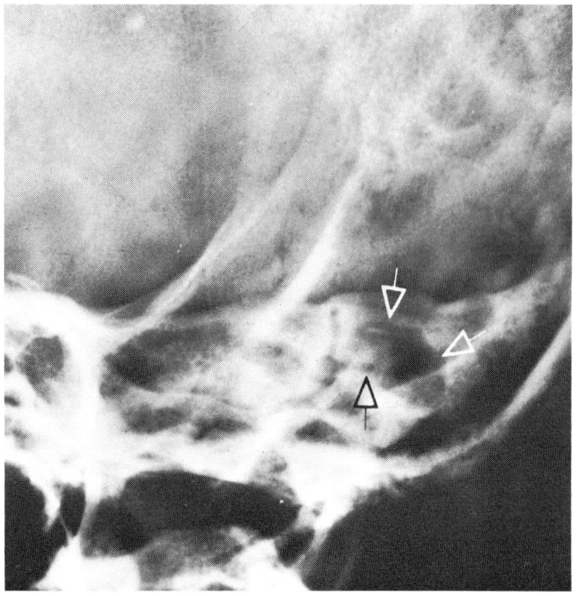

Fig. 19-28. Cholesteatoma. This patient, a 25-year-old woman, with a long history of chronic otitis media on the involved side, had large lucency (white open arrows) in the tympano-antral area (Stenvers view), which proved to be a large cholesteatoma. Antrum measures 16 mm in diameter, which is above the normal limits of 12 mm. Black open arrow indicates lateral semicircular canal extending laterally from the vestibule. Its lateral margin is indistinct and somewhat lucent. These changes suggest some pressure erosion of this canal by the cholesteatoma. Ossicles are not visualized.

continue their normal desquamative process. Since there is no drainage from the inclusion, the desquamative products accumulate and an enlarging secondary cholesteatoma results. As the cholesteatoma increases in size, the adjacent bony structures, such as the ossicular chain, attic, antrum, and tympanum, are eroded by local pressure.

Since more than 95% of cholesteatomas are visible on otologic examination, the roentgenographic studies in most cases serve to define the size and extent of the lesion rather than to make the diagnosis. On rare occasions, such as in congenital ear malformations in which the tympanic membrane is not visible or in primary cholesteatoma not located in the tympanum, an otologic diagnosis is impossible. In these instances the roentgenographic examination is necessary for the diagnosis.

The earliest roentgenographic sign of a secondary cholesteatoma is partial to complete destruction of the bony projection, which represents the innermost portion of the roof of the external auditory canal (Brünner and Sandberg, 1970). This projection of bone, called the drum spur or bony bridge, also forms the lateral wall of the epitympanic recess or attic. It appears as a sharp downward and medial extension of dense bone and is best evaluated by standard roentgenograms in the Chaussé III projection (Chaussé, 1950; Sansregret, 1963). The destruction of the drum spur usually occurs close to the attachment of the superior portion of the tympanic membrane. Minor erosions of the drum spur caused by a cholesteatoma or granulation tissue may be demonstrated only if tomographic cuts are made at 1 mm intervals and compared with the normal side. This roentgenographic technique is the procedure of choice to examine the bone in this disease.

As the cholesteatoma expands, additional bony changes take place. Extension of the cholesteatoma into the epitympanic recess and the mastoid antrum enlarges these structures (Brünner et al., 1966) (Figs. 19-28 to 19-30). (The aditus ad antrum, or passage between the attic and antrum, has no well-defined borders and is not roentgenographically visible.) The antrum is normally cone-shaped with a base superiorly and measures no more than 12 mm. The two antra are usually symmetric in size and shape. Enlargement of the mastoid antrum, indicating a large cholesteatoma (MacMillan, 1936), is rarely seen today since this lesion is being diagnosed earlier. A soft-tissue mass within the tympanic cavity (Fig. 19-31) or evidence of destruction or demineralization of portions or all of the ossicular chain may also be noted on roentgenograms. These changes caused by cholesteatomas are indistinguishable roentgenographically

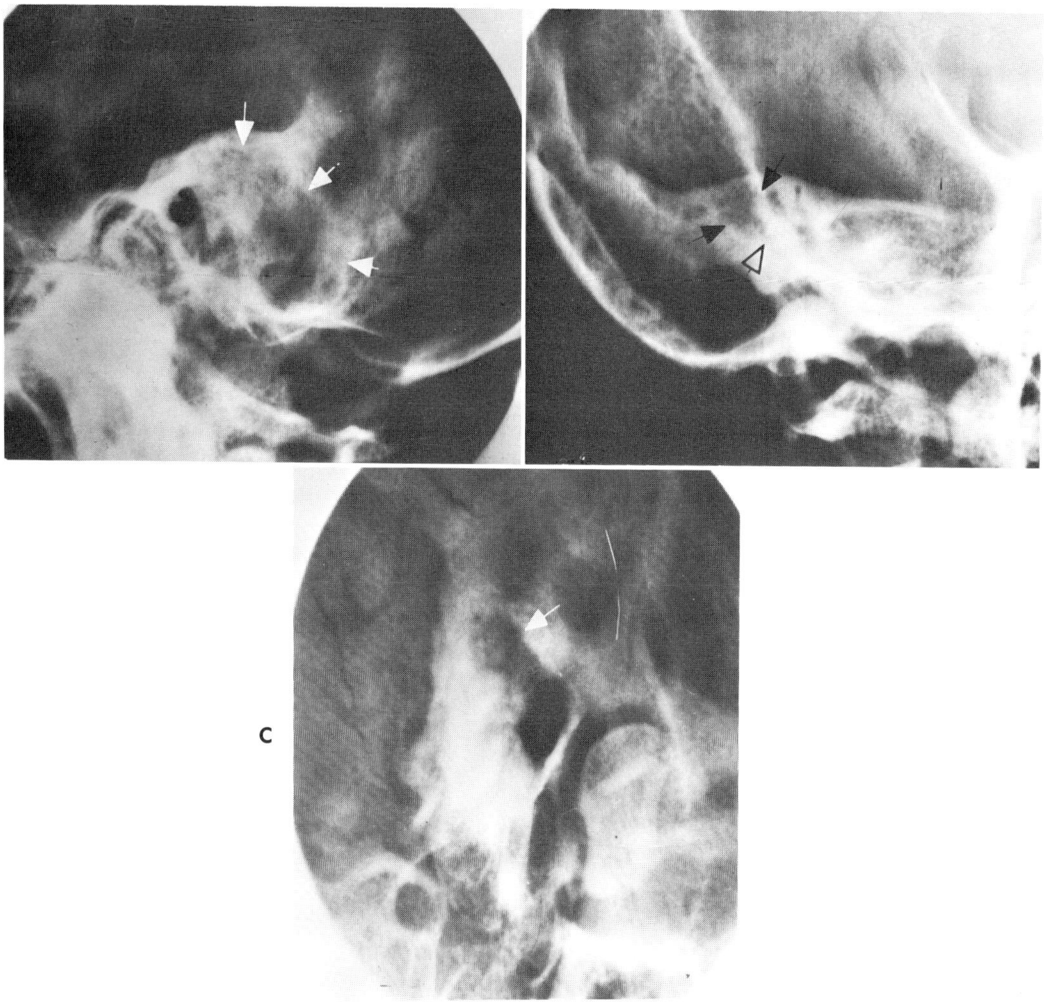

Fig. 19-29. Cholesteatoma. Long history of otitis media with drainage. **A,** Law view shows a large lucent defect (white arrows), extending posteriorly from the region of the antrum and involving most of the underpneumatized sclerotic mastoid bone. **B,** Stenvers view shows a large defect in the antrum (solid black arrows). Thinning of bone overlying the semicircular canal (open black arrow) suggests the presence of a labyrinth fistula, which was later proved surgically. **C,** Mayer view shows destruction of the epitympanic area and erosion upward into the antral area (white arrow). No ossicles are visible, which indicates extensive destruction by the cholesteatoma.

from severe involvement of the tympanic cavity by granulation tissue secondary to chronic inflammation. Either cholesteatoma or granulation tissue may erode the lateral semicircular canal, leading to a fistula. This complication may be identifiable roentgenographically by the loss of the normal sclerotic bone that surrounds the canal (Rovsing and Jensen, 1968) (Fig. 19-26). Standard frontal and lateral views, however, may not be sufficient to identify this lesion. Therefore a basal or axial view, which places the entire lateral edge of the semicircular canal in profile on one film, is the projection of choice if the fistula is suspected clinically.

Trauma

Fractures

Fractures of the temporal bone may accompany any severe head injury, especially if the blow strikes the lateral posterior aspect of the skull. Plain roentgenograms are positive, however, in only 25% to 30% of petrous pyramid fractures diagnosed clinically on the basis of blood in the tympanic cavity, hearing loss, or clinical evidence of damage to the facial nerve. A much higher percentage of these fractures may be diagnosed with the aid of pleuridirectional laminagraphy.

Fractures of the squamous temporal bone are very

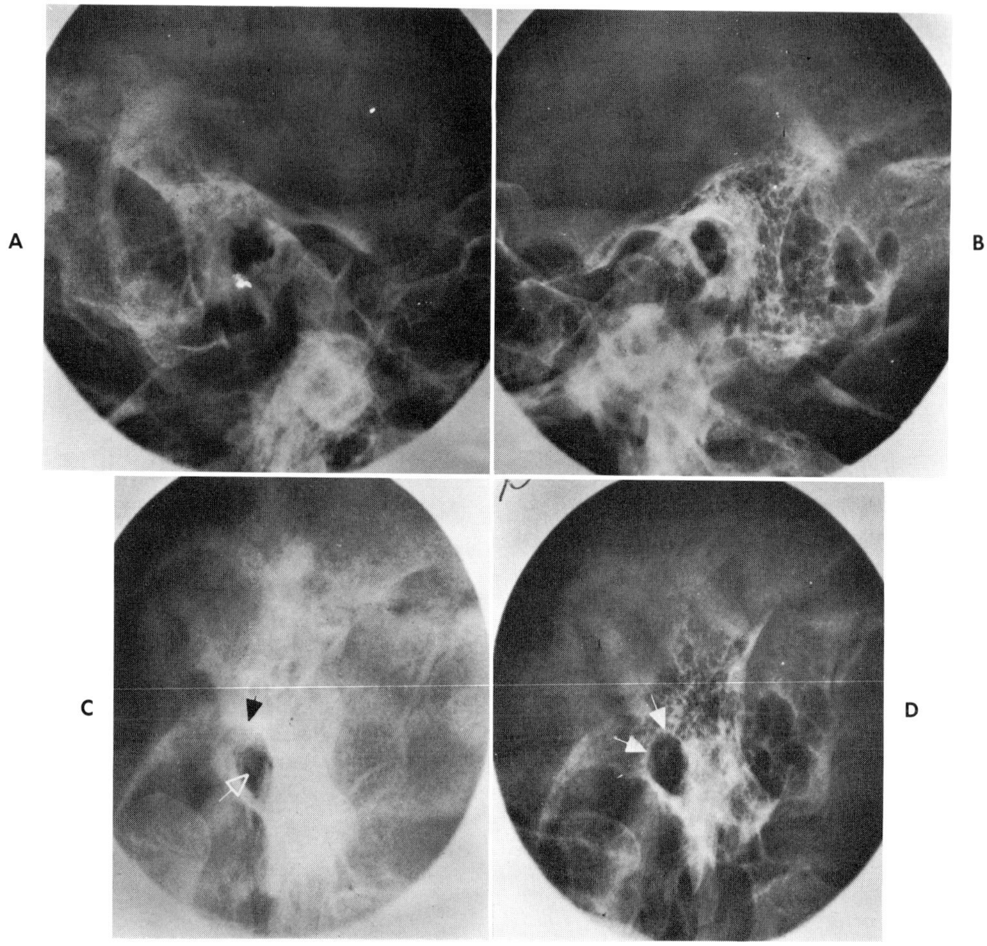

Fig. 19-30. Cholesteatoma. This patient had a 25-year history of drainage with perforation of the tympanic membrane. **A,** Law view shows the petromastoid region underpneumatized and sclerotic. Enlargement of the antrum is not demonstrated. **B,** Normal left side, for comparison with **A. C,** Mayer view shows the mastoid and petromastoid regions sclerotic. Epitympanic recess (black arrow) is widened, with loss of its anterior margin. Malleus is identified (open white arrow) projecting into the canal. **D,** Mayer view of normal side, for comparison, shows the epitympanic recess sharply demarcated (white arrows). Ossicular shadows are well seen.

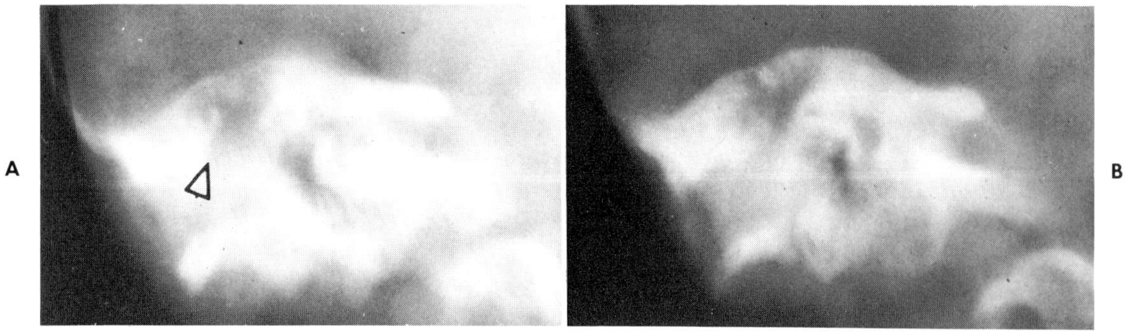

Fig. 19-31. Cholesteatoma. **A,** Polytome laminagram, frontal projection, shows a large soft-tissue mass filling the medial external canal (under arrowhead) and the tympanum (medial to arrowhead). This was a large cholesteatoma. Arrow indicates erosion of bone of the external auditory canal—attic border (the drum spur)—hallmark of a cholesteatoma. **B,** Section slightly posterior to **A** again shows absence of the drum spur.

A

B

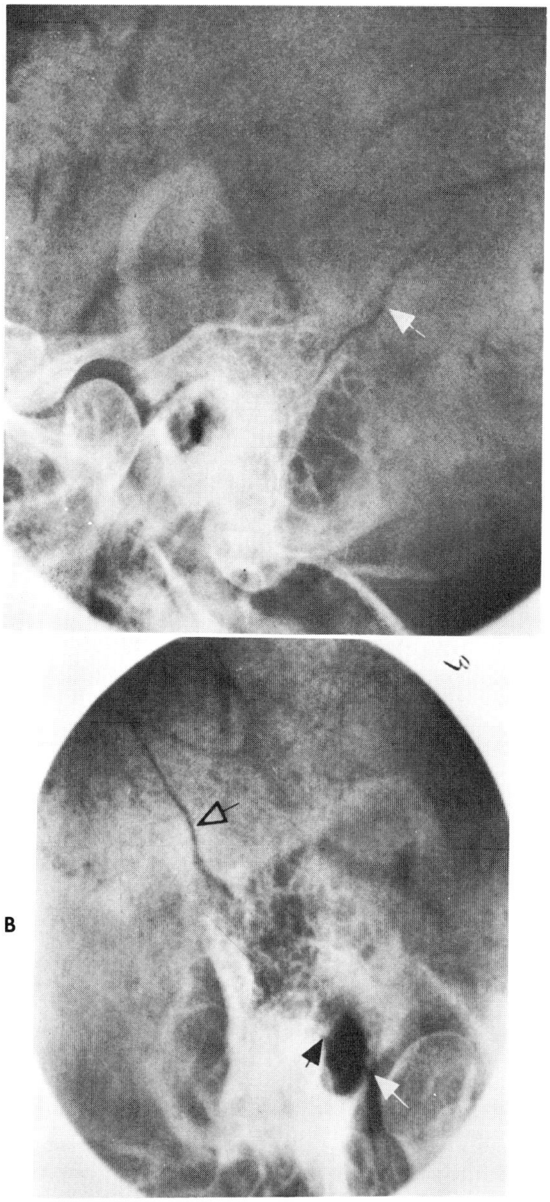

Fig. 19-32. Fracture. **A,** Law view of temporal bone shows a longitudinal fracture line (arrow) extending inferiorly from the squamous portion into the upper area of the mastoid process of the temporal bone. Note some clouding of the mastoid air cells, presumably secondary to hemorrhage. **B,** Mayer-Owen view shows the fracture (open black arrows) extending through the upper portion of the mastoid process, involving both the posterior (solid black arrow) and the anterior (white arrow) walls of the external auditory canal. Extension of this fracture medially into remainder of the temporal bone would constitute a longitudinal fracture.

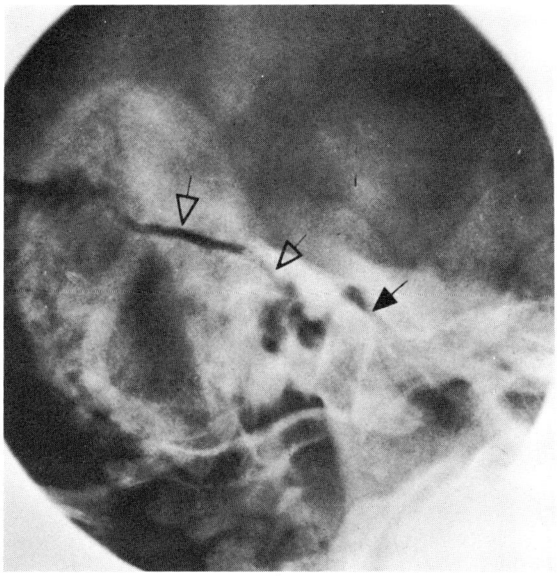

Fig. 19-33. Fracture. Angled lateral view shows a wide fracture line (open arrows) extending across the superior part of the mastoid portion of the temporal bone and involving the external auditory canal superiorly. For orientation, black arrow indicates the condylar process of the mandible seated in the mandibular fossa.

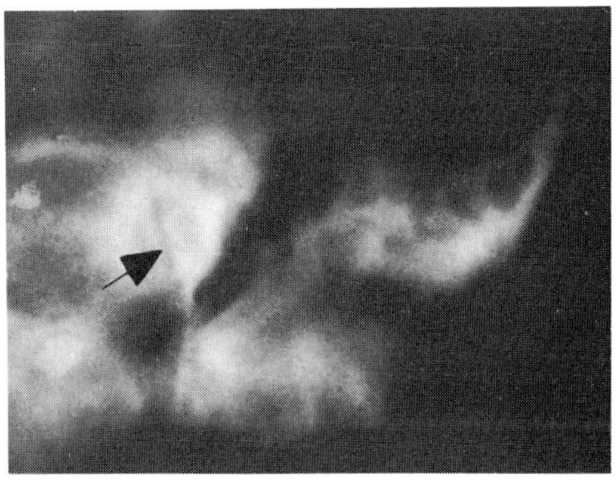

Fig. 19-34. Fracture. Polytome laminagram, frontal projection, at level of the cochlea shows a fracture line (black arrow) through the cochlea. This is an example of a transverse fracture through the petrous pyramid. It was difficult to identify on the plain films.

common (Figs. 19-32 and 19-33) and are discussed in Chapter 39. Depending on the relation of the fracture to the axis of the petrous pyramid, fractures of the remaining temporal bone can be divided into three categories: transverse, longitudinal, and complex. Transverse fractures cross the longitudinal axis of the petrous bone (Fig. 19-34), and longitudinal fractures (Figs. 19-35 and 19-36) are parallel to this axis (Kaseff, 1969). Transverse fractures are the type most often seen on plain films. Although most transverse fractures are just lateral to or through the labyrinth, they may occur as far medially as the internal auditory canal. Fractures that involve the more lateral aspect of the petrous pyramid are usually longitudinal or complex. The longitudinal fractures may be divided into the

A

B

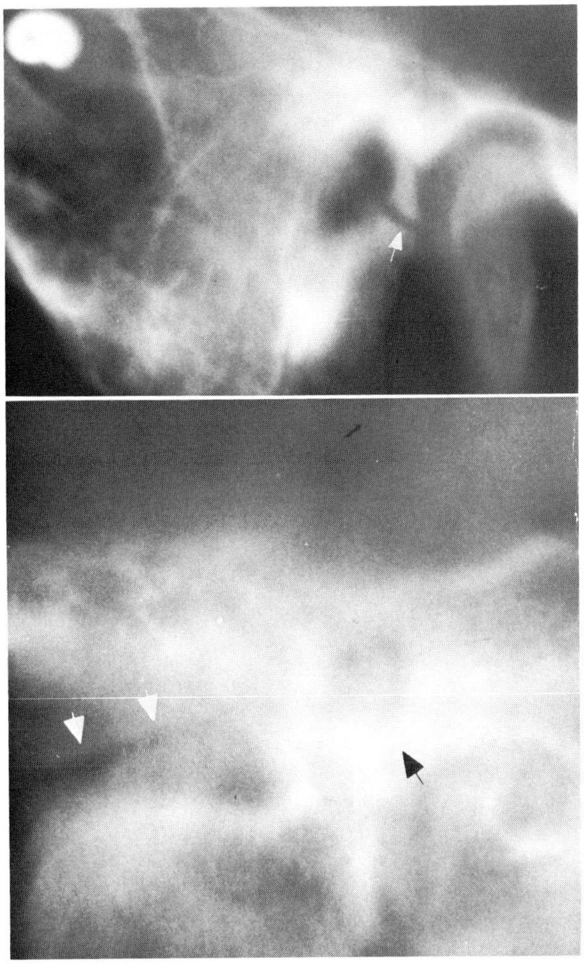

Fig. 19-35. Fracture. **A,** Polytome laminagram of the external auditory canal and mastoid tip at level of the condylar process, lateral projection, shows a sharply defined fracture line (arrow) extending through the anterior wall of the external auditory canal. **B,** Polytome laminagram, frontal projection, shows extent of the longitudinal fracture line (white arrows) in the anterior wall of the external auditory canal. Black arrow indicates cochlear shadow for orientation.

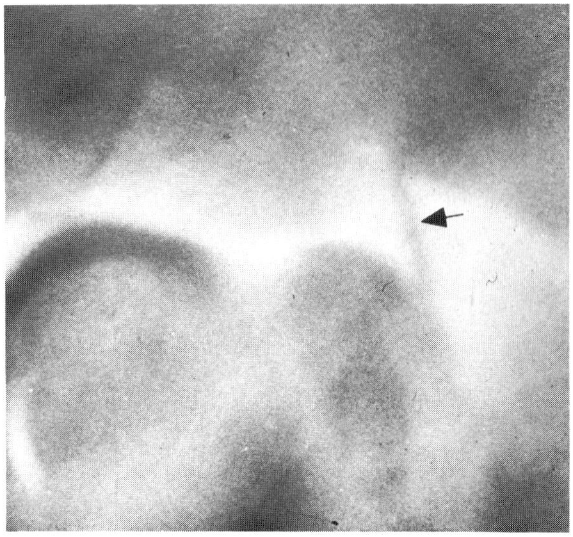

Fig. 19-36. Fracture. Polytome laminagram of the temporal bone at level of the condylar process (viewer's left) of mandible, lateral projection, shows a vertical fracture line (arrow) extending from the roof of the external auditory canal superiorly through the floor of the cranial cavity. Other fractures were present.

anterior and the posterior types (Harwood-Nash, 1970). The anterior type is associated with a fracture of the anterior parietotemporal regions and usually extends along the anterior aspect of the petrous bone through the tegmen tympani to the region of the labyrinth capsule. The posterior type of longitudinal fracture is usually associated with a fracture of the posterior parietal bone and involves the superior mastoid complex and the posterior and superior portions of the petrous bone. This type may also converge on the labyrinth complex. Harwood-Nash (1970) has indicated that, although longitudinal fractures may cross the semicircular canals, the vestibule remains uninvolved and the cochlea is seldom involved. More medially the fractures may extend from the region of the labyrinth either along the roof of the eustachian tube or to one of the nearby foramina, the foramen lacerum, the jugular foramen, or the internal auditory meatus. Those that affect the internal auditory meatus also involve the posterior fossa. The anterior longitudinal fractures tend to extend to the facial canal in the anterior part of its horizontal portion. The posterior longitudinal fractures more often involve the facial canal in the upper part of its vertical portion.

Complex fractures of the temporal bone may have longitudinal and transverse components, and there may be considerable fragmentation of the petrous bone.

Ossicular disruption

Severe head injury may also result in disruption of the ossicular chain, usually caused by dislocation of the incus or malleus, rarely the stapes (Figs. 19-37 and 19-38). The incudomalleolar or incudostapedial joints may be separated. This type of injury classically causes an acute hearing loss of about 60 decibels. The most common dislocation is superolateral and posterior displacement of the incus. Ossicular dislocations are best seen in the lateral pleuridirectional laminagram (Potter, 1969; Wright et al., 1969) (Fig. 19-39); but if severe, they sometimes can be shown on the frontal laminagrams (Fig. 19-40). Comparison of the involved side with the normal side is especially helpful in these cases. Slight dislocations or disarticulations may not be evident roentgenographically, even with superb lamina-

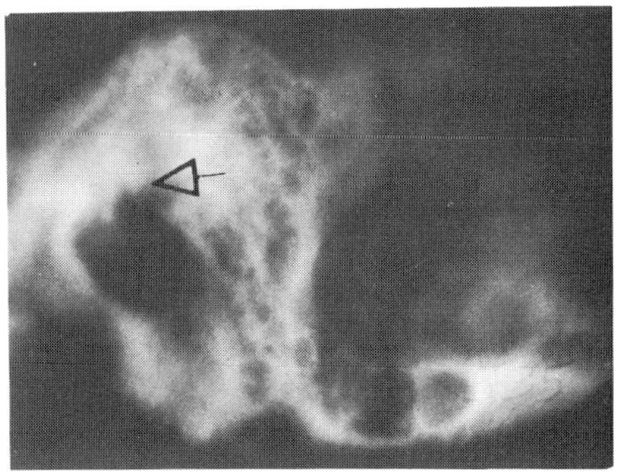

Fig. 19-37. Ossicular dislocation. Polytome laminagram of the petrous bone at level of the malleus and incus, lateral projection, shows slight dislocation of the incus (arrow). Incus is slightly inferior, and its long process slightly posterior, to the normal position.

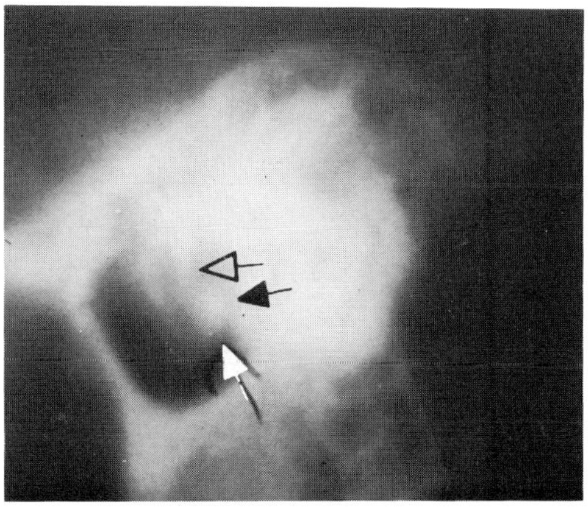

Fig. 19-39. Ossicular dislocation. Polytome laminagram of the temporal bone, lateral projection, shows normal position of the long process of the incus (open arrow). Patient had suffered acute hearing loss after head trauma. Note the fracture through the anterior wall of the external auditory canal. There is a bony fragment (between solid white and solid black arrows), which resulted from a posterior tympanic fracture. This bony fragment is wedged anteriorly into the long process of the incus, causing malfunction. Restoration of hearing followed surgical correction.

A

B

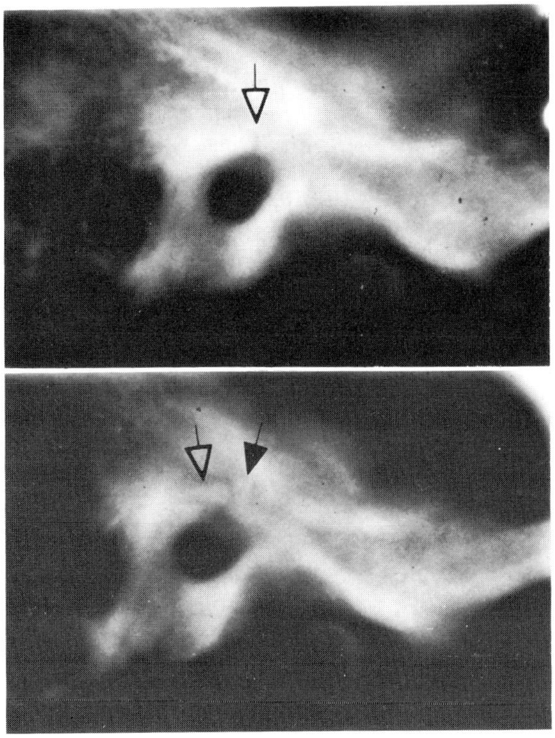

Fig. 19-38. Fracture and dislocation of ossicular chain. A, Polytome laminagram of the temporal bone at level of the external auditory canal, lateral projection, shows a fracture (arrow) extending through the roof of the external auditory canal. B, Polytome laminagram, lateral projection, with the cut several millimeters medial to A. Incus (open arrow) is so situated that its long process projects posteriorly. Note the relatively normal position of the malleus (solid arrow).

graphic sections. In these cases, if deafness is an immediate result of the trauma but fracture or ossicular chain dislocation is not shown, exploration of the middle ear may be necessary.

Fractures of facial nerve canal

Facial nerve paresis may result from a fracture of the temporal bone (Jongkees, 1965). The nerve can be injured anywhere along its course but is most commonly affected in the descending portion of the canal. The entire bony facial canal should be evaluated with both anteroposterior and lateral laminagraphy. Longitudinal fractures tend to involve either the horizontal or the vertical portions of the facial nerve canal. Transverse fractures that extend through the middle ear cavity may involve the facial nerve canal in its horizontal portion medial to the tympanic cavity. All fractures near the facial nerve canal should be carefully evaluated. A fragment from one of these fractures may cause facial nerve compression, and decompression may be necessary. Even if the facial nerve has been severed completely, surgical repair may result in eventual recovery. Occasionally disruption of the canal of the facial nerve may be seen without any clinical evidence of abnormality of function of the nerve within it.

External canal fracture

In severe head injury the external auditory canal is often involved by fracture (Figs. 19-35, 19-38, and

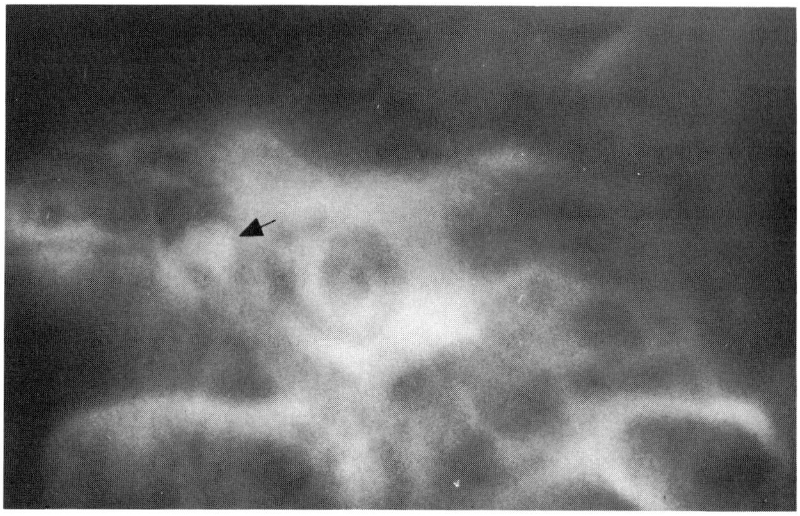

Fig. 19-40. Ossicular dislocation. Polytome laminagram at level of the cochlea, frontal projection, shows density representing the ossicular mass (arrow) somewhat enlarged and relatively more superior and laterally placed than normal. This is due to rotation of the head of the incus to a lateral and superior position. On the lateral view, relationship of the ossicular chain was relatively normal.

19-40). The fracture may extend into the mandibular fossa or extend superiorly to involve the floor of the middle cranial fossa. The associated swelling and hematoma around the external auditory canal may be shown roentgenographically when the air shadow in the external canal is narrowed as compared with that on the opposite side.

Cerebrospinal fluid fistula (otorrhea)

Discharge of the cerebrospinal fluid from the ear, otorrhea, indicates an abnormal connection or channel between the subarachnoid space and the external auditory canal. A fracture line, connecting the middle or external ear with the subarachnoid space directly above or behind it, is the most common cause. If the cerebrospinal fluid fistula is medial to the tympanic membrane, the membrane must also be perforated to allow the cerebrospinal fluid to escape. Otherwise the cerebrospinal fluid will drain through the eustachian tube into the nose, resulting in rhinorrhea. These fistulae are usually caused by fracture after severe head injury, but rarely they may result from surgery, congenital defects, or other temporal bone lesions. Most posttraumatic fistulae close spontaneously (Raaf, 1967); but if they persist, the location of the leak may be correctly determined by tomography. Intrathecal dye studies may be useful, but these can cause an allergic reaction. Isotopic cisternography is often helpful in the evaluation of these fistulae. Closure of a persistent leak is important since the retrograde influx of bacteria may cause recurrent meningitis. Pneumocephalus, caused by air leaking intracranially from the middle ear, can be shown by plain roentgenograms; and its site of origin accurately evaluated by laminagraphy. If the fracture line extends through the labyrinth, a fistula between it and the middle ear may develop.

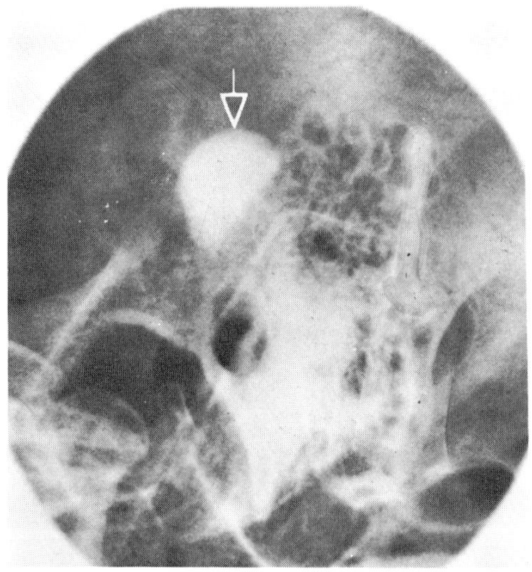

Fig. 19-41. Osteoma. Law projection shows area of increased density (arrow) on lateral aspect of the temporal bone just above the external auditory canal. This represents the typical roentgenographic appearance of an osteoma.

Neoplasms

Temporal bone tumors may be divided into those that involve the external ear, the middle ear, the inner

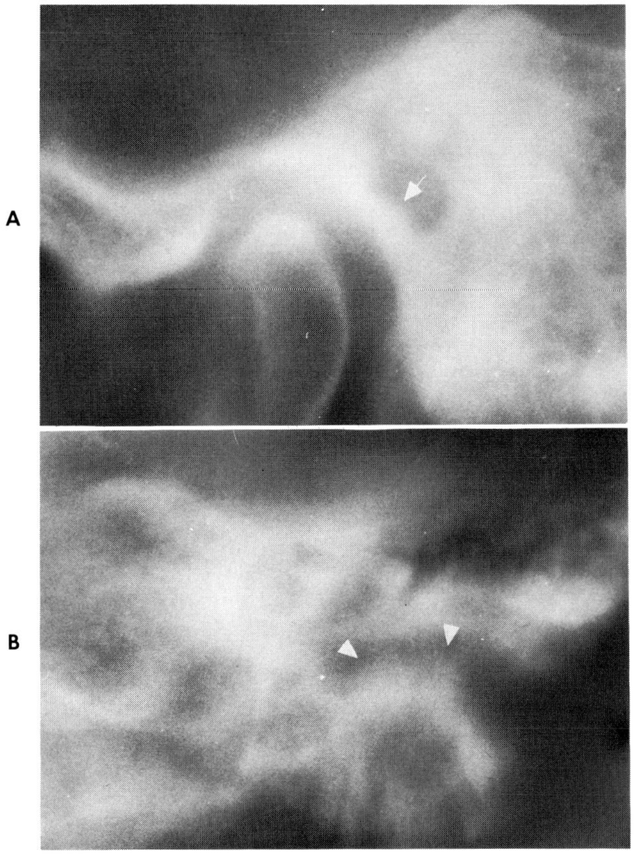

Fig. 19-42. Osteoma. **A,** Laminagraphic section through external auditory canal, lateral projection, shows inward bulge (arrow) from the anteroinferior aspect of the canal. **B,** Laminagram, frontal projection, shows a rounded density (arrowheads) arising from floor of the external auditory canal. This osteoma caused obstructive and irritative changes in the skin of the external canal, leading to mild chronic drainage.

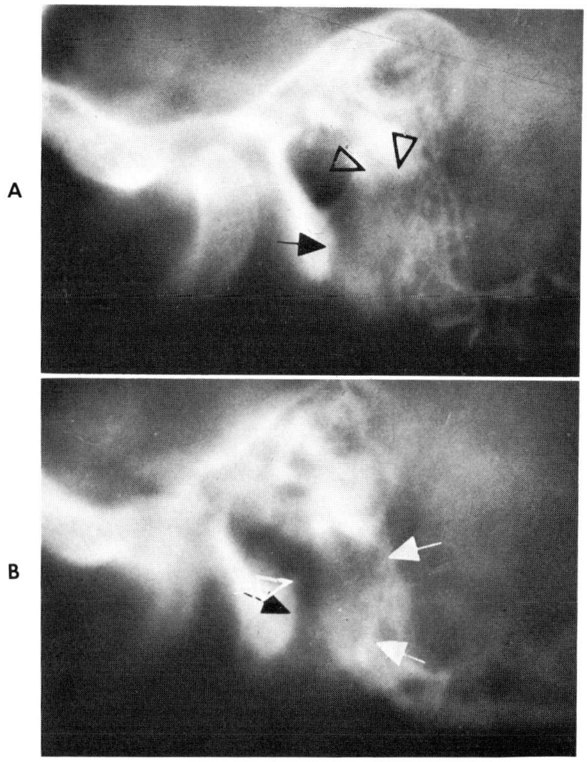

Fig. 19-43. Neurilemmoma of descending portion of facial canal. **A,** Polytome laminagram, lateral projection, shows large lucent defect just behind the external auditory canal. A portion of the facial canal is slightly widened (between open arrowheads). Smoothness of the erosive defect (black arrow) suggests a benign lesion. **B,** Laminagraphic section just medial to **A** shows posterior (solid white arrows), anterior (black arrow), and superior (open white arrow) extent of the expansile tumor. A neurilemmoma arising from the seventh nerve was easily removed surgically. The patient had presented with facial palsy.

ear, the internal auditory canal, and the apex of the petrous temporal bone. Many larger tumors involve more than one of the structures.

External ear

Benign tumors

Osteoma. This is the most common benign tumor of the external ear. It is easily recognized roentgenographically as a sharply defined area of increased density, often extending into the external canal (Figs. 19-41 and 19-42). Osteomas may decrease hearing slightly by partially obstructing the drainage of debris from the external auditory canal. Such an obstruction may lead to a chronic external otitis, which usually resolves completely after the tumor is removed. Osteomas may also be present in the mastoid region, and occasionally they will encroach on the facial canal, causing facial nerve paresis. The roentgenographic findings of a well-demarcated area of radiodensity and increased thickness are the same as those of an osteoma in the external ear.

Lipoma. Lipomas of the external ear are uncommon and do not produce significant roentgenographic changes.

Eosinophilic granuloma. This tumor may cause areas of patchy, irregular destruction of the external canal simulating malignant neoplasm.

Facial nerve sheath tumor. These tumors, usually neurilemmomas, may present in the auditory canal, after breaking through the descending portion of the facial canal (Fig. 19-43).

Malignant tumors. Malignant tumors of the external ear may be primary or secondary. When secondary, they may reach the external canal by direct spread of a contiguous lesion or as a distant metastasis. The radiographic changes in malignant temporal bone tumors

A

B

C

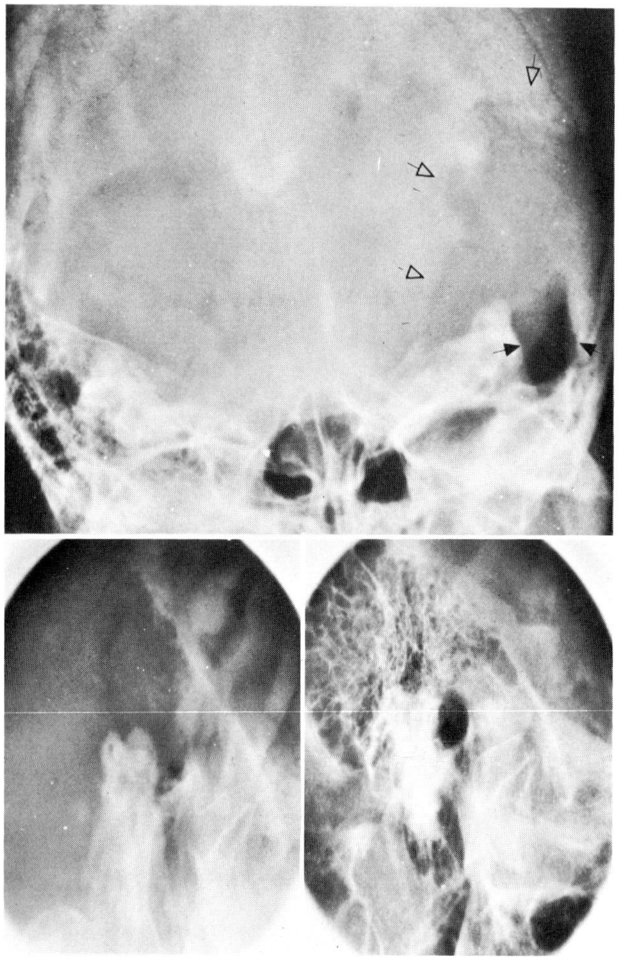

Fig. 19-44. Squamous cell carcinoma arising in or near the external auditory canal. **A,** Towne view shows defect secondary to a previous mastoidectomy (black arrows). In addition, external portion of the temporal bone is demineralized, with destruction extending posteriorly (open arrows) to involve the occipital bone. **B,** Mayer view shows extensive destruction of the lateral aspect of the petrous pyramid. **C,** Normal side, for comparison with **B.**

are the same as in other bones (Fig. 19-44). The bone usually shows irregular areas of osteolytic destruction. Occasionally a slow-growing infiltrating lesion of the periosteum may cause bony sclerosis. A soft-tissue mass may project into the external auditory canal. Roentgenographic studies are mainly of value to determine the extent of involvement rather than the nature of the lesion.

Middle ear

Benign tumors

Glomus tumor. Glomus tumors (chemodectomas) are the most common benign neoplasm in the middle ear. Although histologically benign, they are aggressive

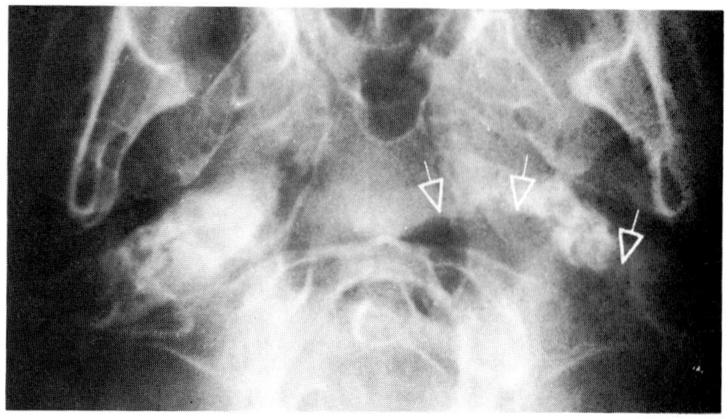

Fig. 19-45. Glomus jugulare tumor. Axial view of skull shows large destructive lesion in the inferomedial aspect of the petrous pyramid on the left (arrows). This defect represents the classic appearance of a glomus jugulare tumor in this projection.

by virtue of their local invasiveness. They arise in the receptor organs on the promontory in the hypotympanum and in the jugular fossa in the superior portion of the jugular bulb. These tumors usually present clinically as reddish purple masses behind the tympanic membrane. They usually cause hearing loss and an annoying bruit. Chemodectomas are extremely vascular, and serious bleeding may result from attempts to remove them surgically or even from a simple biopsy.

Although these tumors are usually easily diagnosed clinically, their size and location can be accurately defined by radiographic views (Eraso, 1961; Di Chiro, et al., 1964; Strickler, 1966).

GLOMUS JUGULARE TUMOR. These tumors arise in chemoreceptor organs in the jugular fossa. When seen behind the tympanic membrane, they have usually spread superiorly and laterally from the jugular fossa through the inferior surface of the petrous pyramids. At this stage they usually show irregularly marginated enlargement of the jugular foramen and an irregular destructive process in the inferior aspect of the midpetrous pyramid (Rice and Holman, 1963) (Figs. 19-45 and 19-46). On the lateral laminagram the spicule of bone common to the anterior margin of the jugular foramen and the posterior margin of the carotid canal, the caroticojugular spine, is completely destroyed if the tumor is large (Fig. 19-8). As the tumor grows through the tympanic cavity, it distorts or destroys the ossicular chain. Late in the course of growth, it may extend into the posterior fossa to present as a low cerebellopontine angle tumor. The glomus jugulare frequently invades the internal jugular vein and can then be seen by retrograde jugular venography as an intraluminal mass (Fig. 19-47). In other cases the jugular vein may show circumferential constriction by surrounding tumor. Carotid

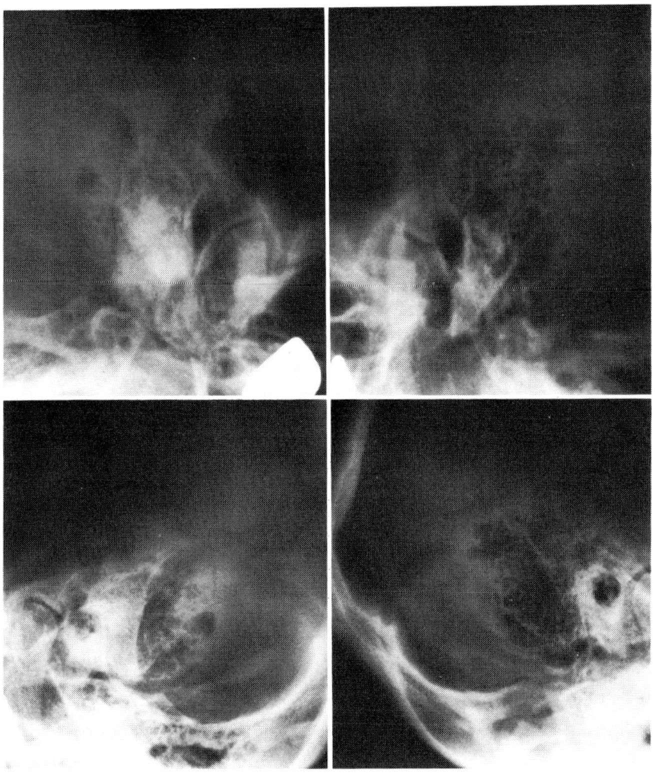

Fig. 19-46. Glomus jugulare tumor. **A,** Mayer-Owen view shows mastoid clouded secondary to a destructive lesion obstructing the mastoid cells and middle ear. Note the lack of definition just beneath the external auditory canal. **B,** Normal side, for comparison. **C,** Law view shows marked clouding of the mastoid, suggesting mastoiditis. **D,** Normal side, for comparison.

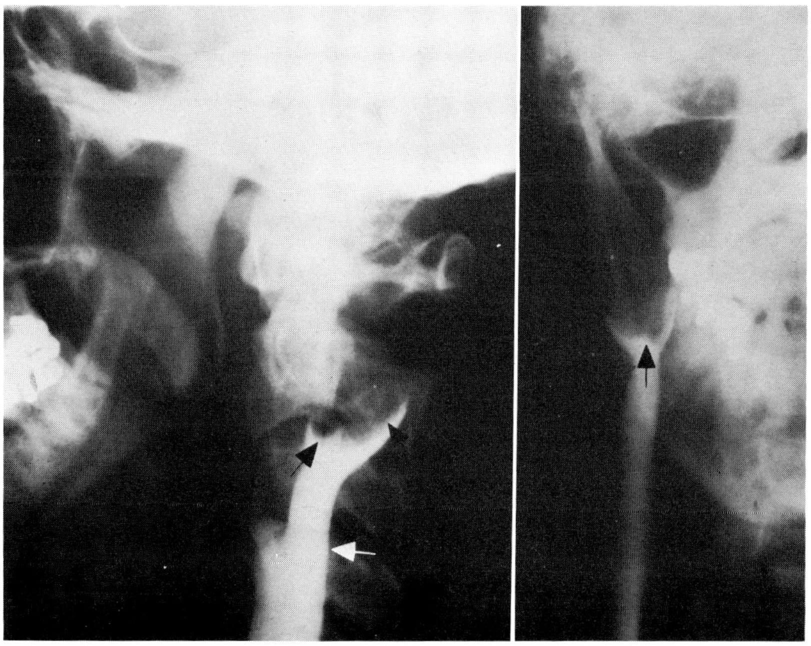

Fig. 19-47. Glomus jugulare tumor. Retrograde jugular venogram. **A,** Lateral view. **B,** Frontal view. Inferior segment of the jugular vein is normal (white arrow). Cephalad flow of contrast is abruptly terminated superiorly. Glomus jugulare tumor projects into the lumen as a large lucent filling defect (black arrows).

angiography is extremely important in the roentgenographic evaluation of glomus jugulare tumors. (See Chapter 58.) Selective external carotid arteriography reveals numerous feeding branches, primarily the ascending pharyngeal artery, supplying a characteristic dense coarsely reticular tumor stain (Hawkins, 1966). Subtraction techniques are particularly helpful to outline these vascular neoplasms. Larger tumors may receive contributions from meningeal branches of the vertebral and internal carotid arteries. Although demonstration of a massive lesion may discourage surgical procedures, extremely large lesions, even those extending into the jugular vein, have been successfully removed.

GLOMUS HYPOTYMPANICUM TUMOR. Chemodectomas, or glomus tumors, arising in the hypotympanicum are usually smaller at the time of diagnosis because they can be seen on otologic examination at a relatively early stage. Unlike glomus jugulare tumors, these lesions are more easily and safely eradicated by extensive temporal bone surgery (House, 1968). Glomus hypotympanicum tumors are differentiated from the glomus jugulare tumors by the absence of significant bone destruction in the region of the jugular foramen. Significant bone destruction from a lesion primarily confined to the tympanic cavity is unusual. The caroticojugular spine remains intact. A soft-tissue mass in the tympanic cavity is usually shown on laminagraphy. Selective external carotid angiography with subtraction techniques reveals a faint blush in the tympanic area if the tumor is large enough (Fig. 19-48).

A

B

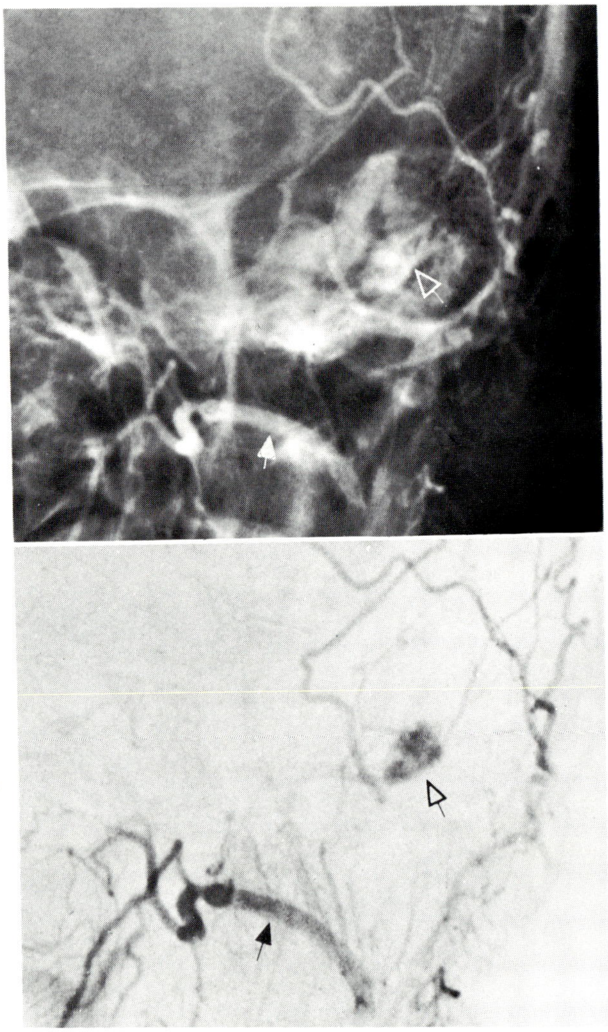

Fig. 19-48. Glomus hypotympanicum tumor. Patient had presented with hearing loss and bruit. A reddish pulsatile mass was seen behind the eardrum. Plain films did not reveal destructive changes in the petrous pyramid. **A,** Selective external carotid arteriogram (Stenvers projection) shows faint area of contrast accumulation (open arrow) inferolateral to the vestibule. For orientation, internal maxillary artery is indicated by white arrow. Orbital rim can also be seen. **B,** Subtraction image of same film shows the tumor (open arrow) in the tympanum more clearly. Internal maxillary artery is indicated by solid arrow.

Neurilemmoma. Neurilemmomas may arise on the cranial nerves that pass through the pars nervosa of the jugular foramen. Regardless of the nerve involved, the clinical presentation is usually one of the variants of the jugular foramen syndrome (Brünner et al., 1963). These tumors cause sharply defined enlargement of the jugular foramen, which indicates pressure erosion. (See Chapter 16.) Neurilemmomas of the seventh (facial) nerve are rare. They may develop anywhere along the course of the facial nerve but are most common in the descending portion of the canal of the nerve (Shambaugh et al., 1969). They may also be found in the internal auditory canal (Brünner et al., 1963).

Malignant tumors. The most common malignant tumor of the middle ear is the squamous cell carcinoma (Tucker, 1965). Adenocarcinoma is less common, and sarcoma is rare. Malignant tumors of the middle ear and mastoid cause irregularly marginated lucent defects that involve various amounts of bone, without evidence of sclerosis (Fig. 19-49). A soft-tissue mass may obliterate the tympanic cavity and cause increased density in this region (Fig. 19-50). Carcinoma of the middle ear may extend upward into the cranial cavity through the superior or the posterior wall of the petrous pyramid. Anterior spread to the sphenoid bone across the petrosphenoid fissure is usually associated with destruction of the sphenoid spine. Malignant tumors may also extend laterally into the external auditory canal. In these cases it may be difficult to determine the exact site of origin. Roentgenographic examination of these tumors is important for the determination of the extent of the lesion if radical surgery is contemplated.

Both benign and malignant tumors may cause increased density of the pneumatized areas of the tempor-

A

B

C

D

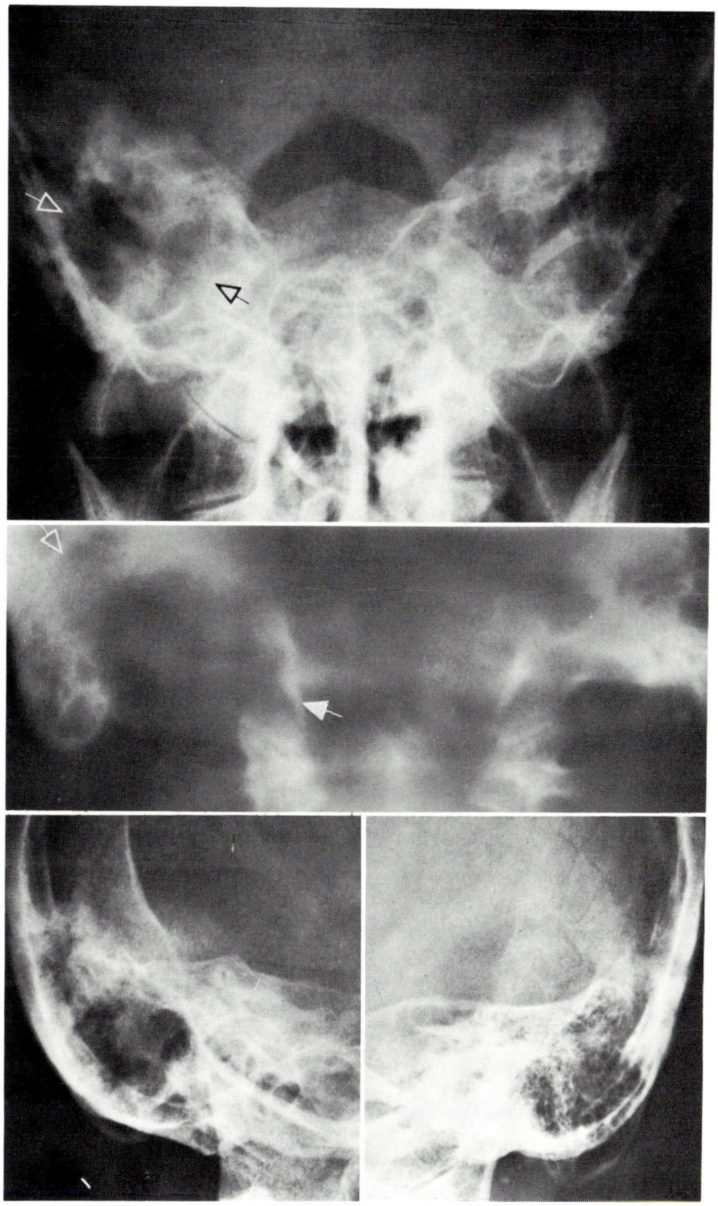

Fig. 19-49. Carcinoma of middle ear. Patient had presented with bleeding and discharge from the external auditory canal. **A,** Towne view shows large lucent defect (arrows) on the undersurface of the petrous temporal bone obliterating most of the landmarks in this region. Ossicles are probably faintly seen but are deformed and displaced laterally. Cochlea and vestibule are intact. **B,** Polytome laminagram, frontal projection, shows extent of the destructive lesion in the inferior aspect of the petrous pyramid. Lesion involves the occipital condyle (solid arrow) and the mastoid (open arrow). **C,** Stenvers view shows bony destruction that affected the middle ear, petrous pyramid, and mastoid region. **D,** Normal side, for comparison.

A

B

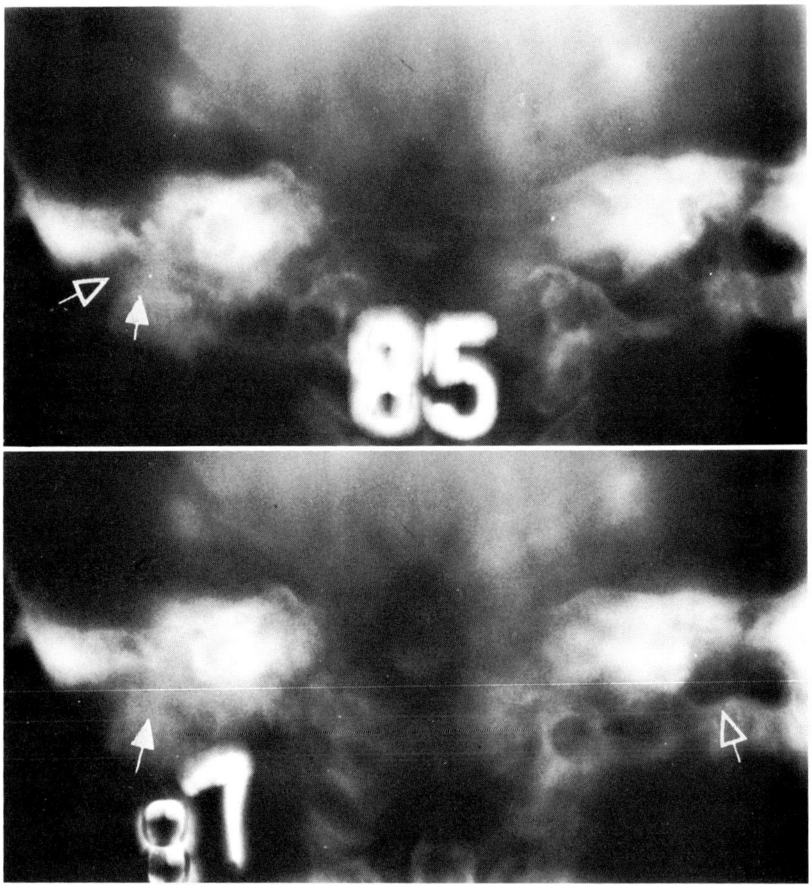

Fig. 19-50. Squamous cell carcinoma of middle ear. Patient had complained of decreased hearing. **A,** Laminagram of petrous bone, frontal projection, shows soft-tissue density obliterating the right tympanic cavity (solid arrow). The soft-tissue density extends laterally into the external auditory canal through the tympanic membrane (open arrow). Bony structures appear intact on this projection. **B,** Laminagram 2 mm anterior to **A** shows destruction of the medial floor of the external auditory canal (solid arrow). Compare with the normal left side (open arrow).

al bone. The increased density, which mimics mastoiditis, results from local infiltration of the tumor obstructing the drainage areas of the mastoid (Fig. 19-46).

Inner ear

Primary tumors, both benign and malignant, arising in or close to the inner ear structures, are rare. Congenital cholesteatoma is occasionally seen in this area, as are metastases from the lung, breast, thyroid, or kidney. Benign or malignant tumors arising in the middle ear may extend to involve the inner ear structures. Large acoustic neuromas may cause bony erosion adjacent to the inner ear structures. Occasionally meningiomas arising in the meninges adjacent to the inner ear structures involve the labyrinth.

Internal auditory canal. Tumors of this region include acoustic neuroma, facial nerve neuroma arising within the internal auditory canal, and meningioma.

Acoustic neuroma. The most common tumor of the inner ear is the acoustic neuroma or neurilemmoma, which arises from the Schwann cells investing the eighth cranial nerve as the nerve enters the internal auditory canal. About 8% of all intracranial tumors are acoustic neurilemmomas, and 95% of these originate within the canal. The other 5% arise from the nerve where it lies within the cerebellopontine angle cistern proximal to the canal. Very few acoustic neuromas are entirely within the internal auditory canal. The great majority project into the cerebellopontine angle cisterns. Occasionally intracanalicular tumors may be seen in neurofibromatosis; these may be bilateral.

Patients with acoustic neuromas present hearing loss, tinnitus, and unsteadiness. Intracranial extension may

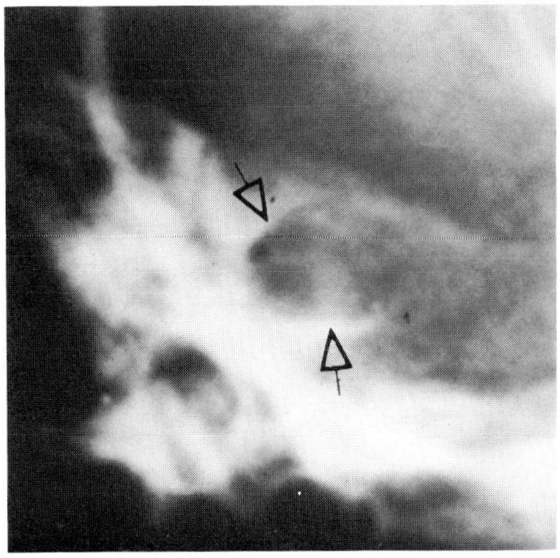

Fig. 19-51. Acoustic neuroma. Stenvers view shows internal auditory canal with marked funneling. This finding is characteristic of large eighth nerve tumors seen in any frontal projection, including the transorbital, Stenvers, and Towne views.

cause pressure on the cerebellum, brainstem, or fifth cranial nerve. Fifth nerve dysfunction usually indicates that the tumor is at least 2.5 to 3 cm in diameter. Eventually the tumor may extend down to compress the ninth and tenth cranial nerves as they cross the angle cistern to enter the pars nervosa of the jugular foramen. Tumors arising within the internal auditory canal enlarge it. The superoinferior height of the internal auditory canal should measure within 1.5 mm of the same portion of the opposite canal. The length of the two canals, measured from the vestibule to the sharply defined medial terminations of the canals, should not differ by more than 2.5 mm on the two sides. Any canal with a superoinferior measurement 2 mm or more larger than the normal side should be considered abnormal when the clinical findings suggest an acoustic neuroma. A posterior wall 3 mm or more shorter than the normal side also indicates abnormality (Valvassori, 1969). The most noticeable roentgenographic change caused by these tumors is erosion of the superior and posterior lips of the porus acusticus (MacMillan, 1969) (Figs. 19-51 to 19-56).

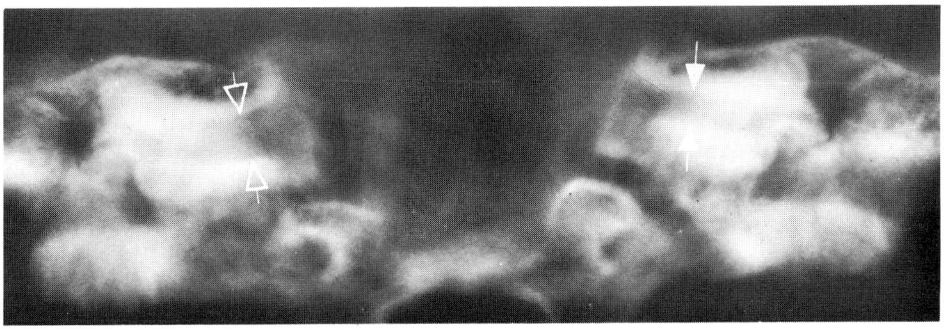

Fig. 19-52. Acoustic neuroma. Polytome laminagram, frontal projection, shows right canal (open arrows) diffusely larger than normal left canal (solid arrows). Note the shortening of the posterior wall on the right as compared to that on the left.

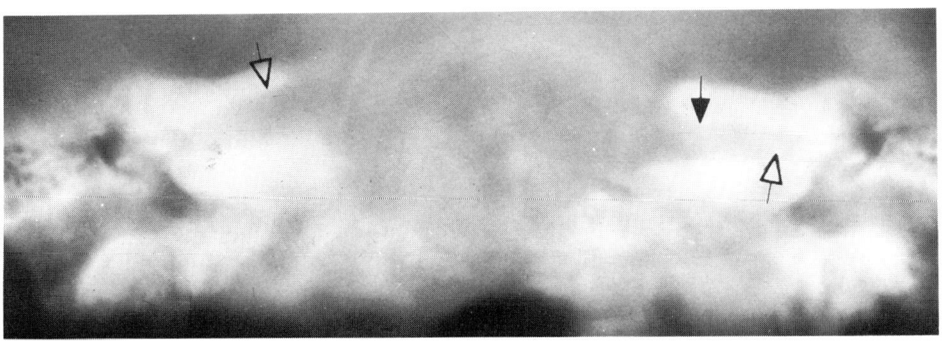

Fig. 19-53. Acoustic neuroma. Left canal is normal in size and, more importantly, shows a downward curve of the medial portion of the roof (solid arrow). Falciform crest (open arrow in left canal) is visible. On the right, there is slight funneling of the medial end of the canal and also loss of the normal downward curve of the roof (open arrow).

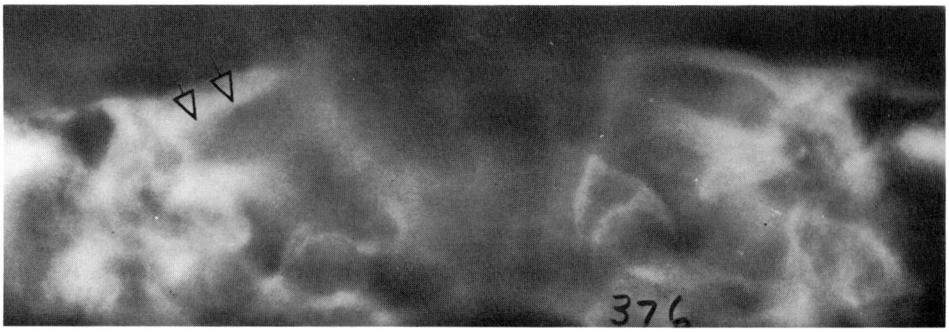

Fig. 19-54. Acoustic neuroma. Funneling and enlargement. More marked enlargement of the canal is seen here than in previous examples. Marked funneling is also noted, as evidenced by the continued upward slant of the roof (arrows). Left canal is normal.

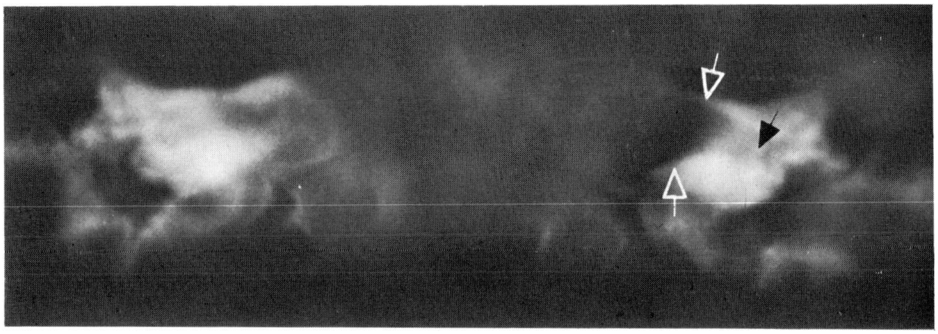

Fig. 19-55. Acoustic neuroma. Falciform crest is faintly seen (solid arrow). Porus acusticus (open arrows) is markedly widened, and the entire canal has a funnel shape. Some inferior erosion, which is less common, is present.

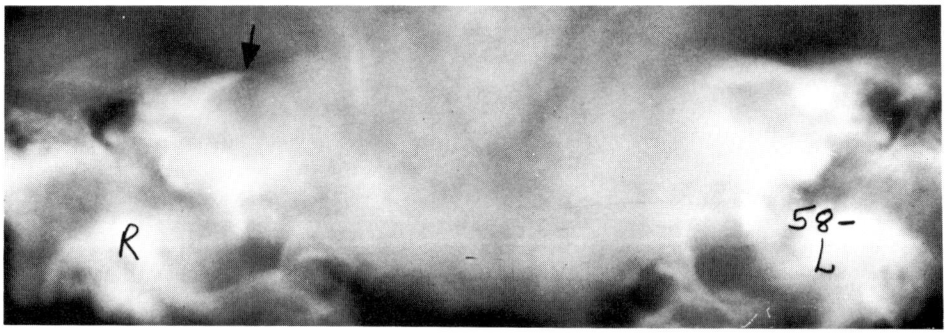

Fig. 19-56. Acoustic neuroma. Marked enlargement of the canal. Entire right canal shows sharply defined enlargement with marked thinning of the superomedial wall (arrow). This finding indicates a large tumor in the cerebellopontine angle.

At first there is only loss of definition of the bony margins. Later the superior cortical margin of the porus acusticus is displaced away from the central axis of the internal auditory canal, leading to funneling of the canal. Most acoustic neuromas arise from the superior vestibular branch of the eighth nerve. The falciform crest is therefore almost always destroyed or rarely displaced downward by acoustic neuromas (Valvassori and Pierce, 1964). The earliest roentgenographic changes of intracanalicular tumors consist of erosive enlargement of the central part of the internal auditory canal (Fig. 19-57) with a relatively normal appearance of the medial end of the canal.

As the tumor enlarges, erosion of the posterior and superior walls of the canal continues. Shortening of the roof and the posterior wall of the canal is also noted

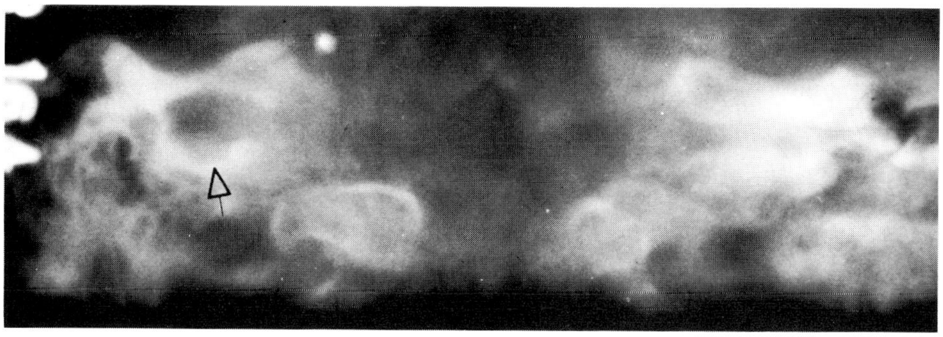

Fig. 19-57. Acoustic neuroma. Intracanalicular. Floor of internal auditory canal is displaced downward on the right (arrow). This displacement is the result of a tumor that was largely intracanalicular with only a few millimeters extending into the cerebellopontine cistern.

A

B

C

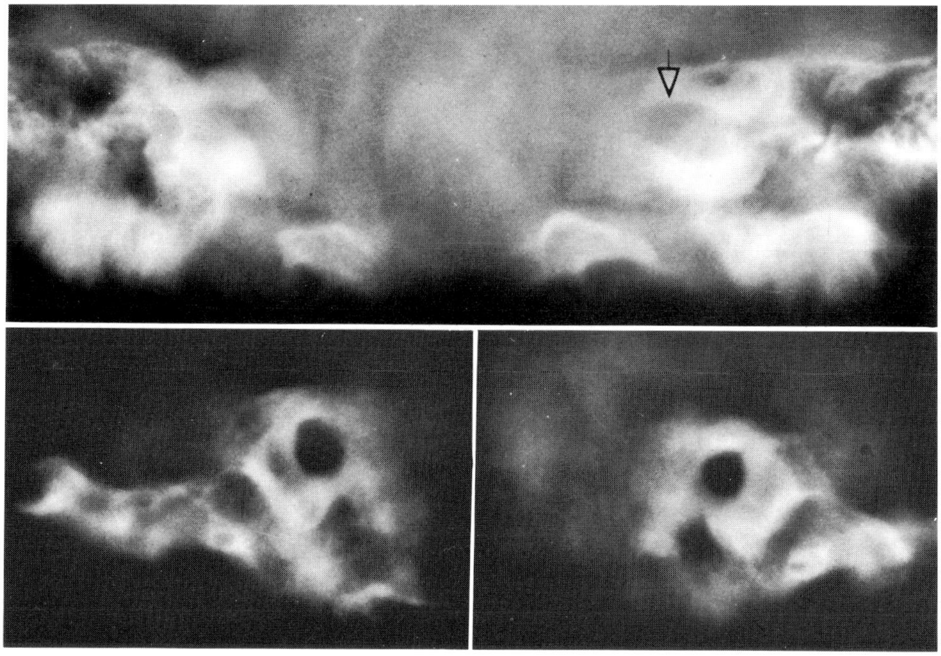

Fig. 19-58. Acoustic neuroma. Largely intracanalicular, with about 6 mm extending into the cerebellopontine angle cistern. **A,** Polytome laminagram, frontal projection, shows characteristic enlargement of the left canal (arrow). **B,** Polytome laminagram of internal auditory canal, lateral projection, shows the canal distinctly enlarged. **C,** Normal canal, for comparison.

(Taveras and Wood, 1964). Erosion of the posterior margin or enlargement of the internal auditory canal may also be shown in lateral projections (Fig. 19-58), particularly when the normal and abnormal sides are compared. Axial views may demonstrate an increase in the anteroposterior measurement of the internal auditory canal as well as posterior funneling (Fig. 19-59). Very large tumors may cause extensive erosion with shortening of the tip of the petrous pyramid (Fig. 19-60) (Towne, 1926).

A common variation in the appearance of the internal auditory canal is referred to as the patulous canal. On cursory examination this canal resembles the bone changes produced by an intracanalicular neoplasm. However, the condition is usually bilateral, which should suggest the correct diagnosis (Fig. 19-61). The patulous canal appears to be frequent in patients with a sensorineural hearing loss of undefined etiology.

Pantopaque cisternography combined with Polytome laminagraphy is a useful diagnostic technique to delineate clearly the canal and the nerves that traverse the canal. Lesions of the nerve within the canal that are as small as 2 or 3 mm in diameter may be identified

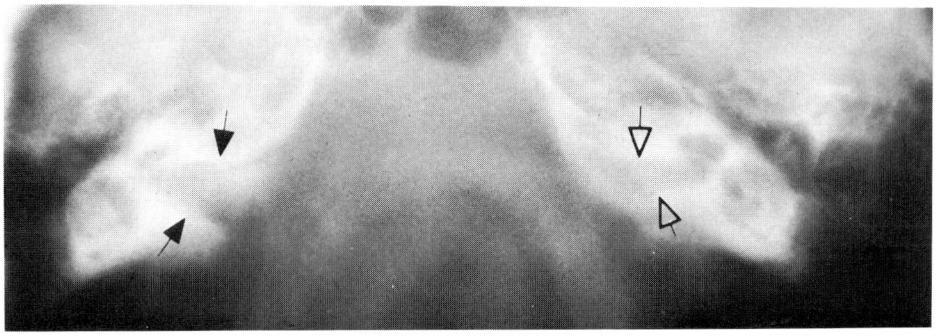

Fig. 19-59. Acoustic neuroma. Polytome laminagram, axial or basal projection, shows right internal auditory canal (solid arrows) markedly enlarged, with erosion of the posterior wall. Canal on the left (open arrows) is normal.

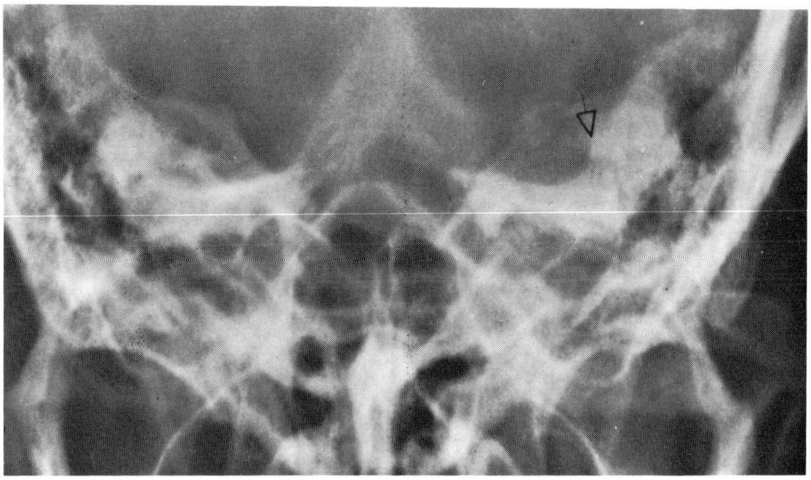

Fig. 19-60. Acoustic neuroma. Towne view shows erosion of petrous pyramid not characteristic of acoustic neuroma. This tumor apparently originated in the cisternal portion of the nerve rather than in the porus acusticus. Note the sharp erosive margin (arrow).

by this method (Hitselberger and House, 1968). Tumors filling the porus acusticus are shown by a rounded indentation in the oily contrast medium. Failure to fill the canal is highly suggestive of the presence of a tumor. Unusually small canals, such as seen in adult Pyle's disease, may not fill by this technique, probably because all the available space is taken up by the nerves and associated tissue.

Facial nerve neuroma. Neuromas of the facial nerve are extremely rare but may cause an erosion similar to that of an acoustic neuroma.

Meningioma. Meningiomas in the internal auditory canal may cause erosion in the region of the canal. The erosion usually extends to involve the adjacent posterior surface of the petrous temporal bone.

Vascular lesion. Vascular lesions may erode the internal auditory canal, causing it to have a funnel-shaped appearance. The anterior inferior cerebellar artery often loops in the porus acusticus. Arteriovenous malformation or occlusive disease causing enlargement or tortuosity of this loop may lead to erosion of the porus acusticus (Fig. 19-62). If an aneurysm is present where the internal auditory artery originates, it may cause erosion of the canal. This diagnosis can be confirmed by vertebral angiography.

The following diagnostic work-up is preferred by us in the evaluation of lesions involving the internal auditory canals: in the presence of unequivocally enlarged internal auditory canals, vertebral angiography should be used first; arterial displacements and tumor stain usually adequately outline the larger tumors that are present when prominent bony changes are seen (Olsson, 1953); less definite enlargement of the canal is probably best evaluated by Pantopaque cisternography (Scanlan, 1964); pneumoencephalography combined with tomography permits a detailed analysis of the cerebellopontine angle cisterns, brainstem, and adjacent structures.

A

B

C

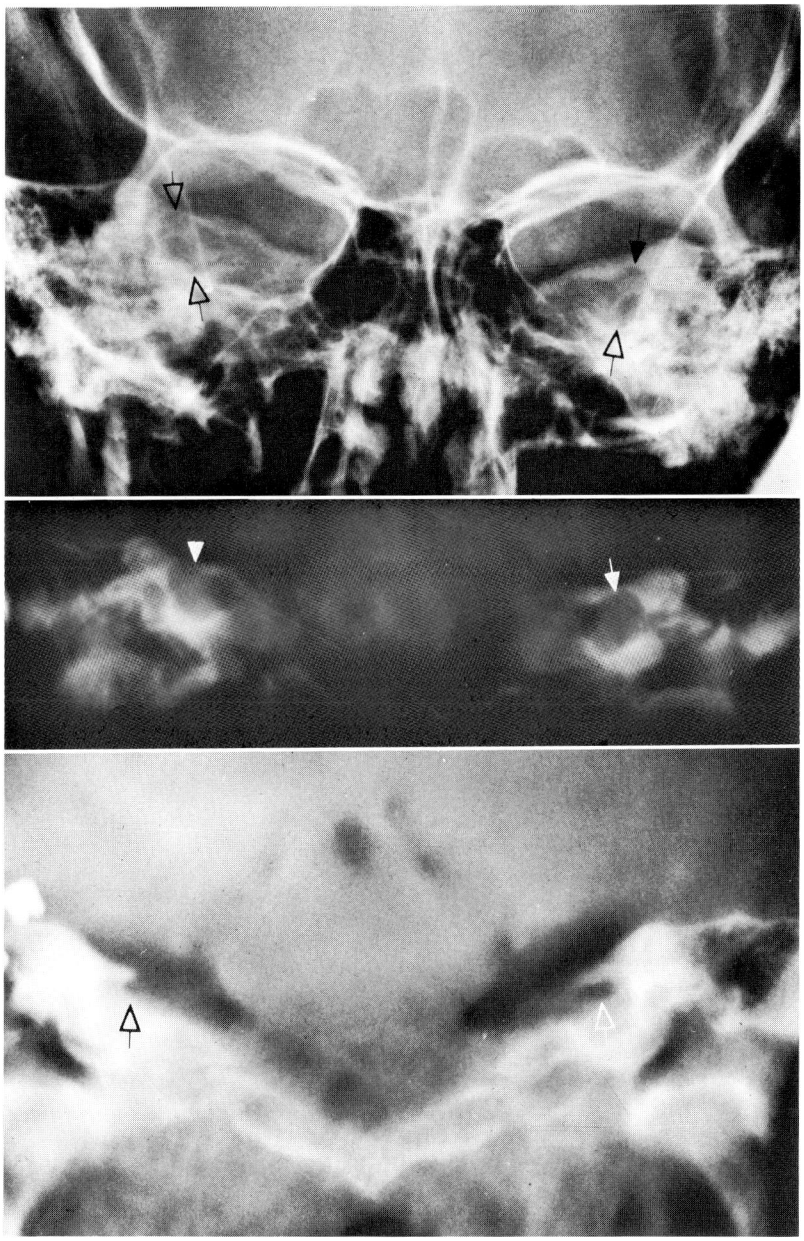

Fig. 19-61. Patulous canals. A 22-year-old music student had sensorineural hearing loss bilaterally. **A,** Transorbital view shows both internal auditory canals with marked degree of central bulge (between arrows). No bony erosion is seen. **B,** Polytome laminagram shows shape of the enlarged canals (arrows). **C,** Polytome laminagram of pneumoencephalogram in the erect position shows both angle cisterns capacious. Small amount of air (arrows) extends into the canals.

Petrous apex. The apex of the petrous temporal bone may be eroded by neuromas of the fifth nerve, meningiomas of the Gasserian cavity, epidermoids adjacent to the apex of the petrous temporal bone (Fig. 19-63), intracavernous aneurysm of the carotid artery (Fig. 19-64), or chordomas (Takahashi et al., 1967).

Otosclerosis

Otosclerosis is a disease that involves the labyrinth. In it scattered foci of spongy bone are laid down in the labyrinth capsule. The etiology of this process is not known although a definite predilection for women and a hereditary tendency have been noted; but the true incidence of the lesion remains a mystery. The incidence

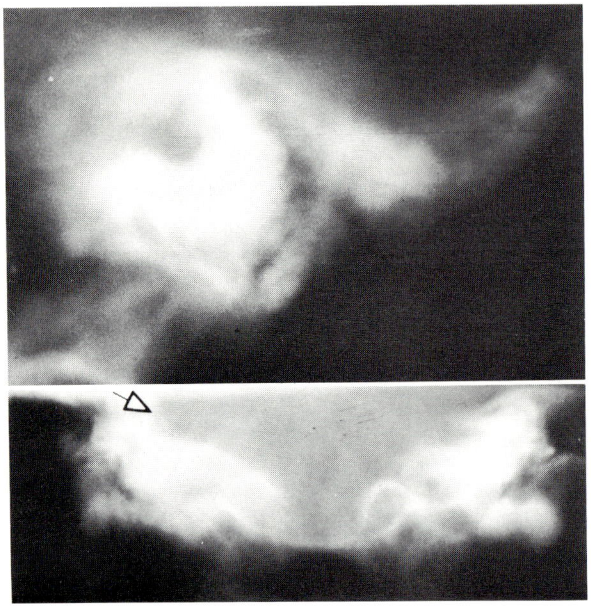

Fig. 19-62. Congenital hypoplasia of cervical carotid and vertebral arteries in young girl. **A,** Polytome laminagram, lateral projection, shows posterior aspect of internal auditory canal eroded. **B,** Polytome laminagram, frontal projection, shows right internal auditory canal funnel shaped (arrow). At angiography these changes were shown to result from collateral vessels traversing the angle cistern, bypassing the hypoplastic carotid and vertebral arteries.

varies in different races. Otosclerosis is usually bilateral but not symmetric.

At first, as the new bone is laid down, dissolution of the enchondral bony structure takes place, with replacement by spongy new bone. This active stage is called otospongiosis. Later, in the mature stage of the disease, the spongy bone becomes less active, recalcified, and then quite dense.

The foci of otosclerotic bone tend to originate in the *fissula ante fenestram,* a cleft extending from the middle ear to the vestibule. This occurs in a large segment of the population; but in only 15% to 20% of persons with otosclerotic changes does the disease spread to involve the cochlea. This may be asymptomatic. If the foci involve the oval window and fixation of the stapes footplate takes place, conductive hearing loss results. Less frequently foci of otosclerotic bone develop away from the fissula in other portions of the labyrinth capsule.

Clinically the patient, usually a young adult, presents with tinnitus and chronic progressive conductive or sensorineural hearing loss. A family history of otosclerosis, or at least of hearing loss, is often noted. The cause of the tinnitus is not clear. After some progression, hearing loss is arrested and remains unchanged for many years. Active foci of otospongiotic bone are more fre-

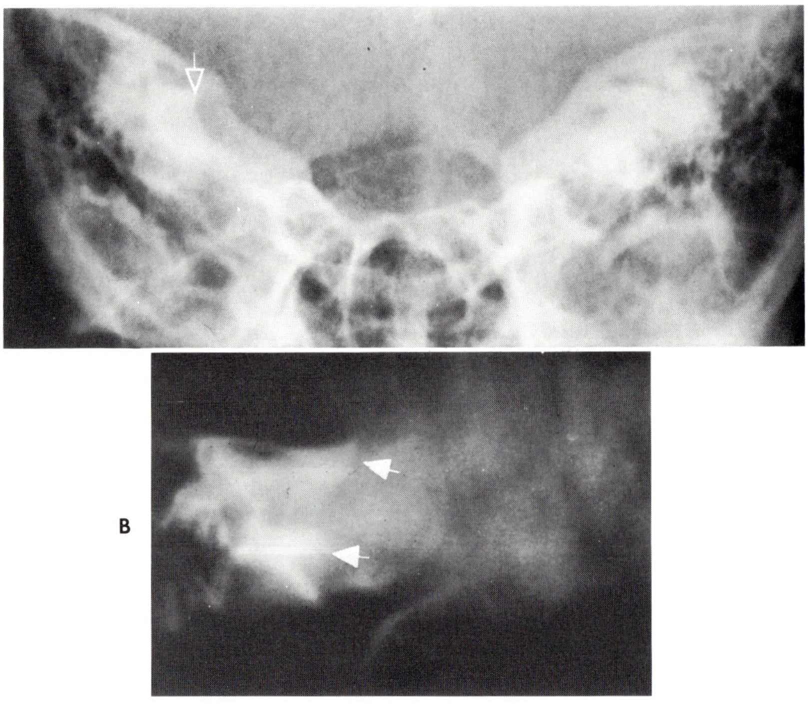

Fig. 19-63. Epidermoid cyst in cerebellopontine angle. **A,** Towne view shows right petrous pyramid eroded lateral to the midportion of the internal auditory canal (arrow). This appearance is similar to that of Fig. 19-60. **B,** Polytome laminagram, frontal projection, shows tip of petrous pyramid with sharply demarcated erosion just lateral to the posterior wall of the porus acusticus (arrows).

quent in younger persons. Patients with osteogenesis imperfecta have an increased incidence of otosclerosis, but the relationship between these diseases is unknown (Altmann, 1962; Shambaugh, 1967).

The otologic surgeon usually establishes the diagnosis by an evaluation of the hearing loss and by otoscopic identification of a positive Schwartze sign, a reddening of the promontory seen through the tympanic membrane. Although a hearing aid may benefit many patients, several operations have been designed to improve the hearing in patients with otosclerosis. One of these operations, infrequently used today, is fenestration, in which an opening is made in the horizontal semicircular canal. Another is stapedectomy, in which various portions of the stapes are removed and replaced with wire or plastic prostheses.

Radiologists have only recently become involved in the evaluation of patients with otosclerosis (Valvassori,

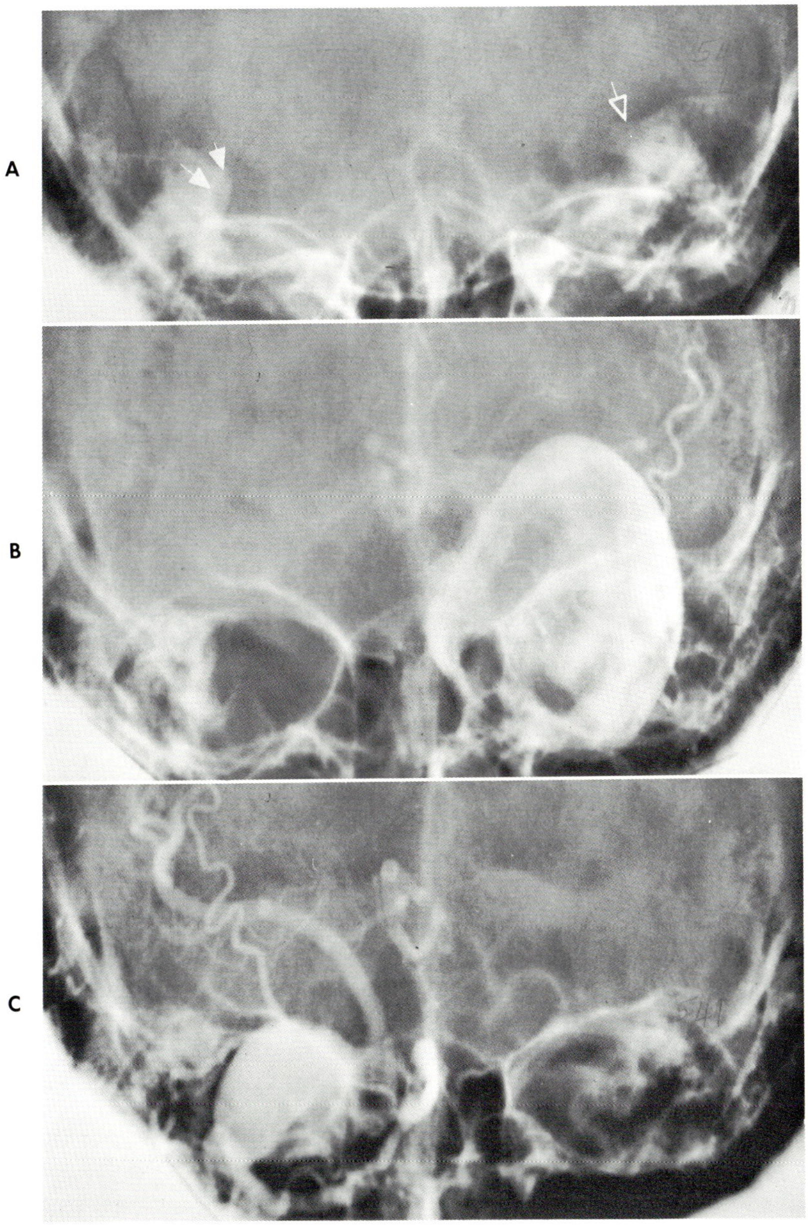

Fig. 19-64. Bilateral petrous pyramid erosion by cavernous internal carotid aneurysms. **A,** Towne view shows extensive erosion of both petrous pyramids (arrows), suggesting either bilateral acoustic neuroma or other large cerebellopontine angle cistern lesions. **B,** Left common carotid arteriogram, frontal projection. **C,** Right brachial arteriogram, frontal projection. Large intracavernous carotid aneurysms are present bilaterally.

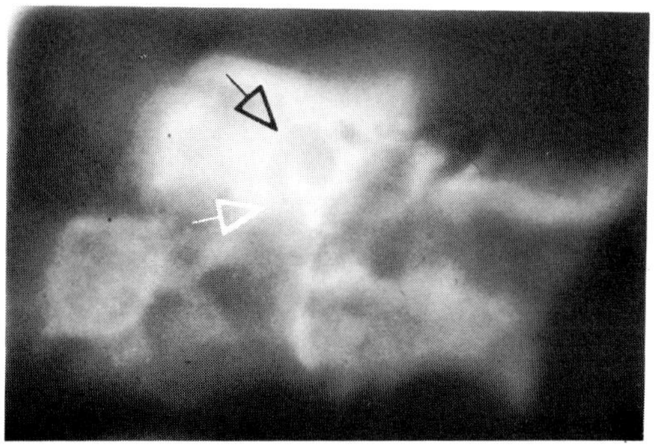

Fig. 19-65. Otosclerosis—spongiotic phase. Polytome laminagram, frontal projection, shows cochlea (black arrow) normally outlined until the basal turn is reached. At this point (white arrow) there is marked demineralization and loss of anatomic contour of the remainder of the cochlea comprising the basal turn.

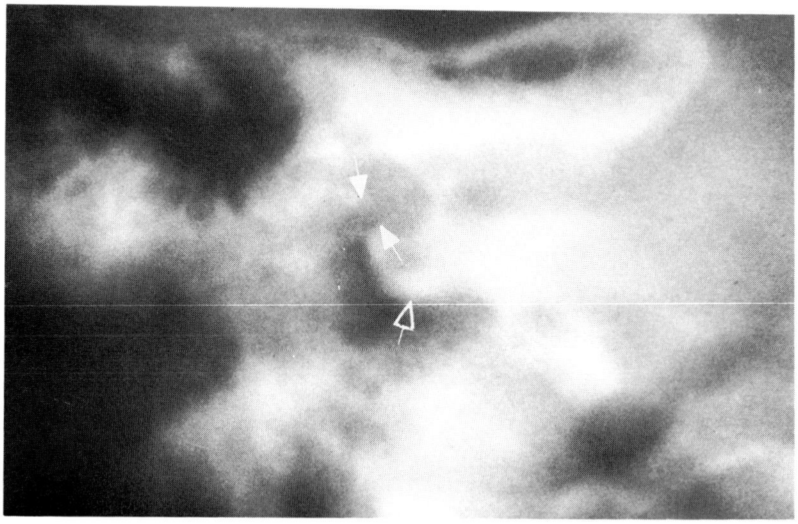

Fig. 19-66. Otosclerosis—mixed phase. Polytome laminagram, frontal projection, shows basal turn of the cochlea increased in density and irregular (open arrow). Oval window (between solid arrows) is widened. This indicates that sclerotic phase involves the cochlea whereas spongiotic phase involves the vestibular window.

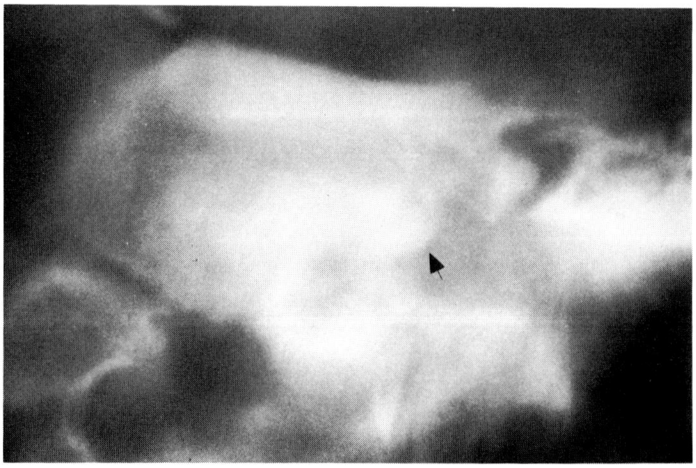

Fig. 19-67. Otosclerosis—sclerotic phase. Polytome laminagram, frontal projection, shows entire cochlea with marked increase in density so that the spiral lamina cannot be identified. Basal turn has a lumpy appearance (arrow). Wire prosthesis placed after stapedectomy is faintly seen, extending from the incus to a very poorly visualized oval window. (See Fig. 19-70.)

1965). Until the development of hypocycloidal laminagraphy, inadequate delineation of the ear structures did not allow evaluation of the regions commonly involved by otosclerosis. Even with the more sensitive laminagraphic units, the diagnosis is not certain unless involvement of the oval (vestibular) window is extensive.

Because the two windows need to be examined carefully, the radiographic technique must be superior. The most useful projections are the straight anteroposterior view and the anteroposterior view with the head rotated 15° to 20° toward the side of involvement (Valvassori, 1966). This latter position brings the oval window into profile. Laminagraphic sections must be obtained through these structures at 1 mm intervals. Coning should restrict the field to the middle and inner ear structures. The roentgenographic findings in otosclerosis are consistent with the pathologic abnormality (Brünner et al., 1966). First, when there is spongiotic involvement of the bone, small lucent areas may be

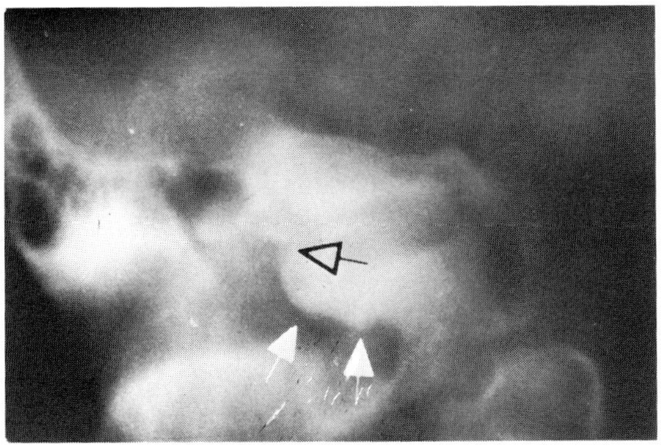

Fig. 19-68. Otosclerosis—sclerotic phase. Polytome laminagram, frontal projection, shows basal turn of the cochlea irregular and increased in density (solid arrows). Height of the vestibular (oval) window (open arrow) is diminished. Original film showed stapes footplate thickening; but this is difficult to reproduce.

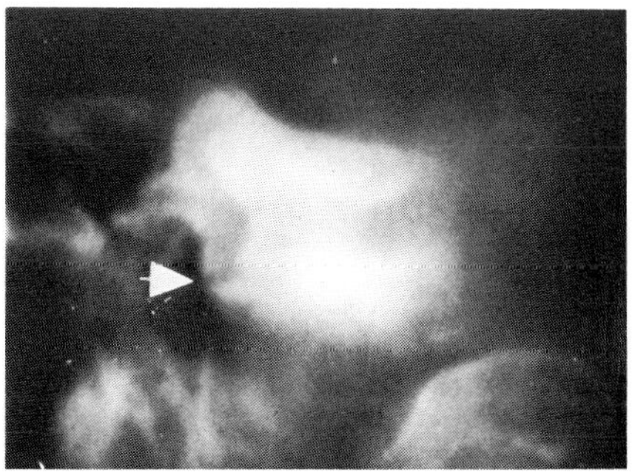

Fig. 19-69. Otosclerosis—fenestral. Polytome laminagram, frontal projection, shows both the oval and the round windows (arrow) narrowed. Cochlea is dense. These findings indicate sclerotic fenestral and cochlear otosclerosis.

A

B

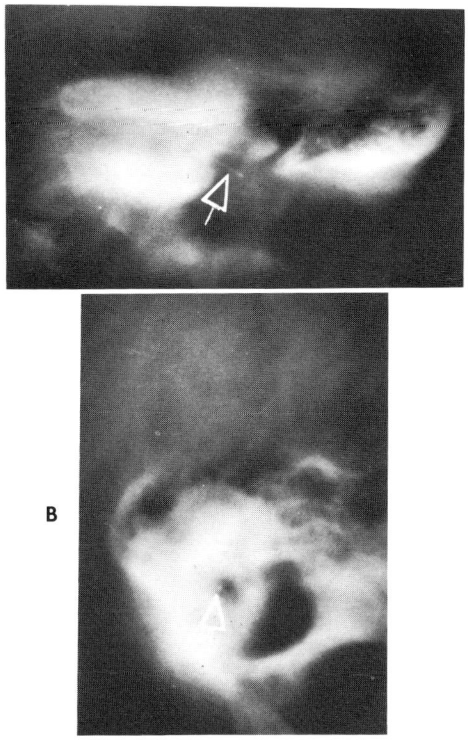

Fig. 19-70. Otosclerosis—after stapedectomy and prosthesis insertion. **A,** Polytome laminagram, frontal projection, shows faint wire prosthesis (arrow) extending from the long process of the incus medially to the markedly sclerosed and narrowed oval window. Cochlea is dense. **B,** Polytome laminagram, lateral projection, shows faint wire prosthesis (arrow) almost end-on as it extends to the vestibular window. Lucency surrounding the wire prosthesis is the vestibule.

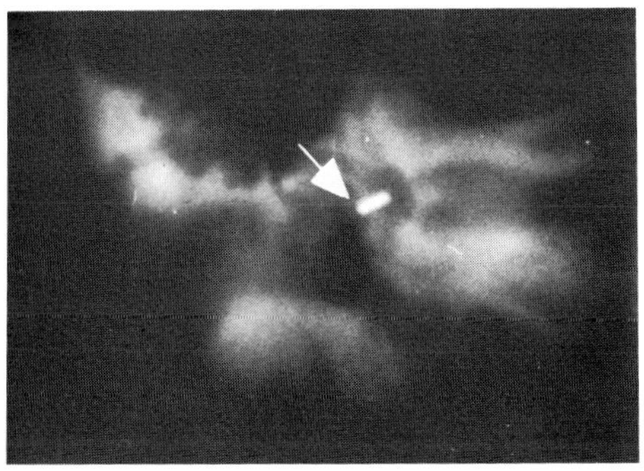

Fig. 19-71. Otosclerosis—after stapedectomy and prosthesis insertion. Polytome laminagram, frontal projection, shows rather bulky metallic strut (arrow) originally placed in vestibular window. At this time, most of the prosthesis rests within the vestibule, an incorrect position.

scattered throughout the cochlea (Fig. 19-65). The oval window, which normally is from 1.5 to 2 mm in its superoinferior diameter, may be widened (Jensen et al., 1966) (Fig. 19-66). These changes suggest that normal enchondral bone has been resorbed or replaced by spongy bone. Later, as these foci mature, the overall bony density may increase (Fig. 19-67). Because of the increased density, the task of distinguishing between the margins of the cochlea and the surrounding bone may be difficult. By this time the windows may be narrowed and their rims increased in thickness (Vignaud et al., 1965). Thickening of the stapes footplate may be seen occasionally (Liliequist, 1968). Failure to delineate the oval window on technically superior films is quite suggestive of the diagnosis (Figs. 19-68 and 19-69).

Most often the radiologist is consulted for confirmation of the diagnosis and to determine the extent of involvement in the oval window and cochlea in patients in whom surgery is being considered. Roentgenographic studies may also be of value to assess the prognosis in a patient whose hearing loss is the result of otosclerosis. The position and location of the prosthesis after stapedectomy may also be demonstrated (Fig. 19-70). Occasionally the prosthesis may be malpositioned or may project completely through the oval window into the vestibule (Fig. 19-71). Roentgenographic examinations may also demonstrate other disease processes complicating otosclerosis, such as inflammatory changes.

Paget's disease

Paget's disease affecting the temporal bone may be associated with basilar invagination (Fig. 19-72). The

A

B

C

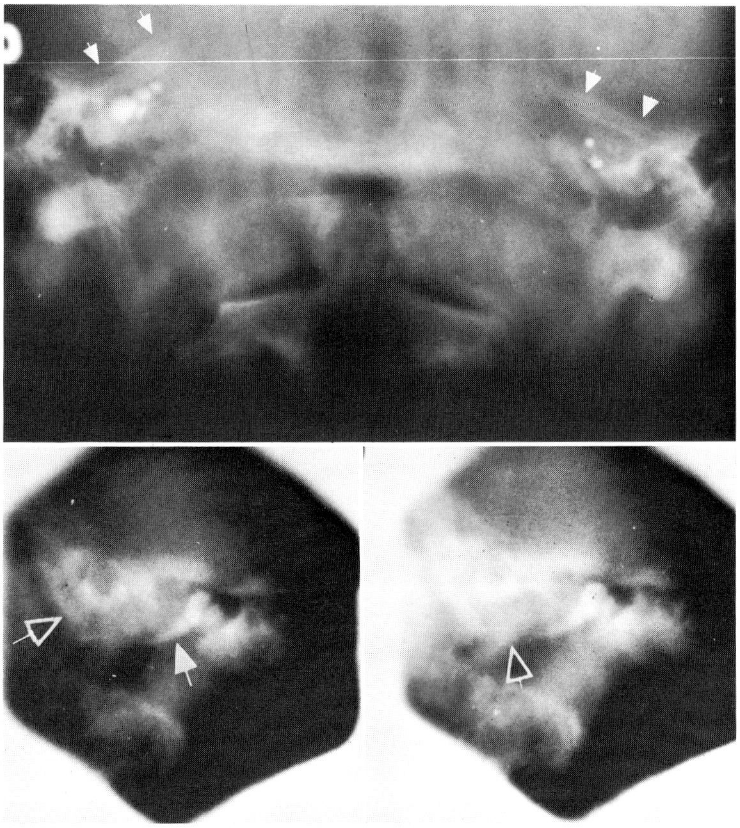

Fig. 19-72. Paget's disease. Basilar invagination and labyrinthine demineralization. **A,** Frontal Polytome of the base of the skull. Marked upward angulation of the medial petrous pyramids (arrows) results from softening of the skull base by involvement with Paget's disease. **B,** Polytome laminagram, frontal projection, shows extensive spotty demineralization of labyrinth structures (open arrow). Long process of the incus extending medially (solid arrow) is well seen. **C,** Polytome laminagram 1 mm posterior to **B** again shows extensive demineralization of the cochlea (arrow). This type of demineralization may be difficult to differentiate from spongiotic involvement by otosclerosis. Whereas otosclerosis usually remineralizes, labyrinthine changes of Paget's disease rarely do.

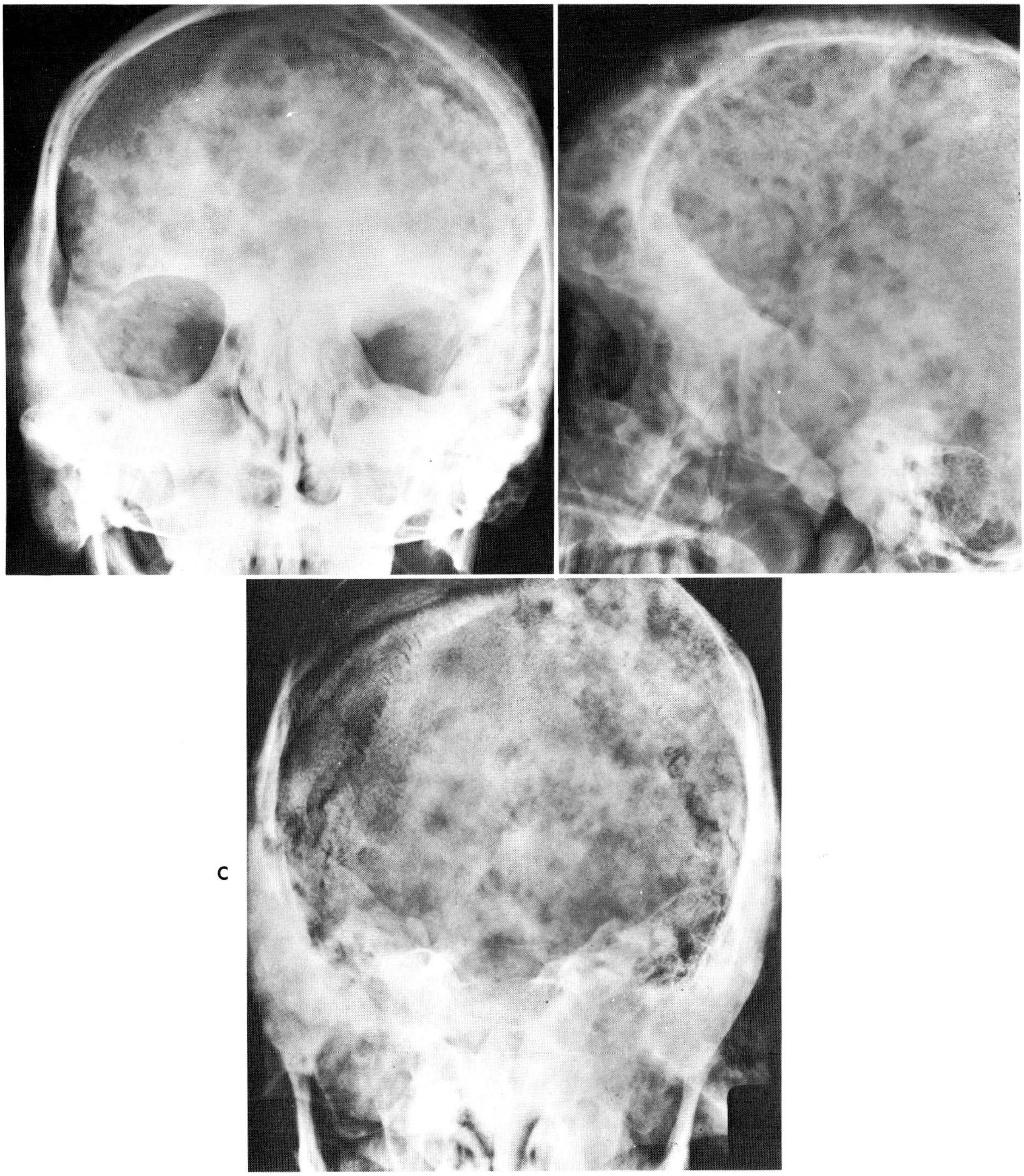

Fig. 19-73. Fibrous dysplasia. **A,** Caldwell view. **B,** Lateral view. **C,** Towne view. Petrous temporal bones are extensively involved by fibrous dysplasia. Bones are markedly thickened, with focal areas of spotty radiolucency. Both the labyrinth and the internal auditory canals, less involved by the disease, are fairly well seen.

labyrinth also may be involved in Paget's disease (Gussen, 1970). Increased lucency of these structures results as the labyrinth is replaced by the new abnormal pagetoid bone (Fig. 19-72). This involvement is usually extensive, generalized, and less focal than that seen with otosclerosis (Petasnick, 1967). The pagetoid bone may cause fixation of the stapes, producing a clinical picture similar to that seen with otosclerosis. The internal auditory canal may be narrowed, secondary to thickening of the petrous portion of the temporal bone, when it is involved by Paget's disease. In contradistinction to otosclerosis, pagetoid changes usually remain roentgenographically lucent.

Meniere's disease

Meniere's disease (endolymphatic hydrops) is diagnosed clinically. Patients with this disease usually complain of vertigo, nausea, vomiting, hearing loss (usually unilateral), and tinnitus. There may also be a sensation of fullness and pressure in the ear. Audiometry reveals a neural type of hearing loss, often with recruitment. Overproduction or underabsorption of endolymphatic fluid, causing increased pressure in the endolymphatic portion of the labyrinth, is suggested as a possible cause (Anson, 1969). Roentgenographic procedures are most often performed to exclude the diagnosis of other lesions, especially acoustic neuroma. Recent studies in Meniere's disease suggest that an evaluation of the endolymphatic drainage system (i.e., the vestibular aqueduct) (Shambaugh et al., 1964) may be useful. Sometimes this aqueduct is sclerosed and obstructed by an overgrowth of its bony surroundings, probably because of fibrosis. Delineation of a normal vestibular aqueduct does not exclude the presence of Meniere's disease. This particular evaluation needs further study before its usefulness can be ascertained.

Histiocytosis X

Histiocytosis X may involve the petrous bone and resembles neoplastic disease in that irregular lucent destructive areas without any identifying characteristics are seen. If the patient has known histiocytosis X lesions elsewhere in the body, the diagnosis can be suggested. Otherwise the extent of the lesion may be delineated so that adequate biopsy tissue can be obtained for histologic proof.

Fibrous dysplasia

Fibrous dysplasia may rarely cause hearing loss through involvement of the petrous temporal bone because of occlusion of the external auditory canal (Cohen and Rosenwasser, 1969) (Fig. 19-73). Usually, if this type of lesion is monostotic, a biopsy must be performed to obtain a definitive diagnosis (Fluur and Soderberg, 1966).

Osteopetrosis

Osteopetrosis may involve the bone but is not related to any neurologic abnormality (Myers and Stool, 1969).

Congenital malformation of ear

To understand congenital ear malformations, knowledge of the embryonic development of the structures of the ear is helpful (Anson and Donaldson, 1967;

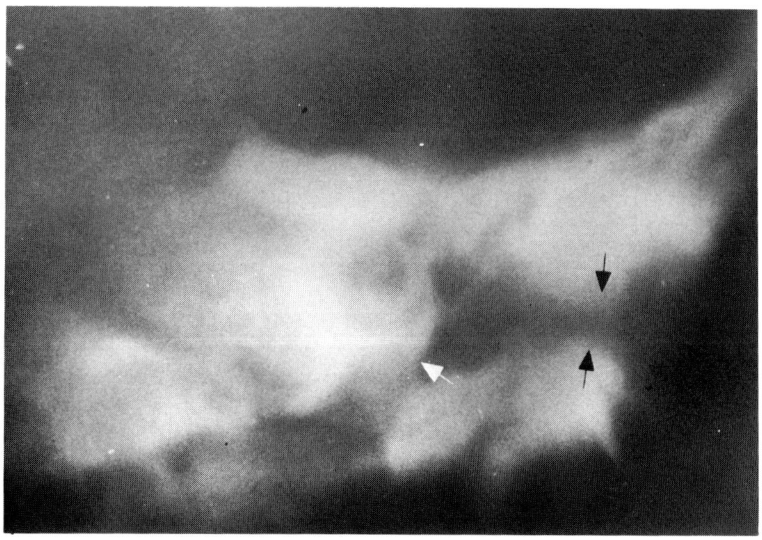

Fig. 19-74. Treacher-Collins syndrome (mandibulofacial dysostosis). Polytome laminagram, frontal projection, shows external auditory canal (between black arrows) narrowed or atretic. Cochlea is indicated by white arrow.

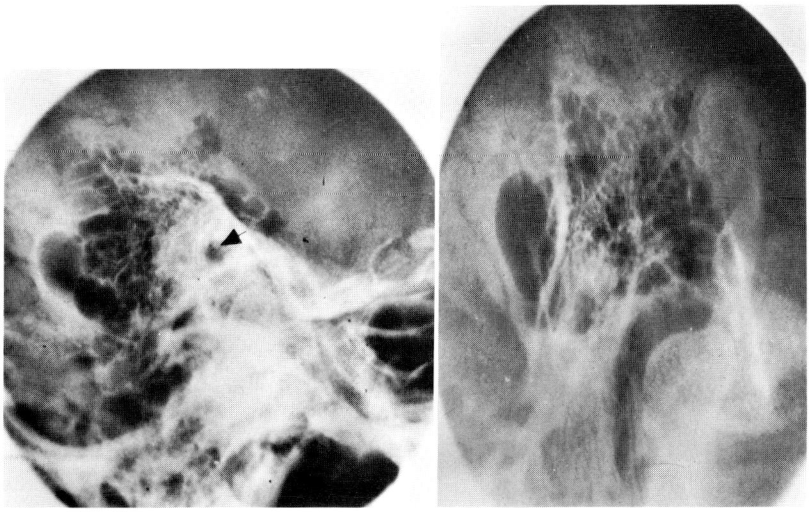

Fig. 19-75. Congenital absence of external auditory canals. **A,** Law view and, **B,** Mayer view of petrous temporal bones. External auditory canal is not visible. Internal auditory canal (arrow) is seen in **A.** These films illustrate the possibility of diagnosing this entity on plain films. In general, however, they are not useful to evaluate the complexity of the malformation.

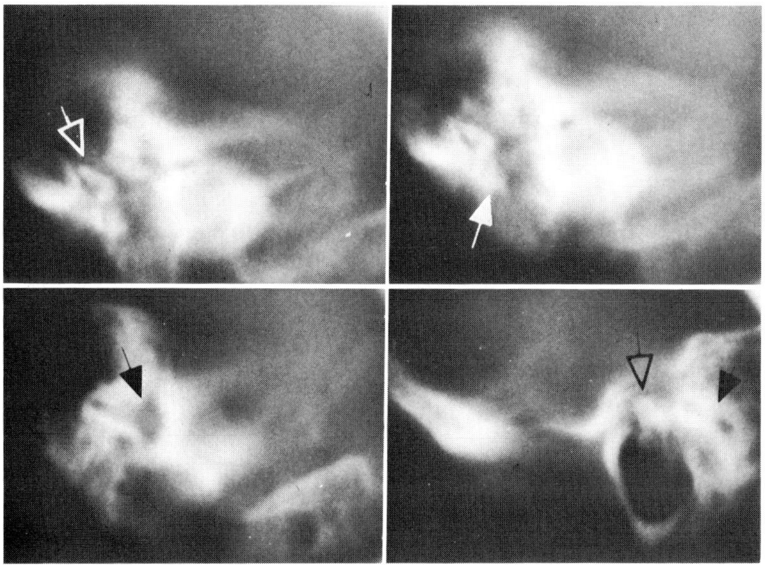

Fig. 19-76. Congenital malformation. **A,** Polytome laminagram, frontal projection, shows unusual configuration of the ossicular chain (arrow) in relation to the epitympanic recess. No external auditory canal is identifed. **B,** Large thick bony plate (arrow) extends inferiorly and almost completely obliterates connection of the middle ear to the outside, except for a bony cleft (just medial to arrow). **C,** Medial aspect of lateral semicircular canal (arrow) is enlarged where it joins the vestibule. This finding indicates an abnormality of the labyrinth structures and diminishes the likelihood of good results from surgery on the external ear malformation. **D,** Polytome laminagram, lateral projection, shows ossicles (open arrow) normally placed, although the malleus (immediately beneath arrow) is somewhat higher in position than the incus. Lateral semicircular canal (solid arrow) is somewhat more obliquely placed than normal.

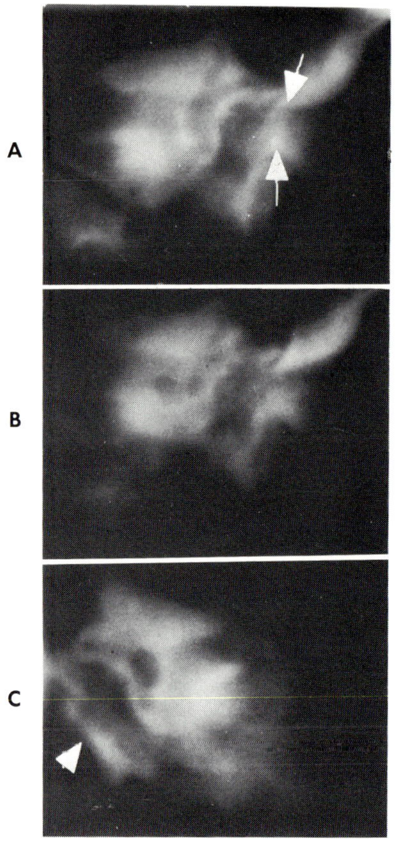

Fig. 19-77. Congenital malformation and atresia of the external ear. **A,** Polytome laminagram, left temporal bone, frontal projection, shows external auditory canal (between arrows) markedly narrowed. A useful external canal is still present, however. Labyrinthine malformation is shown by unusual upward swing of the lateral semicircular canal. **B,** Polytome section 2 mm anterior to **A** again shows narrow and shortened external auditory canal. A small ossicular head is faintly visualized in the epitympanic recess. **C,** Polytome laminagram, right temporal bone, frontal projection, shows bony plate (arrow) completely blocking access to the middle ear from the outside. No external auditory canal structures are present. Again, the superior surface of the semicircular canal is slanted somewhat superiorly.

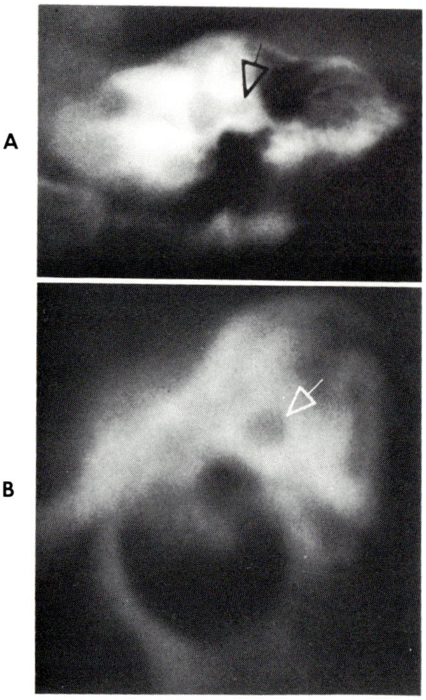

Fig. 19-78. Congenital malformation. **A,** Polytome laminagram, frontal projection, shows external auditory canal markedly deformed. Lateral semicircular canal (arrow) is large and bulbous. **B,** Polytome laminagram, lateral projection, shows bulbous lateral semicircular canal (arrow), seen end-on, probably not representing a canal but rather a bud extending laterally from the vestibule.

Shambaugh, 1967). (See earlier discussion of developmental anatomy.)

As described, the development of the inner ear is separate from that of the rest of the temporal bone. The reason for coexistent significant abnormalities of the middle ear and outer ear, without involvement of the sensorineural apparatus, is easily understood. The malformed ear is the result of defective development during embryonic growth, and its appearance indicates when growth was arrested. Commonly malformation of the auricle, bony atresia of the external meatus, and malformation of the incus and malleus are seen together. The mandible in such malformations also may be poorly developed since it originates from the first branchial groove and arch, as does the external ear. One particular alienation of growth that includes the mandible leads to the Treacher-Collins deformity, or mandibulofacial dysostosis (Fazen et al., 1967) (Fig. 19-74). (See Chapter 26.) This deformity entails downward slanting of the eyes, notching of the lower eyelid, shortening of the mandible, and associated defects of the ear. The severity of the defect of the outer ear varies considerably, and the clinical appearance is related only to the time of cessation of embryonic growth.

Clinical diagnosis of congenital malformation of the external ear is simple. The extent of the middle ear involvement is best indicated by the degree of failure of development of the auricle. The goal of the radiologist is to help define the severity of involvement (James et al., 1964). The thickness of the lateral bony plate between the tympanic cavity and the auricle must be determined, and the anatomic integrity of the sensorineural apparatus assessed (Frey, 1965). Ossicular abnormalities are common. So-called block ossicles are often seen. Identification of even grossly normal ossicles may be important to the surgeon, who can often

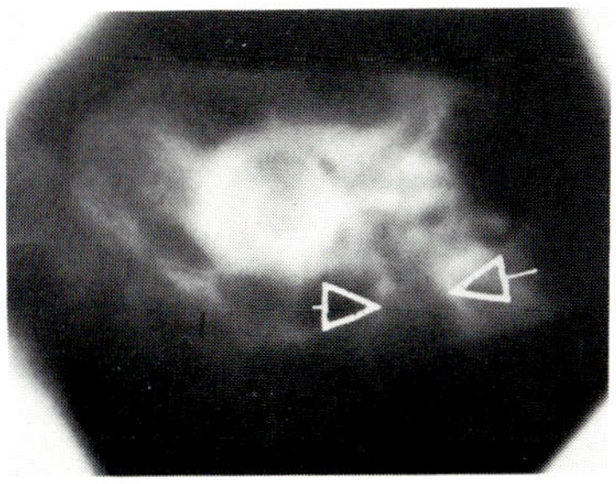

Fig. 19-79. Congenital malformation. Patient with deformed external ear had rudimentary external canal (arrows) extending almost straight caudad from the middle ear.

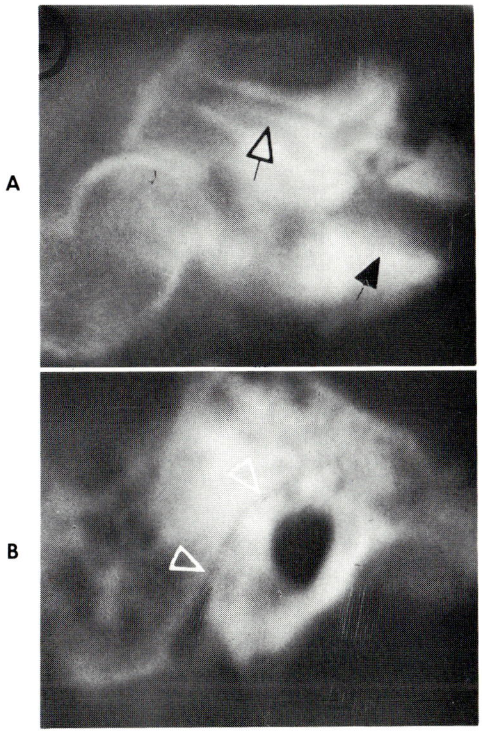

Fig. 19-80. Adult craniometaphyseal dysplasia (Pyle's disease). **A,** Polytome laminagram, frontal projection, shows external and internal auditory canals markedly narrowed (solid arrow). Note the rather thick falciform crest (open arrow) in the internal canal. Density of the visualized bone is increased. Ossicles are well seen. **B,** Polytome laminagram, lateral projection, shows facial canal (arrowheads) markedly narrowed throughout its course. No facial nerve paresis was evident clinically, however.

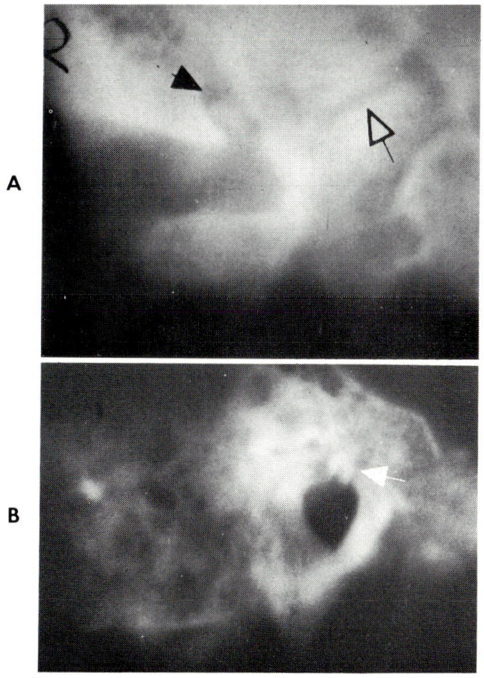

Fig. 19-81. Adult craniometaphyseal dysplasia (Pyle's disease). Patient is a cousin of the one in Fig. 19-80. **A,** Polytome laminagram, frontal projection, shows internal auditory canal (open arrow) and external canal markedly narrowed. Epitympanic recess (solid arrow) is small, tightly confining the ossicles. Note the overall increased density and thickness of the bone. (Neither of the internal auditory canals shown in Figs. 19-80 and 19-81 could be filled with Pantopaque.) Evidently, soft tissue and nerves completely filled the canal. **B,** Polytome laminagram, lateral projection, shows well the malleus and incus (arrow). Their position and relationship appear to be normal.

partially repair the deformed ossicular chain (Brucher et al., 1968). The postoperative mechanical efficiency of this arrangement may be low, but some gain in hearing may result. If the sensorineural apparatus is anatomically abnormal, reconstructive surgery is useless since no hearing can be reclaimed in this situation (Jensen, 1968). Rarely a congenital cholesteatoma may accompany a malformation of the ear. Identification of this process aids considerably in planning the procedure for reconstruction.

The ear is subject to a variety of malformations, ranging from the simple skin web across the external auditory canal, or a minor abnormality of the ossicular chain, to complete absence of the inner and outer ear structures (Jensen and Rovsing, 1968). Pure ossicular malformations are uncommon but should be considered whenever congenital hearing loss is present without significant meatal stenosis. If these patients reach adult life undiagnosed, it may be difficult to distinguish this abnormality from otosclerosis. The abnormalities in congenital malformation of the ear are (in ascending order of severity): skin web without other abnormality, ossicular chain abnormality, meatal stenosis with intact canal, meatal stenosis with bony plate, complete absence of the middle and outer ear structures, and total absence of the sensorineural apparatus (Cliff et al., 1969).

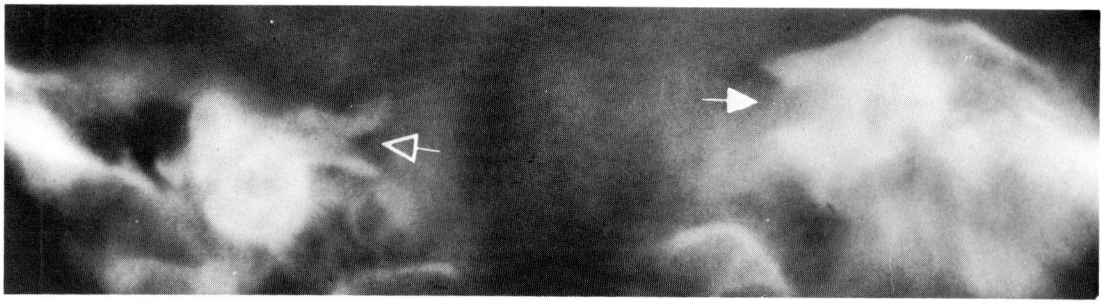

Fig. 19-82. von Recklinghausen's disease—unusual manifestation. Right internal auditory canal (open arrow) is markedly narrowed or atretic. Left canal (solid arrow) appears normal. Patient had systemic neurofibromatosis and was deaf in the right ear.

Some of these changes are illustrated in Figs. 19-75 to 19-79.

Other developmental abnormalities affecting the temporal bone include adult craniometaphyseal dysplasia (adult Pyle's disease) (Figs. 19-80 and 19-81) and von Recklinghausen's disease. The former causes increased density of the bone and underdevelopment of the bony foramina, which may lead to compression of the nerves traversing these openings. The compression commonly causes paresis of the seventh and eighth cranial nerves; and the increased bony density and decreased size of the opening may be well shown roentgenographically. The latter may result in underdevelopment of the temporal bone, with resultant narrowing of the internal auditory canal (Fig. 19-82).

REFERENCES

Altmann, F.: The temporal bone in osteogenesis imperfecta congenita, Arch. Otolaryng. **75**:486-497, 1962.

Anson, B. J.: Endolymphatic hydrops, Arch. Otolaryng. **89**: 70-84, 1969.

Anson, B. J., and Donaldson, J. A.: The surgical anatomy of the temporal bone and ear, Philadelphia, 1967, W. B. Saunders Co.

Baker, H. L., Jr.: Myelographic examination of the posterior fossa with positive contrast media, Radiology **81**:791-801, 1963.

Baron, S. H.: Herniation of brain into the mastoid cavity, Arch. Otolaryng. **90**:779-785, 1969.

Brosnan, M. L.: Primary cholesteatomas of the temporal bone, Arch. Otolaryng. **86**:363-366, 1967.

Brucher, J. A., Rumbaugh, C. L., and Stroud, M. H.: Some radiographic and clinical observations in bony atresia of the external auditory canal, Laryngoscope **78**:216-226, 1968.

Brünner, S.: Roentgen anatomy of the temporal bone using the polytome, Seminars Roentgen. **4**:118-121, 1969.

Brünner, S., Petersen, Ø., and Sandberg, L.: Tomography in cholesteatoma of the temporal bone, Amer. J. Roentgen. **97**: 588-596, 1966.

Brünner, S., Petersen, Ø., and Stoksteld, P.: Laminagraphy of the temporal bone, Amer. J. Roentgen. **86**:281-291, 1961.

Brünner, S., Petersen, Ø., and Stoksteld, P.: Tomography of the facial canal in non-rheumatic facial palsy, Acta Radiol. [Diagn.] **1**:90-95, 1963.

Brünner, S., Rovsing, H., and Jensen, J.: Tomographic changes in otosclerosis, Acta Radiol. [Diagn.] **4**:632-638, 1966.

Brünner, S., and Sandberg, L. E.: Tomography in cholesteatoma and chronic otitis media, Arch. Otolaryng. **91**:560-567, 1970.

Chaussé, C.: Trois incidences pour l'examen du rocher, Acta Radiol. **34**:274-287, 1950.

Cliff, M. M., Laypayowker, M. S., and Woloshin, H. J.: Congenital abnormalities of the temporal bone, Seminars Roentgen. **4**:122-128, 1969.

Cohen, A., and Rosenwasser, H.: Fibrous dysplasia of the temporal bone, Arch. Otolaryng. **89**:447-459, 1969.

Compere, W. E., and Valvassori, G. E.: Radiographic atlas of the temporal bone, American Academy of Ophthalmology and Otolaryngology, St. Paul, Minn., 1964, H. M. Smyth Co., Inc.

Di Chiro, G., Fisher, R. L., and Nelson, K. B.: The jugular foramen, J. Neurosurg. **21**:447-460, 1964.

Eraso, S. T.: Roentgen-clinical diagnosis of glomus jugulare tumor: four cases and a new radiographic technique, Radiology **77**:252-256, 1961.

Etter, L. E., Cross, L. C., and Stuart, M. J.: Roentgenography and roentgenology of the middle ear and mastoid process, Springfield, Ill., 1965, Charles C Thomas, Publisher.

Etter, L. E., and Cross, L. C.: Normal and pathologic roentgen anatomy of the middle ear and mastoid process, Amer. J. Roentgen. **90**:1143-1155, 1963.

Fazen, L. D., Elmore, J., and Nadler, H. L.: Mandibulo-facial dysostosis, Amer. J. Dis. Child. **113**:405-410, 1967.

Fluur, E., and Soderberg, G.: Monostotic fibrous dysplasia (ossifying fibroma) of the mastoid, J. Laryng. **80**:678-680, 1966.

Frey, K. W.: Tomography of malformations of the labyrinth, Fortschr. Roentgenstr. **102**:1-13, 1965.

Gussen, R.: Early Paget's disease of labyrinthine capsule, Arch. Otolaryng. **91**:341-365, 1970.

Harwood-Nash, D. C.: Fractures of the petrous and tympanic parts of the temporal bone in children: a tomographic study of 35 cases, Amer. J. Roentgen. **110**:598-607, 1970.

Hawkins, T. D.: Radiological investigation of glomus jugulare tumors, Acta Radiol. **5**:201-210, 1966.

Hitselberger, W. E., and House, W. F.: Polytome-pantopaque: a technique for the diagnosis of small acoustic tumors, J. Neurosurg. **29**:214-217, 1968.

Holugh, J. V. D.: Restoration of hearing loss after head trauma, Ann. Otol. **78**:210-226, 1969.

House, W. F.: Glomus tympanicum tumors, Arch. Otolaryng. **87**:550-554, 1968.

James, J. A., Penry, J. B., and Ross, F. G.: Tomography and atresia of the external auditory meatus, Brit. J. Radiol. **37**:511-525, 1964.

Jensen, J.: Tomography of the internal ear in deaf children: radiological demonstration of congenital malformation, Rev. Mex. Radiol. **22**:1-3, 1968.

Jensen, J., and Rovsing, H.: Tomography in congenital malformation of the middle ear, Radiology **90**:268-275, 1968.

Jensen, J., Rovsing, H, and Brünner, S.: Tomography of the inner ear and otosclerosis, Brit. J. Radiol. **39**:669-672, 1966.

Jongkees, L. B: Facial paralysis complicating skull trauma, Arch. Otolaryng. **81**:518-522, 1965.

Kaseff, L. G: Tomographic evaluation of trauma to the temporal bone, Radiology **93**:321-327, 1969.

Liliequist, B: Roentgenologic changes in otosclerosis, Acta Radiol. [Diagn.] **7**:129-139, 1968.

MacMillan, A. S.: Cholesteatoma in chronic otitis media, Amer. J. Roentgen. **36**:747-750, 1936.

MacMillan, A. S.: Radiologic diagnosis of neuro-otological problems by conventional radiology, Arch. Otolaryng. **89**:52-57, 1969.

MacPherson, R. I., and Dunbar, J. S.: The radiology of mastoid disease in infants and children, J. Canad. Ass. Radiol. **16**: 0-58, 1965.

Mayer, E. G.: Technic of roentgenologic examination of temporal bone, Radiology **7**:306-317, 1926.

Mazzoni, A., and Hansen, C. C.: Surgical anatomy of the arteries of the internal auditory canal, Arch. Otolaryng. **91**: 128-135, 1970.

Myers, E. N., and Stool, S.: Temporal bone in osteopetrosis, Arch. Otolaryng. **89**:460-469, 1969.

Olsson, O.: Vertebral angiography in the diagnosis of acoustic nerve tumors, Acta Radiol. **39**:265-272, 1953.

Owen, G. R.: Simplified method of producing axial view of Mayer in chronic mastoiditis and attic cholesteatoma, Amer. J. Roentgen. **57**:260-263, 1947.

Pendergrass, E. P., Schaeffer, J. P., and Hodes, P. J.: The head and neck in roentgen diagnosis, Springfield, Ill., 1956, Charles C Thomas, Publisher.

Petasnick, J. P.: Tomography of the temporal bone in Paget's disease, Rev. Mex. Radiol. **21**:299-303, 1967.

Potter, G. D.: Trauma to the temporal bone, Seminars Roentgen. **4**:143-150, 1969.

Raaf, J.: Post-traumatic CSF leaks, Arch. Surg. **95**:648-651, 1967.

Rice, R. P., and Holman, C. B.: Roentgenographic manifestations of tumors of the glomus jugulare, Amer. J. Roentgen. **89**:1201-1208, 1963.

Rovsing, H., and Jensen, J.: Tomographic visualization of labyrinthine fistula, Radiology **90**:261-267, 1968.

Runström, G.: Roentgenological study of acute and chronic otitis media, Acta Radiol., supp. 17, pp. 1-88, 1933.

Sansregret, A.: Technique for the study of the middle ear with special reference to cholesteatoma, Amer. J. Roentgen. **90**: 1156-1166, 1963.

Scanlan, R. L.: Positive contrast medium in the diagnosis of acoustic neuroma, Arch. Otolaryng. **80**:698-706, 1964.

Shambaugh, G. E., Jr.: Surgery of the ear, ed. 2, Philadelphia, 1967, W. B. Saunders Co.

Shambaugh, G. E., Jr., Arenberg, I. K., Barney P. L., and Valvassori, G. E.: Facial neurilemmomas. A study of four diverse cases, Arch. Otolaryng. **90**:7 2-755, 1969.

Shambaugh, G. E., Jr., Clemis, J. O., and Arenberg, I. K.: Endolymphatic duct and sac in Meniere's disease, Arch. Otolaryng. **89**:816-825, 1964.

Stenvers, H. W.: Roentgenology of os petrosum, Arch. Radiol. Electr. **22**:97-119, 1917.

Strickler, J. M.: New and simple techniques for demonstration of the jugular foramen, Amer. J. Roentgen. **97**:601-606, 1966.

Takahashi, M., Wilson, G., and Hanafee, W.: The significance of the petrosal vein in the diagnosis of C.P. angle tumors, Radiology **89**:834-840, 1967.

Taveras, J. M., and Wood, E.: Diagnostic neuroradiology, Baltimore, 1964, The Williams & Wilkins Co.

Towne, E. B.: Erosion of petrous bone by acoustic nerve tumor demonstrated by roentgen ray, Arch. Otolaryng. **4**:515-519, 1926.

Tucker, W. N.: Cancer of the middle ear: review of 89 cases, Cancer **18**:642-650, 1965.

Valvassori, G. E.: Otosclerosis—a new challenge to roentgenology, Amer. J. Roentgen. **94**:566-574, 1965.

Valvassori, G. E.: Interpretation of radiographic findings in cochlear otosclerosis, Otorinolaryng. **75**:572-583, 1966.

Valvassori, G. E.: The abnormal internal auditory canal: diagnosis of acoustic neuroma, Radiology **92**:449-459, 1969.

Valvassori, G. E., and Pierce, R. H.: The normal internal auditory canal, Amer. J. Roentgen. **92**:1232-1241, 1964.

Vignaud, J., Danic, J., Lichtenberg, R., and Sudaker, J.: New research in radio-otology. I. Radiography of the stapes, II. Tomographic aspects of the oval window in otosclerosis, J. Radiol. Electr. **46**:129-134, 1965.

Wright, J. W., Taylor, D E., and Bizal, J. A.: Tomography and the vulnerable incus, Ann. Otol. **78**:263-279, 1969.

Index

G

J

N

T